# EARLY NUTRITION AND LONG-TERM HEALTH

# EARLY NUTRITION AND LONG-TERM HEALTH

## Mechanisms, Consequences, and Opportunities

## SECOND EDITION

*Edited by*

### JOSE M. SAAVEDRA
*Johns Hopkins University, School of Medicine, Baltimore, MD, United States*

### ANNE M. DATTILO
*Nutrition Research and Practice Service, Hollywood, FL, United States*

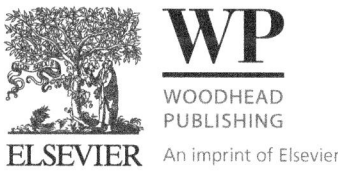

**WP**
WOODHEAD
PUBLISHING

ELSEVIER  An imprint of Elsevier

Woodhead Publishing is an imprint of Elsevier
50 Hampshire Street, 5th Floor, Cambridge, MA 02139, United States
The Boulevard, Langford Lane, Kidlington, OX5 1GB, United Kingdom

ISBN: 978-0-12-824389-3 (print)
ISBN: 978-0-12-824405-0 (online)

For information on all Woodhead publications
visit our website at https://www.elsevier.com/books-and-journals

*Publisher:* Nikki P. Levy
*Acquisitions Editor:* Megan R. Ball
*Editorial Project Manager:* Clark M. Espinosa
*Production Project Manager:* Anitha Sivaraj
*Cover Designer:* Christian J. Bilbow

Typeset by STRAIVE, India

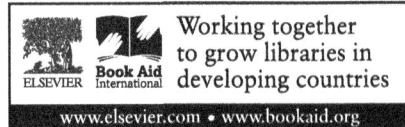

Working together
to grow libraries in
developing countries

www.elsevier.com • www.bookaid.org

# Contents

## 5. Early nutrition: Effects of specific nutrient intake on growth, development, and long-term health

Ricardo Closa-Monasterolo, Joaquin Escribano Subias, Veronica Luque Moreno, and Natalia Ferré Pallas

## 6. Early-life nutrition and neurodevelopment

Sarah E. Cusick and Michael K. Georgieff

## 7. Effects of infant allergen/immunogen exposure on long-term health outcomes

Doerthe A. Andreae and Anna Nowak-Wegrzyn

## 8. Eating development in young children: The complex interplay of developmental domains

Erin Sundseth Ross

## 9. Impact of early nutrition on gut microbiota: Effects on immunity and long-term health

Kirsi Laitinen, Kati Mokkala, and Marko Kalliomäki

# II

# Early nutrition and development of non-communicable diseases

## 11. Early life nutrition and its effect on the development of obesity and type-2 diabetes

Mark H. Vickers

## 12. Early nutrition and development of cardiovascular disease

Tricia L. Hart, Kristina S. Petersen, and Penny M. Kris-Etherton

## 13. Early nutrition and the development of allergic diseases

Edward G.A. Iglesia, David M. Fleischer, and Elissa M. Abrams

## 14. Early nutrition and its effect on the development of celiac disease

Carlo Catassi and Elena Lionetti

# III

## Promoting long-term health: Taking action in the first 1000 days

## 21. Programming long-term health: Nutrition and diet in infants aged 6 months to 1 year

Hermann Kalhoff and Mathilde Kersting

## 22. Developing science-based dietary guidelines for infants and toddlers

Lynda M. O'Neill and Jennifer Orlet Fisher

# Contributors

**Elissa M. Abrams**   University of Manitoba, Winnipeg, MB, Canada

**Carlo Agostoni**   Fondazione IRCCS Ca' Granda Ospedale Maggiore Policlinico, Pediatric Unit, Milano, Italy

**Doerthe A. Andreae**   Allergy and Immunology, Department of Dermatology, University of Utah, Salt Lake City, UT, United States

**Cristiana Berti**   Fondazione IRCCS Ca' Granda Ospedale Maggiore Policlinico, Pediatric Unit, Milano, Italy

**Zulfiqar A. Bhutta**   Centre for Global Child Health, The Hospital for Sick Children, Toronto, ON, Canada; Institute of Global Health and Development, Aga Khan University, Karachi, Pakistan

**Mark A. Burton**   School of Human Development and Health, Faculty of Medicine, University of Southampton, Southampton, United Kingdom

**Carlo Catassi**   Department of Pediatrics, Marche Polytechnic University, Ancona, Italy

**Ricardo Closa-Monasterolo**   Pediatrics, Nutrition and Development Research Unit, Universitat Rovira i Virgili, IISPV, Tarragona, Spain

**Sarah E. Cusick**   Department of Pediatrics, Medical School, University of Minnesota, Minneapolis, MN, United States

**Anne M. Dattilo**   Nutrition Research and Practice Service, Hollywood, FL, United States

**Joaquin Escribano Subias**   Pediatrics, Nutrition and Development Research Unit, Universitat Rovira i Virgili, IISPV; Hospital Universitari Sant Joan de Reus, Tarragona, Spain

**Natalia Ferré Pallas**   Pediatrics, Nutrition and Development Research Unit, Universitat Rovira i Virgili, IISPV, Tarragona, Spain

**Jennifer Orlet Fisher**   Temple University, Center for Obesity Research and Education, Philadelphia, PA, United States

**David M. Fleischer**   Children's Hospital of Colorado, University of Colorado School of Medicine, Aurora, CO, United States

**Michael K. Georgieff**   Department of Pediatrics, Medical School, University of Minnesota, Minneapolis, MN, United States

**Maria Lorella Giannì**   Department of Clinical Sciences and Community Health, University of Milan; Fondazione IRCCS Ca' Granda Ospedale Maggiore Policlinico, NICU, Milan, Italy

**Keith M. Godfrey**   NIHR Southampton Biomedical Research Centre, University of Southampton and University Hospital Southampton NHS Foundation Trust; MRC Lifecourse Epidemiology Centre, University of Southampton, Southampton, United Kingdom

**Anat Guz-Mark**   Institute of Gastroenterology, Nutrition and Liver Diseases, Schneider Children's Medical Center of Israel, Petach Tikva; Sackler Faculty of Medicine, Tel-Aviv University, Tel-Aviv, Israel

**Tricia L. Hart**   Penn State University, University Park, PA, United States

**Edward G.A. Iglesia**   Vanderbilt University Medical Center, Nashville, TN, United States

**Hermann Kalhoff**   Pediatric Clinic, Dortmund; Research Institute of Child Nutrition, University Clinic Bochum, Bochum, Germany

**Marko Kalliomäki**   Department of Clinical Medicine, University of Turku, Turku, Finland

**Mathilde Kersting**   Research Institute of Child Nutrition, University Clinic Bochum, Bochum, Germany

**Penny M. Kris-Etherton** Penn State University, University Park, PA, United States

**Harrie N. Lafeber** Department of Pediatrics and Neonatology, Amsterdam UMC, location Vrije Universiteit Amsterdam and location University of Amsterdam, Emma Children's Hospital; Amsterdam Reproduction and Development (AR&D), Amsterdam, The Netherlands

**Kirsi Laitinen** Institute of Biomedicine, University of Turku, Turku, Finland

**Zohra S. Lassi** Robinson Research Institute, University of Adelaide, Adelaide, SA, Australia

**Karen A. Lillycrop** Biological Sciences, University of Southampton, Southampton, United Kingdom

**Elena Lionetti** Department of Pediatrics, Marche Polytechnic University, Ancona, Italy

**Veronica Luque Moreno** Pediatrics, Nutrition and Development Research Unit, Universitat Rovira i Virgili, IISPV, Tarragona, Spain

**Kati Mokkala** Institute of Biomedicine, University of Turku, Turku, Finland

**Daniela Morniroli** Department of Clinical Sciences and Community Health, University of Milan, Milan, Italy

**Fabio Mosca** Department of Clinical Sciences and Community Health, University of Milan; Fondazione IRCCS Ca' Granda Ospedale Maggiore Policlinico, NICU, Milan, Italy

**Anna Nowak-Wegrzyn** Allergy and Immunology, Department of Pediatrics, NYU Grossman School of Medicine, Hassenfeld Children, New York, NY, United States; Department of Pediatrics, Gastroenterology and Nutrition, Collegium Medicum, University of Warmia and Mazury, Olsztyn, Poland

**Lynda M. O'Neill** Nestlé Research Center, Lausanne, Switzerland

**Emily Oken** Division of Chronic Disease Research Across the Lifecourse (CoRAL), Department of Population Medicine, Harvard Medical School/Harvard Pilgrim Health Care Institute; Department of Nutrition, T. H. Chan Harvard School of Public Health, Boston, MA, United States

**Zahra A. Padhani** Division of Women and Child Health, Aga Khan University, Karachi, Pakistan

**Wei Perng** Department of Epidemiology, Colorado School of Public Health; Lifecourse Epidemiology of Adiposity and Diabetes (LEAD) Center, University of Colorado Anschutz Medical Campus, Aurora, CO, United States

**Kristina S. Petersen** Penn State University, University Park, PA; Texas Tech University, Lubbock, TX, United States

**Erin Sundseth Ross** Feeding Fundamentals, LLC, Thornton; Department of Pediatrics, University of Colorado School of Medicine, Denver, CO, United States

**Charlotte A. Ruys** Department of Pediatrics and Neonatology, Amsterdam UMC, location Vrije Universiteit Amsterdam and location University of Amsterdam, Emma Children's Hospital; Amsterdam Reproduction and Development (AR&D), Amsterdam, The Netherlands

**Jose M. Saavedra** Johns Hopkins University, School of Medicine, Baltimore, MD, United States

**Rehana A. Salam** Division of Women and Child Health, Aga Khan University, Karachi, Pakistan

**Silvia Salvatore** Pediatric Department, Hospital "F. Del Ponte," University of Insubria, Varese, Italy

**Raanan Shamir** Institute of Gastroenterology, Nutrition and Liver Diseases, Schneider Children's Medical Center of Israel, Petach Tikva; Sackler Faculty of Medicine, Tel-Aviv University, Tel-Aviv, Israel

**Monique van de Lagemaat** Department of Pediatrics and Neonatology, Amsterdam UMC, location Vrije Universiteit Amsterdam and location University of Amsterdam, Emma Children's Hospital; Amsterdam Reproduction and Development (AR&D), Amsterdam, The Netherlands

**Chris H.P. van den Akker** Department of Pediatrics and Neonatology, Amsterdam UMC, location Vrije Universiteit Amsterdam and location University of Amsterdam, Emma Children's Hospital; Amsterdam Reproduction and Development (AR&D), Amsterdam, The Netherlands

**Johannes B. van Goudoever** Department of Pediatrics and Neonatology, Amsterdam UMC, location Vrije Universiteit Amsterdam and location University of Amsterdam, Emma Children's Hospital; Amsterdam Reproduction and Development (AR&D), Amsterdam, The Netherlands

**Yvan Vandenplas** Vrije Universiteit Brussel, UZ Brussel, KidZ Health Castle, Brussels, Belgium

**Mark H. Vickers** Liggins Institute, University of Auckland, Auckland, New Zealand

**Giulia Vizzari** Department of Clinical Sciences and Community Health, University of Milan, Milan, Italy

# Foreword

These days, with so much communication becoming virtual and digital, I have become very selective about which books I feel I need in hardcover in my library. Allow me a moment to recount to you why *Early Nutrition and Long-Term Health: Mechanisms, Consequences, and Opportunities* is one of the few books that reside on the shelf next to my desk.

Most of my career has been devoted to nutrition over the life cycle, so I needed a succinct and authoritative source of information on infants and toddler nutrition. I found it when the first edition of this book first came out. It became an old friend that I frequently consulted and needed nearby.

The pace of change in nutrition science and pediatrics is accelerating so rapidly today that it is difficult to stay up to date. This makes it vital to disseminate the evidence about what we know is sound nutrition science for infants and children as widely as possible among the practitioners of today and those in training. This second edition is particularly welcome since that is exactly the book's goal. It succeeds masterfully in compiling today's major developments about the influence of nutrition in early life on long-term health.

This book is outstanding for several reasons. The editors, Dr. Jose M. Saavedra, a distinguished clinical pediatric gastroenterologist with global experience, and Dr. Anne M. Dattilo, a clinical nutrition researcher and superb pediatric dietitian, bring deep knowledge, commitment, and experience to bettering infant and child health. They supplemented their own contributions by drawing on their extensive contacts throughout the world to attract several dozen international experts who have distilled what is known on each specific topic into authoritative, readable, and actionable chapters.

This new edition is a treat to read. It remains grounded in basic and clinical science, retains a life cycle approach, and emphasizes developmental processes that fits well with the life course approach to health and disease that animates our thinking today. It also provides a welcome global perspective. In addition, it now includes new cutting-edge chapters on topics such as epigenetics, cardiovascular disease, the microbiome and the gut-brain axis, and neurodevelopment. There is also an excellent new chapter on science-based dietary guidelines for infants and toddlers. The chapters include learning objectives, future trends and research, and additional sources of information that make this book ideal for both academic settings and practitioners.

The book takes us all the way from pregnancy through consideration of the consequences of actions early on upon later health. Part I covers nutrition in early life and focuses on biological mechanisms and their impact on long-term health. It includes a summary of maternal and fetal nutritional needs, breastfeeding, body composition, developmental nutrition, topics such as neurodevelopment, the microbiome, and the role of epigenetics. Part II covers nutrition and the development of several noncommunicable diseases, including, allergic disease, celiac disease, the gut-brain axis, functional gastrointestinal disorders, obesity, type 2 diabetes, and cardiovascular disease. Part III is devoted to promoting long-term health by acting in the first 1000 days of life. Attention returns to prenatal and preterm infant nutrition, establishing and maintaining healthy parent feeding practices and infant eating patterns in early life and through to obesity prevention. Each of the expanded and updated chapters is written by individuals who are world authorities on their topics.

I have learned much from both Dr. Saavedra and Dattilo's book on this topic of major scientific and societal relevance. I urge you to join me in applauding their ability to translate their extensive knowledge of the relevant research into clinical recommendations that make practical sense in reading this excellent book.

*Johanna T. Dwyer*
Schools of Medicine and Friedman School of Nutrition Science and Policy, Tufts University, Medford, MA, United States; Frances Stern Nutrition Center, Tufts Medical Center, Boston, MA, United States

# PART I

# Nutrition in early life: Mechanisms and impact on long term health

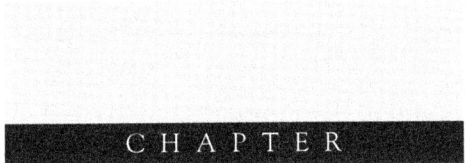

# 1

# Nutrition in the first 1000 days of life: Society's greatest opportunity

*Jose M. Saavedra[a] and Anne M. Dattilo[b]*

[a]Johns Hopkins University, School of Medicine, Baltimore, MD, United States [b]Nutrition Research and Practice Service, Hollywood, FL, United States

## 1.1 Introduction

The first edition of "Early Nutrition and Long-Term Health" (Saavedra and Dattilo, 2017), published 5 years ago, was our initial effort to compile and discuss key elements of the relationship between nutrition in early life and its life-long consequences, as well as the mechanisms mediating this relationship. We noted that progress had been made over the last few decades in several measures of health and nutrition globally, particularly in the reduction of infant mortality, and some markers of undernutrition. We also discussed the rise in non-communicable diseases, how they have moved closer to center stage as the fastest growing threat to our society's health, and how low-income countries and populations disproportionately bear the burden of both under- and overnutrition. Overall, the positive and negative trends in the nutritional landscape for children have not greatly changed over the past 5 years. Some progress has been made, but multiple gaps remain, and new threats have emerged, resulting in new opportunities and challenges for nutrition and health professionals in clinical and public health arenas working with infant and young child populations. We review here the current nutrition and health landscape, the emerging challenges and threats, and the new knowledge that can enable continued progress in improving long-term health by enhancing the nutrition of children.

## 1.2 Nutrition and health in today's global landscape

Some of the gains in child health and nutrition made in the latter part of the past millennium have continued. Globally, the prevalence of stunting and wasting have decreased significantly, to its lowest levels ever, and obesity has continued increasing. National survey data from 50 low- and middle-income countries from 2000 to 2015 show that the global prevalence of low birthweight declined from 17.5% to 14.6%, an average annual reduction rate of 1.23%. The prevalence of undernutrition (stunting and/or wasting) decreased from 56% to 46.1% in low-income countries and from 26.6% to 22% in middle-income countries (Victora et al., 2021). From 2000 to 2020, joint malnutrition estimates from UNICEF, WHO, and the World Bank showed significant improvements in undernutrition. In children below 5 years of age, the prevalence of stunting dropped from 33.1% to 22% in the last 20 years. Today, the global estimate of wasting among children under 5 years is at 6.7%. While progress is noted, for the year 2020, this still translates into 150 million children under 5 years of age who are stunted and 45.4 million who are wasted. In addition, the global prevalence of children with overweight has slightly increased from 5.4% to 5.7%, standing today at 38.9 million who are overweight (UNICEF, 2021). In 1 estimate, by 2030, 90 million children, or 22% of 2- to 4-year-olds, will be overweight (Kharas et al., 2018). Given these trends, a 2017 estimate suggests that this year, 2022, the world will have swung to having more children and adolescents that are obese, rather than moderately and severely underweight (NCD-RisC, 2017). Today, at least one in three children under 5 years of age is undernourished or overweight. However, about one in two children under 5 suffer micronutrient deficiencies or "hidden hunger." Independently, or in combination, deficiencies of vitamin A, iron, folic acid, zinc, and iodine have grave short- and long-term consequences. These include increased risk of mortality, morbidity, blindness, anemia, poor linear growth and cognitive development, suboptimal learning and school performance, and ultimately lower productivity and wages in adulthood (UNICEF, 2019).

Meanwhile, the disparities have persisted. These small gains in undernutrition and the increases in overweight and obesity in infants and young children continue to show significant global and local unequal distribution by country and household income. In high-income countries, the prevalence of childhood obesity has stabilized within some groups, yet continued to accelerate in others, particularly in minority and underserved child populations. Based on data through 2020 for children under 5 years of age, 94% of children with stunting, 97% of those with wasting, and 75% of those overweight lived in Asia and Africa (UNICEF, 2021). The triple burden of undernutrition (stunting and wasting), overnutrition (overweight and obesity), and micronutrient deficiencies, primarily affecting low-income and disadvantaged populations, remains a threat to progress.

Nearly 20 years ago, the World Health Assembly (WHA) endorsed a comprehensive implementation plan for maternal, infant, and young child nutrition, specifying nutrition targets for 2025 (WHO, 2012). These were published in 2014 and included reducing anemia in women of reproductive age, reducing low birth weight, increasing breastfeeding rates, reducing wasting and stunting, and halting the increase in childhood overweight (WHO, 2014). The Global Nutrition Report, an initiative comprised of global institutions and multiple stakeholders, has published in-depth assessments of the state of global nutrition since 2014, measuring progress toward the WHA/WHO nutrition targets for 2025. In their 2021 report, of the 194 countries assessed, 105 (54%) are on track to meet the target for childhood overweight, 27% are on track to meet stunting, and 29% to meet wasting targets. However, anemia reduction in women of reproductive age and low birth weight have shown almost no progress. Hardly any country is on track to meet targets for halting the rise of obesity and diabetes or reducing salt intake. Dietary intake, worldwide, driven by low consumption of fruits and vegetables and rising consumption of red meat and sugar-sweetened beverages have not improved over the last decade (GNR, 2021). The report concluded that significant additional investments will be needed to accelerate progress and meet nutrition targets, as well as to overcome the impact of the COVID-19 pandemic.

## 1.3 COVID-19

In the first edition of "Early Nutrition and Long-Term Health" (Saavedra and Dattilo, 2017), we also noted that despite progress against some nutrition challenges, "emerging pathogens continue to be threats to global health, and improvements in child survival and health have not been equally distributed." These threats, unfortunately, have materialized. Since the initial cases reported in China in November of 2019, with the SARS-CoV-2 virus, which causes coronavirus disease 2019 (COVID-19), the infection has swept through the globe, causing more than 5 million deaths in 2 years, and fatalities continue to amass. Although truly extraordinary progress in technology and vaccinology produced life-saving preventive vaccines in record time, the unequal distribution of these and the unequal pre-pandemic vulnerability of underserved populations of the world will have long-term repercussions.

It is not yet clear when the COVID-19 pandemic will stabilize or subside, and how the emergence of new mutation-driven variants of the virus will affect the epidemiology of the disease. What is clear is that it has had an immediate and will have a long-lasting impact on global nutrition. COVID-19 has brought about a drop in agricultural production, as well as challenges related to processing, transportation, travel and trade restrictions, loss of employment, reduced incomes, and higher prices—all of which will affect the food supply and ultimately the double burden of malnutrition and obesity. The World Food Program estimated that the number of people facing acute food insecurity was expected to rise from 135 in 2019 to 265 million in 2020 as a result of the economic impact of COVID-19 (WFP, 2021). Early in the pandemic, UNICEF estimated that there would be a 30% overall reduction in essential nutrition services coverage, reaching 75% to 100% in some countries already facing humanitarian crises leading to significant increases in child wasting and mortality, particularly for those under 5 years of age in low-income countries. Estimates in 2020 suggest that there could be a 14.3% increase in the prevalence of moderate or severe wasting among children under 5 years of age due to COVID-19 which would translate to an additional estimated 6.7 million children with wasting in 2020, compared with projections before the pandemic (Headey et al., 2020; UNICEF, 2020). The Global nutrition report 2021 also highlighted that additional investment will be needed to meet WHO/WHA nutrition targets for 2025 due to the impact of the COVID-19 pandemic. On average, US$10.8 billion additional financing, annually between 2022 and 2030, may be needed to meet only four targets (stunting, wasting, maternal anemia, and breastfeeding), allowing for the impacts of COVID-19. Previous estimates (for 2016–2025) were an additional US$7 billion annually (GNR, 2021). Thus, the impact of the COVID-19 pandemic on food systems, the economy, and nutrition and health services worldwide is leading to food insecurity. This will have a significant and long-lasting effect on the progress to combat undernutrition.

In addition, there is reason to expect that the diet quality of children will be adversely affected and compounded by decreased physical activity due to changes in schooling, inactivity from lockdowns and quarantines, and potentially increasing obesity rates in middle- and high-income countries, especially among vulnerable groups (Campbell and Wood, 2021).

Preliminary surveys in Europe show significant disruptions in nutrition and lifestyle habits due to COVID-19, with increases in intake of less nutrient-dense foods, increased snacking, and greater inactivity (Zemrani et al., 2021). Studies within the United States have reported lower breastfeeding rates among infants born during the pandemic, compared to infants with similar geographic and family characteristics born before 2019 (Koleilat et al., 2021). Higher use of unresponsive parent feeding behaviors associated with COVID-19 has been documented as emerging (Loth et al., 2022) and increased rates of weight gain among school-age children (Wu et al., 2021) are becoming more apparently linked to the pandemic. In infected adults, overweight is a significant predictor of complications from COVID-19, increasing the risk for severe disease, hospitalization, need for intensive care, and death. Higher mortality rates are significantly associated with higher rates of obesity across countries (World Obesity Federation, 2021), which raises the issue of "nutritional preparedness" in facing future infectious threats. While the relatively low infectivity of the virus in children has directly affected them less, it is clear the social and economic fall-out of the COVID-19 pandemic will increase their short- and long-term nutrition and other health-related risks, especially in the most vulnerable populations (Crowder et al., 2021). The actual effects of the pandemic so far have not been yet quantified and the ongoing impact will need to be continuously assessed, but for many, undernutrition and overnutrition rates will inevitably rise.

## 1.4 Nutrition as a determinant of health

Independent of the effects of the COVID-19 pandemic, the backdrop persists. Although the number of children with obesity may soon overtake those with chronic and acute undernutrition, the long-term consequences of both remain and are a cumulative burden to society. Previous causes of mortality and poor health have been replaced by an epidemic of non-communicable diseases (NCDs), particularly cardiovascular diseases, diabetes, cancers, and chronic respiratory diseases, leading to disabilities, premature death, and dramatically impacting healthcare costs which impact the economic burden of the nations. All NCDs, including heart disease, stroke, cancer, diabetes, and chronic lung disease, are collectively responsible for almost 70% of all deaths worldwide. Almost three-quarters of all NCD deaths occur in low- and middle-income countries (WHO, 2021a).

Nutrition is the most critical underlying and mechanistic factor for most NCDs. The consequences of NCDs can be better understood by their effects on overall disease risk factors which affect the global population, and in turn, increase the risk of mortality and disability. The Global Burden of Disease (GBD) is an effort from a consortium of more than 7000 researchers, which tracks death and disability associated with more than 350 diseases and injuries in 195 countries. The GBD 2019 study is the most comprehensive worldwide observational epidemiologic study to date (Global Burden of Disease (GBD) 2019 Risk Factors Collaborators, 2020). Of the 10 highest risks associated with the highest number of deaths worldwide, 6 are nutrition-related: high blood pressure, high plasma glucose, high BMI, high LDL cholesterol, child and maternal malnutrition, and "dietary risks" (e.g., low fruit and vegetables, high sugar-sweetened beverages, and high salt intake). The other four include tobacco, alcohol, air pollution, and kidney dysfunction. In females, high systolic blood pressure was the first, and dietary risks are the second most common risk factor associated with death. The third was high fasting glucose. In males, following tobacco use, high systolic blood pressure and dietary risks are the second and third most common risks associated with death. Globally, for both sexes, high BMI alone was a risk factor associated with 5 million deaths a year. Dietary risks were associated with 7.94 million yearly deaths and elevated fasting glucose with 6.5 million deaths. Thus, the direct and indirect effects of under and overnutrition are the main drivers of mortality worldwide.

The GBD also reflects trends in mortality associated with undernutrition versus overnutrition from 1990 to 2019. The greatest declines in associated deaths were linked to improvements in child growth failure, household air pollution, unsafe water, and sanitation. The most significant increases were associated with high fasting plasma glucose and high BMI, as well as ambient pollution and drug use. These conditions are not only linked to increased mortality but also disability, measured in disability-adjusted-life-years (DALYs). In 1990, child wasting, low birth weight, and prematurity were the 1st, 2nd, and 3rd causes of DALYs, considering all ages. Today they are the 11th, 4th, and 6th, respectively. On the flipside, in 1990, high BMI, high fasting glucose, and high cholesterol were the 16th, 11th, and 18th causes of disability. Today, they rank 5th, 3rd, and 8th. So, considering all age groups, overnutrition is the highest contributor to disability and high BMI is, by far, the fastest-growing risk for disability worldwide.

For children, however, despite improvements, malnutrition persists. And for children aged 0–9 years, the three leading risk factors for attributable DALYs were all related to undernutrition, including child wasting and micronutrient deficiencies (Global Burden of Disease (GBD) 2019 Risk Factors Collaborators, 2020). As it is clear to everyone, undernutrition and overnutrition risks can coexist within the same country, the same community, and the same household. Thus, nutrition-related factors remain the most common and strongest determinants of global mortality and disability; they affect all ages and reflect the global socioeconomic disparities.

## 1.5 The long-term impact of early nutrition

As we discussed in the first edition of this book, the ultimate origin of nutrition-related health consequences may seem straightforward: a deficit of energy, macro-, and/or micronutrients in a way that does not meet the body's requirements, and/or an excess of energy consumed versus that expended. The potential solutions appear deceptively simple to address since they are linked to only two modifiable risk factors, namely an unhealthy diet and/or a lack of physical activity. However, the timing of nutritional imbalances (excesses or deficits) in specific periods of the life cycle (conception to old age), and the environmental, behavioral, social, and economic context in which these happen can drive, complicate, and compound the problem. The ultimate solution, as discussed below, will require a whole of society approach in improving the diets and lifestyles of individuals.

It is intuitive to assume that early events experienced by an individual have consequences much later in life. Some of these experiences start before birth. The concept that the nutritional status in utero is associated with long-term chronic disease grew from David Barker's observations in the 1980s, suggesting that adult ischemic heart disease can be explained, in part, by intrauterine nutrition (Barker, 2007). The last several decades have seen an explosion in the study and understanding of the mechanisms to explain the relationships between early life events and their long-term consequences in multiple aspects of nutrition, health, disease, and well-being. It is now well accepted that permanent structural and functional changes, during gestation, result in disease in later life. This concept has expanded significantly beyond these original observations that many chronic diseases originate from developmental changes in fetal and early postnatal life. The developmental origins of health and disease (DOHaD) is a construct frequently used to describe these phenomena (International society for developmental origins of health and disease, 2015).

"Nutritional programming," in the first 1000 days, is described as the process and mechanisms by which nutrition-related dietary intake and behaviors and the environment during pregnancy and the first 2 years determine health and risk of disease in later life. Key mechanistic variables affecting the long-term consequences of nutrition-related events include the timing (e.g., pre- and postconceptional maternal nutrition, early, and late postnatal nutrition), and the type of nutrition-related events (under- and overnutrition).

This Book explores the multiple facets of the relationship between nutrition in early life and long-term health. Consequences of early nutrition imbalances, the various sensitive windows of growth and development in the life cycle affected by these imbalances, the potential mechanisms in play and approaches to addressing these excesses or deficits to improve health are included. We summarize below these highlights and the chapters in which these are addressed.

## 1.5.1 Programming influences

### 1.5.1.1 Prenatal influences

Early nutrient deficits and excesses during sensitive developmental windows have long-lasting consequences, particularly on metabolic, neurocognitive, and immunologic functions—commonly referred to as "early programming" (Lassi et al., 2022; Vickers, 2022; Cusick and Georgieff, 2022; Closa-Monasterolo et al., 2022; Andreae and Nowak-Węgrzyn, 2022; Perng and Oken, 2022). The first of these sensitive periods is gestation, which is influenced by maternal nutritional status at the time of conception. Pre-pregnancy maternal malnutrition is a major risk factor for maternal, fetal, and neonatal health complications, and has a profound effect on fetal and infant growth. Preconceptional obesity is also associated with stillbirths, neonatal and infant mortality, cesarean section, preterm birth, cleft palate, and macrosomia. Although various nutrition interventions addressing micronutrient deficiencies have shown a positive impact on maternal, birth, and infant outcomes, the effect of these interventions on growth in later childhood and non-communicable disease in adulthood remain to be better studied (Lassi et al., 2022). Individual nutrient deficits, or excesses, have specific structural and functional effects, which vary depending on timing relative to various sensitive developmental windows. Such is the case with micronutrients during pregnancy, particularly, deficits of folate, iron, iodine, zinc, polyunsaturated fatty acids (PUFAs) (Closa-Monasterolo et al., 2022; Lassi et al., 2022; Perng and Oken, 2022).

Markers of maternal nutrition, particularly preconception BMI, weight gain during pregnancy, and gestational glucose control can significantly modify risks for later metabolic disease in the offspring. Interestingly, both under and overnutrition in utero lead to increased risk of later obesity in children. Observational studies show that maternal obesity, gestational diabetes, and excessive weight gain during pregnancy are associated with later increased adiposity, obesity, type 2 diabetes, and cardiovascular disease (Lassi et al., 2022; Perng and Oken,

2022; Vickers, 2022; Hart et al., 2022). Gestational undernutrition and lower birth weight are also associated with increased adiposity, obesity, and increased cardiovascular risk (Hart et al., 2022; Lassi et al., 2022; Perng and Oken, 2022; Vickers, 2022). The mechanisms are still being elucidated, but these observations suggest adaptive responses reflecting a mismatch between prenatal and postnatal nutritional environments. Some of these phenomena may be mediated through changes in the hypothalamic pituitary axis, insulin secretion and sensing, and vascular responsiveness resulting from nutritional challenges in utero, which may in part result from epigenetic processes, discussed further below. Increasing evidence also indicates that the nutrition of both mother and father are determinant factors of future disease risk, and that the underlying mechanism by which alterations in early-life nutrition can induce phenotypic changes in offspring involves the altered epigenetic regulation of genes (Burton et al., 2022; Vickers, 2022).

Preterm infants reflect similar paradoxes regarding effects of early under- and overnutrition. Compared to those infants born at term, 20% to 45% of very preterm infants have suboptimal growth and neurodevelopment, including cognitive, motor, and behavioral problems in childhood and adolescence. Many of these are attributable to nutrient deficits in their immediate postnatal life. However, as young adults with a relatively normal body mass index, they show decreased lean mass and increased central adiposity (van de Lagemaat et al., 2022). For a long time, nutritional care of premature infants has focused on approximating intrauterine growth rates and providing nutrients for catch-up growth and potentially improving neurodevelopment. However, achieving accelerated catch-up growth may be accompanied by long-term metabolic costs, increasing risks for excess adiposity, and later cardiovascular risks. There seems to be a delicate balance between supporting somatic and neurocognitive development and risking later metabolic-related morbidities, the mechanisms of which need to be better understood (Gianni et al., 2022; van de Lagemaat et al., 2022).

### 1.5.1.2 Breastfeeding and complementary foods

For the early months of life, exclusive breastfeeding remains the ideal form of nutrition. The short-term benefits of breastfeeding, namely protection from gastrointestinal, respiratory and middle ear infections, and necrotizing enterocolitis are well established, and in lower income countries associated with decreased mortality (Guz-Mark and Shamir, 2022). Beneficial long-term outcomes including allergy, autoimmune disorders, and neoplasia are apparent and have been reported. Studies comparing breastfeeding to infant formula are observational and have unavoidable confounders and limitations, for which causality remains difficult to ascertain. The beneficial effect of breastfeeding compared to infant formula on adiposity, overweight, and obesity in older childhood or adolescence has the same limitations; however, the evidence is stronger to favor a protective effect of breastfeeding. The evidence remains weak for assertions of benefits related to the duration of breastfeeding. There are multiple mechanisms by which breastfeeding may limit obesity risk, including compositional differences (particularly low protein content than infant formulas, adipokines, and factors that modulate the infant microbiota, such as human milk oligosaccharides). Finally, there is growing evidence that bottle-feeding per se and its associated caretaker bottle-feeding behaviors (Dattilo, 2022) may contribute to overweight or obesity risk (Guz-Mark and Shamir, 2022; Berti and Agostoni, 2022; Saavedra, 2022).

The timing of introduction to complementary solid foods may play a role. After 6 months of age, it becomes difficult for infants that exclusively breastfeed to meet nutrient needs (especially energy, protein, iron, zinc, and some fat-soluble vitamins) (Kalhoff and Kersting, 2022). However, offering infants solid foods below 4 months of age is not ideal from the developmental point of view (Berti and Agostoni, 2022; Kalhoff and Kersting, 2022; Ross, 2022), and although studies on this include numerous confounders, there is consistent evidence indicating that complementary food introduction before 4 months increases the risk of overweight and obesity in childhood. In the first 2 years of age, excess energy intake, in part related to high dietary energy density, with low intake of fruits and vegetables, and high intake of foods and beverages with added sugar, as well as excess protein intakes, are also consistently associated with risk for childhood obesity. In addition, factors outside the diet appear to be of significance in increasing obesity risk, such as sleep duration, "screen time," and active play or physical activity. The development of healthy eating habits is critical in supporting an infant's self-regulation and avoiding excesses. Parental lack of attention to "hunger and satiety cues" and responsive feeding behaviors are significantly associated with obesity risks. On the other hand, parental adoption of specific feeding behaviors in the first 2 years of life (e.g., responsiveness to hunger and satiety cues, considerations with bottle use, avoidance of using of food to soothe an infant, attention to pressuring/restrictive practices, and repeated opportunity with novel foods) can positively influence a child's dietary intake and indices of body weight or rate of weight gain. Holistic parenting education programs are needed to address these modifiable factors (Berti and Agostoni, 2022; Dattilo, 2022; Saavedra, 2022.)

Experts agree that easy to adopt dietary strategies and guidelines can help caregivers and parents with the complexities of infant and young childhood nutrition and feeding (Kalhoff and Kersting, 2022; O'Neill and Orlet-Fisher, 2022; Ross, 2022). However, there is no universal consensus on the optimal approach to developing food-based guidelines for complementary feeding. Evidence-based quantitative dietary guidelines are limited, and some guidelines, after being translated into menus and analyzed for energy and key nutrients, fall short of recommendations for iron, zinc, calcium, vitamin D, and potassium (O'Neill and Orlet-Fisher, 2022). Fortunately, dietary reference values for energy and key nutrients can be met, using various methodologies, including linear programming, for the development of food-based dietary guidelines for infants and young children from 6 through 24 months of age (Kalhoff and Kersting, 2022; O'Neill and Orlet-Fisher, 2022). Most dietary guidelines today are directed to older children and adults, and few high-income countries developed specific dietary guidance for infants below 2 years of age. The United States published dietary guidelines for infants for the first time in 2020 (NAS, 2020).

Dietary intake of infants, beginning at birth, not only defines the adequacy of energy, macro, and micronutrient intakes that influences growth and development but also affects the development of food preferences (Ross, 2022; Berti and Agostoni, 2022). The first 2 years of life are also characterized by the establishment of dietary patterns that are synchronic with the infant's rapid developmental changes, including the development of self-feeding skills. Newborns have innate reflexes for feeding and a complex set of developmental skills (visual, tactile, taste and other sensory input, as well as fine and gross motor, and oral-motor skills) that come into play and require integration by the infant and parent, for eventual development of the child's independent eating habits (Ross, 2022; Berti and Agostoni, 2022).

## 1.5.2 Key long-term outcomes

### 1.5.2.1 Neurodevelopment and cognition

It has been thoroughly documented that protein-energy malnutrition, as well as specific micronutrient deficiencies in infancy and childhood, can cause irreversible damage to a child's neurodevelopment and long-term physical growth, leading to lifelong stunting, greater susceptibility to infection, diminished capacity to learn, poor school performance, and loss of earning potential (Closa-Monasterolo et al., 2022; Cusick and Georgieff, 2022). Over the last decade, there has been a greater understanding of the mechanisms by which key nutrients like choline, folate, B12, polyunsaturated fatty acids, iodine, iron, and zinc affect brain structure and function, especially during gestation and perinatal period (Lassi et al., 2022; Perng and Oken, 2022). These include epigenetic modifications of critical structural and functional genes that can have life-long impact if the nutritional deficiency coincides with a period of peak brain growth (Cusick and Georgieff, 2022). In infant and toddlers, at least four micronutrients have been directly associated with neurodevelopment during early to middle childhood: iodine, zinc, vitamin B12, and iron. It is important to note that most often these deficiencies can be multiple, and its effects on neurocognition are also influenced and compounded by chronic or inflammatory/infectious stimuli and disadvantages that frequently coexist in populations, particularly in low-income settings. Obesity has also been associated with impaired cognition. Possible mechanisms include altered brain structure, leptin/insulin regulation, oxidative stress, cerebrovascular function, blood-brain barrier, inflammation, and decreased motor performance associated with a degraded musculoskeletal system (John et al., 2017; Schwarzenberg et al., 2018).

### 1.5.2.2 Obesity and cardiovascular disease

Among the long-term consequences of early nutrition imbalances, obesity and cardiovascular risks are today the greatest contributors to the increase in NCD's and global morbidity and mortality. As mentioned earlier, outside of tobacco, alcohol use, and air pollution, all the other 10 highest risk factors associated with deaths and disability worldwide are nutrition related (Global Burden of Disease (GBD) 2019 Risk Factors Collaborators, 2020). And while their development includes heritable genetic components, they seem in a very large measure dependent on potentially modifiable risk factors (Saavedra, 2022; Hart et al., 2022). In addition to the risks of overweight and obesity associated with maternal and gestational nutritional events, overnutrition in infancy and childhood, particularly the consumption in early life of diets inadequately high in energy, excess protein, and particularly excess sugar, sodium, and saturated fat also have long-term consequences, leading to inappropriate metabolic responses, changes in body composition, and increased risk of overweight, obesity, and NCDs in later life (Berti and Agostoni, 2022; Closa-Monasterolo et al., 2022; Hart et al., 2022; Kalhoff and Kersting, 2022; Perng and Oken, 2022; Saavedra, 2022).

The basic underlying cause of obesity and overweight and their related NCDs are ultimately an imbalance between energy consumed and energy expended in an individual. Therefore, theoretically, overweight and obesity are largely preventable. However, the individual level of risk for the development of this imbalance (i.e., dietary intake in quality and quantity vs energy expenditure) and the type and level of phenotypic expression of the imbalance (i.e., as adiposity and other metabolic dysregulation) are dependent on multiple factors. Some factors (e.g., physiologic control of appetite and individual behaviors) (Berti and Agostoni, 2022; Dattilo, 2022) can influence individual intake and be themselves shaped by environmental influences (e.g., social, educational, and cultural). Other factors are less evident or "visible," including genetic influence on metabolic and immunologic responses. And as discussed further below, diet and environmental influences can lead to epigenetic phenomena that, without changing our genes, modify gene expression and thus alter metabolic and inflammatory responses that are expressed as adiposity and cardiovascular disease. So, while the basic equation is simple, the variables that modify it are innumerable, and this has made it difficult to identify and pinpoint the many multiple factors, discussed below, which explain individual and populational risks. In fact, it is remarkable how much progress has been made, no matter how much we still do not know.

A number of dietary factors in the first years of life, particularly associated with increased risk of childhood obesity, have been described. The short-term effect of imbalances in infancy, particularly excess energy consumption leading to increased adiposity and accelerated weight gain, are easily detected. However, the relationship of specific dietary exposures to long-term risks are much more complicated due to the multiple confounders that accumulate over time. In addition, detailed surveys of national or global dietary intakes for infants and children are sparse, mostly from high-income countries, and focus mostly on older children (Rippin et al., 2019; CDC, 2020). Global databases including infants have slightly improved in their reach in the last decades; however, most have focused on breastfeeding rates and time of introduction of solid foods (WHO, 2021b) with less comprehensive country data available to assess indicators of dietary intake or quality (GNR, 2021).

### 1.5.2.3 Allergy and immune disorders

The prevalence of allergic conditions has continued to rise globally, and foods are the most common allergens for infants. In addition, early development of allergy-related conditions (e.g., atopic dermatitis) is strongly associated with subsequent development of other allergies (asthma or gastrointestinal allergic disorders) in later life (Hill et al., 2018). Data so far does not show a consistent relationship between prenatal maternal allergen exposure or breastfeeding and allergy risk; thus, there is no consistent evidence for specific modifications to the maternal diet during pregnancy or lactation for reducing allergic risk (Andreae and Nowak-Węgrzyn, 2022; Iglesia et al., 2022). Given that cow's milk is a common food allergen, hydrolyzed formulas have been developed to decrease risk associated with introduction of cow's milk to infants who are not exclusively breastfed. There is evidence that compared to intact cow's milk protein formulas, specific whey protein hydrolyzed infant formulas may decrease risk of atopic dermatitis and wheezing until 20 years of age, especially in infants with a family history (Gappa et al., 2020). But not all hydrolyzed products are immunogenically equivalent, so the broad use of any hydrolyzed milk formula product is not recommended for allergy prevention.

The timing of introduction of potential allergens in complementary feeding appears to play a role. Historically, it was thought that delaying the introduction of potential allergens (including cow's milk, eggs, peanuts, and tree nuts) past the usual complementary food introduction time of about 6 months, all the way to past a year of age, might decrease risk of allergies. It is clear today that "early" introduction may in fact promote the development of tolerance to potential allergenic foods, namely egg and peanut. There is consensus today that around 6 months of life, though not before 4 months of life, egg and peanut be introduced in the general population, independent of family allergic risk, and not to deliberately delay introduction of other allergens (for which there is less available data). The effect of other nutrition or dietary factors in modifying the development of allergy, including vitamin D supplementation or polyunsaturated fatty acid ingestion, remains unclear (Andreae and Nowak-Węgrzyn, 2022; Iglesia et al., 2022). Breastfeeding has also been studied as a potential factor in the development of celiac disease but has not shown to influence its development. And similarly, the timing of introduction of gluten, between 4 months and 2 years of age does not seem to consistently affect the occurrence of celiac disease. Whether the quantity of gluten introduced at different times in the first years of life has an influence is still unclear (Catassi and Lionetti, 2022).

### 1.5.3 Emerging mechanisms of programming

#### 1.5.3.1 Epigenetics

Nutritional imbalances and their consequences are expected to vary depending on the genetic construct of individuals. However, genetic variants account only for a minimal part of the heritability of complex medical conditions, such as metabolic conditions, overweight, and cardiovascular disease. Therefore, an even greater level of recent interest has focused on other factors and mechanisms which affect the expression of these nutritional imbalances in individuals and populations. One such mechanism is epigenetic phenomena (processes that modulate gene expression without change to nucleotide sequences in our DNA, but determine when and where a gene is expressed). Exposure to, or deficits of, specific nutrients at certain periods of development, as well as ingestion of toxins and exposure to other environmental factors such as pollutants, can have significant effect on the health outcomes related to nutrition. Early life nutrition can thus "program" metabolic pathways for life, in part through epigenetic modification of genes that regulate metabolic processes (Burton et al., 2022).

Gene expression can be influenced by several types of modifications. Methylation (the addition of a methyl ($CH_3$) group to the DNA strand) and histone modifications (the acetylation, methylation, and other changes to histones, which are proteins that provide the structural support to chromosomes) can modify and control gene expression. Nutrients can reverse or promote epigenetic phenomena, thereby modifying the expression of critical genes associated with physiologic and pathologic processes, including embryonic development. Dietary exposures or deficits during critical periods, including micronutrients like folate, high fat diets, or polyunsaturated fatty acids are associated with these epigenetic changes. Much of the research to date is preclinical, in animal models, supported by observational clinical studies showing epigenetic changes (e.g., patterns of methylation in humans). Epigenetic dysregulation appears to operate in several components with obesity and type 2 diabetes, including altered appetite regulation, insulin signaling, changes in adipogenesis, and inflammatory processes. High fat or sugar diets are also associated with methylation and histone modification. Epigenetic mechanisms affecting placental transport of nutrients may partially explain the relationship between maternal nutrition and fetal linear growth. And animal studies, supported by clinical observations, also suggest that epigenetic changes due to nutritional deficits (such as iron, folate, choline, and other nutrients), at specific developmental periods, may be associated with long-term neuro-cognitive consequences. Epigenetic changes may also help explain the transgenerational effect of metabolic changes passed on from mothers and fathers to their offspring (Cusick and Georgieff, 2022; Burton et al., 2022; Vickers, 2022).

Increasing our understanding of epigenetic mechanisms that lead to metabolic, inflammatory, and neurodevelopmental programming, the nutritional factors that trigger them and the critical developmental windows in which they occur will help to guide and improve nutritional strategies for prevention of disease and chronic conditions.

### 1.5.3.2 Microbial environment and the intestinal microbiota

Another major intermediary between nutrition, physiology, and health is our bacterial environment. Our microbiota—the collection of microorganisms in constant contact with our skin, respiratory tract, and particularly in our gut, and the factors which modulate it (e.g., how we are born, our diet, antibiotics) are major determinants of immunologic, metabolic, and neural pathways and responses, and play a critical role in infant development (Yang et al., 2016; Laitinen et al., 2022).

Disturbances in the composition of the microbiota from that typically detected in healthy individuals (dysbiosis), has been linked to many conditions. These include infectious risks (necrotizing enterocolitis, gastrointestinal, and respiratory infections), immune-related conditions (allergy, celiac disease, and leukemia), and metabolic disease (including overweight and obesity). The intestinal microbiota is a critical determinant of an infant's immune development, as it "trains" the gut-associated lymphoid tissue—the largest immune organ of the body. The intestinal microbiota also signals the central nervous system via neuro-endocrine pathways (the gut-brain axis) and appears to affect metabolic functions directly, through energy salvage in the gut, or indirectly, through hormonal and neurotransmitter pathways that can modify intake (Yang et al., 2016; Ratsika et al., 2021).

Microbial colonization of the gut occurs in an exponential manner immediately following birth and the profile of the microbiota is modulated by multiple factors, including the immediate environmental microbial exposure (maternal microbiota, hospital, household members, pets, rural vs urban environment, etc.). However, two factors that have the greatest influence on an infant's developing microbiota include birth mode (cesarean vs vaginal delivery) and what the newborn is fed (breastfeeding vs a breastmilk substitute). Human milk contains bacteria, as well as specific factors that modulate the infant's microbiota, such as human milk oligosaccharides. Children who are born by cesarean section and/or do not breastfeed have varying degrees of dysbiosis (Laitinen et al., 2022). Dysbiosis has been associated with allergy (Andreae and Nowak-Węgrzyn, 2022), celiac disease (Catassi and Lionetti, 2022), overweight and obesity (Saavedra, 2022), and functional gastrointestinal disorders (Salvatore and Vandenplas, 2022). Increasingly, there is evidence for the role of dysbiosis in inflammatory responses that mediate the development of cardiovascular disease later in life. The association, still mostly observational, between obesity risk following antibiotic use perinatally and in infancy further reinforces the potential mechanistic role that dysbiosis may have in the development of obesity (Saavedra, 2022). The use of prebiotics and probiotics, to improve the profile of infant microbiota, as an approach to address allergic conditions and celiac disease has shown mixed results (Laitinen et al., 2022). Dysbiosis has also been associated with alterations of the gut-brain axis and is a factor in the pathophysiology of functional gastrointestinal disorders (e.g., infant colic, constipation, and regurgitation). Specific probiotics have shown positive results in improving signs and symptoms of infant colic (Salvatore and Vandenplas, 2022).

# 1.6 The first 1000 days, a window of opportunity

The effect of nutrition in the first 1000 days on the health and ultimate productivity of individuals is profound. As discussed earlier, poor nutrition increases health risks and disabilities and decreases the neurocognitive potential of children. And not only undernutrition, but maternal and childhood obesity may also negatively impact neurodevelopment (Schwarzenberg et al., 2018). It is difficult to recover from these early effects and deficits later in life. In addition, the impact of poor nutrition early in life can transcend generations. The malnourished female infants of today (with under or overnutrition) can perpetuate the cycle of nutrition-related NCDs and increased mortality and disability in their offspring. Thus, early nutrition impacts the contribution of individuals to society's current and future progress and well-being.

Over the last five to six decades, early nutrition has been increasingly recognized as a key driver and marker of development, and global efforts have dramatically improved child nutrition, education, health, and survival worldwide. In the 1800s, 40% to 50% of children did not survive to age 5, in 1900 this figure was 36%, in 2017 it is 4%. In many ways, now is the best time for children to be alive (Roser et al., 2019; Clark et al., 2020). However, this means that on average, 15,000 children below 5 years of age die each day (Roser et al., 2019). Half of these deaths are attributable to malnutrition (WHO, 2021c). A major contributing factor in morbidity and mortality in undernourished infants and young children are micronutrient deficiencies, which are less "visible" than wasting or stunting, and thus called "hidden hunger." Today, "hidden hunger" may be a greater contributor to disabilities than stunting or wasting alone (Lenaerts and Demont, 2021). So, challenges remain, and additional threats are emerging, which jeopardize children's nutrition. Social and economic disparities persist, and in many areas of the world, they have worsened. The prevalence of wasting has decreased, but high stunting rates persist and have been tougher to overcome. Overweight and obesity continue to rise, mostly in low- and middle-income countries. The effects and costs of the consequent rise in NCDs will materialize in years to come, further compounding nutritional disparities.

On the one hand, meeting the challenge of providing adequate nutrition, overcoming under- and overnutrition given the current environmental and socioeconomic contextual hurdles, and shaping dietary habits in early life may seem difficult or overwhelming. However, the challenge is also our greatest opportunity.

Because the effects of early nutrition are profound and long lasting, the cumulative effect of "getting it right" in early life can ultimately be the greatest return on the investment for society. Pregnancy and the first 2 years of life—the first 1000 days of life—provide a unique window of opportunity for halting persistent malnutrition and the epidemic of NCDs. Environmental, social, and economic changes are needed to allow access and affordability of healthy foods to families, and efforts have yielded progress. In addition, much can be done in the immediate environment of infants and children, by parents and caregivers. The early years are a period of remarkable plasticity in humans, which allows programming of metabolic, immunologic, and cognitive functions, as well as behavioral and dietary intake patterns. This can and needs to be shaped by parents and caregivers. To accomplish this, education in nutrition at multiple levels, but especially to parents will be needed. And this provides additional opportunities for effective intervention. Gestation and infancy are the life periods when parents are most eager to learn and apply educational and other opportunities granted to them to benefit their offspring. Finally, attention and prioritization of nutrition in the first 1000 days may not only enhance the health and lives of individuals but is also an opportunity to reduce disparities in health, education, earning potential, and increase the gross domestic product (GDP) of countries, thus breaking the intergenerational cycle of poverty (Thousand Days, 2016; GNR, 2021).

## 1.7  Investing in early life nutrition

Long-term survival of the species has been a good reason in itself to argue for adequate nourishment of offspring. Human moral and ethical imperatives, which have developed over millennia, have provided societies additional reasons for prioritizing infant nutrition, child-rearing, and well-being over other human activities. In the last few centuries, the scientific understanding that many early life events and deficits may be long lasting and irreversible and can add to long-term personal, communal, and societal burdens has furthered the argument for infant nutrition. Over the last century, a major driver of the focus on the first 1000 days of life is the thoroughly documented scientific understanding that early investments in children's health, education, and development have benefits that compound throughout an individual's lifetime and for society as a whole. This bolsters the rationale for economic investment in this early period of life. The economic argument for investing in children's health and education is irrefutable and is characterized by high benefit-cost ratios (Clark et al., 2020). A recent World Bank report further articulates the case further. As opposed to other investments for development, the returns on investments in early life nutrition are durable, inalienable, and portable. They are "durable because investments made during the critical 1000-day window of opportunity last a lifetime without ever needing to be replenished. Inalienable and portable because they belong to that child no matter what and wherever she or he goes" (Shekar et al., 2017).

Specific estimates of returns on nutrition intervention in early life are hard to come by. In part, because nutrition cuts across and influences so many other aspects of individuals' lives: growth, development, health, education, and well-being. Most estimates on investment returns that relate to nutrition are combined with maternal and infant health, and reasonably, include access to health care interventions. Most are also focused on undernutrition, not on overweight or obesity (Clark et al., 2020; Shekar et al., 2017). An assessment of returns in key aspects of maternal, newborn, and child health, for which nutrition was a cross-cutting theme, showed that increasing investments by just $5 per person per year, up to 2035, in 74 high-burden countries could yield up to 9 times that value in economic and social benefits. The returns include greater gross domestic product growth, through improved productivity, and prevention of deaths, primarily in children under 5 years of age (Stenberg et al., 2014).

A more recent report estimated the costs necessary to invest in high-impact nutrition-specific interventions to achieve the WHA global nutrition targets for stunting, anemia in women, exclusive breastfeeding, and the scaling up of the treatment of severe wasting among young children. Such investment, $70 billion over 10 years (2015–2015 estimates), could reduce 265 million cases of anemia in women, 65 million cases of stunting, 91 million children would be treated for severe wasting, and 105 million additional infants would be exclusively breastfed during the first 6 months of life, over 10 years. This would yield between $4 and

$35 in economic returns, per dollar invested, "making investing in early nutrition one of the best value-for-money development actions" (Shekar et al., 2017). The investments needed for meeting these maternal, infant, and young child targets to overcome undernutrition (2022–2030) were recently reevaluated by the Global Nutrition Report Initiative. Of the $70 billion estimated in 2017 needed to close the financing gap during 2016–2025, extending the needs to meet targets by 2030 would require an additional US$97 billion over the 2022–2030 period. However, the total economic gains to society of investing in nutrition could reach US$5.7 trillion a year by 2030 (GNR, 2021).

On the other hand, the cost of inaction can be enormous. Looking retrospectively, and using height as a proxy measure, the annual loss in GDP associated with inadequate nutrition has been estimated to be as much as 12% in poor countries, primarily related to the effect of undernutrition on cognition. Due to the gains made in stunting, worldwide annual productivity losses associated with undernutrition fell from around 12% in 1900 to about 6% in 2000. Without nutrition improvements, world GDP would have averaged 8% lower over the century (Horton and Steckel, 2011).

There is still too little data and research on estimating the economic cost-benefit and developing specific investment cases for obesity prevention and control. However, cost estimates of obesity and its consequences can help quantify the scope of the economic impact and thus assess the potential benefit of interventions. For example, estimates of obesity-attributed health care costs in Latin America range from 0.1% to 14% of total health care expenditures, depending on the country and study (Milliken and Ellis, 2018). In the United States, the estimated life-time direct medical cost of a 10-year-old child with obesity, compared with a similar child with normal weight, allowing for weight gain in adulthood, is between $12,000 and $19,000 (Finkelstein et al., 2014).

Despite the need for economic evaluations of obesity prevention in early childhood, the research is still very limited (Döring et al., 2016).

## 1.8 Tackling the challenges to improve early life nutrition

The need for global efforts that include all relevant stakeholders to improve global and individual nutrition is clear. At a very basic level, the objective is to meet and balance nutrient requirements and intake to support all aspects of health and well-being (including growth and development in children). Nutrient requirements will be greatly determined by biologic and physiologic needs and intrapersonal factors but also influenced by environmental factors. In addition, intake will be affected by interpersonal and intergroup relations at multiple levels and in varying degrees, including relationships with others in the home, community, social organizations (such as schools), the private sector, government and policy, and international and global organizations. Various social-ecological models have been used to describe these relationships, dependencies, and interactions, to guide public health decisions (Ayala-Marín et al., 2020; Golden and Earp, 2012). Thus, work to improve nutrition, independent of the degree of interactive phenomena, and causal relations between these factors require participation and/or interventions targeting both individuals and stakeholders in these multiple environmental levels of influence.

### 1.8.1 Food systems and environmental threats

Intake will also be determined by the access and affordability of food available to individuals. Food systems have evolved dramatically for humans since foraging was their primary source of sustenance, from the discovery of cooking and processing, all the way to the highly complex and interdependent food systems in existence today. Agriculture and production, distribution, processing, marketing, retail sales, preparation, consumption, and waste disposal or recirculation are all critical environmental components of food systems which determine food security and the ultimate intake of nutrients (FAO, 2018). The Food and Agriculture Organization of the UN and many others call for a "sustainable food system that delivers food security and nutrition for all, in such a way that the economic, social, and environmental bases to generate food security and nutrition for future generations is not compromised." This means that "food systems need to be profitable throughout (economic sustainability), have broad-based benefits for society (social sustainability), and have a positive or neutral impact on the natural environment (environmental sustainability)" (FAO, 2018, 2021). It is increasingly urgent that approaches to address food security account for the interaction between food systems and climate change. Climate change impacts all components of food systems, and the consequences of climate change are likely to disproportionately impact low-income populations, exacerbating disparities. Conversely, food systems contribute to climate change. It is estimated that they account for one-third of all greenhouse gas emissions (Mirzabaev et al., 2021). Tackling this will require that individuals, countries, governments, and public and private enterprise collaborate.

Today, socioeconomic interactions in food systems are present in a world where undernutrition and obesity coexist, suggesting that both are a consequence of similar drivers and similar interests and relationships between multiple stakeholders (e.g., individuals, families, communities, the commercial private sector, government, etc.). Alternative approaches and models to address multiple sector relationships and individuals are being proposed. Food systems themselves have been proposed as a socioecological system in which its socioeconomic and natural dynamics reinforce specific nutritional outcomes (Golden et al., 2021; Wells et al., 2021). The threats to our food systems related to future infectious diseases will also need to be considered in forging a way forward. COVID-19 has awakened current generations to the importance of preparedness for pandemics (WFP, 2021). And undernutrition as well as overweight and obesity decrease our protection from infectivity and increase complications from infections. Food production is affected by climate change, and it is also responsible for 20% to 30% of global greenhouse gas emissions. We can no longer look at the relationship of climate change to food and health as distant or indirect (Binns et al., 2021). Scientific stewardship, political commitment, and prioritizing investments will require that all stakeholders play a part.

### 1.8.2 Multiple stakeholder involvement and its challenges

While the need to invest in nutrition in early life has long been recognized by academia, government, non-government organizations (NGOs), and the private sector, earlier international and global efforts focused on child disease and survival. Work and commitments to child nutrition and well-being have taken shape over the last 10 years. As mentioned earlier, in 2012, the WHA endorsed a comprehensive implementation plan for Maternal, Infant, and Young Child Nutrition, focusing on specific nutrition targets (WHO, 2012). These were published in 2014 and included reducing anemia in women of reproductive age, reducing low birth weight, increasing rates of breastfeeding, reducing wasting and stunting, and halting the increase in childhood overweight (WHO, 2014). The progress toward these was discussed earlier. In 2014, the Second International Conference on Nutrition (ICN2) was jointly organized by the Food and Agriculture Organization of the United Nations and the World Health Organization. It endorsed two outcome documents, committing world leaders to establish national policies aimed at eliminating malnutrition in all its forms, including hidden hunger, and transforming food systems to make nutritious diets available to all (Amoroso, 2016).

In 2015, 193 Member States of the United Nations adopted the 2030 Agenda for Sustainable Development and its 17 Sustainable Development Goals (SDGs), as global objectives to guide the actions of the international community over the next 15 years (2016–2030). A major component of these was to "end hunger, achieve food security and improved nutrition, and promote sustainable agriculture" with two specific nutrition-related goals: SDG 2 (Zero Hunger) and SDG 3 (Good Health and wellbeing), also noting that nutrition has a role to play in achieving other goals of the 2030 Agenda, including those related to poverty, health, education, social protection, gender, water, work, growth, inequality, and climate change (United Nations, 2015). And in 2016, the United Nations General Assembly endorsed the ICN2 outcome documents. It proclaimed the years 2016–2025 as the United Nations Decade of Action on Nutrition and called for an effort by all relevant stakeholders: individuals, families, communities, NGOs, academia, voluntary associations, industry, and the private sector. Goals were identified to address "the need to eradicate hunger and prevent all forms of malnutrition worldwide, particularly undernourishment, stunting, wasting, underweight, and overweight in children under 5 years of age and anemia in women and children, among other micronutrient deficiencies, as well as reverse the rising trends in overweight and obesity and reduce the burden of diet-related non-communicable diseases in all age groups." As such, nutrition was firmly placed at the heart of the development agenda and recognition that transformed food systems have a fundamental role to play in promoting healthy diets and improving nutrition. The achievement of the Sustainable Development (SDGs) will only be met when much greater political focus is devoted to improving nutrition, as nutrition is both an input and an outcome of sustainable development (United Nations, 2016). That same year the WHA welcomed the report of the Commission on Ending Childhood Obesity (WHO, 2016) and its six recommendations to address the obesogenic environment and critical periods in the life course to tackle childhood obesity. The plan to guide countries in implementing the Commission's recommendations was welcomed by the WHA in 2017.

Lack of data, competing interests, and lack of coordination of multiple sectors, among other factors, has hindered the participation and collaboration of needed stakeholders. Over the last decade, not with challenges, efforts have been made to join efforts and develop working partnerships. The Scaling up Nutrition Movement, launched in 2010, brought together governments, United Nations agencies, businesses, donors, civil society organizations, and individuals "in a collective mission to uphold the right to good food and nutrition" (Scaling Up Nutrition, 2021).

The Global Alliance for Improved Nutrition started more than a decade ago has worked toward making good nutrition desirable, available, and affordable by encouraging "…helping food systems generate positive nutrition for all people, especially the most vulnerable, mobilizing private investment and businesses large and small," and working with governments and local organizations to enable them to shift policy in favor of nutritious diets (GAIN, 2021). New efforts are helping bring transparency and hopefully collaboration between sectors. Independent organizations like Access to Nutrition Foundation are developing tools that track, rate, and make public their contribution of the largest food and beverage companies and their performance in addressing obesity, diet-related chronic diseases, and undernutrition (ATNI, 2021). These and other multisectoral partnerships have slowly but continually grown to tackle nutrition challenges, and all continue to emphasize the period of the first 1000 days as critical to their work and investments.

### 1.8.3 Infant nutrition is a driver and a marker of progress

As opposed to adults who have different levels of independence and can modulate external influences in making dietary choices, infants are entirely dependent on their mothers and caregivers for their nutrition. Therefore, they are subject to each and all the environmental, social, and ecologic forces acting upon them. This partially explains why infant survival, nutrition, and health are sensitive markers of the progress and the speed of progress of societies. Since 2000, upper-middle-income countries have reduced their stunting prevalence by more than two-thirds, while low-income and low-middle-income countries only achieved a decrease of one-third. High-middle-income countries decreased stunting by two-thirds, low-middle by 28%, and low-income countries made no progress. And there has been no progress to stem the rate of overweight in nearly 20 years in any country by income group (UNICEF, 2021). Infant and child nutrition will always be major determinants of the future burden of disease and will continue to be a marker of the progress made to improve the health and well-being of nations. The state of child nutrition is the best reflection of society's image. Efforts to tackle the complex challenge of nutrition in early life have slowly emerged and improved outcomes for many individuals, in all periods of the human life cycle. Progress is undeniable, but slower and more disparate than we all would like.

## 1.9 Conclusions

The nutrition of infants and children has been a marker of development, for families, communities, nations, and society. Tremendous progress in improving child survival, wasting, and stunting has been made over the last 50 years, although millions of children are still wasted and remain stunted. Infants and children have also experienced a rapid shift to increasing rates of overweight and obesity. These have increased faster than the decrease in undernutrition, leading to the double burden of disease in most of the world, and exacerbating the disparities between the higher and lower economic levels of society.

Most of the global burden of disease and disability and the cost to society are related to poor nutrition. And much of this burden has its origins in what and how an individual is provided nutrition during gestation and the first 2 years of life. This book explores the mechanisms, consequences, and opportunities associated with early life nutrition, which underscore the enormous potential that investing in early life nutrition has at an individual and societal level.

What food an infant is provided is highly influenced by multiple layers of environmental influences and influencers, so improving infant and child nutrition will require a whole of society approach. Engagement and commitment of all sectors of society will be needed to facilitate access and affordability of food. However, much of *what* and most of *how* an infant is nourished is still parental and caregiver dependent. So much can be accomplished by educating parents on the factors they can still control, and by taking advantage of the dependency and plasticity of early life to shape the immune, metabolic, cognitive, and behavioral future of that individual.

As opposed to other investments in development, investing in the first 1000 days have a life-long effect, and benefits of these investments remain with the individual for life, wherever they live. Thus, compared to all other commitments we can make to improve health and wellness of individuals, investing in early child nutrition, aside being a moral and ethical imperative will provide the greatest economic and social returns to society.

# References

Access to Nutrition Index: (ATNI), 2021. Global Index. Available from: https://www.accesstonutrition.org. (Accessed 15 November 2021).

Amoroso, L., 2016. The second international conference on nutrition: implications for hidden hunger. World Rev. Nutr. Diet. 115, 142–152. https://doi.org/10.1159/000442100. Epub 2016 May 19 27197665.

Andreae, D., Nowak-Węgrzyn, A., 2022. Effects of infant allergen/immunogen exposure on long-term health. In: Saavedra, J.M., Dattilo, A.M. (Eds.), Early Nutrition and Long-Term Health: Mechanisms, Consequences, and Opportunities. Elsevier, Oxford (Chapter 7).

Ayala-Marín, A.M., Iguacel, I., Miguel-Etayo, P., Moreno, L.A., 2020. Consideration of social disadvantages for understanding and preventing obesity in children. Front. Public Health 8, 423. https://doi.org/10.3389/fpubh.2020.00423. 32984237. PMC7485391.

Barker, D.J., 2007. The origins of the developmental origins theory. J. Intern. Med. 261 (5), 412–417.

Berti, C., Agostoni, C., 2022. Establishing healthy eating patterns in infancy. In: Saavedra, J.M., Dattilo, A.M. (Eds.), Early Nutrition and Long-Term Health: Mechanisms, Consequences, and Opportunities. Elsevier, Oxford (Chapter 19).

Binns, C.W., Lee, M.K., Maycock, B., Torheim, L.E., Nanishi, K., Duong, D.T.T., 2021. Climate change, food supply, and dietary guidelines. Annu. Rev. Public Health 42, 233–255. https://doi.org/10.1146/annurev-publhealth-012420-105044. Epub 2021 Jan 26 33497266.

Burton, M.A., Godfrey, K.M., Lillycrop, K.A., 2022. Early nutrition and its effect on the development of obesity. In: Saavedra, J.M., Dattilo, A.M. (Eds.), Early Nutrition and Long-Term Health: Mechanisms, Consequences, and Opportunities. Elsevier, Oxford (Chapter 10).

Campbell, H., Wood, A.C., 2021. Challenges in feeding children posed by the COVID-19 pandemic: a systematic review of changes in dietary intake combined with a dietitian's perspective. Curr Nutr Rep. 10 (3), 155–165. https://doi.org/10.1007/s13668-021-00359-z. 33993426. PMC8123103.

Catassi, C., Lionetti, E., 2022. Early nutrition and its effect on the development of celiac disease. In: Saavedra, J.M., Dattilo, A.M. (Eds.), Early Nutrition and Long-Term Health: Mechanisms, Consequences, and Opportunities. Elsevier, Oxford (Chapter 14).

Center for disease control and Prevention (CDC), 2020. National Health and Nutrition Examination Survey (NHANES). https://www.cdc.gov/nchs/nhanes/nhanes_products.htm. (Accessed 15 November 2022).

Clark, H., Coll-Seck, A.M., Banerjee, A., Peterson, S., Dalglish, S.L., Ameratunga, S., Balabanova, D., Bhan, M.K., Bhutta, Z.A., Borrazzo, J., Claeson, M., Doherty, T., El-Jardali, F., George, A.S., Gichaga, A., Gram, L., Hipgrave, D.B., Kwamie, A., Meng, Q., Mercer, R., Narain, S., Nsungwa-Sabiiti, J., Olumide, A.O., Osrin, D., Powell-Jackson, T., Rasanathan, K., Rasul, I., Reid, P., Requejo, J., Rohde, S.S., Rollins, N., Romedenne, M., Singh Sachdev, H.,

Saleh, R., Shawar, Y.R., Shiffman, J., Simon, J., Sly, P.D., Stenberg, K., Tomlinson, M., Ved, R.R., Costello, A., 2020. A future for the wworld'schildren? A WHO-UNICEF lancet commission. Lancet 395 (10224), 605–658. https://doi. org/10.1016/S01406736(19)32540-1. Epub 2020 Feb 19. Erratum in: Lancet. 2020 May 23;395(10237):1612 32085821.

Closa-Monasterolo, R., Escribano Subías, J., Luque Moreno, V., Ferré, P.N., 2022. Early nutrition: effects of specific nutrient intake on growth, development, and long-term health. In: Saavedra, J.M., Dattilo, A.M. (Eds.), Early Nutrition and Long-Term Health: Mechanisms, Consequences, and Opportunities. Elsevier, Oxford (Chapter 5).

Crowder, S.L., Beckie, T., Stern, M., 2021. A review of food insecurity and chronic cardiovascular disease: implications during the COVID-19 pandemic. Ecol. Food Nutr. 60 (5), 596–611. https://doi.org/10.1080/03670244.2021. 1956485. 34617867.

Cusick, S.E., Georgieff, M.K., 2022. Early life nutrition and neurodevelopment. In: Saavedra, J.M., Dattilo, A.M. (Eds.), Early Nutrition and Long-Term Health: Mechanisms, Consequences, and Opportunities. Elsevier, Oxford (Chapter 6).

Dattilo, A.M., 2022. Early parent feeding behaviors to promote long-term health. In: Saavedra, J.M., Dattilo, A.M. (Eds.), Early Nutrition and Long-Term Health: Mechanisms, Consequences, and Opportunities. Elsevier, Oxford (Chapter 20).

Döring, N., Mayer, S., Rasmussen, F., Sonntag, D., 2016. Economic evaluation of obesity prevention in early childhood: methods, limitations and recommendations. Int. J. Environ. Res. Public Health 13 (9), 911. https://doi. org/10.3390/ijerph13090911. 27649218. PMC5036744.

Finkelstein, E.A., Graham, W.C., Malhotra, R., 2014. Lifetime direct medical costs of childhood obesity. Pediatrics 133 (5), 854–862. https://doi.org/10.1542/peds.2014-0063. Epub 2014 Apr 7 24709935.

Food and Agriculture Organization (FAO), 2018. Sustainable Food Systems. Concept and Framework. https://www. fao.org/3/ca2079en/CA2079EN.pdf. (Accessed 15 November 2021).

Food and Agriculture Organization (FAO), 2021. Food Systems. https://www.fao.org/food-systems/en/. (Accessed 15 November 2021).

Gappa, M., Filipiak-Pittroff, B., Libuda, L., von Berg, A., Koletzko, S., et al., 2020. Long-term effects of hydrolyzed formulae on atopic diseases in the GINI study. Allergy. https://doi.org/10.1111/all.14709.

Gianni, M.L., Morniroli, D., Vizzari, G., Mosca, F., 2022. Early nutrition: effects on iinfants'growth and body composition. In: Saavedra, J.M., Dattilo, A.M. (Eds.), Early Nutrition and Long-Term Health: Mechanisms, Consequences, and Opportunities. Elsevier, Oxford (Chapter 4).

Global Alliance for Improved Nutrition (GAIN), 2021. https://www.gainhealth.org/homepage. (Accessed 15 November 2021).

Global Burden of Disease (GBD) 2019 Risk Factors Collaborators, 2020. Global burden of 87 risk factors in 204 countries and territories, 1990–2019: a systematic analysis for the Global Burden of Disease Study 2019. Lancet 396 (10258), 1223–1249. https://doi.org/10.1016/S0140-6736(20)30752-2. 33069327. PMC7566194 https://www. healthdata.org/gbd/2019.

Global Nutrition Report (GNR), 2021. https://globalnutritionreport.org. (Accessed 15 November 2021).

Golden, S.D., Earp, J.A., 2012. Social ecological approaches to individuals and their contexts: twenty years of health education & behavior health promotion interventions. Health Educ. Behav. 39 (3), 364–372. https://doi. org/10.1177/1090198111418634. Epub 2012 Jan 20 22267868.

Golden, C.D., Gephart, J.A., Eurich, J.G., McCauley, D.J., Sharp, M.K., Andrew, N.L., Seto, K.L., 2021. Social ecological traps link food systems to nutritional outcomes. Glob. Food Sec. 30, 100561. https://doi.org/10.1016/j. gfs.2021.100561. Accessed 15 November 2021.

Guz-Mark, A., Shamir, R., 2022. Long-term health outcomes of breastfeeding. In: Saavedra, J.M., Dattilo, A.M. (Eds.), Early Nutrition and Long-Term Health: Mechanisms, Consequences, and Opportunities. Elsevier, Oxford (Chapter 3).

Hart, T.L., Petersen, K.S., Kris-Etherton, P.M., 2022. Early nutrition and development of cardiovascular disease. In: Saavedra, J.M., Dattilo, A.M. (Eds.), Early Nutrition and Long-Term Health: Mechanisms, Consequences, and Opportunities. Elsevier, Oxford (Chapter 12).

Headey, D., Heidkamp, R., Osendarp, S., Ruel, M., Scott, N., Black, R., Shekar, M., Bouis, H., Flory, A., Haddad, L., Walker, N., 2020. Standing together for nutrition consortium. Impacts of COVID-19 on childhood malnutrition and nutrition-related mortality. Lancet 396 (10250), 519–521. https://doi.org/10.1016/S0140-6736(20)31647-0. Epub 2020 Jul 27 32730743. PMC7384798.

Hill, D.A., Grundmeier, R.W., Ramos, M., Spergel, J.M., 2018. Eosinophilic esophagitis is a late manifestation of the allergic march. J. Allergy Clin. Immunol. Pract. 6 (5), 1528–1533. https://doi.org/10.1016/j.jaip.2018.05.010. Accessed 15 November 2021.

Horton, S., Steckel, R.H., 2011. Global Economic Losses Attributable to Malnutrition 1900–2000 and Projections to 2050. Assessment Paper, Copenhagen Consensus on Human Challenges. https://www.copenhagenconsensus.com/sites/default/files/malnutrition.pdf. (Accessed 15 November 2021).

Iglesia, E.G.A., Fleischer, D.M., Abrams, E.M., 2022. Early nutrition and the development of allergic diseases. In: Saavedra, J.M., Dattilo, A.M. (Eds.), Early Nutrition and Long-Term Health: Mechanisms, Consequences, and Opportunities. Elsevier, Oxford (Chapter 13).

International society for developmental origins of health and disease, 2015. DOHAD. Available from: https://dohadsoc.org/wp-content/uploads/2015/11/DOHaD-Society-Manifesto-Nov-17-2015.pdf. (Accessed 15 November 2021).

John, C.C., Black, M.M., Nelson 3rd., C.A., 2017. Neurodevelopment: the impact of nutrition and inflammation during early to middle childhood in low-resource settings. Pediatrics 139 (Suppl 1), S59–S71. https://doi.org/10.1542/peds.2016-2828H. PMID: 28562249; PMCID: PMC5694688.

Kalhoff, H., Kersting, M., 2022. Programming long-term health: nutrition and diet in infants aged 6 months to 1 year. In: Saavedra, J.M., Dattilo, A.M. (Eds.), Early Nutrition and Long Term Health: Mechanisms, Consequences, and Opportunities. Elsevier, Oxford (Chapter 21).

Kharas, H., McArthur, J.W., Rasmussen, K., September 2018. How many people will the world leave behind? Assessing Current Trajectories on the sustainable development goals. In: Global Economy & Development Working Paper 123. The Brookings Institution.

Koleilat, M., Whaley, S.E., Clapp, C., 2021. The impact of COVID-19 on breastfeeding rates in a low- ncome population. Breastfeed. Med. https://doi.org/10.1089/bfm.2021.0238. Epub ahead of Print. 34870454.

Laitinen, K., Mokkala, K., Kalliomäki, M., 2022. Impact of early nutrition on intestinal microbiota: effects on immunity and long-term health. In: Saavedra, J.M., Dattilo, A.M. (Eds.), Early Nutrition and Long-Term Health: Mechanisms, Consequences, and Opportunities. Elsevier, Oxford (Chapter 9).

Lassi, Z.S., Padhani, Z.A., Salam, R.A., Bhutta, Z.A., 2022. Prenatal nutrition and nutrition in pregnancy: effects on long-term growth and development. In: Saavedra, J.M., Dattilo, A.M. (Eds.), Early Nutrition and Long-Term Health: Mechanisms, Consequences, and Opportunities. Elsevier, Oxford (Chapter 16).

Lenaerts, B., Demont, M., 2021. The global burden of chronic and hidden hunger revisited: new panel data evidence spanning 1990-2017. Glob. Food Sec. 28. https://doi.org/10.1016/j.gfs.2020.100480, 100480. 33738187. PMC7937785.

Loth, K.A., Ji, Z., Wolfson, J., Berge, J.M., Neumark-Sztainer, D., Fisher, J.O., 2022. COVID-19 pandemic shifts in food-related parenting practices within an ethnically/racially and socioeconomically diverse sample of families of preschool-aged children. Appetite 168, 105714. https://doi.org/10.1016/j.appet.2021.105714. 34619241. PMC8503935. Epub 2021 Oct 5.

Milliken, O.V., Ellis, V.L., 2018. Development of an investment case for obesity prevention and control: perspectives on methodological advancement and evidence. Rev. Panam. Salud Publica 42. https://doi.org/10.26633/RPSP.2018.62. PMID: 31093090; PMCID: PMC6385999, e62.

Mirzabaev, A., Olsson, L., Bezner Kerr, R., Pradhan, P., Guadalupe, M., Ferre, R., Lotze-Campen, H.M., May 2021. climate change and food systems. In: Research Partners of the Scientific Group for the Food Systems Summit. United Nations Food Systems Summit Brief. https://sc-fss2021.org/. (Accessed 15 November 2021).

National Academies of Sciences, Engineering, and Medicine (NAS), 2020. Feeding Infants and Children from Birth to 24 Months: Summarizing Existing Guidance. The National Academies Press, Washington, DC, https://doi.org/10.17226/25747.

NCD Risk Factor Collaboration (NCD-RisC), 2017. Worldwide trends in body-mass index, underweight, overweight, and obesity from 1975 to 2016: a pooled analysis of 2416 population-based measurement studies in 128·9 million children, adolescents, and adults. Lancet 390 (10113), 2627–2642. https://doi.org/10.1016/S0140-6736(17)32129-3. Epub 2017 Oct 10 29029897. PMC5735219.

O'Neill, L., Orlet-Fisher, J., 2022. Developing science based dietary guidelines for infants and toddlers. In: Saavedra, J.M., Dattilo, A.M. (Eds.), Early Nutrition and Long-Term Health: Mechanisms, Consequences, and Opportunities. Elsevier, Oxford (Chapter 22).

Perng, W., Oken, E., 2022. Programming long-term health: maternal and fetal nutrition and diet needs. In: Saavedra, J.M., Dattilo, A.M. (Eds.), Early Nutrition and Long-Term Health: Mechanisms, Consequences, and Opportunities. Elsevier, Oxford (Chapter 2).

Ratsika, A., Codagnone, M.C., O'Mahony, S., Stanton, C., Cryan, J.F., 2021. Priming for life: early life nutrition and the microbiota-gut-brain axis. Nutrients 13 (2), 423. https://doi.org/10.3390/nu13020423. 33525617. PMC7912058.

Rippin, H.L., Hutchinson, J., Jewell, J., Breda, J.J., Cade, J.E., 2019. Child and adolescent nutrient intakes from current national dietary surveys of European populations. Nutr. Res. Rev. 32 (1), 38–69. https://doi.org/10.1017/S0954422418000161. Epub 2018 Nov 3 30388967. PMC6536833.

Roser, M., Ritchie, H., Dadonaite, B., 2019. Child and Infant Mortality. Our World Data. https://ourworldindata.org/child-mortality#child-mortality-around-the-world-since-1800. (Accessed 15 November 2021).

Ross, E., 2022. Eating development in young children: understanding the complex interplay of developmental domains. In: Saavedra, J.M., Dattilo, A.M. (Eds.), Early Nutrition and Long Term Health: Mechanisms, Consequences, and Opportunities. Elsevier, Oxford (Chapter 8).

Saavedra, J.M., 2022. Early nutrition and its effect on the development of obesity. In: Saavedra, J.M., Dattilo, A.M. (Eds.), Early Nutrition and Long-Term Health: Mechanisms, Consequences, and Opportunities. Elsevier, Oxford (Chapter 18).

Saavedra, J.M., Dattilo, A.M., 2017. In: Saavedra, J.M., Dattilo, A.M. (Eds.), Early Nutrition and Long-Term Health: Mechanisms, Consequences, and Opportunities. Elsevier, Oxford.

Salvatore, S., Vandenplas, Y., 2022. Early nutrition and its effect on the development of functional gastrointestinal disorders. In: Saavedra, J.M., Dattilo, A.M. (Eds.), Early Nutrition and Long-Term Health: Mechanisms, Consequences, and Opportunities. Elsevier, Oxford (Chapter 15).

Scaling Up Nutrition (SUN), 2021. Strategy 3.0. 2021–2025. https://reliefweb.int/report/world/scaling-nutrition-sun-movement-strategy-30-2021-2025. (Accessed 15 November 2021).

Schwarzenberg, S.J., Georgieff, M.K., Committee On Nutrition, 2018. Advocacy for improving nutrition in the first 1000 Days to support childhood development and adult health. Am. Acad. Pediatr. 141 (2). https://doi.org/10.1542/peds.2017-3716, e20173716 (Epub 2018 Jan 22. PMID: 29358479).

Shekar, M., Kakietek, J., Eberwein, D., Julia, Walters, D., 2017. An Investment Framework for Nutrition: Reaching the Global Targets for Stunting, Anemia, Breastfeeding, and Wasting. Directions in Development-Human Development;World Bank. © World Bank, Washington, DC. https://openknowledge.worldbank.org/handle/10986/26069. License: CC BY 3.0 IGO.

Stenberg, K., Axelson, H., Sheehan, P., Anderson, I., Gülmezoglu, A.M., Temmerman, M., Mason, E., Friedman, H.S., Bhutta, Z.A., Lawn, J.E., Sweeny, K., Tulloch, J., Hansen, P., Chopra, M., Gupta, A., Vogel, J.P., Ostergren, M., Rasmussen, B., Levin, C., Boyle, C., Kuruvilla, S., Koblinsky, M., Walker, N., de Francisco, A., Novcic, N., Presern, C., Jamison, D., Bustreo, F., 2014. Advancing social and economic development by investing in women's and children's health: A new Global Investment Framework. The Lancet 383 (9925), 1333–1354. https://doi.org/10.1016/S0140-6736(13)62231-X.

Thousand Days, 2016. Why 1000 days? Available from: http://thousanddays.org/the-issue/why-1000-days/. (Accessed 15 November 2021).

United Nations (UN), 2015. Transforming our World: The 2030 Agenda for Sustainable Development. United Nations. A/RES/70/1, New York. https://sdgs.un.org/2030agenda.

United Nations (UN), 2016. Calling attention to chronic hunger. In: General Assembly Decides 2016 2025 Will Be Decade of Action on Nutrition. General Assembly Plenary, Seventieth Session, 90th Meeting, April 2016. https://www.un.org/press/en/2016/ga11770.doc.htm. (Accessed 15 November 2021).

United Nations Children's Fund (UNICEF), 2019. The State of the World's Children 2019. Children, Food and Nutrition: Growing Well in a Changing World. UNICEF, New York. ISBN: 978-92-806-5003-7.

United Nations Children's Fund (UNICEF), 2020. Child Nutrition and COVID-19. https://www.unicef.org/press-releases/unicef-additional-67-million-children-under-5-could-suffer-wasting-year-due-covid-19. (Accessed 15 November 2021).

United Nations Children's Fund (UNICEF), 2021. In: World Health Organization, International Bank for Reconstruction and Development/The World Bank (Eds.), Levels and Trends in Child Malnutrition: Key Findings of the 2021 Edition of the Joint Child Malnutrition Estimates. World Health Organization, Geneva. https://www.who.int/publications/i/item/9789240025257. (Accessed 15 November 2021).

van de Lagemaat, M., Ruys, C.A., Lafeber, H.N., van Goudoever, J.B., van den Akker, C.H.P., 2022. Addressing nutritional needs in preterm infants to promote long-term health. In: Saavedra, J.M., Dattilo, A.M. (Eds.), Early Nutrition and Long-Term Health: Mechanisms, Consequences, and Opportunities. Elsevier, Oxford (Chapter 17).

Vickers, M.H., 2022. Early life nutrition and its effect on the development of type-2 diabetes. In: Saavedra, J.M., Dattilo, A.M. (Eds.), Early Nutrition and Long-Term Health: Mechanisms, Consequences, and Opportunities. Elsevier, Oxford (Chapter 11).

Victora, C.G., Christian, P., Vidaletti, L.P., Gatica-Domínguez, G., Menon, P., Black, R.E., 2021. Revisiting maternal and child undernutrition in low-income and middle-income countries: variable progress towards an unfinished agenda. Lancet 397 (10282), 1388–1399. https://doi.org/10.1016/S0140 6736(21)00394-9. Epub 2021 Mar 7 33691094.

Wells, J.C.K., Marphatia, A.A., Amable, G., Siervo, M., Friis, H., Miranda, J.J., Haisma, H.H., Raubenheimer, D., 2021. The future of human malnutrition: rebalancing agency for better nutritional health. Glob. Health 17 (1), 119. https://doi.org/10.1186/s12992-021-00767-4. PMID: 34627303; PMCID: PMC8500827.

World Food Program (WFP), 2021. COVID-19 Will Double Number of People Facing Food Crises Unless Swift Action is Taken. https://www.wfp.org/news/covid-19-will-double-number-people-facing-food-crises-unless-swift-action-taken. (Accessed 15 November 2021).

World Health Organization (WHO), 2012. 65th World Health Assembly WHA, Geneva, 21-26, May 2012.

World Health Organization (WHO), 2014. Global Nutrition Targets 2025: Policy Brief Series (WHO/NMH/NHD/14.2). Geneva, 2014. https://www.who.int/publications/i/item/WHO-NMH-NHD-14.2. (Accessed 15 November 2021).

World Health Organization (WHO), 2016. Report of the Commission on Ending Childhood Obesity. Geneva, Switzerland. ISBN 978 92 4 151006 6 (NLM classification: WS 130 Available from http://apps.who.int/iris/bitstream/10665/204176/1/9789241510066_eng.pdf. (Accessed 15 November 2021).

World Health Organization (WHO), 2021b. Nutrition. Infant and Young Child Feeding Data by Country. https://apps.who.int/nutrition/databases/infantfeeding/countries/en/index.html.

World Health Organization (WHO), 2021c. Malnutrition. https://www.who.int/en/news-room/fact-sheets/detail/malnutrition. Accessed 15 November 2021.

World Health Organization (WHO), 2021a. Non-Communicable Diseases. https://www.who.int/health-topics/noncommunicable-diseases#tab=tab_1. Accessed 15 November 2021.

World Obesity Federation, March 2021. COVID-19 and Obesity: The 2021 Atlas. https://www.worldobesity.org/resources/resource-library/covid-19-and-obesity-the-2021-atlas. (Accessed 15 November 2021).

Wu, A.J., Aris, I.M., Hivert, M.F., Rocchio, C., Cocoros, N.M., Klompas, M., Taveras, E.M., 2021. Association of Changes in obesity prevalence with the COVID-19 pandemic in youth in Massachusetts. JAMA Pediatr. https://doi.org/10.1001/jamapediatrics.2021.5095. Epub ahead of print 34901998.

Yang, I., Corwin, E.J., Brennan, P.A., Jordan, S., Murphy, J.R., Dunlop, A., 2016. The infant microbiome: implications for infant health and neurocognitive development. Nurs. Res. 65 (1), 76–88. https://doi.org/10.1097/NNR.0000000000000133. 26657483. PMC4681407.

Zemrani, B., Gehri, M., Masserey, E., Knob, C., Pellaton, R., 2021. A hidden side of the COVID-19 pandemic in children: the double burden of undernutrition and overnutrition. Int. J. Equity Health 20 (1), 44. https://doi.org/10.1186/s12939-021-01390-w. PMID: 33482829; PMCID: PMC7820834.

# Programming long-term health: Maternal and fetal nutritional and dietary needs

*Wei Perng[a,b] and Emily Oken[c,d]*

[a]Department of Epidemiology, Colorado School of Public Health, University of Colorado Anschutz Medical Campus, Aurora, CO, United States [b]Lifecourse Epidemiology of Adiposity and Diabetes (LEAD) Center, University of Colorado Anschutz Medical Campus, Aurora, CO, United States [c]Division of Chronic Disease Research Across the Lifecourse (CoRAL), Department of Population Medicine, Harvard Medical School/Harvard Pilgrim Health Care Institute, Boston, MA, United States [d]Department of Nutrition, T. H. Chan Harvard School of Public Health, Boston, MA, United States

## CHAPTER LEARNING OBJECTIVES

- Become familiar with current recommendations for maternal dietary needs during three distinct timeframes: from the time of conception through 12 weeks gestation (*periconceptional*), during gestation (*pre-natal*), and the 6 months to 1 year after delivery (*post-natal*).

- Understand the roles of specific micro- and macronutrients in fetal growth and development, as well as their long-term effects on health outcomes in offspring

- Identify gaps in current knowledge and novel areas of inquiry, including the re-emergence of certain micronutrient deficiencies (e.g., iodine), the need for more studies assessing maternal dietary patterns, and a recent push to understand how the placenta may modulate the relationship between maternal nutritional status and offspring outcomes.

## 2.1 Introduction

The notion that experiences in early life affect health in adulthood was most famously promoted by David Barker in the 1980s, following observations of inverse associations of birthweight—a marker of the in utero nutritional environment—with ischemic heart disease mortality among British men (Barker et al., 1989). The field has since grown beyond the original emphasis on fetal programming via the in utero milieu to a broader conceptualization captured by the developmental origins of health and disease (DOHaD) hypothesis, which posits that a range of perinatal and early-life exposures and experiences have life-long health consequences. Early nutrition is now established as a determinant of future chronic disease risk, with cardiovascular and metabolic illnesses being the most widely studied. In fact, the importance of good nutrition in pregnancy and infancy has become the focal point of domestic and international programs promoting health and well-being, including the Bill and Melinda Gates *Global Development Initiative for Nutrition* (Bill and Melinda Gates Foundation, n.d.), *Feed the Future* (Feed the Future, n.d.), *The B-24 Project* (Raiten et al., 2014), and *1000 days* (1000 Days, n.d.). Additionally, for the first time, guidelines for nutrition during pregnancy was included in the Dietary Guidelines for Americans 2020 (Dietary Guidelines Advisory Committee, 2020).

In this chapter we describe nutritional needs and requirements, the relevance of dietary patterns, and gaps in knowledge surrounding diet during the pre- and perinatal periods in relation to later-life disease risk, specifically cardiometabolic and neurodevelopmental outcomes (*nota bene*, we do not address atopic outcomes in detail here as that area has its own rich literature). We focus on maternal nutritional status and intake because the mother is the source of all nutrition for the fetus and most of the nutrition for a breastfeeding infant. We consider three time periods: (1) around the time of conception (*periconceptional*), (2) during gestation *(pre-natal)*, and (3) the 6 months to 1 year after delivery (*post-natal*).

Fig. 2.1 displays maternal and fetal dietary needs during each of the three periods with the corresponding developmental and physiological processes portrayed in parallel. While not all nutrients listed in the Figure have been linked to long-term offspring health outcomes, **Sections 2.2–2.4** summarize existing evidence for nutrients that have been implicated in long-term health of offspring. **Section 2.5** highlights gaps in knowledge and makes suggestions for future research, and **Section 2.6** provides a brief synopsis of the chapter and makes broad recommendations for practice.

## 2.2 Periconceptional nutritional and dietary needs

The periconceptional period comprises the 3 months before conception through approximately 12 weeks gestation. Critical developmental stages that take place during this timeframe include implantation, placentation, and embryogenesis, each of which may be affected by the gravida's health history, current health, and diet. Table 2.1 summarizes current daily intake recommendations for reproductive-aged women according to the National Academy of Sciences Institute of Medicine Food & Nutrition Board (Institute of Medicine Food and Nutrition Board, 2006).

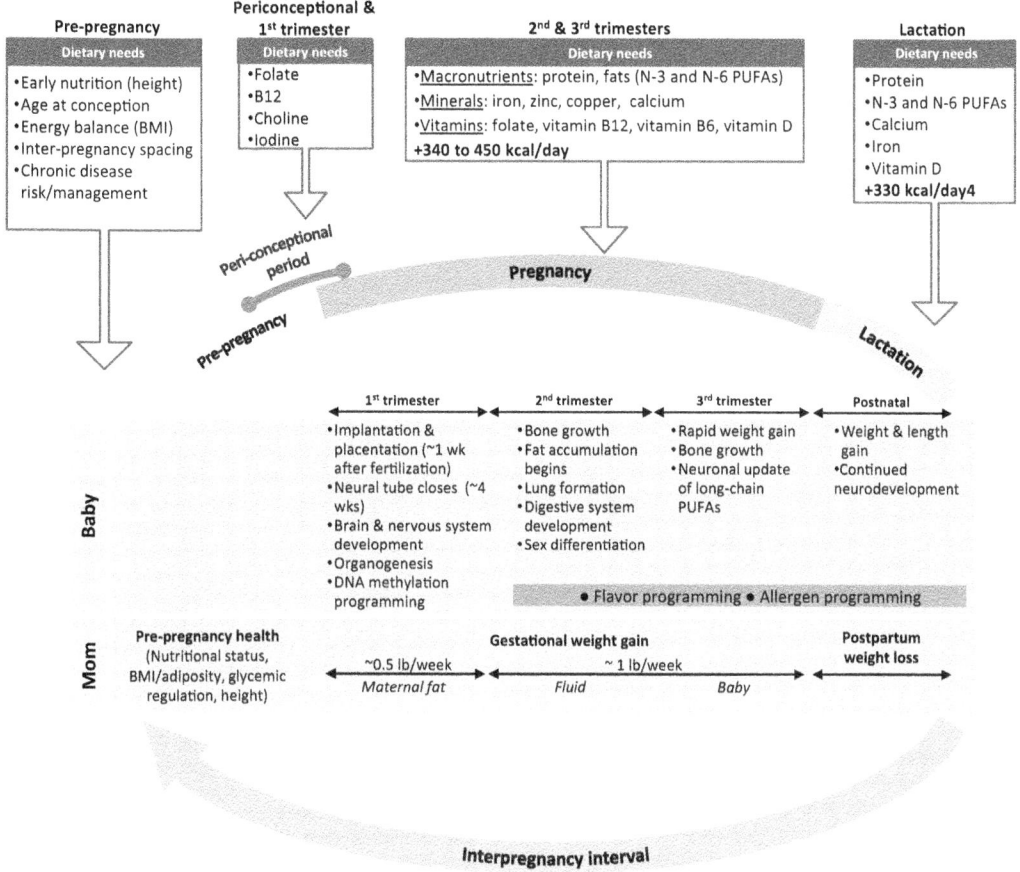

**FIG. 2.1** Maternal and child dietary needs during the periconceptional period, gestation, and post-natally.

Outreach efforts to promote optimal dietary habits and other lifestyle behaviors focus on all reproductive-aged women because up to half of pregnancies are unplanned, and so it remains important for all women who could become pregnant to be aware of the recommendations. A large body of literature focuses on the necessity of these nutrients for healthy birth outcomes (Gardiner et al., 2008; Mcardle and Ashworth, 1999; Ramakrishnan et al., 2012), but few have been studied in relation to long-term offspring outcomes. In this section, we discuss the influence of pre-pregnancy nutritional status - both under- and overnutrition - on health of offspring, followed by what is currently known for specific nutrients.

## 2.2.1 Undernutrition

Animal models indicate that overall, or global, undernutrition around the time of conception can influence maternal endocrine and metabolic processes early in pregnancy (Todd et al., 2009; Jaquiery et al., 2012). These alterations can affect the supply and utilization of available nutrients for the fetus, potentially leading to permanent changes in offspring

**TABLE 2.1**    Recommendations for daily dietary needs during the periconceptional period, pregnancy, and lactation.

| | Recommended daily allowance (RDA) | | |
|---|---|---|---|
| | Periconceptional[a] | Pregnancy | Post-partum/lactation |
| **Vitamins** | | | |
| Folic Acid | 400 µg | 600 µg | 500 µg |
| Vitamin B6 | 1.3 mg | 1.9 mg | 2 mg |
| Vitamin B12 | 2.4 µg | 2.6 µg | 2.8 µg |
| Vitamin A | 500 µg (1665 IU) | 750 µg (2500 IU) | 390 µg (1300 IU) |
| Vitamin D | 15 µg (600 IU) | 15 µg (600 IU) | 15 µg (600 IU) |
| Vitamin E | 7.5 mg (11.3 IU) | 15 mg (22.5 IU) | 19 mg (28.5 IU) |
| **Minerals** | | | |
| Calcium | 14–18 y: 1300 mg | 14–18 y: 1300 mg | 14–18 y: 1300 mg |
| | 19–50 y: 1000 mg | 19–50 y: 1000 mg | 19–50 y: 1000 mg |
| Iron | 18 mg | 27 mg | 9 mg |
| Zinc | 12 mg | 15 mg | 19 mg |
| Iodine | 220 µg | 220 µg | 290 µg |
| Fluoride | 3 mg (AI) | 3 mg (AI) | 3 mg (AI) |
| **Macronutrients** | | | |
| Carbohydrates | 130 g | 175 g | 210 g |
| Protein | 45 g | 71 g | 71 g |
| Fat | ND | ND | ND |
| Trans fatty acids | ND | ND | ND |
| Essential fatty acids | | | |
| N-6 Linoleic acid | 12 g (AI) | 13 g (AI) | 13 g (AI) |
| N-3 Linolenic acid | 1.1 g (AI) | 1.4 g (AI) | 1.3 g (AI) |

*AI*: adequate intake—the recommended average daily intake level based on observed or experimentally determined approximations or estimates of nutrient intake by a group (or groups) of apparently healthy people assumed to be adequate; used when RDA cannot be determined.
*IU*: international units.
*ND*: not determined.
*RDA*: recommended daily allowance—the average daily dietary nutrient intake level that is sufficient to meet the nutrient requirements of nearly all (97%–98%) healthy individuals in a particular life stage and gender group.
[a] *RDA values are for reproductive-aged women, particularly those considering getting pregnant.*
*Institute of Medicine Dietary Reference Intake report, Institute of Medicine Food and Nutrition Board, 2006. Dietary reference intake: the essential guide to nutrient requirements. In: Otten, J.J., Hellwig, J.P., Meyers, L. D. (Eds.). National Academy of Sciences, Washington, D.C.*

phenotype. In humans, there has been little empirical research on periconceptional diet in relation to long-term offspring health outcomes, although maternal height and weight status are widely used as crude proxies for nutritional status. Shorter maternal height, an indicator of poor early-life nutrition, has been correlated with offspring morbidity including childhood mortality, stunting, wasting, and anemia (Subramanian et al., 2009; Ozaltin et al., 2010). While there is inarguably, a strong genetic component in the height/health correlation between parents and offspring, Gray et al. were able to examine relations of parental height with offspring cardiovascular outcomes in both the mother and father. Using prospectively collected data for 2306 offspring from 1456 couples in the Scotland Mid-span Family Study, the investigators found that shorter parents had offspring with lower high-density lipoprotein (HDL) cholesterol, and greater risk of coronary heart disease at 30–59 years (Gray et al., 2012). Because the associations were stronger for maternal than paternal height, these results support the possibility that intrauterine mechanisms, rather than genetics, underlie the observed relations.

Historical famines also provide a lens to examine the influence of acute malnutrition prior to and during pregnancy on long-term offspring outcomes. For example, the unfortunate circumstances that led to the "Hunger Winter" of 1944–45 in the Netherlands enabled researchers to examine consequences of famine during different pregnancy time points on a variety of mental and physical outcomes later in life (Lumey et al., 2007). Although researchers have not detected an effect of famine exposure during gestation on adult cognition or mental health (Stein et al., 1972), Painter et al. reported that persons conceived at the peak of famine, and thus exposed in the first and second trimesters, were slightly heavier at birth and had greater overall and central adiposity than their unexposed same-sex siblings (Painter et al., 2005), a phenomenon that is possibly mediated by DNA methylation (Heijmans et al., 2008). This finding is in contrast to persons exposed to famine later in gestation, who had lower birthweight but also lower obesity risk later in life (Painter et al., 2005). While these findings shed light on long-term consequences of severe malnutrition at conception and early in gestation, the results are likely not generalizable to relatively well-nourished modern-day populations and may also be fraught with unmeasured confounding and survival bias with loss of the more poorly growing fetuses. For mostly practical reasons, the majority of contemporary studies on nutritional deficits during pregnancy have focused on the second and/or third trimester, by which time organogenesis has been completed (more on this topic in **Section 2.3**). Considering that the basic structures of the central nervous system are formed between 3 and 5 weeks of pregnancy, nutrient imbalances during this timeframe could have long-lasting consequences for neurocognitive function, and thus understanding effects of periconceptional diet/nutritional status on long-term offspring health is an urgent area of research. We further discuss the implications of specific nutrient deficiencies in **Section 2.2.3**.

## 2.2.2 Overnutrition

Maternal overnutrition, typically assessed as excess total energy intake, having obesity and/or type 2 diabetes prior to and entering pregnancy (Perng et al., 2019a) is a growing problem worldwide (Flegal et al., 2012; Finucane et al., 2011). Further, maternal adiposity and hyperglycemia—even below thresholds for clinical obesity or diabetes—during the periconceptional period are related to a host of pregnancy and birth complications like gestational diabetes, hypertensive disorders, neural tube defects, pre-term delivery, stillbirth, and macrosomia (Dixit and Girling, 2008), and also have long-term implications for offspring adiposity (Yu et al., 2013; Perng et al., 2014) and metabolic disease risk (Hochner et al., 2012; Fraser et al., 2011; Perng et al., 2014; Francis et al., 2021). Of particular concern are overweight women who consume excess calories and have poor diet quality and therefore insufficient intake of important micronutrients (Rifas-Shiman et al., 2009), necessitating careful assessment of nutrition in this group in order to make appropriate recommendations for dietary intake.

The underlying biological mechanisms linking maternal periconceptional overnutrition to offspring adiposity and cardiometabolic risk remain unclear, but animal experiments indicate that the relationship extends beyond shared genetics and lifestyle. In rodents, diet-induced maternal obesity before pregnancy altered offspring adipocyte metabolism to favor hypertrophy and promotes hyperphagic feeding behavior via alterations in satiety centers of the brain (Begum et al., 2013; Samuelsson et al., 2008; Bringhenti et al., 2013; Howie et al., 2009). A study of maternal-fetal macaque pairs identified differences in metabolite profiles of offspring born to obese vs lean dams independent of dietary intake during breeding and pregnancy, suggesting a specific role of maternal weight status before pregnancy on metabolic programming in offspring (Cox et al., 2009).

Recent in vitro studies nested within human cohorts shed light on specific mechanistic pathways that may link maternal obesity to offspring outcomes. An analysis of pluripotent mesenchymal stem cells harvested from cord blood of a subset of women in the Healthy Start Study (a Colorado pre-birth cohort) found evidence of altered β-catenin pathways and differential expression of genes involved in myocyte growth, amino acid synthesis, and oxidative stress in exclusively among women with obesity (Boyle et al., 2017, 2016; Baker et al., 2017b,a; Shapiro et al., 2016a). Such findings suggest that maternal obesity may "program" offspring health through an effect on the physiology and function of pluripotent stem cells that differentiate into all other biological tissues in the offspring.

As research in this area continues, we note that in addition to improving mechanistic knowledge of how maternal periconceptional nutritional status influences offspring health, growing evidence that maternal nutritional status before pregnancy makes an independent contribution to offspring health could serve as a powerful motivator for women to eat healthfully not just during pregnancy, but also before conception.

## 2.2.3 Nutrients

### 2.2.3.1 Iron

The relevance of iron and iron status in pregnant women has recently resurfaced, with an emphasis on the need to re-evaluate thresholds for assessing of anemia, iron deficiency, and iron-deficiency anemia during pregnancy in pregnant women (O'brien and Ru, 2017) and potentially among all reproductive-aged women given the detrimental effects of iron deficiency on key physiological processes that occur during early pregnancy, such as placentation (Young et al., 2010).

Iron deficiency remains a concern in several countries worldwide. In resource-poor settings, women may have anemia when they enter pregnancy because of inadequate food intake and/or infection. Hand-in-hand with the issue of underweight, anemia is still a prominent public health concern, with prevalence estimates of 30% and 42% for non-pregnant and pregnant women worldwide, respectively (World Health Organization, n.d.). Even in developed settings like the U.S., anemia is a persistent issue that affects 3.8%–6.5% of reproductive-aged women (Le, 2016). While there is little literature on the impact of anemia before pregnancy on long-term offspring outcomes, one study of 405 Chinese women found that pre-pregnancy anemia corresponded with reduced fetal growth (Ronnenberg et al., 2004). The authors further noted that although anemia was an important predictor of pregnancy outcomes in their study sample, preconception iron-deficiency anemia had a particularly strong association with birthweight—i.e., infants born to women with preconception iron-deficiency anemia and adequate B-vitamin status weighed on average 241 g less than those born to women without periconceptional anemia (Ronnenberg et al., 2004). Such findings raise the question of whether iron status entering pregnancy has an independent effect on infant growth, perhaps by influencing hormone synthesis (Allen, 2001).

It is important to bear in mind that, like most nutrients, iron exhibits a U-shaped risk curve. The adverse effects of iron deficiency during early life (i.e., pre-natal period, infancy) on neurobehavioral outcomes were well-described (Lozoff et al., 2006). However, as a divalent metal, iron has potential to react in inorganic reactions that can damage components of the cell. Accordingly, researchers have raised concern regarding the need for careful assessment of population-level iron status to avoid applying across-the-board iron supplementation programs in well-nourished populations (Georgieff et al., 2019).

### 2.2.3.2 Folate

Folate, a water-soluble B-vitamin, has been the single most thoroughly investigated nutrient with respect to maternal periconceptional nutritional status and long-term offspring health. Intervention trials as well as observational studies provide strong evidence that periconceptional folate intake of at least 400 µg daily is protective against fetal neural tube defects (NTDs) (Pitkin, 2007; De-Regil et al., 2010), as well as limb, cardiac, and urinary tract defects (Willett and Stampfer, 2001). However, as we discuss in more detail in **Section 2.3.4**, some concern exists that folate supplementation throughout pregnancy may confer risks in some populations.

### 2.2.3.3 Iodine

Iodine is a key component of thyroid hormones crucial for brain and neurological development, and thus, maternal iodine status starting in the periconceptional period is likely relevant for offspring neurodevelopment given that much of the primordium of the brain and spinal cord forms between the 17th and 30th day after fertilization. Although widespread iodine deficiency is less common in the modern era of salt iodization, even women in industrialized settings may be at risk for insufficient intake (Andersson et al., 2012). Data from the 2001–06 National Health and Nutrition Examination Survey (NHANES) (Perrine et al., 2010) and a recent scoping review (Panth et al., 2019) revealed that despite the initial success of salt iodine fortification in the 1920s to combat endemic iodine deficiency, the issue is re-emerging and at least partially attributable to the growing popularity of sea salts and other non-iodized salts (Maalouf et al., 2015).

It is well-known that severe iodine deficiency during gestation may result in mental retardation and cretinism (Zimmermann, 2012). Mild-to-moderate deficiency might also have discernible effects on offspring cognition. A small prospective study in healthy women found that children of mothers with serum free thyroxine levels below the 10th percentile of the sample ($< 10.4$ pmol/L; $n = 22$), at 12 weeks gestation, a condition likely to have been caused by insufficient iodine, exhibited deficits in psychomotor development in offspring at 10 months of age (Pop et al., 1999). Among 1040 U.K. mother–child dyads from the Avon Longitudinal Study of Parents and Children (ALSPAC), Bath et al. examined the relation between maternal urinary iodine concentrations at approximately 10 weeks gestation with offspring IQ at 8 years (Bath et al., 2013). The investigators found that children of women with mild-to-moderate iodine deficiency (iodine-to-creatinine ratio < 150 μg/g) were more likely to be in lowest quartile for verbal IQ (odds ratio [OR]: 1.58 [95% CI: 1.09, 2.30]), reading accuracy (OR: 1.69 [95% CI: 1.15, 2.49]), and reading comprehension (OR: 1.54 [95% CI: 1.06, 2.23]), than those whose mothers were not deficient (Bath et al., 2013). Moreover, the authors observed a worsening trend in cognitive outcomes with decreasing maternal iodine status (Bath et al., 2013). Taken together, these findings highlight the importance of adequate iodine intake in reproductive-aged women and the need for higher vigilance regarding this issue in pre-natal clinics.

### 2.2.3.4 Vitamin D

Vitamin D is a class of pleiotropic secosteroid hormones that has well-known classical functions in calcium uptake and bone metabolism. In addition, Vitamin D facilitates uptake of iron, magnesium, phosphate, and zinc. In humans, the two most important compounds in this group are vitamin D2 and vitamin D3, the latter of which is synthesized in the skin with adequate sun exposure.

Recent work highlights additional actions of this micronutrient in a variety of cell types, including as a modulator of implantation and placentation during early pregnancy (Ganguly et al., 2018). Given that these processes occur within the first 7–8 days of fertilization and are implicated in the etiology adverse pregnancy outcomes like gestational diabetes, pre-eclampsia, fetal growth restriction, and pre-term delivery (Shin et al., 2010; Kelly et al., 2009), understanding the association between women's vitamin D status entering pregnancy and risk of such complications is crucial. Yet, the relationship between maternal diet and placental physiology/function is difficult to study given that placental tissue is difficult to obtain and generally not assessed until after delivery. Accordingly, deciphering when specific nutrients are most relevant to placental function requires inference from in vitro studies and animal models that may not entirely reflect the sequence of physiological events in vivo. Large collaborative efforts like the Human Placenta Project (U.S. Department of Health and Human Services, n.d.) are instrumental to addressing some of these gaps in literature as researchers develop new non-invasive tools capable of studying the organ in real time in order to understand how it develops and functions throughout pregnancy.

## 2.3 Nutrition during pregnancy

While the consequences of inadequate caloric and/or nutrient intake during pregnancy have historically been the focus of DOHaD research (Barker et al., 1989, 1993; Barker and Osmond, 1986), it is becoming clear that serious long-term health consequences also result from nutrient imbalance, even when total caloric intake is more than sufficient to meet the demands of pregnancy. In this section, we introduce the relevance of total energy intake and macronutrient balance during pregnancy, followed by the importance of specific nutrients.

The demand for energy and nutrients increases during pregnancy. For well-nourished women, only a small number of additional calories are required due to natural adaptations such as increased metabolic efficiency and reduced physical activity (DuFour and Sauther, 2002). Although the exact increase in energy needed during pregnancy depends on plurality and the woman's pre-pregnancy weight status, the Academy of Nutrition and Dietetics provides guidelines for additional caloric needs of an additional 340 cal per day during the second trimester, and up to 450 additional calories per day during the third trimester (Academy of Nutrition and Dietetics, 2013) to reflect current National Academy of Medicine recommendations for gestational weight gain (Institute of Medicine, 2009) which are displayed in Table 2.2.

Total caloric intake, derived from the macronutrients protein, carbohydrate, and fat, is a key determinant of gestational weight gain. While weight gain is not a dietary factor per se, it is a direct consequence of energy balance and could influence long-term offspring health through intrauterine mechanisms.

## 2.3.1 Low energy intake and inadequate gestational weight gain

The fetus needs macronutrients for growth, and not surprisingly, there is an overall linear relationship between maternal gestational weight gain and fetal growth (Oken, 2009). In many cases, poor gestational weight gain—especially in the latter half of pregnancy—is associated with fetal growth restriction as well as greater risk of premature birth. However, there is a complex interaction between nutritional status entering pregnancy and that during pregnancy; for some obese women, pregnancy outcomes may actually be optimized at weight gains lower than the recommended amount, or even with weight loss (Oken et al., 2009).

Inadequate gain is especially prevalent in developing settings where women are malnourished and either do not have access to sufficient food, or have a high physical work demand. Even in developed settings, inadequate gain is experienced by about 10% of women, and is especially concerning among women with low pre-pregnancy BMI, adolescents, or those who experience major psychosocial stressors (Iom National Research Council Committee, 2009).

**TABLE 2.2**  National Academy of Medicine recommendations for gestational weight gain according to pre-pregnancy BMI categories.

|  | Range of recommended weight gain (kg) |
| --- | --- |
| Pre-pregnancy BMI |  |
| Underweight ($< 18.5 \, kg/m^2$) | 12.5–18.0 |
| Normal weight ($18.5–24.9 \, kg/m^2$) | 11.5–16.0 |
| Overweight ($25–29.9 \, kg/m^2$) | 7.0–11.5 |
| Obese ($\geq 30 \, kg/m^2$) | 5.0–9.0 |

*Institute of Medicine, 2009. The National Academies collection: reports funded by National Institutes of Health. In: Rasmussen, K.M., Yaktine, A.L. (Eds.) Weight Gain During Pregnancy: Reexamining the Guidelines. National Academies Press (US) National Academy of Sciences, Washington (DC).*

Women also may consciously restrict their food intake during pregnancy on the premise that smaller infants carry a lower risk of delivery complications in settings where operative deliveries are unavailable or unsafe (Brems and Berg, 1988). Restricted intrauterine growth, which may be consequent to low maternal energy intake and inadequate gestational weight gain—but also to other causes such as maternal smoking, chronic disease, or environmental pollutants—is associated with lower attained height, weight, and BMI in offspring. However, even though babies born small are at lower risk for overall obesity, they have higher risk for metabolic illnesses including hypertension (Leon et al., 1996), diabetes (Lithell et al., 1996; Hales et al., 1991; Valdez et al., 1994), and cardiovascular disease (Eriksson et al., 2001) at any given BMI, potentially through altered patterns of fat accumulation (Hong and Chung, 2018).

Inadequate gestational weight gain is a particular concern in countries undergoing the nutrition transition, which is characterized by a shift in traditional, healthier dietary patterns to a high-fat, high-protein Western diet. Because the nutrition transition is accompanied by urbanization and economic development, all of which result in a more sedentary lifestyle, it is a key contributor to obesity-related disease (Popkin, 2006). In these settings, mothers may be undernourished, manifest by low height or weight, but their children are subsequently exposed to a changing environment with ample availability of processed foods and sugar-sweetened beverages, with fewer opportunities for habitual physical activity (Yang and Huffman, 2013). This combination often leads to rapid weight gain during childhood and adolescence, which itself is a risk factor for metabolic disease especially among individuals who were also small at birth (Fabricius-Bjerre et al., 2011; Fagerberg et al., 2004; Ekelund et al., 2006).

In addition to cardiovascular and metabolic outcomes, inadequate weight gain during pregnancy may have long-term consequences for other organ systems. Among 5000 well-nourished mother–child pairs in the U.K., offspring of women who gained less than the recommended amount of weight during pregnancy had lower measures of cognitive development at 4 years, and were more likely to achieve sub-optimal final-examination results at age 16 years, as compared to children whose mothers gained adequate weight (Gage et al., 2013). The investigators also observed a modest linear trend between weight gain during pregnancy and offspring cognitive outcomes at both time points, supporting a small but positive effect of weight gain during pregnancy on educational attainment. Such findings present a dilemma in light of evidence that lower gestational weight gain, especially in obese mothers, is associated with healthier offspring cardiovascular profiles as we detail in the next section. These trade-offs emphasize the complexity of the relationship between optimal nutrition and weight gain during pregnancy.

### 2.3.2 High energy intake and excessive gestational weight gain

At the other end of the spectrum, maternal overnutrition leads to excess gestational weight gain, which increases offspring risk of obesity and metabolic dysregulation. A wealth of research demonstrates that higher gestational weight gain predicts offspring adiposity at birth (Deierlein et al., 2011; Starling et al., 2015), in childhood (Oken et al., 2007; Perng et al., 2014), adolescence (Oken et al., 2008), and adulthood (Hochner et al., 2012). Many of these studies were able to establish this association independently of mother's pre-pregnancy weight, and maternal/child shared environmental and lifestyle characteristics. Excess gestational weight gain is also correlated with a cluster of pernicious metabolic risk factors in offspring, including elevated blood pressure, insulin resistance, and altered adipocytokine profile (Dello Russo et al., 2013; Fraser et al., 2011; Perng et al., 2014). In some cases, these associations were independent of the concurrent adiposity in the offspring. In addition to the total amount of weight gain during pregnancy, the timing of weight gain may also have repercussions. Greater gestational weight gain during the first trimester has also been linked to larger birth size (Ruchat et al., 2016; Zheng et al., 2019), and higher offspring adiposity (Margerison-Zilko et al., 2012; Hivert et al., 2016) and biomarkers of cardiometabolic risk during childhood (Karachaliou et al., 2015), suggesting that interventions aimed at moderating weight gain early in pregnancy could benefit both the mother and infant.

### 2.3.3 Macronutrients

Studies going back several decades have investigated the relations of maternal macronutrient intake with offspring health by linking historical information on diet during pregnancy to cardiovascular traits in adult offspring. In a study of 253 Scottish adults whose mothers participated in a survey of diet during late pregnancy, Campbell et al. identified two dietary trends related to high blood pressure in offspring at 40 years of age: consumption of < 50 g animal protein per day along with high carbohydrate intake in late pregnancy; and consumption of > 50 g animal protein per day along with low carbohydrate intake in late pregnancy (Campbell et al., 1996). In another study, Sheill et al. followed over 600 offspring of a Scottish women who were encouraged to eat a pound of meat per day during pregnancy while avoiding carbohydrate-rich foods in an effort to reduce preeclampsia, with intakes of 10 foods summarized in these women's antenatal records (Shiell et al., 2001). Around 30 years of age, offspring blood pressure was highest among those whose mothers reported eating the highest amount of meat and fish in late pregnancy. In the subset of offspring who participated in more detailed biochemical analyses, maternal meat and fish intake in late pregnancy was also associated with plasma cortisol concentrations (Herrick et al., 2003). In another study using ration records from the Dutch Famine, Roseboom et al. estimated nutrient intakes for women who were pregnant during the famine and found an inverse relation between the ratio of protein-to-carbohydrate intake and offspring blood pressure at 50 years (Roseboom et al., 2001). These data are crude by current standards for nutritional epidemiology, but the results are intriguing and suggest that a balance in macronutrient intake during pregnancy is important to offspring health.

A few studies in contemporary cohorts indicate that macronutrient composition of a pregnant woman's diet influences her child's cardiovascular health, although current evidence is piecemeal and at times, contradictory. In an analysis of 1040 mother-infant dyads in the Healthy Start study, Crume et al. found that higher intake of macronutrients other than protein—namely, total fat, saturated fat, unsaturated fat, and total carbohydrates—was associated with higher directly measured neonatal fat mass, independent of the woman's pre-pregnancy BMI (Crume et al., 2016). Such findings suggest that higher maternal intake of fats and carbohydrates contributes to neonatal adiposity. Yet in the Aarhus Birth Cohort in Denmark, Maslova et al. reported a positive association between maternal protein intake during pregnancy and offspring obesity at age 20 years that was robust to adjustment for concurrent carbohydrate intake, pre-pregnancy BMI, and post-natal risk factors for obesity (Maslova et al., 2014).

In a study of 2026 Filipino adolescents from the Cebu Longitudinal Health and Nutrition Survey, Adair et al. found an inverse relation of mother's percent of dietary energy from proteins with systolic blood pressure (SBP) in adolescent boys, which is consistent with animal models that document elevated blood pressure in offspring of rats fed a protein-deficient diet during pregnancy (Langley and Jackson, 1994). Among girls, the authors found an inverse relation of mother's percentage calories from fat with both systolic and diastolic blood pressure (Adair et al., 2001). The finding observed in boys is consistent with the earlier observations of Roseboom et al., who found evidence for an inverse association between the ratio of protein to carbohydrates in maternal diet during the third trimester and offspring blood pressure (Roseboom et al., 2001).

Although fewer studies have assessed carbohydrate intake directly (and those that have observed null associations with offspring cardiometabolic outcomes (Maslova et al., 2014)), maternal plasma glucose concentrations during pregnancy (a reflection of both carbohydrate intake as well as the gravida's physiology) has been consistently associated with larger offspring size and adiposity across the lifecourse. This relationship was first recognized in the 1950s as 'Pedersen's hypothesis,' and has since been observed in several historical and contemporary cohorts that noted robust associations of maternal glycemia during pregnancy not only with offspring adiposity and a range of cardiometabolic disease precursors (Perng et al., 2020). To list a few examples: maternal glucose levels across all of pregnancy, even in the absence of diagnosed diabetes, were associated with directly measured fat mass in the Healthy Start study at birth (Crume et al., 2015), as well as with biomarkers of glucose-insulin homeostasis during early childhood independent of the child's prior or concurrent adiposity levels (Francis et al., 2021); mid-pregnancy oral glucose challenge test glucose levels correlated with higher birthweight among 6854 non-diabetic pregnancies in Texas (Yogev et al., 2005); and higher mid-pregnancy oral glucose tolerance test glucose levels was associated with higher birthweight among > 25,000 mother-infant pairs in the Hyperglycemia and Adverse Pregnancy Outcomes (HAPO) study (Metzger et al., 2008). Together, these findings emphasize the relevance of degree and timing of maternal hyperglycemia as determinants of offspring adiposity and metabolic profile. The extent to which maternal glycemic regulation during pregnancy may be influenced by diet quality, independent of total energy intake, requires systematic studies in diverse groups of women.

Of note, the majority of human literature on the effect of maternal hyperglycemia on offspring adiposity have focused on women with gestational diabetes mellitus (GDM), and most (Jovanovic-Peterson et al., 1991; Combs et al., 1992; Major et al., 1998) but not all (Romon et al., 2001) studies indicate that hyperglycemia correlates with greater neonatal adiposity. However, two meta-analyses concluded that the evidence for an association between pre-existing diabetes or gestational diabetes and offspring adiposity during childhood is inconsistent (Philipps et al., 2011; Kim et al., 2011). Reasons for the discrepancies included not accounting for maternal weight status, which is a major determinant of both gestational diabetes and offspring adiposity (though some have argued that adjusting for maternal weight status represents an over-adjustment given the shared pathways between maternal adiposity and hyperglycemia (Perng et al., 2019b)); use of offspring BMI, a crude indicator of body size, rather than direct measures of adiposity; and the possibility that relationship between maternal glycemia during pregnancy and offspring adiposity vary by lifestage—for example, Silverman et al. noted that offspring of mothers with diabetes may be larger at birth and again during the school-age years, but not as toddlers (Silverman et al., 1998). Furthermore, there may be sex differences: among 958 women in Project Viva, a U.S. pre-birth cohort, Regnault et al. examined maternal gestational glucose tolerance during pregnancy with offspring adiposity during mid-childhood (Regnault et al., 2013). The authors found that male offspring of women with gestational diabetes had 1.89 kg (95% CI: 0.33, 3.45) higher total fat mass than those of normoglycemic mothers, with a similar trend observed for DXA trunk-to-peripheral fat mass, a measure of central adiposity. On the other hand, female offspring of women with intermediate glucose intolerance had higher DXA fat mass (2.23 kg [95% CI: 0.12, 4.34]) than those of normoglycemic mothers but not GDM (− 1.25 kg [95% CI: − 3.13, 0.63]) but were not different from those whose mothers had intermediate glucose intolerance. The authors speculated that the sex-specific differences might be due to differences in glycemic sensitivity in utero. Specifically, male fetuses may be more responsive to the woman's current diet and metabolism (Eriksson et al., 2010) potentially through differential placental function (Rosenfeld, 2015), whereas females appear to be more influenced by a woman's diet and health across the life course (Van Abeelen et al., 2011). An important caveat to keep in mind when interpreting findings from studies of glucose tolerance is that it is not possible to delineate the effects of glucose itself, from consequences related to poor maternal glycemic control including concurrent perturbations in other fuels like free fatty acids, and vasculopathy. Future work including in animal models may help parse out these associations.

As mentioned earlier, emerging human data suggest a key role for the placenta in modulating the relationship between maternal diet and offspring health outcomes especially given that this organ may upregulate macronutrient transport to the fetus in response to maternal nutritional status (Diaz et al., 2014). In an analysis of protein abundance and phosphorylation in placental villus samples collected from a subsample of women in the Healthy Start study, Keleher et al. identified several signaling pathways associated with offspring adiposity during early childhood, including those involved in IGF-1 gene expression, GSK3β phosphorylation, the ratio of phosphorylated to total JNK2, and PGC-1α abundance (Keleher et al., 2021). Given that the placenta is essentially a "gatekeeper" of nutrient exchange between the mother and fetus and thus plays a vital role in fetal growth and development, such findings lay the groundwork for future studies to examine the relationship between maternal nutritional status before and during pregnancy with these placental signaling pathways.

### 2.3.4 Micronutrients

In addition to research on effects of global food and macronutrient intake, there is a growing body of literature investigating associations with specific nutrients via dietary intake assessments and biomarkers of nutrient status. While several micronutrients are essential to fetal growth and pregnancy outcomes (Fig. 2.1), this section focuses on evidence regarding those that have been associated with long-term offspring outcomes.

#### 2.3.4.1 B-vitamins

Consistent dietary intake of the B-vitamins during gestation is essential to normal physiological development. The importance of these micronutrients stems from their role in one-carbon metabolism, the fundamental biochemical process that provides the methyl group in all mammalian DNA methylation reactions. Successful completion of the one-carbon cycle requires an adequate supply of the methyl-donors, folate and choline, as well as the methylation cofactors, vitamin B12, vitamin B6, vitamin B2, and zinc. A deficiency or imbalance in these micronutrients could directly influence DNA methylation and consequently, gene expression (Johnson et al., 2003; Lee et al., 2010). Currently, the literature points toward two main categories of long-term offspring outcomes associated with maternal B-vitamin status during pregnancy: cardiometabolic health and cognitive function.

Animal models indicate that the availability of B-vitamins in utero lead to differences in DNA methylation in offspring that have lasting effects on cardiovascular and metabolic health. In the Agouti mouse model, pregnant dams supplemented with vitamin B12, betaine, choline, and folic acid gave birth to leaner offspring with higher methylation of a metastable epiallele involved in cardiovascular phenotype (Dolinoy et al., 2007). Similarly, ewes fed a diet deficient in folate, vitamin B12, and methionine during pregnancy gave birth to offspring with hypomethylated genomic landmarks that were also fatter, had higher blood pressure, and more likely to be insulin resistant as adults (Sinclair et al., 2007). In humans, some inference has been made from the Dutch Famine Cohort that exposure to extreme undernutrition during pregnancy, which likely includes deficiencies in the B-vitamins, corresponds with both greater metabolic disease risk in adulthood as well as aberrant methylation of genes involved in relevant disease pathways (Painter et al., 2005). While this conclusion remains speculative as it is not possible to separate effects of micronutrient deficiencies from global malnutrition, it points toward the need to pay special attention to vegan/vegetarian women who are at higher risk for certain B-vitamin deficiencies.

Studies from modern-day populations have raised concerns about possible unintended adverse effects of universal pre-natal folic acid supplementation since the wide-spread folic acid fortification of wheat flour in over 80 countries beginning in the 1990s (Food Fortification Initiative, n.d.). Specifically, while folic acid is protective against neural tube defects, it may have adverse effects on metabolic health of offspring, especially among women with poor vitamin B12 status. This concern arose from an observational study in Pune, India, where Yajnik et al. found that higher maternal erythrocyte folate concentrations during the second trimester predicted adiposity and insulin resistance in offspring at 6–8 years of age, with the highest levels of insulin resistance occurring among those whose mothers had both high folate and low vitamin B-12 status (Yajnik et al., 2008). These findings were corroborated by a rodent experiment which demonstrated that supplementation with folate during pregnancy increased body fat and insulin resistance in male offspring, especially when paired with a high-fat diet (Huang et al., 2014). While additional work in populations with other nutritional profiles is necessary to confirm these findings, they cast a cautionary light on current across-the-board folic acid fortification in most countries.

DNA methylation is also involved in several processes responsible for proper development and functioning of the central nervous system, including myelination, monoamine neurotransmitter production, and dendritic arborization (Selhub et al., 2000). Inadequate intake of methyl-donor nutrients is associated with impaired neurocognitive performance in children (Dror and Allen, 2008; Black, 2008). For example, longitudinal investigations in children (Bhate et al., 2008) and adolescents (Louwman et al., 2000; Gewa et al., 2009) found inverse associations of vitamin B12 status with measures of neurocognitive performance. Because a great deal of the abovementioned central nervous system development occurs in utero, maternal methyl-donor status during pregnancy could be particularly relevant to later-life behavioral and cognitive outcomes. Researchers have observed that low folate intake during the first trimester is associated with behavioral problems in offspring during toddlerhood (Roza et al., 2010) and in the school-age years (Schlotz et al., 2010). Some literature also hints that maternal methyl-donor micronutrient intake during pregnancy influences offspring cognition, but the message is less cohesive. Villamor et al. found that higher intake of folate during the first trimester was associated with higher scores on the PPVT-III, a test of receptive language that predicts overall intelligence, at 3 years of age in U.S. children (Villamor et al., 2012). However, by 7 years of age, none of these nutrients were associated with offspring cognitive outcomes except for choline, which was only modestly related better visual memory (Boeke et al., 2013). Because cognitive development is fluid, especially during adolescence, and post-natal influences may blunt pre-natal effects, future studies are necessary to understand associations with offspring cognitive outcomes over a longer period of time.

### 2.3.4.2 Polyunsaturated fatty acids

Two types of essential polyunsaturated fatty acids (PUFAs), the omega-3s (N-3) and the omega-6s (N-6), play critical roles in growth and development. The N-3 and N-6 families are derived from the precursors 18:3 N-3 alpha-linolenic acid (ALA) and 18:2 N-6 linoleic acid (LA), respectively. As the primary 18-carbon member of the N-3 series, ALA can be desaturated and elongated into eicosapentaenoic acid (EPA) and docosahexaenoic acid (DHA). Through a shared enzymatic pathway, LA (the main 18-carbon N-6 PUFA) is converted to gamma-linolenic acid (GLA), dihomo-gamma-linolenic acid (DGLA), and arachidonic acid (AA). Some of the long-chain PUFAs can be oxidized to produce eicosanoids, which are hormone-like signaling molecules involved in important biological processes including inflammation and cell differentiation. Because the N-3 and N-6 PUFA families compete for the same enzymes in their processing they have interactive and possibly opposing actions with respect to some physiological outcomes. For example, animal models suggest that some N-6 PUFAs, such as AA, may stimulate inflammation and adipogenesis (Massiera et al., 2003), while the N-3 series (e.g., EPA and DHA) may reduce fat mass through amelioration of inflammation (Cintra et al., 2012). Given the relevance of inflammation to diverse physiological pathways, it is not surprising that maternal PUFA status is associated with pregnancy outcomes as well as long-term health outcomes of the offspring.

A large body of research has focused on the relationship between maternal PUFA status and/or intake with offspring neurodevelopment. The potential beneficial effects of PUFAs on neurocognitive development likely transpire from rapid incorporation of N-3 DHA and the N-6 AA into nervous tissue of brain and retina during the second half of pregnancy (Dobbing and Sands, 1973). Indeed, animal studies show that deprivation of N-3 PUFAs during gestation leads to visual and behavioral deficits that cannot be reversed with post-natal supplementation (Nesheim and Yaktine, 2007). However, a 2018 Cochrane systematic review and meta-analysis of 70 randomized trials comparing marine N-3 interventions via foods and/or supplements with placebo or no marine N-3 fatty acid intervention during pregnancy found a protective effect against preterm birth (< 37 gestational weeks) and early pre-term birth (< 34 gestational weeks), but no significant differences with respect to multiple aspects of childhood development including cognition, attention, behavior, vision, language, hearing, and motor skills (Middleton et al., 2018). The relatively null findings for the developmental outcomes may be related to the fact that fish are the primary natural source of elongated N-3 fatty acids. While high in N-3 PUFAs, fish may also be relatively high in mercury, a neurotoxin that has deleterious effects on the central nervous system during gestation (Harada, 1995; Amin-Zaki et al., 1974). However, data from several observational cohorts show positive associations between pre-natal fish intake and offspring cognition, despite subclinical but measurable detrimental effects of mercury exposure (Strain et al., 2012; Oken et al., 2008; Daniels et al., 2004; Hibbeln et al., 2007). In 2014, the U.S. Environmental Protection Agency and Food and Drug Administration issued advice for pregnant women (or those likely to become pregnant) to limit their overall consumption of seafood to two to three servings per week (US Food And Drug Administration, 2014). Shortly thereafter, the 2015 Dietary Guidelines Advisory Committee conducted a risk/benefit analysis of pre-natal exposure to the beneficial and harmful components of seafood and concluded that the neurodevelopmental risks of not eating fish exceeded the risks of eating moderate amounts of fish. While the 2015 Dietary Guidelines confirm earlier recommendations by the FDA and EPA that pregnant and breastfeeding women should avoid long-lived fish high in methyl mercury content (i.e., tilefish, shark, swordfish, king mackerel), many handbooks provided by clinicians still advise limiting consumption of low-mercury fish and seafood to two servings per week, which may discourage women from eating fish altogether (Oken et al., 2003).

Beyond the potential positive effects of maternal N-3 PUFA status on offspring neurodevelopmental outcomes, several studies have noted a protective role of N-3PUFAs on obesity risk. In the Project Viva cohort ($n \sim 1100$), Donahue et al. found inverse associations of maternal N-3 EPA+DHA dietary intake during mid-pregnancy with offspring subcutaneous fat (0.31 mm [95% CI: 0.04, 0.58] lower subscapular + triceps skinfolds sum per 1 SD maternal DHA+EPA intake) and obesity risk at 3 years (OR: 0.68 [95% CI: 0.50, 0.92] per 1 SD maternal DHA+EPA intake), with similar trends EPA+DHA cord blood plasma levels (Donahue et al., 2011). A subsequent study in the same cohort (Maslova et al., 2018) found inverse associations of cord plasma DHA levels with adiposity indicators and leptin at age 3 years that were particularly strong among children whose mothers had isolated hyperglycemia during pregnancy. The authors also noted that higher maternal intakes of DHA+EPA and fish were associated with lower adiponectin in offspring during early childhood but not in mid-childhood, suggesting a transient effect of pre-natal PUFA status on obesity-related health outcomes in offspring that may be modified by maternal glycemia. Although observational findings suggest a beneficial effect of pre-natal N-3 PUFA status, randomized controlled trials evaluating the effect of maternal N-3 PUFA supplementation on offspring adiposity have been inconsistent (Muhlhausler et al., 2010). Further, an analysis comparing obesity-related biomarkers (i.e., non-fasting serum lipid and glucose) among 4-year-old children whose mothers were part of a randomized trial of pre-natal DHA supplementation in Mexico (Gutierrez-Gomez et al., 2017) found no differences between the intervention and control groups.

On the other hand, pre-natal N-6 PUFA status is associated with higher offspring adiposity. For instance, a study of 293 mother–child pairs in the U.K. reported a positive correlation between total maternal plasma N-6 PUFAs during late pregnancy and offspring fat mass at 4 and 6 years (0.18 kg [95% CI: 0.07, 0.30] and 0.18 kg [95% CI: 0.06, 0.29] higher total fat mass per 1 SD maternal plasma N-6 at 4 years and 6 years, respectively) (Moon et al., 2013). These findings make sense given the pro-inflammatory and pro-adipogenic properties of N-6 PUFAs (Massiera et al., 2003).

The body of literature to date exemplifies not only the broad physiological processes affected by N-3 and N-6 PUFAs, and but also emphasizes a need to evaluate N-3 and N-6 PUFA status in pregnant women (in particular, inadequate intake or deficiencies in N-3 PUFAs) in order to better understand both the short- and long-term implications of inadequate or excessive intake of these nutrients on maternal and offspring health outcomes. Additionally, there is need for additional research to clarify whether there are differences in offspring health outcomes with respect to the source of PUFAs (e.g., from supplements vs marine fish).

### 2.3.4.3 *Vitamin D*

As mentioned earlier, Vitamin D is a class of secosteroids that enhances intestinal absorption of several minerals, the primary one being calcium. Accordingly, the most widely-recognized function of vitamin D is skeletal development—in fact, a woman's serum concentration of 25-hydroxyvitamin D [25(OH)D] during pregnancy is strongly correlated with her child's 25(OH)D status at birth, and infants of women who are vitamin D deficient experience depleted vitamin D concentrations in utero and are born with low stores (Zeghoud et al., 1997). Results from a small study of 50 newborns suggest that such children have lower bone mass at birth than those with adequate vitamin D status (Weiler et al., 2005). There is also longitudinal evidence that a woman's vitamin D status during pregnancy influences offspring bone density in childhood (Javaid et al., 2006) and adulthood (Zhu et al., 2014). In a 2020 systematic review, Jensen et al. (2020) identified seven prospective cohort studies that examined associations of maternal dietary and lifestyle characteristics, including pre-natal vitamin D concentration, with bone density indices in offspring. The results indicated that high concentrations of maternal vitamin D; low fat intake; and high intakes of calcium, phosphorus, and magnesium may increase the bone mineral density in offspring at the age of 16 years.

Vitamin D also plays a role in immune function, since its receptor is present in cells of the immune system, including T-cells, activated B-cells, and dendritic cells (Provvedini et al., 1983). Initial evidence implicating vitamin D in allergic disease came from studies showing an association between a polymorphism in the vitamin D receptor gene and asthma in both adults and children (Raby et al., 2004; Poon et al., 2004). Subsequently, two prospective studies showed an inverse relation of maternal intake of vitamin D during pregnancy with wheezing illnesses in offspring in early childhood (Devereux et al., 2007; Camargo et al., 2007). Similar trends have been observed for asthma as well: in a prospective study of 44,825 Danish mother–child pairs, children of women with the highest vs lowest quintile of total vitamin D intake during mid-pregnancy were about 25% less likely to have asthma at 7 years (Q5 vs Q1 OR: 0.74 [95% CI: 0.56, 0.96]) (Maslova et al., 2013).

Observational findings of an inverse relationship between pre-natal vitamin D status and offspring asthma risk laid the groundwork for the Vitamin D Antenatal Asthma Reduction Trial (VDAART), a randomized, double-blind, placebo-controlled trial of vitamin D supplementation in pregnant women to determine whether such supplementation can prevention development of asthma and allergies in the offspring (Litonjua et al., 2014). In 2020, Lu et al. found that vitamin D sufficiency (25[OH]D level $\geq$ 30 ng/mL) during early and/or late pregnancy among VDAART mothers with asthma corresponded with markedly lower offspring risk of asthma or recurrent wheeze by age 3 years (i.e., adjusted odds ratios of 0.36 to 0.56; $P$-trend < 0.05), with a sustained effect through the age of 6 years. Such findings suggest a protective effect of adequate vitamin D levels on offspring risk of asthma, even among those with genetic predisposition. Whether the beneficial effect of adequate maternal vitamin D status on offspring bone density and asthma-related outcomes is causal or a reflection of sociodemographic and lifestyle characteristics is a topic of ongoing discussion (Curtis et al., 2018) for which definitive answers require long-term follow-up of mother–child pairs from high-quality randomized placebo controlled trials like VDAART, and the UK-based MAVIDOS trial (Moon et al., 2016).

### 2.3.4.4 *Calcium*

Calcium plays important roles in bone mineralization and functions as a signal for many cellular processes. Observations of an inverse association between calcium intake and blood pressure in rats (Belizan et al., 1981), children (Gillman et al., 1992), non-pregnant adults (Belizan et al., 1983a), and pregnant women (Belizan et al., 1983b) has spurred curiosity regarding whether maternal calcium intake during pregnancy reduces offspring blood pressure. In a study of 936 mother–child pairs, each 500-mg increment in maternal supplemental calcium intake during pregnancy corresponded with 3 mmHg (95% CI: − 4.9, − 1.1) lower offspring SBP at 6 months (Gillman et al., 2004); however, there were no associations with offspring blood pressure at a 3-year follow-up (Bakker et al., 2008), leading the authors to speculate that the influence of maternal calcium intake might be only short-term, or could disappear in early childhood only to re-appear in later ages, as animal models indicate that the effects of pre-natal calcium status increase with offspring age (Bergel and Belizan, 2002). Yet, in a randomized controlled trial of 389 children in the Gambia, maternal calcium supplementation of 1500 mg/day from 20 weeks of gestation onwards had no effect on offspring blood pressure at 5–10 years of age (Hawkesworth et al., 2010).

Calcium supplementation is relatively simple and cost-effective intervention that may reduce offspring risk of hypertension, as well as risk of hypertensive disorders during pregnancy for the mother—see systematic review by Imdad et al. (2011) and a relatively recent retrospective cohort study of > 11,000 Bangladeshi women that found a 45% lower risk of pregnancy induced hypertension among women who consumed at least 500 mg/day for at least 6 months of pregnancy (Khanam et al., 2018). Thus, there is growing interest in the extent to which calcium supplementation during pregnancy or intake of calcium-rich foods (e.g., 4–5 servings/day of low-fat dairy foods in Be Healthy in Pregnancy (BHIP) randomized controlled trial (Perreault et al., 2018)) imparts beneficial effects on offspring cardiovascular health in the long term.

### 2.3.4.5 *Iron*

Iron is an essential micronutrient for oxygen transport that is also involved in catalytic activity of a variety of enzymes. In the fetus, iron plays an important role in hemoglobin production and is integral to brain development (Mcardle et al., 2006). Iron deficiency is the most common nutrient deficiency worldwide, affecting up to half of pregnant women in Western societies (Bergmann et al., 2002). The short-term effects of iron deficiency during pregnancy include greater risk of preterm delivery (Bánhidy et al., 2011), and adverse effects on placental structure and function (Gambling and Mcardle, 2004), both of which may have long-term implications for offspring health via fetal organ development.

Animal models suggest that maternal iron deficiency during pregnancy leads to hypertension in offspring (Crowe et al., 1995; Gambling et al., 2003) possibly through alterations in renal development (Lisle et al., 2003), but evidence in humans remains inconclusive. In a study of 1167 US mother–child dyads, Belfort et al. explored the associations of maternal iron intake and two biomarkers of iron status, hemoglobin, and mean corpuscular volume, during the first and second trimesters with offspring blood pressure at 3 years (Belfort et al., 2008). Interestingly, the iron status biomarkers were not associated with offspring blood pressure, although positive associations were observed with maternal iron intake (Belfort et al., 2008). These null results are in agreement with a two studies from ALSPAC, which found no relations between maternal hemoglobin levels or iron intake during pregnancy dietary with offspring vascular outcomes at 7 (Brion et al., 2008) or 10 years among (Alwan et al., 2014). A possible explanation for the null findings is that the abovementioned studies took place in developed countries among generally well-nourished women with low prevalence of iron deficiency. Future work in less well-nourished populations might uncover potential links between iron deficiency and offspring vascular traits.

Maternal iron status has also been implicated in offspring cognitive development, as it is required for myelination and neurotransmitter synthesis (McCann and Ames, 2007). In a systematic review of trials investigating the effect of iron-supplementation during pregnancy and infancy on later-life mental and psychomotor performance (Szajewska et al., 2010), only two studies assessed the effect of pre-natal iron supplementation: one evaluated offspring outcomes at 4 years of age (Zhou et al., 2006), and the other examined offspring at 6–8 years of age in the same population (Parsons et al., 2008). At both time points, there was no difference in IQ between the iron and placebo groups, but the percentage of children with teacher-rated abnormal behavior was higher in the intervention group at 6–8 years (relative risk of iron vs placebo: 3.7 [95% CI: 1.06, 12.91]) (Szajewska et al., 2010). While these results are worrisome and point toward the need for updated studies of iron status in pregnant women in order to identify those who may benefit from iron supplementation as well as iron-replete women for whom additional supplementation may have adverse effects (O'brien and Ru, 2017; Friedrisch and Friedrisch, 2017), the high attrition rate (> 50%) and wide confidence intervals warrant additional work to confirm these findings.

In an attempt to update evidence on the effects of nutritional interventions—including iron supplementation—during early life on mental performance and psychomotor development of children, in 2019 Chmielewska et al. searched MEDLINE and The Cochrane Database of Systematic reviews for relevant studies published since 2009 and found no new evidence regarding pre-natal iron supplementation, and limited evidence suggesting that iron supplementation of infants may positively influence the psychomotor development of children, although it did not seem to affect mental development or behavior (Chmielewska et al., 2019). Caution is needed when interpreting current evidence, as many trials had methodological limitations, including small sample sizes, high attrition rates and no intention-to-treat analyses. Thus, while current evidence regarding the effects of supplementation with iron on neurocognitive and behavioral development is inconclusive, adequately powered high-quality randomized controlled trials are needed to further clarify the effects of iron supplementation—both alone, and with other nutrients—on child neurodevelopment.

## 2.4 Nutrition during the post-natal period

Although maternal nutritional status before and during pregnancy is undeniably important to the developing fetus, the post-natal period is also a relevant time frame for long-term health– not only for the neonate, but also for the mother and her future pregnancies. This section focuses on maternal nutritional needs during the post-natal period as they influence offspring development and chronic disease risk. Other chapters in this book address effects of infant diet, including breastfeeding, parental feeding style, and intake of specific nutrients, on long-term health outcomes.

In this section, we discuss maternal diet during lactation and its effects on milk quality and long-term offspring outcomes. We also highlight the importance of maternal post-partum weight change with respect to its associations with milk quality, infant growth, and the health of subsequent pregnancies.

### 2.4.1 Maternal diet during lactation

Recent years have seen a growing appreciation of the importance of breastfeeding for optimum infant growth and development. Because maternal diet affects breast milk quality (Allen, 2005), there has been increased effort to understand the relationship between maternal diet– in particular, micronutrient intake or status—and breast milk nutrient content. Breast milk concentrations of certain nutrients, namely vitamin A, vitamin D, vitamin B-6, vitamin B-12, folate, iodine, and fatty acids (Dawodu and Tsang, 2012; Allen, 2012; Azizi and Smyth, 2009; Lonnerdal, 1986; Innis, 2014), vary by maternal dietary intake and nutritional status, and could thereby impact offspring development through breastfeeding. There has been particular interest in the effects of maternal N-3 and N-6 long chain polyunsaturated fatty acid (LC-PUFA) intake during lactation on breast milk composition and offspring growth and development (Innis, 2014) as human milk content is especially sensitive to maternal lipid status (Brenna et al., 2007; Kent et al., 2006; Insull et al., 1959; Koletzko et al., 1992). Maternal breast milk lipid content (particularly LC-PUFAs (Pedersen et al., 2012; Much et al., 2013)) has been correlated with some offspring outcomes later in life, including early growth (Ellsworth et al., 2020), body composition (Pedersen et al., 2012; Much et al., 2013) and cognition (Lauritzen et al., 2005; Jensen et al., 2005, 2010; Cheatham et al., 2011). Similar work has been done regarding vitamin D via maternal supplementation during lactation (Oberhelman et al., 2013; Wagner et al., 2006; Hollis and Wagner, 2004; Czech-Kowalska et al., 2014), with results generally indicating that high daily doses—e.g., 5000 IU/day (Oberhelman et al., 2013) or 6400 IU/day (Wagner et al., 2006)—were necessary to increase vitamin D levels in breast milk and circulating levels in the infant.

Two major challenges in understanding the impact of maternal diet during lactation on long-term offspring health involve (1) separating the effects of the nutrient of interest from the overall milk nutrient composition, particularly when the offspring outcome is assessed after the period of exclusive breast feeding, and (2) isolating the effects of maternal diet during lactation from the effect of maternal nutritional status and condition during the pre-natal period. Overcoming the first hurdle will require a more comprehensive assessment of breast milk nutrient content in relation to the mother's dietary intake through observational (Lonnerdal, 1986) or experimental designs (Hoppu et al., 2012), and careful adjustment for offspring diet other than breast milk. However, teasing out the specific influence of breast milk quality from that of nutritional exposures in utero may prove difficult in human populations; experimental animal studies with controlled diets during pregnancy, or studies comparing health outcomes in siblings who were breastfed vs formula-fed could provide insight on this matter.

## 2.4.2 Maternal weight change

In well-nourished populations, the post-natal period is a crucial time not only for the woman's own cardiometabolic trajectory, but also health of the neonate and any future offspring. Most women lose weight after pregnancy, retaining an average of 0.5–1.5 kg at 6–18 months post-partum (Gunderson and Abrams, 2000) compared to their pre-pregnancy weight. However, a non-negligible minority (13%–20%) retain a substantial amount of weight, typically parameterized as a weight at 6 or 12 months post-partum that is at least 5 kg greater than pre-pregnancy weight (Gunderson, 2009). This is worrisome because excess weight after childbirth tends to be deposited centrally as metabolically active fat (Smith et al., 1994). Additionally, failure to lose pregnancy weight within the first year after delivery could lead to long-term obesity (Rooney and Schauberger, 2002) and contribute to development of obesity-related illnesses like heart disease and diabetes (Rooney et al., 2005).

Since most women give birth more than once, excess weight from a previous pregnancy could adversely affect the next one. Although it is difficult to infer causality from observational cohort studies, a clever study of inter-pregnancy weight change and pregnancy outcomes provides an example of how observational data may be analyzed to provide causal support for the adverse effect of weight gain before pregnancy (Villamor and Cnattingius, 2006). Using data from 151,025 Swedish women, Villamor and Cnattingius investigated how change in pre-pregnancy BMI from the first to the second pregnancies corresponded with risk of adverse outcomes during the second pregnancy (Villamor and Cnattingius, 2006). As compared to women whose BMI remained stable from the first to second pregnancy (change of − 1.0 to 0.9 BMI units), those who gained 3 or more BMI had greater risk of preeclampsia (1.78 [95% CI: 1.52, 2.08]), gestational hypertension (1.76 [95% CI: 1.39, 2.23]), gestational diabetes (2.09 [95% CI: 1.68, 2.61]), C-section delivery (1.32 [95% CI: 1.22, 1.44]), stillbirth (1.63 [95% CI: 1.20, 2.21]), and large-for-gestational-age birth (1.87 [95% CI: 1.72, 2.04]). Importantly, the risk of adverse outcomes was linearly related to the amount of inter-pregnancy weight gain, and was apparent even among women with a normal pre-pregnancy BMI, suggesting that even modest increases in BMI before pregnancy could result in perinatal complications (Villamor and Cnattingius, 2006). These findings emphasize the importance of limiting post-partum weight retention not only for the mother, but also for the health of future offspring.

Post-partum weight loss also should be considered with the offspring in mind. On the one hand, weight loss may be helpful for lactation success among overweight and obese women since excess adiposity interferes with the normal hormonal cascades necessary for successful lactogenesis (Rasmussen and Kjolhede, 2004). On the other hand, the energy needed for milk production is provided by maternal diet and tissue reserves, leading to some concern over the impact of weight loss on lactation success. An older study conducted among 45 well-nourished lactating women monitored milk production, dietary intake, and body composition for 4 months post-partum to examine the interrelations of these maternal variables. The authors reported that gradual weight reduction (approximately 12 lbs. in 4 months), and significant decreases in maternal energy intake (2334 kcal/day in the first month vs 2092 kcal/day in the fourth month) were compatible with successful lactation and infant growth (Butte et al., 1984). These preliminary conclusions were corroborated by a 2013 Cochrane Review evaluating the effect of diet, exercise, or both for weight reduction and breastfeeding performance in women after childbirth (Amorim Adegboye and Linne, 2013). The authors concluded that diet and exercise in combination appeared to be the most effect ways to achieve post-partum weight loss, with no adverse effects on milk volume or plasma prolactin concentration or infant length and weight gain. However, because there were only four trials that assessed the influence of these interventions among breastfeeding women, and this meta-analysis has not been recently updated, additional work is required to confirm the safety of diet or exercise, or both, for both mother and baby.

## 2.5  Conclusions

Growing evidence shows that nutrition during pre- and early post-natal life has important ramifications for long-term health. The epidemiological, animal, and in vitro evidence discussed in this chapter highlight the importance of achieving a healthy weight and obtaining adequate (but not excessive) levels of B-vitamins, iron, and iodine prior to pregnancy. During pregnancy, women should be encouraged to follow current guidelines for weight gain and caloric intake, while eating a balanced diet with adequate iodine, iron, calcium, polyunsaturated fatty acids, and B-vitamins. During the post-natal period, literature indicates that focus on maternal weight loss could benefit both mother and child in the long run. Although additional research is needed to clarify mechanisms and address gaps in knowledge, current evidence indicates that nutrition just before conception, during gestation, and in the months after birth can have profound influences on an individual's long-term health. Considering that these aforementioned timeframes are also key junctures when women not only regularly access the healthcare system, but also may be more receptive to making lifestyle changes, dissemination of knowledge into public conversations, education campaigns, and clinical recommendations could have measurable impacts on population health.

## 2.6  Future trends and research

While advances in the field of DOHaD offer new and exciting perspectives that shed light on disease etiology and possible prevention strategies, there are still numerous areas of uncertainty and several avenues in need of additional investigation. This section discusses current gaps in knowledge and avenues for future research.

In addition to burgeoning areas of research mentioned earlier, such as the need to elucidate the role of the placenta in the relationship between maternal nutritional status and offspring health outcomes and disaggregation of the effects of post-natal feeding habits from that of in utero exposures, we describe some additional areas that are ripe with opportunity for future research in this section. First, there remains a need to address the question of causality in studies of maternal nutritional status and long-term offspring health. That is to say, do the associations in observational studies represent true relationships, or are they artifacts of unmeasured confounding? Taking the example of the consistently observed correlation between maternal pre-pregnancy obesity and offspring adiposity, skeptics have posted that the association is merely due to genetic factors and/or shared lifestyle and environmental characteristics between the mother and child. Some examples of clever study designs that could rule out confounding and help disentangle the amalgam of contributions captured by pre-pregnancy weight status include studies using fathers as a "negative control", examining maternal-offspring BMI associations between sibling pairs (Branum et al., 2011) and Mendelian randomization studies using genetic variants associated with obesity as an instrumental variable for maternal adiposity (Lawlor et al., 2008).

Second, there is ample room for further work involves understanding the timing of nutritional exposures. Most early life environmental factors, nutritional status included, do not exist in discrete time windows, and their effects may carry across more than one of the early-life periods described in this chapter. So far, we have relied on historical famines, animal models, and statistical methods to distill independent effects of nutritional factors in specific time early-life periods. Perhaps improvements in dietary and biomarker assessment would enable more detailed characterization of nutritional status during distinct windows of development. In particular, additional studies exploring the role of maternal periconceptional nutritional status in programming long-term offspring outcomes are warranted. The Dutch Famine has enabled researchers to examine long-term health effects of severe global maternal malnutrition around the time of conception, but findings from this cohort represent consequences of extreme undernutrition that may not be generalizable to most present day populations. As mentioned in the previous section, it is also difficult to isolate the influence of maternal nutritional status during the periconceptional environment from that of the intrauterine environment as the two are inextricably linked. A set of animal experiments were able to tease out the specific effect of the periconceptional environment on offspring body fat accumulation patterns by transplanting fertilized eggs from two groups of rats, obese rodents fed a high-fat diet (HF) and lean rodents fed a low-fat diet (LF) to foster dams fed a regular commercial diet (Wu et al., 1998, 1999). The authors found that parental diet at the time of conception had a direct influence on offspring adiposity (Wu et al., 1998, 1999). Despite the fact that gestation for both experimental groups took place in unexposed dams, offspring of HF rodents had greater adiposity than those of LF parents, highlighting the unique influence of periconceptional nutritional exposures. In humans, an analysis of developmental characteristics of oocytes from women at a fertility clinic unveiled distinct phenotypic differences between oocytes of overweight or obese women and their normal weight counterparts, including smaller size, reduced glucose consumption, altered amino acid metabolism, and higher endogenous triglyceride levels (Leary et al., 2015). Although these are pre-implantation differences, such phenotypic characteristics suspected to be part of the reason why heavier women suffer infertility and could also contribute to the adverse outcomes observed in offspring of overweight or obese women. Future work taking advantage of data from in vitro fertilization (IVF) clinics might be able to quantify differences in offspring health with respect to the periconceptional environment by comparing long-term health outcomes of children conceived in different types of IVF culture media.

Third, there is the issue of toxicants, which may travel with specific nutrients or dietary patterns (e.g., mercury and the PUFAs in fish) and could be the upstream cause of changes—including detrimental effects on breastmilk supply (Kasper et al., 2016)—that otherwise appear to be nutritionally mediated. For example, a mouse experiment demonstrated that administration of bisphenol-A (BPA), an endocrine disruptor found in common food packaging materials, early in gestation led to glucose intolerance and increased plasma insulin levels during pregnancy (Alonso-Magdalena et al., 2010). Although this finding was not recapitulated in a small human study (Robledo et al., 2013), it serves as an illustration of how a common toxicant found in foods, as opposed to the food itself or related dietary patterns, could drive development of metabolic issues. This notion highlights the need for interdisciplinary awareness and careful consideration of other environmental factors that could influence disease development under the guise of nutrition.

Fourth, despite the relatively large body of research on maternal diet during pregnancy, the majority of work has focused on specific nutrients. Elucidating the role of individual nutrients provides insight on biological mechanisms, but the human diet does not consist of isolated nutrients. Rather, we eat meals consisting of a variety of foods with complex combinations of nutrients that are likely to interact. Thus, the field of nutritional epidemiology has shifted focus toward evaluating dietary patterns to parallel nutrients and foods typically consumed in combination (Hu, 2002). To date, a few studies have examined maternal dietary patterns during pregnancy with long-term offspring outcomes. In ALSPAC, Shaheen et al. identified five dietary patterns - "health conscious," "traditional," "processed," "vegetarian," and "confectionary," but found that none of the dietary patterns predicted asthma or related atopic outcomes after controlling for confounders (Shaheen et al., 2009). There has also been growing interest in assessing adherence to a priori dietary patterns, rather than characterizing naturally-occurring dietary patterns in a specific study population that may not be relevant to other populations. For example, lower maternal diet quality via a lower Healthy Eating Index score based on U.S. Dietary Guidelines has been linked to offspring adiposity (Sen et al., 2018; Chatzi et al., 2017; Leermakers et al., 2017; Dhana et al., 2018; Zhu et al., 2019; Tahir et al., 2019; Chia et al., 2018; Günther et al., 2019) and metabolic risk (Stefan et al., 2017; Henderson et al., 2019; Shapiro et al., 2016b) across diverse populations. Given that assessments of diet quality like the HEI are also associated with pregnancy outcomes (e.g., higher HEI score during early pregnancy was associated with lower blood glucose levels and lower risk of preeclampsia among women in Project Viva (Rifas-Shiman et al., 2009)), development, assessment, and translation of such diet scores into regular dietary habits has potential to improve maternal health, pregnancy outcomes, and long-term offspring health.

Fifth, a promising arena for future research builds on the concept of early flavor learning. The flavors of foods in the maternal diet are found in the amniotic fluid surrounding the fetus, and growing evidence demonstrates that a preference for these flavors persist into infancy, and possibly childhood and adulthood. In mouse models, investigators have identified changes in the olfactory bulb glomeruli in offspring that correspond with in utero exposure to odorants and metabolites of the mother's diet. Todrank et al. reported that the olfactory bulb glomeruli of mice pups whose mothers had eaten a flavor-supplemented chow were significantly larger than glomeruli of pups whose mothers had eaten a standard flavor chow. Further, at post-natal day 20, the pups also demonstrated clear preferences for the odorants to which they had been exposed pre-natally (Todrank et al., 2011). In humans, some studies have demonstrated that infants exhibit discernible reactions to certain flavors (e.g., carrot) that directly parallel what their mothers ate during pregnancy and lactation (Mennella et al., 2001). While the concept of flavor learning may not directly affect long-term offspring outcomes, they may have indirect benefits in promoting diverse and healthful diets throughout life, and could be used to motivate behavioral change in pregnant women which, by itself, may have the potential to shift dietary habits of offspring (Trout and Wetzel-Effinger, 2012). While this is an empowering concept, behavioral changes can be difficult to come by and other factors, such as cost and availability of fresh foods, are hurdles to healthy eating in many populations.

In addition to the above, there are a number of budding topics on diet during pregnancy that are not necessarily nutritional needs, but have implications for offspring health nonetheless. Sugar-sweetened beverages (SSB) have received press as a culprit of obesity (Harvard School of Public Health: The Nutrition Source, n.d.). Some longitudinal evidence suggests that SSB intake before (Chen et al., 2012) and during (Chen et al., 2009) pregnancy increases risk of gestational diabetes, which may predispose offspring greater adiposity (Regnault et al., 2013). On the other hand, anecdotal concerns have been raised regarding use of artificial-sweeteners, such as those included in diet beverages and numerous foods, in pregnant women. Yet, there is very little published work on this topic. One study using data from the Danish National Birth Cohort found that consumption of artificially-sweetened carbonated beverages during mid-pregnancy predicted offspring risk of asthma and allergic rhinitis during childhood (Maslova et al., 2013). Animal data suggest that consumption of artificial sweeteners might result in alterations in the intestinal microbiome that promote glucose intolerance (Suez et al., 2014). Such findings are highly relevant in light of new evidence from non-human primates that the maternal imprint on offspring microbiome—include those due to maternal dietary intake during pregnancy—is long-lasting (Ma et al., 2014) and potentially irreversible (Pace et al., 2018). It is also worth mentioning that many sugar- or artificially sweetened beverages also include caffeine, and therefore studies should also take into consideration the pharmacokinetics of caffeine metabolism as this substance has been linked to fetal growth restriction (Care Study Group, 2008) and subsequent risk of obesity in offspring during childhood (Li et al., 2015; Voerman et al., 2016).

## Sources of additional information

- Periconceptional period:
  - The *American Journal of Obstetrics and Gynecology* published a report from the Centers for Disease Control and Prevention (CDC) on preconception care efforts (Gardiner et al., 2008), with a lay summary on the web: http://www.cdc.gov/preconception/index.html (Centers for Disease Control and Prevention, n.d.).
  - The American Pregnancy Association provides information on pre-pregnancy diet for increasing fertility, and key food groups and nutrients to focus on to optimize health of the woman during pregnancy as well as health of the developing fetus (American Pregnancy Association, n.d.).
- During gestation:
  - The USDA's website on Nutrition During Pregnancy summarizes current guidelines for nutrient needs of pregnant women (U.S. Department of Agriculture, n.d.), and also includes the report from a 2020 workshop when the Food and Nutrition Board of the National Academies convened to explore new evidence relevant to nutrition during pregnancy (The National Academies of Sciences Engineering and Medicine, n.d.).

- The 2020 scientific report of Dietary Guidelines for Americans is an excellent resource as pregnant women are included in this document (Dietary Guidelines Advisory Committee, 2020).
- Post-natal:
  - Raiten et al.'s executive summary in the *American Journal of Clinical Nutrition* summarizes provides in-depth information on nutritional needs during infant development (Raiten et al., 2014).
  - The National Academies of Sciences, Engineering and Medicine includes information on the most recent evidence regarding nutrition during lactation from the above-mentioned Food and Nutrition Board of the National Academies 2020 workshop (The National Academies of Sciences Engineering and Medicine, n.d.).

## References

1000 Days http://www.thousanddays.org/, n.d. Available: [Accessed March 5th 2021].

Academy of Nutrition and Dietetics, 2013. Healthy Weight During Pregnancy. [Online]. Available https://www.eatright.org/health/pregnancy/prenatal-wellness/healthy-weight-during-pregnancy. Accessed March 5th 2021.

Adair, L.S., Kuzawa, C.W., Borja, J., 2001. Maternal energy stores and diet composition during pregnancy program adolescent blood pressure. Circulation 104, 1034–1039.

Allen, L.H., 2001. Biological mechanisms that might underlie iron's effects on fetal growth and preterm birth. J. Nutr. 131, 581s–589s.

Allen, L.H., 2005. Multiple micronutrients in pregnancy and lactation: an overview. Am. J. Clin. Nutr. 81, 1206s–1212s.

Allen, L.H., 2012. B vitamins in breast milk: relative importance of maternal status and intake, and effects on infant status and function. Adv. Nutr. 3, 362–369.

Alonso-Magdalena, P., Vieira, E., Soriano, S., Menes, L., Burks, D., Quesada, I., Nadal, A., 2010. Bisphenol A exposure during pregnancy disrupts glucose homeostasis in mothers and adult male offspring. Environ. Health Perspect. 118, 1243–1250.

Alwan, N.A., Cade, J.E., Greenwood, D.C., Deanfield, J., Lawlor, D.A., 2014. Associations of maternal iron intake and hemoglobin in pregnancy with offspring vascular phenotypes and adiposity at age 10: findings from the Avon longitudinal study of parents and children. PLoS One 9, e84684.

American Pregnancy Association. Preconception Nutrition. [Online]. Available https://americanpregnancy.org/getting-pregnant/preconception-nutrition-70950/, n.d. Accessed March 5th 2021.

Amin-Zaki, L., Elhassani, S., Majeed, M.A., Clarkson, T.W., Doherty, R.A., Greenwood, M., 1974. Intra-uterine methylmercury poisoning in Iraq. Pediatrics 54, 587–595.

Amorim Adegboye, A.R., Linne, Y.M., 2013. Diet or exercise, or both, for weight reduction in women after childbirth. Cochrane Database Syst. Rev. 7, Cd005627.

Andersson, M., Karumbunathan, V., Zimmermann, M.B., 2012. Global iodine status in 2011 and trends over the past decade. J. Nutr. 142, 744–750.

Azizi, F., Smyth, P., 2009. Breastfeeding and maternal and infant iodine nutrition. Clin. Endocrinol. (Oxf) 70, 803–809.

Baker 2nd, P.R., Patinkin, Z., Shapiro, A.L., De La Houssaye, B.A., Woontner, M., Boyle, K.E., Vanderlinden, L., Dabelea, D., Friedman, J.E., 2017a. Maternal obesity and increased neonatal adiposity correspond with altered infant mesenchymal stem cell metabolism. JCI Insight 2.

Baker 2nd, P.R., Patinkin, Z.W., Shapiro, A.L.B., De La Houssaye, B.A., Janssen, R.C., Vanderlinden, L.A., Dabelea, D., Friedman, J.E., 2017b. Altered gene expression and metabolism in fetal umbilical cord mesenchymal stem cells correspond with differences in 5-month-old infant adiposity gain. Sci. Rep. 7, 18095.

Bakker, R., Rifas-Shiman, S.L., Kleinman, K.P., Lipshultz, S.E., Gillman, M.W., 2008. Maternal calcium intake during pregnancy and blood pressure in the offspring at age 3 years: a follow-up analysis of the project viva cohort. Am. J. Epidemiol. 168, 1374–1380.

Bánhidy, F., Ács, N., Puhó, E.H., Czeizel, A.E., 2011. Iron deficiency anemia: pregnancy outcomes with or without iron supplementation. Nutrition 27, 65–72.

Barker, D.J., Osmond, C., 1986. Infant mortality, childhood nutrition, and ischaemic heart disease in England and Wales. Lancet 1, 1077–1081.

Barker, D.J., Winter, P.D., Osmond, C., Margetts, B., Simmonds, S.J., 1989. Weight in infancy and death from ischaemic heart disease. Lancet 2, 577–580.

Barker, D.J., Gluckman, P.D., Godfrey, K.M., Harding, J.E., Owens, J.A., Robinson, J.S., 1993. Fetal nutrition and cardiovascular disease in adult life. Lancet 341, 938–941.

Bath, S.C., Steer, C.D., Golding, J., Emmett, P., Rayman, M.P., 2013. Effect of inadequate iodine status in UK pregnant women on cognitive outcomes in their children: results from the Avon longitudinal study of parents and children (ALSPAC). Lancet 382, 331–337.

Begum, G., Davies, A., Stevens, A., Oliver, M., Jaquiery, A., Challis, J., Harding, J., Bloomfield, F., White, A., 2013. Maternal undernutrition programs tissue-specific epigenetic changes in the glucocorticoid receptor in adult offspring. Endocrinology 154 (12), 4560–4569.

Belfort, M.B., Rifas-Shiman, S.L., Rich-Edwards, J.W., Kleinman, K.P., Oken, E., Gillman, M.W., 2008. Maternal iron intake and iron status during pregnancy and child blood pressure at age 3 years. Int. J. Epidemiol. 37, 301–308.

Belizan, J.M., Pineda, O., Sainz, E., Menendez, L.A., Villar, J., 1981. Rise of blood pressure in calcium-deprived pregnant rats. Am. J. Obstet. Gynecol. 141, 163–169.

Belizan, J.M., Villar, J., Pineda, O., Gonzalez, A.E., Sainz, E., Garrera, G., Sibrian, R., 1983a. Reduction of blood pressure with calcium supplementation in young adults. JAMA 249, 1161–1165.

Belizan, J.M., Villar, J., Zalazar, A., Rojas, L., Chan, D., Bryce, G.F., 1983b. Preliminary evidence of the effect of calcium supplementation on blood pressure in normal pregnant women. Am. J. Obstet. Gynecol. 146, 175–180.

Bergel, E., Belizan, J.M., 2002. A deficient maternal calcium intake during pregnancy increases blood pressure of the offspring in adult rats. BJOG 109, 540–545.

Bergmann, R.L., Gravens-Muller, L., Hertwig, K., Hinkel, J., Andres, B., Bergmann, K.E., Dudenhausen, J.W., 2002. Iron deficiency is prevalent in a sample of pregnant women at delivery in Germany. Eur. J. Obstet. Gynecol. Reprod. Biol. 102, 155–160.

Bhate, V., Deshpande, S., Bhat, D., Joshi, N., Ladkat, R., Watve, S., Fall, C., De Jager, C.A., Refsum, H., Yajnik, C., 2008. Vitamin B12 status of pregnant Indian women and cognitive function in their 9-year-old children. Food Nutr. Bull. 29, 249–254.

Bill & Melinda Gates Foundation. Nutrition: Strategy Overview. [Online]. Available http://www.gatesfoundation.org/What-We-Do/Global-Development/Nutrition, n.d. Accessed March 5th 2021.

Black, M.M., 2008. Effects of vitamin B12 and folate deficiency on brain development in children. Food Nutr. Bull. 29, S126–S131.

Boeke, C.E., Gillman, M.W., Hughes, M.D., Rifas-Shiman, S.L., Villamor, E., Oken, E., 2013. Choline intake during pregnancy and child cognition at age 7 years. Am. J. Epidemiol. 177, 1338–1347.

Boyle, K.E., Patinkin, Z.W., Shapiro, A.L., Baker 2nd, P.R., Dabelea, D., Friedman, J.E., 2016. Mesenchymal stem cells from infants born to obese mothers exhibit greater potential for adipogenesis: the healthy start BabyBUMP project. Diabetes 65, 647–659.

Boyle, K.E., Patinkin, Z.W., Shapiro, A.L.B., Bader, C., Vanderlinden, L., Kechris, K., Janssen, R.C., Ford, R.J., Smith, B.K., Steinberg, G.R., Davidson, E.J., Yang, I.V., Dabelea, D., Friedman, J.E., 2017. Maternal obesity alters fatty acid oxidation, AMPK activity, and associated DNA methylation in mesenchymal stem cells from human infants. Mol. Metab. 6, 1503–1516.

Branum, A.M., Parker, J.D., Keim, S.A., Schempf, A.H., 2011. Prepregnancy body mass index and gestational weight gain in relation to child body mass index among siblings. Am. J. Epidemiol. 174, 1159–1165.

Brems, S., Berg, A., 1988. "Eating Down" During Pregnancy: Nutrition, Obstetric and Cultural Considerations in the Third World. Discussion Paper Prepared for the ACC/ACN. World Bank, Population, Health and Nutrition Division, Washington, DC.

Brenna, J.T., Varamini, B., Jensen, R.G., Diersen-Schade, D.A., Boettcher, J.A., Arterburn, L.M., 2007. Docosahexaenoic and arachidonic acid concentrations in human breast milk worldwide. Am. J. Clin. Nutr. 85, 1457–1464.

Bringhenti, I., Moraes-Teixeira, J.A., Cunha, M.R., Ornellas, F., Mandarim-De-Lacerda, C.A., Aguila, M.B., 2013. Maternal obesity during the preconception and early life periods alters pancreatic development in early and adult life in male mouse offspring. PLoS One 8, e55711.

Brion, M.J., Leary, S.D., Smith, G.D., Mcardle, H.J., Ness, A.R., 2008. Maternal anemia, iron intake in pregnancy, and offspring blood pressure in the Avon Longitudinal Study of Parents and Children. Am. J. Clin. Nutr. 88, 1126–1133.

Butte, N.F., Garza, C., Stuff, J.E., Smith, E.O., Nichols, B.L., 1984. Effect of maternal diet and body composition on lactational performance. Am. J. Clin. Nutr. 39, 296–306.

Camargo Jr., C.A., Rifas-Shiman, S.L., Litonjua, A.A., Rich-Edwards, J.W., Weiss, S.T., Gold, D.R., Kleinman, K., Gillman, M.W., 2007. Maternal intake of vitamin D during pregnancy and risk of recurrent wheeze in children at 3 y of age. Am. J. Clin. Nutr. 85, 788–795.

Campbell, D.M., Hall, M.H., Barker, D.J., Cross, J., Shiell, A.W., Godfrey, K.M., 1996. Diet in pregnancy and the offspring's blood pressure 40 years later. Br. J. Obstet. Gynaecol. 103, 273–280.

Care Study Group, 2008. Maternal caffeine intake during pregnancy and risk of fetal growth restriction: a large prospective observational study. BMJ 337, a2332.

Centers for Disease Control and Prevention, n.d. Before Pregnancy. [Online]. Available: https://www.cdc.gov/preconception/index.html [Accessed March 5th 2021].

Chatzi, L., Rifas-Shiman, S.L., Georgiou, V., Joung, K.E., Koinaki, S., Chalkiadaki, G., Margioris, A., Sarri, K., Vassilaki, M., Vafeiadi, M., Kogevinas, M., Mantzoros, C., Gillman, M.W., Oken, E., 2017. Adherence to the Mediterranean diet during pregnancy and offspring adiposity and cardiometabolic traits in childhood. Pediatr. Obes. 12, 47–56.

Cheatham, C.L., Nerhammer, A.S., Asserhoj, M., Michaelsen, K.F., Lauritzen, L., 2011. Fish oil supplementation during lactation: effects on cognition and behavior at 7 years of age. Lipids 46, 637–645.

Chen, L., Hu, F.B., Yeung, E., Willett, W., Zhang, C., 2009. Prospective study of pre-gravid sugar-sweetened beverage consumption and the risk of gestational diabetes mellitus. Diabetes Care 32, 2236–2241.

Chen, L., Hu, F.B., Yeung, E., Tobias, D.K., Willett, W.C., Zhang, C., 2012. Prepregnancy consumption of fruits and fruit juices and the risk of gestational diabetes mellitus: a prospective cohort study. Diabetes Care 35, 1079–1082.

Chia, A.R., Tint, M.T., Han, C.Y., Chen, L.W., Colega, M., Aris, I.M., Chua, M.C., Tan, K.H., Yap, F., Shek, L.P., Chong, Y.S., Godfrey, K.M., Fortier, M.V., Lee, Y.S., Chong, M.F., 2018. Adherence to a healthy eating index for pregnant women is associated with lower neonatal adiposity in a multiethnic Asian cohort: the growing up in Singapore towards healthy outcomes (GUSTO) study. Am. J. Clin. Nutr. 107, 71–79.

Chmielewska, A., Dziechciarz, P., Gieruszczak-Białek, D., Horvath, A., Pieścik-Lech, M., Ruszczyński, M., Skórka, A., Szajewska, H., 2019. Effects of prenatal and/or postnatal supplementation with iron, PUFA or folic acid on neurodevelopment: update. Br. J. Nutr. 122, S10–S15.

Cintra, D.E., Ropelle, E.R., Moraes, J.C., Pauli, J.R., Morari, J., Souza, C.T., Grimaldi, R., Stahl, M., Carvalheira, J.B., Saad, M.J., Velloso, L.A., 2012. Unsaturated fatty acids revert diet-induced hypothalamic inflammation in obesity. PLoS One 7, e30571.

Combs, C.A., Gunderson, E., Kitzmiller, J.L., Gavin, L.A., Main, E.K., 1992. Relationship of fetal macrosomia to maternal postprandial glucose control during pregnancy. Diabetes Care 15, 1251–1257.

Cox, J., Williams, S., Grove, K., Lane, R.H., Aagaard-Tillery, K.M., 2009. A maternal high-fat diet is accompanied by alterations in the fetal primate metabolome. Am. J. Obstet. Gynecol. 201 (3), 281.e1–281.e9.

Crowe, C., Dandekar, P., Fox, M., Dhingra, K., Bennet, L., Hanson, M.A., 1995. The effects of anaemia on heart, placenta and body weight, and blood pressure in fetal and neonatal rats. J. Physiol. 488 (Pt 2), 515–519.

Crume, T.L., Shapiro, A.L., Brinton, J.T., Glueck, D.H., Martinez, M., Kohn, M., Harrod, C., Friedman, J.E., Dabelea, D., 2015. Maternal fuels and metabolic measures during pregnancy and neonatal body composition: the healthy start study. J. Clin. Endocrinol. Metabol. 100, 1672–1680.

Crume, T.L., Brinton, J.T., Shapiro, A., Kaar, J., Glueck, D.H., Siega-Riz, A.M., Dabelea, D., 2016. Maternal dietary intake during pregnancy and offspring body composition: the healthy start study. Am. J. Obstet. Gynecol. 215, 609.e1–609.e8.

Curtis, E.M., Moon, R.J., Harvey, N.C., Cooper, C., 2018. Maternal vitamin D supplementation during pregnancy. Br. Med. Bull. 126, 57–77.

Czech-Kowalska, J., Latka-Grot, J., Bulsiewicz, D., Jaworski, M., Pludowski, P., Wygledowska, G., Chazan, B., Pawlus, B., Zochowska, A., Borszewska-Kornacka, M.K., Karczmarewicz, E., Czekuc-Kryskiewicz, E., Dobrzanska, A., 2014. Impact of vitamin D supplementation during lactation on vitamin D status and body composition of mother-infant pairs: a MAVID randomized controlled trial. PLoS One 9, e107708.

Daniels, J.L., Longnecker, M.P., Rowland, A.S., Golding, J., 2004. Fish intake during pregnancy and early cognitive development of offspring. Epidemiology 15, 394–402.

Dawodu, A., Tsang, R.C., 2012. Maternal vitamin D status: effect on milk vitamin D content and vitamin D status of breastfeeding infants. Adv. Nutr. 3, 353–361.

Deierlein, A.L., Siega-Riz, A.M., Adair, L.S., Herring, A.H., 2011. Effects of pre-pregnancy body mass index and gestational weight gain on infant anthropometric outcomes. J. Pediatr. 158, 221–226.

Dello Russo, M., Ahrens, W., De Vriendt, T., Marild, S., Molnar, D., Moreno, L.A., Reeske, A., Veidebaum, T., Kourides, Y.A., Barba, G., Siani, A., 2013. Gestational weight gain and adiposity, fat distribution, metabolic profile, and blood pressure in offspring: the IDEFICS project. Int. J. Obes. (Lond) 37, 914–919.

De-Regil, L.M., Fernandez-Gaxiola, A.C., Dowswell, T., Pena-Rosas, J.P., 2010. Effects and safety of periconceptional folate supplementation for preventing birth defects. Cochrane Database Syst. Rev., Cd007950.

Devereux, G., Litonjua, A.A., Turner, S.W., Craig, L.C., McNeill, G., Martindale, S., Helms, P.J., Seaton, A., Weiss, S.T., 2007. Maternal vitamin D intake during pregnancy and early childhood wheezing. Am. J. Clin. Nutr. 85, 853–859.

Dhana, K., Zong, G., Yuan, C., Schernhammer, E., Zhang, C., Wang, X., Hu, F.B., Chavarro, J.E., Field, A.E., Sun, Q., 2018. Lifestyle of women before pregnancy and the risk of offspring obesity during childhood through early adulthood. Int. J. Obes. (Lond) 42, 1275–1284.

Diaz, P., Powell, T.L., Jansson, T., 2014. The role of placental nutrient sensing in maternal-fetal resource allocation. Biol. Reprod. 91, 82.

Dietary Guidelines Advisory Committee, 2020. Scientific Report of the 2020 Dietary Guidelines Advisory Committee: Advisory Report to the Secretary of Agriculture and the Secretary of Health and Human Services. Agricultural Research Service. U.S. Department of Agriculture, Washington D.C.

Dixit, A., Girling, J.C., 2008. Obesity and pregnancy. J. Obstet. Gynaecol. 28, 14–23.

Dobbing, J., Sands, J., 1973. Quantitative growth and development of human brain. Arch. Dis. Child. 48, 757–767.

Dolinoy, D.C., Huang, D., Jirtle, R.L., 2007. Maternal nutrient supplementation counteracts bisphenol A-induced DNA hypomethylation in early development. Proc. Natl. Acad. Sci. U. S. A. 104, 13056–13061.

Donahue, S.M., Rifas-Shiman, S.L., Gold, D.R., Jouni, Z.E., Gillman, M.W., Oken, E., 2011. Prenatal fatty acid status and child adiposity at age 3 y: results from a US pregnancy cohort. Am. J. Clin. Nutr. 93, 780–788.

Dror, D.K., Allen, L.H., 2008. Effect of vitamin B12 deficiency on neurodevelopment in infants: current knowledge and possible mechanisms. Nutr. Rev. 66, 250–255.

DuFour, D.L., Sauther, M.L., 2002. Comparative and evolutionary dimensions of the energetics of human pregnancy and lactation. Am. J. Hum. Biol. 14, 584–602.

Ekelund, U., Ong, K., Linne, Y., Neovius, M., Brage, S., Dunger, D.B., Wareham, N.J., Rossner, S., 2006. Upward weight percentile crossing in infancy and early childhood independently predicts fat mass in young adults: the Stockholm Weight Development Study (SWEDES). Am. J. Clin. Nutr. 83, 324–330.

Ellsworth, L., Perng, W., Harman, E., Das, A., Pennathur, S., Gregg, B., 2020. Impact of maternal overweight and obesity on milk composition and infant growth. Matern. Child Nutr. 16, e12979.

Eriksson, J.G., Forsen, T., Tuomilehto, J., Osmond, C., Barker, D.J., 2001. Early growth and coronary heart disease in later life: longitudinal study. BMJ 322, 949–953.

Eriksson, J.G., Kajantie, E., Osmond, C., Thornburg, K., Barker, D.J., 2010. Boys live dangerously in the womb. Am. J. Hum. Biol. 22, 330–335.

Fabricius-Bjerre, S., Jensen, R.B., Faerch, K., Larsen, T., Molgaard, C., Michaelsen, K.F., Vaag, A., Greisen, G., 2011. Impact of birth weight and early infant weight gain on insulin resistance and associated cardiovascular risk factors in adolescence. PLoS One 6, e20595.

Fagerberg, B., Bondjers, L., Nilsson, P., 2004. Low birth weight in combination with catch-up growth predicts the occurrence of the metabolic syndrome in men at late middle age: the atherosclerosis and insulin resistance study. J. Intern. Med. 256, 254–259.

Feed the Future http://www.feedthefuture.gov/, n.d. Available: [Accessed March 5th 2021].

Finucane, M.M., Stevens, G.A., Cowan, M.J., Danaei, G., Lin, J.K., Paciorek, C.J., Singh, G.M., Gutierrez, H.R., Lu, Y., Bahalim, A.N., Farzadfar, F., Riley, L.M., Ezzati, M., 2011. National, regional, and global trends in body-mass index since 1980: systematic analysis of health examination surveys and epidemiological studies with 960 country-years and 9.1 million participants. Lancet 377, 557–567.

Flegal, K.M., Carroll, M.D., Kit, B.K., Ogden, C.L., 2012. Prevalence of obesity and trends in the distribution of body mass index among US adults, 1999-2010. JAMA 307, 491–497.

Food Fortification Initiative, n.d. Overview: What We Do. [Online]. Available: https://www.ffinetwork.org/our-work [Accessed March 5th 2021].

Francis, E.C., Dabelea, D., Ringham, B.M., Sauder, K.A., Perng, W., 2021. Maternal blood glucose level and offspring glucose-insulin homeostasis: what is the role of offspring adiposity? Diabetologia 64, 83–94.

Fraser, A., Tilling, K., Macdonald-Wallis, C., Hughes, R., Sattar, N., Nelson, S.M., Lawlor, D.A., 2011. Associations of gestational weight gain with maternal body mass index, waist circumference, and blood pressure measured 16 y after pregnancy: the Avon Longitudinal Study of Parents and Children (ALSPAC). Am. J. Clin. Nutr. 93, 1285–1292.

Friedrisch, J.R., Friedrisch, B.K., 2017. Prophylactic iron supplementation in pregnancy: a controversial issue. Biochem. Insights 10, 1178626417737738.

Gage, S.H., Lawlor, D.A., Tilling, K., Fraser, A., 2013. Associations of maternal weight gain in pregnancy with offspring cognition in childhood and adolescence: findings from the Avon Longitudinal Study of Parents and Children. Am. J. Epidemiol. 177, 402–410.

Gambling, L., Mcardle, H.J., 2004. Iron, copper and fetal development. Proc. Nutr. Soc. 63, 553–562.

Gambling, L., Dunford, S., Wallace, D.I., Zuur, G., Solanky, N., Srai, S.K., Mcardle, H.J., 2003. Iron deficiency during pregnancy affects postnatal blood pressure in the rat. J. Physiol. 552, 603–610.

Ganguly, A., Tamblyn, J.A., Finn-Sell, S., Chan, S.Y., Westwood, M., Gupta, J., Kilby, M.D., Gross, S.R., Hewison, M., 2018. Vitamin D, the placenta and early pregnancy: effects on trophoblast function. J. Endocrinol. 236, R93–r103.

Gardiner, P.M., Nelson, L., Shellhaas, C.S., Dunlop, A.L., Long, R., Andrist, S., Jack, B.W., 2008. The clinical content of preconception care: nutrition and dietary supplements. Am. J. Obstet. Gynecol. 199, S345–S356.

Georgieff, M.K., Krebs, N.F., Cusick, S.E., 2019. The benefits and risks of iron supplementation in pregnancy and childhood. Annu. Rev. Nutr. 39, 121–146.

Gewa, C.A., Weiss, R.E., Bwibo, N.O., Whaley, S., Sigman, M., Murphy, S.P., Harrison, G., Neumann, C.G., 2009. Dietary micronutrients are associated with higher cognitive function gains among primary school children in rural Kenya. Br. J. Nutr. 101, 1378–1387.

Gillman, M.W., Oliveria, S.A., Moore, L.L., Ellison, R.C., 1992. Inverse association of dietary calcium with systolic blood pressure in young children. JAMA 267, 2340–2343.

Gillman, M.W., Rifas-Shiman, S.L., Kleinman, K.P., Rich-Edwards, J.W., Lipshultz, S.E., 2004. Maternal calcium intake and offspring blood pressure. Circulation 110, 1990–1995.

Gray, L., Davey Smith, G., Mcconnachie, A., Watt, G.C., Hart, C.L., Upton, M.N., Macfarlane, P.W., Batty, G.D., 2012. Parental height in relation to offspring coronary heart disease: examining transgenerational influences on health using the west of Scotland Midspan family study. Int. J. Epidemiol. 41, 1776–1785.

Gunderson, E.P., 2009. Childbearing and obesity in women: weight before, during, and after pregnancy. Obstet. Gynecol. Clin. North Am. 36, 317–332. ix.

Gunderson, E.P., Abrams, B., 2000. Epidemiology of gestational weight gain and body weight changes after pregnancy. Epidemiol. Rev. 22, 261–274.

Günther, J., Hoffmann, J., Spies, M., Meyer, D., Kunath, J., Stecher, L., Rosenfeld, E., Kick, L., Rauh, K., Hauner, H., 2019. Associations between the prenatal diet and neonatal outcomes—a secondary analysis of the cluster-randomised gelis trial. Nutrients 11.

Gutierrez-Gomez, Y., Stein, A.D., Ramakrishnan, U., Barraza-Villarreal, A., Moreno-Macias, H., Aguilar-Salinas, C., Romieu, I., Rivera, J.A., 2017. Prenatal docosahexaenoic acid supplementation does not affect nonfasting serum lipid and glucose concentrations of offspring at 4 years of age in a follow-up of a randomized controlled clinical trial in Mexico. J. Nutr. 147, 242–247.

Hales, C.N., Barker, D.J., Clark, P.M., Cox, L.J., Fall, C., Osmond, C., Winter, P.D., 1991. Fetal and infant growth and impaired glucose tolerance at age 64. BMJ 303, 1019–1022.

Harada, M., 1995. Minamata disease: methylmercury poisoning in Japan caused by environmental pollution. Crit. Rev. Toxicol. 25, 1–24.

Harvard School of Public Health: The Nutrition Source, n.d. Sugary Drinks and Obesity Fact Sheet. [Online]. Available: http://www.hsph.harvard.edu/nutritionsource/sugary-drinks-fact-sheet/ [Accessed March 5th 2021].

Hawkesworth, S., Sawo, Y., Fulford, A.J., Goldberg, G.R., Jarjou, L.M., Prentice, A., Moore, S.E., 2010. Effect of maternal calcium supplementation on offspring blood pressure in 5- to 10-y-old rural Gambian children. Am. J. Clin. Nutr. 92, 741–747.

Heijmans, B.T., Tobi, E.W., Stein, A.D., Putter, H., Blauw, G.J., Susser, E.S., Slagboom, P.E., Lumey, L.H., 2008. Persistent epigenetic differences associated with prenatal exposure to famine in humans. Proc. Natl. Acad. Sci. U. S. A. 105, 17046–17049.

Henderson, M., Van Hulst, A., Von Oettingen, J.E., Benedetti, A., Paradis, G., 2019. Normal weight metabolically unhealthy phenotype in youth: do definitions matter? Pediatr. Diabetes 20, 143–151.

Herrick, K., Phillips, D.I., Haselden, S., Shiell, A.W., Campbell-Brown, M., Godfrey, K.M., 2003. Maternal consumption of a high-meat, low-carbohydrate diet in late pregnancy: relation to adult cortisol concentrations in the offspring. J. Clin. Endocrinol. Metab. 88, 3554–3560.

Hibbeln, J.R., Davis, J.M., Steer, C., Emmett, P., Rogers, I., Williams, C., Golding, J., 2007. Maternal seafood consumption in pregnancy and neurodevelopmental outcomes in childhood (ALSPAC study): an observational cohort study. Lancet 369, 578–585.

Hivert, M.-F., Rifas-Shiman, S.L., Gillman, M.W., Oken, E., 2016. Greater early and mid-pregnancy gestational weight gains are associated with excess adiposity in mid-childhood. Obesity (Silver Spring) 24, 1546–1553.

Hochner, H., Friedlander, Y., Calderon-Margalit, R., Meiner, V., Sagy, Y., Avgil-Tsadok, M., Burger, A., Savitsky, B., Siscovick, D.S., Manor, O., 2012. Associations of maternal prepregnancy body mass index and gestational weight gain with adult offspring cardiometabolic risk factors: the Jerusalem Perinatal Family Follow-up Study. Circulation 125, 1381–1389.

Hollis, B.W., Wagner, C.L., 2004. Vitamin D requirements during lactation: high-dose maternal supplementation as therapy to prevent hypovitaminosis D for both the mother and the nursing infant. Am. J. Clin. Nutr. 80, 1752s–8s.

Hong, Y.H., Chung, S., 2018. Small for gestational age and obesity related comorbidities. Ann. Pediatr. Endocrinol. Metab. 23, 4–8.

Hoppu, U., Isolauri, E., Laakso, P., Matomäki, J., Laitinen, K., 2012. Probiotics and dietary counselling targeting maternal dietary fat intake modifies breast milk fatty acids and cytokines. Eur. J. Nutr. 51, 211–219.

Howie, G.J., Sloboda, D.M., Kamal, T., Vickers, M.H., 2009. Maternal nutritional history predicts obesity in adult offspring independent of postnatal diet. J. Physiol. 587, 905–915.

Hu, F.B., 2002. Dietary pattern analysis: a new direction in nutritional epidemiology. Curr. Opin. Lipidol. 13, 3–9.

Huang, Y., He, Y., Sun, X., He, Y., Li, Y., Sun, C., 2014. Maternal high folic acid supplement promotes glucose intolerance and insulin resistance in male mouse offspring fed a high-fat diet. Int. J. Mol. Sci. 15, 6298–6313.

Imdad, A., Jabeen, A., Bhutta, Z.A., 2011. Role of calcium supplementation during pregnancy in reducing risk of developing gestational hypertensive disorders: a meta-analysis of studies from developing countries. BMC Public Health 11 (Suppl 3), S18.

Innis, S.M., 2014. Impact of maternal diet on human milk composition and neurological development of infants. Am. J. Clin. Nutr. 99, 734s–41s.

Institute of Medicine, 2009. The national academies collection: reports funded by National Institutes of Health. In: Rasmussen, K.M., Yaktine, A.L. (Eds.), Weight Gain During Pregnancy: Reexamining the Guidelines. National Academies Press (US), National Academy of Sciences, Washington (DC).

Institute of Medicine Food & Nutrition Board, 2006. In: Otten, J.J., Hellwig, J.P., Meyers, L.D. (Eds.), Dietary reference intake: the essential guide to nutrient requirements. National Academy of Sciences, Washington, D.C.

Insull Jr., W., Hirsch, J., James, T., Ahrens Jr., E.H., 1959. The fatty acids of human milk. II. Alterations produced by manipulation of caloric balance and exchange of dietary fats. J. Clin. Invest. 38, 443–450.

Iom National Research Council Committee, 2009. The national academies collection: reports funded by National Institutes of Health. In: Rasmussen, K.M., Yaktine, A.L. (Eds.), Weight Gain During Pregnancy: Reexamining the Guidelines. National Academies Press (US), National Academy of Sciences, Washington (DC).

Jaquiery, A.L., Oliver, M.H., Honeyfield-Ross, M., Harding, J.E., Bloomfield, F.H., 2012. Periconceptional undernutrition in sheep affects adult phenotype only in males. J. Nutr. Metab. 2012, 123610.

Javaid, M.K., Crozier, S.R., Harvey, N.C., Gale, C.R., Dennison, E.M., Boucher, B.J., Arden, N.K., Godfrey, K.M., Cooper, C., 2006. Maternal vitamin D status during pregnancy and childhood bone mass at age 9 years: a longitudinal study. Lancet 367, 36–43.

Jensen, C.L., Voigt, R.G., Prager, T.C., Zou, Y.L., Fraley, J.K., Rozelle, J.C., Turcich, M.R., Llorente, A.M., Anderson, R.E., Heird, W.C., 2005. Effects of maternal docosahexaenoic acid intake on visual function and neurodevelopment in breastfed term infants. Am. J. Clin. Nutr. 82, 125–132.

Jensen, C.L., Voigt, R.G., Llorente, A.M., Peters, S.U., Prager, T.C., Zou, Y.L., Rozelle, J.C., Turcich, M.R., Fraley, J.K., Anderson, R.E., Heird, W.C., 2010. Effects of early maternal docosahexaenoic acid intake on neuropsychological status and visual acuity at five years of age of breast-fed term infants. J. Pediatr. 157, 900–905.

Jensen, K.H., Riis, K.R., Abrahamsen, B., Händel, M.N., 2020. Nutrients, diet, and other factors in prenatal life and bone health in Young adults: a systematic review of longitudinal studies. Nutrients 12.

Johnson, M.A., Hawthorne, N.A., Brackett, W.R., Fischer, J.G., Gunter, E.W., Allen, R.H., Stabler, S.P., 2003. Hyperhomocysteinemia and vitamin B-12 deficiency in elderly using Title IIIc nutrition services. Am. J. Clin. Nutr. 77, 211–220.

Jovanovic-Peterson, L., Peterson, C.M., Reed, G.F., Metzger, B.E., Mills, J.L., Knopp, R.H., Aarons, J.H., 1991. Maternal postprandial glucose levels and infant birth weight: the diabetes in Early Pregnancy Study. The National Institute of Child Health and Human Development—diabetes in Early Pregnancy Study. Am. J. Obstet. Gynecol. 164, 103–111.

Karachaliou, M., Georgiou, V., Roumeliotaki, T., Chalkiadaki, G., Daraki, V., Koinaki, S., Dermitzaki, E., Sarri, K., Vassilaki, M., Kogevinas, M., Oken, E., Chatzi, L., 2015. Association of trimester-specific gestational weight gain with fetal growth, offspring obesity and cardio-metabolic traits in early childhood. Am. J. Obstet. Gynecol. 212 (4), 502.e1.

Kasper, N., Peterson, K.E., Zhang, Z., Ferguson, K.K., Sánchez, B.N., Cantoral, A., Meeker, J.D., Téllez-Rojo, M.M., Pawlowski, C.M., Ettinger, A.S., 2016. Association of Bisphenol A exposure with breastfeeding and perceived insufficient milk supply in Mexican women. Matern. Child Health J. 20, 1713–1719.

Keleher, M.R., Erickson, K., Smith, H.A., Kechris, K.J., Yang, I.V., Dabelea, D., Friedman, J.E., Boyle, K.E., Jansson, T., 2021. Placental insulin/IGF-1 signaling, PGC1α, and inflammatory pathways are associated with metabolic outcomes at 4-6 years of age: the ECHO Healthy Start Cohort. Diabetes, db200902.

Kelly, R., Holzman, C., Senagore, P., Wang, J., Tian, Y., Rahbar, M.H., Chung, H., 2009. Placental vascular pathology findings and pathways to preterm delivery. Am. J. Epidemiol. 170, 148–158.

Kent, J.C., Mitoulas, L.R., Cregan, M.D., Ramsay, D.T., Doherty, D.A., Hartmann, P.E., 2006. Volume and frequency of breastfeedings and fat content of breast milk throughout the day. Pediatrics 117, e387–e395.

Khanam, F., Hossain, B., Mistry, S.K., Mitra, D.K., Raza, W.A., Rifat, M., Afsana, K., Rahman, M., 2018. The association between daily 500 mg calcium supplementation and lower pregnancy-induced hypertension risk in Bangladesh. BMC Pregnancy Childbirth 18, 406.

Kim, S.Y., England, J.L., Sharma, J.A., Njoroge, T., 2011. Gestational diabetes mellitus and risk of childhood overweight and obesity in offspring: a systematic review. Exp. Diabetes Res. 2011, 541308.

Koletzko, B., Thiel, I., Abiodun, P.O., 1992. The fatty acid composition of human milk in Europe and Africa. J. Pediatr. 120, S62–S70.

Langley, S.C., Jackson, A.A., 1994. Increased systolic blood pressure in adult rats induced by fetal exposure to maternal low protein diets. Clin. Sci. (Lond.) 86, 217–222 (discussion 121).

Lauritzen, L., Jorgensen, M.H., Olsen, S.F., Straarup, E.M., Michaelsen, K.F., 2005. Maternal fish oil supplementation in lactation: effect on developmental outcome in breast-fed infants. Reprod. Nutr. Dev. 45, 535–547.

Lawlor, D.A., Timpson, N.J., Harbord, R.M., Leary, S., Ness, A., McCarthy, M.I., Frayling, T.M., Hattersley, A.T., Smith, G.D., 2008. Exploring the developmental overnutrition hypothesis using parental-offspring associations and FTO as an instrumental variable. PLoS Med. 5, e33.

Le, C.H.H., 2016. The prevalence of anemia and moderate-severe anemia in the US population (NHANES 2003-2012). PLoS One 11, e0166635.

Leary, C., Leese, H.J., Sturmey, R.G., 2015. Human embryos from overweight and obese women display phenotypic and metabolic abnormalities. Hum. Reprod. 30, 122–132.

Lee, J.E., Jacques, P.F., Dougherty, L., Selhub, J., Giovannucci, E., Zeisel, S.H., Cho, E., 2010. Are dietary choline and betaine intakes determinants of total homocysteine concentration? Am. J. Clin. Nutr. 91, 1303–1310.

Leermakers, E.T.M., Tielemans, M.J., Van Den Broek, M., Jaddoe, V.W.V., Franco, O.H., Kiefte-De Jong, J.C., 2017. Maternal dietary patterns during pregnancy and offspring cardiometabolic health at age 6 years: the generation R study. Clin. Nutr. 36, 477–484.

Leon, D.A., Koupilova, I., Lithell, H.O., Berglund, L., Mohsen, R., Vagero, D., Lithell, U.B., Mckeigue, P.M., 1996. Failure to realise growth potential in utero and adult obesity in relation to blood pressure in 50 year old Swedish men. BMJ 312, 401–406.

Li, D.K., Ferber, J.R., Odouli, R., 2015. Maternal caffeine intake during pregnancy and risk of obesity in offspring: a prospective cohort study. Int. J. Obes. (Lond) 39, 658–664.

Lisle, S.J., Lewis, R.M., Petry, C.J., Ozanne, S.E., Hales, C.N., Forhead, A.J., 2003. Effect of maternal iron restriction during pregnancy on renal morphology in the adult rat offspring. Br. J. Nutr. 90, 33–39.

Lithell, H.O., Mckeigue, P.M., Berglund, L., Mohsen, R., Lithell, U.B., Leon, D.A., 1996. Relation of size at birth to non-insulin dependent diabetes and insulin concentrations in men aged 50-60 years. BMJ 312, 406–410.

Litonjua, A.A., Lange, N.E., Carey, V.J., Brown, S., Laranjo, N., Harshfield, B.J., O'connor, G.T., Sandel, M., Strunk, R.C., Bacharier, L.B., Zeiger, R.S., Schatz, M., Hollis, B.W., Weiss, S.T., 2014. The Vitamin D Antenatal Asthma Reduction Trial (VDAART): rationale, design, and methods of a randomized, controlled trial of vitamin D supplementation in pregnancy for the primary prevention of asthma and allergies in children. Contemp. Clin. Trials 38, 37–50.

Lonnerdal, B., 1986. Effects of maternal dietary intake on human milk composition. J. Nutr. 116, 499–513.

Louwman, M.W., Van Dusseldorp, M., Van De Vijver, F.J., Thomas, C.M., Schneede, J., Ueland, P.M., Refsum, H., Van Staveren, W.A., 2000. Signs of impaired cognitive function in adolescents with marginal cobalamin status. Am. J. Clin. Nutr. 72, 762–769.

Lozoff, B., Beard, J., Connor, J., Barbara, F., Georgieff, M., Schallert, T., 2006. Long-lasting neural and behavioral effects of iron deficiency in infancy. Nutr. Rev. 64, S34–S43. discussion S72-91.

Lumey, L.H., Stein, A.D., Kahn, H.S., Van Der Pal-De Bruin, K.M., Blauw, G.J., Zybert, P.A., Susser, E.S., 2007. Cohort profile: the Dutch Hunger Winter families study. Int. J. Epidemiol. 36, 1196–1204.

Ma, J., Prince, A.L., Bader, D., Hu, M., Ganu, R., Baquero, K., Blundell, P., Alan Harris, R., Frias, A.E., Grove, K.L., Aagaard, K.M., 2014. High-fat maternal diet during pregnancy persistently alters the offspring microbiome in a primate model. Nat. Commun. 5, 3889.

Maalouf, J., Barron, J., Gunn, J.P., Yuan, K., Perrine, C.G., Cogswell, M.E., 2015. Iodized salt sales in the United States. Nutrients 7, 1691–1695.

Major, C.A., Henry, M.J., De Veciana, M., Morgan, M.A., 1998. The effects of carbohydrate restriction in patients with diet-controlled gestational diabetes. Obstet. Gynecol. 91, 600–604.

Margerison-Zilko, C.E., Shrimali, B.P., Eskenazi, B., Lahiff, M., Lindquist, A.R., Abrams, B.F., 2012. Trimester of maternal gestational weight gain and offspring body weight at birth and age five. Matern. Child Health J. 16, 1215–1223.

Maslova, E., Hansen, S., Jensen, C.B., Thorne-Lyman, A.L., Strom, M., Olsen, S.F., 2013a. Vitamin D intake in mid-pregnancy and child allergic disease - a prospective study in 44,825 Danish mother-child pairs. BMC Pregnancy Childbirth 13, 199.

Maslova, E., Strom, M., Olsen, S.F., Halldorsson, T.I., 2013b. Consumption of artificially-sweetened soft drinks in pregnancy and risk of child asthma and allergic rhinitis. PLoS One 8, e57261.

Maslova, E., Rytter, D., Bech, B.H., Henriksen, T.B., Rasmussen, M.A., Olsen, S.F., Halldorsson, T.I., 2014. Maternal protein intake during pregnancy and offspring overweight 20 y later. Am. J. Clin. Nutr. 100, 1139–1148.

Maslova, E., Rifas-Shiman, S.L., Olsen, S.F., Gillman, M.W., Oken, E., 2018. Prenatal n-3 long-chain fatty acid status and offspring metabolic health in early and mid-childhood: results from Project Viva. Nutr. Diabetes 8, 29.

Massiera, F., Saint-Marc, P., Seydoux, J., Murata, T., Kobayashi, T., Narumiya, S., Guesnet, P., Amri, E.Z., Negrel, R., Ailhaud, G., 2003. Arachidonic acid and prostacyclin signaling promote adipose tissue development: a human health concern? J. Lipid Res. 44, 271–279.

Mcardle, H.J., Ashworth, C.J., 1999. Micronutrients in fetal growth and development. Br. Med. Bull. 55, 499–510.

Mcardle, H.J., Andersen, H.S., Jones, H., Gambling, L., 2006. Fetal programming: causes and consequences as revealed by studies of dietary manipulation in rats—a review. Placenta 27 (Suppl A), S56–S60.

McCann, J.C., Ames, B.N., 2007. An overview of evidence for a causal relation between iron deficiency during development and deficits in cognitive or behavioral function. Am. J. Clin. Nutr. 85, 931–945.

Mennella, J.A., Jagnow, C.P., Beauchamp, G.K., 2001. Prenatal and postnatal flavor learning by human infants. Pediatrics 107, E88.

Metzger, B.E., Lowe, L.P., Dyer, A.R., Trimble, E.R., Chaovarindr, U., Coustan, D.R., Hadden, D.R., Mccance, D.R., Hod, M., McIntyre, H.D., Oats, J.J., Persson, B., Rogers, M.S., Sacks, D.A., 2008. Hyperglycemia and adverse pregnancy outcomes. N. Engl. J. Med. 358, 1991–2002.

Middleton, P., Gomersall, J.C., Gould, J.F., Shepherd, E., Olsen, S.F., Makrides, M., 2018. Omega-3 fatty acid addition during pregnancy. Cochrane Database Syst. Rev. 11, Cd003402.

Moon, R.J., Harvey, N.C., Robinson, S.M., Ntani, G., Davies, J.H., Inskip, H.M., Godfrey, K.M., Dennison, E.M., Calder, P.C., Cooper, C., 2013. Maternal plasma polyunsaturated fatty acid status in late pregnancy is associated with offspring body composition in childhood. J. Clin. Endocrinol. Metab. 98, 299–307.

Moon, R.J., Harvey, N.C., Cooper, C., D'angelo, S., Crozier, S.R., Inskip, H.M., Schoenmakers, I., Prentice, A., Arden, N.K., Bishop, N.J., Carr, A., Dennison, E.M., Eastell, R., Fraser, R., Gandhi, S.V., Godfrey, K.M., Kennedy, S., Mughal, M.Z., Papageorghiou, A.T., Reid, D.M., Robinson, S.M., Javaid, M.K., 2016. Determinants of the maternal 25-hydroxyvitamin D response to vitamin D supplementation during pregnancy. J. Clin. Endocrinol. Metab. 101, 5012–5020.

Much, D., Brunner, S., Vollhardt, C., Schmid, D., Sedlmeier, E.M., Bruderl, M., Heimberg, E., Bartke, N., Boehm, G., Bader, B.L., Amann-Gassner, U., Hauner, H., 2013. Breast milk fatty acid profile in relation to infant growth and body composition: results from the INFAT study. Pediatr. Res. 74, 230–237.

Muhlhausler, B.S., Gibson, R.A., Makrides, M., 2010. Effect of long-chain polyunsaturated fatty acid supplementation during pregnancy or lactation on infant and child body composition: a systematic review. Am. J. Clin. Nutr. 92, 857–863.

Nesheim, M., Yaktine, A., 2007. Seafood Choices: Balancing Benefits and Risks. The National Academies Press, Washington DC.

Oberhelman, S.S., Meekins, M.E., Fischer, P.R., Lee, B.R., Singh, R.J., Cha, S.S., Gardner, B.M., Pettifor, J.M., Croghan, I.T., Thacher, T.D., 2013. Maternal vitamin D supplementation to improve the vitamin D status of breast-fed infants: a randomized controlled trial. Mayo Clin. Proc. 88, 1378–1387.

O'brien, K.O., Ru, Y., 2017. Iron status of North American pregnant women: an update on longitudinal data and gaps in knowledge from the United States and Canada. Am. J. Clin. Nutr. 106, 1647S–1654S.

Oken, E., 2009. Maternal and child obesity: the causal link. Obstet. Gynecol. Clin. North Am. 36, 361–377. ix-x.

Oken, E., Kleinman, K.P., Berland, W.E., Simon, S.R., Rich-Edwards, J.W., Gillman, M.W., 2003. Decline in fish consumption among pregnant women after a national mercury advisory. Obstet. Gynecol. 102, 346–351.

Oken, E., Taveras, E.M., Kleinman, K.P., Rich-Edwards, J.W., Gillman, M.W., 2007. Gestational weight gain and child adiposity at age 3 years. Am. J. Obstet. Gynecol. 196, 322.e1–8.

Oken, E., Radesky, J.S., Wright, R.O., Bellinger, D.C., Amarasiriwardena, C.J., Kleinman, K.P., Hu, H., Gillman, M.W., 2008a. Maternal fish intake during pregnancy, blood mercury levels, and child cognition at age 3 years in a US cohort. Am. J. Epidemiol. 167, 1171–1181.

Oken, E., Rifas-Shiman, S.L., Field, A.E., Frazier, A.L., Gillman, M.W., 2008b. Maternal gestational weight gain and offspring weight in adolescence. Obstet. Gynecol. 112, 999–1006.

Oken, E., Kleinman, K.P., Belfort, M.B., Hammitt, J.K., Gillman, M.W., 2009. Associations of gestational weight gain with short- and longer-term maternal and child health outcomes. Am. J. Epidemiol. 170, 173–180.

Ozaltin, E., Hill, K., Subramanian, S.V., 2010. Association of maternal stature with offspring mortality, underweight, and stunting in low- to middle-income countries. JAMA 303, 1507–1516.

Pace, R.M., Prince, A.L., Ma, J., Belfort, B.D.W., Harvey, A.S., Hu, M., Baquero, K., Blundell, P., Takahashi, D., Dean, T., Kievit, P., Sullivan, E.L., Friedman, J.E., Grove, K., Aagaard, K.M., 2018. Modulations in the offspring gut microbiome are refractory to postnatal synbiotic supplementation among juvenile primates. BMC Microbiol. 18, 28.

Painter, R.C., Roseboom, T.J., Bleker, O.P., 2005. Prenatal exposure to the Dutch famine and disease in later life: an overview. Reprod. Toxicol. 20, 345–352.

Panth, P., Guerin, G., Dimarco, N.M., 2019. A review of iodine status of women of reproductive age in the USA. Biol. Trace Elem. Res. 188, 208–220.

Parsons, A.G., Zhou, S.J., Spurrier, N.J., Makrides, M., 2008. Effect of iron supplementation during pregnancy on the behaviour of children at early school age: long-term follow-up of a randomised controlled trial. Br. J. Nutr. 99, 1133–1139.

Pedersen, L., Lauritzen, L., Brasholt, M., Buhl, T., Bisgaard, H., 2012. Polyunsaturated fatty acid content of mother's milk is associated with childhood body composition. Pediatr. Res. 72, 631–636.

Perng, W., Gillman, M.W., Mantzoros, C.S., Oken, E., 2014. A prospective study of maternal prenatal weight and offspring cardiometabolic health in midchildhood. Ann. Epidemiol. 24, 793–800.

Perng, W., Oken, E., Dabelea, D., 2019a. Developmental overnutrition and obesity and type 2 diabetes in offspring. Diabetologia 62, 1779–1788.

Perng, W., Oken, E., Dabelea, D., 2019b. Developmental overnutrition and offspring obesity and type 2 diabetes. Diabetologia 62 (10), 1779–1788.

Perng, W., Hockett, C.W., Sauder, K.A., Dabelea, D., 2020. In utero exposure to gestational diabetes mellitus and cardiovascular risk factors in youth: a longitudinal analysis in the EPOCH cohort. Pediatr. Obes. 15, e12611.

Perreault, M., Atkinson, S.A., Mottola, M.F., Phillips, S.M., Bracken, K., Hutton, E.K., Xie, F., Meyre, D., Morassut, R.E., Prapavessis, H., Thabane, L., Team, B.S., 2018. Structured diet and exercise guidance in pregnancy to improve health in women and their offspring: study protocol for the be healthy in pregnancy (BHIP) randomized controlled trial. Trials 19, 691.

Perrine, C.G., Herrick, K., Serdula, M.K., Sullivan, K.M., 2010. Some subgroups of reproductive age women in the United States may be at risk for iodine deficiency. J. Nutr. 140, 1489–1494.

Philipps, L.H., Santhakumaran, S., Gale, C., Prior, E., Logan, K.M., Hyde, M.J., Modi, N., 2011. The diabetic pregnancy and offspring BMI in childhood: a systematic review and meta-analysis. Diabetologia 54, 1957–1966.

Pitkin, R.M., 2007. Folate and neural tube defects. Am. J. Clin. Nutr. 85, 285s–288s.

Poon, A.H., Laprise, C., Lemire, M., Montpetit, A., Sinnett, D., Schurr, E., Hudson, T.J., 2004. Association of vitamin D receptor genetic variants with susceptibility to asthma and atopy. Am. J. Respir. Crit. Care Med. 170, 967–973.

Pop, V.J., Kuijpens, J.L., Van Baar, A.L., Verkerk, G., Van Son, M.M., De Vijlder, J.J., Vulsma, T., Wiersinga, W.M., Drexhage, H.A., Vader, H.L., 1999. Low maternal free thyroxine concentrations during early pregnancy are associated with impaired psychomotor development in infancy. Clin. Endocrinol. (Oxf) 50, 149–155.

Popkin, B.M., 2006. Global nutrition dynamics: the world is shifting rapidly toward a diet linked with noncommunicable diseases. Am. J. Clin. Nutr. 84, 289–298.

Provvedini, D.M., Tsoukas, C.D., Deftos, L.J., Manolagas, S.C., 1983. 1,25-dihydroxyvitamin D3 receptors in human leukocytes. Science 221, 1181–1183.

Raby, B.A., Lazarus, R., Silverman, E.K., Lake, S., Lange, C., Wjst, M., Weiss, S.T., 2004. Association of vitamin D receptor gene polymorphisms with childhood and adult asthma. Am. J. Respir. Crit. Care Med. 170, 1057–1065.

Raiten, D.J., Raghavan, R., Porter, A., Obbagy, J.E., Spahn, J.M., 2014. Executive summary: evaluating the evidence base to support the inclusion of infants and children from birth to 24 mo of age in the dietary guidelines for Americans—"the B-24 Project". Am. J. Clin. Nutr. 99, 663s–91s.

Ramakrishnan, U., Grant, F., Goldenberg, T., Zongrone, A., Martorell, R., 2012. Effect of women's nutrition before and during early pregnancy on maternal and infant outcomes: a systematic review. Paediatr. Perinat. Epidemiol. 26 (Suppl 1), 285–301.

Rasmussen, K.M., Kjolhede, C.L., 2004. Prepregnant overweight and obesity diminish the prolactin response to suckling in the first week postpartum. Pediatrics 113, e465–e471.

Regnault, N., Gillman, M.W., Rifas-Shiman, S.L., Eggleston, E., Oken, E., 2013. Sex-specific associations of gestational glucose tolerance with childhood body composition. Diabetes Care 36, 3045–3053.

Rifas-Shiman, S.L., Rich-Edwards, J.W., Kleinman, K.P., Oken, E., Gillman, M.W., 2009. Dietary quality during pregnancy varies by maternal characteristics in Project Viva: a US cohort. J. Am. Diet. Assoc. 109, 1004–1011.

Robledo, C., Peck, J.D., Stoner, J.A., Carabin, H., Cowan, L., Koch, H.M., Goodman, J.R., 2013. Is bisphenol-A exposure during pregnancy associated with blood glucose levels or diagnosis of gestational diabetes? J. Toxicol. Environ. Health A 76, 865–873.

Romon, M., Nuttens, M.C., Vambergue, A., Verier-Mine, O., Biausque, S., Lemaire, C., Fontaine, P., Salomez, J.L., Beuscart, R., 2001. Higher carbohydrate intake is associated with decreased incidence of newborn macrosomia in women with gestational diabetes. J. Am. Diet. Assoc. 101, 897–902.

Ronnenberg, A.G., Wood, R.J., Wang, X., Xing, H., Chen, C., Chen, D., Guang, W., Huang, A., Wang, L., Xu, X., 2004. Preconception hemoglobin and ferritin concentrations are associated with pregnancy outcome in a prospective cohort of Chinese women. J. Nutr. 134, 2586–2591.

Rooney, B.L., Schauberger, C.W., 2002. Excess pregnancy weight gain and long-term obesity: one decade later. Obstet. Gynecol. 100, 245–252.

Rooney, B.L., Schauberger, C.W., Mathiason, M.A., 2005. Impact of perinatal weight change on long-term obesity and obesity-related illnesses. Obstet. Gynecol. 106, 1349–1356.

Roseboom, T.J., Van Der Meulen, J.H., Van Montfrans, G.A., Ravelli, A.C., Osmond, C., Barker, D.J., Bleker, O.P., 2001. Maternal nutrition during gestation and blood pressure in later life. J. Hypertens. 19, 29–34.

Rosenfeld, C.S., 2015. Sex-specific placental responses in fetal development. Endocrinology 156, 3422–3434.

Roza, S.J., Van Batenburg-Eddes, T., Steegers, E.A., Jaddoe, V.W., Mackenbach, J.P., Hofman, A., Verhulst, F.C., Tiemeier, H., 2010. Maternal folic acid supplement use in early pregnancy and child behavioural problems: the generation R study. Br. J. Nutr. 103, 445–452.

Ruchat, S.M., Allard, C., Doyon, M., Lacroix, M., Guillemette, L., Patenaude, J., Battista, M.C., Ardilouze, J.L., Perron, P., Bouchard, L., Hivert, M.F., 2016. Timing of excessive weight gain during pregnancy modulates newborn anthropometry. J. Obstet. Gynaecol. Can. 38, 108–117.

Samuelsson, A.M., Matthews, P.A., Argenton, M., Christie, M.R., McConnell, J.M., Jansen, E.H., Piersma, A.H., Ozanne, S.E., Twinn, D.F., Remacle, C., Rowlerson, A., Poston, L., Taylor, P.D., 2008. Diet-induced obesity in female mice leads to offspring hyperphagia, adiposity, hypertension, and insulin resistance: a novel murine model of developmental programming. Hypertension 51, 383–392.

Schlotz, W., Jones, A., Phillips, D.I., Gale, C.R., Robinson, S.M., Godfrey, K.M., 2010. Lower maternal folate status in early pregnancy is associated with childhood hyperactivity and peer problems in offspring. J. Child Psychol. Psychiatry 51, 594–602.

Selhub, J., Bagley, L.C., Miller, J., Rosenberg, I.H., 2000. B vitamins, homocysteine, and neurocognitive function in the elderly. Am. J. Clin. Nutr. 71, 614s–620s.

Sen, S., Rifas-Shiman, S.L., Shivappa, N., Wirth, M.D., Hebert, J.R., Gold, D.R., Gillman, M.W., Oken, E., 2018. Associations of prenatal and early life dietary inflammatory potential with childhood adiposity and cardiometabolic risk in project viva. Pediatr. Obes. 13, 292–300.

Shaheen, S.O., Northstone, K., Newson, R.B., Emmett, P.M., Sherriff, A., Henderson, A.J., 2009. Dietary patterns in pregnancy and respiratory and atopic outcomes in childhood. Thorax 64, 411–417.

Shapiro, A.L., Boyle, K.E., Dabelea, D., Patinkin, Z.W., De La Houssaye, B., Ringham, B.M., Glueck, D.H., Barbour, L.A., Norris, J.M., Friedman, J.E., 2016a. Nicotinamide promotes adipogenesis in umbilical cord-derived mesenchymal stem cells and is associated with neonatal adiposity: the healthy start BabyBUMP project. PLoS One 11, e0159575.

Shapiro, A.L., Kaar, J.L., Crume, T.L., Starling, A.P., Siega-Riz, A.M., Ringham, B.M., Glueck, D.H., Norris, J.M., Barbour, L.A., Friedman, J.E., Dabelea, D., 2016b. Maternal diet quality in pregnancy and neonatal adiposity: the Healthy Start Study. Int. J. Obes. (Lond) 40, 1056–1062.

Shiell, A.W., Campbell-Brown, M., Haselden, S., Robinson, S., Godfrey, K.M., Barker, D.J., 2001. High-meat, low-carbohydrate diet in pregnancy: relation to adult blood pressure in the offspring. Hypertension 38, 1282–1288.

Shin, J.S., Choi, M.Y., Longtine, M.S., Nelson, D.M., 2010. Vitamin D effects on pregnancy and the placenta. Placenta 31, 1027–1034.

Silverman, B.L., Rizzo, T.A., Cho, N.H., Metzger, B.E., 1998. Long-term effects of the intrauterine environment. The Northwestern University Diabetes in Pregnancy Center. Diabetes Care 21 (Suppl 2), B142–B149.

Sinclair, K.D., Allegrucci, C., Singh, R., Gardner, D.S., Sebastian, S., Bispham, J., Thurston, A., Huntley, J.F., Rees, W.D., Maloney, C.A., Lea, R.G., Craigon, J., Mcevoy, T.G., Young, L.E., 2007. DNA methylation, insulin resistance, and blood pressure in offspring determined by maternal periconceptional B vitamin and methionine status. Proc. Natl. Acad. Sci. U. S. A. 104, 19351–19356.

Smith, D.E., Lewis, C.E., Caveny, J.L., Perkins, L.L., Burke, G.L., Bild, D.E., 1994. Longitudinal changes in adiposity associated with pregnancy. The CARDIA Study. Coronary artery risk development in young adults study. JAMA 271, 1747–1751.

Starling, A.P., Brinton, J.T., Glueck, D.H., Shapiro, A.L., Harrod, C.S., Lynch, A.M., Siega-Riz, A.M., Dabelea, D., 2015. Associations of maternal BMI and gestational weight gain with neonatal adiposity in the Healthy Start Study. Am. J. Clin. Nutr. 101, 302–309.

Stefan, N., Schick, F., Häring, H.-U., 2017. Causes, characteristics, and consequences of metabolically unhealthy normal weight in humans. Cell Metab. 26, 292–300.

Stein, Z., Susser, M., Saenger, G., Marolla, F., 1972. Nutrition and mental performance. Science 178, 708–713.

Strain, J.J., Davidson, P.W., Thurston, S.W., Harrington, D., Mulhern, M.S., McAfee, A.J., Van Wijngaarden, E., Shamlaye, C.F., Henderson, J., Watson, G.E., Zareba, G., Cory-Slechta, D.A., Lynch, M., Wallace, J.M., Mcsorley, E.M., Bonham, M.P., Stokes-Riner, A., Sloane-Reeves, J., Janciuras, J., Wong, R., Clarkson, T.W., Myers, G.J., 2012. Maternal Pufa status but not prenatal methylmercury exposure is associated with children's language functions at age five years in the Seychelles. J. Nutr. 142, 1943–1949.

Subramanian, S.V., Ackerson, L.K., Davey Smith, G., John, N.A., 2009. Association of maternal height with child mortality, anthropometric failure, and anemia in India. JAMA 301, 1691–1701.

Suez, J., Korem, T., Zeevi, D., Zilberman-Schapira, G., Thaiss, C.A., Maza, O., Israeli, D., Zmora, N., Gilad, S., Weinberger, A., Kuperman, Y., Harmelin, A., Kolodkin-Gal, I., Shapiro, H., Halpern, Z., Segal, E., Elinav, E., 2014. Artificial sweeteners induce glucose intolerance by altering the gut microbiota. Nature 514, 181–186.

Szajewska, H., Ruszczynski, M., Chmielewska, A., 2010. Effects of iron supplementation in nonanemic pregnant women, infants, and young children on the mental performance and psychomotor development of children: a systematic review of randomized controlled trials. Am. J. Clin. Nutr. 91, 1684–1690.

Tahir, M.J., Haapala, J.L., Foster, L.P., Duncan, K.M., Teague, A.M., Kharbanda, E.O., McGovern, P.M., Whitaker, K.M., Rasmussen, K.M., Fields, D.A., Jacobs Jr., D.R., Harnack, L.J., Demerath, E.W., 2019. Higher maternal diet quality during pregnancy and lactation is associated with lower infant weight-for-length, body fat percent, and fat mass in early postnatal life. Nutrients 11, 632.

The National Academies of Sciences Engineering and Medicine, n.d. Nutrition During Pregnancy and Lactation: Exploring New Evidence. [online]. Washington D.C. available: https://www.nap.edu/resource/25841/interactive/?utm_source=HMD%20Email%20List&utm_campaign=3d698de117-ncpf-pw-Dec1_COPY_01&utm_medium=email&utm_term=0_211686812e-3d698de117-180574845&mc_cid=3d698de117&mc_eid=& [accessed march 5th 2021].

Todd, S.E., Oliver, M.H., Jaquiery, A.L., Bloomfield, F.H., Harding, J.E., 2009. Periconceptional undernutrition of ewes impairs glucose tolerance in their adult offspring. Pediatr. Res. 65, 409–413.

Todrank, J., Heth, G., Restrepo, D., 2011. Effects of in utero odorant exposure on neuroanatomical development of the olfactory bulb and odour preferences. Proc. Biol. Sci. 278, 1949–1955.

Trout, K.K., Wetzel-Effinger, L., 2012. Flavor learning in utero and its implications for future obesity and diabetes. Curr. Diab. Rep. 12, 60–66.

U.S. Department of Agriculture, n.d. Nutrition During Pregnancy. [Online]. Available: https://www.nal.usda.gov/fnic/nutrition-during-pregnancy [Accessed March 5th 2021].

U.S. Department of Health and Human Services, 2021. Human Placenta Project. (Online). Available: https://www.nichd.nih.gov/research/supported/HPP/default [Accessed January 5th 2021].

US Food And Drug Administration, 2014. Fish: What Pregnant Women and Parents Should Know. Online, US Department of Health and Human Services. Available: http://www.fda.gov/Food/FoodborneIllnessContaminants/Metals/ucm393070.htm [Accessed March 5th 2021].

Valdez, R., Athens, M.A., Thompson, G.H., Bradshaw, B.S., Stern, M.P., 1994. Birthweight and adult health outcomes in a biethnic population in the USA. Diabetologia 37, 624–631.

Van Abeelen, A.F., De Rooij, S.R., Osmond, C., Painter, R.C., Veenendaal, M.V., Bossuyt, P.M., Elias, S.G., Grobbee, D.E., Van Der Schouw, Y.T., Barker, D.J., Roseboom, T.J., 2011. The sex-specific effects of famine on the association between placental size and later hypertension. Placenta 32, 694–698.

Villamor, E., Cnattingius, S., 2006. Interpregnancy weight change and risk of adverse pregnancy outcomes: a population-based study. Lancet 368, 1164–1170.

Villamor, E., Rifas-Shiman, S.L., Gillman, M.W., Oken, E., 2012. Maternal intake of methyl-donor nutrients and child cognition at 3 years of age. Paediatr. Perinat. Epidemiol. 26, 328–335.

Voerman, E., Jaddoe, V.W.V., Gishti, O., Hofman, A., Franco, O.H., Gaillard, R., 2016. Maternal caffeine intake during pregnancy, early growth, and body fat distribution at school age. Obesity 24, 1170–1177.

Wagner, C.L., Hulsey, T.C., Fanning, D., Ebeling, M., Hollis, B.W., 2006. High-dose vitamin D3 supplementation in a cohort of breastfeeding mothers and their infants: a 6-month follow-up pilot study. Breastfeed. Med. 1, 59–70.

Weiler, H., Fitzpatrick-Wong, S., Veitch, R., Kovacs, H., Schellenberg, J., McCloy, U., Yuen, C.K., 2005. Vitamin D deficiency and whole-body and femur bone mass relative to weight in healthy newborns. CMAJ 172, 757–761.

Willett, W.C., Stampfer, M.J., 2001. Clinical practice. What vitamins should I be taking, doctor? N. Engl. J. Med. 345, 1819–1824.

World Health Organization, 2021. Vitamin and Mineral Nutrition Information System (VMNIS): Global anaemia prevalence and number of individuals affected. [Online]. Available: http://www.who.int/vmnis/anaemia/prevalence/summary/anaemia_data_status_t2/en/ [Accessed March 5th 2021].

Wu, Q., Mizushima, Y., Komiya, M., Matsuo, T., Suzuki, M., 1998. Body fat accumulation in the male offspring of rats fed high-fat diet. J. Clin. Biochem. Nutr. 25, 71–79.

Wu, Q., Mizushima, Y., Komiya, M., Matsuo, T., Suzuki, M., 1999. The effects of high-fat diet feeding over generations on body fat accumulation associated with lipoprotein lipase and leptin in rat adipose tissues. Asia Pac. J. Clin. Nutr. 8, 46–52.

Yajnik, C.S., Deshpande, S.S., Jackson, A.A., Refsum, H., Rao, S., Fisher, D.J., Bhat, D.S., Naik, S.S., Coyaji, K.J., Joglekar, C.V., Joshi, N., Lubree, H.G., Deshpande, V.U., Rege, S.S., Fall, C.H.D., 2008. Vitamin B12 and folate concentrations during pregnancy and insulin resistance in the offspring: the Pune Maternal Nutrition Study. Diabetologia 51, 29–38.

Yang, Z., Huffman, S.L., 2013. Nutrition in pregnancy and early childhood and associations with obesity in developing countries. Matern. Child Nutr. 9 (Suppl 1), 105–119.

Yogev, Y., Langer, O., Xenakis, E.M., Rosenn, B., 2005. The association between glucose challenge test, obesity and pregnancy outcome in 6390 non-diabetic women. J. Matern. Fetal Neonatal Med. 17, 29–34.

Young, M.F., Pressman, E., Foehr, M.L., Mcnanley, T., Cooper, E., Guillet, R., Orlando, M., McIntyre, A.W., Lafond, J., O'brien, K.O., 2010. Impact of maternal and neonatal iron status on placental transferrin receptor expression in pregnant adolescents. Placenta 31, 1010–1014.

Yu, Z., Han, S., Zhu, J., Sun, X., Ji, C., Guo, X., 2013. Pre-pregnancy body mass index in relation to infant birth weight and offspring overweight/obesity: a systematic review and meta-analysis. PLoS One 8, e61627.

Zeghoud, F., Vervel, C., Guillozo, H., Walrant-Debray, O., Boutignon, H., Garabedian, M., 1997. Subclinical vitamin D deficiency in neonates: definition and response to vitamin D supplements. Am. J. Clin. Nutr. 65, 771–778.

Zheng, W., Huang, W., Zhang, Z., Zhang, L., Tian, Z., Li, G., Zhang, W., 2019. Patterns of gestational weight gain in women with overweight or obesity and risk of large for gestational age. Obes. Facts 12, 407–415.

Zhou, S.J., Gibson, R.A., Crowther, C.A., Baghurst, P., Makrides, M., 2006. Effect of iron supplementation during pregnancy on the intelligence quotient and behavior of children at 4 y of age: long-term follow-up of a randomized controlled trial. Am. J. Clin. Nutr. 83, 1112–1117.

Zhu, K., Whitehouse, A.J., Hart, P.H., Kusel, M., Mountain, J., Lye, S., Pennell, C., Walsh, J.P., 2014. Maternal vitamin D status during pregnancy and bone mass in offspring at 20 years of age: a prospective cohort study. J. Bone Miner. Res. 29, 1088–1095.

Zhu, Y., Hedderson, M.M., Sridhar, S., Xu, F., Feng, J., Ferrara, A., 2019. Poor diet quality in pregnancy is associated with increased risk of excess fetal growth: a prospective multi-racial/ethnic cohort study. Int. J. Epidemiol. 48, 423–432.

Zimmermann, M.B., 2012. The effects of iodine deficiency in pregnancy and infancy. Paediatr. Perinat. Epidemiol. 26 (Suppl 1), 108–117.

# Long-term health outcomes of breastfeeding

*Anat Guz-Mark[a,b] and Raanan Shamir[a,b]*

[a]Institute of Gastroenterology, Nutrition and Liver Diseases, Schneider Children's Medical Center of Israel, Petach Tikva, Israel [b]Sackler Faculty of Medicine, Tel-Aviv University, Tel-Aviv, Israel

## CHAPTER LEARNING OBJECTIVES

– Breastfeeding is the natural and desired exclusive feeding for infants up to 6 months of age. Partial breastfeeding is recommended as long as mutually desired by the child and the mother.

– Long-term health benefits of breastfeeding are difficult to establish, and current knowledge is mostly based on observational studies.

– There is evidence for mild neurocognitive advantage for breastfed infants beyond infancy.

– There is evidence that breastfeeding during infancy is negatively associated with childhood obesity.

– There is a trend for some protective role of breastfeeding against childhood hematogenic malignancies.

## 3.1 Introduction

Breastfeeding is considered universally as the natural and desired mode of infant feeding. Exclusive breastfeeding up to the age of 6 months is recommended by pediatric professional organizations worldwide, while partial breastfeeding is also encouraged, and continuation of breastfeeding is preferred as long as mutually desired by the mother and infant (Agostoni et al., 2009; AAP, 2012). Short-term health benefits, which are spread across populations worldwide, are numerous and include mostly reduction of infection rates during infancy, mainly gastrointestinal, otitis media and lower respiratory tract infections, prevention of necrotizing enterocolitis in preterm babies (Ip et al., 2007), and reduction in infant mortality, mainly from infectious disease (Victora et al., 2016). In terms of public health, support of breastfeeding is cost-effective and may contain great potential economic benefits (Bartick and Reinhold, 2010). Besides the health benefits of breastfeeding to both infants and mothers, it is also a social and psychological interaction, with complex influences that may extend far beyond the measured medical and health overt outcomes. While most comparable researches report short-term outcomes during or immediately after the period of breastfeeding, long-term evidence of health benefits are scarce and much more difficult to prove. As breastfeeding is the gold standard for infants' nutrition, randomized control trials are ethically inappropriate to conduct; hence, existing evidence rely mainly on observational data. Such observational studies could be subjected to various confounders that might influence the comparisons to non-breastfed infants, including environmental exposures, parental intelligence and education, socioeconomic status, as well as mother-infant attachment (Peñacoba and Catala, 2019) and psychological factors. Furthermore, environmental factors existing at the time of breastfeeding may be different when the long-term outcomes of breastfeeding are measured many decades later.

PROBIT (Promotion of Breastfeeding Intervention Trial) was a nested controlled study (Kramer et al., 2001) that evaluated the effect of the Baby-Friendly Hospital Initiative training (World Health Organization and United Nations Children's Fund, 1989) on breastfeeding duration, exclusivity, and health outcomes. The follow-up and changes in outcome over two decades are fascinating, but the study compared a population with a rate of 43.3% exclusive breastfeeding at 3 months versus a control population with a 6.4% breastfeeding rate, thus studying the effect of the initiative but not of breastfeeding per se.

This being said, taking the various limitations into account, available literature on the long-term outcomes of breastfed babies is of great importance and reviewed hereby.

## 3.2 Neurodevelopment

The effect of breastfeeding on a child's intelligence has been a focus of research for decades. A plethora of studies published in the previous century reported higher scores in cognitive function tests in breastfed versus formula-fed children. A meta-analysis of 11 comparative studies published in 1999 (Anderson et al., 1999) have shown an adjusted pooled increment of 3.16 points in intelligence quotient (IQ) among children and adolescents who were breastfed as infants compared to children who were formula-fed. Before the adjustments for socioeconomic status, maternal education, and IQ, the difference was as high as 5.32 IQ points. Newer studies used a more strict criteria of adjustments for maternal covariates and especially maternal intelligence rather than education, with pooled analysis that demonstrated a reduction of the positive effect on children's cognitive performance to a non-significant difference between breastfed and non-breastfed subjects (Der et al., 2006). The wide variation of results between studies seems to be affected by environmental and maternal confounders that are associated with most of the effects of breastfeeding on children's neurodevelopment (Walfisch et al., 2013). However, other analyses that did control for maternal IQ still showed a more modest but significant breastfeeding benefit of 2.62 IQ points (Horta et al., 2015a). The positive effect in the later meta-analysis was diminished when comparison was made between studies of older children and adolescents (aged 10–19 years) and studies of younger age, evaluated as 1.92 points of IQ in the older age group (Horta et al., 2015a). Even so, studies conducted among adult participants also demonstrate adjusted positive effects of breastfeeding on adult intelligence (Mortensen et al., 2002).

The positive effect of breastfeeding on cognitive performance was shown to be associated with the duration of breastfeeding during infancy in some studies (Mortensen et al., 2002), with a slightly higher impact of breastfeeding on intelligence score among children breastfed for longer than 6 months (Hou et al., 2021). One recent study demonstrated a beneficial effect on IQ in children breastfed for at least 1 month compared to less than 1 month, but could not demonstrate any dose-response effect in longer periods of breastfeeding (Strøm et al., 2019). A large prospective cohort examining different aspects of cognitive ability at the age of 7 years demonstrated a positive association between breastfeeding duration and higher intelligence score, but no difference in the memory and learning assessments (Belfort et al., 2013). Another recent study of 9 to 10 years old children, showed a correlation between duration of breastfeeding and later cognitive performance in general ability scores, but no significant association in executive function and memory (Lopez et al., 2021).

In the vulnerable population of preterm and very low birth weight infants, consumption of human milk showed a persistent beneficial effect on mental and psychomotor developmental indices. In 1992, Lucas et al. documented an 8.3-point advantage in IQ in preterm babies who received human milk compared to formula (Lucas et al., 1992). The early study by Anderson et al. further showed that low-birth-weight infants had larger IQ differences (between breastfed and formula-fed subjects) than normal-birth-weight infants, suggesting that "premature infants derive more benefits in cognitive development from breast milk than do full-term infants"(Anderson et al., 1999). The amount of breastmilk consumed by preterm infants in the neonatal intensive care unit was further associated with mental and psychomotor developmental indices (Vohr et al., 2007). In another study of preterm babies who were evaluated for IQ and brain size during the period of adolescence, the percentage of breastmilk consumption was significantly correlated with verbal IQ for the whole study group and was correlated to all IQ scores and brain volume among adolescent boys (Isaacs et al., 2010).

The association between breastfeeding and brain structure in later life was demonstrated in other studies, showing a correlation with cortical thickness in parietal lobules (Kafouri et al., 2013) and increased white matter development in frontal regions (Deoni et al., 2013).

The effect of human milk on neurodevelopment was presumed to be influenced by fatty acids uniquely available in human milk and moderated by fatty acyl desaturase 2 (FADS2) genetic variant involved in the control of fatty acid pathways (Caspi et al., 2007). However, later studies failed to support the association between FADS2 polymorphism and the effect on cognitive function (Steer et al., 2010; Martin et al., 2011). A different line of support to the theory of fatty acids importance in modulating neurodevelopment of breastfed infants is suggested by a study that demonstrated a greater beneficial effect of breastfeeding on childhood cognition in women who consumed two or more servings of fish per week (Belfort et al., 2013). Following this theory, the supplementation of long-chain polyunsaturated fatty acids (LCPUFA) to term and preterm formula-fed infants has been a focus of many heterogeneous studies, with no clear long-term beneficial effect on neurodevelopmental outcomes (Moon et al., 2016; Jasani et al., 2017).

It seems that although the positive effect of breastfeeding on cognitive development is strongly supported by the literature, a causal relation is still difficult to establish (Agostoni et al., 2009), while complex environmental confounders are probably associated with the observed beneficial effects.

## 3.3  Obesity, type 2 diabetes, and cardiovascular risk factors

The association between breastfeeding and reduced risk of childhood obesity was observed in many studies and meta-analyses over the last few decades (Owen et al., 2005). The duration of breastfeeding was shown to be inversely associated with the risk of overweight and obesity in later life, with a dose-response effect (Harder et al., 2005; Yan et al., 2014). However, as for all outcomes of breastfeeding, there are numerous possible confounders that are difficult to overcome and may influence growth and obesity risk other than the content of breastmilk itself, including cultural, psychological, dietary, and lifestyle preferences in families that promote breastfeeding. The adjustments to major confounding factors, including maternal obesity and smoking and socioeconomic class, were shown to markedly reduce the inverse association between breastfeeding and BMI (Owen et al., 2005). Breastfeeding may also lower the risk of childhood obesity by allowing infants to self-regulate their energy intake (Dewey, 2003). Nonetheless, there is a different growth pattern in the breastfed infant, as reflected in a plethora of studies as well as in the WHO growth standards (Grummer-Strawn et al., 2010; WHO Multicentre Growth Reference Study Group and De Onis, 2006), identifying slower growth trajectories during the first months of life in breastfed compared to formula-fed babies. The results of different studies and meta-analyses on the risk of later obesity are diverse. Some failed to demonstrate a significant clear association between breastfeeding and risk of later obesity, after controlling for confounders (Patro-Gołąb et al., 2016), while others showed a pooled reduction in the prevalence of overweight or obesity of 13% (Horta et al., 2015b). In the PROBIT trial, the late effects of breastfeeding promotion intervention were assessed, including growth trajectories and adiposity at the age of 16 years. In this nested-control study, no reduction in adolescence overweight or obesity was observed (Martin et al., 2017). Furthermore, the prevalence of overweight/obesity was significantly higher among this intervention group. On the contrary, there is evidence in some contemporary longitudinal cohorts for a reverse association between breastfeeding and the risk of obesity later in childhood (Hummel et al., 2021). With the abundance of different studies on this topic, a recent umbrella review has emphasized that in light of the conflicting results of different meta-analyses, the causality of association between breastfeeding and reduced risk for obesity later in life remains unclear at the moment (Agostoni et al., 2019).

As for the risk of type 2 diabetes, early studies suggested a protective effect of breastfeeding, with a pooled odds ratio of 0.61 compared to formula-fed subjects (Owen et al., 2006), but confounders could not be ruled out. Other studies evaluating insulin resistance in school-aged children and adolescents (Lawlor et al., 2005) have found no significant effect of breastfeeding after controlling for confounding variables. The 2016 meta-analysis found only restricted evidence for a reduced risk for type 2 diabetes (odds ratio of 0.65, with a confidence interval of 0.49–0.86) (Victora et al., 2016). These contradicting findings are in line with the commentary published by the European Society for Paediatric Gastroenterology Hepatology and Nutrition committee of nutrition, suggesting that "the potential for breastfeeding to contribute to reduction of later obesity development, and its possible effects on type 2 diabetes should be explored in more detail" (Agostoni et al., 2009).

Some studies reported lower blood pressure in infants and children who were breastfed compared to formula-fed. Suggested mechanisms include low sodium content in human milk compared to some infant formulas, as well as the presence of LCPUFA in human milk. Yet, a wide heterogenicity was found among studies reporting the association between blood pressure and infant feeding, and the long-term effect was unclear (Owen et al., 2003). A meta-analysis of breastfeeding effects on blood pressure in later life showed some favorable benefit that was not statistically significant when only large studies were considered (>1000 subjects) (Martin et al., 2005c). The same trend was observed in a more recent meta-analysis, with a mild decrease in systolic blood pressure appearing in only small studies and becoming non-significant in large studies (Horta et al., 2015b; Victora et al., 2016).

Low blood cholesterol levels in adulthood were also associated with a history of breastfeeding, although the magnitude of the effect was minimal. The hypothesis regarding this phenomenon is the relatively high content of cholesterol in human milk affecting early metabolic programming by down-regulation of hydroxymethylglutaryl coenzyme A (HMG-CoA) (Wong et al., 1993). The difference in cholesterol levels between breastfed and formula-fed subjects varies in several heterogenic pieces of research and was evaluated as 0.05–0.15 mmol/L in meta-analyses (Horta et al., 2015b; Owen et al., 2008).

Although some of these aforementioned studies may suggest some minor reduction of blood pressure or cholesterol levels in individuals who were breastfed in infancy, strong evidence is lacking, and the effects of confounders are difficult to control.

The only available observational study among adults reported a higher incidence of coronary heart disease among 45 to 59 years old men who were breastfed in infancy, with no evidence of a duration-response effect (Martin et al., 2005a). There are currently no high-quality studies supporting any sustained protective effect of breastfeeding against cardiovascular morbidity and mortality later in life (Owen et al., 2011; Agostoni et al., 2009).

## 3.4 Allergy and autoimmunity

Exclusive breastfeeding during the first months of life has been associated with short-term reductions in atopic dermatitis, eczema, and wheezing (Greer et al., 2008; Muraro et al., 2004). Since early studies reporting this phenomenon, other studies provided conflicting results, with most showing a more significant effect in at-risk infants (Agostoni et al., 2009). Some of the controversy involves potential biases in the observational studies, including genetic differences between groups, as well as reverse causality. Nonetheless, the evidence for a sustained, *long-lasting* effect of breastfeeding on allergy prevention is lacking (Ip et al., 2007; Agostoni et al., 2009; Victora et al., 2016). In the PROBIT trial, although the incidence of atopic dermatitis during the first year of life was lower in the intervention group (breastfeeding promotion) compared to the control group, at 6.5 years of age, there were no longer differences in allergic symptoms and in skin prick tests between the groups (Kramer et al., 2007). Other observational studies also failed to present a significant association between breastfeeding and allergy beyond the period of infancy (Björkstén et al., 2011; Lodge et al., 2015). Although breastfeeding is recommended in all children, there is insufficient data to recommend breastfeeding as a method to prevent food allergy, as stated by the European Academy of Allergy and Clinical Immunology (EAACI) guidelines (Halken et al., 2021).

Breastfeeding was claimed to be negatively associated with various autoimmune diseases, including celiac disease, type 1 diabetes, and inflammatory bowel disease (AAP, 2012).

The pooled protective effect against type 1 diabetes described in previous studies was weak at the most and influenced by a great variation between studies and potential confounding factors (Cardwell et al., 2012). The Environmental Determinants of Diabetes in the Young (TEDDY) study investigated infants with genetic susceptibility for type 1 diabetes in a large prospective cohort. In a follow-up to a median age of 8.3 years published recently (Hummel et al., 2021), breastfeeding duration was not associated with a lower risk of either islet auto-antibodies or tissue transglutaminase autoantibodies.

Lack of breastfeeding was found to be associated with inflammatory bowel disease in several retrospective cohorts (Lautenschlager et al., 2020; Preda et al., 2019; Piovani et al., 2019), limited by their methodological quality. Overall, the evidence linking breastfeeding and inflammatory IBD is inconclusive (Güngör et al., 2019) and more high-quality research is needed.

As for celiac disease, early epidemiological studies reported a protective role of breast-feeding against the development of celiac disease in later childhood (Akobeng et al., 2006). These observations were also supported by a policy statement on breastfeeding by the American Academy of Pediatrics (AAP) in 2012 (AAP, 2012), suggesting a pro-tective effect of breastfeeding at the time of gluten introduction. However, more recent studies from the last decade have found contradictory results, and a meta-analysis pub-lished in 2015 showed no significant effect of breastfeeding on the risk of developing celiac disease (Szajewska et al., 2015). In the prospective PreventCD study, infants at high risk for celiac disease were randomized to introduction of gluten at the age of 4 or 6 months, preferably when still being breastfed. The results published in 2014 showed that breast-feeding, whether exclusive or partial and whether it was ongoing during gluten introduc-tion, did not significantly influence the development of celiac disease (Vriezinga et al., 2014). Interestingly, a recent study from the same cohort performed microbiota analysis of breastmilk samples, and found differences between microbial species in milk from moth-ers whose children went on to develop celiac disease, compared to those that remained healthy (Benítez-Páez et al., 2020). The CELIPREV study, which was another prospective interventional study published in 2014 and in which breastfeeding was not the primary outcome, also demonstrated no significant association between breastfeeding and the de-velopment of celiac disease (Lionetti et al., 2014). In the recent TEDDY cohort mentioned earlier, no association between breastfeeding and later development of celiac serology was demonstrated (Hummel et al., 2021).

## 3.5 Malignancies

One of the main proven short-term effects of breastfeeding is protection against early-life infections (Agostoni et al., 2009; Victora et al., 2016). Following the theory that breastfeed-ing may modulate infants' immune system in early life, the effect of breastfeeding on the development of malignancies has been of great interest (Maia Rda and Wünsch Filho, 2013). Some studies suggested a negative association between breastfeeding and malignancies, with an early meta-analysis demonstrating a lower risk of childhood leukemia and Hodgkin's lymphoma in children who were breastfed compared to formula-fed (Investigators, 2001). Both short-term and prolonged breastfeeding (longer and shorter than 6 months) were fur-ther associated with reduced risk of childhood acute myeloblastic and lymphoblastic leuke-mias (Kwan et al., 2004). For all types of cancers, both in childhood (Martin et al., 2005b) and adulthood (Martin et al., 2005d), pooled results of studies were found to be inconclusive. More recent studies have shown variables results for childhood leukemia, with both meta-analyses published in 2007 and 2015 still supporting a protective role of breastfeeding (Ip et al., 2007; Amitay and Keinan-Boker, 2015). However, studies' heterogenicity in the definition of breastfeeding duration, as well as potential confounders, still remain a substantial concern in the interpretation and implementation of the results. A recent meta-analysis evaluated the dose-response effect of breastfeeding and suggested a non-linear dose-response relationship in the protection against childhood leukemia (Su et al., 2021). The inverse association was also demonstrated for childhood neuroblastoma; however, no association was found with other types of cancer (Su et al., 2021).

## 3.6 Conclusions

The scientific ability to appreciate long-term outcomes of breastfeeding, in high-quality research, is limited. As randomized controlled trials are impractical, all available data are strictly observational, mostly retrospective, with various potential confounders limiting the interpretation of causality, as mentioned hereby. There is currently only limited evidence regarding the long-term benefits of breastfeeding, and it is mostly based on observations from resource-rich populations.

Given these limitations, the current knowledge supports the use of breastfeeding as the natural and desirable mode of infant feeding on the basis of short-term benefits (not discussed in this chapter), together with social, psychological, cultural, financial, and theoretical advantages.

Individuals who were breastfed perform better in cognitive and developmental assessments, as reviewed in this chapter. This consistent neurocognitive mild advantage may reflect a long-term benefit of human milk or breastfeeding, but could also be influenced by other contributing factors that are difficult to fully adjust for in observational studies. The same applies to childhood obesity, which appears to be negatively associated with breastfeeding during infancy. The role of early metabolic programming and the influence of breastfeeding on these early life processes should further be clarified. Other cardiovascular risk factors could not be associated at the moment to breastfeeding according to current studies.

The effects of breastfeeding on the immune system and its development are fascinating. As infants who are breastfed experience lower incidence of infections, other diseases that involve the immune system could also be potentially affected. Furthermore, the important effects of breastfeeding on the microbiota, not discussed here, may provide significant contribution to later health outcomes as the plasticity of the infants' microbiota is diminished in later years (Vu et al., 2021). There is a trend of some protective role of breastfeeding against childhood hematogenic malignancies that might in part be attributed to infections and immune load in early life. Allergic and autoimmune diseases were also claimed to be associated with history of breastfeeding in early studies, but results of contemporary research are contradictory, and no association has consistently been proven. Although the limitations of research regarding the long-term benefits of breastfeeding should be acknowledged, healthcare professionals should continue to protect, promote, and support breastfeeding (Agostoni et al., 2009; Victora et al., 2016; AAP, 2012).

## 3.7 Future research trends

More long-term contemporary cohorts are needed to better appreciate the effects of breast-feeding later in life. As it seems that the research will continue to be based on observational studies due to ethical considerations discussed earlier, there is a role for *prospective* large population-based cohorts that will be able to identify and better control for confounders. Research in low-resource countries is also rising these days and could shed more light on the effects of breastfeeding in deprived populations.

Human breast milk *composition* analysis is of great importance, and research focusing on human milk specific factors will probably lead in the upcoming years including metabolomics of human milk, urine, stools, and blood when available. Furthermore, analysis of human milk microbiota, changes in gut microbiota, including analysis of intestinal microbiota rather than examining stool only, and extending the research to the virome and fungal populations will provide a more comprehensive assessment of the possibility of long-term effect of our gut "biome." These combined research tools will enable to examine the long-lasting effects on the child's immune system, early metabolic programming, and hopefully the long-term effect later in life.

## Sources of additional information

World Health Organization (WHO): https://www.who.int/health-topics/breastfeeding
Centers for Disease Control and Prevention (CDC): https://www.cdc.gov/breastfeeding/index.htm
American Academy of Pediatrics (AAP): https://www.aap.org/en/patient-care/breastfeeding/

## References

AAP, 2012. Breastfeeding and the use of human milk. Pediatrics 129, e827–e841.

Agostoni, C., Braegger, C., Decsi, T., Kolacek, S., Koletzko, B., Michaelsen, K.F., Mihatsch, W., Moreno, L.A., Puntis, J., Shamir, R., Szajewska, H., Turck, D., Van Goudoever, J., 2009. Breast-feeding: a commentary by the ESPGHAN committee on nutrition. J. Pediatr. Gastroenterol. Nutr. 49, 112–125.

Agostoni, C., Guz-Mark, A., Marderfeld, L., Milani, G.P., Silano, M., Shamir, R., 2019. The long-term effects of dietary nutrient intakes during the first 2 years of life in healthy infants from developed countries: an umbrella review. Adv. Nutr. 10, 489–501.

Akobeng, A.K., Ramanan, A.V., Buchan, I., Heller, R.F., 2006. Effect of breast feeding on risk of coeliac disease: a systematic review and meta-analysis of observational studies. Arch. Dis. Child. 91, 39–43.

Amitay, E.L., Keinan-Boker, L., 2015. Breastfeeding and childhood leukemia incidence: a meta-analysis and systematic review. JAMA Pediatr. 169, e151025.

Anderson, J.W., Johnstone, B.M., Remley, D.T., 1999. Breast-feeding and cognitive development: a meta-analysis. Am. J. Clin. Nutr. 70, 525–535.

Bartick, M., Reinhold, A., 2010. The burden of suboptimal breastfeeding in the United States: a pediatric cost analysis. Pediatrics 125, e1048–e1056.

Belfort, M.B., Rifas-Shiman, S.L., Kleinman, K.P., Guthrie, L.B., Bellinger, D.C., Taveras, E.M., Gillman, M.W., Oken, E., 2013. Infant feeding and childhood cognition at ages 3 and 7 years: effects of breastfeeding duration and exclusivity. JAMA Pediatr. 167, 836–844.

Benítez-Páez, A., Olivares, M., Szajewska, H., Pieścik-Lech, M., Polanco, I., Castillejo, G., Nuñez, M., Ribes-Koninckx, C., Korponay-Szabó, I.R., Koletzko, S., Meijer, C.R., Mearin, M.L., Sanz, Y., 2020. Breast-milk microbiota linked to celiac disease development in children: a pilot study from the PreventCD cohort. Front. Microbiol. 11, 1335.

Björkstén, B., Aït-Khaled, N., Innes Asher, M., Clayton, T.O., Robertson, C., 2011. Global analysis of breast feeding and risk of symptoms of asthma, rhinoconjunctivitis and eczema in 6-7 year old children: ISAAC phase three. Allergol Immunopathol (Madr) 39, 318–325.

Cardwell, C.R., Stene, L.C., Ludvigsson, J., Rosenbauer, J., Cinek, O., Svensson, J., Perez-Bravo, F., Memon, A., Gimeno, S.G., Wadsworth, E.J., Strotmeyer, E.S., Goldacre, M.J., Radon, K., Chuang, L.M., Parslow, R.C., Chetwynd, A., Karavanaki, K., Brigis, G., Pozzilli, P., Urbonaite, B., Schober, E., Devoti, G., Sipetic, S., Joner, G., Ionescu-Tirgoviste, C., De Beaufort, C.E., Harrild, K., Benson, V., Savilahti, E., Ponsonby, A.L., Salem, M., Rabiei, S., Patterson, C.C., 2012. Breast-feeding and childhood-onset type 1 diabetes: a pooled analysis of individual participant data from 43 observational studies. Diabetes Care 35, 2215–2225.

Caspi, A., Williams, B., Kim-Cohen, J., Craig, I.W., Milne, B.J., Poulton, R., Schalkwyk, L.C., Taylor, A., Werts, H., Moffitt, T.E., 2007. Moderation of breastfeeding effects on the IQ by genetic variation in fatty acid metabolism. Proc. Natl. Acad. Sci. U. S. A. 104, 18860–18865.

Deoni, S.C., Dean 3rd, D.C., Piryatinsky, I., O'Muircheartaigh, J., Waskiewicz, N., Lehman, K., Han, M., Dirks, H., 2013. Breastfeeding and early white matter development: a cross-sectional study. Neuroimage 82, 77–86.

Der, G., Batty, G.D., Deary, I.J., 2006. Effect of breast feeding on intelligence in children: prospective study, sibling pairs analysis, and meta-analysis. BMJ 333, 945.

Dewey, K.G., 2003. Is breastfeeding protective against child obesity? J. Hum. Lact. 19, 9–18.

Greer, F.R., Sicherer, S.H., Burks, A.W., 2008. Effects of early nutritional interventions on the development of atopic disease in infants and children: the role of maternal dietary restriction, breastfeeding, timing of introduction of complementary foods, and hydrolyzed formulas. Pediatrics 121, 183.

Grummer-Strawn, L.M., Reinold, C., Krebs, N.F., 2010. Use of World Health Organization and CDC growth charts for children aged 0-59 months in the United States. MMWR Recomm. Rep. 59, 1–15.

Güngör, D., Nadaud, P., Dreibelbis, C., Lapergola, C.C., Wong, Y.P., Terry, N., Abrams, S.A., Beker, L., Jacobovits, T., Järvinen, K.M., Nommsen-Rivers, L.A., O'Brien, K.O., Oken, E., Pérez-Escamilla, R., Ziegler, E.E., Spahn, J.M., 2019. Infant milk-feeding practices and diagnosed celiac disease and inflammatory bowel disease in offspring: a systematic review. Am. J. Clin. Nutr. 109, 838s–851s.

Halken, S., Muraro, A., De Silva, D., Khaleva, E., Angier, E., Arasi, S., Arshad, H., Bahnson, H.T., Beyer, K., Boyle, R., Du Toit, G., Ebisawa, M., Eigenmann, P., Grimshaw, K., Hoest, A., Jones, C., Lack, G., Nadeau, K., O'mahony, L., Szajewska, H., Venter, C., Verhasselt, V., Wong, G.W.K., Roberts, G., 2021. EAACI guideline: preventing the development of food allergy in infants and young children (2020 update). Pediatr. Allergy Immunol. 32, 843–858.

Harder, T., Bergmann, R., Kallischnigg, G., Plagemann, A., 2005. Duration of breastfeeding and risk of overweight: a meta-analysis. Am. J. Epidemiol. 162, 397–403.

Horta, B.L., Loret De Mola, C., Victora, C.G., 2015a. Breastfeeding and intelligence: a systematic review and meta-analysis. Acta Paediatr. 104, 14–19.

Horta, B.L., Loret De Mola, C., Victora, C.G., 2015b. Long-term consequences of breastfeeding on cholesterol, obesity, systolic blood pressure and type 2 diabetes: a systematic review and meta-analysis. Acta Paediatr. 104, 30–37.

Hou, L., Li, X., Yan, P., Li, Y., Wu, Y., Yang, Q., Shi, X., Ge, L., Yang, K., 2021. Impact of the duration of breastfeeding on the intelligence of children: a systematic review with network Meta-analysis. Breastfeed. Med. 16, 687–696.

Hummel, S., Weis, A., Bonifacio, E., Agardh, D., Akolkar, B., Aronsson, C.A., Hagopian, W.A., Koletzko, S., Krischer, J.P., Lernmark, Å., Lynch, K., Norris, J.M., Rewers, M.J., She, J.X., Toppari, J., Uusitalo, U., Vehik, K., Virtanen, S.M., Beyerlein, A., Ziegler, A.G., 2021. Associations of breastfeeding with childhood autoimmunity, allergies, and overweight: the environmental determinants of diabetes in the young (TEDDY) study. Am. J. Clin. Nutr. 114, 134–142.

Ip, S., Chung, M., Raman, G., Chew, P., Magula, N., Devine, D., Trikalinos, T., Lau, J., 2007. Breastfeeding and maternal and infant health outcomes in developed countries. Evid. Rep. Technol. Assess. (Full Rep), 1–186.

Isaacs, E.B., Fischl, B.R., Quinn, B.T., Chong, W.K., Gadian, D.G., Lucas, A., 2010. Impact of breast milk on intelligence quotient, brain size, and white matter development. Pediatr. Res. 67, 357–362.

Jasani, B., Simmer, K., Patole, S.K., Rao, S.C., 2017. Long chain polyunsaturated fatty acid supplementation in infants born at term. Cochrane Database Syst. Rev. 3, Cd000376.

Kafouri, S., Kramer, M., Leonard, G., Perron, M., Pike, B., Richer, L., Toro, R., Veillette, S., Pausova, Z., Paus, T., 2013. Breastfeeding and brain structure in adolescence. Int. J. Epidemiol. 42, 150–159.

Kramer, M.S., Chalmers, B., Hodnett, E.D., Sevkovskaya, Z., Dzikovich, I., Shapiro, S., Collet, J.P., Vanilovich, I., Mezen, I., Ducruet, T., Shishko, G., Zubovich, V., Mknuik, D., Gluchanina, E., Dombrovskiy, V., Ustinovitch, A., Kot, T., Bogdanovich, N., Ovchinikova, L., Helsing, E., 2001. Promotion of breastfeeding intervention trial (PROBIT): a randomized trial in the Republic of Belarus. JAMA 285, 413–420.

Kramer, M.S., Matush, L., Vanilovich, I., Platt, R., Bogdanovich, N., Sevkovskaya, Z., Dzikovich, I., Shishko, G., Mazer, B., 2007. Effect of prolonged and exclusive breast feeding on risk of allergy and asthma: cluster randomised trial. BMJ 335, 815.

Kwan, M.L., Buffler, P.A., Abrams, B., Kiley, V.A., 2004. Breastfeeding and the risk of childhood leukemia: a meta-analysis. Public Health Rep. 119, 521–535.

Lautenschlager, S.A., Fournier, N., Biedermann, L., Pittet, V., Schreiner, P., Misselwitz, B., Scharl, M., Rogler, G., Siebenhüner, A.R., 2020. The influence of breastfeeding, cesarean section, pet animals, and urbanization on the development of inflammatory bowel disease: data from the swiss IBD cohort study. Inflamm Intest Dis 5, 170–179.

Lawlor, D.A., Riddoch, C.J., Page, A.S., Andersen, L.B., Wedderkopp, N., Harro, M., Stansbie, D., Smith, G.D., 2005. Infant feeding and components of the metabolic syndrome: findings from the European youth heart study. Arch. Dis. Child. 90, 582–588.

Lionetti, E., Castellaneta, S., Francavilla, R., Pulvirenti, A., Tonutti, E., Amarri, S., Barbato, M., Barbera, C., Barera, G., Bellantoni, A., Castellano, E., Guariso, G., Limongelli, M.G., Pellegrino, S., Polloni, C., Ughi, C., Zuin, G., Fasano, A., Catassi, C., 2014. Introduction of gluten, HLA status, and the risk of celiac disease in children. N. Engl. J. Med. 371, 1295–1303.

Lodge, C.J., Tan, D.J., Lau, M.X., Dai, X., Tham, R., Lowe, A.J., Bowatte, G., Allen, K.J., Dharmage, S.C., 2015. Breastfeeding and asthma and allergies: a systematic review and meta-analysis. Acta Paediatr. 104, 38–53.

Lopez, D.A., Foxe, J.J., Mao, Y., Thompson, W.K., Martin, H.J., Freedman, E.G., 2021. Breastfeeding duration is associated with domain-specific improvements in cognitive performance in 9-10-year-old children. Front. Public Health 9, 657422.

Lucas, A., Morley, R., Cole, T.J., Lister, G., Leeson-Payne, C., 1992. Breast milk and subsequent intelligence quotient in children born preterm. Lancet 339, 261–264.

Maia Rda, R., Wünsch Filho, V., 2013. Infection and childhood leukemia: review of evidence. Rev. Saude Publica 47, 1172–1185.

Martin, R.M., Ben-Shlomo, Y., Gunnell, D., Elwood, P., Yarnell, J.W.G., Davey Smith, G., 2005a. Breast feeding and cardiovascular disease risk factors, incidence, and mortality: the Caerphilly study. J. Epidemiol. Community Health 59, 121–129.

Martin, R.M., Gunnell, D., Owen, C.G., Smith, G.D., 2005b. Breast-feeding and childhood cancer: a systematic review with metaanalysis. Int. J. Cancer 117, 1020–1031.

Martin, R.M., Gunnell, D., Smith, G.D., 2005c. Breastfeeding in infancy and blood pressure in later life: systematic review and meta-analysis. Am. J. Epidemiol. 161, 15–26.

Martin, R.M., Middleton, N., Gunnell, D., Owen, C.G., Smith, G.D., 2005d. Breast-feeding and cancer: the Boyd Orr cohort and a systematic review with meta-analysis. J. Natl. Cancer Inst. 97, 1446–1457.

Martin, N.W., Benyamin, B., Hansell, N.K., Montgomery, G.W., Martin, N.G., Wright, M.J., Bates, T.C., 2011. Cognitive function in adolescence: testing for interactions between breast-feeding and FADS2 polymorphisms. J. Am. Acad. Child Adolesc. Psychiatry 50, 55–62.e4.

Martin, R.M., Kramer, M.S., Patel, R., Rifas-Shiman, S.L., Thompson, J., Yang, S., Vilchuck, K., Bogdanovich, N., Hameza, M., Tilling, K., Oken, E., 2017. Effects of promoting long-term, exclusive breastfeeding on adolescent adiposity, blood pressure, and growth trajectories: a secondary analysis of a randomized clinical trial. JAMA Pediatr. 171, e170698.

Moon, K., Rao, S.C., Schulzke, S.M., Patole, S.K., Simmer, K., 2016. Longchain polyunsaturated fatty acid supplementation in preterm infants. Cochrane Database Syst. Rev. 12, Cd000375.

Mortensen, E.L., Michaelsen, K.F., Sanders, S.A., Reinisch, J.M., 2002. The association between duration of breastfeeding and adult intelligence. JAMA 287, 2365–2371.

Muraro, A., Dreborg, S., Halken, S., Høst, A., Niggemann, B., Aalberse, R., Arshad, S.H., Berg Av, A., Carlsen, K.H., Duschén, K., Eigenmann, P., Hill, D., Jones, C., Mellon, M., Oldeus, G., Oranje, A., Pascual, C., Prescott, S., Sampson, H., Svartengren, M., Vandenplas, Y., Wahn, U., Warner, J.A., Warner, J.O., Wickman, M., Zeiger, R.S., 2004. Dietary prevention of allergic diseases in infants and small children. Part III: critical review of published peer-reviewed observational and interventional studies and final recommendations. Pediatr. Allergy Immunol. 15, 291–307.

Owen, C.G., Whincup, P.H., Gilg, J.A., Cook, D.G., 2003. Effect of breast feeding in infancy on blood pressure in later life: systematic review and meta-analysis. BMJ 327, 1189–1195.

Owen, C.G., Martin, R.M., Whincup, P.H., Smith, G.D., Cook, D.G., 2005. Effect of infant feeding on the risk of obesity across the life course: a quantitative review of published evidence. Pediatrics 115, 1367–1377.

Owen, C.G., Martin, R.M., Whincup, P.H., Smith, G.D., Cook, D.G., 2006. Does breastfeeding influence risk of type 2 diabetes in later life? A quantitative analysis of published evidence. Am. J. Clin. Nutr. 84, 1043–1054.

Owen, C.G., Whincup, P.H., Kaye, S.J., Martin, R.M., Davey Smith, G., Cook, D.G., Bergstrom, E., Black, S., Wadsworth, M.E., Fall, C.H., Freudenheim, J.L., Nie, J., Huxley, R.R., Kolacek, S., Leeson, C.P., Pearce, M.S., Raitakari, O.T., Lisinen, I., Viikari, J.S., Ravelli, A.C., Rudnicka, A.R., Strachan, D.P., Williams, S.M., 2008. Does initial breastfeeding lead to lower blood cholesterol in adult life? A quantitative review of the evidence. Am. J. Clin. Nutr. 88, 305–314.

Owen, C.G., Whincup, P.H., Cook, D.G., 2011. Breast-feeding and cardiovascular risk factors and outcomes in later life: evidence from epidemiological studies. Proc. Nutr. Soc. 70, 478–484.

Patro-Gołąb, B., Zalewski, B.M., Kołodziej, M., Kouwenhoven, S., Poston, L., Godfrey, K.M., Koletzko, B., Van Goudoever, J.B., Szajewska, H., 2016. Nutritional interventions or exposures in infants and children aged up to 3 years and their effects on subsequent risk of overweight, obesity and body fat: a systematic review of systematic reviews. Obes. Rev. 17, 1245–1257.

Peñacoba, C., Catala, P., 2019. Associations between breastfeeding and mother-infant relationships: a systematic review. Breastfeed. Med. 14, 616–629.

Piovani, D., Danese, S., Peyrin-Biroulet, L., Nikolopoulos, G.K., Lytras, T., Bonovas, S., 2019. Environmental risk factors for inflammatory bowel diseases: an umbrella review of meta-analyses. Gastroenterology 157, 647–659.e4.

Preda, C.M., Manuc, T., Istratescu, D., Louis, E., Baicus, C., Sandra, I., Diculescu, M., Reenaers, C., Van Kemseke, C., Nitescu, M., Tieranu, C., Sandu, C.G., Oprea-Calin, G., Tugui, L., Viziru, S., Ciora, C.A., Gheorghe, L.S., Manuc, M., 2019. Environmental factors in Romanian and Belgian patients with inflammatory bowel disease—a retrospective comparative study. Maedica (Bucur) 14, 233–239.

Steer, C.D., Davey Smith, G., Emmett, P.M., Hibbeln, J.R., Golding, J., 2010. FADS2 polymorphisms modify the effect of breastfeeding on child IQ. PLoS One 5, e11570.

Strøm, M., Mortensen, E.L., Kesmodel, U.S., Halldorsson, T., Olsen, J., Olsen, S.F., 2019. Is breast feeding associated with offspring IQ at age 5? Findings from prospective cohort: lifestyle during pregnancy study. BMJ Open 9, e023134.

Su, Q., Sun, X., Zhu, L., Yan, Q., Zheng, P., Mao, Y., Ye, D., 2021. Breastfeeding and the risk of childhood cancer: a systematic review and dose-response meta-analysis. BMC Med. 19, 90.

Szajewska, H., Shamir, R., Chmielewska, A., Pieścik-Lech, M., Auricchio, R., Ivarsson, A., Kolacek, S., Koletzko, S., Korponay-Szabo, I., Mearin, M.L., Ribes-Koninckx, C., Troncone, R., 2015. Systematic review with meta-analysis: early infant feeding and coeliac disease—update 2015. Aliment. Pharmacol. Ther. 41, 1038–1054.

U.K. Childhood Cancer Study Investigators, 2001. Breastfeeding and childhood cancer. Br. J. Cancer 85, 1685–1694.

Victora, C.G., Bahl, R., Barros, A.J., França, G.V., Horton, S., Krasevec, J., Murch, S., Sankar, M.J., Walker, N., Rollins, N.C., 2016. Breastfeeding in the 21st century: epidemiology, mechanisms, and lifelong effect. Lancet 387, 475–490.

Vohr, B.R., Poindexter, B.B., Dusick, A.M., McKinley, L.T., Higgins, R.D., Langer, J.C., Poole, W.K., 2007. Persistent beneficial effects of breast milk ingested in the neonatal intensive care unit on outcomes of extremely low birth weight infants at 30 months of age. Pediatrics 120, e953.

Vriezinga, S.L., Auricchio, R., Bravi, E., Castillejo, G., Chmielewska, A., Crespo Escobar, P., Kolaček, S., Koletzko, S., Korponay-Szabo, I.R., Mummert, E., Polanco, I., Putter, H., Ribes-Koninckx, C., Shamir, R., Szajewska, H., Werkstetter, K., Greco, L., Gyimesi, J., Hartman, C., Hogen Esch, C., Hopman, E., Ivarsson, A., Koltai, T., Koning, F., Martinez-Ojinaga, E., Te Marvelde, C., Pavic, A., Romanos, J., Stoopman, E., Villanacci, V., Wijmenga, C., Troncone, R., Mearin, M.L., 2014. Randomized feeding intervention in infants at high risk for celiac disease. N. Engl. J. Med. 371, 1304–1315.

Vu, K., Lou, W., Tun, H.M., Konya, T.B., Morales-Lizcano, N., Chari, R.S., Field, C.J., Guttman, D.S., Mandal, R., Wishart, D.S., Azad, M.B., Becker, A.B., Mandhane, P.J., Moraes, T.J., Lefebvre, D.L., Sears, M.R., Turvey, S.E., Subbarao, P., Scott, J.A., Kozyrskyj, A.L., 2021. From birth to overweight and atopic disease: multiple and common pathways of the infant gut microbiome. Gastroenterology 160, 128–144.e10.

Walfisch, A., Sermer, C., Cressman, A., Koren, G., 2013. Breast milk and cognitive development- -the role of confounders: a systematic review. BMJ Open 3, e003259.

WHO Multicentre Growth Reference Study Group, De Onis, M., 2006. WHO child growth standards based on length/height, weight and age. Acta Paediatr. 95, 76–85.

Wong, W.W., Hachey, D.L., Insull, W., Opekun, A.R., Klein, P.D., 1993. Effect of dietary cholesterol on cholesterol synthesis in breast-fed and formula-fed infants. J. Lipid Res. 34, 1403–1411.

World Health Organization, United Nations Children's Fund, 1989. Protecting, Promoting and Supporting Breast-Feeding : The Special Role of Maternity Services / a Joint WHO/UNICEF Statement. World Health Organization, Geneva.

Yan, J., Liu, L., Zhu, Y., Huang, G., Wang, P.P., 2014. The association between breastfeeding and childhood obesity: a meta-analysis. BMC Public Health 14, 1267.

# Early nutrition: Effects on infants' growth and body composition

*Maria Lorella Gianni[a,b], Daniela Morniroli[a], Giulia Vizzari[a], and Fabio Mosca[a,b]*

[a]Department of Clinical Sciences and Community Health, University of Milan, Milan, Italy
[b]Fondazione IRCCS Ca' Granda Ospedale Maggiore Policlinico, NICU, Milan, Italy

## CHAPTER LEARNING OBJECTIVES

- Explore the relationship between early nutrition and later outcomes
- Review the mechanisms through which early growth pattern and body composition can modulate long-term health outcome
- Emphasize the role played by the maternal status on offspring's future health

## 4.1 Introduction

Overwhelming evidence has underlined the major contribution of early growth pattern and body composition development to the modulation of long-term health and neurodevelopmental outcomes (Guilloteau et al., 2009; Isganaitis, 2019; Lucas et al., 1999), implying early nutrition as an underlying mechanism (Fall and Kumaran, 2019).

Fetal development and infancy represent a critical time window during which, due to the plasticity of growing and developing tissues, environmental factors cause long-lasting modifications in phenotype (Barker, 2007; Langley-Evans, 2015). Nutritional deficits and/or excesses, even arising for relatively short periods, may therefore lead to adverse outcomes (Padmanabhan et al., 2016).

The importance of exposure to early environmental stimuli for later health outcomes is conceptualized in the idea of developmental programming (Barker, 2007; Goyal et al., 2019). This concept is particularly relevant for the development of metabolic syndrome, whose prevalence has increased worldwide, involving a great economic burden to the health care system (Panuganti et al., 2020). Strong commitment has been advocated to identify the determinants of growth and the underlining mechanisms responsible for the developmental programming in order to implement policies and interventions to improve nutrition in early life and the well-being of the future generation (Clark et al., 2020).

The purpose of this chapter is to present a review of the available scientific data focusing on the major nutritional determinants of growth and body composition, taking into account the particular characteristics of both term and preterm infants. The importance of maternal nutrition status, in terms of under and overnutrition and within the intergenerational cycle of malnutrition, will also be described.

## 4.2 The importance of a life cycle approach for promoting infants and children health

It is now well understood that, according to the "developmental origins of health and disease" hypothesis, the first 1000 days after conception appear to be a critical time window, since it is a time frame characterized by rapid growth, cellular replication and differentiation, and functional development of organ systems. Hence, exposures during early life to adverse environmental influences, such as an alteration in nutrients availability, permanently modify the body's structure, function, and metabolism, shaping the organism's phenotype and leading to lifelong effects on gene expression (Isganaitis, 2019; Vickers, 2014). Based on the current knowledge, epigenetics has been recognized as the molecular basis of developmental programming, since it provides an explanation for how environmental factors can modify the risk for the development of many common diseases, as reported by several epidemiological studies (Marousez et al., 2019). Remarkably, increasing evidence from experimental models has indicated that the epigenetic changes may be responsible also for transgenerational effects highlighting the need for implementing effective nutritional interventions simultaneously across life stages (Arlinghaus et al., 2018; Lacal and Ventura, 2018) (Fig. 4.1).

The strict relationship between maternal under and overnutrition and suboptimal outcomes in offspring is widely acknowledged, but underlying mechanisms have not been fully elucidated (Lecoutre et al., 2018). The epigenetic changes occurring during prenatal life and early infancy, in terms of interindividual variation in DNA methylation patterns and chromatin remodeling, are strong candidates for mediating the transmission of intergenerational signals. Specifically, three mechanisms have been identified as being involved in modulating epigenetic changes at the level of gene expression, in terms of either up- or down-regulation: gene DNA methylation/demethylation, histone modifications, and noncoding RNAs (Simeoni et al., 2014). Among the environmental factors that can regulate gene expression, nutrients have been reported to be particularly important as potential sources of the methyl groups that take part in the methylation processes and of many cofactors, such as folate, that allow the activation of the DNA-methyltransferases (Rando and Simmons, 2015).

Several epidemiological studies have reported an association among maternal undernutrition, low birth weight, and later increased risk of obesity, diabetes, and cardiovascular disease of the offspring (Ravelli et al., 1999). Consistent with these studies, experimental models have demonstrated how maternal dietary manipulation, such as a low protein isocaloric diet or

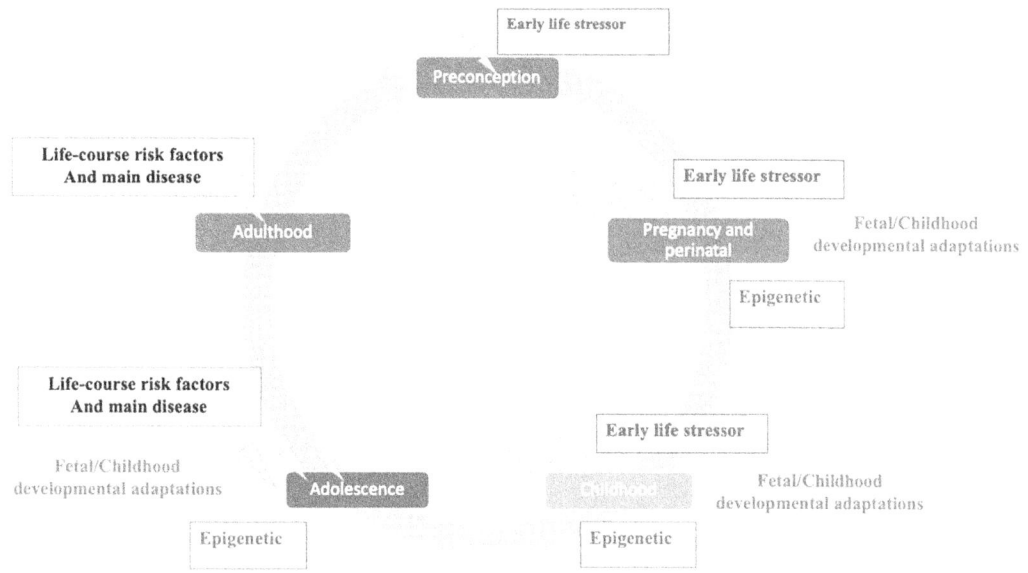

**FIG. 4.1**  Life-cycle model and main factors affecting health of both mother and offspring.

a decrease in the energy intake, negatively impact the hypothalamus-adipose axis development, which plays a key role in regulating energy homeostasis by modulating food intake and energy storage level (Breton, 2013). In addition, maternal undernutrition leads to an increase in size and number of fat cells in the offspring, accompanied by the loss of insulin sensitivity in adipocytes (Breton, 2013; Vickers et al., 2007). Protein restriction has also been associated with increased maternal, fetal, and placental oxidative stress markers (Castro-Rodríguez et al., 2020; Verduci et al., 2021) (Fig. 4.2).

Emerging evidence has indicated that alterations from "optimal" intrauterine growth, not only toward low birth weight but also toward high birth weight, increases the susceptibility to metabolic syndrome in the offspring. In experimental studies, maternal obesity induced by a high-fat diet has been associated with offspring obesity, diabetes, hypertension, fatty liver, behavioral changes, adverse cognitive outcomes, and increased anxiety levels (Castro-Rodríguez et al., 2020) (Fig. 4.2).

Not only excessive gestational weight gain has been associated with higher fat mass at birth and later in childhood but also maternal overweight (body mass index (BMI) 25 kg/m$^2$), which is considered a proxy of maternal nutritional status, has been recognized as an independent risk factor for fetal hyperinsulinemia, elevated birth weight, and body fat (Carlsen et al., 2014; Grieger and Clifton, 2015).

The mechanism underlying the link between maternal obesity and later metabolic disorders has not been clearly elucidated yet. Several studies have suggested that maternal obesity could cause chronic inflammation and oxidative stress. This can result in an impairment of placentation and probably affect fetal metabolism, with special regard to the mechanisms responsible for programming food preferences and/or intake and adipose tissue development. Furthermore, since maternal obesity may be associated with maternal diabetes, insulin

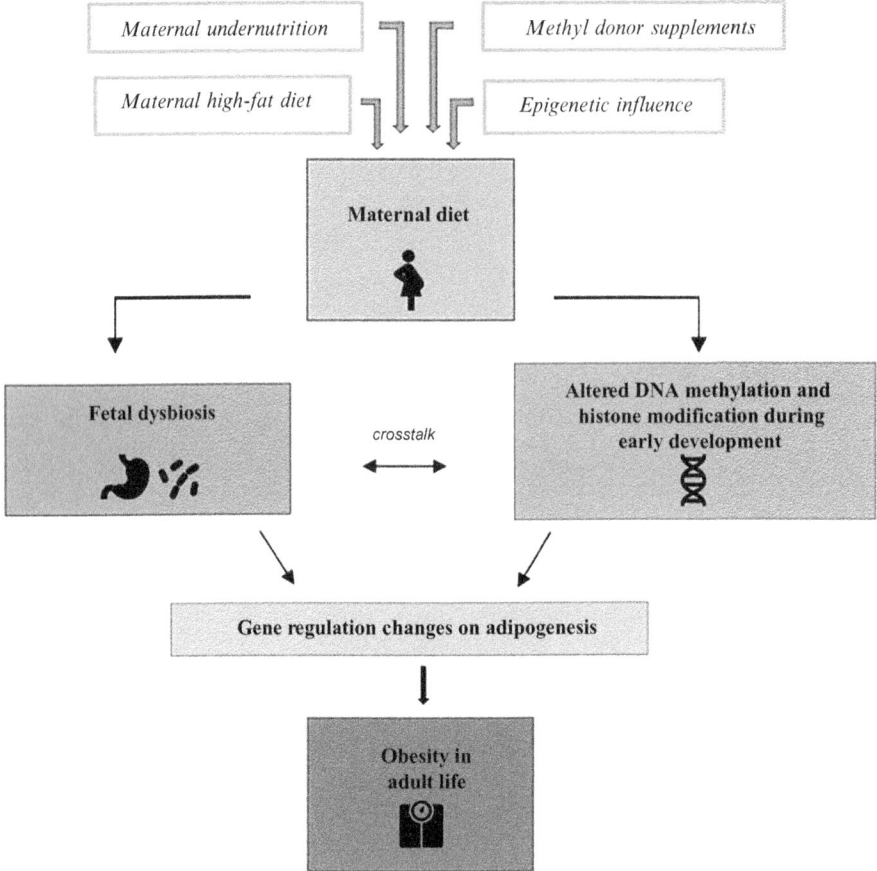

FIG. 4.2    Transmission of intergenerational signals: maternal diets and risk of obesity later in life.

resistance may contribute to the changes in fetal growth and body composition (Parisi et al., 2021; Symonds et al., 2013).

In the last few years, the importance of paternal obesity and undernutrition contribution in affecting offspring health through epigenetic modifications in sperm and alterations in seminal microbiota, fluid hormones, and metabolites has also become clear (Castro-Rodríguez et al., 2020; Hur et al., 2017; Sales et al., 2017).

Much attention has been focused on the gut microbiome disturbances, the so-called "dysbiosis," which has been associated with alteration in immune-mediated, metabolic, and neurodevelopmental disorders signaling pathways, leading to an increased susceptibility for adverse health outcomes (Fig. 4.2). In contrast to the traditional "sterile womb" concept, increasing evidence indicates that the intrauterine environment is already colonized before birth, as suggested by the microbiota detection in the placenta, amniotic fluid, umbilical cord blood, and meconium in healthy gestations (Li, 2018). The specific route of transmission has not been unraveled. However, an entero-mammary pathway has been hypothesized, in which maternal intestinal bacteria are transferred to the mammary gland through the bloodstream, as well as through a dynamic cycling of bacteria from the vagina and maternal skin to infant during delivery and lactation (D'argenio, 2018; Verduci et al., 2021).

During postnatal life, lactation has been increasingly recognized as crucial in continuing the developmental programming already initiated in utero. There is agreement on the long-term health benefits, both for the mother and the infant, associated with breastfeeding, including the reduction in the risk of developing obesity and diabetes (Haschke et al., 2019). However, consistently with what is known about pregnancy, maternal nutritional status appears to induce modifications to the macronutrients and bioactive components of human milk, potentially contributing to the alteration of the mother-infant signaling (Mosca and Gianní, 2017; Picó et al., 2020). Obese mothers could transmit an aberrant microbiome to their infant through lactation, even though the resulting potential metabolic effects have not been clearly elucidated (Verduci et al., 2021). Moreover, human milk of overweight and obese women is characterized by a high content of lactose and fat in colostrum (Leghi et al., 2020). Studies assessing the modifications of breast milk hormones according to maternal nutritional status did not provide consistent results on their role in modeling growth, fat mass deposition, and health outcomes later in life (Mazzocchi et al., 2019).

Within this context, the availability of the "omics" techniques, including proteomics and metabolomics, represents a useful additional tool to identify the potential biomarkers associated with later phenotypes and to monitor the efficacy of tailored preventive interventions (Bardanzellu et al., 2020; Sébédio, 2017).

## 4.3 Programming of growth and body composition of term newborn by early nutrition

In accordance with the World Health Organization, the American Academy of Pediatrics, and the European Society for Pediatric Gastroenterology, Hepatology and Nutrition, breastfeeding represents the normative and unequaled method of feeding infants (Agostoni et al., 2009; Dror and Allen, 2018; Eidelman and Schanler, 2012). Human milk meets the specific infants' nutritional needs, promotes optimal growth, and neurofunctional development, leading to several biological benefits, which are even more pronounced for preterm newborns. These benefits include a reduced risk of developing medical comorbidities during hospitalization (i.e., necrotizing enterocolitis, sepsis, retinopathy of prematurity and bronchopulmonary disease) and non-communicable diseases later in life, such as obesity, type 2 diabetes mellitus, and cardiovascular disease (Agostoni et al., 2013; Harding et al., 2017).

Early nutrition and adequate growth seem to be associated with better later health outcomes. Research has focused on understanding the growth pattern of healthy breastfed infants and gaining further insight into the nutritional and non-nutritional bioactive components of human milk, further exploring how breastmilk composition could be influenced by maternal diet and lifestyle (Verduci et al., 2021).

Moreover, increasing evidence indicates that growth and body composition development of breastfed infants significantly differ from those of formula-fed ones (Agostoni et al., 2009; Gale et al., 2012; Smith et al., 2019; Tahir et al., 2020). The impact of early feeding choices on body composition is even more important when considering later health outcomes, with special regard to the modulation of the risk of developing overweight and obesity (Larqué et al., 2019).

This section will review and discuss infants' growth and factors that could influence body composition during childhood, especially in terms of feeding mode. Some new insights into the nutritional and non-nutritional properties of human milk will also be described. The association between rapid weight gain during infancy and the metabolic syndrome risk will also be addressed.

## 4.4 Early nutrition: Effect on growth and body composition at birth and during weight loss

The first days of life represent a crucial period during which infants experience birth weight loss and a simultaneous change in body composition. Newborns have high energy requirements in order to adapt to extrauterine life, which requires the maintenance of his/her own thermoregulation, fluid balance, and breathing (Regnault et al., 2011). A recent meta-analysis confirmed that fat-free mass and fat mass decrease proportionally to early postnatal weight loss (Wiechers et al., 2019) (Fig. 4.3).

Although the normal physiological weight loss for full-term exclusively breastfed infants has not been defined yet, a weight loss greater than 7%–10% from birth weight is generally accepted as the threshold value indicating the need for intensive breastfeeding evaluation, support, and/or supplementation (Rautava, 2015). Generally, the vast majority of infants lose the most amount of weight within the first 4 days of life (Thulier, 2016). To differentiate a

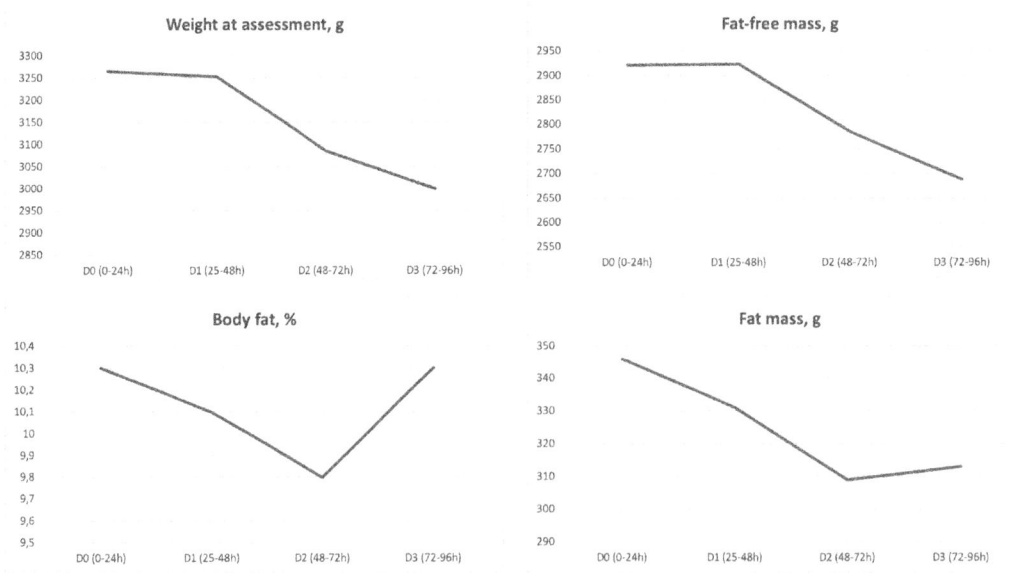

**FIG. 4.3** Body composition changes during postnatal weight loss. *From Wiechers, C., Kirchhof, S., Maas, C., Poets, C.F., Franz, A.R., 2019. Neonatal body composition by air displacement plethysmography in healthy term singletons: a systematic review. BMC Pediatr. 19, 489.*

physiological weight loss from a pathological one, that might signal breastfeeding failure, it is important to evaluate weight nadir and time to regain birth weight (Genna and Notarangelo, 2018). Moreover, excessive weight loss is one of the most important factors that could impair breastfeeding duration. Flaherman et al., in a retrospective cohort study, found that more formula use in the first 25 days after discharge was significantly associated with more weight loss at hospital discharge even if breastfeeding cessation through 1 month did not differ by weight loss trajectory (Flaherman et al., 2017).

There are many risk factors identified for excessive weight loss, among which are higher birth weight, gestational diabetes, and birth by cesarean section. Kelly et al., in a systematic review, suggested that babies born by cesarean section lose more weight in early life than infants born vaginally because of maternal postoperative pain or mobility impairment, maternal intravenous fluid therapy, and postponed time of feeding due to delayed lactogenesis or newborn admission to a neonatal intensive care unit (Eltonsy et al., 2017; Kelly et al., 2020).

Weight loss in the first 4 days of life is due to loss of fat mass and fat-free mass, including body fluids (Roggero et al., 2010). Mode of feeding has been reported to influence the degree of postnatal weight loss. Martens and Romphf found a 3% less weight loss in exclusive formula-fed newborns (2.43% ± 2.12%) in comparison with exclusively breastfed newborns (5.49% ± 2.60%) (Martens and Romphf, 2007). In contrast to these findings, Davanzo et al. reported that weight loss is lower in exclusively breastfed infants than in formula- fed ones (6.7% ± 2.2% vs 7.5% ± 2.4%, respectively) provided that breastfeeding initiation is adequately promoted and supported (Davanzo et al., 2013; Giugliani, 2019). According to these results, breastfeeding does not appear to be a risk factor for greater postnatal weight loss (Giugliani, 2019). On the contrary, the mean time required to regain birth weight appears to be longer in breastfed babies (8.3 days vs 6.5 days, respectively) (Macdonald et al., 2003).

Another determinant of excessive postnatal weight loss is represented by maternal obesity. Regnault et al. found that breastfed infants of obese mothers have a greater risk of excessive weight loss than formula-fed ones (Regnault et al., 2011). For this reason, additional breastfeeding support seems to be necessary for obese mothers to prevent early breastfeeding discontinuation (Regnault et al., 2011). In addition, the authors demonstrated that formula-fed newborns, born to overweight or obese mothers, lose less weight than formula-fed newborns born to underweight mothers (2.6% vs 4.1%, $P = .01$) (Regnault et al., 2011).

## 4.5 Body composition in relation to breastfeeding and formula feeding

The importance of breastfeeding from the very beginning is a cornerstone of scientific knowledge regarding growth and development of newborns. Recent studies have aimed to unravel the mechanisms underlining the beneficial effects associated with breastfeeding (Gianni et al., 2020). Increasing evidence indicates that the less rapid gain in weight for length and the lower absolute weights during the first year of life of breastfeeding infants as compared to formula feeding infants contribute to their reduced risk of developing overweight and obesity in childhood and later in adulthood (Appleton et al., 2018).

According to the most recent findings, not only growth trajectory but also body composition development appears to be implicated in the positive modulation of health outcomes of breastfed infants. A systematic review and meta-analysis of 26 studies (Gale et al., 2012) found a higher fat mass percent and total fat mass content in breastfeeding infants at 3–4 months and 6 months, but these findings were not confirmed at 12 months of life (Gale et al., 2012). The early increased adiposity shown by breastfed infants could be at least partially explained by varying levels of human milk hormones, proteins, and cytokines (Tahir et al., 2020), and may be responsible for a programming effect of early nutrition on intermediary metabolism or appetite regulation. In line with these findings, Tahir et al. demonstrated a lower fat-free mass content and a greater body fat percentage in breastfed infants at 6 months of life (Tahir et al., 2020). Breij et al. showed a positive association between exclusive human milk feeding and subcutaneous fat mass percentage (Breij et al., 2017). On the other hand, Smith et al. argued that the growth pattern in infancy and the subsequent risk of obesity could be related to prenatal exposure to different risk factors, including maternal BMI during pregnancy and maternal smoking. Smith et al. analyzed the body composition of 1583 term babies within the first 72 h after delivery and found that breastfed infants had lower fat mass percentage than exclusively formula-fed infants. Based on these results, the authors hypothesized that prenatal factors, irrespective of the mode of feeding, could influence body composition and later health outcomes (Smith et al., 2019).

## 4.6 Early rapid weight gain and other childhood obesity determinants in full-term infants

In accordance with the Barkers' hypothesis, early life conditions can strongly impact the future life of each individual with lasting consequences on human well-being (Barker, 2007). From this perspective, pregnancy and early life represent sensitive periods during which nutrition and metabolism of both the mother and the fetus/newborn could impact cytogenesis, organogenesis, and metabolic and endocrine responses, thus modulating offsprings' later health outcomes (Koletzko et al., 2019). In particular, maternal nutrition and lifestyle during pregnancy and infant's early nutrition and environment are considered relevant factors related to the development of an infant's adiposity.

The association between pre-pregnancy BMI and gestational weight gain and neonatal and infant adiposity has been well established (Larqué et al., 2019), and greater maternal obesity was associated with lower infant fat-free mass (Gridneva et al., 2018).

Gestational diabetes has been associated with higher neonatal birth weight and fat mass. Moreover, infants born to mothers with gestational diabetes may develop impaired growth and metabolic diseases (Brown et al., 2017). Even though limited evidence has been reported, paternal BMI could also be considered a predictor of infant adiposity, although less strongly than the maternal one (Sørensen et al., 2016).

There is growing interest in evaluating how body composition differs in infants born at the extremes of birth weight. Babies large for gestational age (LGA) generally present a higher birth weight and fat mass percentage and a slower postnatal weight gain when compared to infants born adequate for gestational age (AGA). On the contrary, infants born small for gestational age (SGA), even if they present a lower birth weight and fat mass percentage at birth, show a more rapid postnatal weight gain when compared to infants born AGA (Larqué et al., 2019; Larsson et al., 2019; Roggero et al., 2010). Early rapid postnatal weight and excessive fat mass gain have been associated with an increased risk of later obesity. Ejlerskov et al. conducted a prospective study including 233 children to assess the impact of weight gain through early childhood on body composition development (Ejlerskov et al., 2015). The authors observed that a rapid weight gain from birth to 5 months of age was associated with a high fat mass content at 3 years of age (Ejlerskov et al., 2015). In line with these findings, Chomtho et al. reported that the risk of developing later adiposity seems to be related to rapid weight gain occurring during the first 6 months of life (Chomtho et al., 2008). Moreover, experimental studies have demonstrated that postnatal catch-up growth causes subcutaneous fat remodeling and induces changes in the adipose tissue gene expression (Blüher et al., 2005). On the other hand, the persistence of poor postnatal growth is associated with a higher risk of developing infections, impaired cognitive development, and significant adult height deficit, which needs to be taken into consideration (Longo et al., 2013). Geserick et al. conducted a prospective and retrospective analysis of the course of BMI over time in a population of 51,505 children/adolescents. The authors pointed out that the rate of overweight/obesity in adolescence was higher among children who were born LGA (43.7%) and that the vast majority of obese/overweight adolescents showed the most rapid weight gain during pre-school age (Geserick et al., 2018).

Within this context, it is important to bear in mind that early life risk factors such as maternal obesity, early and rapid weight and fat mass gain, and/or early breastfeeding failure can coexist, generating a cumulative effect as observed by Robinson et al. (2015).

## 4.7 Role of nutrients intake and human milk bioactive compounds as related to infant growth: What's new

Research has focused on gaining further insight into the functions and characteristics of human milk oligosaccharides (HMOs) in light of their importance in the positive modulation of infant's health and development. Specifically, in the last few years, the association between HMOs and infant growth trajectories has been evaluated. Human milk HMOs composition differs from one woman to another and also during the course of lactation. This biodiversity appears to be responsible for driving the impact of HMOs on infant growth and body composition (Berger et al., 2020; Saben et al., 2021). Considering the critical role of HMOs in shaping the infant microbiome, a mediatory role for the infant gut microbiome has been suggested to explain the potential mechanisms underlying infant growth promotion by HMOs (Saben et al., 2021). Alderete et al. analyzed the human milk HMOs composition of 25 breastfeeding mothers and pointed out that higher HMOs diversity at 1 month after delivery was associated with lower total and percentual infant fat mass (Alderete et al., 2015). Lagström et al. reported an inverse association between HMO diversity and lacto-N-neotetraose content with child height and weight z scores during the first 5 years of life, whereas 2′-fucosyllactose concentration was directly associated with child growth (Lagström et al., 2020). Remarkably, greater exposure to 2′-fucosyllactose concentration during the first month of lactation has been related to better infant cognitive development at 24 months of life (Berger et al., 2020).

Recent evidence indicates that maternal pre-pregnancy BMI may affect HMOs composition, further underlining the importance of implementing early nutritional interventions across life stages (Berger et al., 2020; Saben et al., 2020).

The role of polyunsaturated fatty acids (PUFA) in preventing obesity later in life has also been evaluated. Although much progress has been made in this field, the studies obtained so far are still preliminary and require confirmation (Vahdaninia et al., 2019). In light of the association between pre-pregnancy obesity, low n-3 relative to n-6 PUFA status, and altered fetal growth and higher risk of later infant obesity, Monthé-Drèze et al. conducted a pilot double-blind, randomized controlled trial to evaluate the impact of n-3-PUFA supplementation in pregnant obese mothers on fetal growth and body composition development. The authors found that n-3 PUFA supplementation was associated with improved fetal growth, higher birth weight accompanied by a higher fat-free mass deposition, and longer gestation (Monthé-Drèze et al., 2021). These findings need confirmation by larger studies; however, they indicate a potential causal link between maternal obesity and offspring adverse metabolic outcomes, which may have important implications in identifying effective nutritional preventive strategies. The quantity and quality of human milk compounds, especially the protein and amino acids content and composition, also appear to be one of the major determinants of the difference in the rate and quality of growth between breastfed and formula-fed infants (Koletzko et al., 2019). Koletzko et al. conducted a large, multicenter, double-blind, randomized trial including 1138 formula-fed infants, randomized to receive either a low protein or a high protein formula up through the first year of life. The authors demonstrated that the infants fed the high protein formula showed higher weight-for-length z-scores at 6, 12, and 24 months and higher obesity risk at school age. Remarkably, these results indicate the persistent effect of the early protein intake beyond the duration of the intervention (Koletzko et al., 2019). On the contrary, no association between a relatively high-fat diet in infancy and later indices of adiposity has been reported, whereas fat restriction in early life appears to increase the susceptibility to adverse metabolic outcomes in adulthood (Rolland-Cachera et al., 2017).

## 4.8 Influence of early nutrition on preterm infants' growth and body composition. Preterm infants: Time to refine the target?

Preterm infants undergo an impaired development of structure and functions of key organs and systems due to the interruption of the physiological intrauterine organogenesis and exposure to the extrauterine environment at a time when organ plasticity is exceptionally high (Halfon et al., 2017; Msall et al., 2017). As a result, preterm infants are at increased risk of adverse health outcomes, including the development of metabolic syndrome and cognitive impairment, further exacerbated by the occurrence of medical comorbidities (Verduci et al., 2020).

Preterm infants are characterized by high nutritional requirements due to the lower level of nutrients in the body stores at birth, the immaturity of the body systems, the need for rapid postnatal growth, and the occurrence of acute illnesses. Adequate and timely preterm infants' nutritional support has been advocated to avoid malnutrition and limit the occurrence of postnatal growth retardation, thus preventing the need for rapid catch-up growth, which is associated with late adverse metabolic outcomes (Crippa et al., 2020).

It has long been recommended that preterm infants should have a growth pattern, both in terms of growth rates and quality of growth, equal to that of the fetus (Committee on Nutrition, 1985). However, the vast majority of preterm infants are unable to mimic fetal growth (Parlapani et al., 2018) due to their peculiar nutritional and metabolic characteristics and the occurrence of medical comorbidities. The adequacy of fetal growth as a reference for preterm infants' postnatal growth has thus been questioned (Gianni et al., 2016; Villar et al., 2018).

Increasing evidence indicates that the INTERGROWTH-21st Preterm Postnatal Growth Standards, based on the growth of healthy preterm infants who received nutritional care following current guidelines, represent a useful tool in monitoring postnatal preterm infants' growth from 27 weeks to the 64th week of postmenstrual age (Villar et al., 2018). Several studies assessing preterm infant growth during hospital stay have reported a significant reduction of extrauterine growth retardation at discharge when the INTERGROWTH-21st Preterm Postnatal Growth Standards have been implemented (Andrews et al., 2019).

The definition of extrauterine growth retardation is also still under discussion. For many years, many studies have applied the so-called cross-sectional definition (weight below the 10th or 3rd centile or another cut-off at a given time, regardless of birth weight). It has been recently suggested the use of a longitudinal definition, which refers to a weight loss of more than 1 (or 2) standard deviations between birth and a given time (Fenton et al., 2017; Peila et al., 2020) could better relate to long-term auxological and health outcomes. The use of a consensus definition of extrauterine growth retardation could greatly contribute to evaluating the effects of the different nutritional strategies implemented both during hospital stay and after discharge on the long-term outcomes of such vulnerable infants. It could also be useful for clinicians to tailor the nutritional interventions taking into account the balance between growth and the risk of excessive catch-up growth (Fenton et al., 2017; Peila et al., 2020).

A growing number of studies indicate that extrauterine growth retardation of preterm infants is associated with an alteration of body composition when reaching term-corrected age (Gianni et al., 2016). Specifically, it has been reported that, although showing a significantly higher percentage of fat mass (+ 3.06%; 95% CI 0.25–5.88, $P = .03$), probably due to the lower weight (− 590 g; 95% CI 440–750 g, $P < .0001$), they have a moderate lack of absolute fat mass (− 50 g; 95% CI 10–90 g, $P = .02$) and a major lack of fat-free mass (460 g; 95% CI 270–340 g, $P < .001$), in comparison to full-term newborns (Johnson et al., 2012). Fat-free mass gain between birth and hospital discharge has been strongly associated with positive neurodevelopmental outcomes in preterm infants at 12 and 24 months of corrected age. Furthermore, fat-free mass represents a key marker for organ growth and nutritional status (Ramel et al., 2020). The latter findings are even more important when considering the contribution of body composition development to long-term nutritional programming (Parlapani et al., 2018; Wells et al., 2007).

With regard to fat mass distribution, preterm infants at term corrected age have been reported to have increased intra-abdominal adiposity, which positively correlates with the severity of disease experienced during hospital stay (Uthaya et al., 2005). In addition, the intrahepatocellular lipid content, a known risk factor for later cardiovascular disease, appears to be increased in healthy preterm infants at term corrected age and to positively correlate with the early fat intake (Thomas et al., 2008; Vasu et al., 2013). However, Roggero et al. (2015) found that without severe illness during hospital stay, prematurity itself was not associated with an excess of intraabdominal adipose tissue. Moreover, the main difference in fat mass between growth-restricted and AGA newborns is in subcutaneous rather than in intra-abdominal fat (Villar et al., 2017).

This section will address the main nutritional determinants of preterm infants' growth and body composition at hospital discharge and/or at term-corrected age. Growth trajectories and changes in body composition after discharge will also be described. Finally, the available evidence as related to early nutritional programming and later health outcomes will be reviewed.

## 4.9  Early nutritional determinants of growth and body composition of preterm infants

The nutritional care of preterm newborns remains a challenge in clinical practice (Villar et al., 2018). Very low birth weight infants (birth weight ≤ 1500 g) have been reported to develop a major cumulative energy and protein deficit within the fifth postnatal week (Embleton et al., 2001). However, improvements in parenteral and enteral feeding policies have been reported to reduce cumulative nutritional deficits and extrauterine growth retardation during hospital (Loÿs et al., 2013; Roggero et al., 2012).

A decreased weight velocity appears to be associated with a preferential fat mass deposition, as indicated by the finding of a higher fat mass content at term-corrected age in preterm infants with a growth velocity equal or more than 15 g/kg/day during the transition from parenteral to enteral nutrition as compared to those having a growth velocity lower than 15 g/kg/day (Liotto et al., 2020).

These findings support the concept that early fat mass accumulation probably reflects not only the need for adapting to extrauterine life but also a strategy for being protected against potential future decreased nutritional intakes (Lingwood et al., 2020). In line with these results, Lingwood et al. reported that in 50 preterm infants, higher intakes of protein, energy, and carbohydrate were significantly associated with an increase of fat-free mass deposition at 34–37 weeks of postmenstrual age (Lingwood et al., 2020). Ramel et al. found that increased energy and protein administered to 103 very low birth weight infants in the first week after birth and protein intake through the whole neonatal intensive care stay were associated with an increased fat-free mass content at hospital discharge, also after adjustment for early acute and chronic illness (Ramel et al., 2020).

Protein intake is crucial in promoting preterm infants' growth (Gianni et al., 2019; Morlacchi et al., 2018). Power et al. have conducted a prospective cohort study, involving 149 infants born at < 30 weeks of gestation, and pointed out that a higher protein intake (1 g/kg/day higher mean protein intake) in the first month of life was associated with better growth rate during hospital stay (Power et al., 2019). Accordingly, several studies have indicated that each gram per kilogram of protein is associated with weight gain ranging between 3.44 and 4.3 g/kg/day (Ziegler, 2011).

Protein intake cannot be considered irrespective of energy intake. The provision of an adequate energy intake allows for fat-free mass accretion, whereas proteins are oxidized when a lack of energy occurs. On the other hand, once protein intake is sufficient for fat-free mass deposition, additional energy leads to the deposition of fat mass (Dinerstein et al., 2006). Within this context, it is important to consider that preterm infants have higher energy requirements than term ones (Lapillonne et al., 2019) since fat mass deposition increases from 12% at 28 weeks of gestational age to 20% at term. Moreover, the occurrence of medical co-morbidities further increases preterm infants' metabolic requirements (Moltu et al., 2021).

Klevebro et al. reported that every additional 10 kcal/kg/day of energy during the first 6 postnatal days and between days 7 and 27 was associated with higher weight gain on day 7 and a reduced risk of bronchopulmonary dysplasia and any grade of retinopathy of prematurity, respectively (Klevebro et al., 2019).

Human milk feeding, which is strongly recommended as the first choice for enteral feeding in preterm infants, has been reported to be associated with slower weight gain from birth either to discharge or term-corrected age as compared to formula feeding. The improved cognitive outcome of human milk-fed preterm infants, despite the suboptimal weight gain, has been referred to as the "apparent breastfeeding paradox" (Rozé et al., 2012). Increasing evidence indicates that human milk feeding promotes fat-free mass deposition in a dose-dependent manner, thus contributing to the positive recovery of body composition development in preterm infants, which in turn, is associated with better neurodevelopmental outcomes (Ramel et al., 2020). Consistent with these results, Morlacchi et al. reported that preterm infants fed with fortified own mother's milk showed an increased fat-free mass deposition at term-corrected age compared with preterm infants fed with formula (Morlacchi et al., 2016). These findings underline that own mother's milk protein can be utilized for anabolic purposes provided adequate energy is administered.

## 4.10 Growth and body composition of preterm infants' after discharge

Most preterm infants show catch-up growth, defined as reaching a standard deviation score higher than − 2 of the reference population within the first 2 years of life. Specific subgroups of infants born preterm, however, appear to achieve catch-up growth later. Ferguson et al. reported that catch-up growth for length in preterm infants born AGA can occur up to the 18th year of age (Ferguson et al., 2017), whereas Toftlund et al. found out that infants fed unfortified human milk showed a slower catch-up growth as compared to formula-fed infants but extended until 6 years old (Toftlund et al., 2018). Within this context, it is important to bear in mind that the most immature infants, those born with the lowest birth weights and/or SGA and those that have developed comorbidities, are at high risk for persistent growth failure (Da Silva Boguszewski and De Andre Cardoso-Demartini, 2017; Euser et al., 2008).

Regarding body composition development, fat-free mass deficit tends to track after discharge, although studies have reported inconsistent results in relation to the timing of its recovery.

Griffin and Cooke (Griffin and Cooke, 2012) have compared the dynamic changes in body fat over the first year of life between infants born preterm and infants born at term and reported that preterm infants persistently showed a significantly lower percentage of fat mass than term infants at 3 months, at 6 months, and at 12 months (Fig. 4.4).

We have conducted a longitudinal study evaluating body composition in 63 very low birth weight preterm infants at 5 years of age (Giannì et al., 2015). Preterm infants were lighter and shorter than full-term children and exhibited a relative lack of fat-free mass, even after controlling for length, whereas fat mass percentage and content were similar among groups.

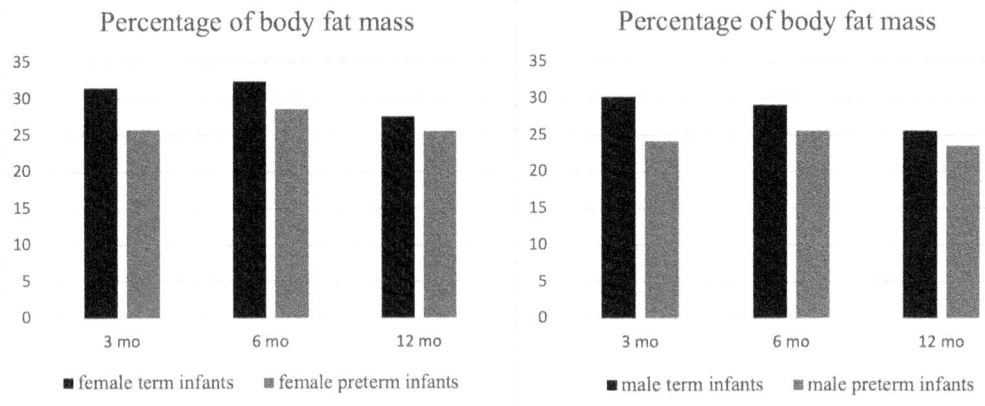

**FIG. 4.4** Changes in body fat over the first year of life between infants born preterm and infants born at term. *From Griffin, I.J., Cooke, R.J., 2012. Development of whole body adiposity in preterm infants. Early Hum. Dev. 88 (Suppl. 1), S19–S24.*

When considering body composition according to gender, preterm boys, but not preterm girls, had a significantly lower fat-free mass index than their peers 22 (12.1±1.1 kg/m vs 13.0±1.0 kg/m, $P < .005$). Consistent with these findings, Fewtrell et al. (Fewtrell et al., 2004) reported a significantly lower fat mass in children born preterm compared with children born at term assessed at ages 8–12 years.

Hamatschek et al. calculated age-specific percentiles, including 110 studies using air displacement plethysmography (2855 preterm and 22,410 term infants), and 28 studies using dual-energy X-ray absorptiometry (1147 preterm and 3542 term infants). The authors confirmed the higher percentage of fat mass in preterm infants assessed at term-corrected age when compared to term infants at birth (16% vs 11%, $P < .001$), whereas at 52 weeks of postmenstrual age, the percentage of fat mass was similar between the two groups, with preterm infants showing 24% and term infants showing 25%. These findings further strengthen the concept that early postnatal life of preterm infants is characterized by a very rapid fat mass accretion, and underlines the importance of measuring body composition also and not only weight gain in order to finely tune the nutritional intervention in preterm infants (Cordova and Belfort, 2020). Contrary to previously published studies, however, the authors found that preterm infants show a catch-up of fat-free mass during the first 6 months. As a result, at 60 weeks of postmenstrual age, fat-free mass content is similar between preterm and term infants (5000 g vs 5100 g, respectively) (Hamatschek et al., 2020).

Since a rapid postnatal gain may be associated with a worse metabolic outcome, the opportunity of providing increased protein and energy, particularly to preterm infants who have developed extrauterine growth retardation, has been questioned (Nuyt et al., 2017; Riskin et al., 2018).

However, evidence is increasing on the usefulness of nutrient enrichment in the post-discharge period. Data actually indicate that, when energy requirements are met, an increased protein intake contributes to the achievement of higher weight paralleled by a preferential deposition of fat-free mass and greater head circumference values (Teller et al., 2016).

Studies assessing the effect of human milk fortification after discharge have reported inconsistent results. Young et al. reported similar growth rates during infancy and neurodevelopmental outcomes at 18 months corrected age in infants fed fortified human milk as compared to infants fed unfortified human milk (Young et al., 2013). However, several authors have reported some benefits with the use of human milk fortification after discharge (Arslanoglu et al., 2019), including better lung function at 6 years (Toftlund et al., 2019), better growth in babies with a birth weight < 1250 g up to 1 year of life (O'Connor et al., 2008), and better visual function (O'Connor et al., 2012). Remarkably, catch-up growth of preterm infants, either born SGA or AGA, appears not to be associated with an increased deposition of fat mass (Cerasani et al., 2020) when they are exclusively human milk fed.

## 4.11  Healthy catch-up growth: The narrow pathway

To which extent the recovery from postnatal growth retardation and the changes in body composition development may affect short- and long-term health outcomes has yet to be fully elucidated. Studies that evaluated the effect of early versus late and rapid versus slow catch-up growth on later health have not provided consistent results, probably due to the lack of established criteria and definitions.

Preterm birth leads to an interruption of organogenesis of multiple organ systems, which takes place during a critical time window in terms of developmental programming (Nuyt et al., 2017; Riskin, 2017; Roggero et al., 2013) (Fig. 4.5).

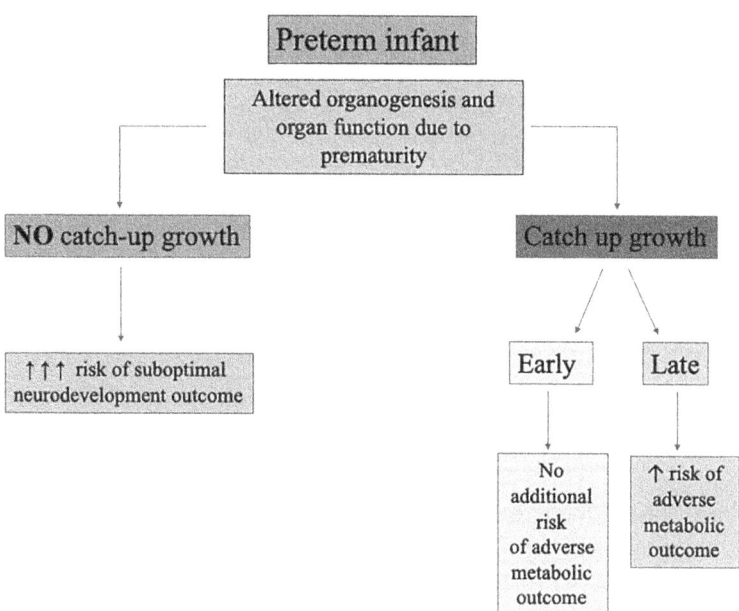

FIG. 4.5   Catch-up growth, a narrow pathway.

Preterm survivors have been reported to be at increased risk for later chronic illnesses, including respiratory, cardiovascular, and neurodevelopment impairment (Crump et al., 2011; D'Onofrio et al., 2013). Yet, the molecular mechanisms underlying the association between prematurity and the increased risk on these complex traits have not been completely clarified. It has been hypothesized that the sudden removal from the intrauterine environment due to premature birth causes stress on infants and leads to modifications in gene expression in the short and long term (Cruickshank et al., 2013). On the other side, it has to be taken into account that many studies have pointed out the importance of early nutritional intervention in order to achieve adequate growth and subsequent neurodevelopment and cognitive outcomes later in life (Schneider and Garcia-Rodenas, 2017). However, concerns regarding the opportunity to promote catch-up growth have arisen, since its achievement may imply a long-term metabolic cost regarding the development of adult morbidities (Crippa et al., 2020).

There is a paucity of studies addressing the potential association of preterm birth independently from the effect of intrauterine growth retardation on later risk of cardiovascular morbidities. Hence, it has not been fully elucidated whether the metabolic consequences of low birth weight due to preterm birth itself may be similar to those associated with low birth weight due to intrauterine growth retardation. However, based on the available evidence, it appears that growth between birth and 12–18 months of corrected age has no negative effect on the risk of developing the metabolic syndrome. In contrast, the occurrence of extrauterine growth retardation is associated with neurodevelopment impairment. On the contrary, growth during late infancy and childhood appears to significantly contribute to adverse later metabolic and cardiovascular outcomes (Lapillonne and Griffin, 2013). Beunders et al. have evaluated the association between postnatal weight gain trajectories and later body composition in 120 infants born very preterm. The authors reported that weight gain during hospital stay was not significantly associated with fat mass content in infancy. In contrast, weight gain following hospital discharge was strongly associated with body composition parameters, both at 2 and 6 months of corrected age, particularly fat mass (Beunders et al., 2020).

Taken all together, these findings underline the importance of the timing of catch-up growth occurrence and suggest that the prevention, when possible, or the limitation of the extrauterine growth retardation is crucial in the positive modulation of the long-term metabolic risk. Clinicians should focus on the identification of a desirable growth target to achieve during hospital stay, according to each infant's birth weight, gestational age, and the development of medical comorbidities, if any, in order to provide the best individualized nutritional approach. Following hospital discharge, the definition of the entity and velocity of catch-up growth and balancing neurodevelopmental and metabolic aspects are crucial in the optimization of long-term health outcomes (Crippa et al., 2020).

## 4.12 Conclusions

A growing body of evidence indicates that early life represents a critical time window in terms of developmental programming. A strict interrelationship between early growth pattern, body composition development, and subsequent health has been reported, implying nutrition as a critical underlying mechanism. Monitoring growth and body composition trajectories may therefore represent a useful tool in identifying infants at highest risk for developing the metabolic syndrome later in life and in monitoring the efficacy of nutritional intervention strategies.

## 4.13 Future trends and research

Future focused research is needed in order to fully understand the specific mechanisms underlying the association between early nutritional determinants of growth and body composition development, and the increased risk of developing later adverse health outcomes. A deeper knowledge of human milk components and the synergistic mechanisms responsible for the beneficial health effects associated with breastfeeding will help gain further insight into the effect of early nutritional interventions on the long-term outcomes, including most of the main areas of adult morbidity. Closing this knowledge gap holds a huge potential for promoting well-being of future generations and will allow clinicians to target specific interventions on the highest risk groups.

## Sources of additional information

**(1)** https://www.aap.org/
**(2)** https://www.espghan.org/guidelines/nutrition/
**(3)** https://www.healthychildren.org/
**(4)** https://www.nutrition.org.uk/
**(5)** https://www.nutritionsociety.org/
**(6)** http://www.nutrition.org/
**(7)** http://www.acog.org/
**(8)** http://www.metabolic-programming.org/
**(9)** https://intergrowth21.tghn.org/

## References

Agostoni, C., Braegger, C., Decsi, T., Kolacek, S., Koletzko, B., Michaelsen, K.F., Mihatsch, W., Moreno, L.A., Puntis, J., Shamir, R., Szajewska, H., Turck, D., Van Goudoever, J., 2009. Breast-feeding: a commentary by the espghan committee on nutrition. J. Pediatr. Gastroenterol. Nutr. 49 (1), 112–125.

Agostoni, C., Baselli, L., Mazzoni, M.B., 2013. Early nutrition patterns and diseases of adulthood: a plausible link? Eur. J. Intern. Med. 24 (1), 5–10.

Alderete, T.L., Autran, C., Brekke, B.E., Knight, R., Bode, L., Goran, M.I., Fields, D.A., 2015. Associations between human milk oligosaccharides and infant body composition in the first 6 mo of life. Am. J. Clin. Nutr. 102, 1381–1388.

Andrews, E.T., Ashton, J.J., Pearson, F., Beattie, R.M., Johnson, M.J., 2019. Early postnatal growth failure in preterm infants is not inevitable. Arch. Dis. Child. Fetal Neonatal Ed. 104 (3), F235–F241.

Appleton, J., Russell, C.G., Laws, R., Fowler, C., Campbell, K., Denney-Wilson, E., 2018. Infant formula feeding practices associated with rapid weight gain: a systematic review. Matern. Child Nutr. 14 (3), e12602.

Arlinghaus, K.R., Truong, C., Johnston, C.A., Hernandez, D.C., 2018. An intergenerational approach to break the cycle of malnutrition. Curr. Nutr. Rep. 7 (4), 259–267.

Arslanoglu, S., Boquien, C.Y., King, C., Lamireau, D., Tonetto, P., Barnett, D., Bertino, E., Gaya, A., Gebauer, C., Grovslien, A., Moro, G.E., Weaver, G., Wesolowska, A.M., Picaud, J.C., 2019. Fortification of human milk for preterm infants: update and recommendations of the European milk bank association (EMBA) working group on human milk fortification. Front. Pediatr. 7 (4), 259–267.

Bardanzellu, F., Puddu, M., Peroni, D.G., Fanos, V., 2020. The human breast milk metabolome in overweight and obese mothers. Front. Immunol. 11, 1533.

Barker, D., 2007. The developmental origins of chronic adult disease. Acta Paediatr. 93, 26–33.

Berger, P.K., Plows, J.F., Jones, R.B., Alderete, T.L., Yonemitsu, C., Poulsen, M., Ryoo, J.H., Peterson, B.S., Bode, L., Goran, M.I., 2020. Human milk oligosaccharide 2'-fucosyllactose links feedings at 1 month to cognitive development at 24 months in infants of normal and overweight mothers. PLoS One 15 (2), e0228323.

Beunders, V.A.A., Roelants, J.A., Hulst, J.M., Rizopoulos, D., Hokken-Koelega, A.C.S., Neelis, E.G., de Fluiter, K.S., Jaddoe, V.W.V., Reiss, I.K.M., Joosten, K.F.M., Vermeulen, M.J., 2020. Early weight gain trajectories and body composition in infancy in infants born very preterm. Pediatr. Obes. 16 (6), e12752.

Blüher, S., Kratzsch, J., Kiess, W., 2005. Insulin-like growth factor I, growth hormone and insulin in white adipose tissue. Best Pract. Res. Clin. Endocrinol. Metab. 19 (4), 577–587.

Breij, L.M., Kerkhof, G.F., De Lucia Rolfe, E., Ong, K.K., Abrahamse-Berkeveld, M., Acton, D., Hokken-Koelega, A.C.S., 2017. Longitudinal fat mass and visceral fat during the first 6 months after birth in healthy infants: support for a critical window for adiposity in early life. Pediatr. Obes. 12, 286–294.

Breton, C., 2013. The hypothalamus-adipose axis is a key target of developmental programming by maternal nutritional manipulation. J. Endocrinol. 216 (2), R19–R31.

Brown, J., Alwan, N.A., West, J., Brown, S., Mckinlay, C.J.D., Farrar, D., Crowther, C.A., 2017. Lifestyle interventions for the treatment of women with gestational diabetes. Cochrane Database Syst. Rev. 5 (5), CD011970.

Carlsen, E.M., Renault, K.M., Nørgaard, K., Nilas, L., Jensen, J.E.B., Hyldstrup, L., Michaelsen, K.F., Cortes, D., Pryds, O., 2014. Newborn regional body composition is influenced by maternal obesity, gestational weight gain and the birthweight standard score. Acta Paediatr. 103, 939–945.

Castro-Rodríguez, D.C., Rodríguez-González, G.L., Menjivar, M., Zambrano, E., 2020. Maternal interventions to prevent adverse fetal programming outcomes due to maternal malnutrition: evidence in animal models. Placenta 102, 49–54.

Cerasani, J., Ceroni, F., De Cosmi, V., Mazzocchi, A., Morniroli, D., Roggero, P., Mosca, F., Agostoni, C., Giannì, M.L., 2020. Human milk feeding and preterm infants' growth and body composition: a literature review. Nutrients 12 (4), 1155.

Chomtho, S., Wells, J.C.K., Williams, J.E., Davies, P.S.W., Lucas, A., Fewtrell, M.S., 2008. Infant growth and later body composition: evidence from the 4-component model. Am. J. Clin. Nutr. 87, 1776–1784.

Clark, H., Coll-Seck, A.M., Banerjee, A., Peterson, S., Dalglish, S.L., Ameratunga, S., Balabanova, D., Bhan, M.K., Bhutta, Z.A., Borrazzo, J., Claeson, M., Doherty, T., El-Jardali, F., George, A.S., Gichaga, A., Gram, L., Hipgrave, D.B., Kwamie, A., Meng, Q., Mercer, R., Narain, S., Nsungwa-Sabiiti, J., Olumide, A.O., Osrin, D., Powell-Jackson, T., Rasanathan, K., Rasul, I., Reid, P., Requejo, J., Rohde, S.S., Rollins, N., Romedenne, M., Singh Sachdev, H., Saleh, R., Shawar, Y.R., Shiffman, J., Simon, J., Sly, P.D., Stenberg, K., Tomlinson, M., Ved, R.R., Costello, A., 2020. A future for the world's children? A WHO–UNICEF–Lancet Commission. Lancet 395 (10224), 605–665.

Committee on Nutrition, 1985. Nutritional needs of low-birth-weight infants. Pediatrics 75, 976–986.

Cordova, E.G., Belfort, M.B., 2020. Updates on assessment and monitoring of the postnatal growth of preterm infants. NeoReviews 21, e98–e108.

Crippa, B.L., Morniroli, D., Baldassarre, M.E., Consales, A., Vizzari, G., Colombo, L., Mosca, F., Giannì, M.L., 2020. Preterm's nutrition from hospital to solid foods: are we still navigating by sight? Nutrients 12 (12), 3646.

Cruickshank, M.N., Oshlack, A., Theda, C., Davis, P.G., Martino, D., Sheehan, P., Dai, Y., Saffery, R., Doyle, L.W., Craig, J.M., 2013. Analysis of epigenetic changes in survivors of preterm birth reveals the effect of gestational age and evidence for a long term legacy. Genome Med. 5 (10), 96. 5. 2013 Oct 18.

Crump, C., Sundquist, K., Sundquist, J., Winkleby, M.A., 2011. Gestational age at birth and mortality in young adulthood. JAMA - J. Am. Med. Assoc. 306, 1233–1240.

D'argenio, V., 2018. The prenatal microbiome: a new player for human health. High-Throughput 7 (4), 38.

D'Onofrio, B.M., Class, Q.A., Rickert, M.E., Larsson, H., Långström, N., Lichtenstein, P., 2013. Preterm birth and mortality and morbidity: a population-based quasi-experimental study. JAMA Psychiat. 70, 1231–1240.

Da Silva Boguszewski, M.C., De Andre Cardoso-Demartini, A., 2017. Growth and growth hormone therapy in short children born preterm. Eur. J. Endocrinol. 176 (3), EJE-16-0482.

Davanzo, R., Cannioto, Z., Ronfani, L., Monasta, L., Demarini, S., 2013. Breastfeeding and neonatal weight loss in healthy term infants. J. Hum. Lact. 29, 45–53.

Dinerstein, A., Nieto, R.M., Solana, C.L., Perez, G.P., Otheguy, L.E., Larguia, A.M., 2006. Early and aggressive nutritional strategy (parenteral and enteral) decreases postnatal growth failure in very low birth weight infants. J. Perinatol. 26, 436–442.

Dror, D.K., Allen, L.H., 2018. Overview of nutrients in humanmilk. Adv. Nutr. 9, 278S–294S.

Eidelman, A.I., Schanler, R.J., 2012. Breastfeeding and the use of human milk. Pediatrics 129, e827–e841.

Ejlerskov, K.T., Christensen, L.B., Ritz, C., Jensen, S.M., Molgaard, C., Michaelsen, K.F., 2015. The impact of early growth patterns and infant feeding on body composition at 3 years of age. Br. J. Nutr. 114, 316–327.

Eltonsy, S., Blinn, A., Sonier, B., DeRoche, S., Mulaja, A., Hynes, W., Barrieau, A., Belanger, M., 2017. Intrapartum intravenous fluids for caesarean delivery and newborn weight loss: a retrospective cohort study. BMJ Paediatr. 1 (1), e000070.

Embleton, N.E., Pang, N., Cooke, R.J., 2001. Postnatal malnutrition and growth retardation: an inevitable consequence of current recommendations in preterm infants? Pediatrics 107, 270–273.

Euser, A.M., De Wit, C.C., Finken, M.J.J., Rijken, M., Wit, J.M., 2008. Growth of preterm born children. Horm. Res. 70 (6), 319–328.

Fall, C.H.D., Kumaran, K., 2019. Metabolic programming in early life in humans. Philos. Trans. R. Soc. Lond. B Biol. Sci. 374 (1770), 20180123.

Fenton, T.R., Chan, H.T., Madhu, A., Griffin, I.J., Hoyos, A., Ziegler, E.E., Groh-Wargo, S., Carlson, S.J., Senterre, T., Anderson, D., Ehrenkranz, R.A., 2017. Preterm infant growth velocity calculations: a systematic review. Pediatrics 139 (3), e20162045.

Ferguson, E.C., Wright, N.P., Gibson, A.T., Carney, S., Wright, A., Wales, J.K., 2017. Adult height of preterm infants: a longitudinal cohort study. Arch. Dis. Child. 102, 503–508.

Fewtrell, M.S., Lucas, A., Cole, T.J., Wells, J.C.K., 2004. Prematurity and reduced body fatness at 8-12 y of age. Am. J. Clin. Nutr. 80, 436–440.

Flaherman, V.J., Schaefer, E.W., Kuzniewicz, M.K., Li, S., Walsh, E., Paul, I.M., 2017. Newborn weight loss during birth hospitalization and breastfeeding outcomes through age 1 month. J. Hum. Lact. 33, 225–230.

Gale, C., Logan, K.M., Santhakumaran, S., Parkinson, J.R.C., Hyde, M.J., Modi, N., 2012. Effect of breastfeeding compared with formula feeding on infant body composition: a systematic review and meta-analysis. Am. J. Clin. Nutr. 95, 656–669.

Genna, C.W., Notarangelo, M., 2018. Differentiating normal newborn weight loss from breastfeeding failure. Clin. Lact. 9, 183–192.

Geserick, M., Vogel, M., Gausche, R., Lipek, T., Spielau, U., Keller, E., Pfäffle, R., Kiess, W., Körner, A., 2018. Acceleration of BMI in early childhood and risk of sustained obesity. N. Engl. J. Med. 379, 1303–1312.

Giannì, M.L., Roggero, P., Piemontese, P., Morlacchi, L., Bracco, B., Taroni, F., Garavaglia, E., Mosca, F., 2015. Boys who are born preterm show a relative lack of fat-free mass at 5 years of age compared to their peers. Acta Paediatr. 104, e119–e123.

Gianni, M.L., Roggero, P., Liotto, N., Taroni, F., Polimeni, A., Morlacchi, L., Piemontese, P., Consonni, D., Mosca, F., 2016. Body composition in late preterm infants according to percentile at birth. Pediatr. Res. 79, 710–715.

Gianni, M.L., Roggero, P., Mosca, F., 2019. Human milk protein vs. formula protein and their use in preterm infants. Curr. Opin. Clin. Nutr. Metab. Care 22 (1), 76–81.

Gianni, M.L., Morniroli, D., Bettinelli, M.E., Mosca, F., 2020. Human milk and lactation. Nutrients 12, 899.

Giugliani, E.R.J., 2019. Growth in exclusively breastfed infants. J. Pediatr. 95 (Suppl 1), 79–84.

Goyal, D., Limesand, S.W., Goyal, R., 2019. Epigenetic responses and the developmental origins of health and disease. J. Endocrinol. 242 (1), T105–T119.

Gridneva, Z., Rea, A., Hepworth, A.R., Ward, L.C., Lai, C.T., Hartmann, P.E., Geddes, D.T., 2018. Relationships between breastfeeding patterns and maternal and infant body composition over the first 12 months of lactation. Nutrients 10 (1), 45.

Grieger, J.A., Clifton, V.L., 2015. A review of the impact of dietary intakes in human pregnancy on infant birthweight. Nutrients 7 (1), 153–178.

Griffin, I.J., Cooke, R.J., 2012. Development of whole body adiposity in preterm infants. Early Hum. Dev. 88 (Suppl 1), S19–S24.

Guilloteau, P., Zabielski, R., Hammon, H., Metges, C., 2009. Adverse effects of nutritional programming during prenatal and early postnatal life, some aspects of regulation and potential prevention and treatments. J. Physiol. Pharmacol. 60 (Suppl 3), 17–35.

Halfon, N., Forrest, C.B., Lerner, R.M., Faustman, E.M., Tullis, E., Son, J., 2017. Life course research agenda (LCRA), version 1.0. In: Handbook of life course health development. Springer International Publishing, pp. 623–645.

Hamatschek, C., Yousuf, E.I., Mollers, L.S., Yiu So, H., Morrison, K.M., Fusch, C., Rochow, N., 2020. Fat and fat-free mass of preterm and term infants from birth to six months: a review of current evidence. Nutrients 12 (2), 288.

Harding, J.E., Cormack, B.E., Alexander, T., Alsweiler, J.M., Bloomfield, F.H., 2017. Advances in nutrition of the newborn infant. Lancet 389 (10079), 1660–1668.

Haschke, F., Binder, C., Huber-Dangl, M., Haiden, N., 2019. Early-life nutrition, growth trajectories, and long-term outcome. Nestle Nutr. Inst. Workshop Ser. 90, 107–120.

Hur, S.S.J., Cropley, J.E., Suter, C.M., 2017. Paternal epigenetic programming: evolving metabolic disease risk. J. Mol. Endocrinol. 58 (3), R159–R168.

Isganaitis, E., 2019. Developmental programming of body composition: update on evidence and mechanisms. Curr. Diab. Rep. 19 (8), 60.

Johnson, M.J., Wootton, S.A., Leaf, A.A., Jackson, A.A., 2012. Preterm birth and body composition at term equivalent age: a systematic review and meta-analysis. Pediatrics 130 (3), e640–e649.

Kelly, N.M., Keane, J.V., Gallimore, R.B., Bick, D., Tribe, R.M., 2020. Neonatal weight loss and gain patterns in caesarean section born infants: integrative systematic review. Matern. Child Nutr. 16 (2), e12914.

Klevebro, S., Westin, V., Stoltz Sjöström, E., Norman, M., Domellöf, M., Edstedt Bonamy, A.K., Hallberg, B., 2019. Early energy and protein intakes and associations with growth, BPD, and ROP in extremely preterm infants. Clin. Nutr. 38, 1289–1295.

Koletzko, B., Godfrey, K.M., Poston, L., Szajewska, H., Van Goudoever, J.B., De Waard, M., Brands, B., Grivell, R.M., Deussen, A.R., Dodd, J.M., Patro-Golab, B., Zalewski, B.M., 2019. Nutrition during pregnancy, lactation and early childhood and its implications for maternal and long-term child health: the early nutrition project recommendations. Ann. Nutr. Metab. 74 (2), 93–106.

Lacal, I., Ventura, R., 2018. Epigenetic inheritance: concepts, mechanisms and perspectives. Front. Mol. Neurosci. 11, 292.

Lagström, H., Rautava, S., Ollila, H., Kaljonen, A., Turta, O., Mäkelä, J., Yonemitsu, C., Gupta, J., Bode, L., 2020. Associations between human milk oligosaccharides and growth in infancy and early childhood. Am. J. Clin. Nutr. 111, 769–778.

Langley-Evans, S.C., 2015. Nutrition in early life and the programming of adult disease: a review. J. Hum. Nutr. Diet. (Suppl 1), 1–14.

Lapillonne, A., Griffin, I.J., 2013. Feeding preterm infants today for later metabolic and cardiovascular outcomes. J. Pediatr., S7. Mosby Inc.

Lapillonne, A., Bronsky, J., Campoy, C., Embleton, N., Fewtrell, M., Fidler Mis, N., Gerasimidis, K., Hojsak, I., Hulst, J., Indrio, F., Molgaard, C., Moltu, S.J., Verduci, E., Domellöf, M., 2019. Feeding the late and moderately preterm infant: a position paper of the European society for paediatric gastroenterology, hepatology and nutrition committee on nutrition. J. Pediatr. Gastroenterol. Nutr. 69, 259–270.

Larqué, E., Labayen, I., Flodmark, C.E., Lissau, I., Czernin, S., Moreno, L.A., Pietrobelli, A., Widhalm, K., 2019. From conception to infancy—early risk factors for childhood obesity. Nat. Rev. Endocrinol. (8), 456–478.

Larsson, A., Ottosson, P., Törnqvist, C., Olhager, E., 2019. Body composition and growth in full-term small for gestational age and large for gestational age Swedish infants assessed with air displacement plethysmography at birth and at 3-4 months of age. PLoS One 14 (5), e0207978.

Lecoutre, S., Petrus, P., Rydén, M., Breton, C., 2018. Transgenerational epigenetic mechanisms in adipose tissue development. Trends Endocrinol. Metab. 29 (10), 675–685.

Leghi, G.E., Netting, M.J., Middleton, P.F., Wlodek, M.E., Geddes, D.T., Muhlhausler, B.S., 2020. The impact of maternal obesity on human milk macronutrient composition: a systematic review and meta-analysis. Nutrients 12 (4), 934.

Li, Y., 2018. Epigenetic mechanisms link maternal diets and gut microbiome to obesity in the offspring. Front. Genet. 9, 342.

Lingwood, B.E., Al-Theyab, N., Eiby, Y.A., Colditz, P.B., Donovan, T.J., 2020. Body composition in very preterm infants before discharge is associated with macronutrient intake. Br. J. Nutr. 123, 800–806.

Liotto, N., Amato, O., Piemontese, P., Menis, C., Orsi, A., Corti, M.G., Colnaghi, M., Cecchetti, V., Pugni, L., Mosca, F., Roggero, P., 2020. Protein intakes during weaning from parenteral nutrition drive growth gain and body composition in very low birth weight preterm infants. Nutrients 12, 1298.

Longo, S., Bollani, L., Decembrino, L., Di Comite, A., Angelini, M., Stronati, M., 2013. Short-term and long-term sequelae in intrauterine growth retardation (IUGR). J. Matern. Neonatal Med. 26, 222–225.

Loÿs, C.M., Maucort-Boulch, D., Guy, B., Putet, G., Picaud, J.C., Haÿs, S., 2013. Extremely low birthweight infants: how neonatal intensive care unit teams can reduce postnatal malnutrition and prevent growth retardation. Acta Paediatr. 102, 242–248.

Lucas, A., Fewtrell, M.S., Cole, T.J., 1999. Fetal origins of adult disease—the hypothesis revisited. BMJ 319, 245.

Macdonald, P.D., Ross, S.R.M., Grant, L., Young, D., 2003. Neonatal weight loss in breast and formula fed infants. Arch. Dis. Child. Fetal Neonatal Ed. 88 (6), F472–F476.

Marousez, L., Lesage, J., Eberlé, D., 2019. Epigenetics: linking early postnatal nutrition to obesity programming? Nutrients 11 (12), 2966.

Martens, P.J., Romphf, L., 2007. Factors associated with newborn in-hospital weight loss: comparisons by feeding method, demographics, and birthing procedures. J. Hum. Lact. 23, 233–241.

Mazzocchi, A., Giannì, M.L., Morniroli, D., Leone, L., Roggero, P., Agostoni, C., De Cosmi, V., Mosca, F., 2019. Hormones in breast milk and effect on infants' growth: a systematic review. Nutrients 11 (8), 1845.

Moltu, S.J., Bronsky, J., Embleton, N., Gerasimidis, K., Indrio, F., Köglmeier, J., de Koning, B., Lapillonne, A., Norsa, L., Verduci, E., Domellöf, M., ESPGHAN committee on nutrition, 2021. Nutritional management of the critically ill neonate: a position paper of the ESPGHAN committ. J. Pediatr. Gastroenterol. Nutr. 73 (2), 274–289.

Monthé-Drèze, C., Sen, S., De Mouzon, S.H., Catalano, P.M., 2021. Effect of omega-3 supplementation in pregnant women with obesity on newborn body composition, growth and length of gestation: a randomized controlled pilot study. Nutrients 13, 1–19.

Morlacchi, L., Mallardi, D., Giannì, M.L., Roggero, P., Amato, O., Piemontese, P., Consonni, D., Mosca, F., 2016. Is targeted fortification of human breast milk an optimal nutrition strategy for preterm infants: an interventional study? J. Transl. Med. 14, 195.

Morlacchi, L., Roggero, P., Giannì, M.L., Bracco, B., Porri, D., Battiato, E., Menis, C., Liotto, N., Mallardi, D., Mosca, F., 2018. Protein use and weight-gain quality in very-low-birth-weight preterm infants fed human milk or formula. Am. J. Clin. Nutr. 107, 195–200.

Mosca, F., Giannì, M.L., 2017. Human milk: composition and health benefits. Pediatr. Med. Chir. 39 (2), 155.

Msall, M.E., Sobotka, S.A., Dmowska, A., Hogan, D., Sullivan, M., 2017. Life course health development outcomes after prematurity: developing a community, clinical, and translational research agenda to optimize health, behavior, and functioning. In: Handbook of Life Course Health Development. Springer International Publishing, pp. 321–348.

Nuyt, A.M., Lavoie, J.C., Mohamed, I., Paquette, K., Luu, T.M., 2017. Adult consequences of extremely preterm birth: cardiovascular and metabolic diseases risk factors, mechanisms, and prevention avenues. Clin. Perinatol. 44 (2), 315–332.

O'Connor, D.L., Khan, S., Weishuhn, K., Vaughan, J., Jefferies, A., Campbell, D.M., Asztalos, E., Feldman, M., Rovet, J., Westall, C., Whyte, H., 2008. Growth and nutrient intakes of human milk-fed preterm infants provided with extra energy and nutrients after hospital discharge. Pediatrics 121, 766–776.

O'Connor, D.L., Weishuhn, K., Rovet, J., Mirabella, G., Jefferies, A., Campbell, D.M., Asztalos, E., Feldman, M., Whyte, H., Westall, C., 2012. Visual development of human milk-fed preterm infants provided with extra energy and nutrients after hospital discharge. J. Parenter. Enteral Nutr. 36, 349–353.

Padmanabhan, V., Cardoso, R.C., Puttabyatappa, M., 2016. Developmental programming, a pathway to disease. Endocrinology 157 (4), 1328–1340.

Panuganti, K.K., Nguyen, M., Kshirsagar, R.K., 2020. Obesity. StatPearls. Internet.

Parisi, F., Milazzo, R., Savasi, V.M., Cetin, I., 2021. Maternal low-grade chronic inflammation and intrauterine programming of health and disease. Int. J. Mol. Sci. 22 (4), 1732.

Parlapani, E., Agakidis, C., Karagiozoglou–Lampoudi, T., 2018. Anthropometry and body composition of preterm neonates in the light of metabolic programming. J. Am. Coll. Nutr. 37 (4), 350–359.

Peila, C., Spada, E., Giuliani, F., Maiocco, G., Raia, M., Cresi, F., Bertino, E., Coscia, A., 2020. Extrauterine growth restriction: definitions and predictability of outcomes in a cohort of very low birth weight infants or preterm neonates. Nutrients 12 (5), 1224.

Picó, C., Reis, F., Egas, C., Mathias, P., Matafome, P., 2020. Lactation as a programming window for metabolic syndrome. Eur. J. Clin. Invest. 51 (5), e13482.

Power, V.A., Spittle, A.J., Lee, K.J., Anderson, P.J., Thompson, D.K., Doyle, L.W., Cheong, J.L.Y., 2019. Nutrition, growth, brain volume, and neurodevelopment in very preterm children. J. Pediatr. 215, 50–55.e3.

Ramel, S.E., Haapala, J., Super, J., Boys, C., Demerath, E.W., 2020. Nutrition, illness and body composition in very low birth weight preterm infants: implications for nutritional management and neurocognitive outcomes. Nutrients 12 (1), 145.

Rando, O.J., Simmons, R.A., 2015. I'm eating for two: parental dietary effects on offspring metabolism. Cell 161 (1), 93–105.

Rautava, S., 2015. Neonatal weight loss and exclusive breastfeeding. Acta Paediatr. 104 (10), 965–966.

Ravelli, A.C.J., Van Der Meulen, J.H.P., Osmond, C., Barker, D.J.P., Bleker, O.P., 1999. Obesity at the age of 50 y in men and women exposed to famine prenatally. Am. J. Clin. Nutr. 70, 811–816.

Regnault, N., Botton, J., Blanc, L., Hankard, R., Forhan, A., Goua, V., Thiebaugeorges, O., Kaminski, M., Heude, B., Charles, M.A., De Agostini, M., Ducimetière, P., Saurel-Cubizolles, M.J., Dargent, P., Fritel, X., Larroque, B., Lelong, N., Marchand, L., Nabet, C., Annesi-Maesano, I., Slama, R., Goua, V., Magnin, G., Schweitzer, M., Foliguet, B., Job-Spira, N., 2011. Determinants of neonatal weight loss in term-infants: specific association with pre-pregnancy maternal body mass index and infant feeding mode. Arch. Dis. Child. Fetal Neonatal Ed. 96 (3), F217–F222.

Riskin, A., 2017. Meeting the nutritional needs of premature babies: their future is in our hands. Br. J. Hosp. Med. 78, 690–694.

Riskin, A., Picaud, J.C., Shamir, R., Braegger, C., Bronsky, J., Cai, W., Campoy, C., Carnielli, V., Darmaun, D., Decsi, T., Domellöf, M., Embleton, N., Fewtrell, M., Fidler Mis, N., Franz, A., Goulet, O., Hartman, C., Hill, S., Hojsak, I., Iacobelli, S., Jochum, F., Joosten, K., Kolaček, S., Koletzko, B., Ksiazyk, J., Lapillonne, A., Lohner, S., Mesotten, D., Mihályi, K., Mihatsch, W.A., Mimouni, F., Mølgaard, C., Moltu, S.J., Nomayo, A., Picaud, J.C., Prell, C., Puntis, J., Riskin, A., Saenz De Pipaon, M., Senterre, T., Shamir, R., Simchowitz, V., Szitanyi, P., Tabbers, M.M., Van Den Akker, C.H.B., Van Goudoever, J.B., Van Kempen, A., Verbruggen, S., Wu, J., Yan, W., 2018. ESPGHAN/ESPEN/ESPR/CSPEN guidelines on pediatric parenteral nutrition: standard versus individualized parenteral nutrition. Clin. Nutr. 37, 2409–2417.

Robinson, S.M., Crozier, S.R., Harvey, N.C., Barton, B.D., Law, C.M., Godfrey, K.M., Cooper, C., Inskip, H.M., 2015. Modifiable early-life risk factors for childhood adiposity and overweight: an analysis of their combined impact and potential for prevention. Am. J. Clin. Nutr. 101, 368–375.

Roggero, P., Giannì, M.L., Orsi, A., Piemontese, P., Amato, O., Moioli, C., Mosca, F., 2010. Neonatal period: body composition changes in breast-fed full-term newborns. Neonatology 97, 139–143.

Roggero, P., Giannì, M.L., Piemontese, P., Amato, O., Agosti, M., Mosca, F., 2012. Effect of nutrition on growth and body composition in infants born preterm. J. Matern. Fetal. Neonatal. Med. 25, 49–52.

Roggero, P., Giannì, M.L., Garbarino, F., Mosca, F., 2013. Consequences of prematurity on adult morbidities. Eur. J. Intern. Med. 24 (7), 624–626.

Roggero, P., Giannì, M.L., Forzenigo, L., Tondolo, T., Taroni, F., Liotto, N., Piemontese, P., Biondetti, P., Mosca, F., 2015. No relative increase in intra-abdominal adipose tissue in healthy unstressed preterm infants at term. Neonatology 107, 14–19.

Rolland-Cachera, M.F., Briend, A., Michaelsen, K.F., 2017. Dietary fat restrictions in young children and the later risk of obesity. Am. J. Clin. Nutr. 105 (6), 1566–1567.

Rozé, J.C., Darmaun, D., Boquien, C.Y., Flamant, C., Picaud, J.C., Savagner, C., Claris, O., Lapillonne, A., Mitanchez, D., Branger, B., Simeoni, U., Kaminski, M., Ancel, P.Y., 2012. The apparent breastfeeding paradox in very preterm infants: relationship between breast feeding, early weight gain and neurodevelopment based on results from two cohorts, EPIPAGE and LIFT. BMJ Open 2 (2), e000834.

Saben, J.L., Sims, C.R., Piccolo, B.D., Andres, A., 2020. Maternal adiposity alters the human milk metabolome: associations between nonglucose monosaccharides and infant adiposity. Am. J. Clin. Nutr. 112, 1228–1239.

Saben, J.L., Sims, C.R., Abraham, A., Bode, L., Andres, A., 2021. Human milk oligosaccharide concentrations and infant intakes are associated with maternal overweight and obesity and predict infant growth. Nutrients 13, 1–16.

Sales, V.M., Ferguson-Smith, A.C., Patti, M.E., 2017. Epigenetic mechanisms of transmission of metabolic disease across generations. Cell Metab. 25 (3), 559–571.

Schneider, N., Garcia-Rodenas, C.L., 2017. Early nutritional interventions for brain and cognitive development in preterm infants: a review of the literature. Nutrients 9 (3), 187.

Sébédio, J.L., 2017. Metabolomics, nutrition, and potential biomarkers of food quality, intake, and health status. In: Advances in Food and Nutrition Research. Academic Press Inc, pp. 83–116.

Simeoni, U., Yzydorczyk, C., Siddeek, B., Benahmed, M., 2014. Epigenetics and neonatal nutrition. Early Hum. Dev. 90, S23–S24.

Smith, H.A., O'B Hourihane, J., Kenny, L.C., Kiely, M., Leahy-Warren, P., Dahly, D.L., Murray, D.M., 2019. Difference between body composition of formula- and breastfed infants at birth. J. Dev. Orig. Health Dis. 10, 616–620.

Sørensen, T.I.A., Ajslev, T.A., Ängquist, L., Morgen, C.S., Ciuchi, I.G., Smith, G.D., 2016. Comparison of associations of maternal peri-pregnancy and paternal anthropometrics with child anthropometrics from birth through age 7 y assessed in the Danish National Birth Cohort. Am. J. Clin. Nutr. 104, 389–396.

Symonds, M.E., Mendez, M.A., Meltzer, H.M., Koletzko, B., Godfrey, K., Forsyth, S., Van Der Beek, E.M., 2013. Early life nutritional programming of obesity: mother-child cohort studies. Ann. Nutr. Metab. 62, 137–145.

Tahir, M.J., Ejima, K., Li, P., Demerath, E.W., Allison, D.B., Fields, D.A., 2020. Associations of breastfeeding or formula feeding with infant anthropometry and body composition at 6 months. Matern. Child Nutr. 17 (2), e13105.

Teller, I.C., Embleton, N.D., Griffin, I.J., van Elburg, R.M., 2016. Post-discharge formula feeding in preterm infants: a systematic review mapping evidence about the role of macronutrient enrichment. Clin. Nutr. 35 (4), 791–801.

Thomas, E.L., Uthaya, S., Vasu, V., McCarthy, J.P., McEwan, P., Hamilton, G., Bell, J.D., Modi, N., 2008. Neonatal intrahepatocellular lipid. Arch. Dis. Child. Fetal Neonatal Ed. 93 (5), F382–F383.

Thulier, D., 2016. Weighing the facts: a systematic review of expected patterns of weight loss in full-term, breastfed infants. J. Hum. Lact. 32 (1), 28–34.

Toftlund, L.H., Halken, S., Agertoft, L., Zachariassen, G., 2018. Catch-up growth, rapid weight growth, and continuous growth from birth to 6 years of age in very-preterm-born children. Neonatology 114, 285–293.

Toftlund, L.H., Agertoft, L., Halken, S., Zachariassen, G., 2019. Improved lung function at age 6 in children born very preterm and fed extra protein post-discharge. Pediatr. Allergy Immunol. 30, 47–54.

Uthaya, S., Thomas, E.L., Hamilton, G., Doré, C.J., Bell, J., Modi, N., 2005. Altered adiposity after extremely preterm birth. Pediatr. Res. 57, 211–215.

Vahdaninia, M., Mackenzie, H., Dean, T., Helps, S., 2019. The effectiveness of ω-3 polyunsaturated fatty acid interventions during pregnancy on obesity measures in the offspring: an up-to-date systematic review and meta-analysis. Eur. J. Nutr. 58 (7), 2597–2613.

Vasu, V., Thomas, E.L., Durighel, G., Hyde, M.J., Bell, J.D., Modi, N., 2013. Early nutritional determinants of intrahepatocellular lipid deposition in preterm infants at term age. Int. J. Obes. (Lond) 37, 500–504.

Verduci, E., Giannì, M.L., Di Benedetto, A., 2020. Human milk feeding in preterm infants: what has been done and what is to be done. Nutrients 12 (1), 44.

Verduci, E., Giannì, M.L., Vizzari, G., Vizzuso, S., Cerasani, J., Mosca, F., Zuccotti, G.V., 2021. The triad mother-breast milk-infant as predictor of future health: a narrative review. Nutrients 13 (2), 486.

Vickers, M.H., 2014. Developmental programming and transgenerational transmission of obesity. Ann. Nutr. Metab. 64 (Suppl 1), 26–34.

Vickers, M.H., Krechowec, S.O., Breier, B.H., 2007. Is later obesity programmed in utero? Curr. Drug Targets 8, 923–934.

Villar, J., Puglia, F.A., Fenton, T.R., Cheikh Ismail, L., Staines-Urias, E., Giuliani, F., Ohuma, E.O., Victora, C.G., Sullivan, P., Barros, F.C., Lambert, A., Papageorghiou, A.T., Ochieng, R., Jaffer, Y.A., Altman, D.G., Noble, A.J., Gravett, M.G., Purwar, M., Pang, R., Uauy, R., Kennedy, S.H., Bhutta, Z.A., 2017. Body composition at birth and its relationship with neonatal anthropometric ratios: the newborn body composition study of the INTERGROWTH-21st project. Nat. Publ. Group 82, 305–316.

Villar, J., Giuliani, F., Barros, F., Roggero, P., Zarco, I.A.C., Rego, M.A.S., Ochieng, R., Gianni, M.L., Rao, S., Lambert, A., Ryumina, I., Britto, C., Chawla, D., Ismail, L.C., Ali, S.R., Hirst, J., Teji, J.S., Abawi, K., Asibey, J., Agyeman-Duah, J., McCormick, K., Bertino, E., Papageorghiou, A.T., Figueras-Aloy, J., Bhutta, Z., Kennedy, S., 2018. Monitoring the postnatal growth of preterm infants: a paradigm change. Pediatrics 141 (2).

Wells, J.C.K., Chomtho, S., Fewtrell, M.S., 2007. Programming of body composition by early growth and nutrition. Proc. Nutr. Soc. 66 (3), 423–434.

Wiechers, C., Kirchhof, S., Maas, C., Poets, C.F., Franz, A.R., 2019. Neonatal body composition by air displacement plethysmography in healthy term singletons: a systematic review. BMC Pediatr. 19, 489.

Young, L., Embleton, N.D., Mccormick, F.M., Mcguire, W., 2013. Multinutrient fortification of human breast milk for preterm infants following hospital discharge. Cochrane Database Syst. Rev. (2), CD004866.

Ziegler, E.E., 2011. Meeting the nutritional needs of the low-birth-weight infant. Ann. Nutr. Metab., 8–18.

# 5

# Early nutrition: Effects of specific nutrient intake on growth, development, and long-term health

*Ricardo Closa-Monasterolo[a], Joaquin Escribano Subias[a,b],
Veronica Luque Moreno[a], and Natalia Ferré Pallas[a]*

[a]Pediatrics, Nutrition and Development Research Unit, Universitat Rovira i Virgili, IISPV,
Tarragona, Spain [b]Hospital Universitari Sant Joan de Reus, Tarragona, Spain

## LEARNING OBJECTIVES

(1) To identify specific critical nutrients during gestation and early infancy that influence healthy growth, development, and long-term health of offspring.

(2) To understand the influence of macronutrients, with focus on protein quantity and fat quality (e.g., long-chain polyunsaturated fatty acids) as they relate to both gestational organ maturation and infant growth and development.

(3) To review mechanisms and impacts of folate, iron, iodine, and zinc nutrition during critical windows of fetal and infant development.

## 5.1 Introduction

Metabolic programming by early nutrition occurs when a nutritional stimulus (by excess or defect) is produced during a critical period (when organs and tissues are growing and developing), modulating the development of the organism to take place at the specific time period, and subsequently "programming" a structure or function that will have long-term health consequences (Barker, 2004; Lucas, 2005). During gestation, the maternal nutritional status may modulate the development of the fetus. In infancy, breastfeeding is the mammalian programmed source providing all of required nutrients and leading to optimal growth and development (Melnik, 2015). However, sooner or later, many infants will be fed through infant formulas or directly to cow's milk, beyond the first year of life. Although breastfeeding is recommended by the World Health Organization (WHO) until the age of 2 years, research focusing on effects of nutrients in formula milks aiming to mimic human milk, and its long-term health effects on the population, has gained strong interest in the last decade. For this reason, in this book chapter, most of the reported evidence will arise from studies performed in formula-fed infants, which address the effect of nutrient supplementation on different health outcomes.

The effects of nutrient intake in early life on long-term health are especially relevant among preterm infants, whom are exposed to an adverse environment when most of their organs and systems are still immature. In this scenario, the organ which has shown to be mostly influenced during the neonatal period among the preterm newborn is the brain (Ramel et al., 2012).

## 5.2 Proteins

In critical periods of growth and development, while tissues, organs, and systems are growing rapidly, one of the main substrates for accelerated growth might be proteins, which act as building blocks. Balanced protein-energy supplementation during pregnancy is associated with better fetal growth and birth outcomes, especially in malnourished women and is associated with an increase on birth weight of about 100 g (95% CI: 56–145 g) (Imdad and Bhutta, 2012). A systematic review assessed the effects of balanced protein-energy supplementation during preconception and pregnancy and found a reduced risk of low birth weight (RR 0.68, 95% CI 0.51–0.92; $N = 522$ in 5 studies), small for gestational age (SGA) birth (RR 0.66, 95% CI 0.49–0.89; $N = 5250$ in 9 studies), and increased birth length (MD 0.16 cm, 95% CI 0.02–0.31; $N = 3698$ in 7 studies), but found non-significant effects on mental development scores at 1 year (MD $-0.74$, 95% CI $-1.95$ to 0.47; $N = 411$ in 1 study) (Vaivada et al., 2017).

The effect of protein and energy supplementation on overall growth in the newborn has been the focus of many studies. A Cochrane Systematic Review (published in 2014 and updated in 2020) comparing low birth weight infants fed with higher versus lower protein content formulas concluded that high protein formulas ($\geq 3.0$ g/kg/day but $< 4.0$ g/kg/day) improved weight gain velocity (Fenton et al., 2014, 2020).

The importance of rapid growth in infancy (i.e., weight gain, linear growth, and head growth) relates to brain development and adiposity. On one hand, improved growth early in infancy has been associated to better neurodevelopment in different studies, and a recent systematic review from Ong et al. (2015) confirmed that improved postnatal weight gain and head circumference was associated to improved neurocognitive outcomes. On the other hand, weight gain velocity early in life has been associated to an increased risk of being overweight and obese in later childhood. A meta-analysis published in 2012 (Weng et al., 2012) confirmed that early rapid weight gain is a factor that increases the likelihood of being overweight in childhood. The UK Millennium Cohort Study quantified that the risk of rapid weight gain during the first year of life (weight for age $z$-score $> 0.67$ SD) may result in fourfold increased risk of being overweight at 3 years. And a meta-analysis of 10 cohorts published in 2012 quantified that each weight gain $z$-score from birth to 1 year increased the risk of being overweight or obese in childhood by 2.5-fold (Druet et al., 2012). These two potential consequences of rapid growth by increasing protein intake, as well as possible effects on other organs and tissues will be developed more extensively from this point.

## 5.2.1 The brain

Protein supply in early infancy has been studied in relation to brain development, mostly in undernourished populations and preterm infants. Observational studies reported that childhood undernutrition has been associated to poorer cognition, behavior, and motor skills later in life; however, there existed the doubt that such relation could be influenced by a lower socioeconomic level (Grantham-McGregor and Baker-Henningham, 2005). Therefore, supplementation studies in undernourished populations provide evidence that protein supplementation early in life improves the brain functioning leading to children and adults with better mental performance (Li et al., 2003; Grantham-McGregor et al., 1991), such as higher intelligence quotients and better school achievement. The time window to improve mental performance in children at the risk of undernutrition has been identified to be as early as possible, that is, late gestation and just after birth (Grantham-McGregor and Baker-Henningham, 2005). Despite these positive results, the magnitude of the effects of nutritional interventions in children younger than 2 years on mental performance seems to be weak, as observed in a meta-analysis by Larson and Yousafzai (2015). Supplementation in undernourished children older than 2 years has shown weak or no effects (Grantham-McGregor and Baker-Henningham, 2005).

Similarly, several studies demonstrate a poorer neurodevelopment in preterm infants, suffering major disabilities, behavioral problems, and motor and learning difficulties with a higher frequency, compared to infants born at term (Cooke, 1991; Powls et al., 1995). Factors influencing those cognitive and motor abilities might be the persistence of arterial duct, periventricular hemorrhages, ventriculomegaly, and any other disturbance of brain growth (Cooke, 2005). In this context, nutrition acquires a special relevance for proper growth. A clinical trial conducted in the United Kingdom investigated the effect of protein and energy supplementation in preterm newborns for approximately 1 month; the results of this study showed that there were less children suffering from cerebral palsy and having low overall and verbal intelligence quotients at 7–8 years if they had received early protein and energy supplementation (Lucas et al., 1998). This study raised the relevance of nutritional management during this critical plastic period of brain growth, in which suboptimal nutrition may not allow a compensation of functional problems by preterm birth.

In summary, protein and energy deficiency or suboptimal intakes during the first months of life in populations with special needs (undernourished and preterm infants) have been associated to a long-term poorer mental performance (ranging from poorer school achievement to major disabilities). However, variations in protein supply within the normal ranges in healthy infants during the first year of life have not affected brain development in a recent clinical trial (Escribano et al., 2016).

## 5.2.2 Adiposity and obesity

The most studied programming mechanism by which protein supply during infancy may affect growth and development is explained by the *"Early Protein Hypothesis."* This hypothesis proposed that a high protein intake in early infancy may result in increased levels of insulin-releasing amino acids, which may in turn stimulate insulin and insulin-like growth factor 1 (IGF-1) secretion and may stimulate the mammalian target of rapamycin complexes signaling, leading to a higher adipogenic activity, increasing the later obesity risk and associated disorders (Koletzko et al., 2009; Wullschleger and Loewith, 2006). The EU Childhood Obesity Project (EU CHOP), a randomized clinical trial (RCT), aimed to study the *"Early Protein Hypothesis."* Formula-fed infants were randomized to be fed either a lower (1.77 and 2.2 g protein/100 kcal) or a higher (2.9 and 4.4 g protein/100 kcal, respectively) protein content formula (the lowest and highest ranges of the recommendations at the time of the study) during the first year of life (Koletzko et al., 2009b). This research was able to demonstrate the "Early Protein Hypothesis" by showing that infants fed with the higher protein formula had faster weight gain during the first 6 months of life and this weight gain was associated to an increased fat mass at 6 months, but not to an increased lean mass at that age (Escribano et al., 2012). Consistently, at 6 months, infants fed with the higher protein content formula had higher serum concentrations of branched-chain amino acids and IGF-1 (Socha et al., 2011), independently of the IGF-1 genetic variants (Rzehak et al., 2013). The higher fatness among infants fed with the higher protein formula remained significant at 6 years of life, supporting a long-term effect of the early protein intake (Totzauer et al., 2018). Body Mass Index (BMI) from children fed with the higher protein content formula was significantly higher at 2 and 6 years compared to the infants fed with the lower protein content formula, and a 50% obesity risk differential at 6 years (Koletzko et al., 2009b; Weber et al., 2014). Moreover, at 6 years, the higher protein group had a twofold higher risk than the lower protein group for excess body fat (adjusted odds ratio: 2.13, P50.019) (Totzauer et al., 2018).

Several systematic reviews have concluded that a lower protein intake during the first months of life (for example, lowering the protein content of infant formulas) reduce the risk of later overweight and obesity in children (Abrams et al., 2015; Patro-Gołąb et al., 2016a,b). Moreover, there are also some indications that protein intake during the complementary feeding period could be also associated with later overweight/obesity (Hörnell et al., 2013; Pearce and Langley-Evans, 2013). One RCT performed in 1-year-old infants who were randomized to consume a formula with lower protein content or cow's milk until the age of 2 years showed a lower fatness among the lower protein intake group infants (Wall et al., 2019). However, specifically well-designed trials, including those that identify a specific quantity or range of protein intakes are necessary to improve the evidence and highlight the window period on which protein intake exerts its effects on later obesity risk.

### 5.2.3 The kidney

The growth and function of the renal system has been shown to be modified by protein supply in different periods of development; protein restriction in animal models during pregnancy lead to offspring with smaller kidneys, with less nephrons and lower renal functioning later in life (Hammond and Janes, 1998; Hoppe et al., 2007). In humans, a study performed in the Generation R cohort in more than 3600 mother and their 6-year-old children pairs found that a higher maternal intake of total and vegetable protein, during the first trimester of pregnancy, was associated with higher creatinine-based eGFR, but not with kidney size (Miliku et al., 2015). In infancy, those fed with higher protein content formulas have bigger kidneys than infants who are fed with lower protein content formulas or breastfed (Escribano et al., 2011). The physiological mechanism to increase kidney size by protein intake may be triple. First, kidney size increases its volume to support the higher need to excrete nitrogen metabolites; kidney growth due to this increased work needs would be reversible. Second, higher protein intakes stimulate IGF-1 secretion, which stimulates kidney growth and body weight gain, and finally, total body weight gain may indirectly promote the growth of the organs to support a higher metabolic work load (Luque et al., 2013).

### 5.2.4 The heart

Evidence that protein intake early in life may lead to cardiac function and structure changes exist. For instance, protein restriction during gestation has been associated with altered left ventricular function in the offspring (Elmes et al., 2007). Also, some authors found associations between protein intake during pregnancy and later blood pressure of the offspring, long-term results were inconclusive (Guardamagna et al., 2012). In infancy and childhood, protein-energy malnutrition has been associated to a reduced left ventricular mass and functioning (Kothari et al., 1992; Ocal et al., 2001; Faddan et al., 2010) and overnutrition has been associated to left ventricular hypertrophy (Moreira et al., 2009). From a physiological point of view, looking at the Early Protein Hypothesis, it can be hypothesized that protein intake could modify heart growth and functioning, since IGF-1 has been shown to mediate cardiac hypertrophy in pathological conditions (Maison et al., 2007).

Results from a subsample of the EU CHOP showed that infants fed with the higher protein content formula during the first year of life had increased cardiac function parameters (such as, ejection and shortening fraction) at 2 years, compared to infants fed with the lower protein formula (Collell et al., 2016). The authors suggested a possible mediation by the IGF-1 axis and hypothesized a prelude of possible cardiac mass hypertrophy, secondary to the increased function. More research aimed to identify the effects of protein intake on later cardiovascular health are necessary. One systematic review revealed that guidelines on nutrition for infants and young children often fail to address long-term outcomes, including the risk of cardiovascular disease or hypertension (Zalewski et al., 2015).

### 5.3 Fats: Long-chain polyunsaturated fatty acids and saturated fats

Fats play a key role in brain development, since they are in very high concentrations in its structure. Because of this, fat deficiency [especially long-chain polyunsaturated fatty acids (LC-PUFAs) but also others such as cholesterol] in critical periods of growth and development may affect the neuronal anatomy and functioning (Ramel and Georgieff, 2014; Georgieff, 2007). LC-PUFAs supplementation or deficiency at different time windows may have different effects, since brain grows and develops by phases. For example, in utero life, from the 18th to the 42nd week of gestation, the majority of axonal and dendritic growth is performed; the synaptic production starts at about the 28th week of gestation and continues until the age of 18 months after birth; the myelination process starts right at the end of the term gestation and is prolonged until late adolescence (Andersen, 2003). Therefore, it is important to differentiate between studies conducted in term or preterm newborns, since the latter are studied during a sensitive time window in which synaptic production of brain development is taking place, whereas full-term infants have had time to more fully develop these processes in utero.

It is worth highlighting that different time periods of nutritional supplementation have to be considered. In parallel to brain growth and development from a structural point of view, different cognitive and behavioral function domains of the human are being developed. However, in any case, it is sensible hypothesizing that any nutritional deficiency and supplementation could influence the neural functioning at any time in childhood, since the brain is growing and its functions and behavioral aspects are developing until the end of the adolescence. LC-PUFAs deficiency and supply effects on brain development and functioning have been extensively reviewed in the literature. The following section will summarize some of the relevant findings.

### 5.3.1  Periconceptional and gestational supply of LC-PUFAs

As LC-PUFAs are basic components in cell membranes and part of the membrane phospholipids in the brain, an appropriate LC-PUFAs supply to the fetus, while the brain is being formed, is crucial. The synthesis of fetal LC-PUFAs is low; therefore, maternal plasma levels of LC-PUFA and placental transfer are critical points for its supply to the fetus (Larque et al., 2012). For this reason, research aims to understand whether maternal intake of LC-PUFAs, and/or supplementation, may be translated into increased maternal plasma levels and to an increased placental transfer.

To find out this question, a study was conducted in pregnant women from the 22nd week of gestation until delivery; women who were supplemented with fish oil [0.5 g DHA and 0.15 g eicosapentaenoic acid (EPA)] were compared to placebo. The investigators observed that fish oil supplementation increased maternal plasma levels of DHA and EPA and cord blood plasma levels of DHA (Krauss-Etschmann et al., 2007). In other words, maternal supply of DHA might be effective on increasing its supply to the fetus. The next question is whether the increased DHA supply to the fetus may have any effect on a child's future development. Several, but not all, studies have reported improved cognitive performance in children associated to higher maternal and cord blood DHA concentrations. One review from Larque et al. (2012) did not find conclusive results associating maternal or cord blood DHA levels and later cognitive improvement in the offspring. However, neonates with mature electroencephalography scores had higher concentrations of DHA in umbilical plasma phospholipids, which may anticipate an improved neurodevelopment from that point in time onward. These authors showed improved results in the Kaufman Assessment Battery for Children among 4-year-old children born to mothers receiving DHA supplements (Helland et al., 2003) and better sequential processing skills among 7-year-old children born to mothers with better DHA plasma levels (Helland et al., 2008).

Conversely, a study published in 2011 did not find a direct association between higher DHA levels in maternal erythrocytes at delivery and cognitive function in the offspring at age 6.5 years assessed by the Kaufman Assessment Battery for Children, but found an association to higher mental processing scores (Campoy et al., 2011). In 2013, Gould et al. (2013) reviewed the effect of maternal supplementation with omega-3 LC-PUFAs and early childhood cognitive and visual development. They found no differences in standardized psychometric test scores for cognitive, language, or motor development between the LC-PUFA-supplemented and control groups. Only cognitive scores were higher among 2–5-year-old children, in whom supplementation resulted in higher Developmental Standard Scores. However, this effect was from two trials they identified having high risk of bias. The conclusion of the systematic review was that the evidence did not conclusively support or refute that omega-3 LC-PUFA supplementation during pregnancy improves cognitive or visual development in the offspring. Similar conclusions were found in a recent systematic review that concluded that n-3 LC-PUFAs administered during pregnancy had no effect on the skills or cognitive development of children in later stages of development (Rangel-Huerta and Gil, 2018).

In summary, maternal supplementation with DHA up to 1 g/day or 2.7 g n-3 LC-PUFAs has not shown any harmful effects in the mother nor in the fetus and newborn (Larque et al., 2012; Koletzko et al., 2007). Supplementation has shown to be effective on increasing supply to the fetus. Overall, associations between maternal DHA supplementation during pregnancy and later cognitive function in children are not conclusive, but do not refute possible improved neurodevelopment.

## 5.3.2 Supplementation with LC-PUFAS to breastfeeding mothers

Human milk is a natural source of LC-PUFAs for the breastfed infant. However, since the human synthesis of LC-PUFAs is low (to be synthesized de novo, conversion of their essential fatty acid precursors is required) (Janssen and Kiliaan, 2014), its concentration in human milk might be influenced by mother's plasma levels.

A first question to answer is whether maternal supplementation during lactation varies LC-PUFAs concentration in breast milk. Several publications confirm that DHA supplementation to lactating woman results in breast milk with higher DHA content (Sherry et al., 2016; Jensen et al., 2000). A second question is whether different LC-PUFAs concentrations in breast milk achieved by maternal supplementation may modulate the infants' plasma concentrations of omega-3 and omega-6 fatty acids. Work published in 2016 (Sherry et al., 2016) confirmed that breast milk and maternal plasma DHA were significantly greater with 200 and 400 mg DHA supplements compared to placebo. Consequently, infant plasma omega 6:3 ratio and arachidonic acid:DHA ratio were significantly greater in the placebo group compared to the DHA supplemented group, resulting in plasmatic infants' LC-PUFAs patterns more "favorable" from a neurodevelopmental point of view. And a third question to answer is whether the transfer of LC-PUFAs from maternal supplementation to breast milk and to infant's plasma is able to affect a child's development. To answer this question, we refer to a Cochrane review, published in 2015. Although some results supported an association between supplementation and child attention at 5 years of age, the Cochrane systematic review concluded that there was no sufficient evidence to support or to refute maternal DHA supplementation during lactation as it did not appear to improve children's neurodevelopment, visual acuity, or growth (Delgado-Noguera et al., 2015). A more recent systematic review performed in 2018 by Rangel-Huerta et al. reached the same conclusions, reporting a lack of effect of n-3 LC-PUFAs supplements to breastfeeding mothers on the cognitive development or their children (Rangel-Huerta and Gil, 2018).

The inconsistent results obtained in different studies may underlie a core rationale to address if there is any long-term effect of DHA maternal supplementation on a child's neurodevelopment. First, the improved structural DHA composition in the brain could prepare this organ for an improved performance throughout infancy. However, the possible benefit in cognitive performance is not detectable early in life. This could be explained by findings that mental performance and skills development is a dynamic process, many other factors as stimulation received are not monitored, and tools for assessing mental performance might not be sensitive enough at an early age range. However, slight effects observed at the age of 5 years may suggest a better preparation of a child's brain that could be translated in higher school performances (for example) later in life.

### 5.3.3 Effects of LC-PUFAs in the preterm infants

Most of the brain growth and synaptic production occurs during the second and third trimesters of in utero life. As such, when preterm infants are born, the nutrition sources they receive are crucial for their brain's development. Omega-3 LC-PUFAs supply has received special attention for their role in brain's structure as well as with the development of the retina, which takes place at the end of gestation.

Several studies have shown the safety of omega-3 LC-PUFAs-supplemented infant formulas for preterm infants, and have also reported that infants fed omega-3 LC-PUFAs-supplemented infant formulas have higher levels of these fatty acids in their erythrocytes (Vanderhoof et al., 1999; Koletzko et al., 2003). Furthermore, several studies have demonstrated that DHA supplementation to preterm infants through infant formula results in benefits for retinal and cognitive development, as shown by findings on electroretinogram activity, visual acuity (SanGiovanni et al., 2000; O'Connor et al., 2001), and developmental outcomes, such as the Bayley motor development index at 12 months and vocabulary comprehension at 14 months (O'Connor et al., 2001).

Although some clinical trials have demonstrated an association between omega-3 LC-PUFAs and different aspects of neurodevelopment at different ages, a Cochrane review and meta-analysis published in 2011 did not show any significant effect of the supplementation when pooling results. It is possible that infants enrolled in the trials were relatively mature and healthy preterm infants, and that the assessment schedule, methodology used, dose, source of supplementation, and fatty acids composition of the control formula varied between trials (Schulzke et al., 2011). More recently, a clinical trial published by Molloy and co-workers concluded that supplementing human milk with DHA at a dose similar to 1% of total fatty acids given in the first months of life to very preterm infants did not appear to benefit visual processing at school age (Molloy et al., 2016).

### 5.3.4 Effects of the LC-PUFAs in term infants

During the first months of life in infants born at term, the brain and the retina are still under formation and growth. It is therefore plausible that LC-PUFAs supplementation through infant formula may support growth and development of cognition and visual acuity.

A Cochrane review that aimed to identify the association between LC-PUFAs and the development of visual acuity and mental performance in infants born at term (Simmer et al., 2011) concluded that the majority of RCT's did not show any consistent beneficial effect of supplementation. Although there is a biological rationale to justify formula milks' supplementation, and it has been shown to be safe, the results obtained by high quality clinical trials do not support the need to supplement routinely to healthy term infants. Further studies that are conducted should consider the depletion status of infants, since probably, infants with the lowest LC-PUFAs concentrations may benefit from supplementation, while well-nourished infants with appropriate fatty acids proportions may not.

## 5.4 Folate

At the beginning of the 1990s, evidence that folic acid supplementation during pregnancy reduced the occurrence of neural tube defects (such as, spina bifida, anencephaly, or encephalocele) appeared. An RCT on periconceptional folic acid supplementation conducted in 33 countries, with more than 1800 women, found a reduction of 72% occurrence of neural tube defects in the infant or fetus (Anon, 1991). A similar clinical trial, conducted in more than 4700 women, replicated the results shortly after (Czeizel and Dudas, 1992).

The mechanism by which folates may affect the central nervous system is by modifying the patterns of methylation of the DNA encoding for development of the brain (Barua et al., 2014a). A recent meta-analysis about DNA methylation in newborns has concluded that it is related to maternal plasma folate levels (Joubert et al., 2016). Interestingly, some of the genes which have been found to be modulated by maternal plasma folate levels were not known to be associated to folic acid biology, but some relate to birth defects other than neural tube defects.

One Cochrane review on periconceptional (defined as before pregnancy and until the first 2 months of pregnancy) folate supplementation from 2010 and 2015 (Maria De-Regil et al., 2010; De-Regil et al., 2015) confirmed that folate supplementation has a strong protective effect against neural tube defects (such as, spina bifida, anencephaly, and encephalocele) in the newborn. In this scenario, periconceptional and infant's folate supplementation have been the focus of research across several decades. Even more, folate supplementation has been the focus of several public health policies as, for example, the folic acid fortification of staple foods, which has been demonstrated to reduce the risk of neural tube defects (Botto et al., 2005; De Wals et al., 2007; Berry et al., 2010).

Besides the association of periconceptional folic acid supplementation with neural tube defects, other birth outcomes have been hypothesized to be influenced. However, a Cochrane review, published in 2013, did not find conclusive evidence of benefit of folic acid supplementation during pregnancy on outcomes, such as preterm birth, deaths, anemia, or predelivery serum folate levels (Lassi et al., 2013). On the contrary, the use of multiple-micronutrient supplements including folic acid plus iron was able to improve some of these outcomes such as prematurity or low birth weight but not perinatal mortality as showed in a Cochrane database published in 2019 (Keats et al., 2019).

The brain develops rapidly during the last trimester of in utero life and the first years of postnatal life (Dobbing, 1981). Therefore, during these periods, the brain is sensitive to key nutritional factors, such as, folate. Although there is clear evidence that periconceptional folic acid supplementation prevents neural tube defects, it was not clear whether folic acid supplementation beyond that period (i.e., during later pregnancy) has any effect on the offspring. Results from the Generation R study (a population-based cohort from Rotterdam, The Netherlands) showed that children born to mothers who did not use folic acid supplements in the first trimester of pregnancy had a higher risk of behavioral problems (OR 1.44; 95% CI 1.12, 1.86) (Roza et al., 2010), as both internalizing and externalizing problems (OR 1.45; 95% CI 1.17, 1.80). More recently, results from the same study showed a modest association between maternal folate concentrations in early pregnancy and fetal head growth (Steenweg-de Graaff et al., 2017).

### 5.4.1 Dosage recommendation

After the first evidence of the association between folic acid during pregnancy and neural tube defects, several recommendations on folic acid supplementation have been stated. In 1992, the United States Public Health Service recommended daily supplementation with 400 µg of folic acid for all women of reproductive age [Centers for Disease Control Prevention (CDC), 1992]. The US Preventive Services Task Force recommends that all women planning a pregnancy take a daily supplement of 400–800 µg (US Preventive Services Task Force, 2009). Similarly, the WHO recommendations, based on the Cochrane review from 2012, supports that women take 400 µg of folic acid from the moment they are trying to conceive and during pregnancy (World Health Organization, 2012). Despite this global recommendation for women at reproductive age, higher amounts (up to 5 µg/day) have been recommended to women at high risk (Moussa et al., 2016).

Finally, recent investigations suggested that supplementation in pregnancy with 5-methyltetrahydrofolate (5-MTHF), the bioactive molecule, instead of folic acid (which is more heat stable and simpler to produce but unactive) could be advantageous because 5-MTHF is immediately active and bioavailable to the mother and fetus and is not influenced by the high prevalent 5-methyltetrahydrofolate reductase gene mutations (Ferrazzi et al., 2020).

### 5.4.2 Potential adverse effects of folic acid supplementation

During recent years, concern has been raised about a potential adverse effect of folic acid over supplementation and some countries have elected not to institute a folic acid fortification program because of concerns of unintended consequences. Apart from the folic acid supplements, there is an increase in the market of multivitamin supplements for prepregnant and pregnant women that include folic acid.

There is a suspicion that maternal folic acid over supplementation during gestation could alter the expression of several genes (Barua et al., 2014b) and could induce aberrant patterns of DNA methylation, playing a mechanistic role in carcinogenesis (by enhancing the progression of established preneoplasic lesions) (Ulrich and Potter, 2006).

Apart from cancer, other concerns related with cognition, hypersensitivity-related outcomes, and thyroid- and diabetes-related disorders have been raised from different studies. For this reason, two separate authoritative bodies (The US National Toxicology Program (NTP) and the Office of Dietary Supplements) convened expert panels to assess the risks from high intakes of folic acid (National Toxocolify Program, 2015; Boyles et al., 2016). In January 2017, the United States Preventative Services Task Force (USPSTF) concluded that "with high certainty the net benefit of daily folic acid supplementation to prevent NTDs in the developing fetus is substantial for women who are planning or capable of pregnancy." Other authoritative organizations have made similar recommendations (Bibbins-Domingo et al., 2017).

# 5.5 Iron

Iron deficiency is very common worldwide (World Health Organization, 2015) and is considered to be one of the most frequent forms of malnutrition (Stoltzfus, 2001, 2003). There are many iron-dependent changes in neurochemistry, neurometabolism, and neuroanatomy during brain development that are prone to induce changes in sensory/motor skills, cognitive/language performance, and social/emotional domains. Therefore, the brain affects behavior and behavior alters the brain (Lozoff and Georgieff, 2006). Early (comprising the fetal period and infancy until 2 years of age) iron deficiency has consistently been shown to be associated to brain development, with effects on both cognition and behavior. Recent knowledge on the effects of iron deficiency or supplementation during gestation and early infancy on child's mental performance is summarized below.

## 5.5.1 Iron supplementation during pregnancy

Iron deficiency is the most common form of nutrient deficiency in pregnant woman, and persistent iron deficiency frequently becomes iron deficiency anemia (IDA). The global prevalence of anemia among pregnant women was estimated to be 38.2% in 2011 (World Health Organization, 2015). Iron deficiency is estimated in low- and middle-income countries with rates that approach 80%, whereas estimated rates in well-resourced countries approach 45% (Georgieff, 2020).

Iron deficiency anemia is considered one of the most important risk factors for maternal and perinatal mortality (Stoltzfus, 2003). Maternal iron deficiency is the most common cause for reduced fetal iron supply (Lozoff and Georgieff, 2006). Fetal brain iron deficiency can also be due to increased fetal iron requirements, with its most common factor to be chronic fetal hypoxia (that increase iron use for erythropoiesis) (Rao and Georgieff, 2002). This clinical situation usually corresponds (among others) to fetal suffering from intrauterine growth restriction. The possible consequences of IDA on pregnancy outcomes are several, such as diminished intellectual capacity, low birth weight, or preterm birth (Steer, 2000; Godfrey et al., 1991; Alwan et al., 2011).

A Cochrane review published in 2015 on the effects of daily oral iron supplementation during pregnancy showed that such supplementation was effective on reducing maternal anemia by 70% and iron deficiency by 57% at term. There were no clear results on maternal infection during pregnancy or maternal mortality (Pena-Rosas et al., 2015a). In relation to the pregnancy outcomes, the Cochrane review on daily oral iron supplementation during pregnancy concluded that low birth weight was prevented by iron supplementation (low quality of evidence). Overall, birth weight was higher among infants from supplemented mothers and preterm birth was prevented in iron-supplemented mothers (both with moderate quality of evidence). Although there was some evidence for neonatal death and congenital anomalies prevention, the quality of the evidence was low (Pena-Rosas et al., 2015a).

Due to this body of evidence, recommendation of maternal iron supplementation for anemia prevention during pregnancy is a common practice. However, adherence to the recommendation of daily supplementation is frequently interrupted because of the side effects of oral iron supplements and the concerns from mothers with adequate iron intakes that they may receive an overdose. For this reason, intermittent supplementation (2–3 times a week on non-consecutive days) has been postulated as a possibly valid preventive intervention. This way of supplementation has been the focus of the Cochrane Reviews as well (Pena-Rosas et al., 2015b).

Findings from the systematic review suggested that intermittent supplementation produced similar maternal and infant outcomes as daily supplementation; however, there were fewer associated side effects and reduced risk of high levels of hemoglobin in mid and late pregnancy. The only disadvantage was that the risk of mild anemia near term was increased among mothers with intermittent regimens compared to mothers with daily recommended regimens. Therefore, the conclusion of the review was that intermittent supplementation was a feasible and effective way of supplementation to pregnant women who are not anemic and have adequate antenatal care. An alternative preventive intervention is the supplementation through micronutrient powders for fortification of foods (Suchdev et al., 2015). More recently, another Cochrane review showed that multiple-micronutrient supplements (including iron and folic acid) in pregnant woman from low- and middle-income countries had better results compared to the iron or acid folic supplementation alone, in terms of reducing premature births, low birth weights, or SGA birth weights (Keats et al., 2019). Therefore, the authors of this review concluded that there are sufficient bases to guide the replacement of iron and folic acid supplements with multiple-micronutrient supplements for pregnant women in low- and middle-income countries.

### 5.5.2 Iron deficiency and supplementation during early infancy

From animal models, it is known that iron deficiency affects the brain through effects on neurotransmitters and myelination (Lozoff and Georgieff, 2006). There is a strong body of evidence showing that infants with iron deficiency (with and without anemia) develop poorly (Lozoff et al., 2006; Grantham-McGregor and Ani, 2001). Different aspects of neurodevelopment are affected by this deficiency, for example, motor development during the first year of life (9–10 months) (Shafir et al., 2008), neuromaturation during the first 2 years of life (Walter, 2003), or cognitive skills, such as attention and object recognition memory at 9 months (Carter et al., 2010). Despite the spontaneous repletion of iron stores by 9 months of age, low neonatal iron status is associated with long-term neurocognitive dysfunctions such as a reduction on recognition memory performance at the age of 3.5–4 years even though the infants are no longer iron deficient (Georgieff, 2020). In addition, infants who suffered iron restriction during pregnancy have a poorer iron status at 9 months of age and thus a higher risk of being iron deficient during infancy and toddlerhood. In turn, this deficiency during the first years of life is associated with slower speed of processing, poorer motor function, and increased social dysfunction during the acute phase of iron deficiency and confers a risk of significant long-term morbidities including depression and anxiety in adulthood (Georgieff, 2020).

A systematic review and meta-analysis published in 2010 about the iron supplementation in non-anemic children, <3 years, found five RCTs showing a beneficial effect of iron supplementation during early life on the Mental Developmental Index of the Bayley Scales of Infant Development at different ages throughout the first 18 months of life. Three of five RCTs showed a beneficial effect of iron supplementation on the Psychomotor Development Index. The meta-analysis of three RCTs ($n = 561$) showed that iron supplementation did not affect children's Mental Developmental Index but showed significant improvement on the Psychomotor Development Index at the age of 12 months. The authors concluded that there was limited evidence, but it suggested that iron supplementation in infants may improve children's psychomotor development, whereas it may not influence their mental development or behavior (Szajewska et al., 2010).

When analyzing this nutritional deficit in relation to infants' neurodevelopment, it appears that infants suffering from anemia might be more likely to be born in a poorer family, receive less stimulation, and possibly may have other nutrient deficits. In this context, an interesting publication from 2013, conducted in Bangladesh, showed that psychosocial stimulation may benefit (in terms of psychomotor and mental development indexes) iron-deficient children (without anemia) but not anemic children, suggesting permanent effects from severe iron deficiency early in life, when the brain is under fast development (Tofail et al., 2013). Several studies have also tested reassessments after supplementation to show persistence of significant differences between children who had suffered from IDA, compared to those who had not. One Cochrane review on the effect of iron supplementation to young children with iron deficiency anemia concluded that there was no convincing evidence that iron treatment had a short-term effect on psychomotor development or cognitive function on young children with IDA. The effect of long-term treatment should be studied (Wang et al., 2013). For example, one study reported long lasting (5–10 years later) effects on cognitive skills of children who had IDA early in infancy (Walter, 2003). Such results suggest a strong programming effect of iron supply in infancy, and reinforce the need of iron deficiency prevention early in life. This prevention should consider that it may not be necessary to have anemia to see an effect. A basic principle of fetal and neonatal iron biology is that iron is prioritized to red cells at the expense of other tissues, including the brain. Therefore, when iron supply does not meet iron demand, the brain may be at risk, even if the infant is not anemic (Lozoff and Georgieff, 2006). In this scenario, it becomes necessary to link the knowledge that very low birth weight has been convincingly associated to a poorer mental performance outcome later in life, shown by lower academic achievement, attention deficits, behavioral problems, and poorer executive functions (Aarnoudse-Moens et al., 2009). Therefore, preventive iron supplementation in infants born preterm or low birth weight may have a possible need. There is evidence that intakes of 2 mg of dietary iron per kilogram daily prevents IDA in low birth weight infants without causing adverse effects, and may reduce the risk of later behavioral problems (Domellof, 2013). However, one systematic review of the literature analyzing the benefits of iron supplementation for low birth weight infants concluded that although supplementation reduced the risk of iron deficiency, there is still no sufficient evidence to make a definitive statement that such supplementation improves growth and neurodevelopmental outcomes (Long et al., 2012).

In summary, iron deficiency during critical periods of brain development (in utero life and first 2 years) may have long-term consequences on cognitive and behavioral skills in children. Since iron deficiency is common worldwide, and more common in low-income settings, such deficiency may have a strong social and economic impact from a public health perspective. Policies to implement preventive supplementation should be studied deeply to avoid overdoses, yet to obtain the maximum benefits.

## 5.6 Iodine

Iodine deficiency has been recognized for many decades and is known to cause cretinism and impaired development and neurocognition in populations with mild deficiency

(Lazarus, 2015). The main iodine source comes from the sea. Historically, it is known that some areas and populations have been iodine deficient. Because iodine supplementation may be an effective way to prevent neurocognitive impairment, in the 1980s, there was a consensus from national and international authorities, and a recommendation from the WHO to provide iodine supplementation through iodized salt, which was called USI (Universal Salt Iodization) (UNICEF-WHO, 1994). In general terms, it seems that salt iodization has been an effective mean to prevent iodine deficiency and goiter (Wu et al., 2002). A review from the WHO reported that of 40 European countries included, it was estimated that the populations of 19 countries had adequate iodine nutrition, 12 had mild iodine deficiency, 1 moderate iodine deficiency, and 8 countries had no sufficient data (Anderson et al., 2007). The review concluded that iodine deficiency remained a public health concern in Europe.

### 5.6.1 Iodine deficiency and supplementation in pregnant women

Iodine deficiency is particularly relevant in pregnancy, since maternal iodine status has been related to brain development in the offspring. The rationale for that association is that iodine is necessary for the production of thyroid hormones, thyroxine and triiodothyronine, which play a very important role in the mechanisms of growth in most of the organs (Bougma et al., 2013). Along with growth in many tissues, thyroid hormones regulate cell migration, differentiation, and myelination in the central nervous system (Manzano et al., 2007). Therefore, with iodine deficiency, metabolism of thyroid hormones is altered resulting in major consequences during critical windows of development (as pregnancy or lactation) (Bougma et al., 2013). In addition, the relationship between maternal iodine deficiency status and pregnancy complications has been also investigated; but a recent systematic review and meta-analysis failed to demonstrate an effect (Nazarpour et al., 2020).

Several studies have reported on the effectiveness of salt iodization to prevent iodine deficiency in pregnant women. In one review, Zimmermann concluded that iodized salt supplementation in pregnant women was effective at improving maternal urinary iodine levels to minimize the increase in thyroid volume during pregnancy and the prevention of increased thyroid volume in the newborn (Zimmermann, 2007).

However, there are more recent publications focusing on historically iodine deficient geographical areas that have become iodine sufficient, following mandatory iodization of table salt (based on studies on school-age children or general population) that reported conflicting results. These recent works have revealed that iodine deficiency is still prevalent among pregnant women, although it has been solved for the general population (Anaforoğlu et al., 2016; Oral et al., 2016).

A systematic review of the literature from 2015 compared urinary iodine concentrations in countries in which iodine salt fortification is mandatory by law or voluntary. This review concluded that although universal salt iodization is the most cost-effective approach to prevent iodine deficiency in pregnant and lactating mothers, urinary iodine concentrations in lactating mothers of most countries either with voluntary programs or in areas with mandatory iodine fortification is still within the iodine deficiency range (Nazeri et al., 2015).

## 5.6.2 Iodine supplementation in pregnant and lactating women and its effects on the offspring

The most important concern of pregnant women being iodine deficient is the possible negative effect on the newborn's brain and mental development. Severe iodine deficiency during pregnancy causes fetal hypothyroxinemia, which during this critical period of brain development may cause an irreversible damage with neurologic negative effects at cognitive and psychomotor level (Thilly et al., 1978; Haddow et al., 1999). There is a consistent body of evidence showing how the mental performance of children born to mothers who are iodine deficient is affected.

A population observational study, conducted in children born to more than 1200 mothers in China, showed that intellectual and motor development of children at 25–30 months of age was associated to abnormalities of maternal thyroid at 16–20 weeks of gestation (Li et al., 2010). Another study published in 2017 showed how suboptimal maternal iodine intakes were associated with impaired child neurodevelopment at 3 years (Abel et al., 2017). In 2013, a systematic review and meta-analysis focused on the relationship between iodine and mental development of children 5 years old and under (Bougma et al., 2013). Results from RCT's on mother's supplementation with iodine indicated an effect size of 0.68 in the offspring's intelligence quotient. Observation studies indicated an even greater effect size (0.46). More recently, a meta-analysis of individual-participant data showed in 6180 mother-child pairs that the maternal iodine/creatinine ratio before the first 14 weeks of gestation was directly correlated with their offspring's mean verbal IQs (Levie et al., 2019).

In summary, there is strong evidence that iodine deficiency during pregnancy results in child's mental and psychomotor delay. Iodine supplementation to pregnant mothers results in improved brain development in the offspring. In addition, it is also worth commenting that a high percentage of lactating women had suboptimal breast milk iodine contents and inadequate intake of iodine from food and supplements. This deficiency could affect the optimal offspring growth and neurological development as young breastfed infants are completely dependent on iodine supplied via breastmilk to ensure sufficient thyroid hormone production (Henjum et al., 2017). In 2017, an RCT aimed to assess if the iodine supplementation to preterm infants was able to improve mental performance at 2 years of age failed to demonstrate a beneficial effect and thus, supplementation to the mother before delivery becomes more relevant (Williams et al., 2017). Although there is consensus on the beneficial effect of universal iodine salt fortification, policies in each country may lead to a systematic or random supplementation of pregnant and lactating mothers, depending on whether this supplementation is mandatory or voluntary. National policies where salt iodization is not mandatory, but only voluntary, should ensure appropriate iodine supplementation to pregnant women.

## 5.7 Zinc

Zinc is a trace mineral involved in RNA and DNA synthesis and methylation (Maret and Sandstead, 2008); therefore, it is an essential element for cellular growth, differentiation, and metabolism. Zinc is present in the brain, bound to proteins, and it is necessary for its structure and functioning (Bhatnagar and Taneja, 2001). Zinc is present in high concentrations in the synaptic vesicles of neurons and takes part in several processes as myelination and release of neurotransmitters. All of this suggests an important role of zinc in the neuronal excitability (Bhatnagar and Taneja, 2001). Even more, some studies revealed that zinc is involved in neurogenesis, which may have implications on brain development, cognition, and behavior (Levenson and Morris, 2011). These mechanisms are highly active during gestational and early neonatal brain development; nutrition in these periods of life could program for later mental performance.

### 5.7.1 Zinc deficiency and supplementation in pregnancy

Animal models of pregnancy, under zinc-deprived diets, have shown effects on activity, behavior, and attention later in the offspring. Even more, animal studies assessing performance later in life after a zinc deprivation during critical periods of brain growth have shown non-reversibility of the damage (Bhatnagar and Taneja, 2001). Other pregnancy outcomes, rather than cognitive function in children, have been assessed after supplementation during gestation. For instance, it has been explored whether zinc supplementation may reduce the risk of preterm delivery and birth weight. A clinical trial published in 2010 found that adding Zn supplementation during pregnancy to routine care of women with a previous preterm delivery had no significant effect on the gestational age at delivery and birth weight but increased the birth head circumference (Danesh et al., 2010). Another clinical trial, conducted in more than 500 pregnant women provided a combined supplementation with iron, folic acid with and without zinc did not show differences in birth weight, head circumference, length, gestational age, preterm delivery, preeclampsia, premature rupture of membranes, nor spontaneous abortion (Zahiri Sorouri et al., 2016). In relation to these outcomes, a Cochrane systematic review was published in 2015 concluding that there was no association between birth weight and prenatal zinc supplementation (Ota et al., 2015).

### 5.7.2 Zinc deficiency and supplementation in infants and children

The prevalence of zinc deficiency throughout childhood is estimated to be high, primarily related to the low consumption of foods high in bioavailable zinc. Estimates suggest a 25% prevalence of zinc deficiency in world's population (Maret and Sandstead, 2006). Zinc supplementation in infants and children has been shown to be beneficial in studies on zinc-deficient children, in terms of growth in prepubertal children (Brown et al., 2002), diarrhea, and pneumonia morbidity in developing countries (Bhutta et al., 1999; Fischer Walker and Black, 2004).

Zinc intake and supplementation in early infancy has been shown to increase the serum/plasma Zn status in infants (Nissensohn et al., 2013). The extent in which these plasma levels affect different parameters are also the focus of study. A recent meta-analysis from the same group found that Zn intake increased growth parameters of infants; however, the magnitude of the effect was small and should be interpreted with caution (Nissensohn et al., 2016). The same group performed another meta-analysis in which they assessed the association between zinc intake and mental and motor development on infants. They found that the effect of Zn supplementation on mental development index changed depending on the dose of supplementation and was not associated with the motor psychomotor index. They concluded that there was no clear effect of Zn supplementation in infants with their mental and motor development. Regarding growth, those authors performed a meta-analysis in children aged 1–8 years and concluded that supplementation between 2 weeks and 12 months had no significant effect on weight gain, height for age, weight for age, and other anthropometric growth outcomes. As the authors commented, one possible explanation for these results was that a great part of the children included in the studies may suffer from different micronutrient deficiencies, and thus zinc supplementation alone was unable to restore an adequate nutritional status (Stammers et al., 2015).

A Cochrane review, similarly, concluded that there are no convincing evidence that zinc supplementation to infants or children results in improved mental or psychomotor development (Gogia and Sachdev, 2012). Although there are indications that zinc intake improves several aspects of executive functions, a meta-analysis failed to show a clear effect of zinc on cognition of children (Warthon-Medina et al., 2015). This lack of evidence about the effects of zinc supplementation is in line with the hypothesis by Stammers et al. (Stammers et al., 2015) about the multiple micronutrient deficiency in infants included in the studies. This is also supported in part by the results observed by Larson et al. in 2015 that found a slightly higher positive effect on mental development when they compared multiple micronutrient supplementations with supplementation of only one micronutrient (Larson and Yousafzai, 2015).

In summary, there is evidence that zinc deficiency results in negative effects on growth, cognitive, and psychomotor development. Although there is evidence that zinc supplementation might be beneficial, and some studies are able to show it, early systematic reviews and meta-analyses failed to demonstrate a convincing effect of zinc supplementation of which may be due to methodological concerns in some of the clinical trials (i.e., multiple deficiencies in the included subjects), subtle effects of zinc supplementation, or difficulty of assessing such little changes by the available tools, such as Bayley scales. Despite these results, a recent Cochrane systematic review that aimed to assess the effectiveness of zinc supplementation on growth promotion and infection prevention in infants younger than 6 months concluded that although zinc was unable to decrease deaths or illness, a positive effect on weight-for-age or weigh-for-length z-scores after 6 months of supplementation was reported (Lassi et al., 2020).

## 5.8 Summary

Through this chapter, we have reviewed a comprehensive body of evidence showing that nutrient deficiencies in critical periods of development (as proteins, omega 3 LC-PUFAs, iron, iodine, and zinc) may lead to alterations in the growth and development of the child. Effects of those deficiencies could be irreversible if produced during pregnancy or in early infancy as well.

Globally, more than 2 billion people are estimated to be deficient in key micronutrients, such as iodine, iron, and zinc, most of them from low-income populations. Some might be deficient in more than one micronutrient and protein at the same time (Abe et al., 2016). Supplementation studies with individual micronutrients during pregnancy (at least in deficient mothers) are beneficial for the brain development of the offspring. However, nutrients do not function alone to stimulate brain development, but they act in harmony at the same moment and also interact with growth factors, which in turn are dependent on adequate nutrient status (as protein or zinc).

A Cochrane review did not find enough evidence to assess the possible effectiveness of improving the maternal and infant's health and development, nor to assess potential adverse effects of multiple-micronutrients supplements on lactating mothers (Abe et al., 2016). However, another Cochrane review assessing the effect of multiple-micronutrients for pregnant woman showed that multiple-micronutrient supplements improve, compared with the individual micronutrient supplementation, some birth outcomes related to later health such as premature birth, low birth weight, or SGA birth (Keats et al., 2019). Therefore, further research aiming to analyze the nutritional status and diet as a whole would really improve the current knowledge of this field.

It is worth highlighting that most of the nutritional deficiencies during pregnancy and early infancy have been associated to brain development. The research aiming to improve brain development through early nutrition is of great importance, since reaching the best mental performance (comprising both cognition and behavior skills) might be directly translated to a benefit on the population in social and economic terms.

## 5.9 Future trends and research

In relation to nutrient supply through infant formulas, a possible future focus of research might be unraveling the possible long-term effects of early protein intake on adiposity and organs function, such as the heart and the kidneys. Even more, the possible effects of protein intake during the second year of life on later obesity risk should be investigated as well.

In relation to LC-PUFAs and micronutrients supplementation, although the worldwide deficiencies are so common, since routine supplementation has not shown consistent beneficial effects of most of the nutrients, one should focus on performing supplementation studies with pregnant women and children who are in a depletion status. Therefore, a further step to move forward shall be looking for fast low-cost methods for nutrient deficiencies screening in pregnancy and early infancy.

And finally, considering that macro and micronutrient deficiencies may happen not in isolation, but multiple deficiencies are usually found in the same subject, diet should be considered in future analyses as a whole, defining what are the dietary patterns that increase the risk of multiple deficiencies with special attention to the effect on brain development.

## Sources of additional information

The Early Nutrition e-Academy (ENeA) is an e-learning platform born from the collaboration of investigators from the field of early nutrition and health. By joining ENeA at http://www.early-nutrition.org/en/enea/, one could receive free of charge CME-accredited training in the area by translating the latest findings from international research collaborations.

## References

Aarnoudse-Moens, C.S.H., Weisglas-Kuperus, N., van Goudoever, J.B., Oosterlaan, J., 2009. Metaanalysis of neurobehavioral outcomes in very preterm and/or very low birth weight children. Pediatrics 124 (2), 717–728.

Abe, S.K., Balogun, O.O., Ota, E., Takahashi, K., Mori, R., 2016. Supplementation with multiple micronutrients for breastfeeding women for improving outcomes for the mother and baby. Cochrane Database Syst. Rev. 2, CD010647.

Abel, M.H., Caspersen, I.H., Meltzer, H.M., Haugen, M., Brandlistuen, R.E., Aase, H., et al., 2017. Suboptimal maternal iodine intake is associated with impaired child neurodevelopment at 3 years of age in the Norwegian mother and child cohort study. J. Nutr. 147 (7), 1314–1324.

Abrams, S.A., Hawthorne, K.M., Pammi, M., 2015. A systematic review of controlled trials of lower-protein or energy-containing infant formulas for use by healthy full-term infants. Adv. Nutr. 6, 178–188.

Alwan, N.A., Greenwood, D.C., Simpson, N.A.B., McArdle, H.J., Godfrey, K.M., Cade, J.E., 2011. Dietary iron intake during early pregnancy and birth outcomes in a cohort of British women. Hum. Reprod. 26 (4), 911–919.

Anaforoğlu, İ., Algun, E., İncecayır, O., Topbas, M., Erdoğan, M.F., 2016. Iodine status among pregnant women after mandatory salt iodisation. Br. J. Nutr. 115 (3), 405–410.

Andersen, S.L., 2003. Trajectories of brain development: point of vulnerability or window of opportunity? Neurosci. Biobehav. Rev. 27, 3–18.

Anderson, M., de Benoist, B., Darnton-Hill, I., Delange, F., 2007. World Health Organization, UNICEF. In: Iodine Deficiency in Europe; A Continuing Public Health Problem. WHO Library Cataloguing-in-Publication D, Geneva, Switzerland.

Anon, 1991. Prevention of neural tube defects: results of the medical research council vitamin study. MRC vitamin study research group. Lancet 338 (8760), 131–137.

Barker, D.J.P., 2004. The developmental origins of adult disease. J. Am. Coll. Nutr. 23 (Suppl. 6), 588S–595S.

Barua, S., Kuizon, S., Junaid, M.A., 2014a. Folic acid supplementation in pregnancy and implications in health and disease. J. Biomed. Sci. BioMed. Cent. 21 (1), 77.

Barua, S., Chadman, K.K., Kuizon, S., Buenaventura, D., Stapley, N.W., Ruocco, F., et al., 2014b. In: Rosenfeld, C.S. (Ed.), Increasing maternal or post-weaning folic acid alters gene expression and moderately changes behavior in the offspring. Public Library of Science, San Francisco, USA. PLoS One, 9 (7), e101674.

Berry, R.J., Bailey, L., Mulinare, J., Bower, C., 2010. Fortification of flour with folic acid. Food Nutr. Bull. 31 (1 Suppl), S22–S35.

Bhatnagar, S., Taneja, S., 2001. Zinc and cognitive development. Br. J. Nutr. 85 (2), s139–s145.

Bhutta, Z.A., Black, R.E., Brown, K.H., Gardner, J.M., Gore, S., Hidayat, A., et al., 1999. Prevention of diarrhea and pneumonia by zinc supplementation in children in developing countries: pooled analysis of randomized controlled trials. Zinc investigators' collaborative group. J. Pediatr. 135 (6), 689–697.

Bibbins-Domingo, K., Grossman, D.C., Curry, S.J., Davidson, K.W., Epling, J.W., Garcia, F.A.R., et al., 2017. Folic acid supplementation for the prevention of neural tube defects: US preventive services task force recommendation statement. JAMA 317, 183–189.

Botto, L.D., Lisi, A., Robert-Gnansia, E., Erickson, J.D., Vollset, S.E., Mastroiacovo, P., et al., 2005. International retrospective cohort study of neural tube defects in relation to folic acid recommendations: are the recommendations working? BMJ 330 (7491), 571.

Bougma, K., Aboud, F.E., Harding, K.B., Marquis, G.S., 2013. Iodine and mental development of children 5 years old and under: a systematic review and meta-analysis. Nutrients 5 (4), 1384–1416.

Boyles, A.L., Yetley, E.A., Thayer, K.A., Coates, P.M., 2016. Safe use of high intakes of folic acid: research challenges and paths forward. Nutr. Rev. 74, 469–474.

Brown, K.H., Peerson, J.M., Rivera, J., Allen, L.H., 2002. Effect of supplemental zinc on the growth and serum zinc concentrations of prepubertal children: a meta-analysis of randomized controlled trials. Am. J. Clin. Nutr. 75 (6), 1062–1071.

Campoy, C., Escolano-Margarit, M.V., Ramos, R., Parrilla-Roure, M., Csabi, G., Beyer, J., et al., 2011. Effects of prenatal fish-oil and 5-methyltetrahydrofolate supplementation on cognitive development of children at 6.5 y of age. Am. J. Clin. Nutr. 94 (6 Suppl), 1880S–1888S.

Carter, R.C., Jacobson, J.L., Burden, M.J., Armony-Sivan, R., Dodge, N.C., Angelilli, M.L., et al., 2010. Iron deficiency anemia and cognitive function in infancy. Pediatrics 126 (2), e427–e434.

Centers for Disease Control Prevention (CDC), 1992. Recommendations for the use of folic acid to reduce the number of cases of spina bifida and other neural tube defects. MMWR Recomm. Rep. 41 (RR-14), 1–7.

Collell, R., Closa-Monasterolo, R., Ferre, N., Luque, V., Koletzko, B., Grote, V., et al., 2016. Higher protein intake increases cardiac function in healthy children. Metabolic programming by infant nutrition: secondary analysis from a clinical trial. Pediatr. Res. 79 (6), 880–888.

Cooke, R.W.I., 1991. Annual audit of three year outcome in very low birth weight infants. Arch. Dis. Child. 63, 295–298.

Cooke, R.W.I., 2005. Perinatal and postnatal factors in very preterm infants and subsequent cognitive and motor abilities. Arch. Dis. Child. Fetal Neonatal Ed. 90 (1), F60–F63.

Czeizel, A.E., Dudas, I., 1992. Prevention of the first occurrence of neural-tube defects by periconceptional vitamin supplementation. N. Engl. J. Med. 327 (26), 1832–1835.

Danesh, A., Janghorbani, M., Mohammadi, B., 2010. Effects of zinc supplementation during pregnancy on pregnancy outcome in women with history of preterm delivery: a double-blind randomized, placebo-controlled trial. J. Matern. Fetal Neonatal Med. 23 (5), 403–408.

De Wals, P., Tairou, F., Van Allen, M.I., Uh, S.-H., Lowry, R.B., Sibbald, B., et al., 2007. Reduction in neural-tube defects after folic acid fortification in Canada. N. Engl. J. Med. 357 (2), 135–142.

Delgado-Noguera, M.F., Calvache, J.A., Bonfill Cosp, X., Kotanidou, E.P., Galli-Tsinopoulou, A., 2015. Supplementation with long chain polyunsaturated fatty acids (LCPUFA) to breastfeeding mothers for improving child growth and development. Cochrane Database Syst. Rev. 7, CD007901.

De-Regil, L.M., Pena-Rosas, J.P., Fernandez-Gaxiola, A.C., Rayco-Solon, P., 2015. Effects and safety of periconceptional oral folate supplementation for preventing birth defects. Cochrane Database Syst. Rev. 12, CD007950.

Dobbing, J., 1981. Nutritional growth restriction and the nervous system. In: Davidson, A.N., Thompson, R.H.S. (Eds.), The Molecular Basis of Neuropathology. Edward Arnold, London, pp. 221–223.

Domellof, M., 2013. Iron and other micronutrient deficiencies in low-birthweight infants. Nestle Nutr. Inst. Workshop Ser. 74, 197–206.

Druet, C., Stettler, N., Sharp, S., Simmons, R.K., Cooper, C., Smith, G.D., et al., 2012. Prediction of childhood obesity by infancy weight gain: an individual-level meta-analysis. Paediatr. Perinat. Epidemiol. 26 (1), 19–26.

Elmes, M.J., Gardner, D.S., Langley-Evans, S.C., 2007. Fetal exposure to a maternal low-protein diet is associated with altered left ventricular pressure response to ischaemia-reperfusion injury. Br. J. Nutr. 98 (1), 93–100.

Escribano, J., Luque, V., Ferre, N., Zaragoza-Jordana, M., Grote, V., Koletzko, B., et al., 2011. Increased protein intake augments kidney volume and function in healthy infants. Kidney Int. Soc. Nephrol. 79 (7), 783–790.

Escribano, J., Luque, V., Ferre, N., Mendez-Riera, G., Koletzko, B., Grote, V., et al., 2012. Effect of protein intake and weight gain velocity on body fat mass at 6 months of age: the EU childhood obesity programme. Int. J. Obes. (Lond) 36, 548–553.

Escribano, J., Luque, V., Canals-Sans, J., Ferre, N., Koletzko, B., Grote, V., Weber, M., Gruszfeld, D., Szott, K., Verduci, E., Riva, E., Brasselle, G., Poncelet, P., 2016. Mental performance in 8 years-old children fed reduced protein content formula during the first year of life: safety analysis of a randomized clinical trial. Br. J. Nutr. 22, 1–9.

Faddan, N.H., El Sayh, K., Shams, H., Badrawy, H., 2010. Myocardial dysfunction in malnourished children. Ann. Pediatr. Cardiol. 3 (2), 113–118.

Fenton, T.R., Premji, S.S., Al-Wassia, H., Sauve, R.S., 2014. Higher versus lower protein intake in formula-fed low birth weight infants. Cochrane Database Syst. Rev. 4, CD003959.

Fenton, T.R., Al-Wassia, H., Premji, S.S., Sauve, R.S., 2020. Higher versus lower protein intake in formula-fed low birth weight infants (review). Cochrane Database Syst. Rev. 6, CD003959.

Ferrazzi, E., Tiso, G., Di Martino, D., 2020. Folic acid versus 5- methyl tetrahydrofolate supplementation in pregnancy. Eur. J. Obstet. Gynecol. Reprod. Biol. 253, 312–319.

Fischer Walker, C., Black, R.E., 2004. Zinc and the risk for infectious disease. Annu. Rev. Nutr. 24, 255–275.

Georgieff, M.K., 2007. Nutrition and the developing brain: nutrient priorities and measurement. Am. J. Clin. Nutr. 85 (2), 614S–620S.

Georgieff, M.K., 2020. Iron deficiency in pregnancy. Am. J. Obstet. Gynecol. 223 (4), 516–524.

Godfrey, K.M., Redman, C.W., Barker, D.J., Osmond, C., 1991. The effect of maternal anaemia and iron deficiency on the ratio of fetal weight to placental weight. Br. J. Obstet. Gynaecol. 98 (9), 886–891.

Gogia, S., Sachdev, H.S., 2012. Zinc supplementation for mental and motor development in children. Cochrane Database Syst. Rev. 12, CD007991.

Gould, J.F., Smithers, L.G., Makrides, M., 2013. The effect of maternal omega-3 (n−3) LCPUFA supplementation during pregnancy on early childhood cognitive and visual development: a systematic review and meta-analysis of randomized controlled trials. Am. J. Clin. Nutr. 97 (3), 531–544.

Grantham-McGregor, S., Ani, C., 2001. A review of studies on the effect of iron deficiency on cognitive development in children. J. Nutr. 131 (2), 649S–668S.

Grantham-McGregor, Baker-Henningham, H., 2005. Review of the evidence linking protein and energy to mental development. Public Health Nutr. 87, 1191–1201.

Grantham-McGregor, S.M., Powell, C.A., Walker, S.P., Himes, J.H., 1991. Nutritional supplementation, psychosocial stimulation, and mental development of stunted children: the Jamaican study. Lancet 338, 1–5.

Guardamagna, O., Abello, F., Cagliero, P., Lughetti, L., 2012. Impact of nutrition since early life on cardiovascular prevention. Ital. J. Pediatr. 38, 73.

Haddow, J.E., Palomaki, G.E., Allan, W.C., Williams, J.R., Knight, G.J., Gagnon, J., et al., 1999. Maternal thyroid deficiency during pregnancy and subsequent neuropsychological development of the child. N. Engl. J. Med. 341 (8), 549–555.

Hammond, K.A., Janes, D.N., 1998. The effects of increased protein intake on kidney size and function. J. Exp. Biol. 201 (13), 2081–2090.

Helland, I.B., Smith, L., Saarem, K., Saugstad, O.D., Drevon, C.A., 2003. Maternal supplementation with very-long-chain n-3 fatty acids during pregnancy and lactation augments children's IQ at 4 years of age. Pediatrics 111 (1), e39–e44.

Helland, I.B., Smith, L., Blomen, B., Saarem, K., Saugstad, O.D., Drevon, C.A., 2008. Effect of supplementing pregnant and lactating mothers with n-3 very-long-chain fatty acids on children's IQ and body mass index at 7 years of age. Pediatrics 122 (2), e472–e479.

Henjum, S., Lilleengen, A.M., Aakre, I., Dudareva, A., Folven Gjengedal, E.L., Meltzer, H.M., et al., 2017. Suboptimal iodine concentration in breastmilk and inadequate iodine intake among lactating women in Norway. Nutrients 9 (7), 643.

Hoppe, C.C., Evans, R.G., Bertram, J.F., Moritz, K.M., 2007. Effects of dietary protein restriction on nephron number in the mouse. Am. J. Physiol. Regul. Integr. Comp. Physiol. 292 (5), R1768–R1774.

Hörnell, A., Lagström, H., Lande, B., Thorsdottir, I., 2013. Protein intake from 0 to 18 years of age and its relation to health: a systematic literature review for the 5th Nordic nutrition recommendations. Food Nutr. Res. 57 (1), 21083.

Imdad, A., Bhutta, Z.A., 2012. Maternal nutrition and birth outcomes: effect of balanced protein-energy supplementation. Paediatr. Perinat. Epidemiol. 26 (suppl 1), 178–190.

Janssen, C.I.F., Kiliaan, A.J., 2014. Long-chain polyunsaturated fatty acids (LCPUFA) from genesis to senescence: the influence of LCPUFA on neural development, aging, and neurodegeneration. Prog. Lipid Res. 53, 1–17.

Jensen, C.L., Maude, M., Anderson, R.E., Heird, W.C., 2000. Effect of docosahexaenoic acid supplementation of lactating women on the fatty acid composition of breast milk lipids and maternal and infant plasma phospholipids. Am. J. Clin. Nutr. 71 (1), 292s–299s.

Joubert, B.R., den Dekker, H.T., Felix, J.F., Bohlin, J., Ligthart, S., Beckett, E., et al., 2016. Maternal plasma folate impacts differential DNA methylation in an epigenome-wide meta-analysis of newborns. Nat. Commun. 7, 10577.

Keats, E.C., Haider, B.A., Tam, E., Bhutta, Z.A., 2019. Multiple-micronutrient supplementation for women during pregnancy (review). Cochrane Database Syst. Rev. 3, CD004905.

Koletzko, B., Sauerwald, U., Keicher, U., Saule, H., Wawatschek, S., Bohles, H., et al., 2003. Fatty acid profiles, antioxidant status, and growth of preterm infants fed diets without or with longchain polyunsaturated fatty acids. A randomized clinical trial. Eur. J. Nutr. 42 (5), 243–253.

Koletzko, B., Cetin, I., Brenna, J.T., 2007. Dietary fat intakes for pregnant and lactating women. Br. J. Nutr. 98 (5), 873–877.

Koletzko, B.R., Von, K., Closa, R., Escribano, J., Scaglioni, S., Giovannini, M., et al., 2009a. Can infant feeding choices modulate later obesity risk? Am J. Clin. Nutr. 89 (5), 1502S–1508S.

Koletzko, B.R., Von, K., Closa, R., Escribano, J., Scaglioni, S., Giovannini, M., et al., 2009b. Lower protein in infant formula is associated with lower weight up to age 2 y: a randomized clinical trial. Am. J. Clin. Nutr. 89, 1836–1845.

Kothari, S., Patel, T., Shetalwad, A., Patel, T., 1992. Left ventricular mass and function in children with severe protein energy malnutrition. Int. J. Cardiol. 35 (1), 19–25.

Krauss-Etschmann, S., Shadid, R., Campoy, C., Hoster, E., Demmelmair, H., Jimenez, M., et al., 2007. Effects of fish-oil and folate supplementation of pregnant women on maternal and fetal plasma concentrations of docosahexaenoic acid and eicosapentaenoic acid: a European randomized multicenter trial. Am. J. Clin. Nutr. 85 (5), 1392–1400.

Larque, E., Gil-Sanchez, A., Prieto-Sanchez, M.T., Koletzko, B., 2012. Omega 3 fatty acids, gestation and pregnancy outcomes. Br. J. Nutr 107 (Suppl), S77–S84.

Larson, L.M., Yousafzai, A.K., 2015. A meta-analysis of nutrition interventions on mental development of children under-two in low- and middleincome countries. Matern. Child Nutr. 13 (1), e12229.

Lassi, Z.S., Salam, R.A., Haider, B.A., Bhutta, Z.A., 2013. Folic acid supplementation during pregnancy for maternal health and pregnancy outcomes. Cochrane Database Syst. Rev. 3, CD006896.

Lassi, Z.S., Kurji, J., Oliveira, C.S., Moin, A., Bhutta, Z.A., 2020. Zinc supplementation for the promotion of growth and prevention of infections in infants less than six months of age. Cochrane Database Syst. Rev. 4 (4), CD010205.

Lazarus, J.H., 2015. The importance of iodine in public health. Environ. Geochem. Health 37 (4), 605–618.

Levenson, C.W., Morris, D., 2011. Zinc and neurogenesis: making new neurons from development to adulthood. Adv. Nutr. 2 (2), 96–100.

Levie, D., Korevaar, T.I.M., Bath, S.C., Murcia, M., Dineva, M., Llop, S., et al., 2019. Association of maternal iodine status with child IQ: a meta-analysis of individual-participant data. J. Clin. Endocrinol. Metab. 104, 5957–5967.

Li, H., Barnhart, H.X., Stein, A.D., Martorell, R., 2003. Effects of early childhood supplementation on the educational achievement of women. Pediatrics 112 (5), 1156–1162.

Li, Y., Shan, Z., Teng, W., Yu, X., Li, Y., Fan, C., et al., 2010. Abnormalities of maternal thyroid function during pregnancy affect neuropsychological development of their children at 25–30 months. Clin. Endocrinol. (Oxf) 72 (6), 825–829.

Long, H., Yi, J.-M., Hu, P.-L., Li, Z.-B., Qiu, W.-Y., Wang, F., et al., 2012. Benefits of iron supplementation for low birth weight infants: a systematic review. BMC Pediatr. 12, 99.

Lozoff, B., Georgieff, M.K., 2006. Iron deficiency and brain development. Semin. Pediatr. Neurol. 13 (3), 158–165.

Lozoff, B., Beard, J., Connor, J., Barbara, F., Georgieff, M., Schallert, T., 2006. Long-lasting neural and behavioral effects of iron deficiency in infancy. Nutr. Rev. 64 (5 Pt. 2), S34–S43.

Lucas, A., 2005. Long-term programming effects of early nutrition—implications for the preterm infant. J. Perinatol. 25 (Suppl. 2), S2–S6.

Lucas, A., Morley, R., Cole, T.J., 1998. Randomised trial of early diet in preterm babies and later intelligence quotient. BMJ 317 (7171), 1481–1487.

Luque, V., Escribano, J., Grote, V., Ferre, N., Koletzko, B., Gruszfeld, D., et al., 2013. Does insulinlike growth factor-1 mediate protein-induced kidney growth in infants? A secondary analysis from a randomised controlled trial. Pediatr. Res. 74 (2), 223–229.

Maison, P., Tropeano, A.I., Quin-Mavier, I., Giustina, A., Chanson, P., 2007. Impact of somatostatin analogs on the heart in acromegaly: a meta-analysis. J. Clin. Endocrinol. Metab. 92 (5), 1743–1747.

Manzano, J., Bernal, J., Morte, B., 2007. Influence of thyroid hormones on maturation of rat cerebellar astrocytes. Int. J. Dev. Neurosci. 25 (3), 171–179.

Maret, W., Sandstead, H.H., 2006. Zinc requirements and the risks and benefits of zinc supplementation. J. Trace Elem. Med. Biol. 20 (1), 3–18.

Maret, W., Sandstead, H.H., 2008. Possible roles of zinc nutriture in the fetal origins of disease. Exp. Gerontol. 43 (5), 378–381.

Maria De-Regil, L., Fernandez-Gaxiola, A.C., Dowswell, T., Pena-Rosas, J.P., 2010. Effects and safety of periconceptional folate supplementation for preventing birth defects. Cochrane Database Syst. Rev. 10, CD007950.

Melnik, B.C., 2015. Milk—a nutrient system of mammalian evolution promoting mTORC1-dependent translation. Int. J. Mol. Sci. 16 (8), 17048–17087.

Miliku, K., Voortman, T., van den Hooven, E.H., Hofman, A., Franco, O.H., Jaddoe, V.W., 2015. First-trimester maternal protein intake and childhood kidney outcomes: the generation R study. Am. J. Clin. Nutr. 102, 123–129.

Molloy, C.S., Stokes, S., Makrides, M., Collins, C.T., Anderson, P.J., Doyle, L.W., 2016. Long-term effect of high-dose supplementation with DHA on visual function at school age in children born at <33 wk gestational age: results from a follow-up of a randomized controlled trial. Am. J. Clin. Nutr. 103 (1), 268–275.

Moreira, A.S.B., Teixeira Teixeira, M., Silveira Osso, F.D., Pereira, R.O., de Oliveira Silva-Junior, G., Garcia de Souza, E.P., et al., 2009. Left ventricular hypertrophy induced by overnutrition early in life. Nutr. Metab. Cardiovasc. Dis. 19 (11), 805–810.

Moussa, H.N., Hosseini Nasab, S., Haidar, Z.A., Blackwell, S.C., Sibai, B.M., 2016. Folic acid supplementation: what is new? Fetal, obstetric, long-term benefits and risks. Future Sci. OA 2 (2), FSO116.

National Toxicology Program, 2015. NTP Monograph: Identifying Research Needs for Assessing Safe Use of High Intakes of Folic Acid. National Toxicology Program, Research Triangle Park, NC. https://ntp.niehs.nih.gov/ntp/ohat/folicacid/final_monograph_508.pdf.

Nazarpour, S., Ramezani Tehrani, F., Behboudi-Gandevani, S., Bidhendi Yarandi, R., Azizi, F., 2020. Maternal urinary iodine concentration and pregnancy outcomes in euthyroid pregnant women: a systematic review and meta-analysis. Biol. Trace Elem. Res. 197 (2), 411–420.

Nazeri, P., Mirmiran, P., Shiva, N., Mehrabi, Y., Mojarrad, M., Azizi, F., 2015. Iodine nutrition status in lactating mothers residing in countries with mandatory and voluntary iodine fortification programs: an updated systematic review. Thyroid 25 (6), 611–620.

Nissensohn, M., Sanchez Villegas, A., Fuentes Lugo, D., Henriquez Sanchez, P., Doreste Alonso, J., Lowe, N.M., et al., 2013. Effect of zinc intake on serum/plasma zinc status in infants: a metaanalysis. Matern. Child Nutr. 9 (3), 285–298.

Nissensohn, M., Sanchez-Villegas, A., Fuentes Lugo, D., Henriquez Sanchez, P., Doreste Alonso, J., Pena Quintana, L., et al., 2016. Effect of zinc intake on growth in infants: a meta-analysis. Crit. Rev. Food Sci. Nutr. 56 (3), 350–363.

O'Connor, D.L., Hall, R., Adamkin, D., Auestad, N., Castillo, M., Connor, W.E., et al., 2001. Growth and development in preterm infants fed long-chain polyunsaturated fatty acids: a prospective, randomized controlled trial. Pediatrics 108 (2), 359–371.

Ocal, B., Unal, S., Zorlu, P., Tezic, H.T., Oguz, D., 2001. Echocardiographic evaluation of cardiac functions and left ventricular mass in children with malnutrition. J. Paediatr. Child Health 37 (1), 14–17.

Ong, K.K., Kennedy, K., Castaneda-Gutierrez, E., Forsyth, S., Godfrey, K.M., Koletzko, B., et al., 2015. Postnatal growth in preterm infants and later health outcomes: a systematic review. Acta Paediatr. 104 (10), 974–986.

Oral, E., Aydogan Mathyk, B., Aydogan, B.I., Acıkgoz, A.S., Erenel, H., Celik Acıoglu, H., et al., 2016. Iodine status of pregnant women in a metropolitan city which proved to be an iodinesufficient area. Is mandatory salt iodisation enough for pregnant women? Gynecol. Endocrinol. 32 (3), 188–192.

Ota, E., Mori, R., Middleton, P., Tobe-Gai, R., Mahomed, K., Miyazaki, C., et al., 2015. Zinc supplementation for improving pregnancy and infant outcome. Cochrane Database Syst. Rev. 2, CD000230.

Patro-Gołąb, B., Zalewski, B.M., Kouwenhoven, S.M., Karaś, J., Koletzko, B., van Goudoever, J.B., et al., 2016a. Protein concentration in milk formula, growth, and later risk of obesity: a systematic review. J. Nutr. 46 (3), 551–564.

Patro-Gołąb, B., Zalewski, B.M., Kołodziej, M., Kouwenhoven, S., Poston, L., Godfrey, J., et al., 2016b. Nutritional interventions or exposures in infants and children aged up to three years and their effects on subsequent risk of overweight, obesity, and body fat: a systematic review of systematic reviews. Obes. Rev. 17 (12), 1245–1257.

Pearce, J., Langley-Evans, S.C., 2013. The types of food introduced during complementary feeding and risk of childhood obesity: a systematic review. Int. J. Obes. (Lond) 37 (4), 477–485.

Pena-Rosas, J.P., De-Regil, L.M., Garcia-Casal, M.N., Dowswell, T., 2015a. Daily oral iron supplementation during pregnancy. Cochrane Database Syst. Rev. 7, CD004736.

Pena-Rosas, J.P., De-Regil, L.M., Gomez Malave, H., Flores-Urrutia, M.C., Dowswell, T., 2015b. Intermittent oral iron supplementation during pregnancy. Cochrane Database Syst. Rev. 10, CD009997.

Powls, A., Botting, N., Marlow, N., Al, E., 1995. Motor impairment in children 12-13 years old with a birth weight of less than 1250g. Arch. Dis. Child. Fetal Neonatal Ed. 72, F62–F66.

Ramel, S.E., Georgieff, M.K., 2014. Preterm nutrition and the brain. World Rev. Nutr. Diet. 110, 190–200.

Ramel, S.E., Demerath, E.W., Gray, H.L., Younge, N., Boys, C., Georgieff, M.K., 2012. The relationship of poor linear growth velocity with neonatal illness and two-year neurodevelopment in preterm infants. Neonatology 102 (1), 19–24.

Rangel-Huerta, O.D., Gil, A., 2018. Effect of omega-3 fatty acids on cognition: an updated systematic review of randomized clinical trials. Nutr. Rev. 76 (1), 1–20.

Rao, R., Georgieff, M.K., 2002. Perinatal aspects of iron metabolism. Acta Paediatr. Suppl. 91 (438), 124–129.

Roza, S.J., van Batenburg-Eddes, T., Steegers, E.A.P., Jaddoe, V.W.V., Mackenbach, J.P., Hofman, A., et al., 2010. Maternal folic acid supplement use in early pregnancy and child behavioural problems: the generation R study. Br. J. Nutr. 103 (3), 445–452.

Rzehak, P., Grote, V., Lattka, E., Weber, M., Gruszfeld, D., Socha, P., et al., 2013. Associations of IGF-1 gene variants and milk protein intake with IGF-I concentrations in infants at age 6 months—results from a randomized clinical trial. Growth Horm. IGF Res. 23 (5), 149–158.

SanGiovanni, J.P., Parra-Cabrera, S., Colditz, G.A., Berkey, C.S., Dwyer, J.T., 2000. Meta-analysis of dietary essential fatty acids and long-chain polyunsaturated fatty acids as they relate to visual resolution acuity in healthy preterm infants. Pediatrics 105 (6), 1292–1298.

Schulzke, S.M., Patole, S.K., Karen, S., 2011. Longchain polyunsaturated fatty acid supplementation in preterm infants. Cochrane Database Syst. Rev. (2), CD000375.

Shafir, T., Angulo-Barroso, R., Jing, Y., Angelilli, M.L., Jacobson, S.W., Lozoff, B., 2008. Iron deficiency and infant motor development. Early Hum. Dev. 84 (7), 479–485.

Sherry, C.L., Oliver, J.S., Marriage, B.J., 2016. Docosahexaenoic acid supplementation in lactating women increases breast milk and plasma docosahexaenoic acid concentrations and alters infant omega 6:3 fatty acid ratio. Prostaglandins Leukot. Essent. Fatty Acids 95, 63–69.

Simmer, K., Patole, S.K., Rao, S.C., 2011. Long-chain polyunsaturated fatty acid supplementation in infants born at term. Cochrane Database Syst. Rev. 12, CD000376.

Socha, P., Grote, V., Gruszfeld, D., Janas, R., Demmelmair, H., Closa-Monasterolo, R., et al., 2011. Milk protein intake, the metabolic-endocrine response, and growth in infancy: data from a randomized clinical trial. Am. J. Clin. Nutr. 94 (6 Suppl), 1776S–1784S.

Stammers, A.L., Lowe, N.M., Medina, M.W., Patel, S., Dykes, F., Pérez-Rodrigo, C., et al., 2015. The relationship between zinc intake and growth in children aged 1-8 years: a systematic review and meta-analysis. Eur. J. Clin. Nutr. 69 (2), 147–153.

Steenweg-de Graaff, J., Roza, S.J., Walstra, A.N., El Marroun, H., Steegers, E.A.P., Jaddoe, V.W.V., et al., 2017. Associations of maternal folic acid supplementation and folate concentrations during pregnancy with foetal and child head growth: the generation R study. Eur. J. Nutr. 56 (1), 65–75. https://doi.org/10.1007/s00394-015-1058-z (Epub ahead of print).

Steer, P.J., 2000. Maternal hemoglobin concentration and birth weight. Am. J. Clin. Nutr. 71 (5 Suppl), 1285S–1287S.

Stoltzfus, R., 2001. Defining iron-deficiency anemia in public health terms: a time for reflection. J. Nutr. 131 (2S–2), 565S–567S.

Stoltzfus, R.J., 2003. Iron deficiency: global prevalence and consequences. Food Nutr. Bull. 24 (4 Suppl), S99–S103.

Suchdev, P.S., Pena-Rosas, J.P., De-Regil, L.M., 2015. Multiple micronutrient powders for home (point-of-use) fortification of foods in pregnant women. Cochrane Database Syst. Rev. 6, CD011158.

Szajewska, H., Ruszczynski, M., Chmielewska, A., 2010. Effects of iron supplementation in nonanemic pregnant women, infants, and young children on the mental performance and psychomotor development of children: a systematic review of randomized controlled trials. Am. J. Clin. Nutr. 91 (6), 1684–1690.

Thilly, C.H., Delange, F., Lagasse, R., Bourdoux, P., Ramioul, L., Berquist, H., et al., 1978. Fetal hypothyroidism and maternal thyroid status in severe endemic goiter. J. Clin. Endocrinol. Metab. 47 (2), 354–360.

Tofail, F., Hamadani, J.D., Mehrin, F., Ridout, D.A., Huda, S.N., Grantham-McGregor, S.M., 2013. Psychosocial stimulation benefits development in nonanemic children but not in anemic, irondeficient children. J. Nutr. 143 (6), 885–893.

Totzauer, M., Luque, V., Escribano, J., Closa-Monasterolo, R., Verdici, E., ReDionigi, A., et al., 2018. Effect of lower versus higher protein content in infant formula through the first year on body composition from 1 to 6 years: follow-up of a randomized clinical trial. Obesity 26, 1203–1210.

Ulrich, C.M., Potter, J.D., 2006. Folate supplementation: too much of a good thing? Cancer Epidemiol. Biomark. Prev. 15 (2), 189–193.

UNICEF-WHO, 1994. Joint committee on health policy. In: World Summit for Children—Mid Decade Goal: Iodine Deficiency Disorders. UNICEF–WHO, Geneva, Switzerland.

US Preventive Services Task Force, 2009. Folic acid for the prevention of neural tube defects: U.S. Preventive Services Task Force recommendation statement. Ann. Intern Med. 150 (9), 626–631.

Vaivada, T., Gaffey, M.F., Bhutta, Z.A., 2017. Promoting early child development with interventions in health and nutrition: a systematic review. Pediatrics 140 (2), e20164308.

Vanderhoof, J., Gross, S., Hegyi, T., Clandinin, T., Porcelli, P., DeCristofaro, J., et al., 1999. Evaluation of a long-chain polyunsaturated fatty acid supplemented formula on growth, tolerance, and plasma lipids in preterm infants up to 48 weeks postconceptional age. J. Pediatr. Gastroenterol. Nutr. 29 (3), 318–326.

Wall, C.R., Hill, R.J., Lovell, A.L., Matsuyama, M., Milne, T., Grant, C.C., et al., 2019. A multicenter, double-blind, randomized, placebo-controlled trial to evaluate the effect of consuming growing up Milk "lite" on body composition in children aged 12-23 mo. Am. J. Clin. Nutr. 109 (3), 576–585.

Walter, T., 2003. Effect of iron-deficiency anemia on cognitive skills and neuromaturation in infancy and childhood. Food Nutr. Bull. 24 (4 Suppl), S104–S110.

Wang, B., Zhan, S., Gong, T., Lee, L., 2013. Iron therapy for improving psychomotor development and cognitive function in children under the age of three with iron deficiency anaemia. Cochrane Database Syst. Rev. 6, CD001444.

Warthon-Medina, M., Moran, V.H., Stammers, A.-L., Dillon, S., Qualter, P., Nissensohn, M., et al., 2015. Zinc intake, status and indices of cognitive function in adults and children: a systematic review and meta-analysis. Eur. J. Clin. Nutr. 69 (6), 649–661.

Weber, M., Grote, V., Closa-Monasterolo, R., Escribano, J., Langhendries, J.P., Dain, E., et al., 2014. Lower protein content in infant formula reduces BMI and obesity risk at school age: follow-up of a randomized trial. Am. J. Clin. Nutr. 99 (5), 1041–1051.

Weng, S.F., Redsell, S.A., Swift, J.A., Yang, M., Glazebrook, C.P., 2012. Systematic review and meta-analyses of risk factors for childhood overweight identifiable during infancy. Arch. Dis. Child. 97 (12), 1019–1026.

Williams, F.L.R., Ogston, S., Hume, R., Watson, J., Stanbury, K., Willatts, P., et al., 2017. Supplemental iodide for preterm infants and developmental outcomes at 2 years: an RCT. Pediatrics 139 (5), e20163703.

World Health Organization, 2012. Guideline: Daily Iron and Folic Acid Supplementation in Pregnant Women. WHO Press, Geneva, Switzerland, pp. 1–32.

World Health Organization, 2015. The Global Prevalence of Anemia in 2011. Switzerland, Geneva, pp. 1–48.

Wu, T., Liu, G.J., Li, P., Clar, C., 2002. Iodised salt for preventing iodine deficiency disorders. Cochrane Database Syst. Rev. (3), CD003204.

Wullschleger, S., Loewith, R.H.M., 2006. TOR signaling in growth and metabolism. Cell 124 (3), 471–484.

Zahiri Sorouri, Z., Sadeghi, H., Pourmarzi, D., 2016. The effect of zinc supplementation on pregnancy outcome: a randomized controlled trial. J. Matern. Fetal Neonatal Med. 29, 2194–2198.

Zalewski, B., Patro, B., Veldhorst, M., Kouwenhoven, S., Crespo-Escobar, P., Calvo-Lerma, J., et al., 2015. Nutrition of infants and young children (1-3 years) and its effect on later health: a systematic review of current recommendations (EarlyNutritrion project). Crit. Rev. Food Sci. Nutr. 57 (3), 489–500.

Zimmermann, M.B., 2007. The impact of iodised salt or iodine supplements on iodine status during pregnancy, lactation and infancy. Public Health Nutr. 10 (12A), 1584–1595.

# 6

# Early-life nutrition and neurodevelopment

## Sarah E. Cusick and Michael K. Georgieff

Department of Pediatrics, Medical School, University of Minnesota, Minneapolis, MN, United States

## CHAPTER LEARNING OBJECTIVES

(1) Identify the stage of life when the developing brain is most vulnerable to environmental stimuli, including nutritional deficiency.

(2) Describe two non-mutually exclusive mechanisms that have been elucidated by preclinical models which help to explain how early-life nutritional deficiencies can lead to poorer long-term brain outcomes.

(3) Explain the relationship between the timing of brain development and nutrient deficiency that determines whether dysfunction is lasting.

(4) List five nutrients that affect brain development for which preclinical evidence of an epigenetic mechanism has been demonstrated.

## 6.1 The developmental origins of health and disease (DOHaD) concept—"In the beginning"

The 1990s marked the onset of formalization and scientific exploration of the concept of the DOHaD (Gluckman and Hanson, 2004). The theory was based on the findings by David Barker's group in England that showed an association between fetal growth restriction and subsequent adult risk of cardiometabolic syndrome. Preclinical, clinical, and epidemiologic studies have since provided biological grounding for the theory, demonstrating that early-life nutrition can "program" metabolic pathways for the lifespan, in part through epigenetic modification of genes that regulate metabolic processes. The discovery of critical or sensitive periods early in life for setting these regulatory processes was key to the theory.

## 6.2 DOHaD, the developing brain, and lifespan brain health

The first decade of the 2000s witnessed the translation of DOHaD principles to the developing brain and the risk of adult neuro- and psychopathologies. Championed largely by the National Institute of Mental Health, there was a realization that many of the identified early-life environmental triggers of adult cardiometabolic diseases such as stress and nutrition also affected the developing brain (reviewed in O'Donnell and Meaney, 2017). Moreover, alterations to those environmental factors in early life were epidemiologically associated with the risk of psychopathologies such as autism, schizophrenia, and depression/anxiety appearing later in life (Insel et al., 2008; Eide et al., 2013; Schmidt et al., 2014). Nutrition and nutrient status have emerged as major environmental drivers of the process. The second decade of the 2000s witnessed a major uptick in original science articles investigating individual nutrients during early life and their impact on brain development across the lifespan.

The late fetal and early postnatal brain has higher metabolic demand than at any time in life (Kuzawa, 1998). Whereas the adult brain consumes 20% of daily delivered energy, a not so inconsiderable number, the neonatal brain consumes 60%. Moreover, the daily energy requirement of the adult on a per kilogram weight basis is only 40% of the neonate. The exceedingly high metabolic requirements relate to the "cost" of structural development in multiple brain regions at that time (Bastian et al., 2016). This development includes some residual neurogenesis and a massive amount of neuronal differentiation and synaptogenesis, particularly in the hippocampus, striatum, cerebellum, and some parts of the cerebral cortex (Thompson and Nelson, 2001). Ultimately, the complexity of dendritic arbors and the strength of connections in neural circuits translate into functional capacity (Bastian et al., 2016). Disruption of metabolic substrates (e.g., nutrients) that support fundamental energy metabolism during this period of rapid growth results in more simplistic arbors, compromised neural circuits, and functions (Jorgenson et al., 2003; Carlson et al., 2009; Bastian et al., 2016).

Several key primary systems are rapidly developing in late fetal and early postnatal life and are at high risk for compromised development during periods of limited substrate availability (Thompson and Nelson, 2001). These primary systems include the hippocampus, myelination, and neurotransmitters, which mediate important primary functions such as recognition memory processing, speed of neural processing, and reward mediation, respectively. Their integrity is key to the neurodevelopmental functioning and advancement of the child (Wachs et al., 2014). However, they also serve as critical scaffolds for later developing systems that support much more complex behaviors such as working memory, reasoning, and attention. The frontal lobe, which is not rapidly developing in late fetal and early postnatal life, nevertheless is dependent on the fidelity of the developing systems mentioned earlier (Wachs et al., 2014). Thus, later-life frontal lobe dysfunction (e.g., ADHD) is a documented consequence of fetal/neonatal malnutrition (Strauss and Dietz, 1998).

## 6.3 Altered early-life nutrition and the cost to society

Nutrient deficiencies at any age, including the fetal and neonatal periods, have the potential to cause acute brain dysfunction. Nutrient repletion in many cases and particularly in the mature brain reverses the brain dysfunction, resulting in no long-term effects. However, nutrient deficiencies in the immature brain can result in brain dysfunction long after the period of deficiency and often despite relatively prompt diagnosis and treatment. An example of long-term effects of early nutrition deficits is the finding that intrauterine growth restriction (IUGR) reduces verbal fluency and overall IQ by seven points, while increasing the risk of ADHD and schizophrenia (Strauss and Dietz, 1998; Eide et al., 2013). Conversely, protein-calorie supplementation of undernourished populations during gestation and in the early postnatal period improves education, job, and social outcomes (Pollitt et al., 1995; Walker et al., 2007). Thus, the long-term effects are the true cost to society of early-life malnutrition in terms of lost productivity and increased mental health problems. One can easily understand how intergenerational poverty and mental health issues are perpetuated by chronic societal and individual malnutrition.

## 6.4 Nutrients and early brain development

All nutrients are important for cell development and function and therefore for brain development. However, certain nutrients have particularly large effects on early brain development, and these are often associated with long-term adult function (Table 6.1). The scientific literature is quite uneven with respect to the long-term effects of these nutrients. In particular, asynchrony can exist between preclinical models and human studies as well as between deficiency versus supplementation studies in humans. The data range from theoretical, that is, a good biological rationale exists but no effects are seen in models or in humans, to understudied at either the preclinical or human level, to wholly synchronous between preclinical models and human studies (Table 6.2).

Nutrient effects on the brain vary based on timing because the brain is a regionalized organ (Kretchmer et al., 1996). Brain regions and processes have unique developmental trajectories (Thompson and Nelson, 2001). Two factors need to be considered when assessing whether a nutrient will have an effect on a brain region. The first is to assess at which age(s) a nutrient is likely to be deficient. The second is to assess whether a given region or process has a requirement for that given nutrient at the age when the nutrient is likely to be in short supply. The intersection of these two factors determines the likely neurobehavioral phenotype, both acutely and long term.

The evidence for long-term effects may be found in preclinical models, human studies, or both. These nutrients can affect neuroanatomy, neurochemistry, and neurophysiology,

TABLE 6.1   Select nutrients with effects on early brain development and later childhood or adult function.

| Macronutrients | Vitamins/cofactors |
|---|---|
| • Protein/IUGR | • Choline |
| • Fats (LC-PUFAs) | • B vitamins (B6, B12) |
| | • Vitamin A |
| | • Vitamin D |

**Micronutrients**
- Iron
- Zinc
- Iodine

**TABLE 6.2**   Nutrients with preclinical evidence of epigenetic modifications affecting long-term brain development.

| Nutrient deficiency | Demonstrated or potential epigenetic mechanism |
| --- | --- |
| **Nutrients with long-lasting effects on brain development and preclinical evidence of epigenetic component** | |
| Protein (IUGR) | • Suppression of hippocampal DUSP5 via alterations to DNA CpG methylation and histone code<br>• Permanent changes to glucocorticoid resistance protein mRNA expression in hippocampus through glucocorticoid receptor's histone acetylation code |
| Iron | • DNA CpG methylation<br>• 5hmC DNA methylation driven by TET methylcytosine dioxygenases<br>• Alteration of histone H3 methylation, histone acetylation, and binding of transcription at the BDNF-IV promotor in the adult hippocampus following gestational/lactational iron deficiency |
| Choline | • Global and gene-specific DNA methylation in rodent brain<br>• Potential methyl donor in context of known long-term histone and DNA CpG methylation alterations induced by iron deficiency |
| B vitamins | • Modification of gene expression through DNA hypomethylation (folate, B12)<br>• Alteration of Stat3 signaling, including increased gene silencing by miR124 in the hippocampus<br>• Pattern change of brain genomic DNA methylation and miRNA activity affected by folate/B12 ratio in pregnancy |
| LC-PUFAs | • Hypermethylation of promotor regions of the nuclear receptor genes Rxr and Ppar, affecting myelin and neurotransmitter system genes<br>• Hypermethylation of BDNF |
| Vitamin A | • Early embryonic effects: Abnormal trimethylation of H3K27 histones that control HOX gene expression required for neural tube closure<br>• Later effects: Reduction of hypothalamic POMC DNA methylation, leading to reduced food intake, body weight and food reward behaviors |
| **Nutrients with long-lasting effects on brain development with plausible, but not demonstrated, epigenetic mechanism** | |
| Iodine | • Hypothyroidism may be associated with DNA methylation and decreases histone acetylation at the GFAP gene promotor with a consequent reduction in GFAP |
| Zinc | • Potential histone methylation and acetylation due to alteration of zinc-finger-containing, multivalent chromatin regulators, e.g., BRPF1. |
| **Nutrient with limited clinical evidence of long-lasting effects on brain development, but demonstrated, plausible epigenetic mechanism** | |
| Vitamin D | Alteration of DNA methylation status, e.g., reduction in aromatase activity involved in brain testosterone synthesis, potentially supporting the prenatal sex steroid theory of autism. |

all of which determine the functioning of the brain. Neuroanatomy includes not only neurons but also the supporting cells, for example, oligodendrocytes, astrocytes, and microglia. Deficiencies of nutrients that affect oxygen consumption rate or protein status will affect neuronal size, dendritic complexity, and synaptogenesis. Neurochemistry refers mostly to the synthesis and activity of neurotransmitters, including neurotransmitter concentrations, receptor density, and re-uptake mechanisms. Nutrients such as iron are crucial for maintaining neurochemical homeostasis, particularly in the monoaminergic (e.g., dopamine and serotonin) and glutamatergic systems (Beard et al., 2006). The brain functions by generating electrical potentials, a process that reflects neuronal metabolism. This neurophysiologic activity is highly metabolic and at risk from deficiencies of substrates (nutrients) that support oxidative metabolism, as well as micronutrients that mediate pre-synaptic neurotransmitter release (Jorgenson et al., 2005; Pisansky et al., 2013).

## 6.5 Mechanisms of long-term dysfunction

The mechanisms of long-term neurobehavioral dysfunction associated with early nutritional status have largely fallen into two, not-mutually exclusive, biological domains: disruption during critical periods of anatomic and functional development and epigenetic modification of synaptic plasticity genes and disease network pathways.

The critical period hypothesis states that interruption of neurodevelopment during a region's critical period of growth results in permanent structural damage to that region (Hensch, 2004). Neurobehavioral deficits result from this disordered regional neuronal structure. While this hypothesis sounds quite deterministic in terms of outcome, developmental cognitive neuroscientists stress that "hard stop" critical periods, as first exemplified in Hubel and Wiesel's experiments with ocular dominant columns (LeVay et al., 1980), are usually the exception in biology, and that many time-dependent developmental processes exhibit more of a sensitive period, rather than a critical period (Bornstein, 1989). Nevertheless, critical periods for certain nutrients during regional neurodevelopment do indeed exist. For example, a critical period for iron has been identified in hippocampal development (Fretham et al., 2012) where neuronal iron deficiency during the period of rapid postnatal growth results in long-term learning and memory deficits. Interesting recent work in the plasticity field is concentrating on whether critical periods can be reopened (Hensch, 2004).

Epigenetic mechanisms represent an exciting area of investigation that is particularly relevant to a number of nutrients (Table 6.2). The ability of nutrients to regulate gene expression through direct mechanisms (e.g., iron-containing histone demethylases) opens a wide array of possibilities for providing mechanisms for long-term effects and for therapeutic options. The developmental timing and permanence/reversibility of epigenetic marks of synaptic plasticity genes and gene networks by early-life nutrients are important areas of ongoing research, ultimately guiding the development of preventive strategies and interventions.

This chapter focuses on the role of early-life nutrition on brain development in humans and the potential epigenetic mechanisms of long-term programming of brain function discovered in preclinical models. Each nutrient that is discussed demonstrates the capacity to affect long-term brain health. A review of the entire literature of each nutrient's effect on each region of the brain is beyond the scope of this chapter. Instead, this chapter focuses on nutrients where clinical studies support the concept of DOHaD effect and where complementary preclinical model data provide evidence of epigenetic modification of chromatin in the brain. The epigenetic modifications that affect brain function alter the regulation of genes involved in synaptic plasticity/efficacy. These can be individual genes, for example, Brain Derived Neurotrophic Factor (BDNF), that have critical roles in neuronal differentiation during development and that are critical for maintenance of adult plasticity, or they can be whole networks of genes responsible for neurobehavioral performance and risk of psychopathology (Tran et al., 2015, 2016; Moody et al., 2017).

A review of all the ways chromatin can be epigenetically modified is also beyond the scope of this review. Instead, we concentrate on nutrients in early life that have been shown to affect the following brain epigenetic processes: DNA CpG methylation, DNA hydroxymethylation, histone methylation/demethylation, histone acetylation, and interfering mRNAs (miRNAs). Importantly, nutrients can induce one or multiple epigenetic processes during development that affect brain function in adulthood (Sable et al., 2014).

## 6.6 Nutrients associated with long-lasting brain outcomes

### 6.6.1 IUGR/protein

#### 6.6.1.1 Clinical studies

Prenatal and early childhood growth, particularly linear growth, which reflects total body protein accretion and thus growth of individual organs including the brain. It predicts school performance and cognition later in life (Miller et al., 2016; Perkins et al., 2017; Alam et al., 2020; Nahar et al., 2020). A growing body of work demonstrates that this linear growth must be supported by adequate maternal nutrition during pregnancy followed by sustained nutrition in the first postnatal year (Spinillo et al., 1993; Pongcharoen et al., 2012; Murray et al., 2015; Wang et al., 2016). Optimal nutritional intake during these periods sets the stage for optimal brain growth and development, while inadequate nutrition during either of these periods endangers that development even in the face of improved nutrition later in childhood.

The timing of this prenatal and first postnatal year is a sensitive period for linear growth, as a proxy for protein accretion has been identified by multiple studies. Growth failure in the fetal period is known as IUGR, often defined as fetal weight less than the 10th percentile for gestational age (Cusick and Georgieff, 2016). Children with IUGR have long-lasting cognitive deficits, including a fivefold greater chance of having poor neurodevelopmental outcomes, including lower verbal ability and novelty preference scores at 2 years of age compared to children without IUGR (Spinillo et al., 1993; Murray et al., 2015; Wang et al., 2016).

The period of vulnerability continues through the first year of life. Length at birth and during the first postnatal year was associated with a higher IQ score at 9 years of age among children living in Thailand, while no measure of growth after 12 months of age was associated with neurodevelopmental outcomes during school-aged years (Pongcharoen et al., 2012). Moreover, a recent analysis that combined data from six low-income countries in the Mal-Ed network revealed that the relationship between stunting (length-for-age Z score more than two standard deviations below the WHO growth standard) and cognition at 5 years of age may be dose-dependent (Nahar et al., 2020). Children who were stunted between 0 and 6 months of age and remained stunted for the first 5 years of life had significantly lower scores of cognitive development at 5 years of age, while no such relationship existed for children whose early stunting resolved or who had late-onset stunting.

A landmark study in Guatemala first demonstrated the critical role of early-life nutrition and protein intake in particular on later brain development (Pollitt et al., 1995). In this study, mothers and children in one village consumed a beverage containing protein and energy twice daily, while mothers and children in another village received a beverage containing energy alone. When assessed in adolescence, those children who had been exposed to the protein-containing beverage early in life had better scores on tests of general intellectual ability compared to children who were exposed to the drink containing energy alone.

A potential epigenetic mechanism affecting placental transport of nutrients may partially explain the relationship between maternal nutrition and fetal linear growth (Castillo-Castrejon et al., 2021). The recent Women First Preconception Maternal Nutrition Trial demonstrated that fetal growth, including linear growth, can be improved with maternal nutritional supplementation, either in the preconceptional period or late in the first trimester. Subsequent study of placental samples of women from Guatemala, where the mean pre-pregnancy BMI was 26.5 and women received preconceptional lipid-based supplementation, and from Pakistan, where the mean pre-pregnancy BMI was 19.8 and women received both lipid-based supplementation and protein supplementation, revealed that lipid-based supplementation activated mTOR and IGF signaling and was associated with improved fetal growth in Pakistani women only. A negative association between DNA methylation of the placental IGF1 gene promoter was found in Guatemalan, but not Pakistani, women and may explain the apparent lack of effect of additional supplementation in the Guatemalan mothers who entered pregnancy with a significantly higher BMI.

### 6.6.1.2 Preclinical studies of epigenetic alterations by IUGR

The effects of IUGR on the developing brain have been studied in multiple preclinical models, including mice, rats, pigs, sheep, and monkeys. IUGR is induced in a variety of ways, including overall nutrient restriction, protein restriction, uterine artery ligation, or maternal temperature manipulation. The evidence from this literature supports the DOHaD concept that early-life growth/nutrient restrictions alter adult brain function. The studies documenting specifically epigenetic mechanisms of the brain have primarily been performed in rodent (Ding and Cui, 2017; Desai et al., 2019) with both gene-specific and genome-wide effects (Grissom and Reyes, 2013; Ding and Cui, 2017; Desai et al., 2019).

IUGR induced by overall maternal nutrient restriction or uterine artery ligation cannot be considered a single nutrient deficiency. The experimental manipulation induces a broad range of nutrient deficiencies as well as inducing fetal stress, which also alters the epigenetic landscape of the brain (Ke et al., 2010, 2011, 2015). The hippocampus appears to be targeted by IUGR, likely because it is rapidly developing during the late fetal/early neonatal period in both humans and rodents. IUGR in rats suppresses brain expression of dual-specificity phosphatase 5 (DUSP5), an important regulator of the growth modulator Erk 1/2, via alterations to DNA CpG methylation and histone code (Ke et al., 2011, 2015). The stress effect of

IUGR on the developing hypothalamic-pituitary-adrenal stress axis is evident from permanent changes to the glucocorticoid receptor's histone acetylation code in the hippocampus, thereby changing the expression of glucocorticoid resistance protein mRNA (Ke et al., 2010).

From a therapeutic standpoint, a diet containing methyl donors has been proposed as a potential nutritional approach to normalize the epigenetic landscape in multiple nutrient deficiencies, including IUGR (Zeisel, 2017). For example, folic acid supplementation of IUGR rats reverses IUGR-induced upregulation of DNMT1 and GAP43 gene expression, returning them toward non-IUGR control values (Ding and Cui, 2017). As noted below, a similar rescue of iron deficiency epigenetic effects has been seen with time-targeted choline supplementation (discussed below).

## 6.6.2 Iron

### 6.6.2.1 Clinical studies

The essential role of iron in neurobehavioral development has been demonstrated by more than three decades of preclinical and clinical research that are remarkably aligned. Reduced metabolism of rodent hippocampal neurons is reflected by deficits in recognition memory in infants born with iron deficiency (Geng et al., 2015, 2020). Impaired neuronal myelination is likely reflected in the slower speed processing documented in infants with iron deficiency (Bastian et al., 2016), while alterations in dopaminergic signaling noted in preclinical models likely lead to changes in socioemotional behavior and more wary, hesitant toddlers (Lozoff et al., 2006; Santos et al., 2018). The fact that iron deficiency is the most common deficiency in the world, affecting nearly two-thirds of the world's children between 6 and 59 months (Walker et al., 2007), underscores the urgent need to address this worldwide burden so that all children can achieve their optimal neurodevelopmental trajectory.

The peak time of brain's need for iron is during the third trimester of pregnancy and the first postnatal year (Cusick and Georgieff, 2016). These are also the periods when dietary iron deficiency is most prevalent in much of the world. If iron is not sufficient during these times, long-lasting dysfunction can occur due to either architectural deficit, for example, impaired hippocampal neuronal metabolism leading to altered hippocampal structure and consequently altered structure of subsequent developing regions of the brain, or epigenetic modification, or both (Christian et al., 2010; Murray-Kolb et al., 2012; Geng et al., 2015, 2020).

Two series of studies in Nepal and China clearly demonstrate the importance of providing supplemental iron at the peak time of brain development for neurobehavioral benefit. And conversely, the lack of effect if iron is not sufficient during this critical window. In Nepal, children of mothers who had received iron prenatally through 12 weeks postpartum had significantly better scores of working memory, inhibitory control, and fine-motor functioning at 7 years of age, regardless of the child, him or herself, having received supplemental iron from 12 to 36 months of age (Christian et al., 2010, 2011). Iron supplementation of children whose mothers received no prenatal iron but who were supplemented themselves with iron from 18 to 36 months of age exhibited no improvement in neurobehavioral tasks at 7 months of age compared to children who were not supplemented themselves and whose mothers were not supplemented (Murray-Kolb et al., 2012).

In China, infants who were born iron-deficient demonstrated poorer recognition memory as measured by auditory-evoked event-related potentials, than non-iron-deficient children (Geng et al., 2015; Angulo-Barroso et al., 2016). However, children who received iron between 6 and 9 months of age had better gross motor scores, regardless of whether their mothers had received prenatal iron. This apparent contrast with the Nepal study exemplifies the importance of considering the timing of iron intervention in tandem with the appropriate brain region or functioning at that time. Motor development relies on cerebellar development, which precedes that of the motor cortex. Motor control shifts from the brainstem and mid-brain to the motor cortex around 3 to 4 months of postnatal age. Early infant, as opposed to maternal, supplementation with iron would directly affect this shift in motor control, as would myelination, which begins around 32 weeks' gestation and continues at a brisk pace during the first 2 years of postnatal life (Thompson and Nelson, 2001).

As with many nutrients, including protein, more iron than required is not necessarily beneficial and may even be harmful. Chilean infants who had been randomly assigned to high- or low-iron formula during infancy underwent neurobehavioral assessment at 10 years of age. Children who had high hemoglobin (> 12.8 g/dL) in infancy and were randomized to receive the high-iron formula had significantly poorer outcomes for spatial memory and visual-motor integration, while infants who had low hemoglobin (< 10.5 g/dL) had significantly better outcomes (Algarín et al., 2013).

### 6.6.2.2 Preclinical studies of epigenetic alterations by iron status

Studies in preclinical models support the DOHaD concept that early-life iron status influences adult brain function (Lozoff et al., 2006; Barks et al., 2019). Iron during gestational and early postnatal development is essential for proper myelination (Ortiz et al., 2004), monoamine neurotransmitter metabolism (Beard et al., 2006), and energy-dependent neuronal structural integrity (Carlson et al., 2009; Bastian et al., 2016). Iron must be supplied during critical periods of neurodevelopment to avoid long-term neurodevelopmental deficits (Fretham et al., 2012). Persistent consequences of early-life iron deficiency in adulthood include abnormal myelin gene expression (Clardy et al., 2006), monoamine neurotransmitter regulation (Unger et al., 2012), and neuronal structure (Carlson et al., 2009; Fretham et al., 2012; Kennedy et al., 2014), all leading to neurobehavioral deficits (Fretham et al., 2012; Unger et al., 2012; Kennedy et al., 2014).

Iron can potentially cause long-term effects by modifying the developing brain's epigenetic landscape through two direct mechanisms; iron-containing and iron-status-responsive histone demethylases named JARIDs (Sengoku and Yokoyama, 2011) and 5-hydroxymethylcytosine (5hmC) DNA methylation driven by TET methylcytosine dioxygenases, which enzymatically convert 5-methylcytosine (5mC) to 5hmC (Tahiliani et al., 2009) and belong to the class of iron- and α-ketoglutarate (αKG)-dependent oxygenases (Zhu et al., 2016). In addition, classic DNA CpG methylation is affected by iron deficiency, although it is unclear whether there is a direct iron-dependent mechanism involved. Gestational-lactational iron deficiency suppresses hippocampal BDNF, a gene susceptible to DNA CpG methylation, in adulthood (Tran et al., 2009) and alters DNA CpG methylation patterns in the developing hippocampus (Lien et al., 2019). Early-life iron deficiency programs adult genome-wide networks related to neural function and psychopathology including schizophrenia, autism, and Alzheimer's Disease

(Tran et al., 2016). Time-targeted supplementation with the methyl donor choline partially reverses the genomic and behavioral abnormalities, providing support for the hypothesis that these findings may be due to changes in the epigenetic landscape (Kennedy et al., 2014, 2018; Tran et al., 2016).

The effect of iron deficiency on histone status of specific genes (e.g., BDNF) that are important for neuronal differentiation during development and functional plasticity in adulthood has been explored in the rat hippocampus (Tran et al., 2015, 2016). Early-life iron deficiency alters histone H3 methylation at the BDNF-IV promotor in the adult hippocampus, largely through persistent increased enrichment of the repressive marks K27me3 and K4me1 accompanied by decreased enrichment of the activation mark K4me3. Histone acetylation and binding of transcription regulators are also reduced at the BDNF promotor site, resulting in overall less BDNF expression in adulthood despite complete restoration of iron status in the early postnatal period (Tran et al., 2015). Choline administration during the period of gestational iron deficiency partially reverses these suppressive effects (Tran et al., 2015, 2016). At the genome-wide level, pathway analysis demonstrates that pre-natal choline administration recovers expression of three Jumanji genes, HDAC, Jarid 1b, Histone H3 and H4, and RNA Polymerase II, suggesting that choline acts through an epigenetic mechanism (Tran et al., 2016).

Gestational-lactational iron deficiency also has a moderate effect on classic DNA CpG methylation status in the developing rat hippocampus, with 229 differentially methylated loci within 108 genes identified. The altered genes code for functional networks regulating neuronal development and cell-to-cell signaling (Lien et al., 2019). Whether these changes in the early postnatal period persist into adulthood has not been assessed. Nevertheless, similar iron deficiency-induced changes to DNA methylation status have been noted in a pig model, providing corroborative evidence of trans-species effects (Schachtschneider et al., 2016). No studies have explored whether 5hmc and iron-dependent TET activity are altered by gestational-lactational iron deficiency in the developing brain, but the question is of more than theoretical value since the brain is one of the most highly enriched organs for TET activity during development (Szulwach et al., 2011).

Overall, there is strong direct and indirect evidence that early-life iron status regulates the expression of critical neurodevelopmental genes and gene networks during development with effects that last into adulthood. Emerging evidence suggests it does so in part through multiple epigenetic processes in which iron is enzymatically involved. These genomic effects last into adulthood and are accompanied by biologically plausible neurobehavioral consequences that parallel neurobehavioral findings in iron-deficient children and adults that were iron deficient as children.

## 6.7 Choline and other methyl compounds

### 6.7.1 Choline

#### 6.7.1.1 Clinical studies

Preclinical literature has supported an integral role for choline in neurodevelopment for many years (see below), but its importance has only recently been demonstrated in clinical studies. Collectively, randomized clinical trials prenatal choline supplementation suggest that a higher dose and use of a more granular region- and/or function test, rather than a global test, are important considerations in designing a study and detecting an effect (Kable et al., 2015; Ross et al., 2016; Caudill et al., 2018; Derbyshire and Obeid, 2020). In a recent double-blind feeding/supplementation study, infants whose mothers received 930 mg rather than 480 mg of choline during the third trimester of pregnancy had faster reaction times throughout the first year of postnatal life (Bahnfleth et al., 2019). These children also performed significantly better on a color-location memory task at 7 years of age. Similarly, maternal supplementation with 900 mg choline and infant supplementation with 600 mg phosphatidylcholine showed better attention and less social withdrawal (Ross et al., 2013, 2016). Finally, 750 mg of prenatal choline improved infant inhibition at 6–12 months of age, but in pregnancies that were affected by alcohol exposure and those that were not (Kable et al., 2015).

The possibility that prenatal choline may ameliorate the hippocampal damage to the brain caused by fetal alcohol exposure is supported by a South African study that found that 6-month-old infants whose mothers were heavy drinkers but received 2 g of choline daily beginning in mid-pregnancy had better visual recognition memory (Jacobson et al., 2018). The benefit to the developing hippocampus with choline in the context of FASD is also evident when choline is given directly to the child. Daily supplementation with 500 mg choline for 9 months to children with FASD improved scores on hippocampally mediated memory tasks among children 2–3 years of age (Wozniak et al., 2015). These benefits persisted, and more emerged 4 years later, with these children exhibited better scores in working memory, nonverbal intelligence, and verbal memory and fewer symptoms of ADHD than children who had received placebo (Wozniak et al., 2020).

## 6.8 Preclinical studies of epigenetic alterations by choline status

Increasing evidence supports the hypothesis that choline plays an important part in the developing brain through epigenetic modifications (Zeisel, 2017). Choline supplementation of rodents during two critical time epochs in hippocampal development, mid-gestation, and postnatally during rapid hippocampal differentiation improves hippocampal structure, electrophysiology, biochemistry, and learning/memory behavior in normal, iron deficient, and fetal alcohol-exposed rats and in mice with genetic mutations that model Rett's Syndrome and Down Syndrome (Meck et al., 1988; Ryan et al., 2008; Moon et al., 2010; Ricceri et al., 2013; Kennedy et al., 2014). While most of these studies did not assess whether the rescue by choline was driven by epigenetic modifications, the fact that the effect was seen across different species and different conditions ranging from toxin exposure to nutrient deficiency to genetic mutations suggests that fundamental biology was being manipulated by choline (Zeisel, 2017). Choline supplementation during mid-gestation decreases global and gene-specific DNA methylation in the rodent brain (Niculescu et al., 2006). Choline's potential role as a methyl donor in the context of known long-term histone and DNA CpG methylation alterations induced by iron deficiency (see above) reinforces the possibility of epigenetic mechanisms at play. Ultimately, the finding that prenatal choline administration partially reverses long-term iron-deficiency-induced changes in histone demethylase regulated gene expression and behavior (see earlier section) lends further biological plausibility for the epigenetic potential of choline (Tran et al., 2015, 2016).

## 6.9 Other methyl compounds

### 6.9.1 B vitamins

#### *6.9.1.1 Clinical studies*

**Folate (B9)**

B vitamins play a critical role in brain development and are required for carbohydrate metabolism, the structure and function of membranes, and the formation of synapses (Prado and Dewey, 2014). The metabolism of folate (vitamin B9) includes multiple one-carbon transfers metabolism that supports purine and thymidine monophosphate biosynthesis and homocysteine remethylation (Naninck et al., 2019; Zheng and Cantley, 2019). Due to its key role in nucleic acid synthesis, folate is required for cell differentiation and proliferation. Deficiency of folate during early pregnancy is an established cause of neural tube defects, including anencephaly and spina bifida (De-Regil et al., 2015). Interventional studies of maternal supplementation and observational studies of maternal folate status or dietary intake and associations with later neurodevelopmental outcomes in early childhood, however, have had varying results (Veena et al., 2010; Campoy et al., 2011; Chatzi et al., 2012; Boeke et al., 2013; van Mil et al., 2014; Catena et al., 2016; Naninck et al., 2019). Structurally, poor prenatal folate status has detrimental effects on global brain development, including smaller total brain volume and predicted poorer performance on the language and visuospatial domains (Saber Cherif et al., 2019).

**Cobalamin (B12)**

Vitamin B12 is required for folate synthesis and serves as a critical cofactor for other enzyme systems. Children with B12 deficiency exhibit poor growth, delayed development, and anemia in observational studies, but relatively few randomized controlled trials of supplementation with B12 alone without other micronutrients have been conducted (Prado and Dewey, 2014). Some, but not all, studies have demonstrated that B12 supplementation of children at risk of B12 deficiency improves motor development (Torsvik et al., 2015; Strand et al., 2020), while 6 months of daily supplementation with B12 marginally improved neurodevelopment in a study of young North Indian children (Kvestad et al., 2015). However, in a large, randomized controlled trial of 600 marginally stunted Nepalese, daily supplementation of vitamin B12 for 1 year did not improve scores of global cognition, growth, or anemia (Strand et al., 2020).

## 6.10 Preclinical studies for folate and B12

The potential methyl donors, folate and B12, induce epigenetic changes in the brain. Folate deficiency in pregnancy is also hypothesized to modify gene expression through DNA hypomethylation, potentially causing long-term detrimental effects on brain development.

Folate supplementation of pregnant women during the second and third trimesters alters DNA methylation of genes related to brain development of their offspring (Caffrey et al., 2018). Like folate, B12 deficiency leads to hypomethylation of DNA. Preclinical models indicate that folate and vitamin B12 deficiencies alter Stat3 signaling, including increased gene silencing by miR124 in the hippocampus, potentially through reversible epigenetic marking (Kerek et al., 2013).

Micronutrients such as folate and B12 often work in concert to induce their effects. Offspring of rat dams exposed to variable deficiencies of folate and B12 during pregnancy exhibit hypomethylation of the brain at birth and hypermethylation in adulthood; findings that could be prevented by supplementation during pregnancy with LC-polyunsaturated fatty acids (LC-PUFAs) (Sable et al., 2014). The dietary ratio of folate and B12 during pregnancy alters the pattern of brain genomic DNA methylation and miRNA activity, with attendant alterations in brain gene expression patterns in the mouse fetus (Mahajan et al., 2019).

These findings illustrate the complexity of interpreting changes to the epigenetic landscape in the fetus and then projecting whether a long-lasting behavioral functional deficit will ensue. To address the critical question of whether maternal-fetal folate status influences the risk of brain dysfunction in adulthood through epigenetic mechanisms, Langie et al. induced folate deficiency in rodent dams and subsequently fed the offspring a high-fat diet to the offspring after weaning (Langie et al., 2013). The adult offspring exposed to this double insult had reduced DNA repair capacity in multiple brain regions accompanied by persistent changes in DNA methylation and DNA-repair gene expression. These brains showed an increased propensity to oxidative DNA damage as adults, which the authors interpreted as a risk for earlier degenerative brain disease. Similarly, adult offspring of mouse dams that were fed a diet low in vitamins B6, B9, and B12 during gestation and lactation had lower levels of hippocampal BDNF accompanied by alterations in the histone mark H3K9me2. The persistent changes in adult brain gene regulation and epigenetic marks were accompanied by significant sociability and social novelty preference behavioral abnormalities (Xu et al., 2021). These studies support the idea that the cost of early-life malnutrition is the life span effect on brain health and that permanent epigenetic marks induced during fetal/neonatal life may underlie those effects.

## 6.10.1 Polyunsaturated fatty acids

### 6.10.1.1 Clinical studies

Clinical studies have demonstrated that PUFAs, specifically the omega-3 fatty acid docosahexaenoic acid (DHA; 6n-3) and the omega-6 fatty acid arachidonic acid (AA; 20:4n-6), play a critical role in cortical visual acuity, signal transduction, brain connectivity, hippocampal development, and myelination of the developing brain (Das and Fams, 2003; Hadders-Algra, 2011; Scholtz et al., 2013; Carlson and Colombo, 2016). These PUFAS are transferred from the mother to the fetal brain primarily during the last trimester of pregnancy and to the infant through breastmilk (Das and Fams, 2003). The substantial amount of PUFAs in breastmilk prompted formula manufacturers in the United States to add DHA and AA to infant formulas beginning in 2001 (Scholtz et al., 2013).

The importance of PUFAS in brain development was first established three decades ago, with improved visual acuity, measured both electrophysiologically and behaviorally, observed in preterm infants who consumed formula supplemented with DHA and AA (Birch et al., 1992; Carlson et al., 1993; Uauy et al., 2001; Carlson and Colombo, 2016). Since then, scores of studies have tested the effect of supplementation with AA in DHA either prenatally or in infancy on neurobehavioral outcomes in infancy and later in childhood, with mixed results (Birch et al., 2010; Colombo et al., 2013; Carlson and Colombo, 2016). One reason for the discordant results may be differences in the time of the start of supplementation, dose, time of neurobehavioral assessment, for example, in infancy or later in childhood, and neurobehavioral test used as the outcome measure. Many studies use tests of global cognition, such as the Bayley Scales of Infant Development or the Mullen Scales, that may be too blunt to detect real differences in circuit-specific function (Verfuerden et al., 2020). By combining several studies with discordant ages, doses, and outcomes, meta-analyses typically compound the problem, most often leading to null results (Barnard et al., 2017).

A recent set of studies from the same group exemplifies the disparate results found with LCPUFA supplementation and later cognition (Colombo et al., 2013, 2019). The KUDOS study was a double-blind, randomized, placebo-controlled trial of 600 mg of daily prenatal DHA supplementation starting at 14.5 weeks' gestation until delivery (Colombo et al., 2019). Mothers who received DHA had fewer preterm births, and their children had improved attention throughout the first 10 months postnatally compared to mothers who received placebo, but prenatal DHA supplementation had no effect on any neurobehavioral outcomes from 10 months through 6 years of age.

However, in a separate study, supplementation of infants with formula containing LC-PUFAs results in no improvement in neurodevelopmental outcomes at 18 months of age, but children who consumed formula with DHA at 32% and 64% of total fatty acids scored significantly better from 3 to 5 years of age on tasks of rule learning and inhibition and on the Weschler Primary Preschool Scales of Intelligence at 6 years of age (Colombo et al., 2013).

## 6.11 Preclinical studies of epigenetic alterations by LC-PUFAs

Studies in preclinical models have long supported the DOHaD concept that early-life LC-PUFA, and perhaps more specifically DHA status, alters adult brain form and function. LC-PUFAs serve multiple functions during early brain development that, if disrupted, likely lead to long-term changes in brain structure. The effects have been particularly seen in the domains of myelination, dopamine neurotransmission, growth factor expression, behavior, and microglial activation (Das and Fams, 2003; Hadders-Algra, 2011; Scholtz et al., 2013; Carlson and Colombo, 2016). DHA is a major nutrient for the developing brain, affecting neuron development and function, as well as astrocyte and brain vasculature function (Basak et al., 2020).

More recent evidence has demonstrated that LC-PUFA status can influence the brain through epigenetic modifications that occur during development. The documented effects largely focus on methylation of the BDNF4 gene (Bhatia et al., 2011; Tyagi et al., 2015) and on genome-wide effects (Maekawa et al., 2017). Gestational deficiency of the two critical LC-PUFAs, AA and DHA, induces an adult schizophrenia phenotype in the mouse (Maekawa et al., 2017). Working memory function is compromised in this model, accompanied by downregulation of myelin integrity and GABA neurotransmission genes in the prefrontal cortex. The promotor regions of the nuclear receptor genes, Rxr and Ppar, which regulate these downstream myelin and neurotransmission system genes, are hypermethylated by the LC-PUFA deficiency, thereby causing the lower gene activity. Reversal of Rxr suppression ameliorates the downstream gene downregulation and restores the normal behavioral phenotype (Maekawa et al., 2017). These mechanistic studies are translatable to studies in humans that show that maternal undernutrition in pregnancy is associated with a higher risk of schizophrenia in the offspring. Specific epigenetic effects by LC-PUFAs on BDNF gene expression during development have also been demonstrated. LC-PUFA supplementation in early life has been shown to protect brain BDNF from hypermethylation and therefore lower expression by a westernized diet introduced in adult life (Tyagi et al., 2015).

### 6.11.1 Iodine and zinc

#### 6.11.1.1 Clinical studies

Whether several nutrients, including iodine and zinc, which are essential for optimal long-term brain development have epigenetic role in brain gene regulation is unclear. Iodine is critical to fetal and infant brain development due to its role in maternal thyroid hormones. Fetal production of T3 is entirely dependent on maternal T4 production in the first trimester and continues to be partially supported by maternal T4 throughout pregnancy (Skeaff, 2011). In areas where severe iodine deficiency is prevalent, iodine supplementation during pregnancy prevents severe iodine deficiency (cretinism) in the infant and improves neurobehavioral outcomes throughout childhood (Skeaff, 2011). Zinc supplementation improves motor development in some studies, but consistent results for either motor or cognitive outcomes have not been observed, either with maternal or child supplementation (Gogia and Sachdev, 2012; Nissensohn et al., 2013; Warthon-Medina et al., 2015). Zinc supplementation of 6-month-old infants in an area of Peru where zinc deficiency was prevalent was associated with better normative information processing and active attention at 12–18 months of age compared to infants who were not supplemented (Colombo et al., 2014) (Cannell, 2017).

## 6.12 Preclinical studies of epigenetic alterations by iodine and zinc

A search of the extant literature does not reveal studies of early-life zinc or iodine deficiency epigenetically targeting either specific neural plasticity genes (e.g., BDNF) or genome-wide networks of neural function or neuropathology. Nevertheless, a plausible epigenetic argument can be made for both.

Iodine is critical for the developing brain because of its role in thyroid hormone synthesis. Thyroid hormones, in turn, regulate multiple aspects of brain development by determining the rate of metabolism of growing cells, including neurons (Bernal, 2005) and astrocytes (Kumar et al., 2018). Glial fibrillary acidic protein (GFAP) indexes astrocyte maturation during neurodevelopment, and its transcriptional regulation is driven by thyroid hormone status via epigenetic mechanisms. Hypothyroidism, which is commonly due to dietary iodine deficiency, increases DNA methylation and decreases histone acetylation at the GFAP gene promotor with a consequent reduction in GFAP expression (Kumar et al., 2018). Structural and behavioral phenotypes induced by this type of epigenetically driven delay in maturation would depend on the timing of the hypothyroidism and, by analogy, of the iodine deficiency.

It has been recognized for over 50 years that zinc is critical for neurodevelopment. Preclinical rodent and monkey models demonstrate that zinc deficiency during fetal and postnatal development reduces brain DNA, RNA, and protein content (Sandstead, 1985), compromises myelination, and alters synaptic neurotransmission (Liu et al., 1992). The major neuronal growth factor, insulin-like growth factor I activity, is compromised by zinc deficiency (McNall et al., 1995). Short- and long-term behavioral abnormalities occur and do not appear to be amenable to postnatal zinc supplementation (Golub et al., 1994; Bhatnagar and Taneja, 2001). The irreversible long-term effects lead to the possibility that epigenetic mechanisms are at play.

DNA methylation is a dynamic process by which the activity is dictated in part by alterations in DNA binding affinity of transcription factors by this epigenetic process, thereby affecting gene transcription rates. Transcription factors with zinc finger DNA binding domains are targets of differential methylation, presenting the possibility that alterations in those binding domains due to zinc deficiency would alter the binding characteristics to target genes important for neurodevelopment, such as EGR1 (Banerjee et al., 2019). Similarly, modifications to histones such as methylation and acetylation may be at risk for zinc deficiency. These processes are dependent on multivalent chromatin regulators, such as BRPF1 (bromodomain- and plan homeodomain-linked PHD), which is a zinc finger-containing protein that both reads epigenetic marks and activates histone acetyltransferases. Fetal deficiency of BRPF1 causes abnormal expression of cortical development genes and significant neurobehavioral abnormalities (You et al., 2015). Zinc metalloenzymes and zinc finger proteins that are involved in DNA methylation and histone modifications are highly dependent on the integrity of their zinc-binding domains (Yusuf et al., 2021). A recent review describes the changes in expression and function of these proteins that can be induced by alterations in zinc status, including zinc deficiency (Yusuf et al., 2021). Although direct evidence implicating early-life dietary zinc deficiency in these potential zinc-dependent epigenetic mechanisms affecting long-term brain function is lacking, nutritional biology appears to strongly point to this area as an area of future research.

### 6.12.1 Vitamins A

#### 6.12.1.1 Clinical studies

Vitamin A and its derivatives are critical in normal embryonic development through regulation of gene expression and neural tube differentiation and patterning in the central nervous system (Tafti and Ghyselinck, 2007). Very few clinical studies link vitamin A supplementation or status specifically with brain outcomes in the child, although poorer vitamin A status has been linked with functioning of the adult brain, including poorer vitamin A status in patients with Alzheimer's disease (Rinaldi et al., 2003).

## 6.13 Preclinical studies of epigenetic effects of vitamin A

Vitamin A (retinol) plays a role in structural brain development, primarily signaling through the retinoic acid receptor and affecting stem cell differentiation into multiple brain cell types. The effects of too little or too much all-trans retinol are thought to occur in part through modulation of the epigenome (Yu et al., 2019). The neural tube, hypothalamus, and pre-frontal cortex are brain regions where vitamin A effects are particularly striking and cause long-term consequences (Sánchez-Hernández et al., 2014; Larsen et al., 2019; Yu et al., 2019). Excess retinol increases the risk of neural tube defects by causing abnormal expression of HOX genes that are critical for neural tube closure. This dysregulation of HOX gene expression during a critical period of neurulation has been shown to be due to retinol-induced abnormal trimethylation of H3K27 histones that control HOX gene expression (Yu et al., 2019). In time contrast to this early embryonic effect of vitamin A on brain epigenetics, later-timed changes in vitamin A status affect a different set of genes through epigenetic mechanisms. Pro-opiomelanocortin (POMC) gene expression in the hypothalamus is important in the regulation of food satiety. Its expression is sensitive to DNA methylation by a host of dietary factors, including vitamin A. Vitamin A supplementation in early postnatal life reduces hypothalamic POMC DNA methylation, leading to reduced food intake, body weight, and food reward behaviors across the lifespan (Sánchez-Hernández et al., 2014). More broadly, excessively high fat-soluble vitamin intake, including vitamins A and D administered during gestation/lactation, causes altered DNA methylation of hypothalamic POMC and hippocampal dopaminergic neurotransmission genes, thereby altering hedonic regulatory pathways implicated in food preference (Sánchez-Hernández et al., 2014).

## 6.13.1 Vitamin D

### 6.13.1.1 *Clinical studies*

Despite preclinical evidence of potential epigenetic mechanisms linking nutrient status to brain outcomes, long-term beneficial effects of vitamin D supplementation have not yet been clearly demonstrated. Some benefit in reducing the symptoms of autism and reducing the incidence of autism with supplementation of mothers already having at least one child with autism has been shown. However, outside of the context of autism, the results of observational studies of maternal or child vitamin D status and association with neurobehavioral outcomes later in childhood have been mixed (Whitehouse et al., 2012; McCarthy et al., 2018; Windham et al., 2019; Chowdhury et al., 2020; Mutua et al., 2020; Specht et al., 2020; Voltas et al., 2020; Melough et al., 2021), and to date, no randomized clinical trials of maternal supplementation with vitamin D have had neurobehavioral development as the primary outcome.

## 6.14 Preclinical studies of epigenetic effects of vitamin D

The effect of vitamin D nutrition during early life on brain development is an emerging subject of preclinical investigations because of epidemiologic associations of maternal vitamin D deficiency with significant developmental psychopathologies, like autism in the offspring. Multiple studies in preclinical models of developmental vitamin D deficiency show negative effects on adult behavior (Eyles et al., 2009; Kesby et al., 2017). While the number of studies exploring the potential of epigenetic modifications in the brain as an explanation for the long-term effects remains quite small, they do demonstrate the ability of vitamin D to alter long-term brain gene expression via alterations to DNA methylation status (Xue et al., 2016; Ali et al., 2020). For example, vitamin D deficiency during gestation hypermethylates the promoter of the aromatase gene involved in brain testosterone synthesis. The subsequent reduction in aromatase activity in the fetal brain results in excessive testosterone in male brains, potentially supporting the prenatal sex steroid theory of autism (Ali et al., 2020).

## 6.15  Conclusions

Many genetic and environmental factors influence brain development and ultimately influence adult brain function. Nutrients represent a class of environmental stimuli that are modifiable by public policy and personalized care. They are particularly critical for brain development in the first 1000 days, which in turn influences the trajectory of brain health across the lifespan. Thus, providing adequate nutrition, particularly by concentrating on nutrients with large effects on early brain development, represents a great opportunity to improve life quality for society. The mechanisms, including epigenetics, by which nutrients exert such a powerful influence on lifespan brain health are being elucidated. Determining the timing and mechanisms of the effects will provide future opportunities for targeted interventions, including nutritional manipulation of the epigenetic landscape of the brain, to promote the healthiest brain health trajectory possible.

## 6.16  Future trends and research

In future, better knowledge of the timing of nutritional deficiency and the corresponding brain region or structure affected, gleaned from developmentally appropriate preclinical models, will guide the selection and timing of appropriate nutrient dosing regimens. The goal will be to leverage knowledge about critical or sensitive periods of brain development to the nutrient to achieve maximal efficacy. Outcome measures of clinical studies aimed at determining whether repletion or supplementation of a given nutrient can improve neurobehavioral outcomes will also need to consider the critical and sensitive periods demonstrated for that nutrient. The assessments will need to index the functions of specific brain regions that were affected rather than relying on global metrics that lack the sensitivity to detect nutrient effects on the brain. These types of assessments, also termed bioindicators, would inform us of the physiologic effect that nutrient is having on the brain.

In the more distant future, an exciting possibility is that nutrients such as choline have the potential to restore brain form and function, potentially through reestablishing a healthy epigenetic landscape that had been negatively altered by a nutrient deficiency. There is great need for adjunct or alternative approaches because many nutrient deficiencies are not addressable in a timely manner, if at all. For example, the practice of screening for iron deficiency via hemoglobin concentration ignores the principle that anemia is the end-stage of the disease and that the brain has already been affected once anemia is diagnosed. The ability of choline, in preclinical models, to reverse the negative effects of iron deficiency anemia even at this late stage, holds promise if the information is translatable for children. This type of workaround solution may also work in situations where nutrient repletion is not feasible or is potentially dangerous, for example, iron therapy where malaria is endemic.

## Sources of additional information

Website for Developmental Origins of Health and Disease: International Society for Developmental Origins of Health and Disease: https://dohadsoc.org

American Academy of Pediatrics Policy Statement on Early Nutrition and Brain Development: Schwarzenberg SJ, Georgieff MK. (2018) Advocacy for improving nutrition in the first 1000 days to support childhood development and adult health. AAP Committee on Nutrition. Pediatrics 141:e20172716.

Review by former National Institutes of Mental Health Director Thomas R. Insel on developmental origins of psychopathology: Bale TL, Baram TZ, Brown AS, Goldstein JM, Insel TR, McCarthy MM, Nemeroff CB, Reyes TM, Simerly RB, Susser ES, Nestler EJ. (2010) Early life programming and neurodevelopmental disorders. Biol Psychiatry 68:314–319.

Review on the role of epigenetics in long-term neurobehavioral deficits: Georgieff MK, Tran PV, Carlson ES. (2018) Developmental origins of psychopathology: Mechanisms, processes and pathways linking the prenatal environment to postnatal outcomes. Development and Psychopathology 30:1063–1086.

Review on nutrition and brain development: Georgieff MK, Ramel SE, Cusick SE. (2018) Nutritional influences on brain development. Acta Paediatr. Aug;107(8):1310–1321. doi: https://doi.org/10.1111/apa.14287. Epub 2018 Mar 22.PMID: 29468731 Review.

## References

Alam, M.A., et al., 2020. Impact of early-onset persistent stunting on cognitive development at 5 years of age: results from a multi-country cohort study. PLoS One 15 (1). https://doi.org/10.1371/journal.pone.0227839, e0227839.

Algarín, C., et al., 2013. Iron-deficiency anemia in infancy and poorer cognitive inhibitory control at age 10 years. Dev. Med. Child Neurol. 55 (5), 453–458. https://doi.org/10.1111/dmcn.12118.

Ali, A.A., et al., 2020. Developmental vitamin D deficiency increases foetal exposure to testosterone. Mol. Autism. 11 (1), 96. https://doi.org/10.1186/s13229-020-00399-2.

Angulo-Barroso, R.M., et al., 2016. Iron supplementation in pregnancy or infancy and motor development: a randomized controlled trial. Pediatrics 137 (4). https://doi.org/10.1542/peds.2015-3547.

Bahnfleth, C., et al., 2019. Prenatal choline supplementation improves child color-location memory task performance at 7 Y of age (FS05-01-19)'. Curr. Dev. Nutr. 3 (Suppl 1). https://doi.org/10.1093/cdn/nzz052.FS05-01-19.

Banerjee, S., Wei, X., Xie, H., 2019. Recursive motif analyses identify brain epigenetic transcription regulatory modules. Comput. Struct. Biotechnol. J. 17, 507–515. https://doi.org/10.1016/j.csbj.2019.04.003.

Barks, A., et al., 2019. Iron as a model nutrient for understanding the nutritional origins of neuropsychiatric disease. Pediatr. Res. 85 (2), 176–182. https://doi.org/10.1038/s41390-018-0204-8.

Barnard, N.D., Willett, W.C., Ding, E.L., 2017. The misuse of meta-analysis in nutrition research. JAMA 318 (15), 1435–1436. https://doi.org/10.1001/jama.2017.12083.

Basak, S., Mallick, R., Duttaroy, A.K., 2020. Maternal docosahexaenoic acid status during pregnancy and its impact on infant neurodevelopment. Nutrients 12 (12). https://doi.org/10.3390/nu12123615.

Bastian, T.W., et al., 2016. Iron deficiency impairs developing hippocampal neuron gene expression, energy metabolism, and dendrite complexity. Dev. Neurosci. 38 (4), 264–276. https://doi.org/10.1159/000448514.

Beard, J.L., et al., 2006. Moderate iron deficiency in infancy: biology and behavior in young rats. Behav. Brain Res. 170 (2), 224–232. https://doi.org/10.1016/j.bbr.2006.02.024.

Bernal, J., 2005. Thyroid hormones and brain development. Vitam. Horm. 71, 95–122. https://doi.org/10.1016/S0083-6729(05)71004-9.

Bhatia, H.S., et al., 2011. Omega-3 fatty acid deficiency during brain maturation reduces neuronal and behavioral plasticity in adulthood. PLoS One 6 (12). https://doi.org/10.1371/journal.pone.0028451, e28451.

Bhatnagar, S., Taneja, S., 2001. Zinc and cognitive development. Br. J. Nutr. 85 (Suppl 2), S139–S145. https://doi.org/10.1079/bjn2000306.

Birch, E.E., et al., 1992. Dietary essential fatty acid supply and visual acuity development. Invest. Ophthalmol. Vis. Sci. 33 (11), 3242–3253.

Birch, E.E., et al., 2010. The DIAMOND (DHA intake and measurement of neural development) study: a double-masked, randomized controlled clinical trial of the maturation of infant visual acuity as a function of the dietary level of docosahexaenoic acid. Am. J. Clin. Nutr. 91 (4), 848–859. https://doi.org/10.3945/ajcn.2009.28557.

Boeke, C.E., et al., 2013. Choline intake during pregnancy and child cognition at age 7 years. Am. J. Epidemiol. 177 (12), 1338–1347. https://doi.org/10.1093/aje/kws395.

Bornstein, M.H., 1989. Sensitive periods in development: structural characteristics and causal interpretations. Psychol. Bull. 105 (2), 179–197. https://doi.org/10.1037/0033-2909.105.2.179.

Caffrey, A., et al., 2018. Gene-specific DNA methylation in newborns in response to folic acid supplementation during the second and third trimesters of pregnancy: epigenetic analysis from a randomized controlled trial. Am. J. Clin. Nutr. 107 (4), 566–575. https://doi.org/10.1093/ajcn/nqx069.

Campoy, C., et al., 2011. Effects of prenatal fish-oil and 5-methyltetrahydrofolate supplementation on cognitive development of children at 6.5 y of age. Am. J. Clin. Nutr. 94 (6 Suppl), 1880S–1888S. https://doi.org/10.3945/ajcn.110.001107.

Cannell, J.J., 2017. Vitamin D and autism, what's new? Rev. Endocr. Metab. Disord. 18 (2), 183–193. https://doi.org/10.1007/s11154-017-9409-0.

Carlson, S.E., Colombo, J., 2016. Docosahexaenoic acid and arachidonic acid nutrition in early development. Adv. Pediatr. 63 (1), 453–471. https://doi.org/10.1016/j.yapd.2016.04.011.

Carlson, S.E., et al., 1993. Visual-acuity development in healthy preterm infants: effect of marine-oil supplementation. Am. J. Clin. Nutr. 58 (1), 35–42. https://doi.org/10.1093/ajcn/58.1.35.

Carlson, S.E., et al., 2009. Iron is essential for neuron development and memory function in mouse hippocampus. J. Nutr. 139 (4), 672–679. https://doi.org/10.3945/jn.108.096354.

Castillo-Castrejon, M., et al., 2021. Preconceptional lipid-based nutrient supplementation in 2 low-resource countries results in distinctly different IGF-1/mTOR placental responses. J. Nutr. 151 (3), 556–569. https://doi.org/10.1093/jn/nxaa354.

Catena, A., et al., 2016. Folate and long-chain polyunsaturated fatty acid supplementation during pregnancy has long-term effects on the attention system of 8.5-y-old offspring: a randomized controlled trial. Am. J. Clin. Nutr. 103 (1), 115–127. https://doi.org/10.3945/ajcn.115.109108.

Caudill, M.A., et al., 2018. Maternal choline supplementation during the third trimester of pregnancy improves infant information processing speed: a randomized, double-blind, controlled feeding study. FASEB J. 32 (4), 2172–2180. https://doi.org/10.1096/fj.201700692RR.

Chatzi, L., et al., 2012. Effect of high doses of folic acid supplementation in early pregnancy on child neurodevelopment at 18 months of age: the mother-child cohort "Rhea" study in Crete, Greece. Public Health Nutr. 15 (9), 1728–1736. https://doi.org/10.1017/S1368980012000067.

Chowdhury, R., et al., 2020. Vitamin D status in early childhood is not associated with cognitive development and linear growth at 6-9 years of age in North Indian children: a cohort study. Nutr. J. 19 (1), 14. https://doi.org/10.1186/s12937-020-00530-2.

Christian, P., et al., 2010. Prenatal micronutrient supplementation and intellectual and motor function in early school-aged children in Nepal. JAMA 304 (24), 2716–2723. https://doi.org/10.1001/jama.2010.1861.

Christian, P., et al., 2011. Preschool iron-folic acid and zinc supplementation in children exposed to iron-folic acid in utero confers no added cognitive benefit in early school-age. J. Nutr. 141 (11), 2042–2048. https://doi.org/10.3945/jn.111.146480.

Clardy, S.L., et al., 2006. Acute and chronic effects of developmental iron deficiency on mRNA expression patterns in the brain. J. Neural Transm. Suppl. 71, 173–196. https://doi.org/10.1007/978-3-211-33328-0_19.

Colombo, J., et al., 2013. Long-term effects of LCPUFA supplementation on childhood cognitive outcomes. Am. J. Clin. Nutr. 98 (2), 403–412. https://doi.org/10.3945/ajcn.112.040766.

Colombo, J., et al., 2014. Zinc supplementation sustained normative neurodevelopment in a randomized, controlled trial of Peruvian infants aged 6-18 months. J. Nutr. 144 (8), 1298–1305. https://doi.org/10.3945/jn.113.189365.

Colombo, J., et al., 2019. The Kansas University DHA Outcomes Study (KUDOS) clinical trial: long-term behavioral follow-up of the effects of prenatal DHA supplementation. Am. J. Clin. Nutr. 109 (5), 1380–1392. https://doi.org/10.1093/ajcn/nqz018.

Cusick, S.E., Georgieff, M.K., 2016. The role of nutrition in brain development: the golden opportunity of the "first 1000 days". J. Pediatr. 175, 16–21. https://doi.org/10.1016/j.jpeds.2016.05.013.

Das, U.N., Fams, 2003. Long-chain polyunsaturated fatty acids in the growth and development of the brain and memory. Nutrition (Burbank, Los Angeles County, Calif.) 19 (1), 62–65. https://doi.org/10.1016/s0899-9007(02)00852-3.

Derbyshire, E., Obeid, R., 2020. Choline, neurological development and brain function: a systematic review focusing on the first 1000 days. Nutrients 12 (6). https://doi.org/10.3390/nu12061731.

De-Regil, L.M., et al., 2015. Effects and safety of periconceptional oral folate supplementation for preventing birth defects. Cochrane Database Syst. Rev. 12, CD007950. https://doi.org/10.1002/14651858.CD007950.pub3.

Desai, M., et al., 2019. Programmed epigenetic DNA methylation-mediated reduced neuroprogenitor cell proliferation and differentiation in small-for-gestational-age offspring. Neuroscience 412, 60–71. https://doi.org/10.1016/j.neuroscience.2019.05.044.

Ding, Y.-X., Cui, H., 2017. Integrated analysis of genome-wide DNA methylation and gene expression data provide a regulatory network in intrauterine growth restriction. Life Sci. 179, 60–65. https://doi.org/10.1016/j.lfs.2017.04.020.

Eide, M.G., et al., 2013. Degree of fetal growth restriction associated with schizophrenia risk in a national cohort. Psychol. Med. 43 (10), 2057–2066. https://doi.org/10.1017/S003329171200267X.

Eyles, D.W., et al., 2009. Developmental vitamin D deficiency causes abnormal brain development. Psychoneuroendocrinology 34 (Suppl 1), S247–S257. https://doi.org/10.1016/j.psyneuen.2009.04.015.

Fretham, S.J.B., et al., 2012. Temporal manipulation of transferrin-receptor-1-dependent iron uptake identifies a sensitive period in mouse hippocampal neurodevelopment. Hippocampus 22 (8), 1691–1702. https://doi.org/10.1002/hipo.22004.

Geng, F., et al., 2015. Impact of fetal-neonatal iron deficiency on recognition memory at 2 months of age. J. Pediatr. 167 (6), 1226–1232. https://doi.org/10.1016/j.jpeds.2015.08.035.

Geng, F., et al., 2020. Timing of iron deficiency and recognition memory in infancy. Nutr. Neurosci., 1–10. https://doi.org/10.1080/1028415X.2019.1704991.

Gluckman, P.D., Hanson, M.A., 2004. Living with the past: evolution, development, and patterns of disease. Science (New York, N.Y.) 305 (5691), 1733–1736. https://doi.org/10.1126/science.1095292.

Gogia, S., Sachdev, H.S., 2012. Zinc supplementation for mental and motor development in children. Cochrane Database Syst. Rev. 12, CD007991. https://doi.org/10.1002/14651858.CD007991.pub2.

Golub, M.S., et al., 1994. Modulation of behavioral performance of prepubertal monkeys by moderate dietary zinc deprivation. Am. J. Clin. Nutr. 60 (2), 238–243. https://doi.org/10.1093/ajcn/60.2.238.

Grissom, N.M., Reyes, T.M., 2013. Gestational overgrowth and undergrowth affect neurodevelopment: similarities and differences from behavior to epigenetics. Int. J. Dev. Neurosci. 31 (6), 406–414. https://doi.org/10.1016/j.ijdevneu.2012.11.006.

Hadders-Algra, M., 2011. Prenatal and early postnatal supplementation with long-chain polyunsaturated fatty acids: neurodevelopmental considerations. Am. J. Clin. Nutr. 94 (6 Suppl), 1874S–1879S. https://doi.org/10.3945/ajcn.110.001065.

Hensch, T.K., 2004. Critical period regulation. Annu. Rev. Neurosci. 27, 549–579. https://doi.org/10.1146/annurev.neuro.27.070203.144327.

Insel, B.J., et al., 2008. Maternal iron deficiency and the risk of schizophrenia in offspring. Arch. Gen. Psychiatry 65 (10), 1136–1144. https://doi.org/10.1001/archpsyc.65.10.1136.

Jacobson, S.W., et al., 2018. Efficacy of maternal choline supplementation during pregnancy in mitigating adverse effects of prenatal alcohol exposure on growth and cognitive function: a randomized, double-blind, placebo-controlled clinical trial. Alcohol. Clin. Exp. Res. 42 (7), 1327–1341. https://doi.org/10.1111/acer.13769.

Jorgenson, L.A., Wobken, J.D., Georgieff, M.K., 2003. Perinatal iron deficiency alters apical dendritic growth in hippocampal CA1 pyramidal neurons. Dev. Neurosci. 25 (6), 412–420. https://doi.org/10.1159/000075667.

Jorgenson, L.A., et al., 2005. Fetal iron deficiency disrupts the maturation of synaptic function and efficacy in area CA1 of the developing rat hippocampus. Hippocampus 15 (8), 1094–1102. https://doi.org/10.1002/hipo.20128.

Kable, J.A., et al., 2015. The impact of micronutrient supplementation in alcohol-exposed pregnancies on information processing skills in Ukrainian infants. Alcohol (Fayetteville, NY) 49 (7), 647–656. https://doi.org/10.1016/j.alcohol.2015.08.005.

Ke, X., et al., 2010. Intrauterine growth retardation affects expression and epigenetic characteristics of the rat hippocampal glucocorticoid receptor gene. Physiol. Genomics 42 (2), 177–189. https://doi.org/10.1152/physiolgenomics.00201.2009.

Ke, X., et al., 2011. Intrauterine growth restriction affects hippocampal dual specificity phosphatase 5 gene expression and epigenetic characteristics. Physiol. Genomics 43 (20), 1160–1169. https://doi.org/10.1152/physiolgenomics.00242.2010.

Ke, X., et al., 2015. IUGR increases chromatin-remodeling factor Brg1 expression and binding to GR exon 1.7 promoter in newborn male rat hippocampus. Am. J. Physiol. Regul. Integr. Comp. Physiol. 309 (2), R119–R127. https://doi.org/10.1152/ajpregu.00495.2014.

Kennedy, B.C., et al., 2014. Prenatal choline supplementation ameliorates the long-term neurobehavioral effects of fetal-neonatal iron deficiency in rats. J. Nutr. 144 (11), 1858–1865. https://doi.org/10.3945/jn.114.198739.

Kennedy, B.C., et al., 2018. Beneficial effects of postnatal choline supplementation on long-term neurocognitive deficit resulting from fetal-neonatal iron deficiency. Behav. Brain Res. 336, 40–43. https://doi.org/10.1016/j.bbr.2017.07.043.

Kerek, R., et al., 2013. Early methyl donor deficiency may induce persistent brain defects by reducing Stat3 signaling targeted by miR-124. Cell Death Dis. 4. https://doi.org/10.1038/cddis.2013.278, e755.

Kesby, J.P., et al., 2017. Developmental vitamin D deficiency alters multiple neurotransmitter systems in the neonatal rat brain. Int. J. Dev. Neurosci. 62, 1–7. https://doi.org/10.1016/j.ijdevneu.2017.07.002.

Kretchmer, N., Beard, J.L., Carlson, S., 1996. The role of nutrition in the development of normal cognition. Am. J. Clin. Nutr. 63 (6), 997S–1001S. https://doi.org/10.1093/ajcn/63.6.997.

Kumar, P., et al., 2018. Mechanisms involved in epigenetic down-regulation of Gfap under maternal hypothyroidism. Biochem. Biophys. Res. Commun. 502 (3), 375–381. https://doi.org/10.1016/j.bbrc.2018.05.173.

Kuzawa, C.W., 1998. Adipose tissue in human infancy and childhood: an evolutionary perspective. Am. J. Phys. Anthropol. (Suppl 27), 177–209. https://doi.org/10.1002/(sici)1096-8644(1998)107:27+<177::aid-ajpa7>3.0.co;2-b.

Kvestad, I., et al., 2015. Vitamin B12 and folic acid improve gross motor and problem-solving skills in young North Indian children: a randomized placebo-controlled trial. PLoS One 10 (6). https://doi.org/10.1371/journal.pone.0129915.

Langie, S.A.S., et al., 2013. Maternal folate depletion and high-fat feeding from weaning affects DNA methylation and DNA repair in brain of adult offspring. FASEB J. 27 (8), 3323–3334. https://doi.org/10.1096/fj.12-224121.

Larsen, R., et al., 2019. The thalamus regulates retinoic acid signaling and development of parvalbumin interneurons in postnatal mouse prefrontal cortex. eNeuro 6 (1). https://doi.org/10.1523/ENEURO.0018-19.2019.

LeVay, S., Wiesel, T.N., Hubel, D.H., 1980. The development of ocular dominance columns in normal and visually deprived monkeys. J. Comp. Neurol. 191 (1), 1–51. https://doi.org/10.1002/cne.901910102.

Lien, Y.-C., et al., 2019. Dysregulation of neuronal genes by fetal-neonatal iron deficiency anemia is associated with altered DNA methylation in the rat hippocampus. Nutrients 11 (5). https://doi.org/10.3390/nu11051191.

Liu, H., et al., 1992. Effects of maternal marginal zinc deficiency on myelin protein profiles in the suckling rat and infant rhesus monkey. Biol. Trace Elem. Res. 34 (1), 55–66. https://doi.org/10.1007/BF02783898.

Lozoff, B., et al., 2006. Long-lasting neural and behavioral effects of iron deficiency in infancy. Nutr. Rev. 64 (5 Pt 2), S34–S43. discussion S72-91 https://doi.org/10.1301/nr.2006.may.s34-s43.

Maekawa, M., et al., 2017. Polyunsaturated fatty acid deficiency during neurodevelopment in mice models the prodromal state of schizophrenia through epigenetic changes in nuclear receptor genes. Transl. Psychiatry 7 (9). https://doi.org/10.1038/tp.2017.182, e1229.

Mahajan, A., et al., 2019. Effect of imbalance in folate and vitamin B12 in maternal/parental diet on global methylation and regulatory miRNAs. Sci. Rep. 9 (1), 17602. https://doi.org/10.1038/s41598-019-54070-9.

McCarthy, E.K., et al., 2018. Antenatal vitamin D status is not associated with standard neurodevelopmental assessments at age 5 years in a well-characterized prospective maternal-infant cohort. J. Nutr. 148 (10), 1580–1586. https://doi.org/10.1093/jn/nxy150.

McNall, A.D., Etherton, T.D., Fosmire, G.J., 1995. The impaired growth induced by zinc deficiency in rats is associated with decreased expression of the hepatic insulin-like growth factor I and growth hormone receptor genes. J. Nutr. 125 (4), 874–879. https://doi.org/10.1093/jn/125.4.874.

Meck, W.H., Smith, R.A., Williams, C.L., 1988. Pre- and postnatal choline supplementation produces long-term facilitation of spatial memory. Dev. Psychobiol. 21 (4), 339–353. https://doi.org/10.1002/dev.420210405.

Melough, M.M., et al., 2021. Maternal plasma 25-hydroxyvitamin D during gestation is positively associated with neurocognitive development in offspring at age 4-6 years. J. Nutr. 151 (1), 132–139. https://doi.org/10.1093/jn/nxaa309.

Miller, S.L., Huppi, P.S., Mallard, C., 2016. The consequences of fetal growth restriction on brain structure and neurodevelopmental outcome. J. Physiol. 594 (4), 807–823. https://doi.org/10.1113/JP271402.

Moody, L., Chen, H., Pan, Y.-X., 2017. Early-life nutritional programming of cognition-the fundamental role of epigenetic mechanisms in mediating the relation between early-life environment and learning and memory process. Adv. Nutr. 8 (2), 337–350. https://doi.org/10.3945/an.116.014209.

Moon, J., et al., 2010. Perinatal choline supplementation improves cognitive functioning and emotion regulation in the Ts65Dn mouse model of down syndrome. Behav. Neurosci. 124 (3), 346–361. https://doi.org/10.1037/a0019590.

Murray, E., et al., 2015. Differential effect of intrauterine growth restriction on childhood neurodevelopment: a systematic review. BJOG Int. J. Obstet. Gynaecol. 122 (8), 1062–1072. https://doi.org/10.1111/1471-0528.13435.

Murray-Kolb, L.E., et al., 2012. Preschool micronutrient supplementation effects on intellectual and motor function in school-aged Nepalese children. Arch. Pediatr. Adolesc. Med. 166 (5), 404–410. https://doi.org/10.1001/archpediatrics.2012.37.

Mutua, A.M., et al., 2020. Vitamin D status is not associated with cognitive or motor function in pre-school Ugandan children. Nutrients 12 (6). https://doi.org/10.3390/nu12061662.

Nahar, B., et al., 2020. Early childhood development and stunting: findings from the MAL-ED birth cohort study in Bangladesh. Matern. Child Nutr. 16 (1). https://doi.org/10.1111/mcn.12864, e12864.

Naninck, E.F.G., Stijger, P.C., Brouwer-Brolsma, E.M., 2019. The importance of maternal folate status for brain development and function of offspring. Adv. Nutr. 10 (3), 502–519. https://doi.org/10.1093/advances/nmy120.

Niculescu, M.D., Craciunescu, C.N., Zeisel, S.H., 2006. Dietary choline deficiency alters global and gene-specific DNA methylation in the developing hippocampus of mouse fetal brains. FASEB J. 20 (1), 43–49. https://doi.org/10.1096/fj.05-4707com.

Nissensohn, M., et al., 2013. Effect of zinc intake on mental and motor development in infants: a meta-analysis. Int. J. Vitam. Nutr. Res. 83 (4), 203–215. https://doi.org/10.1024/0300-9831/a000161.

O'Donnell, K.J., Meaney, M.J., 2017. Fetal origins of mental health: the developmental origins of health and disease hypothesis. Am. J. Psychiatry 174 (4), 319–328. https://doi.org/10.1176/appi.ajp.2016.16020138.

Ortiz, E., et al., 2004. Effect of manipulation of iron storage, transport, or availability on myelin composition and brain iron content in three different animal models. J. Neurosci. Res. 77 (5), 681–689. https://doi.org/10.1002/jnr.20207.

Perkins, J.M., et al., 2017. Understanding the association between stunting and child development in low- and middle-income countries: next steps for research and intervention. Soc. Sci. Med. 193, 101–109. https://doi.org/10.1016/j.socscimed.2017.09.039. 1982.

Pisansky, M.T., et al., 2013. Iron deficiency with or without anemia impairs prepulse inhibition of the startle reflex. Hippocampus 23 (10), 952–962. https://doi.org/10.1002/hipo.22151.

Pollitt, E., et al., 1995. Nutrition in early life and the fulfillment of intellectual potential. J. Nutr. 125 (4 Suppl), 1111S–1118S. https://doi.org/10.1093/jn/125.suppl_4.1111S.

Pongcharoen, T., et al., 2012. Influence of prenatal and postnatal growth on intellectual functioning in school-aged children. Arch. Pediatr. Adolesc. Med. 166 (5), 411–416. https://doi.org/10.1001/archpediatrics.2011.1413.

Prado, E.L., Dewey, K.G., 2014. Nutrition and brain development in early life. Nutr. Rev. 72 (4), 267–284. https://doi.org/10.1111/nure.12102.

Ricceri, L., De Filippis, B., Laviola, G., 2013. Rett syndrome treatment in mouse models: searching for effective targets and strategies. Neuropharmacology 68, 106–115. https://doi.org/10.1016/j.neuropharm.2012.08.010.

Rinaldi, P., et al., 2003. Plasma antioxidants are similarly depleted in mild cognitive impairment and in Alzheimer's disease. Neurobiol. Aging 24 (7), 915–919. https://doi.org/10.1016/s0197-4580(03)00031-9.

Ross, R.G., et al., 2013. Perinatal choline effects on neonatal pathophysiology related to later schizophrenia risk. Am. J. Psychiatry 170 (3), 290–298. https://doi.org/10.1176/appi.ajp.2012.12070940.

Ross, R.G., et al., 2016. Perinatal phosphatidylcholine supplementation and early childhood behavior problems: evidence for CHRNA7 moderation. Am. J. Psychiatry 173 (5), 509–516. https://doi.org/10.1176/appi.ajp.2015.15091188.

Ryan, S.H., Williams, J.K., Thomas, J.D., 2008. Choline supplementation attenuates learning deficits associated with neonatal alcohol exposure in the rat: effects of varying the timing of choline administration. Brain Res. 1237, 91–100. https://doi.org/10.1016/j.brainres.2008.08.048.

Saber Cherif, L., et al., 2019. Methyl donor deficiency during gestation and lactation in the rat affects the expression of neuropeptides and related receptors in the hypothalamus. Int. J. Mol. Sci. 20 (20). https://doi.org/10.3390/ijms20205097.

Sable, P., et al., 2014. Maternal micronutrient imbalance alters gene expression of BDNF, NGF, TrkB and CREB in the offspring brain at an adult age. Int. J. Dev. Neurosci. 34, 24–32. https://doi.org/10.1016/j.ijdevneu.2014.01.003.

Sánchez-Hernández, D., et al., 2014. Increasing vitamin A in post-weaning diets reduces food intake and body weight and modifies gene expression in brains of male rats born to dams fed a high multivitamin diet. J. Nutr. Biochem. 25 (10), 991–996. https://doi.org/10.1016/j.jnutbio.2014.05.002.

Sandstead, H.H., 1985. W.O. Atwater memorial lecture. Zinc: essentiality for brain development and function. Nutr. Rev. 43 (5), 129–137. https://doi.org/10.1111/j.1753-4887.1985.tb06889.x.

Santos, D.C.C., et al., 2018. Timing, duration, and severity of iron deficiency in early development and motor outcomes at 9 months. Eur. J. Clin. Nutr. 72 (3), 332–341. https://doi.org/10.1038/s41430-017-0015-8.

Schachtschneider, K.M., et al., 2016. Impact of neonatal iron deficiency on hippocampal DNA methylation and gene transcription in a porcine biomedical model of cognitive development. BMC Genomics 17 (1), 856. https://doi.org/10.1186/s12864-016-3216-y.

Schmidt, R.J., et al., 2014. Maternal intake of supplemental iron and risk of autism spectrum disorder. Am. J. Epidemiol. 180 (9), 890–900. https://doi.org/10.1093/aje/kwu208.

Scholtz, S.A., Colombo, J., Carlson, S.E., 2013. Clinical overview of effects of dietary long-chain polyunsaturated fatty acids during the perinatal period. Nestle Nutr. Inst. Workshop Ser. 77, 145–154. https://doi.org/10.1159/000351397.

Sengoku, T., Yokoyama, S., 2011. Structural basis for histone H3 Lys 27 demethylation by UTX/KDM6A. Genes Dev. 25 (21), 2266–2277. https://doi.org/10.1101/gad.172296.111.

Skeaff, S.A., 2011. Iodine deficiency in pregnancy: the effect on neurodevelopment in the child. Nutrients 3 (2), 265–273. https://doi.org/10.3390/nu3020265.

Specht, I.O., et al., 2020. Neonatal vitamin D levels and cognitive ability in young adulthood. Eur. J. Nutr. 59 (5), 1919–1928. https://doi.org/10.1007/s00394-019-02042-0.

Spinillo, A., et al., 1993. Infant neurodevelopmental outcome in pregnancies complicated by gestational hypertension and intra-uterine growth retardation. J. Perinat. Med. 21 (3), 195–203. https://doi.org/10.1515/jpme.1993.21.3.195.

Strand, T.A., et al., 2020. Effects of vitamin B12 supplementation on neurodevelopment and growth in Nepalese infants: a randomized controlled trial. PLoS Med. 17 (12). https://doi.org/10.1371/journal.pmed.1003430, e1003430.

Strauss, R.S., Dietz, W.H., 1998. Growth and development of term children born with low birth weight: effects of genetic and environmental factors. J. Pediatr. 133 (1), 67–72. https://doi.org/10.1016/s0022-3476(98)70180-5.

Szulwach, K.E., et al., 2011. 5-hmC-mediated epigenetic dynamics during postnatal neurodevelopment and aging. Nat. Neurosci. 14 (12), 1607–1616. https://doi.org/10.1038/nn.2959.

Tafti, M., Ghyselinck, N.B., 2007. Functional implication of the vitamin A signaling pathway in the brain. Arch. Neurol. 64 (12), 1706. https://doi.org/10.1001/archneur.64.12.1706.

Tahiliani, M., et al., 2009. Conversion of 5-methylcytosine to 5-hydroxymethylcytosine in mammalian DNA by MLL partner TET1. Science (New York, N.Y.) 324 (5929), 930–935. https://doi.org/10.1126/science.1170116.

Thompson, R.A., Nelson, C.A., 2001. Developmental science and the media. Early brain development. Am. Psychol. 56 (1), 5–15. https://doi.org/10.1037/0003-066x.56.1.5.

Torsvik, I.K., et al., 2015. Motor development related to duration of exclusive breastfeeding, B vitamin status and B12 supplementation in infants with a birth weight between 2000-3000 g, results from a randomized intervention trial. BMC Pediatr. 15, 218. https://doi.org/10.1186/s12887-015-0533-2.

Tran, P.V., et al., 2009. Long-term reduction of hippocampal brain-derived neurotrophic factor activity after fetal-neonatal iron deficiency in adult rats. Pediatr. Res. 65 (5), 493–498. https://doi.org/10.1203/PDR.0b013e31819d90a1.

Tran, P.V., et al., 2015. Fetal iron deficiency induces chromatin remodeling at the Bdnf locus in adult rat hippocampus. Am. J. Physiol. Regul. Integr. Comp. Physiol. 308 (4), R276–R282. https://doi.org/10.1152/ajpregu.00429.2014.

Tran, P.V., et al., 2016. Prenatal choline supplementation diminishes early-life Iron deficiency-induced reprogramming of molecular networks associated with behavioral abnormalities in the adult rat Hippocampus. J. Nutr. 146 (3), 484–493. https://doi.org/10.3945/jn.115.227561.

Tyagi, E., et al., 2015. Interactive actions of Bdnf methylation and cell metabolism for building neural resilience under the influence of diet. Neurobiol. Dis. 73, 307–318. https://doi.org/10.1016/j.nbd.2014.09.014.

Uauy, R., et al., 2001. Essential fatty acids in visual and brain development. Lipids 36 (9), 885–895. https://doi.org/10.1007/s11745-001-0798-1.

Unger, E.L., et al., 2012. Behavior and monoamine deficits in prenatal and perinatal iron deficiency are not corrected by early postnatal moderate-iron or high-iron diets in rats. J. Nutr. 142 (11), 2040–2049. https://doi.org/10.3945/jn.112.162198.

van Mil, N.H., et al., 2014. Determinants of maternal pregnancy one-carbon metabolism and newborn human DNA methylation profiles. Reproduction (Cambridge, England) 148 (6), 581–592. https://doi.org/10.1530/REP-14-0260.

Veena, S.R., et al., 2010. Higher maternal plasma folate but not vitamin B-12 concentrations during pregnancy are associated with better cognitive function scores in 9- to 10- year-old children in South India. J. Nutr. 140 (5), 1014–1022. https://doi.org/10.3945/jn.109.118075.

Verfuerden, M.L., et al., 2020. Effect of long-chain polyunsaturated fatty acids in infant formula on long-term cognitive function in childhood: a systematic review and meta-analysis of randomised controlled trials. PLoS One 15 (11). https://doi.org/10.1371/journal.pone.0241800, e0241800.

Voltas, N., et al., 2020. Effect of vitamin D status during pregnancy on infant neurodevelopment: the ECLIPSES study. Nutrients 12 (10). https://doi.org/10.3390/nu12103196.

Wachs, T.D., et al., 2014. Issues in the timing of integrated early interventions: contributions from nutrition, neuroscience, and psychological research. Ann. N. Y. Acad. Sci. 1308, 89–106. https://doi.org/10.1111/nyas.12314.

Walker, S.P., et al., 2007. Child development: risk factors for adverse outcomes in developing countries. Lancet (London, England) 369 (9556), 145–157. https://doi.org/10.1016/S0140-6736(07)60076-2.

Wang, Y., Fu, W., Liu, J., 2016. Neurodevelopment in children with intrauterine growth restriction: adverse effects and interventions. J. Matern. Fetal. Neonatal. Med. 29 (4), 660–668. https://doi.org/10.3109/14767058.2015.1015417.

Warthon-Medina, M., et al., 2015. Zinc intake, status and indices of cognitive function in adults and children: a systematic review and meta-analysis. Eur. J. Clin. Nutr. 69 (6), 649–661. https://doi.org/10.1038/ejcn.2015.60.

Whitehouse, A.J.O., et al., 2012. Maternal serum vitamin D levels during pregnancy and offspring neurocognitive development. Pediatrics 129 (3), 485–493. https://doi.org/10.1542/peds.2011-2644.

Windham, G.C., et al., 2019. Newborn vitamin D levels in relation to autism spectrum disorders and intellectual disability: a case-control study in California. Autism Res. 12 (6), 989–998. https://doi.org/10.1002/aur.2092.

Wozniak, J.R., et al., 2015. Choline supplementation in children with fetal alcohol spectrum disorders: a randomized, double-blind, placebo-controlled trial. Am. J. Clin. Nutr. 102 (5), 1113–1125. https://doi.org/10.3945/ajcn.114.099168.

Wozniak, J.R., et al., 2020. Four-year follow-up of a randomized controlled trial of choline for neurodevelopment in fetal alcohol spectrum disorder. J. Neurodev. Disord. 12 (1), 9. https://doi.org/10.1186/s11689-020-09312-7.

Xu, P., et al., 2021. Behavioral changes and brain epigenetic alterations induced by maternal deficiencies of B vitamins in a mouse model. Psychopharmacology (Berl) 238 (4), 1213–1222. https://doi.org/10.1007/s00213-021-05766-2.

Xue, J., et al., 2016. Maternal vitamin D depletion alters DNA methylation at imprinted loci in multiple generations. Clin. Epigenetics 8, 107. https://doi.org/10.1186/s13148-016-0276-4.

You, L., et al., 2015. Deficiency of the chromatin regulator BRPF1 causes abnormal brain development. J. Biol. Chem. 290 (11), 7114–7129. https://doi.org/10.1074/jbc.M114.635250.

Yu, J., et al., 2019. Reduced H3K27me3 leads to abnormal Hox gene expression in neural tube defects. Epigenetics Chromatin 12 (1), 76. https://doi.org/10.1186/s13072-019-0318-1.

Yusuf, A.P., et al., 2021. Zinc metalloproteins in epigenetics and their crosstalk. Life (Basel, Switzerland) 11 (3). https://doi.org/10.3390/life11030186.

Zeisel, S., 2017. Choline, other methyl-donors and epigenetics. Nutrients 9 (5). https://doi.org/10.3390/nu9050445.

Zheng, Y., Cantley, L.C., 2019. Toward a better understanding of folate metabolism in health and disease. J. Exp. Med. 216 (2), 253–266. https://doi.org/10.1084/jem.20181965.

Zhu, X., et al., 2016. Role of Tet1/3 genes and chromatin remodeling genes in cerebellar circuit formation. Neuron 89 (1), 100–112. https://doi.org/10.1016/j.neuron.2015.11.030.

# Effects of infant allergen/immunogen exposure on long-term health outcomes

*Doerthe A. Andreae[a] and Anna Nowak-Wegrzyn[b,c]*

[a]Allergy and Immunology, Department of Dermatology, University of Utah, Salt Lake City, UT, United States [b]Allergy and Immunology, Department of Pediatrics, NYU Grossman School of Medicine, Hassenfeld Children, New York, NY, United States [c]Department of Pediatrics, Gastroenterology and Nutrition, Collegium Medicum, University of Warmia and Mazury, Olsztyn, Poland

## CHAPTER LEARNING OBJECTIVES: LIST 3–5 LEARNING OBJECTIVES FOR ACADEMIC USE OF CHAPTER

(1) To describe the environmental risk factors for development of atopic disease

(2) To compare strategies for prevention of food allergy

(3) To identify the long-term health effects of dietary factors in infancy and early childhood

## 7.1 Introduction

Allergic diseases (asthma, food allergy, atopic dermatitis (AD), and allergic rhinitis) are the sixth leading cause of chronic diseases in the US Asthma costs the US economy more than $80 billion annually in medical expenses, missed work and school days, and deaths (Nurmagambetov et al., 2018; Nurmagambetov and Krishnan, 2019). Food allergy annual cost is estimated at $24 billion, whereas AD and allergic rhinitis cost approximately $5 billion each. Asthma and food allergy can result in acute reactions leading to fatalities. The prevalence of allergic diseases has increased in the United States over the past two decades, indicating the importance of the modifiable environmental factors exerting epigenetic effects over the hereditary predisposition to produce immunoglobulin E (IgE) antibodies (atopy). The presence of atopy in early childhood has broad and long-lasting implications that impact health far beyond the early years.

Childhood AD has increased worldwide, and the International Study of Asthma and Allergies in Childhood estimates a prevalence from 0.9% to 22% in children aged 6 to 7 years (Odhiambo et al., 2009; Williams et al., 2008). It has been described that atopy early in life, usually manifested as AD, will progress to other diseases of the atopic family, termed the atopic march. A population-based birth cohort showed that manifestation of AD before 1.5 years of age was associated with persistent wheezing by 6 years of age (Stern et al., 2008). Similarly, the presence of AD in infancy has been linked to the presence of allergic rhinitis by the age of 12 years (Ballardini et al., 2014). Over the past decades, the prevalence of food allergies has continued to rise, and food allergies now represent a major public health problem (Jones and Burks, 2017). A recent cross-sectional survey study of US adults estimated that 10.8% of adults report to be food allergic (Gupta et al., 2019), while parent-reported food allergy in the pediatric population was 1 in 12 (Gupta et al., 2018). Clinical food allergy confirmed by oral food challenges was seen in 10% of the infants in a large trial in Australia (Osborne et al., 2011). As seen with other atopic diseases, the prevalence of food allergy continues to increase. Genetic factors alone cannot explain the significant and continued increase in food allergy prevalence in both pediatric and adult children. Additional factors, mainly environmental, are being considered and investigated. As this significant increase in food allergy prevalence has been more pronounced in western countries and urban settings, the investigation of contributing factors might help develop targeted interventions to prevent the development of food allergies early in life (Allen and Koplin, 2019). A clear understanding of the differences in environmental exposures, especially in early life, in children with and without food allergies is paramount to develop strategies for primary prevention. In this chapter, we will review allergen/immunogen exposure in infancy and early childhood with a focus on the development of allergic diseases as well as their impact on other areas of health and well-being.

## 7.2 Mechanisms of sensitization and tolerance to proteins, and timing of introduction of food allergens

### 7.2.1 Distinction between immunogenic and allergenic chemicals and molecules

To discuss the concept of food introduction and development of tolerance versus allergy, a definition of the terms immunogenic and allergic proteins and molecules are important. Proteins and molecules that are immunogenic stimulate the cellular and/or humoral immune system and elicit specific immune responses like lymphocyte proliferation and antibody production. Allergenic proteins and molecules also stimulate the immune system and lead to lymphocyte proliferation and antibody production, however, restricted to pathological allergic responses. The pathological response to food proteins and molecules can be classified into three categories. The categories are based on the role of the IgE antibody. Immediate, IgE-mediated allergic reactions are classified as Type I hypersensitivity reactions. The mechanisms underlying type I hypersensitivity reactions have been extensively studied and are well understood. IgE-mediated food allergy is a classic representative of IgE-mediated atopic diseases (Sicherer and Sampson, 2018; Lopes and Sicherer, 2020). Food allergies with cell-mediated, non-IgE-mediated mechanisms include Food Protein-Induced Enterocolitis Syndrome,

Food Protein-Induced Allergic Proctocolitis, and Food Protein-Induced Enteropathy. These non-IgE-mediated food allergies are often exclusively or predominantly affecting the GI tract (Caubet et al., 2017). A combination of IgE-mediated and cell-mediated mechanisms in food-related atopic diseases can be seen in AD and Eosinophilic Esophagitis (EoE) (Tham and Leung, 2019; Sugita and Akdis, 2020; Davis and Rothenberg, 2016). A summary of atopic diseases presenting as food allergies and sensitivities can be found in Table 7.1.

The complex mechanisms at play that prevent the development of food sensitization and allergy and lead to permanent oral tolerance are remarkable, especially in the light of near constant exposure to allergens starting at birth.

### 7.2.2 Oral tolerance

Oral tolerance to food proteins was first described over 100 years ago by Wells and Osborne. Their experiments showed that guinea pigs did not develop anaphylaxis to proteins that were present in their diet in large amounts (Wells and Osborne, 1911). These experiments have paved the way for the understanding and definition of oral tolerance. The body, specifically the gastrointestinal system, is constantly exposed to proteins, both self and foreign. The differentiation between harmful foreign and innocuous foreign proteins is paramount for the well-being and survival of the organism. Oral tolerance was defined by Chase in 1946 as the active inhibition of immune responses to antigens that have been ingested previously (Chase, 1946). It characterizes the non-responsiveness of the organism, specifically in the gut-associated lymphoid tissue to non-harmful foreign proteins (Shu et al., 2019). Over the past decade, increasing understanding of the development of oral tolerance has informed clinical trials aiming to achieve sustained unresponsiveness to innocuous foreign proteins that had elicited an allergic reaction in an organism.

Ingested food antigens are digested into proteins and amino acids with the help of mechanical force and digestive enzymes (Gan et al., 2018). This degradation of the ingested antigens in combination with the presence of a physical barrier between the gastrointestinal lumen and the bloodstream is contributing to oral tolerance of foreign proteins and antigens (Chehade and Mayer, 2005). Multiple types of immune cells are found in the single epithelial cell layer, most importantly T effector and regulatory cells, B cells, γδ T cells, phagocytes, and antigen-presenting cells that contribute to recognition and clearance of antigens in the intestinal system. Within minutes after ingestion, the food antigens are detected in the epithelium and lamina propria (LP) (Goubier et al., 2008). It has been recognized that the immune system is constantly surveying for unknown molecules, and the development of oral tolerance involves both humoral and cellular mechanisms. CD103$^+$ dendritic cells (DCs) are residing in LP and Peyer's patches from where they engage in active sampling and capturing of food antigens (Schulz et al., 2009) and transport into mesenteric lymph nodes where they are presented to antigen-specific regulatory CD4$^+$ T-cells. A model of step-wise induction of oral tolerance has been proposed by Hadis and colleagues in 2011 (Hadis et al., 2011) with regulatory T lymphocytes (Tregs) developing in the mesenteric lymph nodes followed by migration into the gut and local expansion. CD103$^+$ DC induce Tregs (iTregs) by a mechanism dependent on TGF-β, retinoic acid, and indoleamine-2,3-dioxygenase (IDO), and IL-10 (which are produced by CD103$^+$ DC). This mechanism is assumed to be critical in contributing to the development of tolerance in mesenteric lymph nodes (Coombes et al., 2007). The activated

**TABLE 7.1**    Summary of atopic diseases.

| | Characteristic presentation | Mechanism/pathogenesis | Diagnosis |
|---|---|---|---|
| Atopic dermatitis | Pruritic, relapsing eczematous dermatitis<br>Typically affected areas:<br>• Infancy: scalp, cheeks, trunk, and extremities<br>• Early childhood: flexural areas<br>• Adolescence and adulthood: hands and feet (Simon et al., 2019) | *Mixed IgE/non-IgE mediated*<br>Multifactorial<br>• Skin barrier dysfunction<br>• Environmental factors<br>• Genetic predisposition<br>• Immune dysfunction<br>Key mechanism: compromise to integrity of skin barrier, crucial role of fillaggrin in stratum corneum structure and formation<br>Traditional view: imbalance of T cells, mainly T helper cell types 1, 2, 17, and 22 as well as regulatory T cells (Guttman-Yassky et al., 2017) | Visual inspection of the skin, clinical history including family history and triggering factors |
| IgE-mediated food allergy | Acute cutaneous (urticarial), respiratory (wheezing, coughing, and throat tightness), gastrointestinal (vomiting and diarrhea), and cardiovascular (hypotension) symptoms. | IgE-mediated<br>Cross-linking of IgE molecules results in mediator release from mast cells and basophils | • Skin testing<br>• Specific IgE testing<br>• Component testing<br>• Gold standard is oral food challenge |
| Proctocolitis | Chronic inflammatory response and macroscopic bleeding of the rectum and distal colon<br>– Food protein-induced proctitis/proctocolitis (affecting rectum and colon)<br>– Food protein-induced enteropathy (affecting the small bowl)<br>– Food protein-induced enterocolitis syndrome (affecting the entire gastrointestinal tract) | *Non-IgE mediated*<br>Mechanism not known | Symptoms usually resolve within 3 days when the causing allergen is removed from the infant's or the mother's (for breastfed infants) diet |
| Food protein-induced enterocolitis syndrome | Projectile and repetitive vomiting with onset in 1–3 h following food ingestion; in a chronic form, diarrhea, intermittent vomiting, and arrested body weight gain, leading to dehydration and hypotension, and even lethargy and shock. | *Non-IgE mediated*<br>Considered to be T-cell mediated but role of T-cells unclear; involvement of proinflammatory cytokines linked TNF-α that alter gut permeability and a decrease in regulatory TGF-β. Humoral mechanisms contributing with changes in specific antibodies and a decrease in specific IgG4. | Improves with intravenous fluids, condition disappears when the causal protein has been eliminated from the diet. |
| Eosinophilic esophagitis | Abdominal pain, nausea, vomiting, regurgitation, food impaction, chest pain, slow eating, preference for soft food textures, and failure to thrive | Non-IgE-mediated<br>T-cell-mediated immune response including proinflammatory mediators and chemoattractants (IL-4, IL-5, and IL-13) that regulate eosinophilic Te | Trial of proton pump inhibitors, esophagoscopy with biopsy |

| Management | Prevalence | Long-term consequences |
| --- | --- | --- |
| • Skin care to repair and preserve healthy barrier using moisturizer and emollients<br>• Topical control of skin inflammation using topical steroids or topical calcineurin inhibitors<br>• Control of pruritus<br>• Managing infections including bacterial superinfection or eczema herpeticum | Pediatric prevalence 10%–20% (Silverberg et al., 2021) | • Bacterial superinfections<br>• Food sensitizations<br>• Impaired quality of life<br>• Impaired sleep<br>• Impaired school performance (Roduit et al., 2017) |
| • Avoidance<br>• Peanut oral immunotherapy<br>• Clinical trials investigating oral and sublingual immunotherapy for additional foods | Pediatric prevalence 8% (Rona et al., 2007; Sicherer and Sampson, 2018)<br>Adult prevalence 5% (Sicherer and Sampson, 2018) | – Limited diet with many nutritional, social, and psychological consequences<br>– Risk of severe reactions |
| Avoidance of the causative allergen | Not established | Reintroduction of milk is successful in 50% of 6 months old and reaches 95% at the age of 9 months. Subsequent development of IgE-mediated food allergy is very rare |
| Avoidance of triggers, rechallenge 18–24 months after last reaction, IV fluids for acute reactions | 15.4/100.000 children (Nowak-Wegrzyn and Spergel, 2017) | Usually outgrown by 3 years of age, but some cases persist into teenage years. |
| Diet: elemental formula or 6–7 food elimination diet, or targeted elimination diet<br>Drugs: no FDA approved treatments are available, systemic or topical corticosteroids, immunomodulators, biologics (anti IL-5)<br>Dilatation: for esophageal stricture | Prevalence 0.05%–0.1% | Nutritional consequences (failure to thrive, nutritional deficits), esophageal changes (remodeling, strictures, fibrosis) |

I. Nutrition in early life: Mechanisms and impact on long term health

and differentiated T-cells upregulate gut homing molecules like α4β7 and the chemokine receptor 9 (CCR9), which results in their return to the LP (Johansson-Lindbom et al., 2005). Gut-homing iTregs are expanded in the LP by $CX3CR1^+$ macrophages expressing IL-10. These iTregs contribute to the antigen-specific suppression of systemic immune responses, including allergic sensitization.

Food allergy and celiac disease are the most prevalent examples of a breach of tolerance leading to sensitization to food antigens. The exact mechanism is not fully understood, but it has been hypothesized that a failure to regulate Tregs may lead to a breakdown of tolerance and resulting sensitization. For example, lower number of peripheral blood Tregs have been found in children with food allergies (Karlsson et al., 2004).

The development of oral tolerance to food antigens has been thought to hinge on multiple dietary factors, including the timing of food introduction, the dose of antigen introduced, and the relative antigenicity of the respective food. Dietary and other adjuvant factors have been noted to promote the generation of Tregs and thus the development of oral tolerance. The critical role of a balanced microbiome T cell regulation and maintenance of oral tolerance has been recognized (Kim et al., 2018) and the lasting consequences of early disruptions have been described (Cox et al., 2014). Dietary factors like fiber content are known to directly influence the intestinal microbiome and, in combination with Vitamin A, have also been found to directly enhance tolerogenic $CD103^+$ DC functions underlining the importance of environmental factors in oral tolerance (Tan et al., 2016). Other microbial factors like *Clostridium* species or *Bacteroides fragilis* polysaccharide A promote the generation of Tregs.

Allergic sensitization, on the other hand, can be triggered by bacterial adjuvants such as *Staphylococcus aureus* enterotoxin B. In general, allergic sensitization has been viewed as a gradual process that starts with increased or altered allergen uptake via the skin or gut, systemic dissemination of the allergen, and presentation of the allergen-derived epitope (Wambre and Jeong, 2018). Genetic factors predisposing to a disrupted skin barrier like loss of function filaggrin mutations can lead to sensitization to food antigens through skin contact, per the so-called dual allergen exposure hypothesis postulated by Gideon Lack (Venkataraman et al., 2014). While exposure to food antigens through the intestinal membranes is generally thought to promote the generation of Tregs and resulting in oral tolerance, intestinal inflammation, on the other hand, can lead to a decrease of Treg differentiation promoted by $CD103^+$ DCs and result in loss of oral tolerance (Laffont et al., 2010). Inflammation in the epithelium leads to a shift in the cytokine milieu toward IL-25, IL-33, and Thymic stromal lymphopoietin, resulting in a Th-2 mediated allergic state (Wambre et al., 2017). Th2-mediated inflammation supports B cell activation and class switching to IgE production. This Th2 rich environment eventually leads to decreased Treg differentiation, resulting in a further shift toward allergic state and loss of oral tolerance.

Oral immunotherapy (OIT) is a therapeutic intervention aimed at restoring or creating the balance of oral tolerance over the allergic state. It is taking advantage of natural mechanisms of tolerance promotion via oral ingestion of allergens. A main mechanism is thought to be at the level of Treg promotion and differentiation. At this time, it is widely accepted that desensitization or sustained unresponsiveness to a previously allergenic food can be achieved. If true and lasting oral tolerance can be reinstated remains to be seen (Berin and Mayer, 2013).

The important role of the microbiome will be discussed in more detail later in the chapter.

## 7.2.3 Allergic sensitization

Through the influence of the genetic and environmental factors, oral tolerance can be breached, and "one man's food can become another man's poison" [Lucretius, Roman poet and philosopher].

As detailed earlier, allergic sensitization results when oral tolerance is breached or fails to develop. Contact with an antigen through inflamed lesional skin (e.g., AD) or inflamed intestinal membranes leads to antigen-specific immune reactions, including generation of antigen-specific T lymphocytes and the production of antigen-specific IgE antibodies by plasma cells and subsequent binding to its high-affinity receptors on the surface of mast cells and basophils.

In the early 2000s, observations of increasing rates of food allergy and sensitization led to the hypothesis that early dietary exposure to food allergens might lead to allergic sensitization due to the immaturity and possibly higher permeability of the intestinal membranes. The American Academy of Pediatrics recommended exclusive breastfeeding until 6 months of age and published recommendations regarding food introduction in infants at high risk for atopic diseases. The recommendation was to delay the introduction of milk-containing foods until after 12 months of age, egg should be introduced only after 24 months of age, and peanut, tree nuts, and seafood introduction should be delayed until the 4th year of life (Fiocchi et al., 2006). However, as discussed further in this chapter, delayed introduction of common food allergens did not reduce the frequency of food allergy and subsequent recommendations have been updated based on the accumulating evidence, to early introduction of common food allergens such as peanut and egg, both to infants at risk as well as infants without known risk factors (Fleischer et al., 2016; Devonshire and Robison, 2019).

Allergic sensitization can occur at different stages of prenatal and postnatal life and might also result in loss of tolerance to previously tolerated antigens.

### 7.2.3.1 *Prenatal sensitization*

While previously it had been thought that the initial contact with foreign protein occurs postnatally and the infant is first exposed to food protein via breast milk, it has now been recognized that the fetus is exposed to intact food proteins in the amniotic fluid (Pastor-Vargas et al., 2016). This first prenatal contact might result in sensitization and reactions to food allergens that have not previously been ingested by the infant. In addition, a recent study has shown the effect of maternally derived IgE predisposing to allergic disease by binding to fetal mast cells (Msallam et al., 2020). This study provides important evidence that sensitization can occur prenatally and results in clinical allergy postnatally.

In general, the placenta plays a crucial role in the development of the fetal immune system. A distinct cytokine/chemokine milieu has been seen in allergic versus non-allergic mothers with increased allergen-induced placental IL-6 and TNF-α in atopic mothers (Abelius et al., 2017). The immune system undergoes different changes during the stages of pregnancy. The placental adhesion site cycles from an inflammatory, Th1-skewed state in the first trimester to an anti-inflammatory, Th2-heavy state in the second trimester, and back to an inflammatory state in preparation for delivery in the third trimester (Mor et al., 2017). It has been recognized that maternal genetic factors, as well as environmental and dietary aspects and their interactions, must be considered in prenatal sensitization. Unfortunately, to date, no conclusive data exist to inform physicians and patients on dietary measures to prevent prenatal and postnatal sensitization. There is a need for placebo-controlled randomized trials investigating the effect of specific diets/foods or nutrients in the maternal diet during pregnancy on the development of allergy in the infant. The allergist plays an important role in counseling families and discussing the lack of conclusive studies and guiding potential nutritional interventions (Pham and Bunyavanich, 2018).

### 7.2.3.2 Early postnatal sensitization

Breast- or formula feeding is thought to be the first contact with foreign food antigens in the newborn. However, modification of the maternal diet during pregnancy did not seem to influence the development of food allergies in the infant later in life, as seen in evidence synthesis of multiple interventional studies following children up to 10 years of age (Netting et al., 2014). Studies in a murine model report no correlation between peanut ingestion during pregnancy and breastfeeding on the development of peanut allergy in the breastfed infant (Järvinen et al., 2015). A distinction has to be made between sensitization via proteins passed through breast milk and symptoms in an already sensitized infant through proteins present in breast milk (Rajani et al., 2020). While for many years the recommendation has been to avoid peanuts and tree nuts in the first 3 years of life, with some recommendations including avoidance during pregnancy, these recommendations have been modified after studies failed to show a correlation between maternal diet and the development of atopic disease (Kramer and Kakuma, 2014). Recommendations published by an expert panel from the American Academy of Pediatrics in 2008 (Greer et al., 2008) and recently updated in 2019 (Greer et al., 2019) conclude that there is a lack of evidence to support maternal dietary restrictions during pregnancy and lactation in order to prevent the development of atopic disease. No trials exist today that systematically study the correlation of maternal diet, breastfeeding, formula feeding, and timing of introduction of food allergens in the development of food allergies. It is thought that breastfeeding while introducing food allergens early might be protective against food allergies (Greer et al., 2019). Moderate intake of all allergenic foods and, in general, a healthy, Mediterranean-style diet is endorsed during pregnancy and breastfeeding.

It is likely that other routes of sensitization like transcutaneous exposure are key factors in the development of food allergy.

### 7.2.3.3 Epicutaneous sensitization

A clear association has been shown between early onset of AD and the development of food allergies (Sugita and Akdis, 2020; Lack et al., 2003). The impaired skin barrier leads to increased transcutaneous passage of antigens and subsequent sensitization. When investigating the causes for significant increases in the rates of peanut allergy, Lack et al. noticed that children with severe AD who used skin care products containing peanut oil showed higher rates of peanut sensitization (Lack et al., 2003). The association of AD with the development of atopic diseases has been recognized as the atopic march (Bantz et al., 2014). A progressive shift into atopic disease, starting with the presence of AD is noted. Multiple factors play into the further progression into atopic sensitization. It was found that about 50% of children with moderate-severe AD had a loss of function mutation of filaggrin and showed increased sensitization to peanut (Brough et al., 2014; Venkataraman et al., 2014). This was also noted in mouse models. Filaggrin-deficient mice showed a Th17-dominant skin inflammation and were susceptible to epicutaneous sensitization (Oyoshi et al., 2009). The clinical findings of transcutaneous sensitization and development of food allergies have also been confirmed in other mouse models. Mice that were epicutaneously challenged to the antigen, developed anaphylaxis in contrast to mice that were orally sensitized to the antigen plus adjuvant and then orally challenged (Bartnikas et al., 2013). The dual allergen hypothesis has been proposed by Gideon Lack as the underlying mechanism for the development of peanut and other food allergies. Repeated exposure of lesional skin to food allergens leads to sensitization and IgE response (Abrams and Sicherer, 2019).

#### 7.2.3.4 Sensitization via food ingestion

The introduction of food proteins as in infant formula or complementary food leads to a change in the infant's gut microbiota, and the relative immaturity of the infant's digestive tract may allow for passage of allergens in a form or amount that will trigger allergic sensitization rather than tolerance. Multiple randomized clinical trials completed over the past decade have added significantly to our understanding of timing and effect of early food introduction. The LEAP (Learning Early About Peanut allergy) trial, which compared early peanut introduction (4–11 months) in high-risk children with AD and egg allergy to withholding peanut protein until 60 months of age (Du Toit et al., 2015) showed a significant protective effect of early introduction and has led to changes in current recommendations. Detailed discussions on the effect of food introduction on the development of food allergies can be found in Section 7.2.5 on Section 7.2.5.3.

### 7.2.4 Reasons for increased sensitization

The rapid increase in food allergies and atopic disorders over the past 35 years, just one generation, cannot be explained by genetic factors alone, and several environmental influences are currently being investigated.

#### 7.2.4.1 Hygiene hypothesis

The hygiene hypothesis was initially introduced by Strachan (Strachan, 1989) to explain the rapid increase of atopic diseases in industrialized countries with a so-called "western lifestyle." Two different paths are named as possible underlying mechanisms. The successful fight against infectious diseases in the last century has significantly decreased bacterial, viral, and parasitic exposure and infection in the pediatric population. This led to the hypothesis that these pathogens shape the immune system, and their absence leads to "self"-reactivity explaining the increase of autoimmunity and atopic diseases.

A second hypothesis being deliberated is the influence of pathogen exposure on accentuating the predominately Th2-biased environment in pregnancy and lead to persistence of a Th2-skewed environment in infancy (McFadden et al., 2015).

It is now recognized that microbial exposures can affect allergic sensitization (Marrs et al., 2013). The influence of delivery mode on the development of food allergy has been of considerable interest, also because an increase in the rate of cesarean sections coincided with an increase in food allergies. A large Finnish registry study has been able to show an 18% increase in the rate of cow's milk (CM) allergy in children born via cesarean section compared to vaginal birth (Metsala et al., 2010).

Birth order and its effect on the development of allergic sensitization has been reviewed, and a significant decrease in food allergies was noted in children with older siblings (Metsala et al., 2010; Koplin et al., 2012). The Healthnuts study from Australia similarly found that attendance of communal childcare institutions and contact with domestic or farm animals protected against allergic reactions to food allergens (Koplin et al., 2012). These points underline the important role of microbial exposure in the development of allergic sensitization early in life.

### 7.2.4.2 Dietary fat hypothesis

Another major change coinciding with the rise in food allergies is the change of the daily diet consumed in industrialized countries. The so-called "Western" diets have favored n-6 (omega 6) fatty acids over n-3 (omega 3) fatty acids (Myles, 2014). The increase in the amount of n-6 fatty acids over n-3 fatty acids in the diet has coincided with the increase of allergic diseases. It has been reported that high concentrations of omega-6 fatty acids predispose to a Th2 phenotype and omega-3 fatty acids suppress cell-mediated immune responses (Miles and Calder, 2017). While it is increasingly understood that the amount and composition of dietary fatty acids have important immunoregulatory effects and influence tolerogenic versus inflammatory responses, due to the lack of comparable clinical trials, no firm recommendations on supplementation have been made (Venter et al., 2019).

### 7.2.4.3 Dietary fiber

Similarly, changes in diet and the amount of consumed fiber are also reflected in the amount of short-chain fatty acids (SCFA), bacterial metabolites that are produced by digestion and fermentation of dietary fiber, and also insoluble starches mainly by anaerobic bacteria in the colon (Tan et al., 2014, 2016; Nagatake and Kunisawa, 2019). Bacterial metabolites play a major role in regulating and controlling various immune pathways. In addition to the intestines, other major effects of SCFA on the immune system were shown to involve DC and macrophage biology in the bone marrow and Th 2 cell responses in the airways (Trompette et al., 2014). Interestingly, one study has shown the presence of commensal microbes in the placenta, where they could exert a direct influence on the developing fetus. However, the direct mechanism has not yet been shown (Aagaard et al., 2014). Similarly, metabolites, such as SCFAs are present in breast milk, where they likely play a role in early shaping of the post-natal immune system (Zheng et al., 2020). A recent study has shown lower levels of SCFA in breast milk of atopic mothers (Stinson et al., 2020). Following the concept that insoluble factors that reach the gastrointestinal tract undigested as prebiotics might prevent the development of allergic disease by stimulating growth and activity of "normal" and "healthy" bacteria, prebiotics have been added to infant formula. The most commonly used prebiotic in infant formula is indigestible oligosaccharide. Positive effects on the intestinal microbiome and immune system have been shown with infant formulas containing short-chain galacto-oligosaccharides (scGOS)/long-chain fructo-oligosaccharides (lcFOS) in a 9:1 ratio, closely resembling human milk composition (Salminen et al., 2020). A Cochrane Review from 2013 has concluded that there is evidence that supplementation of infant formula with prebiotics can prevent eczema (Osborn and Sinn, 2013). Additional studies are needed on whether prebiotics should be universally added to infant formula, just for high-risk infants or not at all (Osborn and Sinn, 2013; Gunaratne et al., 2015). A study investigating high fiber diets in a mouse model was able to show an increase in oral tolerance and decreased levels of food allergy (Tan et al., 2016).

**Microbiome involvement**

In addition to the direct influence of the diet on the immune system, the importance of the human microbiome as an interface between outside exposures and the immune system is increasingly recognized (Bunyavanich and Berin, 2019). The role of the microbiome was first discussed in the hygiene hypothesis in 1989 (Strachan, 1989). The microbiome is now being recognized as a key factor in the development of oral tolerance. The human gastrointestinal tract is inhabited by >1000 different strains of bacteria that coexist and complement capacities or deficiencies of the host by encoding for physiological factors (like enzymes) (Dominguez-Bello et al., 2019). The initial hypothesis of development of allergic disease argued for skewing of the immune response toward a Th2-biased system. However, the concomitant rise of Th1-driven autoinflammatory diseases, such as Crohn's disease and Type I diabetes, and the fact that the presence of parasitic infections that are accompanied by a strong Th2 response, but not by increased risk for allergies, have argued against the exclusive role of this mechanism (Yazdanbakhsh et al., 2002). Studies have shown that microbial diversity and composition differ significantly between subjects with food allergies and non-atopic controls (Thompson-Chagoyan et al., 2010; Björkstén et al., 1999). Mouse models have confirmed that the lack of intestinal microbiota in germ-free mice is associated with Th2 skewing and an increase in IgE responses (Hong et al., 2019). The peri- and postnatal period is a crucial time for shaping the immune system, and early influences may enhance sensitization to foods. The postnatal development of the gut microbiome starts immediately after birth, usually by contact of the newborn with the maternal vaginal flora. In fact, as early as few days of life, newborns who go on to develop allergic sensitization later in life have different composition of gut microbiota compared with newborns who will not develop allergic sensitization (Fujimura et al., 2016). There is a firm evidence that the mode of delivery affects the composition of the gut microbiota (Rutayisire et al., 2016). However, the influence of delivery mode on the development of food allergies is not as strongly associated with subsequent development of food sensitization and allergy (Levin et al., 2020). Swabbing of the newborn mouth and skin with the liquid obtained from the maternal vagina within minutes of birth has been shown to re-align the gut microbiota of infants born via C-section closer to the infants delivered vaginally (Clemente J et al.). An ongoing clinical trial, sponsored by the Immune Tolerance Network (ClinicalTrials.gov Identifier: NCT03567707), will determine if vaginal seeding has the potential to prevent development of sensitization to food allergen(s) at 12 months of age.

### 7.2.4.4 *Effect of the antimicrobial triclosan*

In addition to the presence and absence of bacteria and bacterial metabolites, other environmental agents and toxins likely play an important role in shaping the human microbiome and thus influencing the development of tolerance (Jackson-Browne et al., 2019). Triclosan is a broad-spectrum antimicrobial agent that has been used extensively in the past 20 years in products of daily use like antimicrobial soaps and toothpaste. Triclosan works by blocking an enzyme that is essential for fatty acid synthesis in bacteria (Weatherly and Gosse, 2017). The enzyme blocked by triclosan is not present in humans and therefore the use of triclosan had been considered safe for human consumption. This changed when the importance of the human microbiome was recognized (Sanidad et al., 2019). While prenatal or early life exposure did not show a consistent association with the development of allergic sensitization (Lee-Sarwar et al., 2018), investigations relating urine triclosan levels to allergic sensitization showed an increased risk (Savage et al., 2012). While not being allergenic alone, in a mouse model, triclosan may act as an adjuvant and augments immunomodulatory responses (Marshall et al., 2017).

### 7.2.4.5 Antigen form—The role of food processing

While many of the edible food proteins can be consumed in their natural form, processing of foodstuffs has been practiced since the earliest times. The term food processing encompasses a wide variety of methods, from home processing like peeling, cutting, or cooking to industrialized processing like various chilling, freezing, drying, or heating methods impacting the protein structure and therefore allergenicity of the foods in different ways. It is well known that the allergenicity of food proteins is affected by food processing (Verhoeckx et al., 2015). Heating of fruits and vegetables involved in pollen food allergy syndrome is known to reduce symptoms due to a decrease in IgE binding potential (Bohle et al., 2006). A similar reduction in allergenicity is noted in baked egg and baked milk products. In addition, it has been described that tolerance of egg allergens in the baked form is linked to lower sensitivity to egg in the native form in oral food challenges (Capucilli et al., 2018). Peanut processing and its effect on allergenicity have been very well studied. Structural analyses have shown that roasting peanuts alters the structure of the major peanut allergens leading to increased allergenicity. This structural change can also lead to decreased allergenicity, as seen in boiled peanuts (Zhang et al., 2019). Beyer et al. (2001) demonstrated a significant change in allergenicity or IgE binding capacity in processed peanuts. Peanuts that were boiled in water or fried in vegetable oil showed reduced IgE binding capacity to Ara h1, 2, and 3 than roasted peanuts. Mondoulet et al. (2005) confirmed the finding that boiled peanuts showed lower allergenicity than roasted but also raw peanuts. It has been shown that nonenzymatic browning of the peanuts leads to advanced glycation and thus more potent proteins (Ilchmann et al., 2010). The impact of food processing on allergy depends on the processing methods used, the nature of the protein, and patient sensitivity (Ilchmann et al., 2010).

### 7.2.4.6 Role of vitamin D

It has been reported that the incidence of vitamin D insufficiency has increased twofold over a period of just 10 years from the late 1980s to the early 2000s coinciding with a rise in food allergies (Ginde et al., 2009). Studies with large numbers of participants have shown an association between low vitamin D levels and increased risk of food sensitization (Sharief et al., 2011; Kim et al., 2016). The hypothesis that vitamin D plays an important role in the development of tolerance versus sensitization is supported by studies showing that the season of birth is a risk factor for the development of food allergies, as is living in regions with less ambient UV exposure (Matsui et al., 2019; Vassallo et al., 2010). However, the evidence is not entirely conclusive as select studies are showing that high levels of vitamin D in pregnancy and at birth might be linked to a higher risk for food allergies (Weisse et al., 2013). Additional randomized controlled clinical trials on the effect of vitamin D supplementation on food allergy development are needed (Giannetti et al., 2020).

### 7.2.4.7 *Allergen avoidance*

The hypothesis that early ingestion or avoidance of allergenic food is causing or preventing allergic sensitization has been extensively studied and discussed. As discussed in more detail below, it has become evident that prolonged avoidance of food allergens in high-risk children is resulting in higher rates of sensitization (Du Toit et al., 2015). This is now being reflected in food introduction guidelines. Only limited data are available on the effect of allergen avoidance or exposure in breastfeeding mothers. To date, no specific recommendations for lactating mothers have been made apart from a diet rich in fruits, vegetables, fish, and foods containing vitamin D (Greer et al., 2019).

### 7.2.4.8 *Dual allergen exposure*

#### Nutritional immunomodulation

The hypothesis that the absence/presence of certain nutrients in the diet is predisposing to allergic sensitization has been extensively studied. As detailed earlier, current guidelines have moved away from withholding allergens in the diet to the early introduction of many allergenic foods. This is reflected in the most recent guidelines (Greer et al., 2019). Immunotherapeutic strategies for the treatment and prevention of food allergies have been evaluated. To date, one form of OIT is FDA approved. AR 101 is a form of peanut OIT that was shown to lead to increased tolerance and lower symptoms with peanut exposure (Vickery et al., 2018). Additional forms of immunotherapy for food allergies include sublingual immunotherapy and epicutaneous immunotherapy. Immunotherapy for food allergies to date relies on continuous/daily dosing and leads to an increased threshold of clinical reactivity to the food. Food allergy immunotherapy is not proven to restore complete tolerance.

## 7.2.5 Introduction of food proteins

The discussion regarding introduction of food proteins into the infant's/child's diet includes three broad categories:

**(1)** Breastfeeding, including aspects of the maternal diet
**(2)** Introduction of infant formula, including use of modified formulas (hydrolyzed or partially hydrolyzed formulas or elemental formulas)
**(3)** Introduction of complementary foods (including consideration of timing of allergenic foods)

Because genetic factors are not modifiable, currently, the focus has been on developing sound recommendations for feeding and food introduction strategies to decrease sensitization and clinical allergy.

### 7.2.5.1 *Breastfeeding*

Because of the known benefits of breastfeeding, it is globally recommended as the preferred infant nutrition in the first 4–6 months of life in the absence of other contraindications (Greer et al., 2019).

In 2012 (Section on Breastfeeding, 2012), the American Academy of Pediatrics (AAP) reaffirmed its statement from 2005 (Gartner et al., 2005) recommending exclusive breastfeeding for approximately 6 months of life followed by gradual introduction of complementary foods between 4 and 6 months of life and continuation of breastfeeding until 1 year of age or longer as desired by both mother and child. This is confirmed by a Cochrane review that has been updated since its initial publication (Kramer and Kakuma, 2012). The European Academy of Asthma and Clinical Immunology recommends exclusive breastfeeding for 4–6 months (Muraro et al., 2014). The WHO and UNICEF recommend exclusive breastfeeding for 6 months with supplemental foods only introduced after 6 months of exclusive breastfeeding (https://www.who.int/health-topics/breastfeeding#tab=tab_2, WHO Accessed 4-12-21).

Breastfeeding recommendations continue to be critically reviewed in the light of allergy prevention.

### 7.2.5.2 Formula feeding

As discussed earlier, national and international guidelines recommend exclusive breastfeeding for the first 4–6 months of life for infants at risk of developing allergic disease. At-risk infants are defined as infants who have at least one first-degree relative (sibling or parent) with an atopic condition. Children who are at high risk but cannot be exclusively breastfed during the first 4–6 months of life benefit from delaying CM-based formulas (Urashima et al., 2019). A 2018 Cochrane Review reported no benefit of using hydrolyzed infant formula over breastfeeding but reported a slight benefit of using hydrolyzed infant formula over CM-based formula (Osborn et al., 2018).

The following formulas are commercially available:

*Conventional CM-based formulas*: Conventional CM-based infant formulas contain intact CM proteins and large peptides. CM protein is one of the most common food allergens in infancy.
*Partial whey hydrolysate formulas (pHF-W)*: Partially hydrolyzed whey-based formulas are not considered "hypoallergenic" because they contain large peptides capable of inducing allergic responses. The term hypoallergenic in North America is reserved for therapeutic formulas, and not for formulas for risk reduction for atopic disease. The protein source is the whey component of CM and is broken down into large peptides.
*Extensively hydrolyzed casein or whey-based formulas (eHF-C or eHF-W)*: These formulas undergo extensive hydrolysis or ultrafiltration and contain only small peptides that most children (>90%) with CM allergy will tolerate. Extensively hydrolyzed formulas are generally considered hypoallergenic and appropriate for treatment of atopic disease.
*Soy protein-based formulas* do not contain CM but contain soy proteins.
*Amino acid-based formulas* are closest to being nonallergenic because they do not contain peptides that can be recognized by T or B cells. They are recommended in children with severe allergic disease and prior reactions to extensively hydrolyzed formulas. The disadvantages of amino acid-based formulas is their high cost and bitter taste.

Specific formulas and their effects on the prevention of allergy in the infant at risk have been addressed in randomized controlled clinical trials. Urashima and colleagues recently showed that avoidance of supplementation with CM-based formula for at least the first 3 days of life significantly reduced the development of CM allergy and anaphylaxis (Urashima et al., 2019). Multiple studies have been conducted comparing the use of HF versus CM formulas. A recent meta-analysis synthesizing the evidence of dietary modifications in the prevention of food allergies has also investigated the effect of hydrolyzed infant formulas in the prevention of food allergy (de Silva et al., 2020). When discussing the use of hydrolyzed formulas over CM-based non-hydrolyzed formulas, it is important to consider the study outcome. As detailed later, no strong evidence has been found to date that hydrolyzed formulas help in the prevention of food sensitization; however, a protective effect has been demonstrated for other atopic diseases.

A conclusion drawn from various clinical trials was that the use of partially or extensively hydrolyzed whey or casein infant formulas may not reduce the risk of food sensitization when compared to CM-based formulas. Because of the heterogeneity of the trials and the lack of a clear definition of food allergy, the confidence for this recommendation is low, and robust clinical trials comparing hydrolyzed formulas to CM-based formulas in the prevention of food allergy are needed. Clinical trials investigating the effect of extensively hydrolyzed formulas on prevention of food allergies did not show significant protection from food allergies (Lowe et al., 2011; von Berg et al., 2003; Oldaeus et al., 1997; Mallet and Henocq, 1992). A recent Cochrane review could not find a protective effect of hydrolyzed formulas against the development of CM food allergy when compared to breast milk. Very low quality evidence is cited indicating that the use of hydrolyzed formula compared to CM-based formula might prevent the development of a CM allergy in infants (Osborn et al., 2018).

Little evidence was found that showed the benefit of extensively hydrolyzed formulas over partially hydrolyzed formulas or vice versa (Halken et al., 2000).

The largest study of hydrolyzed infant formula on allergy is a large, randomized, double-blind trial started in the late 1990s comparing three hydrolyzed formulas that differed in protein source (casein or whey) and degree of hydrolysis (partially or extensive) to CM-based formulas during the first 4 months regarding the effect on allergic manifestation and AD (GINI study, GINI non-intervention, and GINI plus) (von Berg et al., 2017). One important finding was a benefit of the use of partially hydrolyzed whey and extensively hydrolyzed casein formulas in the prevention of AD up to 15 years of age (Berg et al., 2010; von Berg et al., 2017). In the 15-year analysis, partially hydrolyzed whey also significantly reduced the cumulative incidence and prevalence of allergic rhinitis and asthma prevalence (von Berg et al., 2016). The 15-year analysis was the first time point to how differences in respiratory outcomes should be confirmed by future studies. The investigators from the GINI study concluded that in high-risk children, early intervention using different hydrolyzed formulas has variable preventative effects on asthma, allergic rhinitis, and eczema up to adolescence. Recently published results from 20 years follow-up that included more than 50% of the study participants showed a preventative effect on asthma for the extensively hydrolyzed formula casein and pHF-W and continued their effect on eczema through adolescence into adulthood. No such effect was noted for e-HF-W (extensively hydrolyzed formula whey) (Gappa et al., 2021).

No role has been found for the use of soy formula over breast milk or other formulas in prevention of allergic disease (Osborn and Sinn, 2004).

In addition to studies investigating the effect of hypoallergenic formulas in not inducing allergic sensitization, the tolerogenic potential of a hydrolyzed whey-based formula has been described. The proteins in the tested formula contained functional T-cell epitopes, which potentially could lead to induction of oral tolerance in children allergic to CM protein (Gouw et al., 2018). This tertiary prevention that aims at targeted interventions to induce development of oral tolerance in children with already established CM allergy.

### 7.2.5.3 Solid foods

In the past, recommendations were to delay complementary feeding until after 6 months of life and avoidance of highly allergenic foods. These recommendations were incited by the concern for increased sensitization through high gut permeability and relative immaturity of the gastrointestinal tract in infants (Halken and Høst, 1996) and based on early cohort studies that had shown that early introduction of solid foods before the age of 4 months increased the risk for eczema up to 2.5-fold (Fergusson et al., 1982; Forsyth et al., 1993; Zutavern et al., 2006) and the risk for food allergy up to 5-fold (Kajosaari and Saarinen, 1983). These recommendations were supported by the AAP Committee on Nutrition and incorporated into feeding principles (Anon, 2000) for infants at risk. The current WHO recommendation from 2001 was not directed at allergy prevention but at reduction of infectious gastrointestinal diseases in developing countries. Based on newer studies, the AAP Committee on Nutrition concluded in 2008 that complementary foods should be introduced no earlier than 4 months of age and no later than 6 months (Agostoni et al., 2008; Greer et al., 2008; Muraro et al., 2004). The WHO guidelines continue recommending exclusive breastfeeding until 6 months for nutritional reasons and prevention of infections leading to a discrepancy between national and WHO guidelines in many countries. Current recommendations by both American and European expert committees are not to introduce solid foods into the infants' diet before 4–6 months of age but then allow gradual introduction of all food groups (Agostoni et al., 2008; Greer et al., 2008; Muraro et al., 2014). This reflects a change from previous guidelines recommending delaying certain allergenic foods in high-risk infants, CM until age 1 year, eggs until age 2 years, and peanuts, tree nuts, fish, and shellfish until age 3 years. This change was implemented after initial reports were published suggesting a disadvantage of delayed introduction of allergens. In 2006, results of a longitudinal birth cohort were published showing an increased risk of wheat allergy in children with delayed introduction of grains until after 6 months of age (Poole et al., 2006). Similarly, in 2008, it was reported that Jewish children living in the United Kingdom had a 10-fold higher prevalence of peanut allergy than Jewish children living in Israel who had early and significant exposure to peanuts in their first year of life. By 9 months of age, 69% of children in Israel were eating peanut compared to only 10% in the United Kingdom (Du Toit et al., 2008). A study on preventing peanut allergy by the LEAP Study Group by early exposure to peanut is further investigating this hypothesis (Du Toit et al., 2013). A recent study investigating the influence of increased food diversity in the first year of life found a protective effect of a diverse diet on asthma, food allergy, and food sensitization (Roduit et al., 2014). These studies support the paradigm shift away from delayed introduction of allergens. The recent randomized trial of early introduction of dietary peanut randomized 640 infants between the ages of 4 and 11 months with severe eczema, egg allergy, or both to consume or avoid peanut until 60 months of age (Du Toit et al., 2015). Severe eczema and egg allergy have been previously identified as risk factors for development of peanut allergy. The primary outcome was the proportion of participants with peanut allergy at 60 months of age. Among the 530 infants in the intention-to-treat population who initially had negative results on the skin-prick test, the prevalence of peanut allergy at 60 months of age was 13.7% in the avoidance group and 1.9% in the consumption group ($P < .001$). Among the 98 participants in the intention-to-treat population who initially had small positive skin test results (1–4 mm wheal diameter), the prevalence of peanut allergy was 35.3% in the avoidance group and 10.6% in the consumption group ($P = .004$). There was no significant difference in the incidence of serious adverse events in children who were ingesting peanut and those avoiding peanut. The early introduction of peanut significantly decreased the frequency of the development of peanut allergy among children at high risk for this allergy and modulated immune responses to peanut. The significant risk reduction observed in this study provides evidence for the benefits of early introduction of dietary peanut in infants with severe eczema and egg allergy. Early introduction of peanut takes advantage of the oral tolerance pathways activated by ingestion that precedes the potential sensitization to peanut via the disrupted skin barrier. This exciting study opens the door to an effective early intervention for the at-risk population. At this time, the optimal practical implementation of the study findings remains to be determined. It is unclear how to translate the study findings to the populations of infants with milder forms of eczema or no eczema and those in the countries where peanut consumption is generally less common than in the United Kingdom, United States, Canada, and Australia (Fleischer et al., 2016). The study enforced regular ingestion of peanut products, either peanut snack or peanut butter, three times per week for 5 years. This may not be practical for many families at large; the absolute minimum of peanut consumption sufficient to maintain tolerance remains to be determined. The EAT trial recruited 1303 exclusively breastfed infants who were 3 months of age and randomly assigned them to the early introduction of 6 allergenic foods (peanut, cooked egg, CM, sesame, whitefish, and wheat; early-introduction group) or to the current practice recommended in the United Kingdom of exclusive breastfeeding to approximately 6 months of age (standard-introduction group). The primary outcome was food allergy to one or more of the six foods between 1 and 3 years of age (Perkin et al., 2016, 2019). The trial did not show the efficacy of early introduction of allergenic foods in an intention-to-treat analysis. In the per-protocol analysis, the prevalence of any food allergy was significantly lower in the early-introduction group than in the standard-introduction group (2.4% vs 7.3%, $P = .01$), as was the prevalence of peanut allergy (0% vs 2.5%, $P = .003$) and egg allergy (1.4% vs 5.5%, $P = .009$); there were no significant effects with respect to milk, sesame, fish, or wheat. The consumption of 2 g per week of peanut or egg-white protein was associated with a significantly lower prevalence of these respective allergies than was less consumption. The early introduction of all six foods was not easily achieved but was safe. Further analysis raised the question of whether the prevention of food allergy by means of early introduction of multiple allergenic foods was dose-dependent. Another randomized, placebo-controlled trial investigated the efficacy and safety of early hen's egg introduction from ages 4 to 6 months to prevent hen's egg allergy in the general population (Bellach et al., 2017). The trial included 4- to 6-month-old infants who were not sensitized against hen's egg, as determined based on specific serum antibodies (IgE). These infants were randomized to receive either verum (egg white powder) or placebo (rice powder) added to the first weaning food three times a week under a concurrent egg-free diet from age 4 to 6 until 12 months. Among 406 screened infants, 23 (5.7%) had hen's egg-specific IgE before randomization. Seventeen of 23 underwent subsequent double-blind, placebo-controlled food challenges, and 16 were confirmed as allergic, including 11 with anaphylactic reactions. At 12 months of age, 5.6% of the children in the verum group were hen's egg sensitized versus 2.6% in the placebo group (primary outcome; relative risk, 2.20; 95% CI, 0.68–7.14; $P = .24$), and 2.1% were confirmed to have hen's egg allergy versus 0.6% in the placebo group (relative risk, 3.30; 95% CI, 0.35–31.32; $P = .35$). The study found no evidence that consumption of hen's egg starting at 4–6 months of age prevents hen's egg sensitization or allergy.

In contrast, it might result in frequent allergic reactions in the community, considering that many 4- to 6-month-old infants were already allergic to hen's egg. Many population-based, prospective birth cohort studies conducted in different countries do not support delayed introduction of solids beyond 4–6 months of age for prevention of allergic disease (Zutavern et al., 2008; Snijders et al., 2008; Du Toit et al., 2008; Joseph et al., 2011; Grimshaw et al., 2013; Luccioli et al., 2014). An Australian population-based cross-sectional study (HealthNuts) was able to show a benefit of introducing cooked egg early in preventing allergic sensitization (Koplin et al., 2010). A UK-based randomized controlled clinical trial that now completed enrollment is investigating if introduction of the six most allergenic foods from as early as 3 months together with continued breastfeeding will reduce the prevalence of food allergies by the age of 3 years (www.eatstudy.co.uk). In addition to timing, the order and nature of food introduction to modify risk using nutritional supplements are being investigated. As described earlier, the modification of the intestinal flora might play an important role in the development of food allergies. Possible nutritional supplements that are being investigated are probiotics and prebiotics and their modulatory effects on the normal gut flora.

### 7.2.5.4 Role of probiotics

The crucial role of the human microbiome in induction and maintenance of oral tolerance to food allergens has been discussed earlier. A difference in the composition of the microbiome between allergic and healthy children has been observed. It has been shown by different epidemiologic studies that the use of probiotic bacteria, bacterial lysates, and prebiotics is associated with protection against chronic inflammatory disease. The use and mechanisms of prebiotics will be reviewed later. Probiotics are defined as live bacteria that naturally colonize the gastrointestinal tract, and their presence in adequate amounts is associated with health benefits for the host (Morelli and Capurso, 2012; Guarner and Schaafsma, 1998). Supplementation of probiotics has been shown to have anti-inflammatory properties together with cytokine changes that might skew toward Th1-biased responses (Heller and Duchmann, 2003; Sudo et al., 1997) and inhibit Th2-biased responses and IgE production. In addition, probiotics were shown to increase secretion of IL-10 and TGF-$\beta$ by upregulating T regulatory cells (Feleszko et al., 2007). Until recently, intervention was geared toward starting supplementation with probiotics in the early postnatal period or very late in pregnancy to influence colonization of the fetal intestines. It has been realized that influence on the fetal microbiome starts much earlier during pregnancy, and studies have investigated the effect on the offspring of prenatal supplementation with probiotics (Boyle et al., 2011). A meta-analysis synthesizing evidence from randomized controlled clinical trials investigating the use of probiotics in infants for primary prevention of allergies found a mild reduction in clinical eczema in infants but insufficient evidence for general recommendation of probiotic supplementation for prevention of allergic disease or food hypersensitivity (Osborn and Sinn, 2007). More recent trials investigating prenatal only, pre- and postnatal, and postnatal only use of probiotics for the prevention of atopic disease or eczema did not find an effect on allergic sensitization. However, follow-up data of one randomized-placebo controlled clinical trial investigating the effect of pre- and postnatal supplementation of probiotics on AD showed decreased disease manifestations after 2–6 years of treatment (Wickens et al., 2008, 2012, 2013).

#### 7.2.5.5 *Role of prebiotics*

Prebiotics are food components that are nondigestible and reach the colon, where they provide nutrition and stimulate growth and activity of bacteria of the normal gut flora. They are commonly added as nutritional supplements like oligosaccharides (Agostoni et al., 2004). Pooling of data from multiple studies in a recently updated Cochrane review showed potential benefit in the prevention of AD, but no conclusive evidence was found regarding prevention of other allergic disease or food allergy (Osborn and Sinn, 2013).

## 7.3 Long-term effect on immunologic/allergic response of introduction of allergen/immunogen exposure in early life

It has been shown that many children with early onset of atopic conditions or sensitizations continue to have other allergic diseases as asthma, AD, food allergies, and allergic rhinitis, also termed the allergic march (Wahn, 2000). Sensitization to allergens in infancy frequently offsets an escalation of allergic problems. Children with early atopy have an increased risk of developing food allergies later in life as has been shown in numerous studies and has been summarized by Du Toit et al. (2016). The risk of atopic diseases progressing to affect additional organs and systems over the course of many years is reflected in the description of EoE as a late manifestation of atopy (Hill et al., 2018).

### 7.3.1 Nutritional consequences of food allergy

Elimination diets are often necessary for the treatment of most of the allergic conditions described earlier, which can lead to severe nutritional deficiencies of macro- and micronutrients if not supervised and monitored adequately. A multitude of reasons is contributing to nutritional problems in children with food hypersensitivities. Children with multiple diagnosed food allergies have a lower intake of total calories and micro- and macronutrients than children without food allergies (Christie et al., 2002). Children with food allergies were reported to be significantly shorter than age-matched controls without food allergies. In children with CM allergy, both height and weight are affected (Mehta et al., 2014). And it has been shown that those nutritional deficiencies during childhood lead to long-term effects in later life. Young adults with IgE-mediated milk allergy on a CM-free diet were found to have decreased bone mineral density and early osteoporosis that was reversible after milk desensitization (Goldberg et al., 2018). Factors that lead to nutritional deficiencies in these children include behavioral issues as picky eating, refusal to take supplemental formula or other supplements to substitute for eliminated foods, economic problems of the affected families to afford the necessary supplemental foods, and other psychosocial factors. Elimination diets should always be supervised by an allergist or gastroenterologist, preferably in collaboration with a nutritionist to avoid severe nutritional consequences as rickets or vitamin and mineral deficiencies.

### 7.3.2 Growth

Weight gain and growth are sensitive markers of adequate nutritional intake, with weight gain being most sensitive to changes in energy intake. Stature can be permanently affected by chronic nutritional deficiencies. Children with food allergies are at greater risk for impaired weight gain and growth than children without food allergies (Christie et al., 2002; Smith et al., 2020), in particular, those with milk allergy. Growth and weight gain of all children should be monitored using growth curves as provided by the WHO for children up to 2 years of age and CDC for children older than 2 years (Kuczmarski et al., 2002; Ogden et al., 2002).

### 7.3.3 Neurodevelopment

In adult patients, it has been shown that atopic disorders can be triggered by psychological factors (Wright, 2005) and on the other hand, atopic disorders are linked to adverse outcomes in cognitive abilities and increased anxiety and depression (Satish et al., 2004; Katz et al., 2010). In children, this relationship is more complex, but an association between atopic disease and adverse outcomes in many areas, including cognitive and neurodevelopment has been shown (Chida et al., 2008). Possible contributing factors that impact development in allergic children are clinical manifestations of the allergy and necessary treatments affecting neurodevelopment (Blaiss, 2004; Meltzer, 2016) and a changed home environment because of parental and patient anxiety (Bollinger et al., 2006). Chronic stress caused by chronic disease may also alter both the immune and central nervous system through effects on the hypothalamic-pituitary-adrenal (HPA) axis (Buske-Kirschbaum et al., 2004). Studies have shown an association between HPA axis dysregulation and behavior, associating elevated cortisol levels to emotional dysregulation and other psychological problems (Gunnar and Donzella, 2002). These observations point to the important interactions between the neuroimmune systems.

### 7.3.4 Social development

In comparison to other chronic disorders, patients with food allergy only experience symptoms intermittently but must maintain a high degree of vigilance to avoid acute reactions. The knowledge that accidental exposure may trigger a severe or even fatal anaphylactic reaction poses a burden on both parents and affected children. Increased anxiety was found in both allergic children and their mothers. It was found that anxiety that results in implementation of safety measures and prevention of exposure is beneficial, but anxiety that leads to excessive restrictions and social withdrawal can be detrimental (Muñoz-Furlong, 2001, 2003). Children who have experienced reaction to a food in the past often become more fearful and may develop an eating disorder (Le et al., 2013). A diagnosis of food or food-associated allergies fundamentally changes the life of most affected families. Daily tasks as grocery shopping and cooking are altered. Attending social events as birthday parties involves strategic planning and preparation. A recent study showed that 10% of families completely banned the allergenic food from their house and 15.3% consumed all meals separately (Polloni et al., 2013). The effect of food allergy on the quality of life of the caregiver was shown to be dependent on additional factors. Families where the child was older at the diagnosis of food allergy has had an anaphylactic reaction, comorbid eczema, or multiple food allergies were found to have more negatively affected quality of life; as well as caregivers with an inaccurate perception of the food allergy or a lower income (Howe et al., 2014). Restricting foods from nonaffected family members, especially if atopic but not food allergic, might lead to development of a food allergy to the restricted food. Allergic teenagers are an especially vulnerable group, as they are assuming more responsibility for their allergies on the one hand, and can engage in risk-taking behaviors on the other (MacKenzie et al., 2010). Various publications have investigated bullying as a frequent problem that is putting adolescent patients at significant physical and emotional risk. It has been shown that many adolescents do not disclose bullying to their parents, further impacting their quality of life (Shemesh et al., 2013; Lieberman et al., 2010). Because of the detrimental effects of bullying, clinicians should routinely ask both patients and parents about bullying and encourage parents to intervene at school if bullying is identified (Annunziato et al., 2014).

## 7.3.5 Nutrition for protection from infections

Infections are a leading cause of morbidity and mortality in infants and young children (Bentley et al., 2018), with acute respiratory infections presenting (to avoid tautology for the next posing) a considerable health burden in developed countries. Upper respiratory tract infections (RTIs) in young children account for more than one-third of pediatric consultations in primary care, according to data for the United Kingdom (Hay et al., 2005) and the United States (Monto, 2002), posing a major burden on healthcare services as well as stress to parents. The highest incidence rates of RTIs occur during the first 2 years of life. A US study showed these young children have an average of six to eight RTIs each year (Monto, 2002).

Population data from high-income countries suggest that approximately one quarter of all children are hospitalized at least once with an infection by the age of 5 years, and 1 in 10 have multiple hospitalizations (Bentley et al., 2018).

Overuse of antibiotics is a global problem, especially in pediatric care. Antibiotics are commonly prescribed for young children with acute RTIs in many countries (Thompson et al., 2013), despite limited evidence of effectiveness. Antibiotics were prescribed in nearly one-quarter of RTI episodes (21.9%), where a burden diary was submitted by parents in the Australian study (Sarna et al., 2016) and in a similar proportion (24.9%) of infectious episodes in the Danish cohort study (Vissing et al., 2018). Furthermore, antibiotics are also prescribed in more than 30% of asthma exacerbations in children, despite antibiotics not currently being recommended in guidelines and demonstrating minimal clinical benefits (Murray et al., 2021).

Breastfeeding has been shown to be protective against infections in young children. A large study including 28 systematic reviews and meta-analyses of associations between breastfeeding and outcomes carried out for *The Lancet* demonstrated that breastfeeding was associated with protection against childhood infections, including RTIs, acute otitis media, and diarrhea in children under 2 years of age (Victora et al., 2016). Children who were breastfed for longer periods had lower infectious morbidity and mortality into the second year of life, and protection against otitis media until 2 years of age and possibly beyond compared to those who were not breastfed or breastfed for shorter periods.

A review of studies conducted in Europe and the United States found that any form of breastfeeding for the first 6 months of life was protective against acute otitis media in children under 2 years of age. Interestingly, "more versus less" breastfeeding was associated with a 33% reduction of acute otitis media (Bowatte et al., 2015). This suggests that mixed milk feeding, which occurs in a large proportion of infants, is also likely to confer protection against infections.

In *the Lancet* review, the authors suggested that important imprinting events might be modulated during breastfeeding (Victora et al., 2016). These events could be mediated directly or through effects on the infant microbiome. The ability of the microbiome to regulate host responses in infancy depends on individual bacterial species, which modulate immune regulation and T-cell polarization as well as metabolic responses and other processes (Victora et al., 2016; Hooper et al., 2012). Human milk contains a variety of bioactive substances with immune-modulatory, anti-inflammatory, and antimicrobial properties that provide protection to infants while their immune system matures (Bowatte et al., 2015). For example, human milk contains a large number of indigestible human milk oligosaccharides (HMOs), which function as prebiotics to support growth of specific bacteria (Gibson et al., 2017). More recently, it has been recognized that human milk also contains both viable and non-viable bacteria, postbiotics, that can affect colonization of the infant gut (Hill et al., 2014; Salminen et al., 2020). In addition to changes mediated through the gut microbiota, breastmilk components, such as HMOs, might directly influence an infant's epigenetic programming (Victora et al., 2016; Verduci et al., 2014).

## 7.3.6 Strategies to influence the gut microbiota and improve immune outcomes

Breastfeeding is important in the prevention and treatment of diseases associated with aberrant patterns of microbial colonization, including infections, underlining the benefit of supporting women to breastfeed their babies. The gut microbiota of formula-fed infants is more diverse compared to breastfed infants and dominated by *Bacteroides*, *Bifidobacteria*, *Staphylococci*, *Escherichia coli*, and *Clostridia* (Szajewska et al., 2017). Abnormal colonization patterns have been associated with long-term effects on immune and metabolic homeostasis. Considering that breastfeeding is the gold standard for infant nutrition, infant formulas that support the establishment of a microbiota resembling that of breastfed infants might improve immune outcomes in infants that cannot be breastfed.

Supplementation of infant formula with prebiotics, Human identical Milk Oligosaccharides (HiMOs), probiotics, or synbiotics (traditionally defined as a combination of a probiotic and a prebiotic) has been used as a nutritional approach to optimize immune responses through modulation of the gut microbiota. This seems to be especially relevant in infants with abnormal colonization patterns, such as infants born via C-section and infants with CMA. In infants with CMA, an appropriate hypoallergenic formula can be used when breastfeeding is not possible or insufficient to help resolve symptoms and support growth and development. Traditionally, hypoallergenic formulas did not contain factors that stimulate gut microbiota development.

Prebiotics and HiMOs are now frequently added to infant milk formula (IMF) to mimic the effects of HMOs and achieve a bifidogenic milieu. Probiotics are live microorganisms which can supplement the bacterial population and reverse the dysbiosis seen in specific target populations.

### 7.3.6.1 The effect of prebiotics and synbiotics on infection outcomes in healthy infants

In healthy infants, feeding with IMF supplemented with a prebiotic mixture of scGOS and lcFOS results in a gut microbiota more similar to infants fed with human milk compared to babies fed with standard formula without scGOS/lcFOS, reviewed in the study by Oozeer 2013 (Oozeer et al., 2013).

Several studies also suggested that the addition of a specific prebiotic mixture scGOS/lcGOS 9:1 to IMF is associated with reduced risk of upper respiratory infections and even achieving an imprinting effect over the long term (Arslanoglu et al., 2007, 2008; Bruzzese et al., 2009). Although the exact mechanism of action is not yet elucidated, it is likely that the immune-modulating effect of this prebiotic mixture is mediated through intestinal microbiota modification.

### 7.3.6.2 The effect of prebiotics and synbiotics on infection outcomes in infants with CMA

Three randomized controlled trials showed that a specific synbiotic mixture (scFOS/lcFOS and *B. breve* M-16V) is able to rebalance gut microbiota in infants with CMA and align it closer in composition and activity to that of healthy breastfed infants (Burks et al., 2015; Candy et al., 2018; Fox et al., 2019).

Several studies have shown fewer RTIs and otitis media (ear infections) (measured as adverse event outcomes) in infants with CMA receiving a hypoallergenic formula with HiMOs (2'FL & LNnT) as well as with the specific synbiotic mixture scFOS/lcFOS and *B. breve* M-16V (Vandenplas et al., 2020; Burks et al., 2015; Candy et al., 2018; Chatchatee et al., 2021). Synbiotic usage was also associated with reduced overall medication use, including antibiotics and antipyretics.

## 7.4 Future trends and research needs

Ongoing research over the past two decades has led to changes and reversals of many practices and recommendations for prevention of food allergies and atopic disease.

### 7.4.1 Breastfeeding/hydrolyzed formula

Based on recommendations from a study conducted over 30 years ago in Finland that showed a protective effect of long exclusive breastfeeding, atopic mothers tend to breastfeed longer than non-atopic mothers (Saarinen et al., 1979). Other birth cohort studies have confirmed this association for asthma and wheezing but not for other atopic disorders (Kull et al., 2010; Silvers et al., 2012; Brew et al., 2012; Sonnenschein-van der Voort et al., 2012). The effect of breastfeeding (duration and exclusivity) on the development of food allergy is not understood in its entirety, and current recommendations are based on multiple factors, including the benefit of breastfeeding in the prevention of infectious diarrhea in many parts of the world and timing of introduction of solids. Of special interest in this context are possible anti-inflammatory properties of breast milk and the influence of maternal diet during pregnancy and lactation, with clear recommendations missing. In children who cannot be exclusively breastfed during the first 4 months of life, the use of HF formula was found to be beneficial over CM (Osborn and Sinn, 2003; Szajewska et al., 2010). However, to our knowledge, no large trials have been conducted examining the use of HF versus breast milk in the prevention of allergic disease for various reasons (Osborn and Sinn, 2003). In infants who are at risk (who have at least one first-degree relative (parent or sibling) with an atopic condition) but cannot be exclusively breastfed during the first 4–6 months of life, "hypoallergenic" formulas (e.g., partially or extensively hydrolyzed whey or casein amino acid-based) were shown to be beneficial over conventional CM-based formulas are currently recommended by both American and European expert committees (Fleischer et al., 2013).

### 7.4.2 Introduction of solids

Early or late introduction of allergens in the infant's diet has been a major focus in preventative research with a paradigm shift over the past years from recommending delaying the introduction of allergenic foods to the current recommendations of gradual introduction of all food groups into the child's diet after 4–6 months (Muraro et al., 2014; Greer et al., 2008; Agostoni et al., 2008). An ongoing trial investigating the effect of early introduction of the six main allergenic foods while continuing breastfeeding on allergic sensitization at 3 years will provide more information and help create guidelines (www.eatstudy.co.uk). Additional longitudinal studies showing the preventative effect of this intervention in the future are needed.

### 7.4.3 Significance of human microbiome

There is increasing evidence that the composition of the human gut microbiome plays a significant role in the development and prevention of allergic disease. Multiple studies over the past decade have shown that the presence and timing of intestinal dysbiosis is a critical factor in the development of allergic sensitization (Bunyavanich and Berin, 2019). Studying the human microbiome in the broader context of environmental exposure, genetic and epigenetic traits is crucial to further understanding of the role of the human microbiome in the development of allergic disease. Studies have evaluated the influence of supplementing probiotics and prebiotics for prevention of atopy (Fiocchi et al., 2012). The perceived low risk and side effect profile lead to common use despite inconsistent evidence for efficacy. However, it is not fully elucidated which bacterial strain is associated with the most clinical benefit. In addition, no strong evidence exists for timing, dose, and duration of supplementation, and additional research is needed here.

### 7.4.4 Environmental factors

As detailed earlier, the increasing prevention of infections and general changes in lifestyle have been implicated in the continued rise in allergic disease. It has been hypothesized that the immune system remains under-challenged, while being continuously exposed to environmental pollution leading to low-grade inflammation (Breiteneder et al., 2019). Climate change is a major threat to health globally. Its impact on the development of allergic diseases is being studied from various aspects (Katelaris and Beggs, 2018). In most regions of the world, an increase in the duration and severity of the pollen season has been noted (Ariano et al., 2010). The effect of these increased pollen counts on the development of food allergies and other allergic diseases like EoE is currently being evaluated. Emerging topics in environmental health research and the impact of allergic diseases include the understanding of the gene-environment interaction and the role of epigenetic changes, as well as the better understanding of additive and summative effects of environmental exposures (Breiteneder et al., 2019). Some environmental factors such as the role of vitamin D deficiency in the development of allergic sensitization have been studied extensively (Sharief et al., 2011; Osborne et al., 2012). Research on other potentially influencing elements is just being started. Very few studies investigating the role of the antimicrobial triclosan have been published, mainly describing possible underlying mechanisms (Savage et al., 2012; Bertelsen et al., 2013; Anderson et al., 2013). Along those lines, the influence and mechanism of environmental toxins and altered proteins must be further investigated.

## 7.4.5 Consequences of food allergies

Even though data are published on nutritional consequences of food allergy like impact on growth and neurodevelopment and the impact on social development, there is a strong need for interventions targeting and preventing these negative consequences in patients with allergies and allergic sensitization.

### Sources of additional information

All major professional societies dealing with patients with allergic diseases have physician and patient information on their websites:

- American Academy of Asthma Allergy and Immunology (AAAAI) [www.aaaai.org]
- American College of Asthma, Allergy, and Immunology (ACAAI) [www.acaai.org]
- World Allergy Organization (WAO) [www.worldallergy.org]
- American Academy of Dermatology (AAD) [www.aad.org]
- American Gastroenterological Association (AGA) [www.gastro.org]

There is a wide array of lay organizations lobbying for patients with allergies:

- Food Allergy Research and Education (FARE) [www.foodallergy.org]
- National Eczema Association [www.nationaleczema.org]
  - GI kids (Patient Association for children with digestive disorders) [http://www. gikids.org/content/5/en/EosinophilicEsophagitis]
- The International FPIES Association [www.fpies.org]
- The FPIES Foundation [http://fpiesfoundation.org]

## References

Aagaard, K., Ma, J., Antony, K.M., Ganu, R., Petrosino, J., Versalovic, J., 2014. The placenta harbors a unique microbiome. Sci. Transl. Med. 6 (237ra65).

Abelius, M.S., Jedenfalk, M., Ernerudh, J., Janefjord, C., Berg, G., Matthiesen, L., Jenmalm, M.C., 2017. Pregnancy modulates the allergen-induced cytokine production differently in allergic and non-allergic women. Pediatr. Allergy Immunol. 28, 818–824.

Abrams, E.M., Sicherer, S., 2019. Cutaneous sensitization to peanut in children with atopic dermatitis: a window to prevention of peanut allergy. JAMA Dermatol. 155, 13–14.

Agostoni, C., Axelsson, I., Goulet, O., Koletzko, B., Michaelsen, K.F., Puntis, J.W., Rigo, J., Shamir, R., Szajewska, H., Turck, D., 2004. Prebiotic oligosaccharides in dietetic products for infants: a commentary by the ESPGHAN committee on nutrition. J. Pediatr. Gastroenterol. Nutr. 39, 465–473.

Agostoni, C., Decsi, T., Fewtrell, M., Goulet, O., Kolacek, S., Koletzko, B., Michaelsen, K.F., Moreno, L., Puntis, J., Rigo, J., Shamir, R., Szajewska, H., Turck, D., van Goudoever, J., 2008. Complementary feeding: a commentary by the ESPGHAN committee on nutrition. J. Pediatr. Gastroenterol. Nutr. 46, 99–110.

Allen, K.J., Koplin, J.J., 2019. What can urban/rural differences in food allergy prevalence tell us about the drivers of food allergy? J. Allergy Clin. Immunol. 143, 554–556.

Anderson, S.E., Franko, J., Kashon, M.L., Anderson, K.L., Hubbs, A.F., Lukomska, E., Meade, B.J., 2013. Exposure to triclosan augments the allergic response to ovalbumin in a mouse model of asthma. Toxicol. Sci. 132, 96–106.

Annunziato, R.A., Rubes, M., Ambrose, M.A., Mullarkey, C., Shemesh, E., Sicherer, S.H., 2014. Longitudinal evaluation of food allergy-related bullying. J Allergy Clin Immunol Pract 2, 639–641.

Anon, 2000. American Academy of Pediatrics. Committee on nutrition. Hypoallergenic infant formulas. Pediatrics 106, 346–349.

Ariano, R., Canonica, G.W., Passalacqua, G., 2010. Possible role of climate changes in variations in pollen seasons and allergic sensitizations during 27 years. Ann. Allergy Asthma Immunol. 104, 215–222.

Arslanoglu, S., Moro, G.E., Boehm, G., 2007. Early supplementation of prebiotic oligosaccharides protects formula-fed infants against infections during the first 6 months of life. J. Nutr. 137, 2420–2424.

Arslanoglu, S., Moro, G.E., Schmitt, J., Tandoi, L., Rizzardi, S., Boehm, G., 2008. Early dietary intervention with a mixture of prebiotic oligosaccharides reduces the incidence of allergic manifestations and infections during the first two years of life. J. Nutr. 138, 1091–1095.

Ballardini, N., Bergström, A., Böhme, M., van Hage, M., Hallner, E., Johansson, E., Söderhäll, C., Kull, I., Wickman, M., Wahlgren, C.F., 2014. Infantile eczema: prognosis and risk of asthma and rhinitis in preadolescence. J. Allergy Clin. Immunol. 133, 594–596.

Bantz, S.K., Zhu, Z., Zheng, T., 2014. The atopic march: progression from atopic dermatitis to allergic rhinitis and asthma. J. Clin. Cell. Immunol. 5, 202.

Bartnikas, L.M., Gurish, M.F., Burton, O.T., Leisten, S., Janssen, E., Oettgen, H.C., Beaupré, J., Lewis, C.N., Austen, K.F., Schulte, S., Hornick, J.L., Geha, R.S., Oyoshi, M.K., 2013. Epicutaneous sensitization results in IgE-dependent intestinal mast cell expansion and food-induced anaphylaxis. J. Allergy Clin. Immunol. 131, 451–460.e1-6.

Bellach, J., Schwarz, V., Ahrens, B., Trendelenburg, V., Aksünger, Ö., Kalb, B., Niggemann, B., Keil, T., Beyer, K., 2017. Randomized placebo-controlled trial of hen's egg consumption for primary prevention in infants. J. Allergy Clin. Immunol. 139, 1591–1599.e2.

Bentley, J.P., Burgner, D.P., Shand, A.W., Bell, J.C., Miller, J.E., Nassar, N., 2018. Gestation at birth, mode of birth, infant feeding and childhood hospitalization with infection. Acta Obstet. Gynecol. Scand. 97, 988–997.

Berg, A., Krämer, U., Link, E., Bollrath, C., Heinrich, J., Brockow, I., Koletzko, S., Grübl, A., Filipiak-Pittroff, B., Wichmann, H.E., Bauer, C.P., Reinhardt, D., Berdel, D., 2010. Impact of early feeding on childhood eczema: development after nutritional intervention compared with the natural course – the GINIplus study up to the age of 6 years. Clin. Exp. Allergy 40, 627–636.

Berin, M.C., Mayer, L., 2013. Can we produce true tolerance in patients with food allergy? J. Allergy Clin. Immunol. 131, 14–22.

Bertelsen, R.J., Longnecker, M.P., Løvik, M., Calafat, A.M., Carlsen, K.H., London, S.J., Lødrup Carlsen, K.C., 2013. Triclosan exposure and allergic sensitization in Norwegian children. Allergy 68, 84–91.

Beyer, K., Morrow, E., Li, X.M., Bardina, L., Bannon, G.A., Burks, A.W., Sampson, H.A., 2001. Effects of cooking methods on peanut allergenicity. J. Allergy Clin. Immunol. 107, 1077–1081.

Björkstén, B., Naaber, P., Sepp, E., Mikelsaar, M., 1999. The intestinal microflora in allergic Estonian and Swedish 2-year-old children. Clin. Exp. Allergy 29, 342–346.

Blaiss, M.S., 2004. Allergic rhinitis and impairment issues in schoolchildren: a consensus report. Curr. Med. Res. Opin. 20, 1937–1952.

Bohle, B., Zwölfer, B., Heratizadeh, A., Jahn-Schmid, B., Antonia, Y.D., Alter, M., Keller, W., Zuidmeer, L., van Ree, R., Werfel, T., Ebner, C., 2006. Cooking birch pollen-related food: divergent consequences for IgE- and T cell-mediated reactivity in vitro and in vivo. J. Allergy Clin. Immunol. 118, 242–249.

Bollinger, M.E., Dahlquist, L.M., Mudd, K., Sonntag, C., Dillinger, L., Mckenna, K., 2006. The impact of food allergy on the daily activities of children and their families. Ann. Allergy Asthma Immunol. 96, 415–421.

Bowatte, G., Tham, R., Allen, K.J., Tan, D.J., Lau, M., Dai, X., Lodge, C.J., 2015. Breastfeeding and childhood acute otitis media: a systematic review and meta-analysis. Acta Paediatr. 104, 85–95.

Boyle, R.J., Ismail, I.H., Kivivuori, S., Licciardi, P.V., Robins-Browne, R.M., Mah, L.J., Axelrad, C., Moore, S., Donath, S., Carlin, J.B., Lahtinen, S.J., Tang, M.L., 2011. Lactobacillus GG treatment during pregnancy for the prevention of eczema: a randomized controlled trial. Allergy 66, 509–516.

Breiteneder, H., Diamant, Z., Eiwegger, T., Fokkens, W.J., Traidl-Hoffmann, C., Nadeau, K., O'Hehir, R.E., O'Mahony, L., Pfaar, O., Torres, M.J., Wang, Y., Zhang, L., Akdis, C.A., 2019. Future research trends in understanding the mechanisms underlying allergic diseases for improved patient care. Allergy 74, 2293–2311.

Brew, B.K., Kull, I., Garden, F., Almqvist, C., Bergström, A., Lind, T., Webb, K., Wickman, M., Marks, G.B., 2012. Breastfeeding, asthma, and allergy: a tale of two cities. Pediatr. Allergy Immunol. 23, 75–82.

Brough, H.A., Simpson, A., Makinson, K., Hankinson, J., Brown, S., Douiri, A., Belgrave, D.C., Penagos, M., Stephens, A.C., Mclean, W.H., Turcanu, V., Nicolaou, N., Custovic, A., Lack, G., 2014. Peanut allergy: effect of environmental peanut exposure in children with filaggrin loss-of-function mutations. J. Allergy Clin. Immunol. 134, 867–875.e1.

Bruzzese, E., Volpicelli, M., Squeglia, V., Bruzzese, D., Salvini, F., Bisceglia, M., Lionetti, P., Cinquetti, M., Iacono, G., Amarri, S., Guarino, A., 2009. A formula containing galacto- and fructo-oligosaccharides prevents intestinal and extra-intestinal infections: an observational study. Clin. Nutr. 28, 156–161.

Bunyavanich, S., Berin, M.C., 2019. Food allergy and the microbiome: current understandings and future directions. J. Allergy Clin. Immunol. 144, 1468–1477.

Burks, A.W., Harthoorn, L.F., van Ampting, M.T., Oude Nijhuis, M.M., Langford, J.E., Wopereis, H., Goldberg, S.B., Ong, P.Y., Essink, B.J., Scott, R.B., Harvey, B.M., 2015. Synbiotics-supplemented amino acid-based formula supports adequate growth in cow's milk allergic infants. Pediatr. Allergy Immunol. 26, 316–322.

Buske-Kirschbaum, A., Fischbach, S., Rauh, W., Hanker, J., Hellhammer, D., 2004. Increased responsiveness of the hypothalamus-pituitary-adrenal (HPA) axis to stress in newborns with atopic disposition. Psychoneuroendocrinology 29, 705–711.

Candy, D.C.A., van Ampting, M.T.J., Oude Nijhuis, M.M., Wopereis, H., Butt, A.M., Peroni, D.G., Vandenplas, Y., Fox, A.T., Shah, N., West, C.E., Garssen, J., Harthoorn, L.F., Knol, J., Michaelis, L.J., 2018. A synbiotic-containing amino-acid-based formula improves gut microbiota in non-IgE-mediated allergic infants. Pediatr. Res. 83, 677–686.

Capucilli, P., Cianferoni, A., Fiedler, J., Gober, L., Pawlowski, N., Ram, G., Saltzman, R., Spergel, J.M., Heimall, J., 2018. Differences in egg and milk food challenge outcomes based on tolerance to the baked form. Ann. Allergy Asthma Immunol. 121, 580–587.

Caubet, J.C., Szajewska, H., Shamir, R., Nowak-Węgrzyn, A., 2017. Non-IgE-mediated gastrointestinal food allergies in children. Pediatr. Allergy Immunol. 28, 6–17.

Chase, M.W., 1946. Inhibition of experimental drug allergy by prior feeding of the sensitizing agent. Proc. Soc. Exp. Biol. Med. 61, 257–259.

Chatchatee, P., Nowak-Wegrzyn, A., Lange, L., Benjaponpitak, S., Chong, K.W., Sangsupawanich, P., van Ampting, M.T.J., Oude Nijhuis, M.M., Harthoorn, L.F., Langford, J.E., Knol, J., Knipping, K., Garssen, J., Trendelenburg, V., Pesek, R., Davis, C.M., Muraro, A., Erlewyn-Lajeunesse, M., Fox, A.T., Michaelis, L.J., Beyer, K., Team, P. S, 2021. Tolerance development in cow's milk-allergic infants receiving amino acid-based formula: a randomized controlled trial. J. Allergy Clin. Immunol. 149, 650–658.e5.

Chehade, M., Mayer, L., 2005. Oral tolerance and its relation to food hypersensitivities. J. Allergy Clin. Immunol. 115, 3–12 (quiz 13).

Chida, Y., Hamer, M., Steptoe, A., 2008. A bidirectional relationship between psychosocial factors and atopic disorders: a systematic review and meta-analysis. Psychosom. Med. 70, 102–116.

Christie, L., Hine, R.J., Parker, J.G., Burks, W., 2002. Food allergies in children affect nutrient intake and growth. J. Am. Diet. Assoc. 102, 1648–1651.

Coombes, J.L., Siddiqui, K.R.R., Arancibia-Cárcamo, C.V., Hall, J., Sun, C.M., Belkaid, Y., Powrie, F., 2007. A functionally specialized population of mucosal CD103+ DCs induces Foxp3+ regulatory T cells via a TGF-β -and retinoic acid-dependent mechanism. J. Exp. Med. 204, 1757–1764.

Cox, L.M., Yamanishi, S., Sohn, J., Alekseyenko, A.V., Leung, J.M., Cho, I., Kim, S.G., Li, H., Gao, Z., Mahana, D., Zárate Rodriguez, J.G., Rogers, A.B., Robine, N., Loke, P., Blaser, M.J., 2014. Altering the intestinal microbiota during a critical developmental window has lasting metabolic consequences. Cell 158, 705–721.

Davis, B.P., Rothenberg, M.E., 2016. Mechanisms of disease of eosinophilic esophagitis. Annu. Rev. Pathol. 11, 365–393.

de Silva, D., Halken, S., Singh, C., Muraro, A., Angier, E., Arasi, S., Arshad, H., Beyer, K., Boyle, R., Du Toit, G., Eigenmann, P., Grimshaw, K., Hoest, A., Jones, C., Khaleva, E., Lack, G., Szajewska, H., Venter, C., Verhasselt, V., Roberts, G., 2020. Preventing food allergy in infancy and childhood: systematic review of randomised controlled trials. Pediatr. Allergy Immunol. 31, 813–826.

Devonshire, A.L., Robison, R.G., 2019. Prevention of food allergy. Allergy Asthma Proc. 40, 450–452.

Dominguez-Bello, M.G., Godoy-Vitorino, F., Knight, R., Blaser, M.J., 2019. Role of the microbiome in human development. Gut 68, 1108–1114.

Du Toit, G., Katz, Y., Sasieni, P., Mesher, D., Maleki, S.J., Fisher, H.R., Fox, A.T., Turcanu, V., Amir, T., Zadik-Mnuhin, G., Cohen, A., Livne, I., Lack, G., 2008. Early consumption of peanuts in infancy is associated with a low prevalence of peanut allergy. J. Allergy Clin. Immunol. 122, 984–991.

Du Toit, G., Roberts, G., Sayre, P.H., Plaut, M., Bahnson, H.T., Mitchell, H., Radulovic, S., Chan, S., Fox, A., Turcanu, V., Lack, G., 2013. Identifying infants at high risk of Peanut allergy: the learning early about Peanut allergy (LEAP) screening study. J. Allergy Clin. Immunol. 131, 135–143.e1-12.

Du Toit, G., Roberts, G., Sayre, P.H., Bahnson, H.T., Radulovic, S., Santos, A.F., Brough, H.A., Phippard, D., Basting, M., Feeney, M., Turcanu, V., Sever, M.L., Gomez Lorenzo, M., Plaut, M., Lack, G., 2015. Randomized trial of peanut consumption in infants at risk for peanut allergy. N. Engl. J. Med. 372, 803–813.

Du Toit, G., Tsakok, T., Lack, S., Lack, G., 2016. Prevention of food allergy. J. Allergy Clin. Immunol. 137, 998–1010.

Feleszko, W., Jaworska, J., Rha, R.D., Steinhausen, S., Avagyan, A., Jaudszus, A., Ahrens, B., Groneberg, D.A., Wahn, U., Hamelmann, E., 2007. Probiotic-induced suppression of allergic sensitization and airway inflammation is associated with an increase of T regulatory-dependent mechanisms in a murine model of asthma. Clin. Exp. Allergy 37, 498–505.

Fergusson, D.M., Horwood, L.J., Shannon, F.T., 1982. Risk factors in childhood eczema. J. Epidemiol. Community Health 36, 118–122.

Fiocchi, A., Assa'ad, A., Bahna, S., 2006. Food allergy and the introduction of solid foods to infants: a consensus document. Ann. Allergy Asthma Immunol. 97, 10–21.

Fiocchi, A., Burks, W., Bahna, S.L., Bielory, L., Boyle, R.J., Cocco, R., Dreborg, S., Goodman, R., Kuitunen, M., Haahtela, T., Heine, R.G., Lack, G., Osborn, D.A., Sampson, H., Tannock, G.W., Lee, B.W., 2012. Clinical use of probiotics in Pediatric allergy (CUPPA): a world allergy organization position paper. World Allergy Organ. J. 5, 148–167.

Fleischer, D.M., Spergel, J.M., Assa'ad, A.H., Pongracic, J.A., 2013. Primary prevention of allergic disease through nutritional interventions. J Allergy Clin Immunol Pract 1, 29–36.

Fleischer, D.M., Sicherer, S., Greenhawt, M., Campbell, D., Chan, E., Muraro, A., Halken, S., Katz, Y., Ebisawa, M., Eichenfield, L., Sampson, H., Lack, G., Du Toit, G., Roberts, G., Bahnson, H., Feeney, M., Hourihane, J., Spergel, J., Young, M., As'aad, A., Allen, K., Prescott, S., Kapur, S., Saito, H., Agache, I., Akdis, C.A., Arshad, H., Beyer, K., Dubois, A., Eigenmann, P., Fernandez-Rivas, M., Grimshaw, K., Hoffman-Sommergruber, K., Host, A., Lau, S., O'Mahony, L., Mills, C., Papadopoulos, N., Venter, C., Agmon-Levin, N., Kessel, A., Antaya, R., Drolet, B., Rosenwasser, L., 2016. Consensus communication on early Peanut introduction and prevention of Peanut allergy in high-risk infants. Pediatr. Dermatol. 33, 103–106.

Forsyth, J.S., Ogston, S.A., Clark, A., Florey, C.D., Howie, P.W., 1993. Relation between early introduction of solid food to infants and their weight and illnesses during the first two years of life. BMJ 306, 1572–1576.

Fox, A.T., Wopereis, H., van Ampting, M.T.J., Oude Nijhuis, M.M., Butt, A.M., Peroni, D.G., Vandenplas, Y., Candy, D.C.A., Shah, N., West, C.E., Garssen, J., Harthoorn, L.F., Knol, J., Michaelis, L.J., Group, A. S, 2019. A specific synbiotic-containing amino acid-based formula in dietary management of cow's milk allergy: a randomized controlled trial. Clin. Transl. Allergy 9, 5.

Fujimura, K.E., Sitarik, A.R., Havstad, S., Lin, D.L., Levan, S., Fadrosh, D., Panzer, A.R., Lamere, B., Rackaityte, E., Lukacs, N.W., Wegienka, G., Boushey, H.A., Ownby, D.R., Zoratti, E.M., Levin, A.M., Johnson, C.C., Lynch, S.V., 2016. Neonatal gut microbiota associates with childhood multisensitized atopy and T cell differentiation. Nat. Med. 22, 1187–1191.

Gan, J., Bornhorst, G.M., Henrick, B.M., German, J.B., 2018. Protein digestion of baby foods: study approaches and implications for infant health. Mol. Nutr. Food Res. 62, 00231.

Gappa, M., Filipiak-Pittroff, B., Libuda, L., von Berg, A., Koletzko, S., Bauer, C.P., Heinrich, J., Schikowski, T., Berdel, D., Standl, M., 2021. Long-term effects of hydrolyzed formulae on atopic diseases in the GINI study. Allergy 76, 1903–1907.

Gartner, L.M., Morton, J., Lawrence, R.A., Naylor, A.J., O'Hare, D., Schanler, R.J., Eidelman, A.I., 2005. Breastfeeding and the use of human milk. Pediatrics 115, 496–506.

Giannetti, A., Bernardini, L., Cangemi, J., Gallucci, M., Masetti, R., Ricci, G., 2020. Role of vitamin D in prevention of food allergy in infants. Front. Pediatr. 8, 447.

Gibson, G.R., Hutkins, R., Sanders, M.E., Prescott, S.L., Reimer, R.A., Salminen, S.J., Scott, K., Stanton, C., Swanson, K.S., Cani, P.D., Verbeke, K., Reid, G., 2017. Expert consensus document: the international scientific Association for Probiotics and Prebiotics (ISAPP) consensus statement on the definition and scope of prebiotics. Nat. Rev. Gastroenterol. Hepatol. 14, 491–502.

Ginde, A.A., Liu, M.C., Camargo Jr., C.A., 2009. Demographic differences and trends of vitamin D insufficiency in the US population, 1988-2004. Arch. Intern. Med. 169, 626–632.

Goldberg, M.R., Nachshon, L., Sinai, T., Epstein-Rigbi, N., Oren, Y., Eisenberg, E., Katz, Y., Elizur, A., 2018. Risk factors for reduced bone mineral density measurements in milk-allergic patients. Pediatr. Allergy Immunol. 29, 850–856.

Goubier, A., Dubois, B., Gheit, H., Joubert, G., Villard-Truc, F., Asselin-Paturel, C., Trinchieri, G., Kaiserlian, D., 2008. Plasmacytoid dendritic cells mediate oral tolerance. Immunity 29, 464–475.

Gouw, J.W., Jo, J., Meulenbroek, L., Heijjer, T.S., Kremer, E., Sandalova, E., Knulst, A.C., Jeurink, P.V., Garssen, J., Rijnierse, A., Knippels, L.M.J., 2018. Identification of peptides with tolerogenic potential in a hydrolysed whey-based infant formula. Clin. Exp. Allergy 48, 1345–1353.

Greer, F.R., Sicherer, S.H., Burks, A.W., 2008. Effects of early nutritional interventions on the development of atopic disease in infants and children: the role of maternal dietary restriction, breastfeeding, timing of introduction of complementary foods, and hydrolyzed formulas. Pediatrics 121, 183–191.

Greer, F.R., Sicherer, S.H., Burks, A.W., 2019. The effects of early nutritional interventions on the development of atopic disease in infants and children: the role of maternal dietary restriction, breastfeeding, hydrolyzed formulas, and timing of introduction of allergenic complementary foods. Pediatrics 143, e20190281.

Grimshaw, K.E., Maskell, J., Oliver, E.M., Morris, R.C., Foote, K.D., Mills, E.N., Roberts, G., Margetts, B.M., 2013. Introduction of complementary foods and the relationship to food allergy. Pediatrics 132, e1529–e1538.

Guarner, F., Schaafsma, G.J., 1998. Probiotics. Int. J. Food Microbiol. 39, 237–238.

Gunaratne, A.W., Makrides, M., Collins, C.T., 2015. Maternal prenatal and/or postnatal n-3 long chain polyunsaturated fatty acids (LCPUFA) supplementation for preventing allergies in early childhood. Cochrane Database Syst. Rev. 2015, CD010085.

Gunnar, M.R., Donzella, B., 2002. Social regulation of the cortisol levels in early human development. Psychoneuroendocrinology 27, 199–220.

Gupta, R.S., Warren, C.M., Smith, B.M., Blumenstock, J.A., Jiang, J., Davis, M.M., Nadeau, K.C., 2018. The public health impact of parent-reported childhood food allergies in the United States. Pediatrics 142, e20181235.

Gupta, R.S., Warren, C.M., Smith, B.M., Jiang, J., Blumenstock, J.A., Davis, M.M., Schleimer, R.P., Nadeau, K.C., 2019. Prevalence and severity of food allergies among US adults. JAMA Netw. Open 2, e185630.

Guttman-Yassky, E., Waldman, A., Ahluwalia, J., Ong, P.Y., Eichenfield, L.F., 2017. Atopic dermatitis: pathogenesis. Semin. Cutan. Med. Surg. 36, 100–103.

Hadis, U., Wahl, B., Schulz, O., Hardtke-Wolenski, M., Schippers, A., Wagner, N., Müller, W., Sparwasser, T., Förster, R., Pabst, O., 2011. Intestinal tolerance requires gut homing and expansion of FoxP3+ regulatory T cells in the lamina propria. Immunity 34, 237–246.

Halken, S., Høst, A., 1996. Prevention of allergic disease. Exposure to food allergens and dietetic intervention. Pediatr. Allergy Immunol. 7, 102–107.

Halken, S., Hansen, K.S., Jacobsen, H.P., Estmann, A., Faelling, A.E., Hansen, L.G., Kier, S.R., Lassen, K., Lintrup, M., Mortensen, S., Ibsen, K.K., Osterballe, O., Host, A., 2000. Comparison of a partially hydrolyzed infant formula with two extensively hydrolyzed formulas for allergy prevention: a prospective, randomized study. Pediatr. Allergy Immunol. 11, 149–161.

Hay, A.D., Heron, J., Ness, A., Team, A. S, 2005. The prevalence of symptoms and consultations in pre-school children in the Avon longitudinal study of parents and children (ALSPAC): a prospective cohort study. Fam. Pract. 22, 367–374.

Heller, F., Duchmann, R., 2003. Intestinal flora and mucosal immune responses. Int. J. Med. Microbiol. 293, 77–86.

Hill, C., Guarner, F., Reid, G., Gibson, G.R., Merenstein, D.J., Pot, B., Morelli, L., Canani, R.B., Flint, H.J., Salminen, S., Calder, P.C., Sanders, M.E., 2014. Expert consensus document. The international scientific Association for Probiotics and Prebiotics consensus statement on the scope and appropriate use of the term probiotic. Nat. Rev. Gastroenterol. Hepatol. 11, 506–514.

Hill, D.A., Grundmeier, R.W., Ramos, M., Spergel, J.M., 2018. Eosinophilic esophagitis is a late manifestation of the allergic march. J Allergy Clin Immunol Pract 6, 1528–1533.

Hong, S.W., Eunju, O., Lee, J.Y., Lee, M., Han, D., Ko, H.J., Sprent, J., Surh, C.D., Kim, K.S., 2019. Food antigens drive spontaneous IgE elevation in the absence of commensal microbiota. Sci. Adv. 5 (eaaw1507).

Hooper, L.V., Littman, D.R., Macpherson, A.J., 2012. Interactions between the microbiota and the immune system. Science 336, 1268–1273.

Howe, L., Franxman, T., Teich, E., Greenhawt, M., 2014. What affects quality of life among caregivers of food-allergic children? Ann. Allergy Asthma Immunol. 113, 69–74.e2.

Ilchmann, A., Burgdorf, S., Scheurer, S., Waibler, Z., Nagai, R., Wellner, A., Yamamoto, Y., Yamamoto, H., Henle, T., Kurts, C., Kalinke, U., Vieths, S., Toda, M., 2010. Glycation of a food allergen by the Maillard reaction enhances its T-cell immunogenicity: role of macrophage scavenger receptor class A type I and II. J. Allergy Clin. Immunol. 125, 175–183.e1-11.

Jackson-Browne, M.S., Henderson, N., Patti, M., Spanier, A., Braun, J.M., 2019. The impact of early-life exposure to antimicrobials on asthma and eczema risk in children. Curr. Environ. Health Rep. 6, 214–224.

Järvinen, K.M., Westfall, J., de Jesus, M., Mantis, N.J., Carroll, J.A., Metzger, D.W., Sampson, H.A., Berin, M.C., 2015. Role of maternal dietary peanut exposure in development of food allergy and oral tolerance. PLoS One 10, e0143855.

Johansson-Lindbom, B., Svensson, M., Pabst, O., Palmqvist, C., Marquez, G., Förster, R., Agace, W.W., 2005. Functional specialization of gut CD103+ dendritic cells in the regulation of tissue-selective T cell homing. J. Exp. Med. 202, 1063–1073.

Jones, S.M., Burks, A.W., 2017. Food allergy. N. Engl. J. Med. 377, 1168–1176.

Joseph, C.L., Ownby, D.R., Havstad, S.L., Woodcroft, K.J., Wegienka, G., Mackechnie, H., Zoratti, E., Peterson, E.L., Johnson, C.C., 2011. Early complementary feeding and risk of food sensitization in a birth cohort. J. Allergy Clin. Immunol. 127, 1203–1210.e5.

Kajosaari, M., Saarinen, U.M., 1983. Prophylaxis of atopic disease by six months' total solid food elimination. Evaluation of 135 exclusively breast-fed infants of atopic families. Acta Paediatr. Scand. 72, 411–414.

Karlsson, M.R., Rugtveit, J., Brandtzaeg, P., 2004. Allergen-responsive CD4+CD25+ regulatory T cells in children who have outgrown cow's milk allergy. J. Exp. Med. 199, 1679–1688.

Katelaris, C.H., Beggs, P.J., 2018. Climate change: allergens and allergic diseases. Intern. Med. J. 48, 129–134.

Katz, P.P., Morris, A., Julian, L., Omachi, T., Yelin, E.H., Eisner, M.D., Blanc, P.D., 2010. Onset of depressive symptoms among adults with asthma: results from a longitudinal observational cohort. Prim. Care Respir. J. 19, 223–230.

Kim, S.H., Ban, G.Y., Park, H.S., Kim, S.C., Ye, Y.M., 2016. Regional differences in vitamin D levels and incidence of food-induced anaphylaxis in South Korea. Ann. Allergy Asthma Immunol. 116, 237–243.e1.

Kim, M., Galan, C., Hill, A.A., Wu, W.J., Fehlner-Peach, H., Song, H.W., Schady, D., Bettini, M.L., Simpson, K.W., Longman, R.S., Littman, D.R., Diehl, G.E., 2018. Critical role for the microbiota in CX(3)CR1(+) intestinal mononuclear phagocyte regulation of intestinal T cell responses. Immunity 49, 151–163.e5.

Koplin, J.J., Osborne, N.J., Wake, M., Martin, P.E., Gurrin, L.C., Robinson, M.N., Tey, D., Slaa, M., Thiele, L., Miles, L., Anderson, D., Tan, T., Dang, T.D., Hill, D.J., Lowe, A.J., Matheson, M.C., Ponsonby, A.L., Tang, M.L., Dharmage, S.C., Allen, K.J., 2010. Can early introduction of egg prevent egg allergy in infants? A population-based study. J. Allergy Clin. Immunol. 126, 807–813.

Koplin, J.J., Martin, P.E., Tang, M.L.K., Gurrin, L.C., Lowe, A.J., Osborne, N.J., Robinson, M.N., Ponsonby, A., Dharmage, S.C., Allen, K.J., 2012. Do factors known to alter infant microbial exposures alter the risk of food allergy and eczema in a population-based infant study? J. Allergy Clin. Immunol. 129, AB231.

Kramer, M.S., Kakuma, R., 2012. Optimal duration of exclusive breastfeeding. Cochrane Database Syst. Rev. 2012, CD003517.

Kramer, M.S., Kakuma, R., 2014. Maternal dietary antigen avoidance during pregnancy or lactation, or both, for preventing or treating atopic disease in the child. Evid. Based Child Health 9, 447–483.

Kuczmarski, R.J., Ogden, C.L., Guo, S.S., Grummer-Strawn, L.M., Flegal, K.M., Mei, Z., Wei, R., Curtin, L.R., Roche, A.F., Johnson, C.L., 2002. 2000 CDC growth charts for the United States: methods and development. Vital Health Stat. 11, 1–190.

Kull, I., Melen, E., Alm, J., Hallberg, J., Svartengren, M., van Hage, M., Pershagen, G., Wickman, M., Bergström, A., 2010. Breast-feeding in relation to asthma, lung function, and sensitization in young schoolchildren. J. Allergy Clin. Immunol. 125, 1013–1019.

Lack, G., Fox, D., Northstone, K., Golding, J., 2003. Factors associated with the development of peanut allergy in childhood. N. Engl. J. Med. 348, 977–985.

Laffont, S., Siddiqui, K.R.R., Powrie, F., 2010. Intestinal inflammation abrogates the tolerogenic properties of MLN CD103+ dendritic cells. Eur. J. Immunol. 40, 1877–1883.

Le, T.M., Zijlstra, W.T., van Opstal, E.Y., Knol, M.J., L'Hoir, M.P., Knulst, A.C., Pasmans, S.G., 2013. Food avoidance in children with adverse food reactions: influence of anxiety and clinical parameters. Pediatr. Allergy Immunol. 24, 650–655.

Lee-Sarwar, K., Hauser, R., Calafat, A.M., Ye, X., O'connor, G.T., Sandel, M., Bacharier, L.B., Zeiger, R.S., Laranjo, N., Gold, D.R., Weiss, S.T., Litonjua, A.A., Savage, J.H., 2018. Prenatal and early-life triclosan and paraben exposure and allergic outcomes. J. Allergy Clin. Immunol. 142, 269–278.e15.

Levin, M.E., Botha, M., Basera, W., Facey-Thomas, H.E., Gaunt, B., Gray, C.L., Kiragu, W., Ramjith, J., Watkins, A., Genuneit, J., 2020. Environmental factors associated with allergy in urban and rural children from the south African food allergy (SAFFA) cohort. J. Allergy Clin. Immunol. 145, 415–426.

Lieberman, J.A., Weiss, C., Furlong, T.J., Sicherer, M., Sicherer, S.H., 2010. Bullying among pediatric patients with food allergy. Ann. Allergy Asthma Immunol. 105, 282–286.

Lopes, J.P., Sicherer, S., 2020. Food allergy: epidemiology, pathogenesis, diagnosis, prevention, and treatment. Curr. Opin. Immunol. 66, 57–64.

Lowe, A.J., Hosking, C.S., Bennett, C.M., Allen, K.J., Axelrad, C., Carlin, J.B., Abramson, M.J., Dharmage, S.C., Hill, D.J., 2011. Effect of a partially hydrolyzed whey infant formula at weaning on risk of allergic disease in high-risk children: a randomized controlled trial. J. Allergy Clin. Immunol. 128, 360–U373.

Luccioli, S., Zhang, Y., Verrill, L., Ramos-Valle, M., Kwegyir-Afful, E., 2014. Infant feeding practices and reported food allergies at 6 years of age. Pediatrics 134 (suppl 1), S21–S28.

MacKenzie, H., Roberts, G., van Laar, D., Dean, T., 2010. Teenagers' experiences of living with food hypersensitivity: a qualitative study. Pediatr. Allergy Immunol. 21, 595–602.

Mallet, E., Henocq, A., 1992. Long-term prevention of allergic diseases by using protein hydrolysate formula in at-risk infants. J. Pediatr. 121, S95–S100.

Marrs, T., Bruce, K.D., Logan, K., Rivett, D.W., Perkin, M.R., Lack, G., Flohr, C., 2013. Is there an association between microbial exposure and food allergy? A systematic review. Pediatr. Allergy Immunol. 24, 311–320.e8.

Marshall, N.B., Lukomska, E., Nayak, A.P., Long, C.M., Hettick, J.M., Anderson, S.E., 2017. Topical application of the anti-microbial chemical triclosan induces immunomodulatory responses through the S100A8/A9-TLR4 pathway. J. Immunotoxicol. 14, 50–59.

Matsui, T., Tanaka, K., Yamashita, H., Saneyasu, K.I., Tanaka, H., Takasato, Y., Sugiura, S., Inagaki, N., Ito, K., 2019. Food allergy is linked to season of birth, sun exposure, and vitamin D deficiency. Allergol. Int. 68, 172–177.

McFadden, J.P., Thyssen, J.P., Basketter, D.A., Puangpet, P., Kimber, I., 2015. T helper cell 2 immune skewing in pregnancy/early life: chemical exposure and the development of atopic disease and allergy. Br. J. Dermatol. 172, 584–591.

Mehta, H., Ramesh, M., Feuille, E., Groetch, M., Wang, J., 2014. Growth comparison in children with and without food allergies in 2 different demographic populations. J. Pediatr. 165, 842–848.

Meltzer, E.O., 2016. Allergic rhinitis: burden of illness, quality of life, comorbidities, and control. Immunol. Allergy Clin. N. Am. 36, 235–248.

Metsala, J., Lundqvist, A., Kaila, M., Gissler, M., Klaukka, T., Virtanen, S.M., 2010. Maternal and perinatal characteristics and the risk of cow's milk allergy in infants up to 2 years of age: a case-control study nested in the Finnish population. Am. J. Epidemiol. 171, 1310–1316.

Miles, E.A., Calder, P.C., 2017. Can early omega-3 fatty acid exposure reduce risk of childhood allergic disease? Nutrients 9, 784.

Mondoulet, L., Paty, E., Drumare, M.F., Ah-Leung, S., Scheinmann, P., Willemot, R.M., Wal, J.M., Bernard, H., 2005. Influence of thermal processing on the allergenicity of peanut proteins. J. Agric. Food Chem. 53, 4547–4553.

Monto, A.S., 2002. Epidemiology of viral respiratory infections. Am. J. Med. 112 (suppl 6A), 4S–12S.

Mor, G., Aldo, P., Alvero, A.B., 2017. The unique immunological and microbial aspects of pregnancy. Nat. Rev. Immunol. 17, 469–482.

Morelli, L., Capurso, L., 2012. FAO/WHO guidelines on probiotics: 10 years later. J. Clin. Gastroenterol. 46 (suppl), S1–S2.

Msallam, R., Balla, J., Rathore, A.P.S., Kared, H., Malleret, B., Saron, W.A.A., Liu, Z., Hang, J.W., Dutertre, C.A., Larbi, A., Chan, J.K.Y., St John, A.L., Ginhoux, F., 2020. Fetal mast cells mediate postnatal allergic responses dependent on maternal IgE. Science 370, 941–950.

Muñoz-Furlong, A., 2001. Living with food allergies: not as easy as you might think. FDA Consum. 35, 40.

Muñoz-Furlong, A., 2003. Daily coping strategies for patients and their families. Pediatrics 111, 1654–1661.

Muraro, A., Dreborg, S., Halken, S., Høst, A., Niggemann, B., Aalberse, R., Arshad, S.H., Berg Av, A., Carlsen, K., Duschén, K., Eigenmann, P., Hill, D., Jones, C., Mellon, M., Oldeus, G., Oranje, A., Pascual, C., Prescott, S., Sampson, H., Svartengren, M., Vandenplas, Y., Wahn, U., Warner, J.A., Warner, J.O., Wickman, M., Zeiger, R.S., 2004. Dietary prevention of allergic diseases in infants and small children. Part I: immunologic background and criteria for hypoallergenicity. Pediatr. Allergy Immunol. 15, 103–111.

Muraro, A., Halken, S., Arshad, S.H., Beyer, K., Dubois, A.E., Du Toit, G., Eigenmann, P.A., Grimshaw, K.E., Hoest, A., Lack, G., O'Mahony, L., Papadopoulos, N.G., Panesar, S., Prescott, S., Roberts, G., de Silva, D., Venter, C., Verhasselt, V., Akdis, A.C., Sheikh, A., 2014. EAACI food allergy and anaphylaxis guidelines. Primary prevention of food allergy. Allergy 69, 590–601.

Murray, C.S., Lucas, S.J., Blakey, J., Kaplan, A., Papi, A., Paton, J., Phipatanakul, W., Price, D., Teoh, O.H., Thomas, M., Turner, S., Papadopoulos, N.G., 2021. A real-life comparative effectiveness study into the addition of antibiotics to the management of asthma exacerbations in primary care. Eur. Respir. J. 58, 2003599.

Myles, I.A., 2014. Fast food fever: reviewing the impacts of the Western diet on immunity. Nutr. J. 13, 61.

Nagatake, T., Kunisawa, J., 2019. Emerging roles of metabolites of ω3 and ω6 essential fatty acids in the control of intestinal inflammation. Int. Immunol. 31, 569–577.

Netting, M.J., Middleton, P.F., Makrides, M., 2014. Does maternal diet during pregnancy and lactation affect outcomes in offspring? A systematic review of food-based approaches. Nutrition 30, 1225–1241.

Nowak-Wegrzyn, A., Spergel, J.M., 2017. Food protein-induced enterocolitis syndrome: not so rare after all! J. Allergy Clin. Immunol. 140, 1275–1276.

Nurmagambetov, T.A., Krishnan, J.A., 2019. What will uncontrolled asthma cost in the United States? Am. J. Respir. Crit. Care Med. 200, 1077–1078.

Nurmagambetov, T., Kuwahara, R., Garbe, P., 2018. The economic burden of asthma in the United States, 2008-2013. Ann. Am. Thorac. Soc. 15, 348–356.

Odhiambo, J.A., Williams, H.C., Clayton, T.O., Robertson, C.F., Asher, M.I., 2009. Global variations in prevalence of eczema symptoms in children from ISAAC phase three. J. Allergy Clin. Immunol. 124, 1251–1258.e23.

Ogden, C.L., Kuczmarski, R.J., Flegal, K.M., Mei, Z., Guo, S., Wei, R., Grummer-Strawn, L.M., Curtin, L.R., Roche, A.F., Johnson, C.L., 2002. Centers for Disease Control and Prevention 2000 growth charts for the United States: improvements to the 1977 National Center for Health Statistics version. Pediatrics 109, 45–60.

Oldaeus, G., Anjou, K., Bjorksten, B., Moran, J.R., Kjellman, N.I.M., 1997. Extensively and partially hydrolysed infant formulas for allergy prophylaxis. Arch. Dis. Child. 77, 4–10.

Oozeer, R., van Limpt, K., Ludwig, T., Ben Amor, K., Martin, R., Wind, R.D., Boehm, G., Knol, J., 2013. Intestinal microbiology in early life: specific prebiotics can have similar functionalities as human-milk oligosaccharides. Am. J. Clin. Nutr. 98, 561S–571S.

Osborn, D.A., Sinn, J., 2003. Formulas containing hydrolysed protein for prevention of allergy and food intolerance in infants. Cochrane Database Syst. Rev. (4), CD003664.

Osborn, D.A., Sinn, J., 2004. Soy formula for prevention of allergy and food intolerance in infants. Cochrane Database Syst. Rev. (3), CD003741.

Osborn, D.A., Sinn, J.K., 2007. Probiotics in infants for prevention of allergic disease and food hypersensitivity. Cochrane Database Syst. Rev. (4), CD006475.

Osborn, D.A., Sinn, J.K., 2013. Prebiotics in infants for prevention of allergy. Cochrane Database Syst. Rev. (3), CD006474.

Osborn, D.A., Sinn, J.K., Jones, L.J., 2018. Infant formulas containing hydrolysed protein for prevention of allergic disease. Cochrane Database Syst. Rev. 10, CD003664.

Osborne, N.J., Koplin, J.J., Martin, P.E., Gurrin, L.C., Lowe, A.J., Matheson, M.C., Ponsonby, A.L., Wake, M., Tang, M.L., Dharmage, S.C., Allen, K.J., 2011. Prevalence of challenge-proven IgE-mediated food allergy using population-based sampling and predetermined challenge criteria in infants. J. Allergy Clin. Immunol. 127, 668–676.e1-2.

Osborne, N.J., Ukoumunne, O.C., Wake, M., Allen, K.J., 2012. Prevalence of eczema and food allergy is associated with latitude in Australia. J. Allergy Clin. Immunol. 129, 865–867 (United States).

Oyoshi, M.K., Murphy, G.F., Geha, R.S., 2009. Filaggrin-deficient mice exhibit TH17-dominated skin inflammation and permissiveness to epicutaneous sensitization with protein antigen. J. Allergy Clin. Immunol. 124, 485–493.e1.

Pastor-Vargas, C., Maroto, A.S., Díaz-Perales, A., Villalba, M., Esteban, V., Ruiz-Ramos, M., de Alba, M.R., Vivanco, F., Cuesta-Herranz, J., 2016. Detection of major food allergens in amniotic fluid: initial allergenic encounter during pregnancy. Pediatr. Allergy Immunol. 27, 716–720.

Perkin, M.R., Logan, K., Tseng, A., Raji, B., Ayis, S., Peacock, J., Brough, H., Marrs, T., Radulovic, S., Craven, J., Flohr, C., Lack, G., 2016. Randomized trial of introduction of allergenic foods in breast-fed infants. N. Engl. J. Med. 374, 1733–1743.

Perkin, M.R., Logan, K., Bahnson, H.T., Marrs, T., Radulovic, S., Craven, J., Flohr, C., Mills, E.N., Versteeg, S.A., van Ree, R., Lack, G., 2019. Efficacy of the enquiring about tolerance (EAT) study among infants at high risk of developing food allergy. J. Allergy Clin. Immunol. 144, 1606–1614.e2.

Pham, M.N., Bunyavanich, S., 2018. Prenatal diet and the development of childhood allergic diseases: food for thought. Curr Allergy Asthma Rep 18, 58.

Polloni, L., Toniolo, A., Lazzarotto, F., Baldi, I., Foltran, F., Gregori, D., Muraro, A., 2013. Nutritional behavior and attitudes in food allergic children and their mothers. Clin. Transl. Allergy 3, 41.

Poole, J.A., Barriga, K., Leung, D.Y., Hoffman, M., Eisenbarth, G.S., Rewers, M., Norris, J.M., 2006. Timing of initial exposure to cereal grains and the risk of wheat allergy. Pediatrics 117, 2175–2182.

Rajani, P.S., Martin, H., Groetch, M., Järvinen, K.M., 2020. Presentation and management of food allergy in breastfed infants and risks of maternal elimination diets. J Allergy Clin Immunol Pract 8, 52–67.

Roduit, C., Frei, R., Depner, M., Schaub, B., Loss, G., Genuneit, J., Pfefferle, P., Hyvärinen, A., Karvonen, A.M., Riedler, J., Dalphin, J.C., Pekkanen, J., von Mutius, E., Braun-Fahrländer, C., Lauener, R., 2014. Increased food diversity in the first year of life is inversely associated with allergic diseases. J. Allergy Clin. Immunol. 133, 1056–1064.

Roduit, C., Frei, R., Depner, M., Karvonen, A.M., Renz, H., Braun-Fahrländer, C., Schmausser-Hechfellner, E., Pekkanen, J., Riedler, J., Dalphin, J.C., von Mutius, E., Lauener, R.P., Hyvärinen, A., Kirjavainen, P., Remes, S., Roponen, M., Dalphin, M.L., Kaulek, V., Ege, M., Genuneit, J., Illi, S., Kabesch, M., Schaub, B., Pfefferle, P.I., Doekes, G., 2017. Phenotypes of atopic dermatitis depending on the timing of onset and progression in childhood. JAMA Pediatr. 171, 655–662.

Rona, R.J., Keil, T., Summers, C., Gislason, D., Zuidmeer, L., Sodergren, E., Sigurdardottir, S.T., Lindner, T., Goldhahn, K., Dahlstrom, J., McBride, D., Madsen, C., 2007. The prevalence of food allergy: a meta-analysis. J. Allergy Clin. Immunol. 120, 638–646.

Rutayisire, E., Huang, K., Liu, Y., Tao, F., 2016. The mode of delivery affects the diversity and colonization pattern of the gut microbiota during the first year of infants' life: a systematic review. BMC Gastroenterol. 16, 86.

Saarinen, U.M., Kajosaari, M., Backman, A., Siimes, M.A., 1979. Prolonged breast-feeding as prophylaxis for atopic disease. Lancet 2, 163–166.

Salminen, S., Stahl, B., Vinderola, G., Szajewska, H., 2020. Infant formula supplemented with biotics: current knowledge and future perspectives. Nutrients 12, 1952.

Sanidad, K.Z., Xiao, H., Zhang, G., 2019. Triclosan, a common antimicrobial ingredient, on gut microbiota and gut health. Gut Microbes 10, 434–437.

Sarna, M., Ware, R.S., Sloots, T.P., Nissen, M.D., Grimwood, K., Lambert, S.B., 2016. The burden of community-managed acute respiratory infections in the first 2-years of life. Pediatr. Pulmonol. 51, 1336–1346.

Satish, U., Streufert, S., Dewan, M., Voort, S.V., 2004. Improvements in simulated real-world relevant performance for patients with seasonal allergic rhinitis: impact of desloratadine. Allergy 59, 415–420.

Savage, J.H., Matsui, E.C., Wood, R.A., Keet, C.A., 2012. Urinary levels of triclosan and parabens are associated with aeroallergen and food sensitization. J. Allergy Clin. Immunol. 130, 453–460.e7.

Schulz, O., Jaensson, E., Persson, E.K., Liu, X., Worbs, T., Agace, W.W., Pabst, O., 2009. Intestinal CD103+, but not CX3CR1+, antigen sampling cells migrate in lymph and serve classical dendritic cell functions. J. Exp. Med. 206, 3101–3114.

Section on Breastfeeding, 2012. Breastfeeding and the use of human milk. Pediatrics 129, e827-41.

Sharief, S., Jariwala, S., Kumar, J., Muntner, P., Melamed, M.L., 2011. Vitamin D levels and food and environmental allergies in the United States: results from the National Health and nutrition examination survey 2005-2006. J. Allergy Clin. Immunol. 127, 1195–1202.

Shemesh, E., Annunziato, R.A., Ambrose, M.A., Ravid, N.L., Mullarkey, C., Rubes, M., Chuang, K., Sicherer, M., Sicherer, S.H., 2013. Child and parental reports of bullying in a consecutive sample of children with food allergy. Pediatrics 131, e10–e17.

Shu, S.A., Yuen, A.W.T., Woo, E., Chu, K.H., Kwan, H.S., Yang, G.X., Yang, Y., Leung, P.S.C., 2019. Microbiota and food allergy. Clin. Rev. Allergy Immunol. 57, 83–97.

Sicherer, S.H., Sampson, H.A., 2018. Food allergy: a review and update on epidemiology, pathogenesis, diagnosis, prevention, and management. J. Allergy Clin. Immunol. 141, 41–58.

Silverberg, J.I., Barbarot, S., Gadkari, A., Simpson, E.L., Weidinger, S., Mina-Osorio, P., Rossi, A.B., Brignoli, L., Saba, G., Guillemin, I., Fenton, M.C., Auziere, S., Eckert, L., 2021. Atopic dermatitis in the pediatric population: a cross-sectional, international epidemiologic study. Ann. Allergy Asthma Immunol. 126, 417–428.e2.

Silvers, K.M., Frampton, C.M., Wickens, K., Pattemore, P.K., Ingham, T., Fishwick, D., Crane, J., Town, G.I., Epton, M.J., 2012. Breastfeeding protects against current asthma up to 6 years of age. J. Pediatr. 160, 991–996.e1.

Simon, D., Wollenberg, A., Renz, H., Simon, H.U., 2019. Atopic dermatitis: collegium internationale allergologicum (CIA) update 2019. Int. Arch. Allergy Immunol. 178, 207–218.

Smith, S.J., Abrams, E.M., Kozyrskyj, A., Becker, A., Protudjer, J.L.P., 2020. Food allergy and growth from late childhood to early adolescence. Ann. Allergy Asthma Immunol. 125, 483–485.

Snijders, B.E., Thijs, C., van Ree, R., van den Brandt, P.A., 2008. Age at first introduction of cow milk products and other food products in relation to infant atopic manifestations in the first 2 years of life: the KOALA birth cohort study. Pediatrics 122, e115–e122.

Sonnenschein-van der Voort, A.M., Jaddoe, V.W., van der Valk, R.J., Willemsen, S.P., Hofman, A., Moll, H.A., de Jongste, J.C., Duijts, L., 2012. Duration and exclusiveness of breastfeeding and childhood asthma-related symptoms. Eur. Respir. J. 39, 81–89.

Stern, D.A., Morgan, W.J., Halonen, M., Wright, A.L., Martinez, F.D., 2008. Wheezing and bronchial hyper-responsiveness in early childhood as predictors of newly diagnosed asthma in early adulthood: a longitudinal birth-cohort study. Lancet 372, 1058–1064.

Stinson, L.F., Gay, M.C.L., Koleva, P.T., Eggesbø, M., Johnson, C.C., Wegienka, G., Du Toit, E., Shimojo, N., Munblit, D., Campbell, D.E., Prescott, S.L., Geddes, D.T., Kozyrskyj, A.L., 2020. Human milk from atopic mothers has lower levels of short chain fatty acids. Front. Immunol. 11, 1427.

Strachan, D.P., 1989. Hay fever, hygiene, and household size. BMJ 299, 1259–1260.

Sudo, N., Sawamura, S., Tanaka, K., Aiba, Y., Kubo, C., Koga, Y., 1997. The requirement of intestinal bacterial flora for the development of an IgE production system fully susceptible to oral tolerance induction. J. Immunol. 159, 1739–1745.

Sugita, K., Akdis, C.A., 2020. Recent developments and advances in atopic dermatitis and food allergy. Allergol. Int. 69, 204–214.

Szajewska, H., Horvath, A., Piwowarczyk, A., 2010. Meta-analysis: the effects of saccharomyces boulardii supplementation on helicobacter pylori eradication rates and side effects during treatment. Aliment. Pharmacol. Ther. 32, 1069–1079.

Szajewska, H., Ruszczyński, M., Szymański, H., Sadowska-Krawczenko, I., Piwowarczyk, A., Rasmussen, P.B., Kristensen, M.B., West, C.E., Hernell, O., 2017. Effects of infant formula supplemented with prebiotics compared with synbiotics on growth up to the age of 12 mo: a randomized controlled trial. Pediatr. Res. 81, 752–758.

Tan, J., McKenzie, C., Potamitis, M., Thorburn, A.N., Mackay, C.R., Macia, L., 2014. The role of short-chain fatty acids in health and disease. Adv. Immunol. 121, 91–119.

Tan, J., McKenzie, C., Vuillermin, P.J., Goverse, G., Vinuesa, C.G., Mebius, R.E., Macia, L., Mackay, C.R., 2016. Dietary fiber and bacterial SCFA enhance oral tolerance and protect against food allergy through diverse cellular pathways. Cell Rep. 15, 2809–2824.

Tham, E.H., Leung, D.Y., 2019. Mechanisms by which atopic dermatitis predisposes to food allergy and the atopic march. Allergy, Asthma Immunol. Res. 11, 4–15.

Thompson, M., Vodicka, T.A., Blair, P.S., Buckley, D.I., Heneghan, C., Hay, A.D., Team, T. P, 2013. Duration of symptoms of respiratory tract infections in children: systematic review. BMJ 347, f7027.

Thompson-Chagoyan, O.C., Vieites, J.M., Maldonado, J., Edwards, C., Gil, A., 2010. Changes in faecal microbiota of infants with cow's milk protein allergy—a Spanish prospective case-control 6-month follow-up study. Pediatr. Allergy Immunol. 21, e394–e400.

Trompette, A., Gollwitzer, E.S., Yadava, K., Sichelstiel, A.K., Sprenger, N., Ngom-Bru, C., Blanchard, C., Junt, T., Nicod, L.P., Harris, N.L., Marsland, B.J., 2014. Gut microbiota metabolism of dietary fiber influences allergic airway disease and hematopoiesis. Nat. Med. 20, 159–166.

Urashima, M., Mezawa, H., Okuyama, M., Urashima, T., Hirano, D., Gocho, N., Tachimoto, H., 2019. Primary prevention of cow's milk sensitization and food allergy by avoiding supplementation with cow's milk formula at birth: a randomized clinical trial. JAMA Pediatr. 173, 1137–1145.

Vandenplas, Y., et al., 2020. Extensively hydrolyzed formula with two human milk oligosaccharides reduces rate of upper respiratory tract infections in infants with cow's milk allergy. In: Late-breaking oral abstract presentation at EAACI Digital Congress. Presented at the EAACI Digital Congress., 2020 Lausanne.

Vassallo, M.F., Banerji, A., Rudders, S.A., Clark, S., Mullins, R.J., Camargo Jr., C.A., 2010. Season of birth and food allergy in children. Ann. Allergy Asthma Immunol. 104, 307–313.

Venkataraman, D., Soto-Ramírez, N., Kurukulaaratchy, R.J., Holloway, J.W., Karmaus, W., Ewart, S.L., Arshad, S.H., Erlewyn-Lajeunesse, M., 2014. Filaggrin loss-of-function mutations are associated with food allergy in childhood and adolescence. J. Allergy Clin. Immunol. 134, 876–882.e4.

Venter, C., Meyer, R.W., Nwaru, B.I., Roduit, C., Untersmayr, E., Adel-Patient, K., Agache, I., Agostoni, C., Akdis, C.A., Bischoff, S.C., Du Toit, G., Feeney, M., Frei, R., Garn, H., Greenhawt, M., Hoffmann-Sommergruber, K., Lunjani, N., Maslin, K., Mills, C., Muraro, A., Pali-Schöll, I., Poulson, L.K., Reese, I., Renz, H., Roberts, G.C., Smith, P., Smolinska, S., Sokolowska, M., Stanton, C., Vlieg-Boerstra, B., O'mahony, L., 2019. EAACI position paper: influence of dietary fatty acids on asthma, food allergy, and atopic dermatitis. Allergy 74, 1429–1444.

Verduci, E., Banderali, G., Barberi, S., Radaelli, G., Lops, A., Betti, F., Riva, E., Giovannini, M., 2014. Epigenetic effects of human breast milk. Nutrients 6, 1711–1724.

Verhoeckx, K.C.M., Vissers, Y.M., Baumert, J.L., Faludi, R., Feys, M., Flanagan, S., Herouet-Guicheney, C., Holzhauser, T., Shimojo, R., van der Bolt, N., Wichers, H., Kimber, I., 2015. Food processing and allergenicity. Food Chem. Toxicol. 80, 223–240.

Vickery, B.P., Vereda, A., Casale, T.B., Beyer, K., Du Toit, G., Hourihane, J.O., Jones, S.M., Shreffler, W.G., Marcantonio, A., Zawadzki, R., Sher, L., Carr, W.W., Fineman, S., Greos, L., Rachid, R., Ibáñez, M.D., Tilles, S., Assa'ad, A.H., Nilsson, C., Rupp, N., Welch, M.J., Sussman, G., Chinthrajah, S., Blumchen, K., Sher, E., Spergel, J.M., Leickly, F.E., Zielen, S., Wang, J., Sanders, G.M., Wood, R.A., Cheema, A., Bindslev-Jensen, C., Leonard, S., Kachru, R., Johnston, D.T., Hampel Jr., F.C., Kim, E.H., Anagnostou, A., Pongracic, J.A., Ben-Shoshan, M., Sharma, H.P., Stillerman, A., Windom, H.H., Yang, W.H., Muraro, A., Zubeldia, J.M., Sharma, V., Dorsey, M.J., Chong, H.J., Ohayon, J., Bird, J.A., Carr, T.F., Siri, D., Fernández-Rivas, M., Jeong, D.K., Fleischer, D.M., Lieberman, J.A., Dubois, A.E.J., Tsoumani, M., Ciaccio, C.E., Portnoy, J.M., Mansfield, L.E., Fritz, S.B., Lanser, B.J., Matz, J., Oude Elberink, H.N.G., Varshney, P., Dilly, S.G., Adelman, D.C., Burks, A.W., 2018. AR101 oral immunotherapy for peanut allergy. N. Engl. J. Med. 379, 1991–2001.

Victora, C.G., Bahl, R., Barros, A.J., França, G.V., Horton, S., Krasevec, J., Murch, S., Sankar, M.J., Walker, N., Rollins, N.C., Group, L. B. S, 2016. Breastfeeding in the 21st century: epidemiology, mechanisms, and lifelong effect. Lancet 387, 475–490.

Vissing, N.H., Chawes, B.L., Rasmussen, M.A., Bisgaard, H., 2018. Epidemiology and risk factors of infection in early childhood. Pediatrics 141, e20170933.

von Berg, A., Koletzko, S., Grubl, A., Filipiak-Pittroff, B., Wichmann, H.E., Bauer, C.P., Reinhardt, D., Berdel, D., German Infant Nutritional, I, 2003. The effect of hydrolyzed cow's milk formula for allergy prevention in the first year of life: the German infant Nutritional intervention study, a randomized double-blind trial. J. Allergy Clin. Immunol. 111, 533–540.

von Berg, A., Filipiak-Pittroff, B., Schulz, H., Hoffmann, U., Link, E., Sußmann, M., Schnappinger, M., Brüske, I., Standl, M., Krämer, U., Hoffmann, B., Heinrich, J., Bauer, C.P., Koletzko, S., Berdel, D., 2016. Allergic manifestation 15 years after early intervention with hydrolyzed formulas—the GINI study. Allergy 71, 210–219.

von Berg, A., Filipiak-Pittroff, B., Krämer, U., Link, E., Heinrich, J., Koletzko, S., Grübl, A., Hoffmann, U., Beckmann, C., Reinhardt, D., Bauer, C.P., Wichmann, E., Berdel, D., 2017. The German infant Nutritional intervention study (GINI) for the preventive effect of hydrolyzed infant formulas in infants at high risk for allergic diseases. Design and selected results. Allergol. Select 1, 28–38.

Wahn, U., 2000. What drives the allergic march? Allergy 55, 591–599.

Wambre, E., Jeong, D., 2018. Oral tolerance development and maintenance. Immunol. Allergy Clin. N. Am. 38, 27–37.

Wambre, E., Bajzik, V., Delong, J.H., O'Brien, K., Nguyen, Q.A., Speake, C., Gersuk, V.H., Deberg, H.A., Whalen, E., Ni, C., Farrington, M., Jeong, D., Robinson, D., Linsley, P.S., Vickery, B.P., Kwok, W.W., 2017. A phenotypically and functionally distinct human T(H)2 cell subpopulation is associated with allergic disorders. Sci. Transl. Med. 9, eaam9171.

Weatherly, L.M., Gosse, J.A., 2017. Triclosan exposure, transformation, and human health effects. J. Toxicol. Environ. Health B Crit. Rev. 20, 447–469.

Weisse, K., Winkler, S., Hirche, F., Herberth, G., Hinz, D., Bauer, M., Röder, S., Rolle-Kampczyk, U., von Bergen, M., Olek, S., Sack, U., Richter, T., Diez, U., Borte, M., Stangl, G.I., Lehmann, I., 2013. Maternal and newborn vitamin D status and its impact on food allergy development in the German LINA cohort study. Allergy 68, 220–228.

Wells, H.G., Osborne, T.B., 1911. The biological reactions of the vegetable proteins. J. Infect. Dis. 8, 66–124.

Wickens, K., Black, P.N., Stanley, T.V., Mitchell, E., Fitzharris, P., Tannock, G.W., Purdie, G., Crane, J., 2008. A differential effect of 2 probiotics in the prevention of eczema and atopy: a double-blind, randomized, placebo-controlled trial. J. Allergy Clin. Immunol. 122, 788–794.

Wickens, K., Black, P., Stanley, T.V., Mitchell, E., Barthow, C., Fitzharris, P., Purdie, G., Crane, J., 2012. A protective effect of lactobacillus rhamnosus HN001 against eczema in the first 2 years of life persists to age 4 years. Clin. Exp. Allergy 42, 1071–1079.

Wickens, K., Stanley, T.V., Mitchell, E.A., Barthow, C., Fitzharris, P., Purdie, G., Siebers, R., Black, P.N., Crane, J., 2013. Early supplementation with lactobacillus rhamnosus HN001 reduces eczema prevalence to 6 years: does it also reduce atopic sensitization? Clin. Exp. Allergy 43, 1048–1057.

Williams, H., Stewart, A., von Mutius, E., Cookson, W., Anderson, H.R., 2008. Is eczema really on the increase worldwide? J. Allergy Clin. Immunol. 121, 947–954.e15.

Wright, R.J., 2005. Stress and atopic disorders. J. Allergy Clin. Immunol. 116, 1301–1306.

Yazdanbakhsh, M., Kremsner, P.G., van Ree, R., 2002. Allergy, parasites, and the hygiene hypothesis. Science 296, 490–494.

Zhang, T., Shi, Y., Zhao, Y., Wang, J., Wang, M., Niu, B., Chen, Q., 2019. Different thermal processing effects on peanut allergenicity. J. Sci. Food Agric. 99, 2321–2328.

Zheng, N., Gao, Y., Zhu, W., Meng, D., Walker, W.A., 2020. Short chain fatty acids produced by colonizing intestinal commensal bacterial interaction with expressed breast milk are anti-inflammatory in human immature enterocytes. PLoS One 15, e0229283.

Zutavern, A., Brockow, I., Schaaf, B., Bolte, G., von Berg, A., Diez, U., Borte, M., Herbarth, O., Wichmann, H.E., Heinrich, J., 2006. Timing of solid food introduction in relation to atopic dermatitis and atopic sensitization: results from a prospective birth cohort study. Pediatrics 117, 401–411.

Zutavern, A., Brockow, I., Schaaf, B., von Berg, A., Diez, U., Borte, M., Kraemer, U., Herbarth, O., Behrendt, H., Wichmann, H.E., Heinrich, J., 2008. Timing of solid food introduction in relation to eczema, asthma, allergic rhinitis, and food and inhalant sensitization at the age of 6 years: results from the prospective birth cohort study LISA. Pediatrics 121, e44–e52.

# Eating development in young children: The complex interplay of developmental domains

*Erin Sundseth Ross*

Feeding Fundamentals, LLC, Thornton, CO, United States; Department of Pediatrics, University of Colorado School of Medicine, Denver, CO, United States

## CHAPTER LEARNING OBJECTIVES

1. To discuss the influence of motor skill development, from birth to 2 years of age, as it relates to infant and young child feeding.

2. To describe how cognitive/language and self-awareness development shape early infant feedings, the transition to solids, and strategies to increase acceptance of novel foods.

3. To identify how sensory components of taste, smell, texture, and the visual representation of food impact how infants and young children learn to eat.

4. To recognize the reciprocal relationship between parent and child interactions at mealtimes and the role of parents, as teachers, in the development of healthy eating behaviors.

## 8.1 Introduction

Newborn infants are born with primitive reflexes to support the transition from intrauterine to extra-uterine life; among the most important are the reflexes that support eating. These reflexes are necessary until the infant has enough experience that they learn how to eat volitionally. The newborn infant is completely reliant upon the parent, and in this age range, all nutrition is in liquid form. Across the first 3 years of life, the responsibility and tasks during feeding transitions from the parent to the child. The child becomes proficient at eating a wide variety of age-appropriate foods. We have some evidence that nutrition influences motor, cognitive, and language developmental milestones (Villar et al., 2020; Khandelwal et al., 2020). However, the relationships between nutrition and achieving developmental milestones appear to be multifactorial (Michels et al., 2017). There is also evidence that suggests a complex interaction of skills and behaviors across developmental domains underlie the child's ability to transition to more complex foods. Skills develop within the gross, fine, and oral motor domains, and influence food preferences. Cognitive development during this timeframe affects how the child perceives their role and assumes their responsibilities within the feeding context. The child and the parent must negotiate this transition in responsibilities. The parent–child interaction during mealtimes is a strong influence on the child's acceptance of new foods and on family mealtimes. Children also increase their awareness and acceptance of various sensory properties of foods. How they experience the sensory inputs of food is another determinant of their willingness to try as well as eat a wide variety of age-appropriate foods.

In general, development in gross, fine, and oral motor skills, as well as within the cognitive arena, is widely thought to support the transition to more complex textures across the first 3 years of life. **Bright Futures in Practice: Nutrition** is a resource for staff working within the Women, Infants and Children US government nutrition organization (Story et al., 2002). This guide recognizes both the environment and the development of infants and children as influences on nutritional status. In fact, the guide specifically states that "the developmental approach, which is based on the unique social and psychological characteristics of each developmental period, is critical for understanding children's and adolescents' attitudes toward food and for encouraging healthy eating behaviors" (p. 5) (Story et al., 2002).

Theoretical models have been proposed that shed light on the complexity within this transition period (Ammon and Etzel, 1977; Wolstenholme et al., 2020). Eating requires coordination of skills across these developmental domains. It is difficult if not impossible to identify exactly what skill is necessary for what part of feeding; this is especially true for textured foods. On the surface, eating is easy—pick up a piece, bring it to the mouth, and chew and swallow the food. But what are the specific skills involved in this activity? Postural stability is a gross motor skill that allows an infant to use their hands for grasping. Eye-hand coordination, fine motor abilities, motor planning, and body awareness/spatial understanding are all interacting during reaching, grasping, and getting the food to the mouth. The sensory system processes what the food looks like, smells like, and feels like, and these inputs influence the decision and the direct actions to pick up the food. The more familiar the food (a cognitive factor), the more likely the child will try the food. Once the food is in the mouth, there is a complex integration of sensory (e.g., tactile and taste) and motor skills (e.g., tongue and jaw movements) that coordinate to track the food within the mouth and appropriately engage the correct motor patterns for chewing. Even after the food is swallowed, data suggest that postingestive feedback may influence preferences for food (Tepper and Barbarossa, 2020). Feeding appears to be easy but requires the ability to coordinate multiple inputs and skills. In addition, the child's increasing autonomy and their interactions with primary caregivers affect their mealtime behaviors.

Children must learn these skills to navigate the transitions in textures, which involve milk-feeds from a bottle or breast through a variety of solid textures. Solids typically begin with a smooth pureed food, and transition to a thicker mash or table foods mashed for the child. Parents then typically introduce meltable, easy to eat foods—also called finger foods or dissolvables (easy-to-chew). They next offer soft cubes or pieces (minced and moist), soft mechanical foods (soft and bite-sized to easy-to-chew), and then hard mechanical (regular) foods. The International Dysphagia Diet Standardization Initiative (IDDSI; https://www.iddsi.org)

has created a standardized definition for textures of foods, included here in "( )". Once a child can successfully manage textures in a single form, mixed texture meals—often called "family meals" round out the basis of the diet.

Parents and professionals both need to understand that eating relies on skill development. And children develop skills within a similar window of time, but not at the exact same time. Wide variations in the achievement of skills (motor, language, feeding, and social) are commonly reported (Cheng et al., 2009; Noller and Ingrisano, 1984). In addition, there is a difference between the emergence and mastery of these skills (Touwen, 1971; Noller and Ingrisano, 1984). Mastery is achieved within 6 months of emergence in only one-half of the infants across a variety of skills (Touwen, 1971; Noller and Ingrisano, 1984). Term and preterm infants achieve the developmental milestones in feeding at a similar age range when age is adjusted for prematurity (Torola et al., 2012). When parents offer foods to preterm infants based on chronological age rather than adjusted age, infants are more likely to lack the developmental skills necessary to manage the foods (Chung et al., 2014). Ex-preterm infants are more likely to reject foods (e.g., pushing foods away, gagging, crying, and holding foods in their mouth and refusing to swallow) if they are not developmentally ready (Chung et al., 2014). However, even healthy term babies may be offered foods for which they are not developmentally ready.

Further evidence that eating is reliant upon the motor, cognitive, and sensory skills comes from the body of literature focused on children with feeding problems. Children with motor, sensory, or cognitive delays/disorders often had problems feeding as infants and toddlers (Seiverling et al., 2019). For instance, children diagnosed with an autism spectrum disorder are at high risk of feeding problems both as infants and as children (Emond et al., 2010; Barnevik Olsson et al., 2013; Seiverling et al., 2018; Adams et al., 2020; Margari et al., 2020; Phillips et al., 2014; Hubbard et al., 2014). In fact, many children with developmental delays are at increased risk of growth and feeding disorders (Phillips et al., 2014; O'neill and Richter, 2013; Benfer et al., 2015; Stanley et al., 2019; Ravel et al., 2020; Osaili et al., 2019; Nordstrøm et al., 2020; Gal et al., 2011; Cooper-Brown et al., 2008; Calis et al., 2008). It is helpful to understand how children learn to eat when we are focusing on what children eat, to better recognize the many factors that influence a child's intake.

## 8.2 Summary of motor skill development

Motor skills develop in the gross motor, fine motor, and oral motor domains. And these skills are rapidly changing, especially in the first 2 years of life. Table 8.1 describes the major milestones for each food texture, within the domains of motor and postural, oral motor, sensory, and parental influences. The ages listed are approximate ranges for the emergence of the skills. These skills are described in greater detail in the following section.

### 8.2.1 Gross motor

A few published studies demonstrate a strong correlation between gross motor skill development and advancing oral motor skills between 5 and 24 months of age (Koda et al., 2006; Telles and Macedo, 2008). For instance, in healthy term infants, the emergence of sitting appears to be a prerequisite for the advancement of oral skills (Telles and Macedo, 2008). Infants whose gross motor and/or language skills occur later frequently show delays in developing

**TABLE 8.1** Developmental skills required to successfully transition through textures during the first 1000 days.

| Source of nutrition | Skills | Typical age ranges |
|---|---|---|
| Breast milk or formula during breast feeding and bottle feeding | **Motor and postural** | Birth through 2–4 months |
| | • Balanced flexion/extension, resulting in slightly flexed extremities, and neck | |
| | • Limited head control. Majority of postural support and head control provided by the feeder as they hold the infant | |
| | • Learns to move against gravity to push up, roll | |
| | • Fine motor skills are limited to a reflexive grasp initially, moving toward reaching and grasping volitionally | |
| | • Visual motor develops with tracking of visual inputs | |
| | **Oral motor** | Birth through 2 months |
| | • Oral movements in vertical plane during breast or bottle feeding | |
| | • Feeding supported by primitive responses (e.g., rooting, sucking, extrusion, and phasic bite) and controlled by a central pattern generator through 2–4 months of age | |
| | • Tongue, jaw, and cheeks in full contact with a vertical compression of all structures | |
| | • Sucking begins with compression, then integrates suction, which increases efficiency | |
| | • Beginning as early as 2 months of age, feeding skills transition to volitional and the infant loses the primitive reflexive motor movements as well as the central pattern generator | Two months through weaning |
| | **Sensory** | |
| | • During formula feeding, sensory inputs remain constant (visual, texture of the bottle, and taste/smell of the formula) | |
| | • During breast milk feeding, and especially with direct breast feeding, sensory inputs vary during the feeding and across the feeding based upon the mother's diet (smell/taste) and the emptying of the breast (texture) | |
| | **Parental interaction** | |
| | • Visual interaction and social engagement during feedings | |
| | • Parents decide when, what, and how to feed the infant | |

| Smooth purees | Motor and postural | Four months |
| | • Begins sitting in a semireclined chair | |
| | • Stable head control supported by body/trunk muscles in a semireclined position | |
| | • Swipes and reaches for objects, initially with two hands and then with one | |
| | • Combines reach and grasp (a two-step motor sequence), using a palmar grasp | |
| | • Brings toys to mouth (a three-step motor sequence), using a palmar grasp | |
| | • Greater awareness of body, as evidenced by grasping of toes and bilateral hand play as well as hands to mouth | |
| | • Moves to a more upright sitting position as they develop better postural stability | |
| | • Independent sitting emerges for brief periods | |
| | • Visual motor develops, as the infant begins to anticipate the spoon with an open mouth, and tongue protrusion may begin with visual presentation of the food | |
| | Oral motor | By 4 months |
| | • Feeding skills transition from primitive responses (with a loss of rooting, phasic biting, extrusion, and sucking driven by the Central Pattern Generators) to volitional movements of latching and sucking | |
| | • Stable head control supports stability as well as mobility of the jaw | |
| | • Upper lip begins to exert pressure on the spoon to clear food | |
| | • Initial difficulty with actively moving the food from the front to the back of the mouth | |
| | • Tongue movements integrate forward-backward movements of the tongue | |
| | • Most of the food is retained in mouth by 6 months | |
| | • Lower jaw grows downward/forward, increasing space in the oral cavity | |
| | • Larynx begins downward movement in neck | |
| | Sensory | Beginning at 5 months of age |
| | • Different visual (color), taste/smell, and texture inputs across feedings. These inputs remain more constant for commercially prepared foods | |
| | • Infants offered with home-made purees will receive varying visual, taste/smell and texture inputs within a feeding | |
| | • More vestibular input during feedings as infants sit more upright and move forward to accept the spoon | |
| | Parental Interaction | |
| | • Turn taking is introduced and reinforced with spoon feeding | |
| | • Positive reinforcement of bites and facial expressions can improve intake | |

*Continued*

**TABLE 8.1** Developmental skills required to successfully transition through textures during the first 1000 days—cont'd

| Source of nutrition | Skills | Typical age ranges |
|---|---|---|
| Meltable or dissolvable solids (Easy to chew) | **Motor and postural** | Six to eight months |
| | • Beginning of independent sitting, with improved head control | |
| | • Begins trunk rotation and weight shifting, allowing exploration of foods on tray | |
| | • Bilateral skill development supports gross motor skills (e.g., transferring toys between hands, crawling) as well as bilateral movements in the mouth | |
| | • Self-feeding typically emerges, requiring raking grasp patterns incorporating voluntary release skills | |
| | • Radial-palmar and radial-digital grasps emerge | |
| | • Visual-motor skills improve with looking for, grasping foods for self-feeding | |
| | **Oral motor** | Four to five months for primitive patterns |
| | • Munching (vertical) pattern of chewing appears | |
| | • Lip closure emerges during chewing and bolus formation | |
| | • Tongue moves laterally when food enters the mouth along the sides of the jaw | |
| | • May break off pieces of meltable foods with gums/pressure | |
| | • Emerging tongue lateralization | |
| | **Sensory** | |
| | • Visual, smell/taste, and tactile all changing with each new food. Auditory input of foods is minimal | |
| | • Within a food (as it is being eaten), the visual, smell/taste and tactile are changing, which requires a constant integration of these sensory inputs | |
| | **Parental interaction** | |
| | • Most families who are using baby-led weaning techniques are offering solid foods | |
| | • Cofeeding emerges | |
| Soft cubes/soft mechanicals (Minced and moist, soft and bite-sized) | **Motor and postural** | Seven to eight months |
| | • Inferior scissor and scissor grasps emerge | |
| | • Pincer grasps (inferior, pincer, and fine pincer) emerge | |
| | • Infant manipulates foods with hands and pulls soft foods apart with both hands, working on bilateral movements and visual-motor skills | |
| | **Oral motor** | Six to eight months of age |
| | • Munching pattern still predominant | |
| | • Lateral jaw movements support diagonal chewing, which may appear with some soft mechanical foods | |
| | • Tongue movements are independent of jaw movements | |
| | • Tongue lateralization (separate from jaw movements) moves foods toward, and holds foods on gums/teeth for chewing | |
| | **Sensory** | |
| | • Visual, smell/taste, and tactile all changing with each new food. Auditory typically is the same across foods | |
| | • Within a food (as it is being eaten), the visual may change. Smell/taste, tactile, and auditory may remain the same (with a single component food) | |
| | **Parental interaction** | |
| | • Some utensil use is introduced, with the parent loading the spoon or fork for the child | |
| | • Parental role modeling improves acceptance and intake | |

| Category | Details | Timing |
|---|---|---|
| Hard mechanicals (Regular) | **Motor and postural** | |
| | • With textured table foods, utensils are often introduced if they have not yet been offered | Ten to twelve months |
| | • Utensils require a body scheme and map to use a tool as an extension of the body | |
| | • Visual motor skills are required to place the utensil into the bowl, or to spear food onto a fork | |
| | **Oral motor** | |
| | • Initially can dip spoon into puree, but limited volume on spoon once it reaches mouth. | By fifteen to eighteen months |
| | • The child puts food onto a spoon or fork with fingers, and then brings to mouth | |
| | • Food is bitten off in larger pieces, or placed in the mouth with a utensil or fingers | |
| | • Food must be moved from the anterior oral cavity to the lateral edge of the teeth/gums | Seven to eight months |
| | • Placement of foods near back of mouth/angle of the jaw improves efficiency of chewing | |
| | • Diagonal and lateral movements begin with single shifts off midline, and slowly combine to reach a true rotary chewing motion | |
| | • Chewing begins with an arrhythmic, poorly graded rotary movement that improves with age. | Emergence of pattern by 8 months |
| | • Foods such as raw vegetables, fruits, legumes, and real meats require a rotary chewing motion that includes a shredding lateral shift of the jaw—the most sophisticated movement of the mouth | |
| | • Rotary chewing improves in coordination for several years | |
| | **Sensory** | |
| | • Visual, smell/taste, tactile, and auditory inputs all change with each new food | |
| | • Within a food (as it is being eaten), all inputs change as well | |
| | **Parental interaction** | |
| | • With emergence of language, children become more autonomous | |
| | • Battles about what to eat, how much to eat is a common complaint of parents | |
| | • Parents have the most control over their child's diet and can influence acceptance of foods through repeated exposure, modeling eating, talking about foods, and positive reinforcement | |
| Cup drinking | **Motor** | |
| | • Able to grasp objects at midline with both hands and bring to mouth with appropriate force while in a sitting position | Eight months |
| | • Able to rotate trunk/body and shift weight, maintaining a stable upright seated position while tilting head backward, engaging posture and balance | |
| | **Oral-motor** | |
| | • Jaw stability precedes lip control during drinking | Ten to twelve months |
| | • Able to create some jaw stability while the cup is at the mouth—typically first through biting on the cup or putting the tongue into the cup | |
| | • Able to draw fluid into the mouth, and then close the lips to prevent spillage | |
| | **Sensory** | |
| | • Over time children learn to drink a variety of flavors from a variety of cups | After twelve to fifteen months |
| | **Parental interaction** | |
| | • Parents often offer spouted sippy cups as they do not like the spill | |
| | • Parents can improve drinking by offering a variety of cups and allowing spills and mess | |

oral skills for eating (Koda et al., 2006). The period of time when self-feeding surpasses being fed by a caregiver coincides, in one study, with the emergence of walking (Koda et al., 2006). Delayed independent walking and timing of the introduction to solids are associated in yet another study (Wang et al., 2019b). Bringing hands to midline is another skill that occurs prior to volitional movement of the tongue toward midline (Telles and Macedo, 2008).

Sitting, grasping, crawling, and walking all have wide ranges of "normal emergence"(Touwen, 1971). Head control and body stability provide a motor base that supports fine motor function of hands and mouth (Telles and Macedo, 2008). Fine motor control and coordination both improve with the strengthening of the proximal musculature of the trunk (Naylor and Morrow, 2001). Between 4 and 9 months of age, there is also a wide variance in "quality" (e.g., sitting while propping with arms compared with sitting upright without support) (Touwen, 1971). Postural stability in sitting is important during chewing. In 12-month-olds there is a backward shift of the trunk, head, and neck during chewing (Stolovitz and Gisel, 1991).

## 8.2.2 Fine motor

Self-feeding improves throughout the second and third years of life (Nakao et al., 1990). Grasping begins with a two-step motor sequence (reach and grasp) and then moves to a three-step motor sequence (reach, grasp, and bring to mouth). Grasping goes through multiple refinements and is influenced by age as well as the size, distance, and texture of the object being grasped (Connolly and Dalgleish, 1989; Touwen, 1971; Berthier and Keen, 2006; Lee et al., 2006; Zaal and Thelen, 2005; Newell et al., 1993; McCarty et al., 1999, 2001; Von Hofsten and Ronnqvist, 1988; Tamura et al., 2000; Erhardt, 1994). Goal-directed reaching is observed as early as 4 months although there is great variability in speed, smoothness of movement, and efficiency across ages. Over the first year of life, there is increasing consistency in reaching quality (Connolly and Dalgleish, 1989).

Eye-hand coordination influences several skills of eating (Carruth and Skinner, 2002). Visual input affects grasping, with the hand starting to close in anticipation of the encounter with the object in infants as young as 5–6 months of age (Von Hofsten and Ronnqvist, 1988). Quality of fine motor behaviors (e.g., coordination) influences 8-month-olds' frequency of manipulation and oral exploration of objects (Kopp, 1974). Visual monitoring of objects increases from 6 to 12 months of age (Connolly and Dalgleish, 1989; Kochukhova and Gredeback, 2010). Grasping is also influenced by the touch and proprioceptive senses. In a study of 189 infants aged 7–21 months, researchers questioned whether infants "saw" or "felt" an object prior to reaching for the object on their arm (Chinn et al., 2019). They found that infants improved their coordination of reaching for objects placed on the opposite arm over time. Overall, 46% of infants looked for the object before reaching, 14% of infants reached for the object before looking for it, and 40% simultaneously looked and reached for the object (Chinn et al., 2019).

Eating with utensils is more difficult than eating with hands (Tamura et al., 2000). The utensil must be integrated into the body awareness—becoming an extension of the hand. The whole body initially moves when bringing the spoon to the mouth (Connolly and Dalgleish, 1989). Movement resulting from food being brought to the mouth changes from a simple movement of the elbow joint to a compound movement in which the shoulder, elbow, forearm, wrist joint, and finger are involved (Tamura et al., 2000). Wrist rotation is used more frequently when filling a spoon after the age of two (Connolly and Dalgleish, 1989).

Reaching and grasping are necessary for developing skills for self-feeding. Children who lack the ability to feed themselves are not able to assume their full responsibility for eating. This may affect their ability to transition to a full range of textures, which may, in turn, affect their dietary variety and consumption. Typically, a child who is unable to feed themselves remains on a liquid and/or pureed diet for an extended period; This restricted diet influences the development of oral skills.

## 8.2.3 Oral motor

Oral skills required for breast and bottle feeding are significantly different from those required to eat semisolid and solid foods. Healthy, term infants are born with a sophisticated repertoire of oral behaviors, controlled by a central pattern generator, that facilitate a rapid transition from intrauterine to extra-uterine life (Widstrom and Thingstrom-Paulsson, 1993; Widstrom et al., 2010; Sheppard and Mysak, 1984; Delaney and Arvedson, 2008; Da Costa et al., 2010; Davies et al., 1988; Selley et al., 1990; Rogers and Arvedson, 2005; Thach, 2007; Miller, 2002). Although primitive responses are present at birth, feeding undergoes a major transition within a window of approximately 2–4 months of age that includes a change in configuration of the oral structures and a loss of primitive responses as eating becomes volitional (Qureshi et al., 2002; Tamura et al., 1998; Delaney and Arvedson, 2008; Tutor and Gosa, 2011; Torola et al., 2012; Sheppard and Mysak, 1984; Widstrom and Thingstrom-Paulsson, 1993; Eishima, 1991).

### *8.2.3.1 Newborn feeding*

During the newborn period, the tongue and jaw move in unison, and the oral cavity and pharynx function as a single unit high in the neck of the infant (Cichero, 2017). Infants have buccal pads that support sucking and suction, and these are reabsorbed around 6 months of age when chewing requires more intraoral space (Dodrill and Gosa, 2015). Over the first 12 months of life, the anatomy changes as the oral skills develop to eat textured foods. Beginning around 3 months of age, the mandible grows downward and forward, increasing the space in the oral cavity and oro-pharynx (Tutor and Gosa, 2012). The infant's palate grows wider and higher from birth through 12 months of age (Le Reverend et al., 2014). By 2–3 years of age, the larynx descends and curve of pharynx is replaced by the clear 90-degree angle between the oropharynx and the nasopharynx (Gosa, 2013; Cichero, 2017).

Tongue and jaw movements are vertical during the initial period of infant feeding (Cichero, 2017; Dodrill and Gosa, 2015). Oral skills necessary for eating smooth pureed foods include a "forward-back" motion to draw the food from the front to the back of the mouth (Stolovitz and Gisel, 1991; Gisel, 1991; Cichero, 2017, 2016). Between 4 and 6 months of age, there is little differentiation of movement between the jaw and the tongue (Ayano et al., 2000). Infants retain most of the food in their mouth by 6 months of age, and use full lip closure to draw pureed food off of the spoon by 8 months of age (Stolovitz and Gisel, 1991; Telles and Macedo, 2008). In fact, lip pressure increases steadily from 5 months to 3 years of age (Chigira et al., 1994). Data from a small study using pureed foods suggest only a small increase in efficiency (time) is seen between 6 and 10 months, implying that skills for eating purees are fully mature by 10 months (Gisel, 1991). However, these foods are typically mashed upward into the palate, rather than manipulated by the tongue laterally.

### 8.2.3.2 Purees

Most studies suggest infants have the skill to eat and enjoy the process of eating purees sometime between 4 and 6 months of age (Kwavnick et al., 1999; Beal, 1957; Mennella et al., 2005; Torola et al., 2012; Brown and Lee, 2010; Lande et al., 2003; Cheng et al., 2009; Schwartz et al., 2011; Coulthard et al., 2010). In the few studies that directly measured oral ability to eat pureed foods, the fact that the majority of infants easily tolerated the food suggests that infants may develop the skill even earlier than offered (Torola et al., 2012; Wasser et al., 2011; Wright et al., 2004). There are old data that suggest infants offered foods very early (e.g., 1–2 months of age) respond with crying, fussing or spitting out the foods; they are willing to accept these foods when offered between 4 and 6 months of age (Beal, 1957). Across several cultures parents frequently introduce pureed foods early. Cereals are typically offered around 3 months, with a range of 1 and 1.5 months to 7 months (Wasser et al., 2011; Kwavnick et al., 1999; Beal, 1957; Caton et al., 2011; Wright et al., 2004; Dubois et al., 1979; Mennella et al., 2005; Lande et al., 2003; Carruth et al., 1997, 2004; Coulthard et al., 2009; Lanigan et al., 2001; Carruth and Skinner, 2002; Wang et al., 2019a). In a study of infants in the United States, approximately 32% of infants are introduced to complementary foods prior to 4 months of age (Chiang et al., 2020). This finding is also replicated in a study of Dutch infants, where 21% were introduced before 4 months (Wang et al., 2019a). One concern is that many infants are not developmentally ready to transition to purees at this young age.

### 8.2.3.3 Textured foods

With the introduction of finger- and table-foods, infants learn to move foods side-to-side in their mouth, chewing the foods while coordinating movements of both their tongue and their jaw (Gisel, 1988b,a, 1991; Gisel et al., 1984, 1986; Schwaab et al., 1986b,a; Stolovitz and Gisel, 1991). The movements of the jaw and tongue become multidirectional as the infant learns to eat these foods (Dodrill and Gosa, 2015). The simplistic movements that were managed by the central pattern generator are replaced by the more complex movements requiring greater cortical input necessary to eat textured foods (Dodrill and Gosa, 2015).

At 8 months, food is pressed into the mouth with the hand, or torn off with the teeth, and there is limited to no involvement of the lips in drawing the food into the mouth (Tamura et al., 2000). By 11 months, the movements of the jaw change to chewing, and the fingers place the foods into the mouth (Tamura et al., 2000). By 15 months of age, the fingers no longer enter the boundary of the mouth, because the teeth and the tongue accept the food at the lips and draw in the piece (Tamura et al., 2000).

The tongue appears to improve in the ability to move the food in the mouth with greater efficiency between 6 months and 4 years of age (Gisel, 1988b,a, 1991; Gisel et al., 1984, 1986; Schwaab et al., 1986b,a; Schwartz et al., 1984b,a; Stolovitz and Gisel, 1991). Between 6 and 24 months, children increasingly move solid textures from one side of the mouth to middle or to the other side and use lip closure during chewing (Stolovitz and Gisel, 1991). Beginning around 10 months of age, the tongue becomes increasingly independent of the movements of the jaw; it can now move foods laterally while the jaw is moving vertically (Stolovitz and Gisel, 1991; Dodrill and Gosa, 2015; Telles and Macedo, 2008).

Chewing requires coordination between antagonistic muscle pairs while activating both lateral and vertical movements (Harris and Coulthard, 2016). Each of these movements plays a different role in chewing, and different foods require different movement patterns (Wilson et al., 2012; Wilson and Green, 2009; Le Reverend et al., 2014; Simione et al., 2018). While jaw opening/closing is observed in 1-month-old infants, true chewing that requires a crushing force and appropriate food placement appear later, between 5 and a half months and 7 and a half months (Sheppard and Mysak, 1984). Infants who lack lateral tongue movements and/or chewing skills usually do not reject foods that require these movements. Rather, they often allow solid textures to melt in their mouths before initiating the swallow or swallow soft pieces whole (Stolovitz and Gisel, 1991; Harris and Mason, 2017). The strength and coordination of the muscles improve significantly between 6 and 24 months, with further improvement during the toddler years (Green et al., 1997; Steeve et al., 2008; Le Reverend et al., 2014; Wilson et al., 2012; Wilson and Green, 2009).

"Munching" involves vertical jaw movements without shifting off midline. This pattern is observable at a median age of 5 months with a range of 4–8 months (Gisel, 1991; Stolovitz and Gisel, 1991; Tamura et al., 2000; Torola et al., 2012). Infants 6–12 months of age often revert to sucking behaviors with purees while they use chewing motions with solids (Gisel, 1991). Lateral and diagonal jaw movements are more evident between 5 and 12 months of age (Telles and Macedo, 2008; Torola et al., 2012; Le Reverend et al., 2014; Wilson et al., 2012; Wilson and Green, 2009). There is a marked decrease in time and chewing cycles for eating solid and viscous foods between 6 months and 2 years, with the majority of improvements seen between 6 and 10 months of age (Gisel, 1988b, 1991; Wilson et al., 2012; Green et al., 1997; Wilson and Green, 2009; Stolovitz and Gisel, 1991; Tamura et al., 2000; Zucker and Hughes, 2020).

However, the texture of food affects the number of cycles observed during chewing as well as the time required for chewing a bite of food (Gisel, 1988b, 1991, 1988a; Stolovitz and Gisel, 1991; Schwaab et al., 1986a). The lack of a standard food with which to test chewing has been cited as a major limitation of what is currently known about the development of mastication (Le Reverend et al., 2014). We do have longitudinal data collected from infants beginning at 9 and continuing through 36 months (Simione et al., 2018). Across this time period, oral skills improved, but the texture of the food significantly influenced which chewing abilities were used (Simione et al., 2018). The force necessary to crush the food, the texture (wet vs dry), and the amount of saliva that was produced, as well as the density of the food all influenced the jaw excursions both vertically and laterally (Simione et al., 2018).

Jaw movements mature further to include a more coordinated, "rotary chew" that involves vertical, diagonal, and rotary movements (Torola et al., 2012; Gisel, 1991; Telles and Macedo, 2008; Wilson et al., 2012; Wilson and Green, 2009). Beginning rotary movements appear at a median of 7–8 months, with a range of 7–10 months (Torola et al., 2012). However, these rudimentary movements are not used functionally at this age. Early chewing is less coordinated and more arrhythmic than mature chewing (Cichero, 2016). In fact, early chewing begins with very little shifting off midline (Wilson and Green, 2009). Coordinated movements of the muscles required for both vertical and diagonal/rotary chewing are well established by 12 months of age but continue to be refined throughout childhood (Green et al., 1997; Telles and Macedo, 2008). Chewing motions between 12 and 36 months of age decrease in variability and increase in efficiency with a decrease in both time and cycles required for chewing (Gisel, 1988b; Wilson et al., 2012). As shown in Fig. 8.1, the jaw begins to show a rotary pattern, characterized eventually by a common point of occlusion and less variability in vertical, horizontal, and diagonal planes.

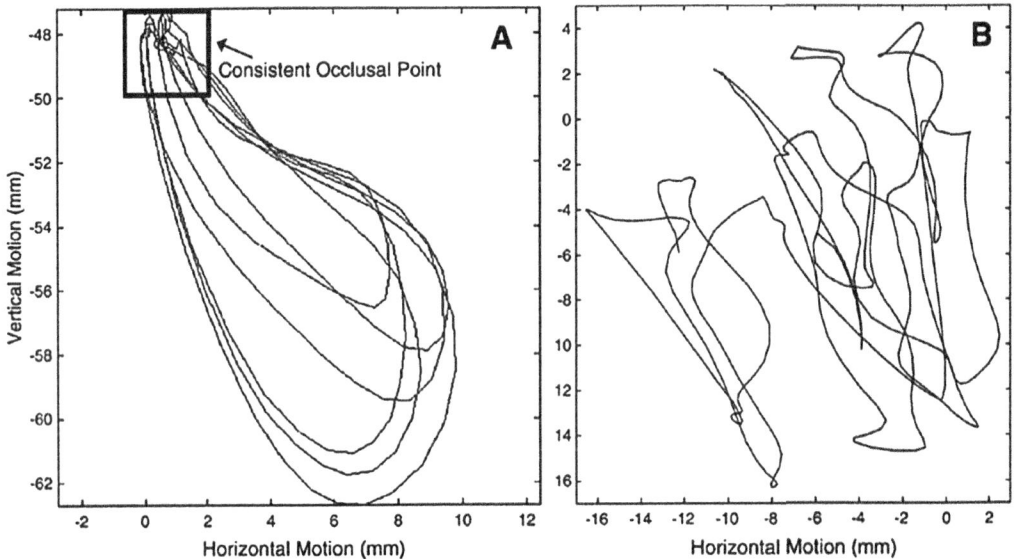

FIG. 8.1   (A) Illustration of the horizontal excursion analysis using a mature chewing sequence. Note the consistent occlusal point. (B) Illustration of the horizontal excursion analysis using a 12-month-old chewing sequence. Note the lack of a consistent occlusal point.

### 8.2.3.4 *Cup drinking*

Although we know quite a bit about infant bottles and breast-feeding skills, much less is known about cup drinking. Specifically, we lack data to show how the tongue moves and manages the bolus during cup drinking (Scarborough et al., 2018). Most of what we know about the ability to drink from a cup is from parent reports. Of course, these studies are highly influenced by the parents' choices. The ability to drink from an open cup is not the same as a parent allowing a child to drink from an open cup. In a parental-report study of children's eating and drinking skills, most (60%) children used cups/glasses with lids from 8 to 20 months of age; most began using cups without lids by 2 years of age (Carruth and Skinner, 2002). Although we know the child must be able to hold and lift the cup to their mouth, the lack of research regarding oral skills engaged during cup drinking is unfortunate. As described earlier, the entire body of the child is engaged during cup drinking.

## 8.3  Summary of cognitive and self-awareness development

A child's behavior during mealtimes and the foods they accept are both influenced by a variety of cognitive/language and self-awareness factors. These factors include how: (1) parents and others talk to children about food; (2) they may be influenced by advertising; (3) they perceive intangible concepts of foods, (4) they learn to share control over the mealtime, and (5) they think and communicate in general (Mura Paroche et al., 2017). Children learn about food through developmental processes such as familiarization, observation, associations, and categorizations (Mura Paroche et al., 2017). Familiarization and observation appear to be the two developmental processes most active in the child under the age of 3. Repeated taste exposure is one way to familiarize the child with the new food. Learning to eat through association has limited data, but it does appear that pairing a novel food with a preferred food may increase likelihood of trying the new food; this exposure may indirectly affect acceptance of the novel food (Hausner et al., 2012). Autonomy and language emerge during this second year of life, and they increasingly influence eating.

There are both intrinsic issues and environmental/parenting issues that affect dietary intake in young infants (Patel et al., 2020; Forestell, 2017; Spahn et al., 2019; Mennella et al., 2017; Spill et al., 2019; Issanchou, 2017). Parents and other adult caregivers can positively influence how infants and young children eat, through role modeling (Dearden et al., 2009; Aboud et al., 2009; Aboud and Akhter, 2011; Blissett et al., 2012; Gregory et al., 2011; Fries and Van Der Horst, 2019; Issanchou, 2017), offering a variety of food and repeatedly exposing a child to novel foods (Lumeng and Cardinal, 2007; Wardle et al., 2003; Guthrie et al., 2000; Birch, 1987; Fries et al., 2017; De Wild et al., 2017; Spill et al., 2019; Issanchou, 2017; Zeinstra et al., 2018; Nekitsing et al., 2019), talking about the food and how much they enjoy eating (Byrne and Nitzke, 2002; Houston-Price et al., 2009a,b; Heath et al., 2010; Lumeng et al., 2008; Uehara, 2000; Edelson et al., 2016; Fries et al., 2017; Moens et al., 2018), and by using positive reinforcement strategies (Aboud and Akhter, 2011; Aboud et al., 2009; Blissett et al., 2012; Dearden et al., 2009; Gregory et al., 2011; Haycraft et al., 2011; Cooke et al., 2011; Drucker et al., 1999; Remington et al., 2012; De Wild et al., 2017; Issanchou, 2017; Moens et al., 2018).

### 8.3.1.1 Cognition and early feedings

Infants communicate and share control during mealtimes, even as a newborn (Caton et al., 2011; Skinner et al., 1998a; Engle and Zeitlin, 1996; Wright et al., 2011, 2006; Van Dijk et al., 2012; Ventura et al., 2019; Ventura, 2017). Infants as young as 1 and a half months use a variety of communication strategies to communicate likes, such as opening their mouth, eating readily, or eating a large volume (Crist and Napier-Phillips, 2001; Skinner et al., 1998b; Van Dijk et al., 2012; Wright et al., 2006; Engle and Zeitlin, 1996). Half of the infants reportedly wean off breastfeeding because of competing awareness of, and interest in exploring, the environment (Clarke and Harmon, 1983). Social interactions influence intake as well. For instance, socializing during bottle feedings increases intake, and toddlers are drawn toward social engagement and anticipate feeding interactions (Kochukhova and Gredeback, 2010; Lumeng et al., 2007; Spegman and Houck, 2005). In an experiment on factors affecting intake, mother-led feeding experiences were compared with infant-led. Infants ate 42% more formula when the mother determined when to start and stop the feeding (Ventura and Mennella, 2017). However, there was a wide range for this outcome, with some infants taking less during maternal-led than infant-led experiences. Greater intakes were predicted by a combination of infant factors (older, more regulatory problems/disorganization, higher positive moods) as well as maternal factors (lower levels of both restrictive and responsive feeding styles) (Ventura and Mennella, 2017).

### 8.3.1.2 Cognition and transitions to solids

Infants increasingly take over control during mealtimes. At the initiation of solid foods, infants and mothers continue learning how to work together, and over a period of time establish behaviors that are more sensitive toward each other and more consistent day to day (Van Dijk et al., 2012, 2009; Young and Drewett, 2000; Harris and Coulthard, 2016). The introduction to solid foods appears to be a crucial time where parents have the most control over offering a variety of foods and encouraging acceptance of a variety of flavors (Spyreli et al., 2019; Nicklaus, 2016a, 2011; Mennella and Trabulsi, 2012; Johnson and Moding, 2020; Ahern et al., 2013). During the weaning time (around 12 months), infants are both partially fed by their caregiver and partially self-fed (Schapiro, 1968; Van Dijk et al., 2012; Young and Drewett, 2000; Crist and Napier-Phillips, 2001; Koda et al., 2006; Spegman and Houck, 2005). Large variations in these two behaviors (accepting food and self-feeding) are seen within a meal, meal-to-meal, and day-to-day (Hittner and Faith, 2012; Young and Drewett, 2000; Parkinson and Drewett, 2001; Van Dijk et al., 2012, 2009; Spegman and Houck, 2005).

Infants as young as 6 months are observing and learning about what is food and what is not. However, in the beginning they rely on observing what their parent eats to determine what is edible (Wertz and Wynn, 2014). This is part of a developmental process of categorization. Children are closer to 18 months of age before they truly understand what is edible independent of observing their parents (Rozin et al., 1986). Social role modeling grows out of this interest in others. Peer role-modeling appears to be an effective way to increase tasting and eating nonpreferred foods after 18 months of age (Birch, 1980; Greenhalgh et al., 2009). By 24 months, the child begins to specifically follow and imitate their mother's behavior during mealtimes (Spegman and Houck, 2005).

Children demonstrate increased autonomy across the 1–3 year period (Spegman and Houck, 2005). How a child thinks about themselves in relation to others influences their food choices (Repacholi and Gopnik, 1997; Haycraft et al., 2011). As children begin to talk, they verbally request preferred and refuse nonpreferred foods. Mothers report that preschoolers exert a great deal of control over both meal and snack foods offered to the entire family (Hoerr et al., 2005; Engle and Zeitlin, 1996; Crist and Napier-Phillips, 2001; Harris et al., 2020). Mealtimes may be perceived as unpleasant as the child exerts their independence. Many parents complain of battling at mealtimes as their children reach preschool age (Harris et al., 2020, 2018).

### 8.3.2 Strategies to increase acceptance of novel foods

Infants are innately drawn to some flavors and typically reject other flavors (to be discussed more fully in the following section). But infants learn through repeated experiences with and exposures to new foods (Nicklaus, 2016b; Caton et al., 2014; Ventura and Worobey, 2013; Zeinstra et al., 2018; Ahern et al., 2013). Most children accept a novel food quickly (within 1–2 bites) when the food is introduced earlier than a year of age. Children 1–3 years of age are reported to be more distractible during eating and show more negative reactions to foods as they get older (Hittner and Faith, 2012). Children begin to reject new foods—a behavior known as neophobia. Neophobia is reported to affect between 12% and 30% of children (Torres et al., 2020; Moding and Stifter, 2016; Kozioł-Kozakowska et al., 2018). Food neophobia may influence dietary intake of micronutrients (Kozioł-Kozakowska et al., 2018; Bell et al., 2018). A child's temperament and their response to novel situations (not just food), as well as the strategies parents use during this time influence the development of neophobia (Moding and Stifter, 2016; An et al., 2020; Yuan et al., 2016; Bell et al., 2018). Food refusals are much more common after the age of 1, and by 3 years of age children often reject both novel and previously liked foods (Birch, 1987; Gisel, 1991; Cashdan, 1998). This may be due to a generalized desire to control their world, which is part of a cognitive developmental phase characterized by the emergence of language. This is important to understand, because parents need to continue to offer the foods and encourage their child to try a taste.

Familiarization and repeated exposures are perhaps the most studied of the developmental processes. And these influences begin even during pregnancy. Data suggest mothers should be encouraged to eat a wide variety of foods while pregnant as well as during lactation, as flavors are transmitted to the fetus and infant through amniotic fluid and human milk, respectively (Forestell, 2017; Spahn et al., 2019; Mennella et al., 2017). Mothers should understand that eating a wide variety of foods/flavors during lactation is beneficial in helping their infant develop a liking for a wider variety of foods and flavors (Mennella et al., 2017; Maier et al., 2008; Ventura, 2017).

Feeding a variety of foods appears to improve intake of both those foods and of novel foods. And this improvement appears to last past the first 2 years of life. In a study of 7-month-old infants, feeding different pureed foods daily increased acceptance of novel foods (Maier et al., 2008). And in a follow-up of these same children at 6 years of age, these children continued to demonstrate this same behavior (Maier-Nöth, 2019; Maier-Nöth et al., 2016). Most children learn to like vegetables through repeated exposures; liking does not appear to be innate (Fisher et al., 2012; Anzman-Frasca et al., 2012; Hausner et al., 2012; Havermans and Jansen, 2007). When allowed to choose, preschool children do not typically choose vegetables during mealtimes (Nicklaus et al., 2005).

It is imperative that adults consider developmental learning processes when considering how to encourage children to eat a wide variety of nutrient-dense foods. Since parents spend the most time with children under the age of 2-years, they need to maximize this time of influence by being good role models as well as repeatedly exposing children to a wide variety of foods. And yet, while most mothers report knowing variety is important, they may not understand how to interact during mealtimes to best encourage tasting (Spyreli et al., 2019).

A fairly successful strategy to help a child learn to eat a nonpreferred vegetable is to have them take a small taste of the food. Parents often use verbal prompts when trying to get their children to eat. Prompts that are encouraging without exerting pressure are associated with increased intake of fruits and vegetables (Edelson et al., 2016). But pressuring and coercive techniques are associated with more refusals in children as young as 16 months of age (Fries et al., 2017; Edelson et al., 2016; An et al., 2020; Kutbi, 2020). This balance between encouraging and becoming coercive is a difficult one for parents and is influenced by their own and their child's temperament. Some children need many more than 2–8 tastes; in fact, some require 6–14 opportunities to taste the vegetable before they indicate that they like it (Anzman-Frasca et al., 2012).

Another strategy is to allow a child to spit the food out after tasting it, which increases their willingness to try the bite (Anzman-Frasca et al., 2012). Data provide initial evidence for the conditioning of flavor preferences based on postingestive consequences, with children preferring foods of higher caloric density (Birch et al., 1990; Johnson et al., 1991; Kern et al., 1993). Pairing a preferred food with a novel food during introduction also appears to have some support as a strategy (Fisher et al., 2012; Hausner et al., 2012; Busick et al., 2008; Havermans and Jansen, 2007). Repeated exposure to taste appears to be the most effective and long-lasting strategy, although other exposures may have some transient affect. Visual and/or olfactory exposures to new foods without combining with other sensory inputs does not appear to have the lasting effect.

Clearly, children's food preferences are forming early in life and become more solidified as the child enters preschool years. Younger children are more easily influenced to try new foods, especially fruits and vegetables (Liem et al., 2010; Northstone et al., 2001). Many children under two are cared for outside their home by professional caregivers, and there are a number of nutrition-based programs designed for preschool-aged children that show promise. Educational programs, especially those that are multisensory, that are offered to parents as well as childcare providers appear to improve the diets and mealtime behaviors of children as early as 6 months of age (Helle et al., 2019; Hodder et al., 2020; Johnson et al., 2019; Tournier et al., 2020; Kähkönen et al., 2018; Nekitsing et al., 2019). In a large study of children within 61 early childhood centers (ECC) in Canada, preschool teachers in 31 ECCs were provided education designed to improve their ability to influence physical activity and healthy eating. While several outcomes were no different between children in the two groups, children in the intervention preschools improved in their locomotor motor skills (based on standardized testing) and increased their intake of fruits and vegetables (Leis et al., 2020). Guidance to adults around how to best encourage food exploration appears to be a worthwhile endeavor given what we know about the formation of preferences within the first 1000 days.

## 8.4 Summary of sensory development

Eating involves the integration of several sensory components, including taste, smell, texture, and the visual representation of the food. These sensory components influence the acceptance, or in some cases the rejection of a food (Duffy and Bartoshuk, 1996; Bartoshuk and Beauchamp, 1994; Nicklaus, 2016a,b). We have data that suggests picky eating may be more common in children with sensory sensitivities (Rodrigues et al., 2020; Steinsbekk et al., 2017). As one example, infants who were perceived as more over-responsive to sensory inputs ate the least amount of the offered food (Coulthard et al., 2016). The basic food flavors (salt, sweet, bitter, sour, and umami) are recognized by the newborn; newborns appear to have some preferences and dislikes even at birth (Mennella and Bobowski, 2015; Cowart et al., 2004). Although infants may reject specific flavors and prefer others, repeated taste exposures appear to modify these innate responses for most children (Nicklaus, 2016b; Caton et al., 2014; Ventura and Worobey, 2013; Zeinstra et al., 2018). The following section describes the basic information regarding salt, sweet, and bitter tastes, as well as how the infant and young child change in their response to sensory inputs across the first 1000 days.

### 8.4.1 Salt exposure

The human newborn clearly detects the presence of saline, and measures of sucking are suppressed relative to water (Beauchamp et al., 1994). However, while infants change their sucking strength, they often eat a similar amount of either salted or unsalted water. This is likely because the sucking response is not under voluntary control in the newborn, as described earlier. By 2.5–4 months of age infants appear indifferent to salt solutions in water and formula compared to plain water (Beauchamp et al., 1994, 1986; Schwartz et al., 2009). By 4 months, a similar solution in formula disrupts sucking patterns, and by 6 months disrupts infant sucking patterns and decreases sucking strength (Beauchamp et al., 1994; Beauchamp and

Engelman, 1991). By 8 months of age, an infant will reject salted formula (Beauchamp et al., 1994). Interestingly, infants appear to react differently to saline than formula. By 4–6.5 months of age, infants and children consume more moderately saline solutions over plain water, but not higher concentrations of saline solutions (Beauchamp et al., 1994, 1986; Schwartz et al., 2011, 2009). While they reject higher saline solutions, the rejection for infants 4–8 months of age is not as pronounced as the rejection by newborns (Beauchamp et al., 1994). There appears to be an interaction with starchy table foods. While infants react with indifference or rejection at 2 months to saline, they show a preference by 6 months of age when they have been exposed to starchy table foods (Stein et al., 2012). A preference for salt over plain water has also been reported at 12 months (Schwartz et al., 2009). Salted vegetables and soup appear to be more accepted than unsalted during the weaning period, and even in toddlers as old as 2 years of age (Beauchamp and Moran, 1984; Beauchamp and Engelman, 1991; Bouhlal et al., 2014).

## 8.4.2 Sucrose exposure

Infants are born preferring sweet over the other flavors. However, they are also influenced by early experiences. Exposure to sweetened water appears to increase liking for sucrose solutions over plain water solutions in 6-month-old infants (Beauchamp and Moran, 1982; Busick et al., 2008; Schwartz et al., 2011). Preference for sucrose relative to water declines in 6-month-old infants not fed sweetened water (Beauchamp and Moran, 1982; Busick et al., 2008). Intake of sucrose in water at 6 months is correlated to intake at 2 years of age (Beauchamp and Moran, 1984). Sucrose has been shown to help children accept an initially disliked juice, even when it is later removed from the juice (Liem and Mennella, 2002; Capaldi and Privitera, 2008).

### 8.4.2.1 Bitter and umami

Bitter taste, which is the flavor profile for many vegetables, appears to be innately disliked by both fetuses and newborns, and the rejection increases in the early months of life (Rosenstein and Oster, 1988; Steiner et al., 2001; Kajiura et al., 1992). Infants typically show dislike but will eat bitter flavors, especially when exposed to them repeatedly (Schwartz et al., 2009). Infants appear to be indifferent to umami flavors (both preference and ingestion) through the first year (Schwartz et al., 2009). However, there is great variability in liking and ingestion of all of the flavors except salty across the first year, limiting the generalizability of these findings (Schwartz et al., 2009).

### 8.4.2.2 Flavors/smells and the influence on learning to eat

Newborn infants are aware and have an ability to discriminate differences in smells and flavors presented even within the first few days of life (Crook, 1978; Beauchamp et al., 1994; Rosenstein and Oster, 1988). This is, in part, because they are exposed to a variety of flavors/ tastes within the uterine environment (Spahn et al., 2019; Varendi et al., 1996). Taste buds develop early on in gestation and begin transmitting information to the nervous system in the last trimester of pregnancy (Forestell, 2017). If they were exposed to flavors during the fetal period because of their mother's consumption, infants preferentially turn toward the same smells (Delaunay-El Allam et al., 2006; Fomon et al., 1983; Varendi et al., 1996; Marlier et al., 1997).

Even newborn infants who have not had any tastes outside of the womb differentiate the basic flavors of sour, bitter, sweet, and umami (Bartoshuk and Beauchamp, 1994). Infants will eat similar amounts of these basic flavors when mixed with water, but will show negative facial expressions with all except the sweet flavors (Rosenstein and Oster, 1988). Facial expressions are interpreted as hedonic indicators of "liking" a food. Many infants will eat a food even though they demonstrate facial expressions (such as squinting, nose wrinkling, a "yuck" or gape face) that a parent might interpret as dislike (Mennella et al., 2016). In addition, the congruence between liking (based upon facial behaviors) and ingesting (volume consumed) is poor below 3 months, but improves steadily between 3 and 12 months (Schwartz et al., 2009). Once again, this is likely due in part to the transition from reflexive sucking to volitional eating described earlier.

Breastmilk flavors and smells are affected by the maternal diet; therefore, breast fed infants are exposed to these same inputs (Mennella and Beauchamp, 1991a,b, 1999; Mennella, 1993, 1997; Hausner et al., 2009; Spahn et al., 2019; Mennella et al., 2017; Ventura, 2017). Infants respond to changes in the flavor of breast milk with changes in their sucking patterns (Mennella and Beauchamp, 1991a,b, 1999; Mennella, 1997, 1993, 2014). Flavors experienced by infants during breastfeeding are recognized when introduced into purees (Mennella and Beauchamp, 1999; Hausner et al., 2010; Mennella et al., 2017). Infants prefer the flavor of breast milk, as shown by a greater acceptance of cereals prepared with breast milk over water (Mennella and Beauchamp, 1997).

Formulas lack the flavor variety seen in breast milk, and therefore formula-fed infants do not experience variations in flavors during feedings. However, much has been learned through a series of experiments using hydrolysate (HCF) formulas. Compared with cow's milk formula and human breast milk (which are both sweeter), HCF formulas have a fairly pronounced bitter/sour taste and a strong odor. Infants fed these formulas appear to develop a preference—one that is brand-specific (Mennella and Beauchamp, 2005). In addition, while infants under 3–4 months of age readily accept HCFs, infants vigorously reject them by 5–6 months of age (Mennella and Beauchamp, 2005). Infants fed HCFs prior to 3–4 months return to the HCF after eating a nonhydrolysate formula with much less difficulty than infants who have never be fed HCFs (Mennella and Beauchamp, 1996, 2005; Mennella et al., 2011). The age of introduction to this type of formula has greater influence than more recent exposure to the formula, indicating a "sensitive period" for these flavor compounds (Mennella and Beauchamp, 1996, 2005; Mennella et al., 2011).

### Complementary foods

Moderately strong evidence suggests that breastfed infants more readily accept a wider variety of foods during the complementary food period (Forestell and Mennella, 2007; Sullivan and Birch, 1994; Hausner et al., 2010; Burnier et al., 2011; Harris and Coulthard, 2016; Ventura, 2017). The foods that a mother eats are typically similar to the foods that she will provide during the introduction to complementary foods. Data suggest that infants will accept flavors that they have been exposed to through the breast milk more readily in foods, but breastfed infants also appear to accept a wider variety of novel flavors (Mennella and Beauchamp, 1999; Mennella et al., 2016, 2009; Mennella and Bobowski, 2015; Mennella, 2014; Mennella and Ventura, 2011; Beauchamp and Mennella, 2011, 2009). Mothers who eat a diet rich in fruits and vegetables expose their infants to these flavors, and may facilitate fruit and vegetable acceptance for their toddlers. However, there does appear to be a dose effect.

Infants who were breastfed exclusively for at least 3 months of age were more likely to eat a wider variety and volume of vegetables as preschoolers (Coulthard et al., 2009). In a different study, only infants breastfed longer than 6 months were less fussy at 4 years of age compared with formula-fed infants (De Barse et al., 2017). Infants also appear to be influenced by the flavor learning from formulas, although the learning seems to be more limited. Infants fed HCFs prefer pureed foods/cereals with a similar bitter/sour flavor palate (Mennella et al., 2006, 2009). With exposure, infants who breastfeed for at least 3 months increase their intake of complementary foods more rapidly than do formula-fed infants (Sullivan and Birch, 1994; Forestell and Mennella, 2007; Maier et al., 2008; Burnier et al., 2011).

Between the ages of 5 and 7 months, most children will accept a majority of foods offered and they do not appear to consistently reject bitter- or sour-tasting foods (Schwartz et al., 2009, 2011). Across the 3–9 months age range, sweet and salty tastes appear to be the most preferred (Sullivan and Birch, 1994; Beauchamp et al., 1986; Schwartz et al., 2009). There is limited evidence that some infants prefer sour tastes, and the liking of sour taste at 18 months is correlated with increased fruit consumption (Blossfeld et al., 2007a). Salty vegetables tend to be more accepted than plain vegetables (Schwartz et al., 2009; Bouhlal et al., 2014). Interindividual variability increases for all flavors except salty (Schwartz et al., 2009; Hausner et al., 2012). Ingestion and liking do not systematically lead to the same conclusions but become more congruent in the first year (Schwartz et al., 2009; Mennella and Beauchamp, 1996). Most infants appear to generalize their acceptance of novel foods when offered variety across and within meals (Maier et al., 2008; Mennella et al., 2008).

Data suggest infants eat more of a novel food after repeated taste experiences with that food, and increased exposure to a variety of food may generalize to novel foods (Mennella et al., 2008; Mennella and Beauchamp, 1997; Sullivan and Birch, 1994; Birch et al., 1998; Wright et al., 2004; Forestell and Mennella, 2007; Busick et al., 2008; Gerrish and Mennella, 2001; Maier et al., 2008). The number of taste exposures is variable during this period (Mennella et al., 2008; Birch, 1998). Some children do not increase their acceptance with each taste, and for the parents of these children the recommendation to "just keep offering it" may be frustrating.

Caton and colleagues suggest there are three basic categories of acceptance for most children. Infants aged 4–38 months from France, the United Kingdom, and Denmark were followed through the introduction to complementary foods. The three primary classifications of acceptance styles included "learners, plate-cleaners, and noneaters" although 23% of children in their study had such variable acceptance patterns that they were classified as "others" (Caton et al., 2014). Most infants (40%) were "learners" and increased steadily in the amount of a novel puree they ate with each exposure. Some infants (21%) did not need repeated exposures and ate >75% of the offered food at every exposure. These infants were considered "plate cleaners." The remaining 16%, were considered "noneaters." Even by the fifth taste exposure, they did not accept more puree and ate <10 g every time. For the parents of these children, repeatedly offering food does not appear to be an effective strategy. The child's behaviors during mealtimes influence their parent's willingness to continue offering a variety of foods to their child. Many infants dislike the first taste but will keep eating the food (Wright et al., 2004; Schwartz et al., 2009). Most parents will stop giving their child food that is repeatedly rejected because they want their child to eat and grow. Parents may also add salt or sugar to the foods to make it "taste better." In one study, the odds of a mother adding these flavors increased between 12 and 24 months as the child got older (Masztalerz-Kozubek et al., 2020).

It is likely that the number of exposures needed when introducing a novel food is between 3 and 14, depending on the child (Johnson and Moding, 2020; Mennella et al., 2016). It typically takes eight to ten exposures to a new food before the parent will see an increase in intake (Forestell, 2017). And yet the average number of exposures to nonpreferred foods is reported to be two to three (Johnson and Moding, 2020; Skinner et al., 2002b).

Prior to 6 months of age, there does not appear to be a lasting benefit to transitioning infants to pureed or textured foods. In a few small randomized controlled trials, infants fed exclusively by breast prior to 6 months were able to transition to a similar variety of pureed foods as those infants introduced to foods at 4 months of age (Cohen et al., 1994, 1995). Data suggest any differences in the variety of foods eaten in the second half of the first year that may be seen in infants offered solids earlier than 6 months of age disappear by 15 months of age (Northstone et al., 2001; Cohen et al., 1995). However, there does appear to be a sensitive period within which solids should be introduced. Children who are not offered any kind of solid foods prior to 10 months of age are more likely to be difficult to feed at 15 months of age, and at increased risk of having a lower variety of foods and eating insufficient volumes of foods at 7 years of age (Coulthard et al., 2009; Northstone et al., 2001). And the texture of food influences the development and use of various chewing motions (Simione et al., 2018).

Children's food preferences are strongly related to their mother's food preferences; likely this is in part due to repeated exposure in the family home (Skinner et al., 2002a,b; Ahern et al., 2013). Food-related variety in the first 2 years strongly influences dietary variety in school-aged children (Skinner et al., 2002a,b; Gregory et al., 2011; Mallan et al., 2016). Even though children are exposed to foods outside of the family home, by 8 years of age their preferences are still primarily formed by what their mother prefers (Skinner et al., 2002a,b).

### 8.4.2.3 Baby-led weaning

Baby-led weaning (BLW) or "auto-weaning" is a strategy whereby parents offer "real" foods (not pureed). The goal is to facilitate the infant self-feeding (Cichero, 2016). Typically, infants are rarely or never offered pureed foods during BLW (Brown and Lee, 2011a). Reported benefits include improved parent–child relationships during mealtimes as the food is shared among all participants, increased infant autonomy and parental responsiveness, and decreased cost (Alvisi et al., 2015; Arden and Abbott, 2015; Brown and Lee, 2011b, 2011a, 2013; Cameron et al., 2012; Utami et al., 2020; Cichero, 2016). Data suggest that infants weaned using this approach are more satiety-responsive and less likely to be overweight (Brown and Lee, 2015; Townsend and Pitchford, 2012). However, it is not clear whether parental characteristics or BLW itself influence this behavior.

There is some evidence that these infants may be offered a wider variety of flavors and textures, which in turn may enhance the quality of the toddler's diet (Brown and Lee, 2011a, 2013; Townsend and Pitchford, 2012; Utami et al., 2020). When an infant rejects a food that is offered during BLW, there appears to be a greater acceptance by the parent that the infant is learning about the food (Arden and Abbott, 2015). Rejection is not seen as "dislike" and parents are more likely to repeatedly offer foods that have been rejected. Six-month-old infants offered home-cooked fruits and vegetables during this time ate more vegetables at 7 years of age. However, in this study the foods were mashed for the infant (Coulthard et al., 2010). In a fairly large study of 2999 infants, children were exposed to fewer textures by mothers who offered only commercially prepared purees (Demonteil et al., 2018). And in a study of 876 infants aged

6–36 months, parents were asked about how they had fed their infant at 6–7 months of age (Fu et al., 2018). Of these infants, 72% were mostly/all spoon-fed, 11% followed a partial BLW approach and a partial spoon-feeding approach, and the remaining 18% were reportedly fully or mostly weaned using BLW. The parents also filled out a food fussiness scale on their child's current eating. Compared with mostly/all spoon-fed infants, those fully or mostly following the BLW approach scored lower on food fussiness scales (Fu et al., 2018).

Healthcare workers do have some concerns regarding BLW. Dietary intake of vegetables and certain nutrients (e.g., iron) reportedly drop off as infants begin to transition off pureed foods and onto textured foods (Johnson and Moding, 2020; Butte et al., 2010). And this is for infants who are given purees and are older when they transition to the family foods than what is seen with BLW. The family diet may be inadequate for the infant and toddler during BLW, and some infants may not have the endurance to eat sufficient amounts (Rowan and Harris, 2012; Cameron et al., 2013; Wright et al., 2011; Daniels et al., 2015; Morison et al., 2016). Parents reportedly do not change their dietary habits when they begin BLW (Rowan and Harris, 2012). Infants fed using the BLW approach have been shown to have diets higher in fat and lower in iron, zinc, and Vitamin B12 (Morison et al., 2016). There does not appear to be a difference in exposure to appropriate, nutrient-dense foods between traditionally weaned infants and BLW infants; the differences seen are in consumption (Rowan et al., 2019). Parents report that 30% of infants fed using BLW have choking or gagging incidents (Cameron et al., 2012; Fangupo et al., 2016). This is likely because the oral skills are transitioning from those adequate for liquids; eating solids of any texture (even pureed) requires learning a new oral-motor pattern. Infants who are offered pureed foods can practice moving the bolus of puree toward the back, and gradually build up movement patterns and strength that will be useful when transitioning to textured foods (Cichero, 2017; Ross, 2016). However, gagging may be a part of normal development as an infant practices novel oral skills. Infants who were spoon-fed had more choking episodes when first introduced to purees with lumps and to finger foods than infants introduced using BLW (Brown, 2018). Modifications to the strict BLW approach have been created in part to decrease the risks of choking. In a study of 206 infants 6–8 months of age, while infants fed using a modified BLW approach gagged more frequently at 6 months of age, they gagged less frequently at 8 months compared with traditionally weaned babies (Fangupo et al., 2016).

Modified BLW approaches have the goal of retaining the best of BLW (shared mealtimes, infant autonomy, and parental responsiveness) while addressing oral skill abilities to eat the offered foods, and nutritional concerns (Daniels et al., 2015; Williams Erickson et al., 2018; Morison et al., 2018). In a small pilot, The Baby-Led Introduction to SolidS (BLISS) study showed fewer foods that were choking hazards and more foods that were rich in iron were offered to babies whose mothers used the BLISS protocol (Cameron et al., 2015). Combining some pureed foods, specifically iron-rich foods that are difficult to offer within a BLW approach (e.g., infants cereals and pureed meats) with modified BLW strategies may be the "best approach" (Theurich et al., 2020; Cichero, 2016). Dietary guidance can also be protective of overweight and controlling feeding practices, and improve responsiveness, as shown in the NOURISH study (Daniels et al., 2012).

### Textured foods

Taste and texture exposures are critical for the development of oral motor skills (Harris and Mason, 2017; Cichero, 2017; Castenmiller et al., 2019). Many parents begin by offering smooth purees, and then transition to purees with some lumps/bumps and soft cubes of foods. Infants 6–12 months of age show more frequent negative expressions to lumpy and diced textures, and appear to enjoy smooth purees; infants 12–24 months of age show more interest in the diced and lumpy textures (Lundy et al., 1998; Blossfeld et al., 2007b). In one study out of France ($n$ = 2999 infants), infants were slowly offered soft/small pieces beginning at 6 months; larger/harder pieces were introduced typically after 13 months of age (Demonteil et al., 2018). Healthy infants are able to eat some finger foods between 5 and 6 months of age (Brown and Lee, 2010; Wright et al., 2010), and approximately 50% of children are offered finger foods before 6 months of age (Wright et al., 2010). The transition from fluid-based nutrition to solid foods requires physiological and anatomical changes to tolerate the new textures in addition to the other allergy, nutrition, and cultural/social considerations (Harris and Mason, 2017; Cichero, 2017; Castenmiller et al., 2019).

Once the child can tolerate foods of a single texture, the next and perhaps final step in texture acceptance is eating mixed textures. Unfortunately, we have little data to guide our practice. In a recent review of the influence of food texture on swallowing, most research has been on modifying textures to support oral feeding in adults with dysphagia (Steele et al., 2015). In fact, the lack of a consistent framework to categorize textures has led to an effort to standardize terminology and definitions in this population (Cichero et al., 2017). This effort is the International Dysphagia Diet Standardization Initiative (IDDSI). However, we know that even typically developing children may refuse foods that "touch each other"; these data have been collected primarily with children over the age of 3 years (Hubbard et al., 2014; Alm et al., 2015). As an example, in a small study of children aged 7–8, 8 of the 12 children reported they avoided foods that were combined or that touched (Alm et al., 2015). In another study of 4–6 year olds ($n$ = 30), children reduced their verbal rating of liking a food when it was in contact with a disliked food compared with a like-like combination; this dislike was more common in females, and the younger the child, the longer their dislike of the "contaminated" food remained (Brown et al., 2012). When exactly food proximity and mixing becomes a source of rejection is not fully understood but appears to be another influencing factor.

## 8.5 Looking at the "whole child": Putting the science to work

Both the parent and the child bring characteristics to the dyad during mealtimes. The parent has innate characteristics (e.g., their temperament), but is also influenced by their skills and abilities as a parent. What do they know about child development in general, and specifically for their own child? Are they able to choose foods that are developmentally appropriate for their child at that time point? Do they understand that a "dislike face" frequently does not interfere with their child's eating of the food, and that repeated exposures for many children will help them learn to like the new food? Do they have appropriate knowledge and skills to respond to their child if their initial strategy does not work? In addition to these factors, parents are affected by the availability of resources. Some families have limited access to fresh food or have limited financial resources to buy foods. They are less likely to keep offering foods that their child repeatedly rejects due to concern about waste, as discussed earlier. Time is also a precious resource for many people in today's world. Stress (family, financial, time) makes it more difficult to focus on being a teacher at the end of the day, especially when your child is not an easy-going, "plate cleaner" or "learner." In developing successful nutrition programs, researchers, and policymakers should consider these parental factors.

This has been a review of the skills and abilities of the child, along with their innate characteristics, that affect their ability to learn about new foods. What is emerging as a key area to study is a better understanding of how the child's reaction in turn influences the parent's behavior. Nutrition research has focused mostly on what the child should be eating, and less on this complex interplay of skills and temperament of the child and the parent. While this has been studied during mealtimes between parents and children who have been diagnosed with a food refusal, it will be helpful to better understand this process in children who are "picky" or "fussy" (Gueron-Sela et al., 2011).

Research teams have often lacked a multidisciplinary focus. Therapists and child developmentalists may have knowledge about the skills necessary for eating a wide variety of age-appropriate foods; nutrition scientists have knowledge about what children should be eating. Given the importance of the first 1000 days on the development of the child as well as the child's eating habits, it is imperative that we invest in more holistic approaches to helping both parents and children embrace their roles during this time. We can help parents and other caregivers more effectively step into their role as teachers. Fig. 8.2 describes the parental

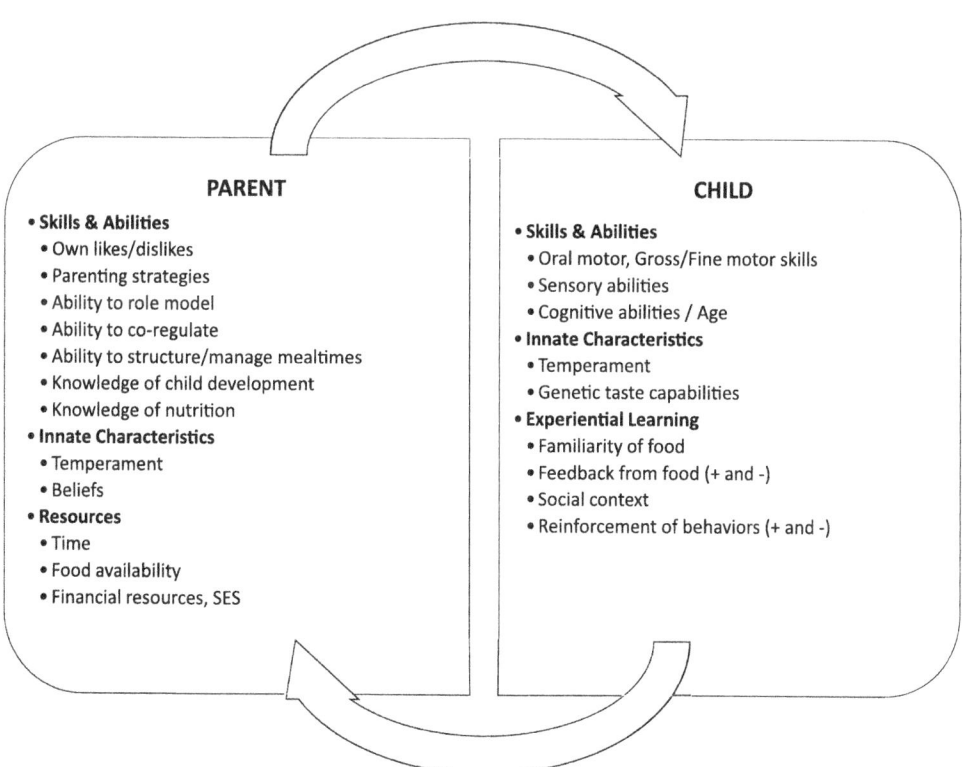

FIG. 8.2 The circular influence during mealtimes. The child and the parent both bring unique skills and characteristics to the feeding experience.

characteristics and the child's characteristics and includes a feedback from the child to the parent that influences both the child's food acceptance and the strategies used by the parent.

Parents understand their role as teachers when it relates to many aspects of infant development. They accept their role when teaching their child to talk or walk. However, they may not be fully aware of (1) the influence of their child's development on their child's food preferences, (2) how to teach their child to eat a wide variety of foods, and/or (3) how to help their child overcome initial rejection when repeated exposures to novel foods is not effective. Clearly many parents would benefit from additional understanding of the infant skills necessary to eat more textured foods, given the high incidence of choking reported by parents during complementary feeding. Currently, many countries are focusing on childhood nutrition. However, the influence of the developmental domains discussed here may not be fully appreciated by parents and healthcare workers alike. When the typical strategies of offering a novel food repeatedly do not work, both need additional, effective strategies to help the developing child learn and grow.

## 8.6 Future trends and additional research needs

These data suggest that this period of the first 1000 days presents a significant opportunity to shape a child's diet. Developmental milestones in gross, fine, and oral motor influence both the ability and the desire to eat certain foods. The same can be said of how the child perceives the sensory experiences when eating (taste, texture, and visual). The child becomes more independent, and how they think about themselves and their world along with parental and societal factors affect their feeding behaviors during mealtimes. The data increasingly demonstrate a bidirectional influence during feedings.

A major confounder of the studies of sensory development in the first 6 months of life continues to be that the infant transitions from sucking that is driven by the central pattern generator, to volitional sucking. Automatic sucking responses may override preferences, which clearly could influence how researchers interpret the development of an infant's taste. For instance, in one study newborn infants initiated and maintained sucking even though they were given sweet, salty, bitter, and sour flavors (Rosenstein and Oster, 1988). The only differentiating factor was facial expression. The expression was relaxed with the sweet flavor and showed distaste across a furrowed brow for the other three stimuli (Rosenstein and Oster, 1988). This developmental transition has not been mentioned in any of the referenced studies. A second confounding factor present in these studies is that preferences are inferred based on the volume ingested by an infant. Flow rate from the bottle may influence how much volume an infant eats during a meal. Flow rate is determined by the bottle nipple/teat characteristics but also by hydrostatic pressures and gravity (Lau and Schanler, 2000). None of these studies used a self-paced, vacuum free bottle. It would be helpful if the factors of (1) reflexive vs volitional sucking, and (2) flow rate could be more clearly controlled in future studies of infant preferences. These factors may partially explain why intersubject variability is high for infants at 3, 6, 9, and 12 months of age (Schwartz et al., 2009).

Our knowledge on the development of oral skills for eating is confounded by the textures of food, which has not been held constant across many of the early studies (Gisel, 1991, 1988a,b; Stolovitz and Gisel, 1991; Le Reverend et al., 2014). And we have data that suggest the food itself affects how the child chews (Simione et al., 2018). Data clearly demonstrate both within-subject and between-subject variations across different foods as well as different eating sessions (Young and Drewett, 2000; Parkinson and Drewett, 2001; Hittner and Faith, 2012; Van Dijk et al., 2012, 2009; Spegman and Houck, 2005). However, much of the data currently available were collected either (1) in a single occasion, or (2) with only one texture of food. We know that the tongue is used to place or keep the food in place between the upper and lower jaw while the jaw moves in vertical, lateral, and diagonal planes. But the tongue is not fully observable during eating (Stolovitz and Gisel, 1991; Gisel, 1988a,b; Green et al., 1997). And as described, data suggest children who lack oral skills often still eat the food; they just do so by swallowing it whole or after it dissolves (Harris and Mason, 2017; Stolovitz and Gisel, 1991). It will be quite a breakthrough when we have data that is able to fully describe what the tongue is doing during chewing as well as during drinking from a cup. This technology along with the use of a standard set of foods and several sessions to observe eating behaviors will help the field more fully understand the emergence of chewing and drinking skills in young children (Le Reverend et al., 2014).

Unfortunately, we still rely heavily on parental report of milestone achievements, and these measures typically lack objective definitions. These report measures often lose the distinction between emergence and proficiency (e.g., crawling with tummy on or off the floor). In addition, the parent may offer food based upon several factors that might include the development of the infant but may be influenced by factors such as culture, the infant's temperament, or their own parental beliefs (Enneman et al., 2009; Mcmeekin et al., 2013; Wright et al., 2004; Carruth et al., 1997; Mennella et al., 2005). An infant may have the ability to eat food but is not offered that food based upon these external factors. This may account for some of the differences seen in studies of oral skill development between preterm and term infants (Torola et al., 2012). And finally, data regarding reaching, grasping, and bringing things to the mouth primarily have been collected using toys, which lack the sensory inputs that food presents. These data show actions are dependent upon texture and size; what would the data show with food?

Observations of parent–child interactions during mealtimes are also frequently conducted in a single occasion. As such, the role of the parent on the child's eating may not accurately reflect the parent's typical behaviors. Parenting "styles" have been described, and associated with an increased risk of a child becoming overweight, although this does not appear to hold true until the child controls their own food selection (Blissett and Haycraft, 2008; Golan and Crow, 2004). Parenting practices such as coercion or pressuring do influence the child's willingness to try foods. Fussy/picky eating in a child who is under the age of 2 may lead to increased use of coercive tactics by parents during mealtimes, which, in turn, leads to more picky eating in the child (Kutbi, 2020; Farrow et al., 2009; Berge et al., 2016; Jansen et al., 2017; Spahn et al., 2019). It is increasingly apparent that this relationship is bidirectional. What other characteristics of the child are influencing the effectiveness of the strategies parents use to encourage a healthy diet?

## 8.6.1 Support for parents during this period

As described, skills develop within a window of time—sometimes the range of skill acquisition is quite large. For typically developing children who may not yet have developed the skills to eat a food that is offered, they may reject the food despite repeated exposures. This is certainly true with children who have even minor developmental delays (Skuse, 1993). The parent, who oftentimes is attempting to follow recommendations from healthcare providers, may not know how to respond if the child's reactions are negative—especially in the case of a choking episode. A parent who offers a food that is not developmentally appropriate may then delay offering these foods even after the child has developed the skill to eat them, because of the fear of choking. Alternatively, if a child has had repeated experiences where they gagged or choked on foods because they had yet to develop the skill to eat those textures, the child may avoid eating foods of similar texture. To make things even more complicated, children need to practice with foods to improve their skill of eating the foods; avoiding giving challenging foods too long also has negative consequences. Most parents are doing their best, but for some children the parents may need more direction to appropriately offer the "just right" challenge of food. Guidance from professionals during this critical time of learning to eat a wide variety of nutritious foods can lead to fewer controlling feeding practices, and improved responsiveness, as shown in the NOURISH study (Daniels et al., 2012). The three classes of foods that require the most sophisticated oral motor skills, and are the most challenging from a sensory standpoint include iron-rich foods (typically meats), fruits, and vegetables. The easiest textures and the most palatable foods to eat are "snack" foods such as cookies, biscuits, fries, and chips. Given all these factors described in this chapter, it should not be surprising that children gravitate toward these easy-to-eat foods, and adults struggle to encourage healthy eating in very young children. This period is one of constant change—in food source, in skill development, in preference development, and in understanding one's place in the world.

## 8.7  Summary

Clearly, experiences in the first 1000 days of life set the stage for healthy eating habits in children. The number of foods eaten as toddlers influences the variety of foods (specifically, fruits and vegetables) eaten as preschoolers (Mallan et al., 2016). When the skills to eat are not fully developed, the child may react poorly to parental attempts at offering a wide variety of foods. Research can focus and incorporate these skill domains that are developing within these first 1000 days. Both researchers and clinicians can develop more effective strategies to improve nutrition, by understanding not only the "what" (e.g., children should eat more fruits and vegetables) but also the "why" (children reject these foods both because of flavor profiles but also because they require the most sophisticated oral motor skills) and the "how" (practical strategies to assist parents in teaching their children the skills for eating a wide variety of age-appropriate foods.)

## Sources of additional information

**General information regarding child development, with an emphasis on feeding and eating skills:** http://www.med.umich.edu/yourchild/topics/feedbaby.htm
**General information regarding cup drinking:**
https://www.cdc.gov/nutrition/infantandtoddlernutrition/mealtime/fingers-spoons-forks-cups.html

**General information about supporting the development of healthy eating habits:** http://ellynsatterinstitute.org/

**General information about what a child should be eating, and general ideas about habits:** http://www.choosemyplate.gov/

**Information regarding children with feeding problems. Includes an interactive questionnaire of typical and concerning feeding behaviors:** www.feedingmatters.org

**Information regarding feeding and swallowing disorders in children:** http://www.asha.org/public/speech/swallowing/Feeding-and-Swallowing-Disorders-in-Children/

**Information on various textures of purees and solids with details for standardization go to the International Dysphagia Diet Standardization Initiative (IDDSI):** https://www.iddsi.org

**Review of chewing development in infancy:**

Le Reverend, B.J., Edelson, L.R., Loret, C., 2014. Anatomical, functional, physiological, and behavioral aspects of the development of mastication in early childhood. Br. J. Nutr., 111, 403–14.

Wilson, E.M., Green, J.R., 2009. The development of jaw motion for mastication. Early Hum. Dev., 85, 303–11.

**Review of sensory development related to eating in infancy:**

Mennella, J.A., Reiter, A.R., Daniels, L.M., 2016. Vegetable and Fruit Acceptance during Infancy: Impact of Ontogeny, Genetics, and Early Experiences. Adv. Nutr. 7, 211S–9S.

**Review of cup drinking skills:**

Scarborough, D., Brink, K.E., Bailey-Van kuren, M., 2018. Open-Cup Drinking Development: A review of the literature. Dysphagia, 33, 293–302.

**Review of How infants and Children learn to eat:**

Mura Paroche, M., CAton, S.J., Vereijken, C., Weenen, H., Houston-Price, C., 2017. How Infants and Young Children Learn About Food: A Systematic Review. Front Psychol. 8, 1046.

**Definitions of food textures**

Puree: typically a smooth consistency, generally a mashed fruit or vegetable, cereal, or dairy product (e.g., yogurt).

Meltable hard solid: A solid, dry formed food that melts in the mouth, using saliva, without pressure. Also known as a dissolvable or "easy to chew".

Soft cube/soft mechanical: A soft, solid food that requires little to no chewing. May be mashed by tongue or gums; does not require teeth to mash sufficiently for swallowing. Also known as "minced and moist" or "soft and bite-sized."

Hard mechanical: Food that requires significant amount of force from the teeth/jaws to break into pieces and swallow. Food often has tendons, fiber, or breaks into sharp-edged pieces. Also known as "regular." Examples include raw fruits and vegetables, solid meats (such as chicken breast), and potato chips.

Mixed texture: Food that includes more than one texture. May include a thin puree background with defined cubes of food within. Examples include sandwiches, pizzas, and pastas with sauce.

# References

Aboud, F.E., Akhter, S., 2011. A cluster-randomized evaluation of a responsive stimulation and feeding intervention in bangladesh. Pediatrics 127, e1191–e1197.

Aboud, F.E., Shafique, S., Akhter, S., 2009. A responsive feeding intervention increases children's self-feeding and maternal responsiveness but not weight gain. J. Nutr. 139, 1738–1743.

Adams, S.N., Verachia, R., Coutts, K., 2020. 'A blender without the lid on': mealtime experiences of caregivers with a child with autism spectrum disorder in South Africa. S. Afr. J. Commun. Disord. 67, e1–e9.

Ahern, S.M., Caton, S.J., Bouhlal, S., Hausner, H., Olsen, A., Nicklaus, S., Moller, P., Hetherington, M.M., 2013. Eating a rainbow. Introducing vegetables in the first years of life in 3 European countries. Appetite 71, 48–56.

Alm, S., Olsen, S.O., Honkanen, P., 2015. The role of family communication and parents' feeding practices in children's food preferences. Appetite 89, 112–121.

Alvisi, P., Brusa, S., Alboresi, S., Amarri, S., Bottau, P., Cavagni, G., Corradini, B., Landi, L., Loroni, L., Marani, M., Osti, I.M., Povesi-Dascola, C., Caffarelli, C., Valeriani, L., Agostoni, C., 2015. Recommendations on complementary feeding for healthy, full-term infants. Ital. J. Pediatr. 41, 36.

Ammon, J.E., Etzel, M.E., 1977. Sensorimotor organization in reach and prehension: a development model. Phys. Ther. 57, 7–14.

An, M., Zhou, Q., Younger, K.M., Liu, X., Kearney, J.M., 2020. Are maternal feeding practices and mealtime emotions associated with toddlers' food neophobia? A follow-up to the DIT-coombe hospital birth cohort in Ireland. Int. J. Environ. Res. Public Health 17.

Anzman-Frasca, S., Savage, J.S., Marini, M.E., Fisher, J.O., Birch, L.L., 2012. Repeated exposure and associative conditioning promote preschool children's liking of vegetables. Appetite 58, 543–553.

Arden, M.A., Abbott, R.L., 2015. Experiences of baby-led weaning: trust, control and renegotiation. Matern. Child Nutr. 11, 829–844.

Ayano, R., Tamura, F., Ohtsuka, Y., Mukai, Y., 2000. The development of normal feeding and swallowing: Showa University study of the feeding function. Int. J. Orofacial Myology 26, 24–32.

Barnevik Olsson, M., Carlsson, L.H., Westerlund, J., Gillberg, C., Fernell, E., 2013. Autism before diagnosis: crying, feeding and sleeping problems in the first two years of life. Acta Paediatr. 102, 635–639.

Bartoshuk, L.M., Beauchamp, G.K., 1994. Chemical senses. Annu. Rev. Psychol. 45, 419–449.

Beal, V.A., 1957. On the acceptance of solid foods, and other food patterns, of infants and children. Pediatrics 20, 448–457.

Beauchamp, G.K., Engelman, K., 1991. High salt intake. Sensory and behavioral factors. Hypertension 17, I176–I181.

Beauchamp, G.K., Mennella, J.A., 2009. Early flavor learning and its impact on later feeding behavior. J. Pediatr. Gastroenterol. Nutr. 48 (Suppl 1), S25–S30.

Beauchamp, G.K., Mennella, J.A., 2011. Flavor perception in human infants: development and functional significance. Digestion 83 (Suppl 1), 1–6.

Beauchamp, G.K., Moran, M., 1982. Dietary experience and sweet taste preference in human infants. Appetite 3, 139–152.

Beauchamp, G.K., Moran, M., 1984. Acceptance of sweet and salty tastes in 2-year-old children. Appetite 5, 291–305.

Beauchamp, G.K., Cowart, B.J., Moran, M., 1986. Developmental changes in salt acceptability in human infants. Dev. Psychobiol. 19, 17–25.

Beauchamp, G.K., Cowart, B.J., Mennella, J.A., Marsh, R.R., 1994. Infant salt taste: developmental, methodological, and contextual factors. Dev. Psychobiol. 27, 353–365.

Bell, L.K., Jansen, E., Mallan, K., Magarey, A.M., Daniels, L., 2018. Poor dietary patterns at 1-5years of age are related to food neophobia and breastfeeding duration but not age of introduction to solids in a relatively advantaged sample. Eat. Behav. 31, 28–34.

Benfer, K.A., Weir, K.A., Bell, K.L., Ware, R.S., Davies, P.S., Boyd, R.N., 2015. Clinical signs suggestive of pharyngeal dysphagia in preschool children with cerebral palsy. Res. Dev. Disabil. 38, 192–201.

Berge, J.M., Trofholz, A., Schulte, A., Conger, K., Neumark-Sztainer, D., 2016. A qualitative investigation of parents' perspectives about feeding practices with siblings among racially/ethnically and socioeconomically diverse households. J. Nutr. Educ. Behav. 48, 496–504.e1.

Berthier, N.E., Keen, R., 2006. Development of reaching in infancy. Exp. Brain Res. 169, 507–518.

Birch, L.L., 1980. Effects of peer models' food choices and eating behaviors on preschoolers food preferences. Child Dev., 489–496.

Birch, L.L., 1987. The role of experience in children's food acceptance patterns. J. Am. Diet. Assoc. 87, S36–S40.

Birch, L.L., 1998. Development of food acceptance patterns in the first years of life. Proc. Nutr. Soc. 57, 617–624.

Birch, L.L., McPhee, L., Steinberg, L., Sullivan, S., 1990. Conditioned flavor preferences in young children. Physiol. Behav. 47, 501–505.

Birch, L.L., Gunder, L., Grimm-Thomas, K., Laing, D.G., 1998. Infants' consumption of a new food enhances acceptance of similar foods. Appetite 30, 283–295.

Blissett, J., Haycraft, E., 2008. Are parenting style and controlling feeding practices related? Appetite 50, 477–485.

Blissett, J., Bennett, C., Donohoe, J., Rogers, S., Higgs, S., 2012. Predicting successful introduction of novel fruit to preschool children. J. Acad. Nutr. Diet. 112, 1959–1967.

Blossfeld, I., Collins, A., Boland, S., Baixauli, R., Kiely, M., Delahunty, C., 2007a. Relationships between acceptance of sour taste and fruit intakes in 18-month-old infants. Br. J. Nutr. 98, 1084–1091.

Blossfeld, I., Collins, A., Kiely, M., Delahunty, C., 2007b. Texture preferences of 12-month-old infants and the role of early experiences. Food Qual. Prefer. 18, 396–404.

Bouhlal, S., Issanchou, S., Chabanet, C., Nicklaus, S., 2014. 'Just a pinch of salt'. An experimental comparison of the effect of repeated exposure and flavor-flavor learning with salt or spice on vegetable acceptance in toddlers. Appetite 83, 209–217.

Brown, A., 2018. No difference in self-reported frequency of choking between infants introduced to solid foods using a baby-led weaning or traditional spoon-feeding approach. J. Hum. Nutr. Diet. 31, 496–504.

Brown, A., Lee, M., 2011a. A descriptive study investigating the use and nature of baby-led weaning in a UK sample of mothers. Matern. Child Nutr. 7, 34–47.

Brown, A., Lee, M., 2011b. Maternal control of child feeding during the weaning period: differences between mothers following a baby-led or standard weaning approach. Matern. Child Health J. 15, 1265–1271.

Brown, A., Lee, M., 2013. An exploration of experiences of mothers following a baby-led weaning style: developmental readiness for complementary foods. Matern. Child Nutr. 9, 233–243.

Brown, A., Lee, M.D., 2015. Early influences on child satiety-responsiveness: the role of weaning style. Pediatr. Obes. 10, 57–66.

Brown, S.D., Harris, G., Bell, L., Lines, L.M., 2012. Disliked food acting as a contaminant in a sample of young children. Appetite 58, 991–996.

Burnier, D., Dubois, L., Girard, M., 2011. Exclusive breastfeeding duration and later intake of vegetables in preschool children. Eur. J. Clin. Nutr. 65, 196–202.

Busick, D.B., Brooks, J., Pernecky, S., Dawson, R., Petzoldt, J., 2008. Parent food purchases as a measure of exposure and preschool-aged children's willingness to identify and taste fruit and vegetables. Appetite 51, 468–473.

Butte, N.F., Fox, M.K., Briefel, R.R., Siega-Riz, A.M., Dwyer, J.T., Deming, D.M., Reidy, K.C., 2010. Nutrient intakes of US infants, toddlers, and preschoolers meet or exceed dietary reference intakes. J. Am. Diet. Assoc. 110, S27–S37.

Byrne, E., Nitzke, S., 2002. Preschool children's acceptance of a novel vegetable following exposure to messages in a storybook. J. Nutr. Educ. Behav. 34, 211–213.

Calis, E.A., Veugelers, R., Sheppard, J.J., Tibboel, D., Evenhuis, H.M., Penning, C., 2008. Dysphagia in children with severe generalized cerebral palsy and intellectual disability. Dev. Med. Child Neurol. 50, 625–630.

Cameron, S.L., Heath, A.L., Taylor, R.W., 2012. Healthcare professionals' and mothers' knowledge of, attitudes to and experiences with, Baby-Led Weaning: a content analysis study. BMJ Open 2.

Cameron, S.L., Taylor, R.W., Heath, A.L., 2013. Parent-led or baby-led? Associations between complementary feeding practices and health-related behaviours in a survey of New Zealand families. BMJ Open 3, e003946.

Cameron, S.L., Taylor, R.W., Heath, A.L., 2015. Development and pilot testing of Baby-Led Introduction to SolidS—a version of Baby-Led Weaning modified to address concerns about iron deficiency, growth faltering and choking. BMC Pediatr. 15, 99.

Capaldi, E.D., Privitera, G.J., 2008. Decreasing dislike for sour and bitter in children and adults. Appetite 50, 139–145.

Carruth, B.R., Skinner, J.D., 2002. Feeding behaviors and other motor development in healthy children (2-24 months). J. Am. Coll. Nutr. 21, 88–96.

Carruth, B.R., Nevling, W., Skinner, J.D., 1997. Developmental and food profiles of infants born to adolescent and adult mothers. J. Adolesc. Health 20, 434–441.

Carruth, B.R., Ziegler, P.J., Gordon, A., Hendricks, K., 2004. Developmental milestones and self-feeding behaviors in infants and toddlers. J. Am. Diet. Assoc. 104, s51–s56.

Cashdan, E., 1998. Adaptiveness of food learning and food aversions in children. Soc. Sci. Inf. 37, 613–632.

Castenmiller, J., De Henauw, S., Hirsch-Ernst, K.I., Kearney, J., Knutsen, H.K., Maciuk, A., Mangelsdorf, I., Mcardle, H.J., Naska, A., Pelaez, C., Pentieva, K., Siani, A., Thies, F., Tsabouri, S., Vinceti, M., Bresson, J.L., Fewtrell, M., Kersting, M., Przyrembel, H., Dumas, C., Titz, A., Turck, D., 2019. Appropriate age range for introduction of complementary feeding into an infant's diet. EFSA J. 17, e05780.

Caton, S.J., Ahern, S.M., Hetherington, M.M., 2011. Vegetables by stealth. An exploratory study investigating the introduction of vegetables in the weaning period. Appetite 57, 816–825.

Caton, S.J., Blundell, P., Ahern, S.M., Nekitsing, C., Olsen, A., Moller, P., Hausner, H., Remy, E., Nicklaus, S., Chabanet, C., Issanchou, S., Hetherington, M.M., 2014. Learning to eat vegetables in early life: the role of timing, age and individual eating traits. PLoS One 9, e97609.

Cheng, S., Maeda, T., Tomiwa, K., Yamakawa, N., Koeda, T., Kawai, M., Ogura, T., Yamagata, Z., 2009. Contribution of parenting factors to the developmental attainment of 9-month-old infants: results from the Japan Children's Study. J. Epidemiol. 19, 319–327.

Chiang, K.V., Hamner, H.C., Li, R., Perrine, C.G., 2020. Timing of introduction of complementary foods - United States, 2016-2018. MMWR Morb. Mortal. Wkly Rep. 69, 1787–1791.

Chigira, A., Omoto, K., Mukai, Y., Kaneko, Y., 1994. Lip closing pressure in disabled children: a comparison with normal children. Dysphagia 9, 193–198.

Chinn, L.K., Hoffmann, M., Leed, J.E., Lockman, J.J., 2019. Reaching with one arm to the other: coordinating touch, proprioception, and action during infancy. J. Exp. Child Psychol. 183, 19–32.

Chung, J., Lee, J., Spinazzola, R., Rosen, L., Milanaik, R., 2014. Parental perception of premature infant growth and feeding behaviors: use of gestation-adjusted age and assessing for developmental readiness during solid food introduction. Clin. Pediatr. (Phila) 53, 1271–1277.

Cichero, J.A.Y., 2016. Introducing solid foods using baby-led weaning vs spoon-feeding: a focus on oral development, nutrient intake and quality of research to bring balance to the debate. Nutr. Bull. 41, 72–77.

Cichero, J.A.Y., 2017. Unlocking opportunities in food design for infants, children, and the elderly: understanding milestones in chewing and swallowing across the lifespan for new innovations. J Texture Stud 48, 271–279.

Cichero, J.A., Lam, P., Steele, C.M., Hanson, B., Chen, J., Dantas, R.O., Duivestein, J., Kayashita, J., Lecko, C., Murray, J., Pillay, M., Riquelme, L., Stanschus, S., 2017. Development of international terminology and definitions for texture-modified foods and thickened fluids used in dysphagia management: the IDDSI framework. Dysphagia 32, 293–314.

Clarke, S.K., Harmon, R.J., 1983. Infant-initiated weaning from the breast in the first year. Early Hum. Dev. 8, 151–156.

Cohen, R.J., Brown, K.H., Canahuati, J., Rivera, L.L., Dewey, K.G., 1994. Effects of age of introduction of complementary foods on infant breast milk intake, total energy intake, and growth: a randomised intervention study in Honduras. Lancet 344, 288–293.

Cohen, R.J., Rivera, L.L., Canahuati, J., Brown, K.H., Dewey, K.G., 1995. Delaying the introduction of complementary food until 6 months does not affect appetite or mother's report of food acceptance of breast-fed infants from 6 to 12 months in a low income, Honduran population. J. Nutr. 125, 2787–2792.

Connolly, K., Dalgleish, M., 1989. The emergence of a tool-using skill in infancy. Dev. Psychol. 25, 894–912.

Cooke, L.J., Chambers, L.C., Anez, E.V., Croker, H.A., Boniface, D., Yeomans, M.R., Wardle, J., 2011. Eating for pleasure or profit: the effect of incentives on children's enjoyment of vegetables. Psychol. Sci. 22, 190–196.

Cooper-Brown, L., Copeland, S., Dailey, S., Downey, D., Petersen, M.C., Stimson, C., Van Dyke, D.C., 2008. Feeding and swallowing dysfunction in genetic syndromes. Dev. Disabil. Res. Rev. 14, 147–157.

Coulthard, H., Harris, G., Emmett, P., 2009. Delayed introduction of lumpy foods to children during the complementary feeding period affects child's food acceptance and feeding at 7 years of age. Matern. Child Nutr. 5, 75–85.

Coulthard, H., Harris, G., Emmett, P., 2010. Long-term consequences of early fruit and vegetable feeding practices in the United Kingdom. Public Health Nutr. 13, 2044–2051.

Coulthard, H., Harris, G., Fogel, A., 2016. Association between tactile over-responsivity and vegetable consumption early in the introduction of solid foods and its variation with age. Matern. Child Nutr. 12 (4), 848–859. https://doi.org/10.1111/mcn.12228.

Cowart, B.J., Beauchamp, G.K., Mennella, J.A., 2004. Development of taste and smell in the neonate. In: Polin, R.A., Fox, W.W., Abman, S.H. (Eds.), Fetal and Neonatal Physiology, third ed. Saunders, Philadelphia.

Crist, W., Napier-Phillips, A., 2001. Mealtime behaviors of young children: a comparison of normative and clinical data. J. Dev. Behav. Pediatr. 22, 279–286.

Crook, C.K., 1978. Taste perception in the newborn infant. Infant Behav. Dev. 1, 52–69.

Da Costa, S.P., Van Der Schans, C.P., Boelema, S.R., Van Der Meij, E., Boerman, M.A., Bos, A.F., 2010. Sucking patterns in fullterm infants between birth and 10 weeks of age. Infant Behav. Dev. 33, 61–67.

Daniels, L.A., Mallan, K.M., Battistutta, D., Nicholson, J.M., Perry, R., Magarey, A., 2012. Evaluation of an intervention to promote protective infant feeding practices to prevent childhood obesity: outcomes of the NOURISH RCT at 14 months of age and 6 months post the first of two intervention modules. Int. J. Obes. (Lond) 36, 1292–1298.

Daniels, L., Heath, A.L., Williams, S.M., Cameron, S.L., Fleming, E.A., Taylor, B.J., Wheeler, B.J., Gibson, R.S., Taylor, R.W., 2015. Baby-Led Introduction to SolidS (BLISS) study: a randomised controlled trial of a baby-led approach to complementary feeding. BMC Pediatr. 15, 179.

Davies, A.M., Koenig, J.S., Thach, B.T., 1988. Upper airway chemoreflex responses to saline and water in preterm infants. J. Appl. Physiol. 64, 1412–1420.

De Barse, L.M., Jansen, P.W., Edelson-Fries, L.R., Jaddoe, V.W.V., Franco, O.H., Tiemeier, H., Steenweg-De Graaff, J., 2017. Infant feeding and child fussy eating: the generation R study. Appetite 114, 374–381.

De Wild, V.W.T., De Graaf, C., Jager, G., 2017. Use of different vegetable products to increase preschool-aged children's preference for and intake of a target vegetable: a randomized controlled trial. J. Acad. Nutr. Diet. 117, 859–866.

Dearden, K.A., Hilton, S., Bentley, M.E., Caulfield, L.E., Wilde, C., Ha, P.B., Marsh, D., 2009. Caregiver verbal encouragement increases food acceptance among Vietnamese toddlers. J. Nutr. 139, 1387–1392.

Delaney, A.L., Arvedson, J.C., 2008. Development of swallowing and feeding: prenatal through first year of life. Dev. Disabil. Res. Rev. 14, 105–117.

Delaunay-El Allam, M., Marlier, L., Schaal, B., 2006. Learning at the breast: preference formation for an artificial scent and its attraction against the odor of maternal milk. Infant Behav. Dev. 29, 308–321.

Demonteil, L., Ksiazek, E., Marduel, A., Dusoulier, M., Weenen, H., Tournier, C., Nicklaus, S., 2018. Patterns and predictors of food texture introduction in French children aged 4-36 months. Br. J. Nutr. 120, 1065–1077.

Dodrill, P., Gosa, M.M., 2015. Pediatric dysphagia: physiology, assessment, and management. Ann. Nutr. Metab. 66 (Suppl 5), 24–31.

Drucker, R.R., Hammer, L.D., Agras, W.S., Bryson, S., 1999. Can mothers influence their child's eating behavior? J. Dev. Behav. Pediatr. 20, 88–92.

Dubois, S., Hill, D.E., Beaton, G.H., 1979. An examination of factors believed to be associated with infantile obesity. Am. J. Clin. Nutr. 32, 1997–2004.

Duffy, V.B., Bartoshuk, L.M., 1996. Sensory factors in feeding. In: Capaldi, E.D. (Ed.), Why We Eat What We Eat : The Psychology of Eating, first ed. American Psychological Association, Washington, DC.

Edelson, L.R., Mokdad, C., Martin, N., 2016. Prompts to eat novel and familiar fruits and vegetables in families with 1-3 year-old children: relationships with food acceptance and intake. Appetite 99, 138–148.

Eishima, K., 1991. The analysis of sucking behaviour in newborn infants. Early Hum. Dev. 27, 163–173.

Emond, A., Emmett, P., Steer, C., Golding, J., 2010. Feeding symptoms, dietary patterns, and growth in young children with autism spectrum disorders. Pediatrics 126, e337–e342.

Engle, P.L., Zeitlin, M., 1996. Active feeding behavior compensates for low interest in food among young Nicaraguan children. J. Nutr. 126, 1808–1816.

Enneman, A., Hernandez, L., Campos, R., Vossenaar, M., Solomons, N.W., 2009. Dietary characteristics of complementary foods offered to Guatemalan infants vary between urban and rural settings. Nutr. Res. 29, 470–479.

Erhardt, R.P., 1994. Developmental hand dysfunction: theory, assessment, and treatment. Pro-Ed, Inc, Austin, TX.

Fangupo, L.J., Heath, A.M., Williams, S.M., Erickson Williams, L.W., Morison, B.J., Fleming, E.A., Taylor, B.J., Wheeler, B.J., Taylor, R.W., 2016. A baby-led approach to eating solids and risk of choking. Pediatrics 138.

Farrow, C.V., Galloway, A.T., Fraser, K., 2009. Sibling eating behaviours and differential child feeding practices reported by parents. Appetite 52, 307–312.

Fisher, J.O., Mennella, J.A., Hughes, S.O., Liu, Y., Mendoza, P.M., Patrick, H., 2012. Offering "dip" promotes intake of a moderately-liked raw vegetable among preschoolers with genetic sensitivity to bitterness. J. Acad. Nutr. Diet. 112, 235–245.

Fomon, S.J., Ziegler, E.E., Nelson, S.E., Edwards, B.B., 1983. Sweetness of diet and food consumption by infants. Proc. Soc. Exp. Biol. Med. 173, 190–193.

Forestell, C.A., 2017. Flavor perception and preference development in human infants. Ann. Nutr. Metab. 70 (Suppl 3), 17–25.

Forestell, C.A., Mennella, J.A., 2007. Early determinants of fruit and vegetable acceptance. Pediatrics 120, 1247–1254.

Fries, L.R., Van Der Horst, K., 2019. Parental feeding practices and associations with children's food acceptance and picky eating. Nestle Nutr. Inst. Workshop Ser. 91, 31–39.

Fries, L.R., Martin, N., Van Der Horst, K., 2017. Parent-child mealtime interactions associated with toddlers' refusals of novel and familiar foods. Physiol. Behav. 176, 93–100.

Fu, X., Conlon, C.A., Haszard, J.J., Beck, K.L., Von Hurst, P.R., Taylor, R.W., Heath, A.M., 2018. Food fussiness and early feeding characteristics of infants following Baby-Led Weaning and traditional spoon-feeding in New Zealand: an internet survey. Appetite 130, 110–116.

Gal, E., Hardal-Nasser, R., Engel-Yeger, B., 2011. The relationship between the severity of eating problems and intellectual developmental deficit level. Res. Dev. Disabil. 32, 1464–1469.

Gerrish, C.J., Mennella, J.A., 2001. Flavor variety enhances food acceptance in formula-fed infants. Am. J. Clin. Nutr. 73, 1080–1085.

Gisel, E.G., 1988a. Chewing cycles in 2- to 8-year-old normal children: a developmental profile. Am. J. Occup. Ther. 42, 40–46.

Gisel, E.G., 1988b. Tongue movements in normal 2- to 8-year-old children: extended profile of an eating assessment. Am. J. Occup. Ther. 42, 384–389.

Gisel, E.G., 1991. Effect of food texture on the development of chewing of children between six months and two years of age. Dev. Med. Child Neurol. 33, 69–79.

Gisel, E.G., Lange, L.J., Niman, C.W., 1984. Chewing cycles in 4- and 5-year-old Down's syndrome children: a comparison of eating efficacy with normals. Am. J. Occup. Ther. 38, 666–670.

Gisel, E.G., Schwaab, L., Lange-Stemmler, L., Niman, C.W., Schwartz, J.L., 1986. Lateralization of tongue movements during eating in children 2 to 5 years old. Am. J. Occup. Ther. 40, 265–270.

Golan, M., Crow, S., 2004. Parents are key players in the prevention and treatment of weight-related problems. Nutr. Rev. 62, 39–50.

Gosa, M., 2013. Infant airway protection mechanisms during swallowing. In: SIG 13 Perspectives on Swallowing and Swallowing Disorders (Dysphagia). vol. 22, pp. 156–160.

Green, J.R., Moore, C.A., Ruark, J.L., Rodda, P.R., Morvee, W.T., Vanwitzenburg, M.J., 1997. Development of chewing in children from 12 to 48 months: longitudinal study of Emg patterns. J. Neurophysiol. 77, 2704–2716.

Greenhalgh, J., Dowey, A.J., Horne, P.J., Fergus Lowe, C., Griffiths, J.H., Whitaker, C.J., 2009. Positive- and negative peer modelling effects on young children's consumption of novel blue foods. Appetite 52, 646–653.

Gregory, J.E., Paxton, S.J., Brozovic, A.M., 2011. Maternal feeding practices predict fruit and vegetable consumption in young children. Results of a 12-month longitudinal study. Appetite 57, 167–172.

Gueron-Sela, N., Atzaba-Poria, N., Meiri, G., Yerushalmi, B., 2011. Maternal worries about child underweight mediate and moderate the relationship between child feeding disorders and mother-child feeding interactions. J. Pediatr. Psychol. 36, 827–836.

Guthrie, C.A., Rapoport, L., Wardle, J., 2000. Young children's food preferences: a comparison of three modalities of food stimuli. Appetite 35, 73–77.

Harris, G., Coulthard, H., 2016. Early eating behaviours and food acceptance revisited: breastfeeding and introduction of complementary foods as predictive of food acceptance. Curr. Obes. Rep. 5, 113–120.

Harris, G., Mason, S., 2017. Are there sensitive periods for food acceptance in infancy? Curr. Nutr. Rep. 6, 190–196.

Harris, H.A., Ria-Searle, B., Jansen, E., Thorpe, K., 2018. What's the fuss about? Parent presentations of fussy eating to a parenting support helpline. Public Health Nutr. 21, 1520–1528.

Harris, H.A., Jansen, E., Rossi, T., 2020. 'It's not worth the fight': fathers' perceptions of family mealtime interactions, feeding practices and child eating behaviours. Appetite 150, 104642.

Hausner, H., Nicklaus, S., Issanchou, S., Molgaard, C., Moller, P., 2009. Breastfeeding facilitates acceptance of a novel dietary flavour compound. Clin. Nutr. 29, 141–148.

Hausner, H., Olsen, A., Moller, P., 2012. Mere exposure and flavour-flavour learning increase 2-3 year-old children's acceptance of a novel vegetable. Appetite 58, 1152–1159.

Havermans, R.C., Jansen, A., 2007. Increasing children's liking of vegetables through flavour-flavour learning. Appetite 48, 259–262.

Haycraft, E., Farrow, C., Meyer, C., Powell, F., Blissett, J., 2011. Relationships between temperament and eating behaviours in young children. Appetite 56, 689–692.

Heath, P., Houston-Price, C., Kennedy, O.B., 2010. Can visual exposure impact on children's visual preferences for fruit and vegetables? Proc. Nutr. Soc. 69, E422.

Helle, C., Hillesund, E.R., Wills, A.K., Øverby, N.C., 2019. Evaluation of an eHealth intervention aiming to promote healthy food habits from infancy -the Norwegian randomized controlled trial Early Food for Future Health. Int. J. Behav. Nutr. Phys. Act. 16, 1.

Hittner, J.B., Faith, M.S., 2012. Typology of emergent eating patterns in early childhood. Eat. Behav. 12, 242–248.

Hodder, R.K., O'brien, K.M., Tzelepis, F., Wyse, R.J., Wolfenden, L., 2020. Interventions for increasing fruit and vegetable consumption in children aged five years and under. Cochrane Database Syst. Rev. 5, Cd008552.

Hoerr, S., Utech, A.E., Ruth, E., 2005. Child control of food choices in Head Start families. J. Nutr. Educ. Behav. 37, 185–190.

Houston-Price, C., Burton, E., Hickinson, R., Inett, J., Moore, E., Salmon, K., Shiba, P., 2009a. Picture book exposure elicits positive visual preferences in toddlers. J. Exp. Child Psychol. 104, 89–104.

Houston-Price, C., Butler, L., Shiba, P., 2009b. Visual exposure impacts on toddlers' willingness to taste fruits and vegetables. Appetite 53, 450–453.

Hubbard, K.L., Anderson, S.E., Curtin, C., Must, A., Bandini, L.G., 2014. A comparison of food refusal related to characteristics of food in children with autism spectrum disorder and typically developing children. J. Acad. Nutr. Diet. 114, 1981–1987.

Issanchou, S., 2017. Determining factors and critical periods in the formation of eating habits: results from the habeat project. Ann. Nutr. Metab. 70, 251–256.

Jansen, P.W., De Barse, L.M., Jaddoe, V.W.V., Verhulst, F.C., Franco, O.H., Tiemeier, H., 2017. Bi-directional associations between child fussy eating and parents' pressure to eat: who influences whom? Physiol. Behav. 176, 101–106.

Johnson, S.L., Moding, K.J., 2020. Introducing hard-to-like foods to infants and toddlers: mothers' perspectives and children's experiences about learning to accept novel foods. Nestle Nutr. Inst. Workshop Ser. 95, 88–99.

Johnson, S.L., McPhee, L., Birch, L.L., 1991. Conditioned preferences: young children prefer flavors associated with high dietary fat. Physiol. Behav. 50, 1245–1251.

Johnson, S.L., Ryan, S.M., Kroehl, M., Moding, K.J., Boles, R.E., Bellows, L.L., 2019. A longitudinal intervention to improve young children's liking and consumption of new foods: findings from the Colorado LEAP study. Int. J. Behav. Nutr. Phys. Act. 16, 49.

Kähkönen, K., Rönkä, A., Hujo, M., Lyytikäinen, A., Nuutinen, O., 2018. Sensory-based food education in early childhood education and care, willingness to choose and eat fruit and vegetables, and the moderating role of maternal education and food neophobia. Public Health Nutr. 21, 2443–2453.

Kajiura, H., Cowart, B.J., Beauchamp, G.K., 1992. Early developmental change in bitter taste responses in human infants. Dev. Psychobiol. 25, 375–386.

Kern, D.L., McPhee, L., Fisher, J., Johnson, S., Birch, L.L., 1993. The postingestive consequences of fat condition preferences for flavors associated with high dietary fat. Physiol. Behav. 54, 71–76.

Khandelwal, N., Mandliya, J., Nigam, K., Patil, V., Mathur, A., Pathak, A., 2020. Determinants of motor, language, cognitive, and global developmental delay in children with complicated severe acute malnutrition at the time of discharge: an observational study from Central India. PLoS One 15, e0233949.

Kochukhova, O., Gredeback, G., 2010. Preverbal infants anticipate that food will be brought to the mouth: an eye tracking study of manual feeding and flying spoons. Child Dev. 81, 1729–1738.

Koda, N., Tachibana, Y., Hirose, T., Yasuda, J., Hinobayashi, T., Minami, T., 2006. Development of eating behavior by Japanese toddlers in a nursery school: relation to independent walking. Percept. Mot. Skills 103, 145–150.

Kopp, C.B., 1974. Fine motor abilities of infants. Dev. Med. Child Neurol. 16, 629–636.

Kozioł-Kozakowska, A., Piórecka, B., Schlegel-Zawadzka, M., 2018. Prevalence of food neophobia in pre-school children from southern Poland and its association with eating habits, dietary intake and anthropometric parameters: a cross-sectional study. Public Health Nutr. 21, 1106–1114.

Kutbi, H.A., 2020. The relationships between maternal feeding practices and food neophobia and picky eating. Int. J. Environ. Res. Public Health 17.

Kwavnick, B.S., Reid, D.J., Joffres, M.R., Guernsey, J.R., 1999. Infant feeding practices in ottawa-carleton: the introduction of solid foods. Can. J. Public Health 90, 403–407.

Lande, B., Andersen, L.F., Baerug, A., Trygg, K.U., Lund-Larsen, K., Veierod, M.B., Bjorneboe, G.E., 2003. Infant feeding practices and associated factors in the first six months of life: the Norwegian infant nutrition survey. Acta Paediatr. 92, 152–161.

Lanigan, J.A., Bishop, J., Kimber, A.C., Morgan, J., 2001. Systematic review concerning the age of introduction of complementary foods to the healthy full-term infant. Eur. J. Clin. Nutr. 55, 309–320.

Lau, C., Schanler, R.J., 2000. Oral feeding in premature infants: advantage of a self-paced milk flow. Acta Paediatr. 89, 453–459.

Le Reverend, B.J., Edelson, L.R., Loret, C., 2014. Anatomical, functional, physiological and behavioural aspects of the development of mastication in early childhood. Br. J. Nutr. 111, 403–414.

Lee, M.H., Liu, Y.T., Newell, K.M., 2006. Longitudinal expressions of infant's prehension as a function of object properties. Infant Behav. Dev. 29, 481–493.

Leis, A., Ward, S., Vatanparast, H., Humbert, M.L., Chow, A.F., Muhajarine, N., Engler-Stringer, R., Bélanger, M., 2020. Effectiveness of the Healthy Start-Départ Santé approach on physical activity, healthy eating and fundamental movement skills of preschoolers attending childcare centres: a randomized controlled trial. BMC Public Health 20, 523.

Liem, D.G., Mennella, J.A., 2002. Sweet and sour preferences during childhood: role of early experiences. Dev. Psychobiol. 41, 388–395.

I. Nutrition in early life: Mechanisms and impact on long term health

Liem, D.G., Zandstra, L., Thomas, A., 2010. Prediction of children's flavour preferences. Effect of age and stability in reported preferences. Appetite 55, 69–75.

Lumeng, J.C., Cardinal, T.M., 2007. Providing information about a flavor to preschoolers: effects on liking and memory for having tasted it. Chem. Senses 32, 505–513.

Lumeng, J.C., Patil, N., Blass, E.M., 2007. Social influences on formula intake via suckling in 7 to 14-week-old-infants. Dev. Psychobiol. 49, 351–361.

Lumeng, J.C., Cardinal, T.M., Sitto, J.R., Kannan, S., 2008. Ability to taste 6-n-propylthiouracil and BMI in low-income preschool-aged children. Obesity (Silver Spring) 16, 1522–1528.

Lundy, B., Field, T., Carraway, K., Hart, S., Malphurs, J., Rosenstein, M., Palaez-Nogueras, M., Colletta, F., Off, D., Hernandez-Reif, M., 1998. Food texture preferences in infants vs toddlers. Early Child Dev. Care 146, 69–85.

Maier, A.S., Chabanet, C., Schaal, B., Leathwood, P.D., Issanchou, S.N., 2008. Breastfeeding and experience with variety early in weaning increase infants' acceptance of new foods for up to two months. Clin. Nutr. 27, 849–857.

Maier-Nöth, A., 2019. Early development of food preferences and healthy eating habits in infants and young children. Nestle Nutr. Inst. Workshop Ser. 91, 11–20.

Maier-Nöth, A., Schaal, B., Leathwood, P., Issanchou, S., 2016. The lasting influences of early food-related variety experience: a longitudinal study of vegetable acceptance from 5 months to 6 years in two populations. PLoS One 11, e0151356.

Mallan, K.M., Fildes, A., Magarey, A.M., Daniels, L.A., 2016. The relationship between number of fruits, vegetables, and noncore foods tried at age 14 months and food preferences, dietary intake patterns, fussy eating behavior, and weight status at age 3.7 years. J. Acad. Nutr. Diet. 116, 630–637.

Margari, L., Marzulli, L., Gabellone, A., De Giambattista, C., 2020. Eating and mealtime behaviors in patients with autism spectrum disorder: current perspectives. Neuropsychiatr. Dis. Treat. 16, 2083–2102.

Marlier, L., Schaal, B., Soussignan, R., 1997. Orientation responses to biological odours in the human newborn. Initial pattern and postnatal plasticity. C. R. Acad. Sci. III 320, 999–1005.

Masztalerz-Kozubek, D., Zielinska, M.A., Rust, P., Majchrzak, D., Hamulka, J., 2020. The use of added salt and sugar in the diet of polish and austrian toddlers. Associated factors and dietary patterns, feeding and maternal practices. Int J Environ Res Public Health, 17.

McCarty, M.E., Clifton, R.K., Collard, R.R., 1999. Problem solving in infancy: the emergence of an action plan. Dev. Psychol. 35, 1091–1101.

McCarty, M.E., Clifton, R.K., Collard, R.R., 2001. The beginnings of tool use in infants and toddlers. Infancy 2, 233–256.

Mcmeekin, S., Jansen, E., Mallan, K., Nicholson, J., Magarey, A., Daniels, L., 2013. Associations between infant temperament and early feeding practices. A cross-sectional study of Australian mother-infant dyads from the NOURISH randomised controlled trial. Appetite 60, 239–245.

Mennella, J.A., 1993. Early flavor experiences: when do they start? Zero Three 14, 1–7.

Mennella, J.A., 1997. Infants' suckling responses to the flavor of alcohol in mothers' milk. Alcohol. Clin. Exp. Res. 21, 581–585.

Mennella, J.A., 2014. Ontogeny of taste preferences: basic biology and implications for health. Am. J. Clin. Nutr. 99, 704S–711S.

Mennella, J.A., Beauchamp, G.K., 1991a. Maternal diet alters the sensory qualities of human milk and the nursling's behavior. Pediatrics 88, 737–744.

Mennella, J.A., Beauchamp, G.K., 1991b. The transfer of alcohol to human milk. Effects on flavor and the infant's behavior. N. Engl. J. Med. 325, 981–985.

Mennella, J.A., Beauchamp, G.K., 1996. Developmental changes in the acceptance of protein hydrolysate formula. J. Dev. Behav. Pediatr. 17, 386–391.

Mennella, J.A., Beauchamp, G.K., 1997. Mothers' milk enhances the acceptance of cereal during weaning. Pediatr. Res. 41, 188–192.

Mennella, J.A., Beauchamp, G.K., 1999. Experience with a flavor in mother's milk modifies the infant's acceptance of flavored cereal. Dev. Psychobiol. 35, 197–203.

Mennella, J.A., Beauchamp, G.K., 2005. Understanding the origin of flavor preferences. Chem. Senses 30 (Suppl 1), i242–i243.

Mennella, J.A., Bobowski, N.K., 2015. The sweetness and bitterness of childhood: Insights from basic research on taste preferences. Physiol. Behav. 152, 502–507.

Mennella, J.A., Trabulsi, J.C., 2012. Complementary foods and flavor experiences: setting the foundation. Ann. Nutr. Metab. 60 (Suppl 2), 40–50.

Mennella, J.A., Ventura, A.K., 2011. Early feeding: setting the stage for healthy eating habits. Nestle Nutr. Workshop Ser. Pediatr. Program. 68, 153–163. discussion 164-8.

Mennella, J.A., Turnbull, B., Ziegler, P.J., Martinez, H., 2005. Infant feeding practices and early flavor experiences in Mexican infants: an intra-cultural study. J. Am. Diet. Assoc. 105, 908–915.

Mennella, J.A., Kennedy, J.M., Beauchamp, G.K., 2006. Vegetable acceptance by infants: effects of formula flavors. Early Hum. Dev. 82, 463–468.

Mennella, J.A., Nicklaus, S., Jagolino, A.L., Yourshaw, L.M., 2008. Variety is the spice of life: strategies for promoting fruit and vegetable acceptance during infancy. Physiol. Behav. 94, 29–38.

Mennella, J.A., Forestell, C.A., Morgan, L.K., Beauchamp, G.K., 2009. Early milk feeding influences taste acceptance and liking during infancy. Am. J. Clin. Nutr. 90, 780S–788S.

Mennella, J.A., Lukasewycz, L.D., Castor, S.M., Beauchamp, G.K., 2011. The timing and duration of a sensitive period in human flavor learning: a randomized trial. Am. J. Clin. Nutr. 93, 1019–1024.

Mennella, J.A., Reiter, A.R., Daniels, L.M., 2016. Vegetable and fruit acceptance during infancy: impact of ontogeny, genetics, and early experiences. Adv. Nutr. 7, 211S–219S.

Mennella, J.A., Daniels, L.M., Reiter, A.R., 2017. Learning to like vegetables during breastfeeding: a randomized clinical trial of lactating mothers and infants. Am. J. Clin. Nutr. 106, 67–76.

Michels, K.A., Ghassabian, A., Mumford, S.L., Sundaram, R., Bell, E.M., Bello, S.C., Yeung, E.H., 2017. Breastfeeding and motor development in term and preterm infants in a longitudinal Us cohort. Am. J. Clin. Nutr. 106, 1456–1462.

Miller, A.J., 2002. Oral and pharyngeal reflexes in the mammalian nervous system: their diverse range in complexity and the pivotal role of the tongue. Crit. Rev. Oral Biol. Med. 13, 409–425.

Moding, K.J., Stifter, C.A., 2016. Temperamental approach/withdrawal and food neophobia in early childhood: concurrent and longitudinal associations. Appetite 107, 654–662.

Moens, E., Goossens, L., Verbeken, S., Vandeweghe, L., Braet, C., 2018. Parental feeding behavior in relation to children's tasting behavior: an observational study. Appetite 120, 205–211.

Morison, B.J., Taylor, R.W., Haszard, J.J., Schramm, C.J., Williams Erickson, L., Fangupo, L.J., Fleming, E.A., Luciano, A., Heath, A.L., 2016. How different are baby-led weaning and conventional complementary feeding? A cross-sectional study of infants aged 6-8 months. BMJ Open 6, e010665.

Morison, B.J., Heath, A.M., Haszard, J.J., Hein, K., Fleming, E.A., Daniels, L., Erickson, E.W., Fangupo, L.J., Wheeler, B.J., Taylor, B.J., Taylor, R.W., 2018. Impact of a modified version of baby-led weaning on dietary variety and food preferences in infants. Nutrients 10.

Mura Paroche, M., Caton, S.J., Vereijken, C., Weenen, H., Houston-Price, C., 2017. How infants and young children learn about food: a systematic review. Front. Psychol. 8, 1046.

Nakao, H., Aoyama, H., Suzuki, T., 1990. Development of eating behavior and its relation to physical growth in normal weight preschool children. Appetite 14, 45–57.

Naylor, A., Morrow, A., 2001. Developmental Readiness of Normal Full Term Infants to Progress From Exclusive Breastfeeding to the Introduction of Complementary Foods: Reviews of the Relevant Literature Concerning Infant Immunologic, Gastrointestinal, Oral Motor and Maternal Reproductive and Lactational Development. Academy for Educational Development, Washington, DC.

Nekitsing, C., Blundell-Birtill, P., Cockroft, J.E., Hetherington, M.M., 2019. Taste exposure increases intake and nutrition education increases willingness to try an unfamiliar vegetable in preschool children: a cluster randomized trial. J. Acad. Nutr. Diet. 119, 2004–2013.

Newell, K.M., McDonald, P.V., Baillargeon, R., 1993. Body scale and infant grip configurations. Dev. Psychobiol. 26, 195–205.

Nicklaus, S., 2011. Children's acceptance of new foods at weaning. Role of practices of weaning and of food sensory properties. Appetite 57, 812–815.

Nicklaus, S., 2016a. Complementary feeding strategies to facilitate acceptance of fruits and vegetables: a narrative review of the literature. Int. J. Environ. Res. Public Health 13.

Nicklaus, S., 2016b. The role of food experiences during early childhood in food pleasure learning. Appetite 104, 3–9.

Nicklaus, S., Boggio, V., Issanchou, S., 2005. Food choices at lunch during the third year of life: high selection of animal and starchy foods but avoidance of vegetables. Acta Paediatr. 94, 943–951.

Noller, K., Ingrisano, D., 1984. Cross-sectional study of gross and fine motor development. Birth to 6 years of age. Phys. Ther. 64, 308–316.

Nordstrøm, M., Retterstøl, K., Hope, S., Kolset, S.O., 2020. Nutritional challenges in children and adolescents with Down syndrome. Lancet Child Adolesc. Health 4, 455–464.

Northstone, K., Emmett, P., Nethersole, F., 2001. The effect of age of introduction to lumpy solids on foods eaten and reported feeding difficulties at 6 and 15 months. J. Hum. Nutr. Diet. 14, 43–54.

O'neill, A.C., Richter, G.T., 2013. Pharyngeal dysphagia in children with Down syndrome. Otolaryngol. Head Neck Surg. 149, 146–150.

Osaili, T.M., Attlee, A., Naveed, H., Maklai, H., Mahmoud, M., Hamadeh, N., Asif, T., Hasan, H., Obaid, R.S., 2019. Physical status and parent-child feeding behaviours in children and adolescents with down syndrome in the United Arab Emirates. Int. J. Environ. Res. Public Health 16.

Parkinson, K.N., Drewett, R.F., 2001. Feeding behaviour in the weaning period. J. Child Psychol. Psychiatry Allied Discip. 42, 971–978.

Patel, M.D., Donovan, S.M., Lee, S.Y., 2020. Considering nature and nurture in the etiology and prevention of picky eating: a narrative review. Nutrients 12.

Phillips, K.L., Schieve, L.A., Visser, S., Boulet, S., Sharma, A.J., Kogan, M.D., Boyle, C.A., Yeargin-Allsopp, M., 2014. Prevalence and impact of unhealthy weight in a national sample of US adolescents with autism and other learning and behavioral disabilities. Matern. Child Health J. 18, 1964–1975.

Qureshi, M.A., Vice, F.L., Taciak, V.L., Bosma, J.F., Gewolb, I.H., 2002. Changes in rhythmic suckle feeding patterns in term infants in the first month of life. Dev. Med. Child Neurol. 44, 34–39.

Ravel, A., Mircher, C., Rebillat, A.S., Cieuta-Walti, C., Megarbane, A., 2020. Feeding problems and gastrointestinal diseases in Down syndrome. Arch. Pediatr. 27, 53–60.

Remington, A., Anez, E., Croker, H., Wardle, J., Cooke, L., 2012. Increasing food acceptance in the home setting: a randomized controlled trial of parent-administered taste exposure with incentives. Am. J. Clin. Nutr. 95, 72–77.

Repacholi, B.M., Gopnik, A., 1997. Early reasoning about desires: evidence from 14- and 18-month-olds. Dev. Psychol. 33, 12–21.

Rodrigues, L., Silverio, R., Costa, A.R., Antunes, C., Pomar, C., Infante, P., Cristina, C., Amado, F., Lamy, E., 2020. Taste sensitivity and lifestyle are associated with food preferences and BMI in children. Int. J. Food Sci. Nutr. 71, 875–883.

Rogers, B., Arvedson, J., 2005. Assessment of infant oral sensorimotor and swallowing function. Ment. Retard. Dev. Disabil. Res. Rev. 11, 74–82.

Rosenstein, D., Oster, H., 1988. Differential facial responses to four basic tastes in newborns. Child Dev. 59, 1555–1568.

Ross, E., 2016. Eating development in young children: understanding the complex interplay of developmental domains. In: Saavedra, J., Dattilo, A. (Eds.), Early Nutrition and Long-Term Health: Mechanisms, Consequences, and Opportunities. Elsevier Ltd, London, UK.

Rowan, H., Harris, C., 2012. Baby-led weaning and the family diet. A pilot study. Appetite 58, 1046–1049.

Rowan, H., Lee, M., Brown, A., 2019. Differences in dietary composition between infants introduced to complementary foods using Baby-led weaning and traditional spoon feeding. J. Hum. Nutr. Diet. 32, 11–20.

Rozin, P., Hammer, L., Oster, H., Horowitz, T., Marmora, V., 1986. The child's conception of food: differentiation of categories of rejected substances in the 16 months to 5 year age range. Appetite 7, 141–151.

Scarborough, D., Brink, K.E., Bailey-Van Kuren, M., 2018. Open-cup drinking development: a review of the literature. Dysphagia 33, 293–302.

Schapiro, S., 1968. Adrenal catecholamine response of the infant rat to insulin-provoked hypoglycemia. Endocrinology 82, 1065–1067.

Schwaab, L.M., Niman, C.W., Gisel, E.G., 1986a. Comparison of chewing cycles in 2-, 3-, 4-, and 5-year-old normal children. Am. J. Occup. Ther. 40, 40–43.

Schwaab, L.M., Niman, C.W., Gisel, E.G., 1986b. Tongue movements in normal 2-, 3-, and 4-year-old children: a continuation study. Am. J. Occup. Ther. 40, 180–185.

Schwartz, J.L., Niman, C.W., Gisel, E.G., 1984a. Chewing cycles in 4- and 5-year-old normal children: an index of eating efficacy. Am. J. Occup. Ther. 38, 171–175.

Schwartz, J.L., Niman, C.W., Gisel, E.G., 1984b. Tongue movements in normal preschool children during eating. Am. J. Occup. Ther. 38, 87–93.

Schwartz, C., Issanchou, S., Nicklaus, S., 2009. Developmental changes in the acceptance of the five basic tastes in the first year of life. Br. J. Nutr. 102, 1375–1385.

Schwartz, C., Chabanet, C., Lange, C., Issanchou, S., Nicklaus, S., 2011. The role of taste in food acceptance at the beginning of complementary feeding. Physiol. Behav. 104, 646–652.

Seiverling, L., Towle, P., Hendy, H.M., Pantelides, J., 2018. Prevalence of feeding problems in young children with and without autism spectrum disorder: a chart review study. J. Early Interv. 40, 335–346.

Seiverling, L., Williams, K.E., Hendy, H.M., Adams, W., Yusupova, S., Kaczor, A., 2019. Sensory Eating Problems Scale (Seps) for children: psychometrics and associations with mealtime problems behaviors. Appetite 133, 223–230.

Selley, W.G., Ellis, R.E., Flack, F.C., Brooks, W.A., 1990. Coordination of sucking, swallowing and breathing in the newborn: its relationship to infant feeding and normal development. Br. J. Disord. Commun. 25, 311–327.

Sheppard, J.J., Mysak, E.D., 1984. Ontogeny of infantile oral reflexes and emerging chewing. Child Dev. 55, 831–843.

Simione, M., Loret, C., Le Révérend, B., Richburg, B., Del Valle, M., Adler, M., Moser, M., Green, J.R., 2018. Differing structural properties of foods affect the development of mandibular control and muscle coordination in infants and young children. Physiol. Behav. 186, 62–72.

Skinner, J., Carruth, B.R., Moran 3rd, J., Houck, K., Schmidhammer, J., Reed, A., Coletta, F., Cotter, F., Ott, D., 1998a. Toddler's food preferences: concordance with family members' preferences. J. Nutr. Educ. 30, 17–22.

Skinner, J.D., Carruth, B.R., Houck, K., Moran 3rd, J., Reed, A., Coletta, F., Ott, D., 1998b. Mealtime communication patterns of infants from 2 to 24 months of age. J. Nutr. Educ. 30, 8–16.

Skinner, J.D., Carruth, B.R., Bounds, W., Ziegler, P., Reidy, K., 2002a. Do food-related experiences in the first 2 years of life predict dietary variety in school-aged children? J. Nutr. Educ. Behav. 34, 310–315.

Skinner, J.D., Carruth, B.R., Wendy, B., Ziegler, P.J., 2002b. Children's food preferences: a longitudinal analysis. J. Am. Diet. Assoc. 102, 1638–1647.

Skuse, D., 1993. Identification and management of problem eaters. Arch. Dis. Child. 69, 604–608.

Spahn, J.M., Callahan, E.H., Spill, M.K., Wong, Y.P., Benjamin-Neelon, S.E., Birch, L., Black, M.M., Cook, J.T., Faith, M.S., Mennella, J.A., Casavale, K.O., 2019. Influence of maternal diet on flavor transfer to amniotic fluid and breast milk and children's responses: a systematic review. Am. J. Clin. Nutr. 109, 1003s–1026s.

Spegman, A.M., Houck, G.M., 2005. Assessing the feeding/eating interaction as a context for the development of social competence in toddlers. Issues Compr. Pediatr. Nurs. 28, 213–236.

Spill, M.K., Johns, K., Callahan, E.H., Shapiro, M.J., Wong, Y.P., Benjamin-Neelon, S.E., Birch, L., Black, M.M., Cook, J.T., Faith, M.S., Mennella, J.A., Casavale, K.O., 2019. Repeated exposure to food and food acceptability in infants and toddlers: a systematic review. Am. J. Clin. Nutr. 109, 978s–989s.

Spyreli, E., McKinley, M.C., Allen-Walker, V., Tully, L., Woodside, J.V., Kelly, C., Dean, M., 2019. "The one time you have control over what they eat": a qualitative exploration of mothers' practices to establish healthy eating behaviours during weaning. Nutrients 11.

Stanley, M.A., Shepherd, N., Duvall, N., Jenkinson, S.B., Jalou, H.E., Givan, D.C., Steele, G.H., Davis, C., Bull, M.J., Watkins, D.U., Roper, R.J., 2019. Clinical identification of feeding and swallowing disorders in 0-6 month old infants with Down syndrome. Am. J. Med. Genet. A 179, 177–182.

Steele, C.M., Alsanei, W.A., Ayanikalath, S., Barbon, C.E.A., Chen, J., Cichero, J.A.Y., Coutts, K., Dantas, R.O., Duivestein, J., Giosa, L., Hanson, B., Lam, P., Lecko, C., Leigh, C., Nagy, A., Namasivayam, A.M., Nascimento, W.V., Odendaal, I., Smith, C.H., Wang, H., 2015. The influence of food texture and liquid consistency modification on swallowing physiology and function: a systematic review. Dysphagia 30, 2–26.

Steeve, R.W., Moore, C.A., Green, J.R., Reilly, K.J., Ruark Mcmurtrey, J., 2008. Babbling, chewing, and sucking: oromandibular coordination at 9 months. J. Speech Lang. Hear. Res. 51, 1390–1404.

Stein, L.J., Cowart, B.J., Beauchamp, G.K., 2012. The development of salty taste acceptance is related to dietary experience in human infants: a prospective study. Am. J. Clin. Nutr. 95, 123–129.

Steiner, J.E., Glaser, D., Hawilo, M.E., Berridge, K.C., 2001. Comparative expression of hedonic impact: affective reactions to taste by human infants and other primates. Neurosci. Biobehav. Rev. 25, 53–74.

Steinsbekk, S., Bonneville-Roussy, A., Fildes, A., Llewellyn, C.H., Wichstrøm, L., 2017. Child and parent predictors of picky eating from preschool to school age. Int. J. Behav. Nutr. Phys. Act. 14, 87.

Stolovitz, P., Gisel, E.G., 1991. Circumoral movements in response to three different food textures in children 6 months to 2 years of age. Dysphagia 6, 17–25.

Story, M., Holt, K., Sofka, D., 2002. Bright Futures in Clinical Practice: Nutrition. National Center for Education in Maternal and Child Health, Rockville, MD.

Sullivan, S.A., Birch, L.L., 1994. Infant dietary experience and acceptance of solid foods. Pediatrics 93, 271–277.

Tamura, Y., Matsushita, S., Shinoda, K., Yoshida, S., 1998. Development of perioral muscle activity during suckling in infants: a cross-sectional and follow-up study. Dev. Med. Child Neurol. 40, 344–348.

Tamura, F., Chigira, A., Ishii, H., Nishikata, H., Mukai, Y., 2000. Assessment of the development of hand and mouth coordination when taking food into the oral cavity. Int. J. Orofacial Myology 26, 33–43.

Telles, M.S., Macedo, C.S., 2008. Relationship between the motor development of the body and the acquisition of oral skills. Pro Fono 20, 117–122.

Tepper, B.J., Barbarossa, I.T., 2020. Taste, nutrition, and health. Nutrients 12.

Thach, B.T., 2007. Maturation of cough and other reflexes that protect the fetal and neonatal airway. Pulm. Pharmacol. Ther. 20, 365–370.

Theurich, M.A., Grote, V., Koletzko, B., 2020. Complementary feeding and long-term health implications. Nutr. Rev. 78, 6–12.

Torola, H., Lehtihalmes, M., Yliherva, A., Olsen, P., 2012. Feeding skill milestones of preterm infants born with extremely low birth weight (ELBW). Infant Behav. Dev. 35, 187–194.

Torres, T.O., Gomes, D.R., Mattos, M.P., 2020. Factors associated with food neophobia in children: systematic review. Rev Paul Pediatr 39, e2020089.

Tournier, C., Bernad, C., Madrelle, J., Delarue, J., Cuvelier, G., Schwartz, C., Nicklaus, S., 2020. Fostering infant food texture acceptance: a pilot intervention promoting food texture introduction between 8 and 15 months. Appetite 158, 104989.

Touwen, B.C., 1971. A study on the development of some motor phenomena in infancy. Dev. Med. Child Neurol. 13, 435–446.

Townsend, E., Pitchford, N.J., 2012. Baby knows best? The impact of weaning style on food preferences and body mass index in early childhood in a case-controlled sample. BMJ Open 2, e000298.

Tutor, J.D., Gosa, M.M., 2011. Dysphagia and aspiration in children. Pediatr. Pulmonol. (online access 3/4/2011).

Tutor, J.D., Gosa, M.M., 2012. Dysphagia and aspiration in children. Pediatr. Pulmonol. 47, 321–337.

Uehara, I., 2000. Transition from novelty to familiarity preference depending on recognition performance by 4-yr.-olds. Psychol. Rep. 87, 837–848.

Utami, A.F., Wanda, D., Hayati, H., Fowler, C., 2020. "Becoming an independent feeder": infant's transition in solid food introduction through baby-led weaning. BMC Proc. 14, 18.

Van Dijk, M., Hunnius, S., Van Geert, P., 2009. Variability in eating behavior throughout the weaning period. Appetite 52, 766–770.

Van Dijk, M., Hunnius, S., Van Geert, P., 2012. The dynamics of feeding during the introduction to solid food. Infant Behav. Dev. 35, 226–239.

Varendi, H., Porter, R.H., Winberg, J., 1996. Attractiveness of amniotic fluid odor: evidence of prenatal olfactory learning? Acta Paediatr. 85, 1223–1227.

Ventura, A.K., 2017. Does breastfeeding shape food preferences? Links to obesity. Ann. Nutr. Metab. 70 (Suppl 3), 8–15.

Ventura, A.K., Mennella, J.A., 2017. An experimental approach to study individual differences in infants' intake and satiation behaviors during bottle-feeding. Child. Obes. 13, 44–52.

Ventura, A.K., Worobey, J., 2013. Early influences on the development of food preferences. Curr. Biol. 23, R401–R408.

Ventura, A.K., Sheeper, S., Levy, J., 2019. Exploring correlates of infant clarity of cues during early feeding interactions. J. Acad. Nutr. Diet. 119, 1452–1461.

Villar, J., Ochieng, R., Staines-Urias, E., Fernandes, M., Ratcliff, M., Purwar, M., Barros, F., Horta, B., Cheikh Ismail, L., Albernaz, E., Kunnawar, N., Temple, S., Giuliani, F., Sandells, T., Carvalho, M., Ohuma, E., Jaffer, Y., Alison Noble, J., Gravett, M., Pang, R., Lambert, A., Bertino, E., Di Nicola, P., Papageorghiou, A., Stein, A., Bhutta, Z., Kennedy, S., 2020. Late weaning and maternal closeness, associated with advanced motor and visual maturation, reinforce autonomy in healthy, 2-year-old children. Sci. Rep. 10, 5251.

Von Hofsten, C., Ronnqvist, L., 1988. Preparation for grasping an object: a developmental study. J. Exp. Psychol. Hum. Percept. Perform. 14, 610–621.

Wang, L., Van Grieken, A., Van Der Velde, L.A., Vlasblom, E., Beltman, M., L'hoir, M.P., Boere-Boonekamp, M.M., Raat, H., 2019a. Factors associated with early introduction of complementary feeding and consumption of non-recommended foods among Dutch infants: the Beeboft study. BMC Public Health 19, 388.

Wang, P., Hao, M., Han, W., Yamauchi, T., 2019b. Factors associated with nutritional status and motor development among young children. Nurs. Health Sci. 21, 323–329.

Wardle, J., Cooke, L.J., Gibson, E.L., Sapochnik, M., Sheiham, A., Lawson, M., 2003. Increasing children's acceptance of vegetables; a randomized trial of parent-led exposure. Appetite 40, 155–162.

Wasser, H., Bentley, M., Borja, J., Davis Goldman, B., Thompson, A., Slining, M., Adair, L., 2011. Infants perceived as "fussy" are more likely to receive complementary foods before 4 months. Pediatrics 127, 229–237.

Wertz, A.E., Wynn, K., 2014. Selective social learning of plant edibility in 6- and 18-month-old infants. Psychol. Sci. 25, 874–882.

Widstrom, A.M., Thingstrom-Paulsson, J., 1993. The position of the tongue during rooting reflexes elicited in newborn infants before the first suckle. Acta Paediatr. 82, 281–283.

Widstrom, A.M., Lilja, G., Aaltomaa-Michalias, P., Dahllof, A., Lintula, M., Nissen, E., 2010. Newborn behaviour to locate the breast when skin-to-skin: a possible method for enabling early self-regulation. Acta Paediatr. 100, 79–85.

Williams Erickson, L., Taylor, R.W., Haszard, J.J., Fleming, E.A., Daniels, L., Morison, B.J., Leong, C., Fangupo, L.J., Wheeler, B.J., Taylor, B.J., Te Morenga, L., Mclean, R.M., Heath, A.M., 2018. Impact of a modified version of baby-led weaning on infant food and nutrient intakes: the bliss randomized controlled trial. Nutrients 10.

Wilson, E.M., Green, J.R., 2009. The development of jaw motion for mastication. Early Hum. Dev. 85, 303–311.

Wilson, E.M., Green, J.R., Weismer, G., 2012. A kinematic description of the temporal characteristics of jaw motion for early chewing: preliminary findings. J. Speech Lang. Hear. Res. 55, 626–638.

Wolstenholme, H., Kelly, C., Hennessy, M., Heary, C., 2020. Childhood fussy/picky eating behaviours: a systematic review and synthesis of qualitative studies. Int. J. Behav. Nutr. Phys. Act. 17, 2.

Wright, C.M., Parkinson, K.N., Drewett, R.F., 2004. Why are babies weaned early? Data from a prospective population based cohort study. Arch. Dis. Child. 89, 813–816.

Wright, C.M., Parkinson, K.N., Drewett, R.F., 2006. How does maternal and child feeding behavior relate to weight gain and failure to thrive? Data from a prospective birth cohort. Pediatrics 117, 1262–1269.

Wright, C.M., Cameron, K., Tsiaka, M., Parkinson, K.N., 2011. Is baby-led weaning feasible? When do babies first reach out for and eat finger foods? Matern. Child Nutr. 7, 27–33.

Young, B., Drewett, R., 2000. Eating behaviour and its variability in 1-year-old children. Appetite 35, 171–177.

Yuan, W.L., Rigal, N., Monnery-Patris, S., Chabanet, C., Forhan, A., Charles, M.A., De Lauzon-Guillain, B., 2016. Early determinants of food liking among 5y-old children: a longitudinal study from the EDEN mother-child cohort. Int. J. Behav. Nutr. Phys. Act. 13, 20.

Zaal, F.T., Thelen, E., 2005. The developmental roots of the speed-accuracy trade-off. J. Exp. Psychol. Hum. Percept. Perform. 31, 1266–1273.

Zeinstra, G.G., Vrijhof, M., Kremer, S., 2018. Is repeated exposure the holy grail for increasing children's vegetable intake? Lessons learned from a Dutch childcare intervention using various vegetable preparations. Appetite 121, 316–325.

Zucker, N.L., Hughes, S.O., 2020. The persistence of picky eating: opportunities to improve our strategies and messaging. Pediatrics 145.

# 9

# Impact of early nutrition on gut microbiota: Effects on immunity and long-term health

*Kirsi Laitinen[a], Kati Mokkala[a], and Marko Kalliomäki[b]*

[a]Institute of Biomedicine, University of Turku, Turku, Finland

[b]Department of Clinical Medicine, University of Turku, Turku, Finland

## LEARNING OBJECTIVES

- To familiarize with features of gut microbiota and factors that impact microbiota colonization of the infant.

- To recognize the role of gut microbiota in the development of infant immune system.

- To apply the information on diet—gut microbiota interactions in the analysis of long-term impacts on human health.

- To review mechanisms explaining the link between the gut microbiota and metabolic disorders.

## 9.1 Introduction

Increasing scientific evidence has emerged in the last decades highlighting the importance of early life events, i.e., during the fetal period and in early infancy, on the later health of the individual. During the critical periods of development, disturbances in the nutritional, hormonal, and/or metabolic environment can evoke permanent changes in the body's structure, physiology, and metabolism; for example, they can contribute to the risk of adulthood diseases (Barker, 2007). There is now convincing evidence demonstrating the critical role of gut microbiota, i.e., microbes residing in the gastrointestinal tract, in many physiological and immunological processes and also in regulating the onset of many diseases. The first microbial contact with the child may already take place during pregnancy. This, along with microbiota colonization in infancy, may be related to the occurrence of later disease through a process called microbial programming. A wide variety of bacteria, viruses, and fungi live in different sites of the human body including skin, respiratory tract, and gut. Here, we focus on the gut microbiota.

The symbiotic host-microbiota interaction is of major significance for human physiology and health (reviewed in Power et al., 2014; Walker and Lawley, 2013). The gut microbiota is known to synthesize vitamins, like vitamin K and some B vitamins, folic acid, and biotin, as well as phytoestrogens. The microbiota also participates in the digestion of food, particularly in handling the non-digestible components like fiber and carbohydrates that reach the colon (20–60 g/d), thereby contributing to energy harvest by the host. Many metabolites are produced by microbiota, including short-chain fatty acids. These compounds are not only important fuels for gut cells but also act in support of gut barrier function and can influence the host's immune functions. The gut microbiota also participates in conferring protection against pathogens in at least three ways: (1) by competition for attachment sites on the mucosa, (2) via the production of antimicrobial compounds, and (3) through the stimulation of the host's defenses.

This chapter will describe the typical composition of the infant's microbiota and its evolution over the first years of life with potential contributing factors in the diet and the environment. Furthermore, the relation of the composition of the microbiota with risk of diseases and the efficacy of microbiota modification by dietary interventions such as the consumption of probiotics along with underlying mechanisms will be discussed.

## 9.2 Composition and stability of the microbiota present in infants from early childhood to adult life

### 9.2.1 General features of the gut microbiota and modern analysis methods

The gut microbiota can be considered as an important multifunctional organ influencing the host's physiology, metabolism, nutrition, neural, and immune system. According to one estimate, the ratio of bacterial cells residing in the human body to actual human cells is around 1 to 1 (Sender et al., 2016). The majority of the bacteria reside in the colon, where more than 1000 different microbial species have been detected (Rajilić-Stojanović and de Vos, 2014), although it is anticipated that more await discovery. This vast number of cells clearly highlights the significance of the gut microbiota in human health.

Recent development in analytical methods has given us deeper insights into both the taxonomic composition and possible functional properties of the gut microbiota. These technical advances have provided further opportunities to investigate the role of the gut microbiota in human health and disease. Many of these novel technologies are based on DNA sequencing; the most widely exploited approach is 16S ribosomal RNA (16S rRNA) sequencing, in which the sequencing of the species-specific 16S rRNA gene allows identification of bacterial species. Whole-genome sequencing is one of the most recent methods; this technique is based on sequencing the entire genome and thus provides not only high-resolution data on the taxonomy but also, as the complete DNA is sequenced, information on the genes and thus insights into the functional capacities of the bacteria can be glimpsed. Data from both these analyses require the application of novel and sophisticated computational and bioinformatics tools, which are constantly being developed.

The composition of the gut microbiota can be characterized based on abundance and diversity. The relative abundance of certain bacteria defines the amount of this bacteria in the microbial community, for example, in the gut. Alpha-diversity is a measure of diversity within the sample, while beta-diversity reveals the variation amongst samples. Alpha-diversity is usually expressed as the number of species richness (number of species) and evenness (the relative abundance of the species). Beta-diversity is mainly based on taxonomic abundances and differences in these profiles between the samples.

The composition and concentration of microbes vary in the different sections of the gastrointestinal tract; in the proximal part (stomach, duodenum, and jejunum), the concentration of bacteria is low (1 − 1000), but it gradually increases (from $10^7$ up to $10^{14}$) toward the distal part (ileum, colon) of the gut. In the proximal part, more aerobic or facultative bacteria are found, whereas in the distal part, there is an abundance of anaerobic bacteria. For example, the typical bacteria found in the proximal sections are two genera: *Lactobacillus* and *Streptococcus*; in the distal parts, the characteristic bacteria include genus *Clostridium*, *Bacteroides*, and *Bifidobacterium*. The most dense bacterial population is found in the large intestine, where the most common phyla are Actinobacteria, Bacteroidetes, Firmicutes, and Proteobacteria (reviewed in Rajilić-Stojanović and de Vos, 2014), with *Bacteroidetes* and *Firmicutes* having the highest abundance (Qin et al., 2010).

## 9.2.2 Microbiota development and stability

While the gut microbiota is exposed to changes due to environmental factors during the whole human lifespan, the most intense development occurs during the first years of life. In adulthood, the microbiota is less plastic and thus more resistant to changes. Although stable, the adult gut microbiota not only differs amongst individuals but even within the same individual. In fact, it is far from clear what actually constitutes a healthy microbiota. However, there is convincing evidence that a diverse microbiota, i.e., a wide variation in bacterial species, may play a role in human health. Several studies have found an association between gut microbiota dysbiosis (i.e., disruption of microbiota homeostasis) with non-communicable diseases, such as obesity, inflammatory bowel disease, metabolic syndrome, and allergies (Huang et al., 2020).

### 9.2.2.1 Colonization of the infant's gut after birth

Meconium is the infant's first feces; it is produced after birth and contains the amniotic fluid ingested in the fetal period in the uterus, and microbial colonization can occur during that time. After birth, the infant's intestine is rapidly colonized by multiple microbes. It has been suggested that immediately after the birth (within 24h), the species diversity is high due to the transfer of microbes from both the mother and the environment, but it gradually decreases depending on the capability of the bacteria to colonize the gut (Ferretti et al., 2018). Thus, in general, the diversity of the early infant microbiota increases gradually.

The major bacteria phyla found in the infant's intestine include Actinobacteria, Bacteroidetes, Firmicutes, and Proteobacteria, and these can be detected already in meconium. The first bacteria to colonize the infant's gut are facultative anaerobes, such as *Enterobacteria*. Next, colonization continues with anaerobic bacteria, such as *Bifidobacterium*, *Bacteroides*, and *Clostridium* (reviewed in Cheng et al., 2016), resulting in a shift in the microbiota community toward

TABLE 9.1   Terminology.

| Terms used in the chapter | |
| --- | --- |
| Microbiota | Microbial community; gut microbiota: microbes in gut |
| Microbiome | Microbiota genomes |
| Probiotics | Live microorganisms that, when administered in adequate amounts, confer a health benefit to the host |
| Dysbiosis | Disruption of microbiota homeostasis/imbalance of microbiota composition |
| Microbiota diversity | Measure of the variety present in the microbial community, e.g., in the human gut. Diversity consists of two components, richness and evenness. Species richness: how many species present, species evenness: the relative abundance of species |
| Gram-negative/gram-positive | Classification of bacteria based on gram-staining |
| Obligate anaerobe | A bacteria living and growing only in the absence of oxygen |
| Facultative anaerobe | A bacteria living and growing in the presence and absence of oxygen |
| 16S rRNA sequencing | DNA sequencing of the 16S rRNA (16S ribosomal ribonucleic acid) gene |
| Metagenomics sequencing | DNA sequencing of the whole genome |

one more typical of the adult gut environment. The colonization process is dependent on multiple factors; however, at 4 months after birth, a high proportion, even as many as 61.2%, of the species are proposed to be common with the infant's mother (Ferretti et al., 2018). Due to changing feeding habits as well as contributions from other environmental factors, the diversity increases, and the microbiota gradually changes in its composition and diversity to resemble that of adults. During the first years, the microbiota stabilizes so that by 3 years of age, it starts to resemble the adult microbiota, however, still being susceptible to alterations mediated by many factors (Table 9.1).

## 9.3   Factors influencing the development of the gut microbiota

### 9.3.1   The composition of the gut microbiota in infants is prone to environmental changes

The gut microbiota varies widely from one individual to another, particularly in children (Yatsunenko et al., 2012). In general, the microbiota of adults is more resilient at resisting change, while its composition in infants is more prone to alterations due to various triggers like diet. Other contributing factors which can influence the infant's microbiota include mode of delivery, gestational length, early feeding practices, as well as maternal characteristics, including the mother's microbiota composition (Fig. 9.1). As stated, the first contact between the infant and bacteria already takes place in the uterus. The domestic environment of the child has also been shown to influence the composition of the child's microbiota, examples being exposure to pets (Nermes et al., 2013) or attendance at a daycare center (Thompson et al., 2015). In addition, antibiotic treatments disrupt and modify the microbiota in specific manner (reviewed in Gibson et al., 2015; Zimmermann and Curtis, 2019), with preterm and

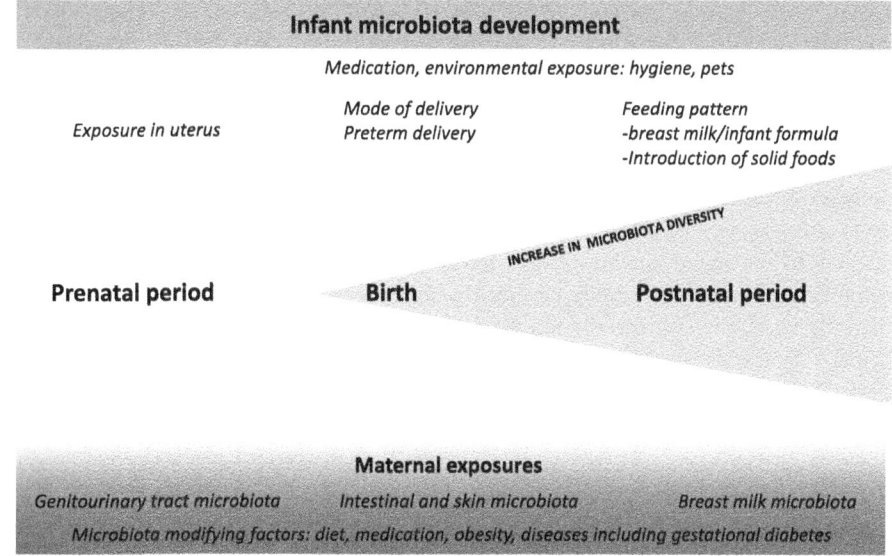

FIG. 9.1    Development of the infant's microbiota and influencing factors.

very low birth weight infants being at the highest risk, as these children often receive antibiotics at a very early stage of their lives. In the longer term, antibiotic administration may influence the evolution of the gut microbiota by reducing the microbial load as well as the microbiota diversity. Evidently, antibiotic treatment may influence human health beyond its specific function, i.e., combatting pathogen-induced infections by modulating the development of the immune defense system. Indeed, antibiotic exposure, particularly during the first 6 months of life or in children administered repeated treatments, has been associated with an increased risk of overweight and obesity in childhood (Rasmussen et al., 2018). Similarly, there is some evidence that early-life antibiotic exposure can increase the risk of food allergy in children (Netea et al., 2019).

Genetics may also influence the composition of the gut microbiota and subsequently the host's metabolism (Goodrich et al., 2014). In a study of dichorionic triplet set, a similar gut microbiota was detected in monozygotic twins, which was distinct from a fraternal sibling at 1 month of age, while the profile had become more uniform amongst the three infants at 12 months of age, highlighting the impact of environmental factors in modulating the microbiota population (Murphy et al., 2015). Overall, the host's genetics explain only a minor proportion of the composition of the gut microbiota and less than that attributable to diet, drugs, and anthropometric characteristics (Rothschild et al., 2018).

## 9.3.2  Diet shapes gut microbiota

There is clear evidence for the impact of diet emerging from studies that have evaluated the composition of the microbiota in different geographical areas like Africa where the diet consists of more vegetables, fruits, and grains and thus is rich in both fiber and starch, while the diets in Western countries are abundant in dairy products and meat. The microbiota composition of southeastern African and northern European infants has been shown to differ (Grześkowiak et al., 2012). Although *Bifidobacteria* were dominant in both areas when the feces of breastfed infants were studied, the *Bacteroides-Prevotella* group was more abundant in 6-month-old Malawian infants' microbiota; furthermore, Clostridium perfringens, as well as Staphylococcus aureus, were detected only in Finnish infants. Similarly, in another study in 1- to 6-year-old children from Italy and Burkina Faso, significant differences in the composition of the microbiota were detected, showing enrichment in Bacteroidetes and depletion of Firmicutes (De Filippo et al., 2010). These studies most likely reflect the evolution of microbiota in response to the composition of the diet as well as hygienic conditions, possibly allowing maximization of energy intake from a high-fiber diet and potentially also protection from diseases. In addition, the change from a traditional African diet that is composed of cereals, legumes, and vegetables by introducing foods of animal origin seemed to evoke changes in the functional profile of the gut microbiota so that it became more suited for the metabolism of animal protein and fat (De Filippo et al., 2017). The effect of diet on the gut microbiota has also been examined by comparing the composition of the gut microbiota in subjects following specific diets such as a gluten-free diet (Sanz, 2010) or a vegetarian or vegan diet, although the evidence has been challenged by some investigators (Trefflich et al., 2020). A controlled feeding study demonstrated changes in the composition of the microbiota within 24 h of initiation of a high-fat and low-fiber or low-fat and high-fiber diet (Wu et al., 2011). In the longer term, the intakes of protein and animal fat were related to the induced growth of *Bacteroides*, whereas the carbohydrate and fiber intake were linked to that of *Prevotella* (Wu et al., 2011). Particular diet patterns may thus associate with distinct combinations of bacteria in the intestine, the so-called enterotypes. Thus, diet may induce modifications in gut microbiota at several levels, namely through the dietary pattern (like Western diet or vegetarian diet), specific foods (whole grain), nutrients (fiber, fat), or food-associated microbes, as reviewed by Graf et al. (2015). Currently, the best known are the impacts of dietary fiber on gut microbiota (Shortt et al., 2018), but more evidence is emerging on the role of dietary fats in modulating the composition of the gut microbiota (Mokkala et al., 2020). A higher intake of fat, particularly saturated fatty acids, has been typically related to an increased Firmicutes to Bacteroidetes ratio and a reduced abundance of *Bifidobacteria*, which potentially could relate to an increased risk for health-related conditions like obesity and type 2 diabetes, thus highlighting the importance of the quality of dietary fat.

With respect to infants, they may be colonized by bacteria through several routes, one source being breast milk. The gut microbiota of breastfed infants has been shown to differ from that of formula-fed infants (Kleessen et al., 1995; Thompson et al., 2015), indicating not only the impact of feeding type but also how a differing diet can influence the infant's microbiota and its development. Regardless of the geographical location (Grześkowiak et al., 2012), *Bifidobacteria* typify the gut microbiota of healthy breastfed infants and point to the presence of *Bifidobacteria* in breast milk (Gueimonde et al., 2007). In a systematic review, 554 bacterial species belonging to 178 genera were identified in breast milk, the most common belonging to four phyla, which are as follows: Proteobacteria, Firmicutes, Actinobacteria, and Bacteroidetes (Togo et al., 2019). There are likely several routes through which bacteria can gain access to breast milk, i.e., from the maternal intestine via the entero-mammary pathway and through retrograde translocation from the infant's mouth or maternal skin and possibly also from the maternal oral cavity (oro-mammary pathway) (Moossavi and Azad, 2020).

In addition to microbes, breast milk also contains many bioactive components, including human milk oligosaccharides (HMOs) that induce gut microbial growth. Indeed the bifidogenic potential of HMOs has been mimicked by adding other prebiotic compounds like fructooligosaccharides (FOS) or galactooligosaccharides to infant formulas (reviewed in Lyons et al., 2020). The composition of breast milk, including microbiota changes throughout lactation, has been investigated (Cabrera-Rubio et al., 2012). *Weissella* and *Leuconostoc* were predominant in colostrum samples, whereas *Veillonella, Leptotrichia,* and *Prevotella* were typical in 1- and 6-month breast milk samples (Cabrera-Rubio et al., 2012). Furthermore, breast milk from obese mothers tended to contain a different and less diverse bacterial community when compared with milk from normal-weight mothers, demonstrating the role of the mother's nutritional status on the microbiota composition of her milk. As a healthy breastfed infant represents a model for optimal infant feeding, this gives rise to the opportunity to supplement infant formula with added probiotics or prebiotics in case the child needs to be fed by infant formula instead of breast milk. A systematic review of the scientific literature found no reason of concern with regard to infant growth or with adverse effects associated with these formulas (Braegger et al., 2011).

There are changes in the composition of an infant's microbiota associated with the cessation of breastfeeding and with the introduction of solid foods. In a five-country study, the proportions of *Bifidobacteria*, *Enterobacteria* and Clostridium difficile, and C. perfringens species decreased, while those of C. coccoides and C. leptum proportions increased (Fallani et al., 2011). In a Danish study, the abundances of certain species, particularly of Bacteroidetes-related species increased, whereas *Bifidobacterium* and *Lactobacillus* species, as well as *Enterobacteriaceae* were reduced (Bergström et al., 2014). Interestingly, the microbiota of infants who had been exclusively breastfed at the time of solid food introduction changed less than the microbiota of non-exclusively breastfed infants (Thompson et al., 2015). In general, the initiation of solid feeding increases species diversity. At weaning, infants are subjected to new dietary exposures which drive changes in the composition and function of the microbiota. For example, there was an increase observed in those genes involved in carbohydrate and pyruvate metabolism which may relate to obtaining energy, but overall, the cessation of breastfeeding appeared to be the major factor explaining the changes in the composition and functional properties of the gut microbiota (Bäckhed et al., 2015). Eventually, the composition of the child's microbiota starts to resemble more that of an adult, but further changes in the developing microbiota still occur until he/she has reached the age of 3 years (Bergström et al., 2014; Yatsunenko et al., 2012).

### 9.3.3 Maternal influence on microbiota development

The development of the infant's microbiota is influenced by many maternal factors. Indeed, as stated earlier, early events are important as mothers provide the first inoculum for the infant. This may occur already in utero and through the umbilical blood during pregnancy. Furthermore, maternal vaginal and gut microbiota may be transferred to the infant at birth, with skin contact also being an important contributor. According to an expert opinion, the uterus is likely to be sterile (i.e., free of microbes detected by a cultivation method), but there are possible incidents of transient presence of microbes, and thus the developing fetus can be subjected to microbial exposures (Blaser et al., 2021). Indeed, bacterial translocation may take place via the amniotic sac and placenta. One proposal has been that the measured DNA fractions identified in the placenta are due either to contamination or to the presence of bacterial DNA in blood leaving the placenta. Although bacteria may be present, it does not seem that the placenta houses a characteristic microbial community. Nonetheless, if the fetus is exposed to small amounts of microbes in utero, this could perhaps influence fetal development, primarily through immunologic mechanisms—a topic for future investigation.

Mode of delivery, whether cesarian or vaginal, also shapes the infant's microbiota (Dominguez-Bello et al., 2010). The initial encounter with microbes may come primarily from the mother or, in case of cesarean section, more extensively from the environment, including the nursing staff. In the study of Dominguez-Bello et al. (2010), it was shown that vaginally delivered infants acquired bacterial communities resembling their own mother's vaginal microbiota (*Lactobacillus, Prevotella, Sneathia* spp.), whereas cesarean section infants were colonized more by skin bacteria (*Staphylococcus, Corynebacterium, and Propionibacterium spp.*). Whether infants born with elective cesarean section would benefit from the transplantation of maternal fecal microbiota is a topic being investigated by some researchers. In a proof of concept study, seven infants received a diluted fecal sample in human milk from their own mothers (Korpela et al., 2020). In a 3-month follow-up, the infants exhibited no adverse effects, and their fecal microbiota showed similarities to vaginally delivered infants. At this point, although "a protocol for oral transplantation of maternal fecal microbiota to newborn infants born by cesarean section" for use in healthy mothers and infants has been published (Helve et al., 2021), there is no consensus on the feasibility of fecal transplantation in this vulnerable group in health care nor on its ultimate benefits. Several other factors like gestational age may influence the infant's microbiota as indicated by differing microbial communities present in the meconium in infants delivered less than or above 33 weeks of gestation (Ardissone et al., 2014) and the relationship of the vaginal microbiota composition with gestational age at delivery (DiGiulio et al., 2015). The vaginal microbiota may contribute to fetal health as indicated by the associations detected between vaginal microbiota and preterm delivery, but the evidence is thus far from conclusive (Peelen et al., 2019).

The maternal nutritional status during pregnancy may influence the development of the gut microbiota in infants. Higher weights and body mass indexes of mothers, as well as excessive weight gain during pregnancy, were related to higher concentrations of *Bacteroides*, *Clostridium*, and *Staphylococcus* and lower concentrations of the *Bifidobacterium* group (Collado et al., 2010). In another study, reduced numbers of *Bacteroides* and *Bifidobacterium* and increased numbers of *Staphylococcus, Enterobacteriaceae, and* Escherichia coli were measured in overweight pregnant women in comparison to normal-weight pregnant women (Santacruz et al., 2010). A higher maternal gestational weight gain was also associated with a lower richness and diversity of the microbiota (Robinson et al., 2017). In addition, if the mother is suffering from gestational diabetes, this may influence her infant's microbiota as measured from saliva and pharyngeal aspirates (Wang et al., 2018), as well as from feces (Crusell et al., 2020; Soderborg et al., 2020). Whether gestational diabetes actually alters maternal gut microbiota is a matter for debate, as reviewed in Hasain et al. (2020); in fact, a recent study applying the metagenomics approach indicated that this was not the case (Mokkala et al., 2021). Koren et al. (2012) described maternal microbiota changes during pregnancy. In the first trimester, the microbiota resembled the composition of healthy non-pregnant subjects, but by the third trimester, the composition had changed, showing signs of microbiota dysbiosis, similar to that encountered in the metabolic syndrome. Furthermore, when compared to overweight women, obese pregnant women have been shown to have dysbiosis and aberrations in many metabolic and inflammatory markers (Houttu et al., 2018).

In the light of the importance of early nutrition programming, it is possible that some epigenetic programming occurs already during pregnancy via the microbiota and its subsequent metabolic effects, one example being epigenetic regulation. Administration of probiotics during pregnancy was shown to reduce DNA methylation of the promoter of the fat mass and obesity-associated (FTO) gene (Vähämiko et al., 2019). This may translate into altered transcription and expression of the FTO gene, which has subsequent impacts on the risk of obesity and metabolic conditions, including type 2 diabetes. This highlights the importance of one modifiable factor, i.e., diet, in regulating gut microbiota with its subsequent metabolic and clinical effects. Although the evidence for this proposal is thus far limited, it does seem plausible that the maternal diet during pregnancy can modify both the mother's and her child's microbiota (Maher et al., 2020). A diet that is in accordance with the dietary guidelines seems to benefit the gut microbiota. This was demonstrated in a study in overweight and obese pregnant women in which an overall healthy diet measured by the diet quality index was shown to relate to a higher gut microbiota diversity (Laitinen and Mokkala, 2019).

There is clear scientific evidence that diet and other environmental factors shape the developing gut microbiota; it is less certain whether these functional changes exert long-term impacts on human physiology and health.

## 9.4 Microbiota effects on (long-term) health

### 9.4.1 Clinical evidence: Microbiota differences detected prior to disease

Early microbiota colonization is important for the development of the immune system and also for immunological tolerance. Disturbances in the development of the gut microbiota in early life may have long-lasting consequences in later life, for example, elevating the individual's risk of non-communicable diseases, such as allergy and obesity.

#### 9.4.1.1 Allergy

Exposure to microorganisms and the establishment of microbiota colonization in early life is essential for the development of the immune system. The lack of an adequate microbial exposure may result in reduced immunological stimulation and subsequent disturbances in the development of the immune system. The onset of allergy has been associated with multiple factors, including caesarian birth, formula feeding, lack of maternal exposure to animals, or consumption of antimicrobial agents when pregnant. All these factors are also known to impact the composition of the microbiota in the infant's gut, thus confirming the importance of microbiota exposure as immunological stimuli and consequently on the later manifestation of allergy.

Many clinical studies have investigated the impact of the composition of gut microbiota in various stages of an infant's life on allergic symptoms in later childhood. A lower diversity of gut microbiota in early life has been shown to associate with an increased risk of childhood atopic diseases (Bisgaard et al., 2011; Abrahamsson et al., 2014a; Wang et al., 2008).

A higher diversity and abundance of butyrate-producing bacteria at 6 months of age were associated with milder symptoms in infants suffering from atopic eczema (Nylund et al., 2015). However, this is at odds with one finding where increased microbiota diversity at 18 months of age was associated with eczema at 2 years of age (Nylund et al., 2013). The impact of decreases or increases in specific bacteria is not clear since the results are conflicting. There are a few studies indicating that there are increased levels of *Clostridium* and decreased levels of *Bifidobacterium* in feces of infants who later developed an allergic disease (Kalliomäki et al., 2001a; Björkstén et al., 2001). In another trial, early colonization with lactobacilli was shown to decrease the risk for allergy (Johansson et al., 2011). The explanation for inconsistent results may be due to the variations not only in the child's age but also in the methods used when feces were collected, as well as associated conditions in children when evaluated.

### 9.4.1.2 Obesity

The role of gut microbiota in obesity and obesity-associated disorders has attracted a considerable amount of interest. The composition of the gut microbiota, both in terms of the diversity and abundance of certain bacteria has been shown to associate with obesity, but it is not clear whether these associations are a cause or a consequence of the condition. Based on results emerging from animal studies, many mechanisms have been proposed to explain how gut microbiota can influence the host's energy metabolism and thus impact the development of obesity. For example, gut bacteria can influence fatty acid metabolism and the storage of energy in the host as they are able to digest polysaccharides and thus increase energy availability. Short-chain fatty acids are bacterial fermentation products, which together with the increased amount of monosaccharides, can be absorbed, resulting in elevated energy storage. Microbiota may suppress the release of fasting-induced adipocyte factor, a lipoprotein lipase inhibitor, increasing lipid storage in adipocytes (Bäckhed et al., 2004). The activity of adenosine monophosphate-activated protein kinase, AMPK, an important enzyme involved in energy homeostasis, may be suppressed by microbiota (Bäckhed et al., 2007), resulting in increased fat deposition. In addition to impacting energy metabolism, microbial metabolites may modify intestinal function by altering the effects of several hormones (peptide YY, (PYY)) (Samuel et al., 2008). These effects are species-dependent and thus make it easier to understand that an abundance of a specific bacterial species can contribute to the host's energy metabolism depending on its capacities, for example, the microbe's ability to harvest energy from the host's diet.

With regard to obesity in infancy, there are a few studies suggesting that alterations in the gut microbiota may precede the development of childhood obesity. The abundance of *Bifidobacterium* during the first year of life was higher in children who were normal weight at age 7 years, whereas a higher *Staphylococcus* abundance was found in those children who became overweight (Kalliomäki et al., 2008). In another study, the BMI Standard Deviation Score at the age of 3 and 52 weeks was associated with a low *Staphylococcus* concentration at the same age (Vael et al., 2011). A higher abundance of Bacteroides fragilis has been correlated with childhood obesity in three studies (Vael et al., 2011; Scheepers et al., 2015; Ignacio et al., 2016). Further, as found in adults, changes in the Firmicutes to Bacteroidetes ratio may associate with childhood obesity (Indiani et al., 2018). Another report found that the gut microbiota at the age of 2 years explained over 50% of the variation in BMI at 12 years of age (Stanislawski et al., 2018).

In adults, obesity has been associated with reduced diversity and richness of the gut microbiota (Turnbaugh et al., 2009; Peters et al., 2018; Liu et al., 2017). Several investigators have demonstrated differences at the phyla level between lean and obese individuals; however, the results are not truly consistent. Some workers have claimed that obese individuals have a lower proportion of Bacteroidetes and a higher proportion of Actinobacteria (Turnbaugh et al., 2009) or Firmicutes (Ley et al., 2006). Nonetheless, there are other reports that there are no such differences in microbiota ratios between obese and lean individuals (Zhang et al., 2009; Duncan et al., 2008; Jumpertz et al., 2011). At the genus and species level, lean women were shown to have a higher prevalence of Lactobacillus plantarum, *Bifidobacterium genus*, Bifidobacterium longum, Clostridium coccoides, and Clostridium leptum when compared to their obese counterparts (Teixeira et al., 2013). In twins discordant for BMI, the *Clostridium cluster IV* diversity correlated inversely with BMI, while Eubacterium ventriosum and Roseburia intestinalis relatives (SCFA producers) correlated positively and relatives of *Oscillospira guillermondii* (a butyrate producer) negatively with the differences in their BMIs (Tims et al., 2013). In another study, obesity was associated with an increased abundance of Bacilli-class and its families *Streptococcaceae* and *Lactobacillaceae*, while there was a lower abundance of *Christensenellaceae*, *Clostridiaceae*, and *Dehalobacteriaceae* (Peters et al., 2018).

Weight loss has been shown to induce alterations into the composition of the microbiota; the proportion of Bacteroidetes increased while that of Firmicutes declined (Ley et al., 2006). A metagenomics analysis detected lower gene counts and bacterial diversity in obese individuals when the impact of sleeve gastrectomy was investigated in young obese and lean individuals. In obese subjects, Bacteroides thetaiotaomicron species were depleted. Interestingly, after sleeve gastrectomy, the microbiota in the previously obese individuals shifted toward that of their lean counterparts, thus suggesting that weight loss by sleeve gastrectomy could restore a healthy microbiota (Liu et al., 2017).

The presence of low-grade inflammation has been suggested to be involved in obesity-associated metabolic disturbances. A metagenomic study investigating the association between low-grade inflammation and obesity (Le Chatelier et al., 2013) demonstrated that the gut microbiota was one potential trigger of the inflammation encountered in obese people. In that study, a low bacterial richness (bacterial gene count) correlated with more inflammatory phenotypes and overall adiposity, insulin resistance, and dyslipidemia. The study group with a low bacterial gene count was also dominated by *Bacteroides* and some *Ruminococcus* species, such as Ruminococcus gnavus. A higher gene richness was associated with Faecalibacterium prausnitzii, *Bifibacterium*, *Lactobacillus*, *Alistipes*, and *Akkermansia*. For example, *Bacteroides* and R. gnavus are considered to be proinflammatory bacteria, whereas *F. praunitzii* is anti-inflammatory, and the association of these bacteria in the above groups support the theory that obesity is associated with the presence of a more proinflammatory microbiota composition.

Although there is emerging evidence linking obesity and overweight with alterations in the composition of the gut microbiota, it is not clear whether the microbiota is the predisposing factor or a consequence of the obese status. In addition, the findings are somewhat inconsistent, this being attributable to several aspects, including the effects of diet and other lifestyle factors. Clearly, a more appropriate way to investigate the role of various bacteria in species level and their function in the development of obesity would be to perform a metagenomic analysis, as this would provide more information on the functional potential of the bacteria than can be obtained from the more widely used taxonomic analyses, for example, 16S rRNA sequencing.

## 9.4.2 Mechanisms: Intestinal permeability, a link between the gut microbiota and metabolic disorders

The intestinal epithelium forms a structural barrier between the intestinal lumen and the body's circulation. The maintenance of intestinal epithelial integrity is essential; first, for preventing the passage of harmful components, such as pathogens, antigens, and food components from coming into contact with the internal environment; and second, for ensuring the physiological exchange of fluid between the lumen and tissues. It is evident that the regulation of this process is important for human health and furthermore, that it can be influenced by many stimuli.

Intestinal integrity plays an important role in the regulation of nutrient intake and defense against pathogens in infancy. For example, alterations in intestinal permeability have been associated with multiple metabolic disorders including obesity and type 2 diabetes. In addition, in infants, an increase in intestinal permeability has been found in the child's allergy to cow's milk (Kalach et al., 2001). At birth, intestinal permeability is high but gradually decreases in response to various factors, including hormones, breast milk, and the production of the mucus layer.

### 9.4.2.1 Structure of the intestinal epithelium

The integrity of the intestinal epithelium is maintained by the interactions between multiple cells and junctions (Fig. 9.2). A single layer of rapidly renewing epithelial cells (turning over every 3–5 days) separates the gut lumen from the underlying lamina propria. The intestinal epithelial stem cells, responsible for the renewal of the intestinal epithelium, are able to develop into many specialized cell types. Absorptive enterocytes are the most abundant (80%) cells originating from the intestinal epithelial cells. Goblet, Paneth, and enteroendocrine cells are secreting cells, goblet cells synthesize and release mucin, and together with Paneth cells also producing antimicrobial peptides. The enteroendocrine cells synthesize several bioactive molecules, such as hormones which exert both local and systemic effects as well as digestive regulators. Microfold cells (M cells), yet another intestinal epithelial cell population, are responsible for the delivery of antigens to the lamina propria. The lamina propria contains immune cells, including macrophages, dendritic cells, plasma cells, and lamina propria lymphocytes (Fig. 9.2) (reviewed in Suzuki, 2013; Turner, 2009).

Adjacent epithelial cells are joined together by junctional complexes (Fig. 9.2). The most common apical complex is the tight junction (TJ), consisting of TJ proteins claudins, zonula occludens (ZO1), occludin, and F-actin. The TJ is responsible for the regulation of paracellular transport, and hence these junctions are an important factor in controlling the flux of intestinal components. Several proteins, i.e., E-cadherin, $\alpha$-catenin 1, $\beta$-catenin, catenin $\delta1$, and F-actin, form the adherent junction, which is located below the TJ. Desmosomes are located below the apical junctions and consist of desmoglein, desmocollin, desmoplakin, and keratin filaments (as reviewed in Turner, 2009).

### 9.4.2.2 Regulation of intestinal integrity by microbiota and diet

Intestinal integrity can be altered in response to various factors such as nutrients, inflammatory factors, certain diseases, and gut bacteria. The regulation occurs through alterations in the function and formation of the TJs. It is evident that the gut microbiota has an important

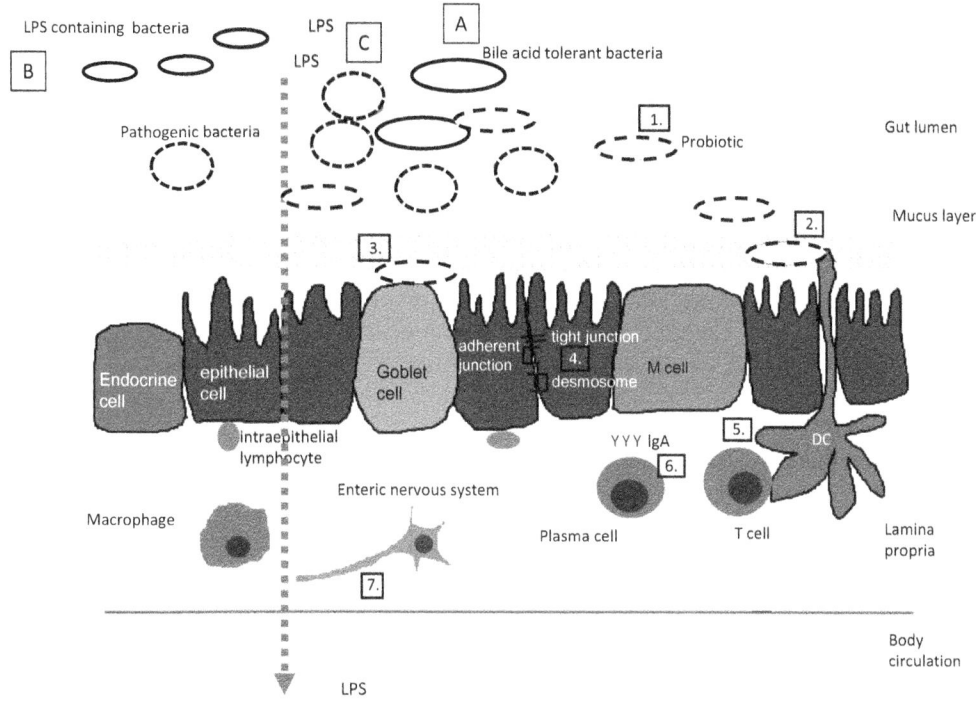

FIG. 9.2   Structure and cells in the intestinal epithelia. Potential routes of action of probiotics are marked with numbers from 1 to 7. These include effects in the gut lumen (1), in the epithelial cell lining (2–4), and below the intestinal epithelium (5–7). Examples of the mechanism by which the dietary intake of fat modifies gut microbiota (A–C): a high fat intake (A) induces an increase in the amounts of bile acids resulting in an increased abundance of bile acid tolerant bacteria, (B) an increase in the abundance of LPS containing bacteria, and (C) an elevated fecal content of LPS, which may be able to gain access to the systemic circulation. Please see the text for details.

role in the homeostasis of intestinal integrity. Several in vitro studies have suggested that treatment with probiotics, for example, *Lactobacilli* and *Bifidobacteria,* can increase intestinal epithelial integrity (Putaala et al., 2008; Anderson et al., 2010), whereas certain pathogenic bacteria may induce detrimental alterations in intestinal integrity, thus increasing intestinal permeability. Pathogenic bacteria may directly bind to epithelial cells, or toxins secreted by these pathogens may function as TJ disturbing factors.

In addition to microbiota, dietary factors are involved in the regulation of intestinal integrity. For example, a high-fat diet (Moreira et al., 2012) and alcohol (Elamin et al., 2013) may precede the appearance of increased intestinal permeability. Certain dietary components, such as eicosapentaenoic acid (EPA), docosahexaenoic acid (DHA) (Li et al., 2008), probiotics (Ulluwishewa et al., 2011), and vitamins, such as vitamins D and A, amino acids glutamine, and arginine (as reviewed in Farré et al., 2020), have been related to intestinal permeability with potential beneficial health effects. However, this evidence has mainly originated either from in vitro tests or from work done in experimental animals. It may also be that at least a part of the impact of diet may occur via the gut microbiota; dietary factors may act as a substrate for growth of beneficial bacteria or for the production of bacterial metabolites, such as butyrate production from fiber. Butyrate, a short-chain fatty acid, is known to be a fuel used by intestinal epithelial cells.

### 9.4.2.3 Intestinal permeability: A link between gut microbiota and metabolic disorders

Intestinal integrity plays a critical role in providing barriers against the passage of harmful intestinal components into the systemic circulation. Bacterial or dietary components may act as antigens should they gain access to the circulation. The increased passage of harmful components, as a result of the increase in intestinal permeability, may trigger an inflammatory response resulting in the development of various metabolic disorders. An example of this kind of response is metabolic endotoxemia, a condition where excessive amounts (i.e., two to three times compared to normal) of the gram-negative bacterial endotoxin, lipopolysaccharide (LPS), are found in the blood (Cani et al., 2007). LPS is a bacterial wall antigen capable of triggering a powerful inflammatory response aimed at eliminating pathogenic bacteria. Metabolic endotoxemia may induce a chronic and elevated inflammatory response, known as a low-grade inflammation (Boroni Moreira and de Cássia Gonçalves Alfenas, 2012). This low-grade inflammation is characterized by increased levels of proinflammatory cytokines, including tumor necrosis factor α, IL-6, IL-1β, and C-reactive protein. These inflammatory factors are capable of regulating various cellular pathways, such as those involved in insulin signaling, and thus they may induce alterations in insulin sensitivity. Low-grade inflammation has been associated with chronic lifestyle-associated metabolic disorders, such as obesity, cardiovascular diseases, type 2 diabetes, and metabolic syndrome in adults. Metabolic endotoxemia, which results from the increase in intestinal permeability and leakage of LPS into the systemic circulation, may thus be a link between gut microbiota and metabolic disorders, since an elevated level of LPS has been found in patients with type 2 diabetes (Jayashree et al., 2014; Creely et al., 2007; Al-Attas et al., 2009; Gomes et al., 2016), nonalcoholic fatty liver disease (Carpino et al., 2020), and has been linked with cardiovascular diseases (Kallio et al., 2015; Battson et al., 2018).

Pregnancy is associated with alterations in metabolic pathways, inflammatory status, and body composition. The inflammatory status in a normal pregnancy resembles the situation of low-grade inflammation. It is not yet clear if obesity and overweight during pregnancy further influence maternal inflammation or whether and how the gut microbiota and intestinal permeability are involved. An increase in intestinal permeability and the passage of bacterial and other components first to the mother's bloodstream and further to the fetus may be one source of microbiota programming of the fetus.

## 9.4.3 Effects of microbiota on the immune system and beyond

### 9.4.3.1 The gut microbiota affects the developing immune and neural systems

The gastrointestinal immune system protects the host from pathogenic microbes while tolerating innocent encounters with foreign antigens such as food and non-pathogenic bacteria. It is essential for immunological homeostasis and health that both of these characteristics of the gut mucosal immune system develop normally in the postnatal phase (Round and Mazmanian, 2009).

Studies with germ-free mice have demonstrated that gut microbial colonization is mandatory for normal postnatal development of the mucosal immune system (Round and Mazmanian, 2009). Mice reared in a sterile environment suffer developmental defects in the number and/or function of many structures, including the formation of intestinal epithelial cells and the capillary network, Peyer's patches, cellular lamina propria, plasma cells in germinal centers, isolated lymphoid follicles, mesenteric lymph nodes, CD8 + intraepithelial lymphocytes, CD4 + lamina propria lymphocytes, intestinal-type 17T helper (Th17) cells, T regulatory cells in mesenteric lymph nodes, immunoglobulin A producing plasma cells, as well as in their expression of antimicrobial peptides (reviewed in Jain and Walker, 2015).

The enteric nervous system is a complex network of neurons and glia that controls several aspects of bowel function such as motility, secretion, and blood flow to enable the appropriate fluid and nutrient absorption and waste elimination. The gastrointestinal physiology is thus tightly controlled by the two layers of interconnected ganglia, the outer myenteric plexus, located between the longitudinal and circular muscle walls of the intestine, and the inner submucosal plexus, located between circular muscle and bowel mucosa (Avetisyan et al., 2015). Both the developing gut microbiota and the immune system exert a major postnatal impact on the formation and function of the enteric neural circuitry (as reviewed by Obata and Pachnis, 2016). Germ-free mice display deficits in gut motility due to their reduced number of enteric neurons. They also have defects in the numbers of enteric glial cells as well as in the excitability of primary afferent neurons in the enteric nervous system (Obata and Pachnis, 2016).

The gut-brain axis refers to the bidirectional biochemical signaling between the gastrointestinal tract, the enteric nervous system, and the central nervous system. The terms microbiota-gut-brain axis and diet-microbiota-gut-brain axis have also been introduced since experimental studies have pointed to the crucial role of diet and especially of the gut microbiota in these complex interactions. Studies in germ-free mice as compared with conventionally reared mice have demonstrated that these animals exhibit numerous changes in their central nervous systems, for example, increases in myelination of the prefrontal cortex, disturbed neurogenesis in the hippocampus, and a more permeable blood–brain barrier, and decreases in the concentration of brain-derived neural factor, in the expression of TJ proteins in blood–brain barrier and in the maturity of microglia (as reviewed by Cryan et al., 2019).

### 9.4.3.2 Microbiota acts on several mechanisms in the developing gut

Maturational signals of microbial colonization are transmitted partly through the pattern recognition receptors of the innate immune system. These receptors detect conserved microbial components termed microbe-associated molecular patterns which are found both in commensals and pathogens (Sellge and Kufer, 2015). Recognition of microbe-associated molecular patterns by neonatal intestinal epithelial cells is needed in order to stimulate the development of the isolated lymphoid follicles that support the maturation of B cells and the subsequent production of secretory immunoglobulin A, the most important immunoglobulin produced by the gut-associated lymphatic tissue. Early, controlled microbial contact with the host's immune system is also thought to facilitate the development of tolerance to non-pathogenic bacteria (Jain and Walker, 2015). In support of the role of this very early host-microbe crosstalk, the expression of Toll-like receptor 4, the receptor for the Gram-negative bacterial product LPS, is high in intestinal epithelial cells at birth, but after the initial microbial contact, its expression is rapidly down-regulated in order to prevent disruption of intestinal homeostasis due to uncontrolled inflammation (Lotz et al., 2006; Chassin et al., 2010).

Dendritic cells in lamina propria make contact with microbial antigens mainly through microfold cells, the specialized epithelial cells found in Peyer's patches in the small intestine and in isolated lymphoid follicles located in the large intestinal mucosa. These antigen-loaded dendritic cells can then induce the T-cell dependent B-cell maturation into immunoglobulin A-producing plasma cells or the maturation of naïve T cells into effector type 1T helper (Th1), type 2T helper (Th2), or Th17 cells or into FOXP3 + T regulatory cells. It is the balance of these proinflammatory and anti-inflammatory cells of the adaptive immune system in the gut-associated lymphatic tissue which seems to be crucial in ensuring immunological homeostasis. A Th1-, Th2-, and Th17-biased immune system has been shown to result in experimental colitis, allergy, and arthritis (Belkaid and Hand, 2014; Mowat, 2018). Different commensals have variable abilities to stimulate the intestinal immune system; their activity is thought to be dependent on their capability to colonize normally sterile sites such as intestinal crypts and the inner mucus layer of the large intestine. On that basis, commensal bacteria proven to have effects on the host's immune system have been classified either as inflammatory commensals (or pathobionts) or immunoregulatory commensals (or autobionts). These bacteria differ from pathogens by representing indigenous gut microbiota as well as from other commensals in their ability to proliferate after disruption of the intestinal homeostasis to stimulate specific immune responses (Palm et al., 2015). For example, an overgrowth of *Enterobacteriaceae* is frequently observed both in patients suffering an enteric infection and in those individuals with inflammatory bowel disease (Knights et al., 2014).

Aryl hydrocarbon receptor (AhR) is a transcription factor that has been shown to provide an important link between the intestinal immune system, diet, and gut microbiota, with this linkage being mediated by tryptophan metabolites (as reviewed in Gao et al., 2018). Two ligands capable of activating the AhR have been isolated from cruciferous vegetables, such as broccoli and cabbage. Moreover, the activation of the AhR by indoles, i.e., bacterial tryptophan metabolites, is needed for the normal postnatal development of lymphoid follicles and intraepithelial lymphocytes (Li et al., 2011; Kiss et al., 2011). Indole-3-aldehyde, an indole derived from tryptophan by bacterial enzymes, is a ligand of the AhR that increases intestinal epithelial integrity via the production of interleukin-22 (Zelante et al., 2013). Tryptophan, an essential amino acid found in various vegetables and fish, is converted to kynurenine by indoleamine 2,3-dioxygenase. Both kynurenine, an indolyl metabolite and a ligand of the AhR, and the enzyme indoleamine 2-3-dioxygenase contribute to the induction of T regulatory cells and immune tolerance (Munn and Mellor, 2013). Interestingly, an experimental study found that intestinal peristalsis was regulated by AhR signaling in enteric neurons (Obata et al., 2020). Moreover, the magnitude of the signaling correlated with the microbial load along the gut, i.e., the greater the microbial load, the more robust the signaling activation in neurons. These findings provide evidence that the AhR functions as a critical biosensor, both in intestinal homeostasis involving epithelial cells and immune cells, as well as in intestinal neuronal circuits, thus linking microbiota and diet closely to the immunological and neural properties of the gut.

## 9.5  Dietary potential to modify gut microbiota

Diet modulation is a compelling approach when attempting to modify the gut microbiota to improve an individual's health. Supplementation of diet with probiotics has a long tradition, and there has been extensive research into these interventions. Also prebiotics have been studied but to a lesser extent. A newer research approach has been to identify the microbiota modulating properties of different fats, mainly long-chain polyunsaturated fatty acids (LC-PUFA). One opportunity to modify gut microbiota is fecal microbiota transplantation (FMT).

### 9.5.1.1  Probiotics

Probiotics are defined as live microorganisms that, when administered in adequate amounts, confer a health benefit on the host (Rijkers et al., 2010). Since allergic disease, especially eczema, and necrotizing enterocolitis have been the two most common clinical conditions evaluated in the prospective probiotic intervention trials conducted so far, this chapter focuses on the preventive effect of probiotics on these diseases.

The first clinical study in the prevention of allergic disease by probiotics was published by our group in 2001 (Kalliomäki et al., 2001b). We recruited a total of 159 pregnant women who had a personal or family history of allergy, i.e., children or a husband with an allergic disease. The participants were randomized to receive either Lactobacillus rhamnosus GG or placebo for 2–4 weeks before delivery. After delivery, the preparation was given either to the infant or consumed by the breastfeeding mother for 6 months. The presence of eczema, either atopic (i.e., eczema associated with antigen-specific immunoglobulin E antibodies) or non-atopic (eczema without such antibodies) at the age of 2 years was the primary outcome of the study. The prevalence of eczema was reduced to half in the probiotic group as compared to children in the placebo group (23% vs 46%). However, there was no preventive impact on atopic sensitization as analyzed by skin prick tests and antigen-specific immunoglobulin E concentrations (Kalliomäki et al., 2001b).

Since then, numerous interventions with probiotics in the prevention of allergy have been carried out. These studies have been reviewed in depth (Wang et al., 2019); the overall conclusion is that probiotics seem to have some preventive effect, although it is moderate at best, in early eczema in high-risk children. However, no impact has been detected against the development of atopic sensitization, food allergy, allergic rhinitis, or asthma. The World Allergy Organization guideline panel suggested the provision of probiotics during pregnancy in women who had a high risk for having an allergic child. The panel suggested probiotic use also in breastfeeding mothers if their infants had a high risk for developing allergy as well as being provided to these high-risk infants (Fiocchi et al., 2015). The panel did not take a stand on which probiotics should be used and at which dose, since there has been extensive variability in these aspects between the trials. The panel stated further that the evidence so far is very low in quality, and several topics should be addressed more carefully in the future. In contrast to the World Allergy Organization, many other prominent medical authorities such as the American Academy of Pediatrics, the European Academy of Allergy and Clinical Immunology, the National Institute of Allergy and Infectious Disease, and the European Society for Pediatric Gastroenterology, Hepatology, and Nutrition do not recommend the use of probiotics for the primary prevention of any form of allergic disease (Wang et al., 2019).

Necrotizing enterocolitis is a multifactorial inflammatory disorder of the intestine that ultimately leads to necrosis of the affected intestine and death. Most of the patients are preterm infants, of which up to 15% may be affected. Necrotizing enterocolitis is a severe disease, with surgical intervention needed in approximately half of the cases, and despite that, the mortality rate may be as high as 15%–30%. Necrotizing enterocolitis is the most common cause of the short bowel syndrome in children, and it is also a risk factor for impairment in neurodevelopment later in childhood (Abrahamsson et al., 2014b). The first clinical studies demonstrating a preventive effect of probiotics in necrotizing enterocolitis date back to the beginning of this millennium (Dani et al., 2002; Costalos et al., 2003). Thereafter several randomized controlled trials with probiotics in preterm babies have been conducted, although necrotizing enterocolitis has not been the primary outcome in all of those studies. A meta-analysis combined data from 34 randomized clinical studies with more than 9000 preterm infants (Bi et al., 2019). According to this analysis, probiotic supplementation prevented necrotizing enterocolitis, gut-associated sepsis, and all-cause mortality in preterm infants. Moreover, a probiotic mixture was found to be more effective than single probiotic strains (Bi et al., 2019). However, it is not yet known whether the preventive effect can also be obtained in extremely low birth weight (less than 1000 g) infants in the subgroup of preterm babies with the highest incidence of necrotizing enterocolitis (AlFaleh and Anabrees, 2014). In contrast, the latest network meta-analysis (containing data of 45 trials with 12,320 participants) concluded that probiotic *Lactobacillus* or *Bifidobacterium* should be combined with a prebiotic in order to achieve the optimal effect on premature infant health (Chi et al., 2021). The third recommendation was given by the European Society for Pediatric Gastroenterology, Hepatology, and Nutrition (based on their own network meta-analysis) in which a conditional recommendation was issued to provide either *L. rhamnosus* GG ATC53103 or the combination of Bifidobacterium infantis Bb-02, Bifidobacterium lactis Bb-12, and Streptococcus thermophilus TH-4 to premature infants for the prevention of necrotizing enterocolitis (van den Akker et al., 2020). These partly incompatible recommendations demonstrate that there are still many mysteries swirling around this topic. Indeed there are still a great many unknowns, e.g., the optimal mixture of probiotic strains, doses, and timing of probiotic intervention. Safety issues both in the short term and long term are also a reason why there needs to be a careful evaluation before embarking on poorly designed trials in these most vulnerable infants. Therefore, large multicenter clinical trials with probiotics on the prevention of necrotizing enterocolitis in preterm babies are urgently needed to address these issues.

### 9.5.1.2 Mechanisms of action

Although the exact effects and fate of swallowed probiotics in the gastrointestinal tract are dependent on several factors (such as genetics and the microbiome of the host and probiotic dose and strains used) and are at least partly unknown, animal studies and trials with different types of immune cells in vitro have revealed numerous potential mechanisms of action by which probiotics may act in the body as illustrated in Fig. 9.2 (reviewed in Suez et al., 2019).

Probiotics can produce bacteriocins and other antibacterial proteins in the gut lumen, where they inhibit the colonization of pathogens and other harmful microbes (1 in Fig. 9.2; Martinez et al., 2015). Probiotics are able to impact cytokine signaling pathways in intestinal epithelial cells (2 in Fig. 9.2; Ganguli et al., 2013). They stimulate goblet cells to secrete mucin, and in that way, they can facilitate mucus production and promote the integrity of the intestinal barrier (3 in Fig. 9.2; Wang et al., 2014). In addition, they strengthen the intestinal epithelial barrier by inducing the production of intercellular TJ proteins (4 in Fig. 9.2; Zhao et al., 2015). Probiotics are further able to induce T cell activation through dendritic cells (5 in Fig. 9.2; Mollna et al., 2015) and also via the production of immunoglobulin A (6 in Fig. 9.2; Holscher et al., 2012). Moreover, they have an impact on intestinal motility mediated through enteral neural cells (7 in Fig. 9.2; Wang et al., 2010). In animal models, probiotics have also been shown to affect signaling to the central nervous system to induce anxiolytic, antidepressant, and nociceptive effects in the host (reviewed by Sarkar et al., 2016). However, human studies have so far failed to demonstrate these kinds of beneficial effects, for example, on stress, cognitive performance, or anxiety (Kelly et al., 2017; Reis et al., 2018).

## 9.5.2 Prebiotics

Another food ingredient that might benefit gut health and subsequently host health is prebiotic. In mid 1990s, prebiotic was first defined by Gibson and Roberfroid as "a non-digestible food ingredient that beneficially affect the host by selectively stimulating the growth and/or activity of one or a limited number of bacteria in the colon and thus improves the host health" (Gibson and Roberfroid, 1995). Since then, the definition was expanded to define prebiotic as "a substrate that is selectively utilized by host microorganisms conferring a health benefit" by the International Scientific Association of Probiotics and Prebiotics (ISAPP). Prebiotics, like inulin and oligofructose, are found in vegetables and fruits including onion, leek, and banana, as well as in grains including rye and wheat, the daily intake being few grams (Moshfegh et al., 1999). Prebiotics are also added to some food and infant formula, the typical substances being fructo-oligosaccharides and galactooligosaccharides.

The benefit of consuming prebiotics arise from their capacity to modify gut microbiota composition. For example, inulin-type fructans (short-chain FOS, oligofructose, and inulin) promote the abundance of *Bifidobacterium*, *Lactobacillus*, and *F. prausnitzii* (Hughes et al., 2021), the bacteria typically considered beneficial for health. Associated health benefits include increased insulin sensitivity and improved lipid profile as well as improvement in laxation (Hughes et al., 2021). The proposed mechanisms for prebiotic action relate to improvement in intestinal barrier function either through modulating gut microbiota composition or directly by regulation of TJ protein expression and distribution (Rose et al., 2021).

The clinical evidence in the studies administering prebiotic to adults or children are limited and reveal only some health benefits, as reviewed by the World Gastroenterology Organization (Guarner et al., 2017). A recent systematic review (De Silva et al., 2020) indicated a small decrease (12%) in the relative risk of food allergy in infants due to consumption of infant formula with prebiotics (oligosaccharides). However, the certainty of the evidence was considered very low (applying standardized GRADE statements). In the systematic review performed by the World Allergy Organization, the risk of asthma or recurrent wheezing was found to be reduced in infants who received prebiotics during the first year of life (Cuello-Garcia et al., 2016). Thus, the panel suggested using prebiotic supplementation in not-exclusively breastfed infants but not in exclusively breastfed infants, and highlighted very low certainty of the prevailing scientific evidence. Another systematic review identified 41 publications on the administration of prebiotic-supplemented infant formula compared with unsupplemented, and concluded that no safety concerns with regard to growth or adverse events were related to their use but the potential benefits related primarily to stool softening (Skórka et al., 2018). In preterm infants, the use of prebiotics may decrease the incidence of sepsis, mortality, and length of hospital stay (Chi et al., 2019).

While prebiotics have the capacity to modulate gut microbiota composition and the prevailing mechanisms exists to yield potential health benefits, the current clinical evidence from the randomized controlled trials is only modest. Some benefits may occur in the prevention of asthma and allergic rhinitis and in the management of preterms.

### 9.5.3 Fecal microbiota transplantation

A novel approach to modify the gut microbiota and treat diseases is FMT. FMT has been performed in patients with recurrent *Clostridioides difficile* diarrhea. In this technique, gut bacteria from a healthy donor is transferred into the gastrointestinal tract to re-establish the healthy bacteria, for example, of patients with severe *C. difficile* diarrhea, a spore-forming bacteria, in which the state of dysbiosis may induce diarrhea. FMT has been in experimental use in some other conditions, for example, ulcerative colitis and irritable bowel syndrome, although with variable results (Green et al., 2020). The use of FMT in other gut microbiota-related human pathological conditions, like obesity and metabolic syndrome, has mainly been investigated in experimental animals. However, one study has reported benefits of FMT in individuals with type 2 diabetes (Vrieze et al., 2012). In general, FMT is considered to be a safe procedure, when the donors are screened to ensure that they are healthy and the procedure follows the recommended practice (for further details see Carlson Jr, 2020).

### 9.5.4 Long-chain polyunsaturated fatty acids

LC-PUFA contribute to human health by multiple pathways. For example, n-3 fatty acids EPA and DHA are suggested to possess anti-inflammatory properties, and therefore their presence may help to combat those pathological conditions associated with inflammation. LC-PUFAs are important during pregnancy both for the development and health outcomes of the infant. Recently, the gut microbiota has been proposed as one link between dietary fat and metabolic effects in the host. Several mechanisms have been proposed to explain how dietary fat, gut microbiota, and host metabolism can interact (as reviewed in Mokkala et al., 2020). These include an increase in the levels of bile acids induced by a high-fat content, with a subsequently increased abundance of bile acid-tolerant bacteria. A high-fat diet may also increase the abundance of LPS containing bacteria and elevate the fecal content of LPS, some of which may be able to gain access to the systemic circulation.

Studies investigating the intake of fish oil, rich in EPA and DHA, in early childhood have detected alterations in gut microbiota composition, but this may be influenced by diet, for example, breastfeeding. Those children born to mothers who had consumed 150 g portions of farmed salmon per week from 20 weeks of pregnancy to delivery, had lower counts of Atobium cluster when compared to a control group. However, this was only seen in formula-fed children and not with exclusively breastfed infants (Urwin et al., 2014). In another study, the intake of fish oil, as compared to sunflower oil, increased the diversity of the gut microbiota and altered the bacterial groups in 18-month-old children, and as described in the earlier study, this change was only evident in children who had stopped breastfeeding before 9 months of age (Andersen et al., 2011).

## 9.6 Conclusions

Based on the vast amount of scientific literature, it is evident that the gut microbiota contributes to human physiology and health. While the microbiota in adults is relatively resilient to change, the infant's gut microbiota is prone to experience changes due to various environmental factors such as the composition of the diet. The evolving microbiota in the developing infant thus offers an opportunity for modification in terms of its composition in such a way that would be beneficial for human health, for example, promoting the healthy development of metabolism as well as the neural and immune systems.

## 9.7 Future trends and research needs

Despite active research in the field, the composition of gut microbiota and its relation to health are still rather poorly defined. More importantly, with regard to human health, the functional capacity that different microbes alone and together in the intestine may exert should be studied in detail. Functional metagenomics and metabolomics combined with other types of omics along with experimental studies aimed at clarifying the mechanisms behind these effects are sorely needed. If the goal is to establish novel dietary approaches for both the prevention and management of non-communicable diseases, then there is a crucial need for well-designed and executed randomized placebo-controlled intervention trials. In addition to traditional dietary interventions, these could include FMT and other gut microbiota related studies as long as strict safety practices are ensured. Finally, it is likely that longitudinal large clinical prospective cohort studies utilizing new techniques of data lakes and data mining would improve our understanding of the numerous ways that the intestinal microbiota can modify our health for better or worse.

## Sources of further information

Cryan, J.F., O'Riordan, K.J., Kowan, C.S.M., Sandhu, K.W., Bastiaanssen, T.F.S., Boehme, M., et al. 2019. The microbiota-gut-brain axis. Physiol. Rev. 99:1877–2013.
Power, S.E., O'Toole, P.W., Stanton, C., Ross, R.P., Fitzgerald, G.F. 2014.
Intestinal microbiota, diet and health. Br. J. Nutr. 111 (3), 387–402.
Suez, J., Zmora, N., Segal, E, Elinav, E., 2019. The pros, cons, and many unknowns of probiotics. Nature. Med. 25, 716–729.
Walker, A.W., Lawley, T.D. 2013. Therapeutic modulation of intestinal dysbiosis. Pharmacol. Res. 69 (1), 75–86.

# References

Abrahamsson, T.R., Jakobsson, H.E., Andersson, A.F., Björkstén, B., Engstrand, L., Jenmalm, M.C., 2014a. Low gut microbiota diversity in early infancy precedes asthma at school age. Clin. Exp. Allergy 44 (6), 842–850.

Abrahamsson, T.R., Rautava, S., Moore, A.M., Neu, J., Sherman, P.M., 2014b. The time for a confirmatory necrotizing enterocolitis probiotics prevention trial in extremely low birth weight infant in North America is now! J. Pediatr. 165 (2), 389–394.

Al-Attas, O.S., Al-Daghri, N.M., Al-Rubeaan, K., da Silva, N.F., Sabico, S.L., Kumar, S., et al., 2009. Changes in endo-toxin levels in T2DM subjects on anti-diabetic therapies. Cardiovasc. Diabetol. 8, 20.

AlFaleh, K., Anabrees, J., 2014. Probiotics for prevention of necrotizing enterocolitis in preterm infants. Cochrane Database Syst. Rev. 4, CD005496.

Andersen, A.D., Mølbak, L., Michaelsen, K.F., Lauritzen, L., 2011. Molecular fingerprints of the human fecal microbiota from 9 to 18 months old and the effect of fish oil supplementation. J. Pediatr. Gastroenterol. Nutr. 53 (3), 303–309.

Anderson, R.C., Cookson, A.L., McNabb, W.C., Kelly, W.J., Roy, N.C., 2010. Lactobacillus plantarum DSM 2648 is a potential probiotic that enhances intestinal barrier function. FEMS Microbiol. Lett. 309 (2), 184–192.

Ardissone, A.N., de la Cruz, D.M., Davis-Richardson, A.G., Rechcigl, K.T., Li, N., Drew, J.C., et al., 2014. Meconium microbiome analysis identifies bacteria correlated with premature birth. PLoS One 9 (3), e90784.

Avetisyan, M., Schill, E.M., Heuckeroth, R.O., 2015. Building a second brain in the bowel. J. Clin. Invest. 125 (3), 899–907.

Bäckhed, F., Ding, H., Wang, T., Hooper, L.V., Koh, G.Y., Nagy, A., et al., 2004. The gut microbiota as an environmental factor that regulates fat storage. Proc. Natl. Acad. Sci. U. S. A. 101 (44), 15718–15723.

Bäckhed, F., Manchester, J.K., Semenkovich, C.F., Gordon, J.I., 2007. Mechanisms underlying the resistance to diet-induced obesity in germ-free mice. Proc. Natl. Acad. Sci. U. S. A. 104 (3), 979–984.

Bäckhed, F., Roswall, J., Peng, Y., Feng, Q., Jia, H., Kovatcheva-Datchary, P., 2015. Dynamics and stabilization of the human gut microbiome during the first year of life. Cell Host Microbe 17 (5), 690–703.

Barker, D.J.P., 2007. The origins of the developmental origins theory. J. Intern. Med. 261, 412–417.

Battson, M.L., Lee, D.M., Weir, T.L., Gentile, C.L., 2018. The gut microbiota as a novel regulator of cardiovascular function and disease. J. Nutr. Biochem. 56, 1–15.

Belkaid, Y., Hand, T.W., 2014. Role of the microbiota in immunity and inflammation. Cell 157 (1), 121–141.

Bergström, A., Skov, T.H., Bahl, M.I., Roager, H.M., Christensen, L.B., Ejlerskov, K.T., et al., 2014. Establishment of intestinal microbiota during early life: a longitudinal, explorative study of a large cohort of Danish infants. Appl. Environ. Microbiol. 80 (9), 2889–2900.

Bi, L., Yan, B., Qang, Q., Li, M., Cui, H., 2019. Probiotic strategies to prevent necrotizing enterocolitis in preterm in-fants: a meta-analysis. Pediatr. Surg. Int. 35, 1143–1162.

Bisgaard, H., Li, N., Bonnelykke, K., Chawes, B.L., Skov, T., Paludan-Müller, G., Stokholm, J., et al., 2011. Reduced diversity of the intestinal microbiota during infancy is associated with increased risk of allergic disease at school age. J. Allergy Clin. Immunol. 128 (3), 646–652.

Björkstén, B., Sepp, E., Julge, K., Voor, T., Mikelsaar, M., 2001 Oct. Allergy development and the intestinal microflora during the first year of life. J. Allergy Clin. Immunol. 108 (4), 516–520.

Blaser, M.J., Devkota, S., McCoy, K.D., Relman, D.A., Yassour, M., Young, V.B., 2021. Lessons learned from the prena-tal microbiome controversy. Microbiome 9 (1), 8. https://doi.org/10.1186/s40168-020-00946-2.

Boroni Moreira, A.P., de Cássia Gonçalves Alfenas, R., 2012. The influence of endotoxemia on the molecular mecha-nisms of insulin resistance. Nutr. Hosp. 27, 382–390.

Braegger, C., Chmielewska, A., Decsi, T., Kolacek, S., Mihatsch, W., Moreno, L., et al., 2011. Supplementation of infant formula with probiotics and/or prebiotics: a systematic review and comment by the ESPGHAN committee on nutrition. J. Pediatr. Gastroenterol. Nutr. 52 (2), 238–250.

Cabrera-Rubio, R., Collado, M.C., Laitinen, K., Salminen, S., Isolauri, E., Mira, A., 2012. The human milk microbiome changes over lactation and is shaped by maternal weight and mode of delivery. Am. J. Clin. Nutr. 96 (3), 544–551.

Cani, P.D., Amar, J., Iglesias, M.A., et al., 2007. Metabolic endotoxemia initiates obesity and insulin resistance. Diabetes 56, 1761–1772.

Carlson Jr., P.E., 2020. Regulatory considerations for fecal microbiota transplantation products. Cell Host Microbe 27 (2), 173–175.

Carpino, G., Del Ben, M., Pastori, D., Carnevale, R., Baratta, F., Overi, D., et al., 2020. Increased liver localization of lipopolysaccharides in human and experimental NAFLD. Hepatology 72 (2), 470–485.

Chassin, C., Kocur, M., Pott, J., Duerr, C.U., Gütle, D., Lotz, M., et al., 2010. miR-146a mediates protective innate immune tolerance in the neonate intestine. Cell Host Microbe 8 (4), 358–368.

Cheng, J., Ringel-Kulka, T., Heikamp-de Jong, I., Ringel, Y., Carroll, I., de Vos, W.M., et al., 2016. Discordant temporal development of bacterial phyla and the emergence of core in the fecal microbiota of young children. ISME J. 4, 1002–1014.

Chi, C., Buys, N., Li, C., Sun, J., Yin, C., 2019. Effects of prebiotics on sepsis, necrotizing enterocolitis, mortality, feeding intolerance, time to full enteral feeding, length of hospital stay, and stool frequency in preterm infants: a meta-analysis. Eur. J. Clin. Nutr. 73, 657–670.

Chi, C., Li, C., Buys, N., Wang, W., Yin, C., Sun, J., 2021. Effects of probiotics in preterm infants: a network meta-analysis. Pediatrics 147 (1), e20200706.

Collado, M.C., Isolauri, E., Laitinen, K., Salminen, S., 2010. Effect of mother's weight on infant's microbiota acquisition, composition, and activity during early infancy: a prospective follow-up study initiated in early pregnancy. Am. J. Clin. Nutr. 92 (5), 1023–1030.

Costalos, C., Skouteri, V., Gounaris, A., Sevastiadou, S., Triandafilidou, A., Ekonomidou, C., et al., 2003. Enteral feeding of premature infants with *Saccharomyces boulardii*. Early Hum. Dev. 74 (2), 89–96.

Creely, S.J., McTernan, P.G., Kusminski, C.M., Fisher, M., Da Silva, N.F., Khanolkar, M., et al., 2007. Lipopolysaccharide activates an innate immune system response in human adipose tissue in obesity and type 2 diabetes. Am. J. Physiol. Endocrinol. Metab. 292, E740-7.

Crusell, M.K.W., Hansen, T.H., Nielsen, T., Allin, K.H., Rühlemann, M.C., Damm, P., et al., 2020. Comparative studies of the gut microbiota in the offspring of mothers with and without gestational diabetes. Front. Cell. Infect. Microbiol. 10. https://doi.org/10.3389/fcimb.2020.536282, 536282 (eCollection 2020).

Cryan, J.F., O'Riordan, K.J., Kowan, C.S.M., Sandhu, K.W., Bastiaanssen, T.F.S., Boehme, M., et al., 2019. The microbiota-gut-brain axis. Physiol. Rev. 99, 1877–2013.

Cuello-Garcia, C.A., Fiocchi, A., Pawankar, R., Yepes-Nuñez, J.J., Morgano, G.P., Zhang, Y., et al., 2016. World allergy organization-McMaster University guidelines for allergic disease prevention (GLAD-P): prebiotics. World Allergy Organ. J. 9 (10). https://doi.org/10.1186/s40413-016-0102-7.

Dani, C., Biadaioli, R., Bertini, G., Martelli, E., Rubaltelli, F.F., 2002. Probiotic feeding in prevention of urinary tract infection, bacterial sepsis and necrotizing enterocolitis in preterm infants. A prospective double-blind study. Biol. Neonate 82 (2), 103–108.

De Filippo, C., Cavalieri, D., Di Paola, M., Ramazzotti, M., Poullet, J.B., Massart, S., et al., 2010. Impact of diet in shaping gut microbiota revealed by a comparative study in children from Europe and rural Africa. Proc. Natl. Acad. Sci. U. S. A. 107 (33), 14691–16696.

De Filippo, C., Di Paola, M., Ramazzotti, M., Albanese, D., Pieraccini, G., Banci, E., et al., 2017. Diet, environments, and gut microbiota. A preliminary investigation in children living in rural and urban Burkina Faso and Italy. Front. Microbiol. 8, 1979.

de Silva, D., Halken, S., Singh, C., Muraro, A., Angier, E., Arasi, S., et al., European Academy of Allergy, Clinical Immunology Food Allergy, Anaphylaxis Guidelines Group, 2020. Preventing food allergy in infancy and childhood: systematic review of randomised controlled trials. Pediatr. Allergy Immunol. 31 (7), 813–826.

DiGiulio, D.B., Callahan, B., McMurdie, J., Costello, P.J., Lyell, E.K., Robaczewska, D.J., et al., 2015. Temporal and spatial variation of the human microbiota during pregnancy. Proc. Natl. Acad. Sci. U. S. A. 112 (35), 11060–11065.

Dominguez-Bello, M.G., Costello, E.K., Contreras, M., Magris, M., Hidalgo, G., Fierer, N., et al., 2010. Delivery mode shapes the acquisition and structure of the initial microbiota across multiple body habitats in newborns. Proc. Natl. Acad. Sci. U. S. A. 107 (26), 11971–11975.

Duncan, S.H., Lobley, G.E., Holtrop, G., Ince, J., Johnstone, A.M., Louis, P., et al., 2008. Human colonic microbiota associated with diet, obesity and weight loss. Int. J. Obes. 32 (11), 1720–1724.

Elamin, E.E., Masclee, A.A., Dekker, J., Jonkers, D.M., 2013. Ethanol metabolism and its effects on the intestinal epithelial barrier. Nutr. Rev. 71, 483–499.

Fallani, M., Amarri, S., Uusijarvi, A., Adam, R., Khanna, S., Aguilera, M., et al., 2011. Determinants of the human infant intestinal microbiota after the introduction of first complementary foods in infant samples from five European centres. Microbiology 157 (Pt 5), 1385–1392.

Farré, R., Fiorani, M., Abdu Rahiman, S., Matteoli, G., 2020. Intestinal permeability, inflammation and the role of nutrients. Nutrients 12 (4), 1185.

Ferretti, P., Pasolli, E., Tett, A., Asnicar, F., Gorfer, V., Fedi, S., et al., 2018. Mother-to-infant microbial transmission from different body sites shapes the developing infant gut microbiome. Cell Host Microbe 24 (1), 133–145.

Fiocchi, A., Pawankar, R., Cuello-Garcia, C., Ahn, K., Al-Hammadi, S., Agarwal, A., et al., 2015. World allergy organization-cMaster guidelines for allergy disease prevention (GLAD-P): probiotics. World Allergy Organ. J. 8 (1), 4.

Ganguli, K., Meng, D., Rautava, S., Lu, L., Walker, W.A., Nanthakumar, N., 2013. Probiotics prevent necrotizing enterocolitis by modulating enterocyte genes that regulate innate immune-mediated inflammation. Am. J. Physiol. Gastrointest. Liver Physiol. 304 (2), G132–G141.

Gao, J., Xu, K., Liu, H., Liu, G., Bai, M., Peng, C., et al., 2018. Impact of the gut microbiota on intestinal immunity mediated by tryptophan metabolism. Front. Cell. Infect. Microbiol. 8, 13.

Gibson, M.K., Crofts, T.S., Dantas, G., 2015. Antibiotics and the developing infant gut microbiota and resistome. Curr. Opin. Microbiol. 31 (27), 51–56.

Gibson, G.R., Roberfroid, M.B., 1995. Dietary modulation of the human colonie microbiota: introducing the concept of prebiotics. J. Nutr. 125, 1401–1412.

Gomes, J.M.G., Costa, J.A., Alfenas, R.C.G., 2016. Metabolic endotoxemia and diabetes mellitus: a systematic review. Metabolism 68, 133–144.

Goodrich, J.K., Waters, J.L., Poole, A.C., Sutter, J.L., Koren, O., Blekhman, R., et al., 2014. Human genetics shape the gut microbiome. Cell 159 (4), 789–799.

Graf, D., Di Cagno, R., Fåk, F., Flint, H.J., Nyman, M., Saarela, M., et al., 2015. Contribution of diet to the composition of the human gut microbiota. Microb. Ecol. Health Dis. 4 (26), 26164.

Green, J.E., Davis, J.A., Berk, M., Hair, C., Loughman, A., Castle, D., et al., 2020. Efficacy and safety of fecal microbiota transplantation for the treatment of diseases other than *Clostridium difficile* infection: a systematic review and meta-analysis. Gut Microbes 12 (1), 1–25.

Grześkowiak, Ł., Collado, M.C., Mangani, C., Maleta, K., Laitinen, K., Ashorn, P., et al., 2012. Distinct gut microbiota in southeastern African and northern European infants. J. Pediatr. Gastroenterol. Nutr. 54 (6), 812–816.

Guarner, F., Sanders, M.E., Eliakim, R., Fedorak, R., Gangl, A., Garisch, J., et al., 2017. World Gastroenterology Organization Global Guidelines: Probiotics and Prebiotics. World Gastroenterology Organization. https://www.worldgastroenterology.org/guidelines/global-guidelines/probiotics-and-prebiotics/probiotics-and-prebiotics-english. (Accessed 15 October 2021).

Gueimonde, M., Laitinen, K., Salminen, S., Isolauri, E., 2007. Breast milk: a source of bifidobacteria for infant gut development and maturation? Neonatology 92 (1), 64–66.

Hasain, Z., Mokhtar, N.M., Kamaruddin, N.A., Mohamed Ismail, N.A., Razalli, N.H., Gnanou, J.V., et al., 2020. Gut microbiota and gestational diabetes mellitus: a review of host-gut microbiota interactions and their therapeutic potential. Front. Cell. Infect. Microbiol. 10, 188.

Helve, O., Dikareva, E., Stefanovic, V., Kolho, K.-L., Salonen, A., de Vos, W.M., Andersson, S., 2021. Protocol for oral transplantation of maternal fecal microbiota to newborn infants born by cesarean section. STAR Protoc. 2 (1), 100271.

Holscher, H.D., Czerkies, L.A., Cekola, P., Litov, R., Benbow, M., Santema, S., et al., 2012. Bifidobacterium lactis Bb12 enhances intestinal antibody response in formula-fed infants: a randomized, double-blind, placebo-controlled trial. J. Parenter. Enter. Nutr. 36 (1 Suppl), 106S–117S.

Houttu, N., Mokkala, K., Laitinen, K., 2018. Overweight and obesity status in pregnant women are related to intestinal microbiota and serum metabolic and inflammatory profiles. Clin. Nutr. 37 (6 Pt A), 1955–1966.

Huang, R., Ju, Z., Zhou, P.K., 2020. A gut dysbiotic microbiota-based hypothesis of human-to-human transmission of non-communicable diseases. Sci. Total Environ. 745, 141030.

Hughes, R.L., Alvarado, D.A., Swanson, K.S., Holscher, H.D., 2021. The prebiotic potential of inulin-type fructans: a systematic review. Adv. Nutr. https://doi.org/10.1093/advances/nmab119, nmab119.

Ignacio, A., Fernandes, M.R., Rodrigues, V.A., Groppo, F.C., Cardoso, A.L., Avila-Campos, M.J., et al., 2016. Correlation between body mass index and faecal microbiota from children. Clin. Microbiol. Infect. (3). 258.e1-8.

Indiani, C.M.D.S.P., Rizzardi, K.F., Castelo, P.M., Ferraz, L.F.C., Darrieux, M., Parisotto, T.M., 2018. Childhood obesity and firmicutes/bacteroidetes ratio in the gut microbiota: a systematic review. Child. Obes. 14 (8), 501–509.

Jain, N., Walker, W.A., 2015. Diet and host-microbial crosstalk in postnatal intestinal immune homeostasis. Diet and host-microbial crosstalk in postnatal intestinal immune homeostasis. Nat. Rev. Gastroenterol. Hepatol. 12 (1), 14–25.

Jayashree, B., Bibin, Y.S., Prabhu, D., Shanthirani, C.S., Gokulakrishnan, K., Lakshmi, B.S., et al., 2014. Increased circulatory levels of lipopolysaccharide (LPS) and zonulin signify novel biomarkers of proinflammation in patients with type 2 diabetes. Mol. Cell. Biochem. 388, 203–210.

Johansson, M.A., Sjögren, Y.M., Persson, J.O., Nilsson, C., Sverremark-Ekström, E., 2011. Early colonization with a group of lactobacilli decreases the risk for allergy at five years of age despite allergic heredity. PLoS One 6 (8), e23031.

Jumpertz, R., Le, D.S., Turnbaugh, P.J., Trinidad, C., Bogardus, C., Gordon, J.I., et al., 2011. Energy-balance studies reveal associations between gut microbes, caloric load, and nutrient absorption in humans. Am. J. Clin. Nutr. 94 (1), 58–65.

Kalach, N., Rocchiccioli, F., de Boissieu, D., Benhamou, P.H., Dupont, C., 2001. Intestinal permeability in children: variation with age and reliability in the diagnosis of cow's milk allergy. Acta Paediatr. 90 (5), 499–504.

Kallio, K.A., Hätönen, K.A., Lehto, M., Salomaa, V., Männistö, S., Pussinen, P.J., et al., 2015. Endotoxemia, nutrition, and cardiometabolic disorders. Acta Diabetol. 52, 395–404.

Kalliomäki, M., Collado, MC., Salminen, S., Isolauri, E., 2008. Early differences in fecal microbiota composition in children may predict overweight. Am. J. Clin. Nutr. 87 (3), 534–538.

Kalliomäki, M., Kirjavainen, P., Eerola, E., Kero, P., Salminen, S., Isolauri, E., 2001a. Distinct patterns of neonatal gut microflora in infants in whom atopy was and was not developing. J. Allergy Clin. Immunol. 107 (1), 129–134.

Kalliomäki, M., Salminen, S., Arvilommi, H., Kero, P., Koskinen, P., Isolauri, E., 2001b. Probiotics in primary prevention of atopic disease: a randomised placebo-controlled trial. Lancet 357 (9262), 1076–1079.

Kelly, J.R., Allen, A.P., Temko, A., Hutch, W., Kennedy, P.J., Farid, N., et al., 2017. Lost in translation? The potential psychobiotic Lactobacillus rhamnosus (JB-1) fails to modulate stress or cognitive performance in healthy male subjects. Brain Behav. Immun. 61, 50–59.

Kiss, E.A., Vonarbourg, C., Kopfmann, S., Hobeika, E., Finke, D., Esser, C., et al., 2011. Natural aryl hydrocarbon receptor ligands control organogenesis of intestinal lymphoid follicles. Science 334 (6062), 1561–1565.

Kleessen, B., Bunke, H., Tovar, K., Noack, J., Sawatzki, G., 1995. Influence of two infant formulas and human milk on the development of the faecal flora in newborn infants. Acta Paediatr. 84 (12), 1347–1356.

Knights, D., Silverberg, M.S., Weersma, R.K., Gevers, D., Dijkstra, G., Huang, H., et al., 2014. Complex host genetics influence the microbiome in inflammatory bowel disease. Genome Med. 6 (12), 107.

Koren, O., Goodrich, J.K., Cullender, T.C., Spor, A., Laitinen, K., Bäckhed, H.K., et al., 2012. Host remodeling of the gut microbiome and metabolic changes during pregnancy. Cell 150 (3), 470–480.

Korpela, K., Helve, O., Kolho, K.L., Saisto, T., Skogberg, K., Dikareva, E., et al., 2020. Maternal fecal microbiota transplantation in infants born by cesarean section rapidly restores normal gut microbial development – a proof of concept study. Cell 183, 1–11.

Laitinen, K., Mokkala, K., 2019. Overall dietary quality relates to gut microbiota diversity and abundance. Int. J. Mol. Sci. 20 (8), 1835.

Le Chatelier, E., Nielsen, T., Qin, J., Prifti, E., Hildebrand, F., Falony, G., 2013. Richness of human gut microbiome correlates with metabolic markers. Nature 500 (7464), 541–546.

Ley, R.E., Turnbaugh, P.J., Klein, S., Gordon, J.I., 2006. Microbial ecology: human gut microbes associated with obesity. Nature 444 (7122), 1022–1023.

Li, Q., Zhang, Q., Wang, M., Zhao, S., Xu, G., Li, J., 2008. N-3 polyunsaturated fatty acids prevent disruption of epithelial barrier function induced by proinflammatory cytokines. Mol. Immunol. 45 (5), 1356–1365.

Li, Y., Innocentin, S., Withers, D.R., Roberts, N.A., Gallagher, A.R., Grigorieva, E.F., 2011. Exogenous stimuli maintain intraepithelial lymphocytes via aryl hydrocarbon receptor activation. Cell 147 (3), 629–640.

Liu, R., Hong, J., Xu, X., Feng, Q., Zhang, D., Gu, Y., et al., 2017. Gut microbiome and serum metabolome alterations in obesity and after weight-loss intervention. Nat. Med. 23 (7), 859–868.

Lotz, M., Gütle, D., Walther, S., Ménard, S., Bogdan, C., Hornef, M.W., 2006. Postnatal acquisition of endotoxin tolerance in intestinal epithelial cells. J. Exp. Med. 203 (4), 973–984.

Lyons, K.E., Ryan, A., Dempsey, E.M., Ross, R.P., Stanton, C., 2020. Breast milk, a source of beneficial microbes and associated benefits for infant health. Nutrients 12 (4), 1039.

Maher, S.E., O'Brien, E.C., Moore, R.L., Byrne, D.F., Geraghty, A.A., Saldova, R., et al., 2020. The association between the maternal diet and the maternal and infant gut microbiome: a systematic review. Br. J. Nutr., 1–29.

Martinez, F.A., Dominguez, J.M., Converti, A., de Souza Oliveira, R.P., 2015. Production of bacteriocidin-like inhibitory substance by Bifidobacterium lactis in skim milk supplemented with additivies. J. Dairy Res. 82 (3), 350–355.

Mokkala, K., Houttu, N., Cansev, T., Laitinen, K., 2020. Interactions of dietary fat with the gut microbiota: evaluation of mechanisms and metabolic consequences. Clin. Nutr. 39 (4), 994–1018.

Mokkala, K., Paulin, N., Houttu, N., Koivuniemi, E., Pellonperä, O., Khan, S., et al., 2021. Metagenomics analysis of gut microbiota in response to diet intervention and gestational diabetes in overweight and obese women: a randomised, double-blind, placebo-controlled clinical trial. Gut 70 (2), 309–318.

Mollna, M.A., Diaz, A.M., Hesse, C., Ginter, W., Gentilini, M.W., Nuñez, G.G., et al., 2015. Immunostimulatory effects triggered by enterococcus faecalis CECT 7121 probiotic strain involve activation of dendritic cells and interferon-gamma production. PLoS One 10 (5), e0127262.

Moossavi, S., Azad, M.B., 2020. Origins of human milk microbiota: new evidence and arising questions. Gut Microbes 12 (1), 1667722.

Moreira, A.P., Texeira, T.F., Ferreira, A.B., Peluzio Mdo, C., Alfenas Rde, C., 2012. Influence of a high-fat diet on gut microbiota, intestinal permeability and metabolic endotoxaemia. Br. J. Nutr. 108 (5), 801–819.

Moshfegh, A.J., Friday, J.E., Goldman, J.P., Ahuja, J.K., 1999. Presence of inulin and oligofructose in the diets of Americans. J. Nutr. 129 (7 Suppl), 1407S–1411S.

Mowat, A.M., 2018. To respond or not to respond – a personal perspective of intestinal tolerance. Nat. Rev. Immunol. 18, 405–415.

Munn, D.H., Mellor, A.L., 2013. Indoleamine 2,3 dioxygenase and metabolic control of immune responses. Trends Immunol. 34 (3), 137–143.

Murphy, K., O'Shea, C.A., Ryan, C.A., Dempsey, E.M., O'Toole, P.W., Stanton, C., et al., 2015. The gut microbiota composition in dichorionic triplet sets suggests a role for host genetic factors. PLoS One 10 (4), e0122561.

Nermes, M., Niinivirta, K., Nylund, L., Laitinen, K., Matomäki, J., Salminen, S., et al., 2013. Perinatal pet exposure, faecal microbiota, and wheezy bronchitis: is there a connection? ISRN Allergy 2013, 827934.

Netea, S.A., Messina, N.C., Curtis, N., 2019. Early-life antibiotic exposure and childhood food allergy: a systematic review. J. Allergy Clin. Immunol. 144 (5), 1445–1448.

Nylund, L., Satokari, R., Nikkilä, J., Rajilić-Stojanović, M., Kalliomäki, M., Isolauri, E., Salminen, S., de Vos, W.M., 2013. Microarray analysis reveals marked intestinal microbiota aberrancy in infants having eczema compared to healthy children in at-risk for atopic disease. BMC Microbiol. 13, 12.

Nylund, L., Nermes, M., Isolauri, E., Salminen, S., de Vos, W.M., Satokari, R., 2015. Sverity of atopic disease inversely correlates with intestinal microbiota diversity and butyrate-producing bacteria. Allergy 70 (2), 241–244.

Obata, Y., Pachnis, V., 2016. The effect of microbiota and immune system on the development and organization of the enteric nervous system. Gastroenterology 151 (5), 836–844.

Obata, Y., Castano, A., Boeing, S., Bon-Frauches, A.C., Fung, C., Fallesen, T., et al., 2020. Regular programming by microbiota regulates intestinal physiology. Nature 578 (7794), 284–289.

Palm, N.W., de Zoete, M.R., Flavell, R.A., 2015. Immune-microbiota interactions in health and disease. Clin. Immunol. 159 (2), 122–127.

Peelen, M.J., Luef, B.M., Lamont, R.F., de Milliano, I., Jensen, J.S., Limpens, J., et al., PREBIC Biomarker Working Group 2014–2018, 2019. The influence of the vaginal microbiota on preterm birth: a systematic review and recommendations for a minimum dataset for future research. Placenta 79, 30–39.

Peters, B.A., Shapiro, J.A., Church, T.R., Miller, G., Trinh-Shevrin, C., Yuen, E., et al., 2018. A taxonomic signature of obesity in a large study of American adults. Sci. Rep. 8 (1), 9749.

Power, S.E., O'Toole, P.W., Stanton, C., Ross, R.P., Fitzgerald, G.F., 2014. Intestinal microbiota, diet and health. Br. J. Nutr. 111 (3), 387–402.

Putaala, H., Salusjärvi, T., Nordström, M., Saarinen, M., Ouwehand, A.C., Bech Hansen, E., et al., 2008. Effect of four probiotic strains and Escherichia coli O157:H7 on tight junction integrity and cyclo-oxygenase expression. Res. Microbiol. 159 (9–10), 692–698.

Qin, J., Li, R., Raes, J., Arumugam, M., Burgdorf, K.S., Manichanh, C., et al., 2010. A human gut microbial gene catalogue established by metagenomic sequencing. Nature 464 (7285), 59–65.

Rajilić-Stojanović, M., de Vos, W.M., 2014. The first 1000 cultured species of the human gastrointestinal microbiota. FEMS Microbiol. Rev. 38 (5), 996–1047.

Rasmussen, S.H., Shrestha, S., Bjerregaard, L.G., Ängquist, L.H., Baker, J.L., Jess, T., et al., 2018. Antibiotic exposure in early life and childhood overweight and obesity: a systematic review and meta-analysis. Diabetes Obes. Metab. 20, 1508–1514.

Reis, D.J., Ilardi, S.S., Punt, S.E.W., 2018. The anxiolytic effect of probiotics: a systematic review and meta-analysis of the clinical and preclinical literature. PLoS One 13, e0199041.

Rijkers, G.T., Bengmark, S., Enck, P., Haller, D., Herz, U., Kalliomäki, M., et al., 2010. Guidance for substantiating the evidence for beneficial effects of probiotics: current current status and recommendations for future research. J. Nutr. 140 (3), 671S–676S.

Robinson, A., Fiechtner, L., Roche, B., Ajami, N.J., Petrosino, J.F., Camargo Jr., C.A., 2017. Association of maternal gestational weight gain with the infant fecal microbiota. J. Pediatr. Gastroenterol. Nutr. 65 (5), 509–515.

Rose, E.C., Odle, J., Blikslager, A.T., Ziegler, A.L., 2021. Probiotics, prebiotics and epithelial tight junctions: a promising approach to modulate intestinal barrier function. Int. J. Mol. Sci. 22 (13), 6729.

Rothschild, D., Weissbrod, O., Barkan, E., Kurilshikov, A., Korem, T., Zeevi, D., et al., 2018. Environment dominates over host genetics in shaping human gut microbiota. Nature 555, 210–215.

Round, J.L., Mazmanian, S.K., 2009. The gut microbiota shapes intestinal immune responses during health and disease. Nat. Rev. Immunol. 9 (5), 313–323.

Samuel, B.S., Shaito, A., Motoike, T., Rey, F.E., Backhed, F., Manchester, J.K., et al., 2008. Effects of the gut microbiota on host adiposity are modulated by the short-chain fatty-acid binding G protein-coupled receptor, Gpr41. Proc. Natl. Acad. Sci. U. S. A. 105 (43), 16767–16772.

Santacruz, A., Collado, M.C., García-Valdés, L., Segura, M.T., Martín-Lagos, J.A., Anjos, T., et al., 2010. Gut microbiota composition is associated with body weight, weight gain and biochemical parameters in pregnant women. Br. J. Nutr. 104 (1), 83–92.

Sanz, Y., 2010. Effects of a gluten-free diet on gut microbiota and immune function in healthy adult humans. Gut Microbes 1 (3), 135–137.

Sarkar, A., Lehto, S.M., Harty, S., Dinan, T.G., Cryan, J.F., Burnet, P.W.J., 2016. Psychobiotics and the manipulation of bacteria-gut-brain signals. Trends Neurosci. 39 (11), 763–781.

Scheepers, L.E., Penders, J., Mbakwa, C.A., Thijs, C., Mommers, M., Arts, I.C., 2015. The intestinal microbiota composition and weight development in children: the KOALA birth cohort study. Int. J. Obes. 39 (1), 16–25.

Sellge, G., Kufer, T.A., 2015. PRR-signaling pathways: learning from microbial tactics. Semin. Immunol. 27 (2), 75–84.

Sender, R., Fuchs, S., Milo, R., 2016. Are we really vastly outnumbered? Revisiting the ratio of bacterial to host cells in humans. Cell 164 (3), 337–340. https://doi.org/10.1016/j.cell.2016.01.013. 26824647.

Shortt, C., Hasselwander, O., Meynier, A., Nauta, A., Fernández, E.N., Putz, P., et al., 2018. Systematic review of the effects of the intestinal microbiota on selected nutrients and non-nutrients. Eur. J. Nutr. 57 (1), 25–49.

Skórka, A., Pieścik-Lech, M., Kołodziej, M., Szajewska, H., 2018. Infant formulae supplemented with prebiotics: are they better than unsupplemented formulae? An updated systematic review. Br. J. Nutr. 119 (7), 810–825.

Soderborg, T.K., Carpenter, C.M., Janssen, R.C., Weir, T.L., Robertson, C.E., Ir, D., et al., 2020. Gestational diabetes is uniquely associated with altered early seeding of the infant gut microbiota. Front. Endocrinol. 11, 603021.

Stanislawski, M.A., Dabelea, D., Wagner, B.D., Iszatt, N., Dahl, C., Sontag, M.K., et al., 2018. Gut microbiota in the first 2 years of life and the association with body mass index at age 12 in a Norwegian birth cohort. MBio 9 (5), e01751-18.

Suez, J., Zmora, N., Segal, E., Elinav, E., 2019. The pros, cons, and many unknowns of probiotics. Nat. Med. 25, 716–729.

Suzuki, T., 2013. Regulation of intestinal epithelial permeability by tight junction. Cell. Mol. Life Sci. 70 (4), 631–659.

Teixeira, T., Grześkowiak, L.M., Salminen, S., Laitinen, K., Bressan, J., Gouveia Peluzio Mdo, C., 2013. Faecal levels of Bifidobacterium and Clostridium coccoides but not plasma lipopolysaccharide are inversely related to insulin and HOMA index in women. Clin. Nutr. 32 (6), 1017–1022.

Thompson, A.L., Monteagudo-Mera, A., Cadenas, M.B., Lampl, M.L., Azcarate-Peril, M.A., 2015. Milk- and solid-feeding practices and daycare attendance are associated with differences in bacterial diversity, predominant communities, and metabolic and immune function of the infant gut microbiome. Front. Cell. Infect. Microbiol. 5, 3.

Tims, S., Derom, C., Jonkers, D.M., Vlietinck, R., Saris, W.H., Kleerebezem, M., et al., 2013. Microbiota conservation and BMI signatures in adult monozygotic twins. ISME J. 7 (4), 707–717.

Togo, A., Dufour, J.-C., Lagier, J.-C., Dubourg, G., Raoult, D., Million, M., 2019. Repertoire of human breast and milk microbiota: a systematic review. Future Microbiol. 14, 623–641.

Trefflich, I., Jabakhanji, A., Menzel, J., Blaut, M., Michalsen, A., Lampen, A., 2020. Is a vegan or a vegetarian diet associated with the microbiota composition in the gut? Results of a new cross-sectional study and systematic review. Crit. Rev. Food Sci. Nutr. 60 (17), 2990–3004.

Turnbaugh, P.J., Hamady, M., Yatsunenko, T., Cantarel, B.L., Duncan, A., Le, R.E., et al., 2009. A core gut microbiome in obese and lean twins. Nature 457 (7228), 480–484.

Turner, J., 2009. Intestinal mucosal barrier function in health and disease 2009. Nat. Rev. Immunol. 9 (11), 799–809.

Ulluwishewa, D., Anderson, R.C., McNabb, W.C., Moughan, P.J., Wells, J.M., Roy, N.C., 2011. Regulation of tight junction permeability by intestinal bacteria and dietary components. J. Nutr. 141 (5), 769–776.

Urwin, H.J., Miles, E.A., Noakes, P.S., Kremmyda, L.S., Vlachava, M., Diaper, N.D., et al., 2014. Effect of salmon consumption during pregnancy on maternal and infant faecal microbiota, secretory IgA and calprotectin. Br. J. Nutr. 111 (5), 773–784.

I. Nutrition in early life: Mechanisms and impact on long term health

Vael, C., Verhulst, S.L., Nelen, V., Goossens, H., Desager, K.N., 2011. Intestinal microflora and body mass index during the first three years of life: an observational study. Gut Pathog. 3 (1), 8.

Vähämiko, S., Laiho, A., Lund, R., Isolauri, E., Salminen, S., Laitinen, K., 2019. The impact of probiotic supplementation during pregnancy on DNA methylation of obesity-related genes in mothers and their children. Eur. J. Nutr. 58 (1), 367–377.

van den Akker, C.H.P., van Goudoever, J.B., Shamir, R., Domellöf, M., Embleton, N.D., Hojsak, I., et al., 2020. Probiotics and preterm infants: a position paper by the ESPGHAN committee on nutrition and the ESPGHAN working group for probiotics and prebiotics. J. Pediatr. Gastroenterol. Nutr. 70 (5), 664–680.

Vrieze, A., Van Nood, E., Holleman, F., Salojärvi, J., Kootte, R.S., Bartelsman, J.F., et al., 2012. Transfer of intestinal microbiota from lean donors increases insulin sensitivity in individuals with metabolic syndrome. Gastroenterology 143 (4), 913–916.e7.

Walker, A.W., Lawley, T.D., 2013. Therapeutic modulation of intestinal dysbiosis. Pharmacol. Res. 69 (1), 75–86.

Wang, M., Karlsson, C., Olsson, C., Adlerberth, I., Wold, A.E., Strachan, D.P., 2008. Reduced diversity in the early fecal microbiota of infants with atopic eczema. J. Allergy Clin. Immunol. 121 (1), 129–134.

Wang, B., Mao, Y.K., Diorio, C., Pasyk, M., Wu, R.Y., Bienenstock, J., et al., 2010. Luminal administration ex vivo of a live Lactobacillus species moderates mouse jejunal motility within minutes. FASEB J. 24 (10), 4078–4088.

Wang, L., Cao, H., Liu, L., Wang, B., Walker, W.A., Agra, S.A., et al., 2014. Activation of epidermal growth factor receptor mediates mucin production stimulated by p40, a Lactobacillus rhamnosus GG-derived protein. J. Biol. Chem. 289 (29), 20234–20244.

Wang, J., Zheng, J., Shi, W., Du, N., Xu, X., Zhang, Y., et al., 2018. Dysbiosis of maternal and neonatal microbiota associated with gestational diabetes mellitus. Gut 67 (9), 1614–1625.

Wang, H.T., Anvari, S., Anagnostou, K., 2019. The role of probiotics in preventing allergic disease. Child. Aust. 6, 24.

Wu, G.D., Chen, J., Hoffmann, C., Bittinger, K., Chen, Y.-Y., et al., 2011. Linking long-term dietary patterns with gut microbial enterotypes. Science 334 (6052), 105–108.

Yatsunenko, T., Rey, F.E., Manary, M.J., Trehan, I., Dominguez-Bello, M.G., Contreras, M., et al., 2012. Human gut microbiome viewed across age and geography. Nature 486 (7402), 222–227.

Zelante, T., Iannitti, R.G., Cunha, C., De Luca, A., Giovannini, G., Pieraccini, G., et al., 2013. Tryptophan catabolites from microbiota engage aryl hydrocarbon receptor and balance mucosal reactivity via interleukin-22. Immunity 39 (2), 372–385.

Zhang, H., DiBaise, J.K., Zuccolo, A., Kudrna, D., Braidotti, M., Yu, Y., 2009. Human gut microbiota in obesity and after gastric bypass. Proc. Natl. Acad. Sci. U. S. A. 106 (7), 2365–2370.

Zhao, H., Zhao, C., Dong, Y., Zhang, M., Wang, Y., Li, F., et al., 2015. Inhibition of miR122a by Lactobacillus rhamnosus GG supernatant increases intestinal occludin expression and protects mice from alcoholic liver disease. Toxicol. Lett. 234 (3), 194–200.

Zimmermann, P., Curtis, N., 2019. The effect of antibiotics on the composition of the intestinal microbiota – a systematic review. J. Inf. Secur. 79 (6), 471–489.

# 10

# Linking nutrition to long-term health: Epigenetic mechanisms

*Mark A. Burton[a], Keith M. Godfrey[b,c], and Karen A. Lillycrop[d]*

[a]School of Human Development and Health, Faculty of Medicine, University of Southampton, Southampton, United Kingdom [b]NIHR Southampton Biomedical Research Centre, University of Southampton and University Hospital Southampton NHS Foundation Trust, Southampton, United Kingdom [c]MRC Lifecourse Epidemiology Centre, University of Southampton, Southampton, United Kingdom [d]Biological Sciences, University of Southampton, Southampton, United Kingdom

## LEARNING OBJECTIVES

- Evaluate the impact of early life nutrition on later health outcomes.

- Describe epigenetic processes and how they regulate gene expression.

- Outline the evidence that nutrition affects later health through modulation of the epigenome.

- Describe how altered epigenetic marks may be used as predictive biomarkers.

## 10.1 Introduction

Non-communicable diseases (NCD) that include obesity, type-2 diabetes (T2D), and cardiovascular disease (CVD) are increasingly prevalent in both high and low-middle income countries, with mortality projected to rise along with economic and social development (Mathers and Loncar, 2006). Such burgeoning rates of NCDs cannot simply be accounted for by genetic factors; rather, the rapid rise in NCDs suggests that environmental factors such as modified nutritional intakes may play critical roles in mediating the increasing rates of NCDs. There is now substantial evidence from both human and animal experimental studies that demonstrate that early life environment, particularly nutrition during key developmental windows, can modulate growth and developmental trajectories, including the programming of far-reaching effects on the risk of developing NCDs during later life (Chen et al., 2016; Godfrey and Barker, 2001; Fleming et al., 2018).

The mechanisms by which early-life environment can influence later phenotypes and long-term disease risk has been suggested to include epigenetic processes. Epigenetic processes can modulate levels of gene expression without a change in the DNA nucleotide sequence (Burdge and Lillycrop, 2010; Ferguson-Smith, 2011; Atlasi and Stunnenberg, 2017), determining when and where a gene is expressed. Modulation of epigenetic processes during specific developmental windows has been shown to induce stable changes in gene expression that can persist throughout the life course, influencing later disease susceptibility (Zhang and Kutateladze, 2018). In this chapter, we will focus on how both maternal and paternal nutrition can alter the epigenome, the proposed mechanisms involved in mediating such effects, and the experimental evidence that such changes are causally involved in determining long-term health and future disease risk.

## 10.1.1 Early-life environment: A determinant of long-term health and non-communicable disease risk

Numerous human epidemiological studies have described associations between an adverse early life environment and subsequent risk of chronic disease. Early-life environment was first proposed to be an important determinant of later disease risk in a Norwegian study, which identified a strong association between undernutrition and poverty during childhood and adolescence followed by later prosperity with the occurrence of CVD during late middle age (Forsdahl, 1977). Studies by Barker and co-workers subsequently demonstrated that, even within the normal birth weight range, lower birth weight was associated with an increased risk of CVD and metabolic syndrome (hypertension, insulin resistance, T2D, dyslipidemia, and obesity) in later life, suggesting that a poor early life environment may influence future disease risk (Barker and Osmond, 1988; Barker et al., 1989, 1993; Hales et al., 1991). The association between low birth weight and later NCD risk was subsequently replicated in numerous mother-offspring cohorts across both high and low-middle income countries (Hanson and Gluckman, 2014; Fall, 2013). In some of these studies, a J- or U-shaped relationship between birth weight and disease risk was seen, with babies born at the highest birth weight also being at increased risk of disease (Ong, 2006; Pettitt and Jovanovic, 2001). In all of these studies, birth weight is thought to be a crude indicator of a suboptimal intrauterine environment compromised through maternal or environmental factors that may include maternal undernutrition or overnutrition, obesity, gestational diabetes, or placental insufficiency (Hanson et al., 2011).

These epidemiological studies providing the first population-based evidence of the importance of the early life environment were followed by studies of the Dutch Hunger Winter, a severe famine which occurred in the Netherlands during the winter of 1944; follow-up of those conceived/born around the time of the famine clearly demonstrated that maternal nutritional intake is a key early life factor that influences the health of the child during later life. Such studies found that individuals whose mothers were exposed to famine periconceptually and during the first trimester of pregnancy exhibited an increased risk of obesity and CVD, whereas individuals whose mothers were exposed during the later stages of gestation showed an increased incidence of insulin resistance and hypertension during later life

(Roseboom et al., 2006; Painter et al., 2005). Comparable findings have now been replicated in a myriad of experimental animal models where nutrition pre, during, and post-pregnancy can be precisely controlled. Such studies have found that feeding a protein-restricted (PR) or globally-restricted diet during pregnancy resulted in offspring with alterations in metabolism and phenotype (Bertram and Hanson, 2001; Burns et al., 1997; Torrens et al., 2008; Langley et al., 1994). For example, maternal PR induced changes in liver structure and function in the offspring (Burns et al., 1997), while in a separate study, maternal PR in F0 mice was shown to induce the transmission of raised blood pressure and endothelial dysfunction to the F2 generation in the absence of dietary challenge in the F1 generation (Torrens et al., 2008).

Given the rapid rise in the consumption of energy-rich diets and the increased incidence of obesity in modern society, recent research has focused on the long-term effect of maternal overnutrition and obesity on the health of the offspring. Such studies have shown that feeding dams diets high in fat or junk food during pregnancy and/or lactation results in offspring which exhibit similar features to human cardio-metabolic disease, including hypertension, dyslipidemia, obesity, and insulin resistance in later life (Samuelsson et al., 2008). Furthermore, maternal obesity induced by dietary intervention in experimental animal models has been shown to lead to the development of diabetes, obesity, elevated blood pressure, fatty liver, and modified offspring behavior (Patel et al., 2015), permanently altering metabolic control processes in the fetus such as changes in the hypothalamic response to leptin and pancreatic beta cell physiology (Patel et al., 2015).

In humans, observational studies have demonstrated that maternal obesity, gestational diabetes, and excessive weight gain during pregnancy are associated with increased risks of coronary heart disease, stroke, obesity, T2D, and asthma in children during later life (Godfrey et al., 2017; Crozier et al., 2010; Voerman et al., 2019). Further epidemiological studies have also suggested that early post-natal environment is also an important developmental window for nutritional programming. Studies in the UK Southampton Women's Survey (SWS) have demonstrated associations between early postnatal exposures with childhood body composition at birth, 4 and 6–7 years (Robinson et al., 2015), with, for example, a short duration of breastfeeding associated with greater childhood adiposity. Studies have also shown that lean mass was greater in children at 4 years of age whose weaning diets complied with infant feeding guidance (diet based on home-prepared foods, fruit, vegetables, and longer breastfeeding duration (Robinson et al., 2009). Furthermore, ongoing follow-up of the Helsinki Birth Cohort Study, a comparison of siblings discordant for duration of breastfeeding has shown that increased BMI and greater % body fat in later life were associated with both short (< 2 months) and long (≥ 8 months) breastfeeding durations (O'Tierney et al., 2009). Subsequent environmental exposures, which include nutritional factors during adolescence and adult life may also modify the risk of disease (Burdge et al., 2009; Yadav et al., 2018). Thus, trajectories of health or disease risk are influenced at various stages of the life course by environmental exposures to determine future health.

## 10.2 Developmental programming of long-term health

The induction of different phenotypes by perturbations in early-life nutrition has been suggested to reflect a predictive adaptive response (PAR) whereby the organism, acting through the process of developmental plasticity, adapts its developmental program in response to environmental cues in early life to aid health and survival during later life (Gluckman et al., 2005). Such tuning of phenotype has potential adaptive value because it adjusts the phenotype to current circumstances and/or matches responses to the predicted later environment. However, when an organism adapts to one environment in utero and is subsequently exposed to a different environment after birth (e.g., from compromised nutritional cues from the mother or placenta, or from rapid environmental change through improved socio-economic conditions and modified diets), a mismatch leaves the organism maladapted to the current environmental stimuli and at risk of future metabolic disease (Bateson et al., 2004; Cleal et al., 2007). A mismatch between prenatal and postnatal environments has been suggested to be central to the burgeoning rates of NCD observed in countries undergoing socioeconomic transition, for example, as populations migrate from rural to more urban areas (Godfrey et al., 2007). In the western world, exposure to energy/sugar-rich or highly processed diets high in trans or saturated fatty acids may be beyond our normal biological adaptive capacity, leading to pathological changes and an increased risk of future disease. Such mismatch is likely to program the risk of metabolic and other NCDs, as articulated by the 'developmental origins' or 'DOHaD' paradigm (Heindel and Vandenberg, 2015). For example, early life may be considered a critical period when both appetite and regulation of energy balance are programmed, leading to lifelong consequences for the risk of altered metabolism, excess adiposity gain, and associated health conditions (Fig. 10.1).

## 10.2.1 Epigenetic regulation of gene expression

Epigenetic processes regulate the expression potential of genes without altering the underlying DNA nucleotide sequence. Epigenetic processes include covalent modifications to DNA in the form of methylation, modifications to the histone proteins, around which the DNA is coiled, and non-coding RNAs (ncRNAs). Together such processes control either access of the transcriptional machinery to underlying DNA sequences, the stability of messenger RNA (mRNA), and/or its translational competence, thereby defining when and where genes are expressed and levels of expression. Epigenetic modifications function as dynamic processes, mediated through epigenetic readers, writers, and erasers (Yang et al., 2016). This reflects the complex interplay between an organism and its environment, enabling cells to fine-tune gene expression based on environmental stimuli in order to meet cellular demands (Moosavi and Motevalizadeh Ardekani, 2016). Such processes may function alone, but the different components of epigenetic regulation often work in concert with each other to determine the epigenetic state of a cell and its expression profile (Kelly et al., 2010).

## 10.2.2 DNA methylation

DNA methylation takes place most commonly when the covalent transfer of a methyl group ($CH_3$) to the $C_5$ position of cytosine occurs, generating 5-methylcytosine. In mammals, the majority of methylated cytosines are located directly next to a guanine, forming cytosine, and guanine nucleotides linked by a phosphate, more commonly annotated as a CpG; DNA methylation may also occur in other genomic contexts (Titcombe et al., 2021). In general, low levels of DNA methylation (hypomethylation) in the promoter or control regions of genes are associated with transcriptional activation and enhanced gene expression, while high levels

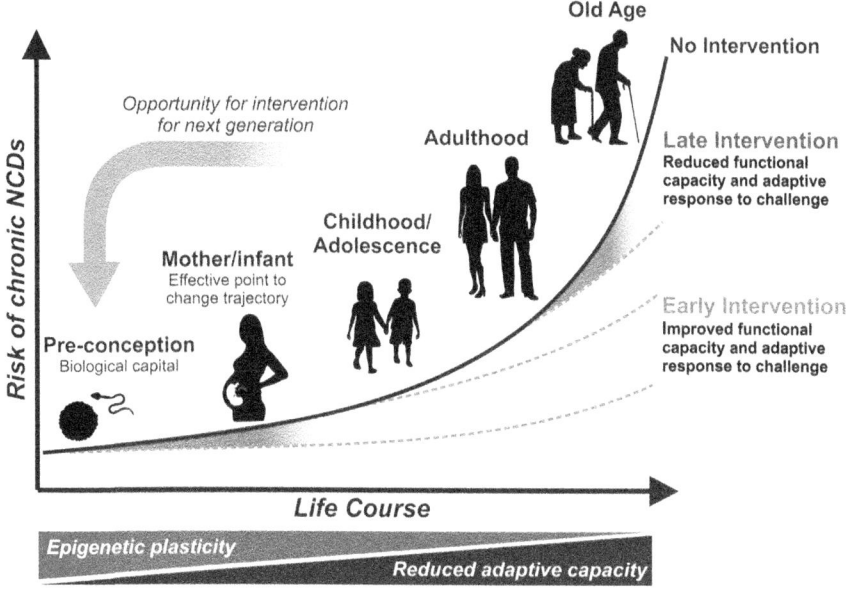

**FIG. 10.1** Shows the conceptual framework for current research into trajectories of NCD risk throughout the life course and windows of opportunity for successful intervention. The risk of NCDs increases across the life course as epigenetic plasticity is reduced and accumulative effects of reduced adaptive capacity to new environmental challenges occur (*gray triangles* showing trajectories). The greatest increase in NCD risk occurs during adult life, but the trajectory is set much earlier, being influenced by factors such as paternal nutritional intake prior to conception or maternal nutritional intake prior to conception and during pregnancy, as well as fetal, infant, and childhood nutritional intake. During early life, timely interventions can have a large effect on later disease risk, with levels of biological capacity for effects becoming less pronounced towards adulthood. Later intervention can remain impactful, especially for vulnerable groups with varying levels of tissue-specific plasticity present during adulthood and old age. Timely intervention during adolescence/adulthood increases biological capital and may have important impacts on the long-term health of the next generation through epigenetic paternal and maternal transmission to offspring . *Adapted from Godfrey, K.M., Costello, P.M., Lillycrop, K.A., 2016. Development, epigenetics and metabolic programming. Nestle Nutr. Inst. Workshop Ser. 85, 71–80.*

of methylation (hypermethylation) are associated with transcriptional repression and gene silencing (Bird and Macleod, 2004). Methylation of CpGs within promoter regions leads to transcriptional repression by either blocking transcription factor binding to DNA, or through recruitment of methyl-CpG binding proteins, which in turn recruit histone-modifying complexes to condense the DNA, restricting transcription factor access to the gene and repressing transcription (Miller and Grant, 2013). Conversely, low levels of methylation allow transcription factors access to underlying nucleotide sequences and subsequent gene activation.

### 10.2.3 Histone modifications and chromatin configuration

In eukaryotic organisms, DNA localized within the nucleus of the cell is coiled around a histone octamer consisting of two copies of each core histone (H2A, H2B, H3, and H4), which forms a unit of chromatin called a nucleosome. Each nucleosome is folded upon itself, forming a solenoid (30 nm fiber) which is then further coiled and compacted to form a 200 nm fiber of compactly packaged DNA (Bannister and Kouzarides, 2011). Although the primary role of histones was previously considered to be essential to reduce the effective size of DNA, it is now clear that histones also play a critical regulatory role in gene expression. Histone proteins contain two domains: a globular domain and an amino tail domain. The amino tail domains are rich in positively charged amino acids which interact with negatively charged DNA and are now known to be subject to a large number of post-translational modifications; these include acetylation, methylation ubiquitination, citrullination, and phosphorylation (Bannister and Kouzarides, 2011). Such modifications can either directly modify chromatin structure or provide binding sites for direct interactions with effector proteins, which bring about distinct cellular processes (Tessarz and Kouzarides, 2014). For example, histone acetyltransferases induce the acetylation of lysine residues located within histone tails, neutralizing the positive charge of the lysine, thereby reducing the interaction of the histone with DNA. This leads to the opening of chromatin, allowing access to the transcriptional machinery and subsequent gene activation. Conversely, histone deacetylases actively remove acetyl groups, restoring the positive charge and leading to a closing down of chromatin structure resulting in gene repression (Turner, 2000).

### 10.2.4 Non-coding RNAs

Approximately 90% of the eukaryotic genome is transcribed; however, only 1%–2% of the genome encodes functional proteins (Morris et al., 2004). RNA species that are transcribed but not translated are classed as ncRNAs. These classes of RNA molecules display remarkable biological diversity and demonstrate the ability to fold into complex structures and interact with DNA targets, proteins as well as other RNAs in order to modulate transcriptional and translational activity (Zampetaki et al., 2018). Functionally important regulatory types of ncRNA, based on their average size, are classified as either small ncRNA (sncRNAs) that are typically less than 200 nucleotides in length and of which the main classes include tRNAs, microRNAs (miRNA), small interfering RNAs (siRNAs), tRNA-derived small RNAs (tsRNAs), piwi RNAs (piRNAs), small nucleolar RNAs (snoRNAs), small nuclear RNAs (snRNAs), extracellular RNA (exRNAs) and small cajal specific RNAs (scaRNAs); or long non-coding RNAs (lncRNA) which are typically greater than 200 nucleotides in length. Micro RNAs, the most studied of the sncRNAs, can induce mRNA degradation or translational repression and, when binding within the promoter region of a gene, induce both DNA methylation and repressive histone modifications resulting in reduced transcriptional activity or even complete repression (Hawkins et al., 2009; Morris et al., 2004; Kim et al., 2008). ncRNAs may also perform regulatory roles after cleavage; for example, tRFs, abundant 14- to 32-nucleotide RNA fragments derived from tRNA have been shown to be involved in transcriptional regulation (Chen et al., 2016; Sharma et al., 2016; Maute et al., 2013; Schimmel, 2018).

ncRNAs have been shown to interact and functionally cooperate either with each other or different classes of ncRNA, leading to synergistic target inhibition (Krek et al., 2005). DNA methylation, histone modification, and ncRNA, therefore work synergistically to regulate gene expression. Studies suggest that DNA methylation may function to consolidate changes in gene expression induced by histone modifications and ncRNA, and that DNA methylation represents the most stable of these epigenetic marks, which is required for long-term persistent repression of gene expression (Fig. 10.2).

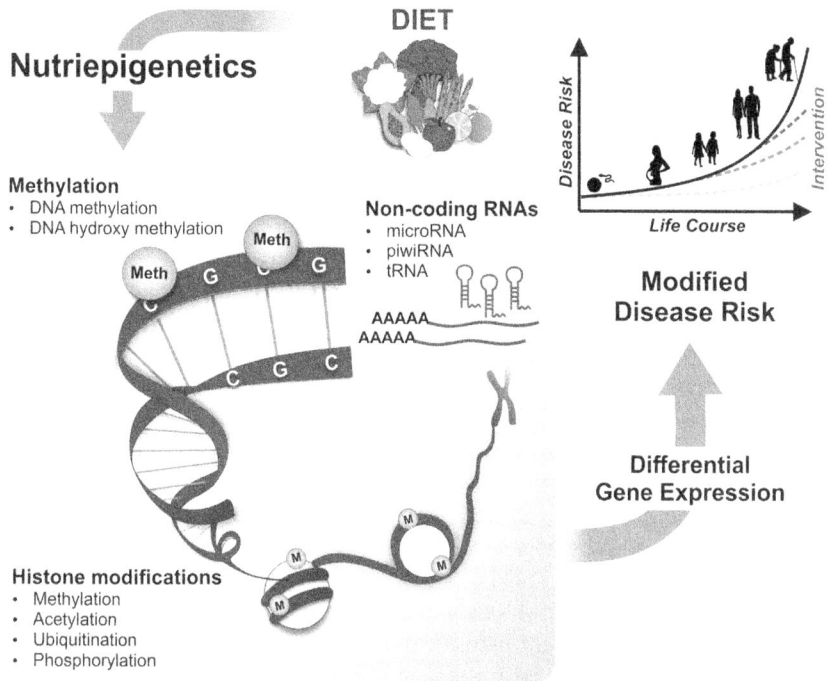

FIG. 10.2   Shows a graphical summary of the interactions between nutrition and the epigenome (nutriepigenom-ics). Changes in dietary intake and levels of metabolites have been shown to modulate epigenetic processes, including DNA methylation, histone modifications, and non-coding RNAs, which regulate whether genes are turned on or off and the levels of expression. Changes in epigenetic processes in response to nutrition and subsequent modulation of gene expression have been shown to modify disease risk. Interventions during specific periods of the life course can alter levels of tissue-specific plasticity and provide effective windows for modulating long-term health.

## 10.2.5  Maternal nutrition as a modifier of the epigenome: Evidence from experimental animal studies

The mechanisms by which maternal diet can induce such long-term phenotypic changes in the offspring have been suggested to include the altered epigenetic regulation of genes. The first demonstration that maternal diet could alter DNA methylation in the offspring came from work on agouti mice. Coat color in agouti mice is determined by the methylation status of an IAP (endogenous retrovirus-like element) retrotransposon upstream of the transcription start site of the *agouti* gene; this acts as a cryptic promoter directing expression of the agouti gene, which encodes for a paracrine signaling protein that induces a switch in melanocytes from the production of black eumelanin to yellow phaeomelanin. Supplementation of the maternal diet of agouti mice with folic acid, vitamin $B_{12}$, choline, and betaine induced a graded shift in coat color of the litter from predominately yellow (agouti) to brown (pseudo-agouti). This shift was accompanied by the hypermethylation of the agouti gene (Wolff et al., 1998).

In models of nutritional programming, there is also evidence of both epigenetic and phenotypic changes in the offspring. For example, feeding pregnant rats a PR diet induced the hypomethylation of the glucocorticoid receptor (GR) and peroxisome proliferator-activated receptor alpha *(Ppar-α)* promoters in livers of both juvenile and adult offspring; this was accompanied by an increase in the expression of the GR and *Pparα* genes and in the metabolic processes that they control (Lillycrop et al., 2007, 2008). In contrast, global dietary restriction during pregnancy induced the hypermethylation of the GR and *Pparα* promoters, as well as a decrease in glucocorticoid receptor and *Pparα* mRNA expression (Gluckman et al., 2007). This demonstrates that the effects of maternal nutrition on the offspring's epigenome and levels of gene expression may be dependent upon the specific nature of the maternal nutritional challenge. Such findings are consistent with the hypothesis that dietary-induced epigenetic changes may provide a mechanism for adapting to an adverse environment.

Maternal HF diets have also been associated with epigenetic and phenotypic changes in the offspring. In offspring from mice fed a HF diet during pregnancy, hypomethylation of the promoter regions of the dopamine reuptake transporter, μ-opioid receptor, and preproenkephalin genes was observed. These are genes specifically linked to reward pathways, and the intake of palatable foods and their hypomethylation was accompanied by increased gene expression in the nucleus accumbens, prefrontal cortex, and hypothalamic brain regions (Vucetic et al., 2010). Maternal high-fat feeding during pregnancy has also been shown to induce a decrease in the expression of fatty acid desaturase 2, the rate-limiting enzyme in polyunsaturated fatty acid (PUFA) synthesis, and alter the methylation of key CpG nucleotides within its promoter in the offspring (Hoile et al., 2013; Kelsall et al., 2012), directly linking HF feeding to modified fatty acid metabolism through epigenetic regulation. In addition, neonatal overfeeding induced by raising rat pups in small litters induced hypermethylation of two CpG dinucleotides within the appetite control gene pro-opiomelanocortin. The two CpG sites hypermethylated are essential for the induction of pro-opiomelanocortin expression by leptin and insulin (Plagemann et al., 2009; Marco et al., 2013). Such studies provide compelling evidence that maternal HF intake during pregnancy alters DNA methylation within offspring leading to long-term alterations in gene expression, metabolism, and feeding behaviors.

Although most studies have focused on the effect of maternal diet on DNA methylation changes in the offspring, there is growing evidence that early life nutrition can also induce persistent changes in both histone modifications and miRNAs. For example, maternal PR has been reported to modulate hepatic miRNA expression with miR-615, miR-124, miR-376b and let-7e shown to be significantly downregulated and miR-708 and miR-879 significantly upregulated in offspring; this was accompanied by altered glucose metabolism in C57BL/6J mice (Zheng et al., 2017). Similarly, a maternal HF diet during pregnancy and lactation has been shown to alter hepatic expression of miRNAs in the adult offspring (Zhang et al., 2009). Furthermore, offspring born to dams fed HF diet developed cardiac hypertrophy and increased extracellular matrix deposition with microarray analysis of cardiac tissue identifying a micro-RNA subset including let-7g, miR-15, miR-21, miR-27a, miR-29c, miR-33, miR-101a, miR-218a, and miR-450a down-regulated in HF diet-exposed animals, which were predicted to regulate transforming growth factor-beta (TGFβ)-mediated remodeling (Siddeek et al., 2019). Maternal PR and HF diets during pregnancy have also been reported to lead to histone modifications. In islet cells, a decrease in hepatic Nuclear factor (HNF) 3a expression in the liver of PR offspring was accompanied by substantial changes in histone modifications at the HNF4a promoter; these included a reduction in Histone H3 lysine 4 (H3K4) methylation, and an increase in H3K9me2 and H3K27me3 (Sandovici et al., 2011), while in offspring from dams fed a HF diet during pregnancy and lactation decreased H3K27me3, H2Ak119ub1 and DNA methylation levels were observed together with a down-regulation of the enhancer of Zeste Homolog 2 (EZH2), and DNMT3B expression in heart tissue (Blin et al., 2020).

## 10.2.6 Maternal nutrition as a modifier of the epigenome: Evidence from human studies

Individuals periconceptually exposed to famine during the Dutch Hunger Winter (Tobi et al., 2009; Heijmans et al., 2008) have been shown to demonstrate differences in levels of DNA methylation. Decreased methylation of the imprinted insulin-like growth factor 2 (IGF2) gene and increased methylation of IL-10, leptin, and ATP-binding cassette A1 genes were observed in genomic DNA isolated from whole blood cells from individuals exposed to famine during early gestation in utero compared with unexposed same-sex siblings (Heijmans et al., 2008). Changes in DNA methylation were only observed when individuals were exposed to famine during early gestation (Tobi et al., 2009). These changes persisted up to 60–70 years after exposure, suggesting the methylome is most susceptible to alterations in maternal diet during the very early stages of development and that such variations in maternal diet can induce persistent epigenetic changes in the offspring that last a lifetime.

Further research by Waterland et al. has identified what has been termed metastable epialleles (ME), which demonstrate an epigenetic state independent of tissue type and are considered vulnerable to transient environmental influences (Rakyan et al., 2002). Altered DNA methylation of ME was identified in individuals conceived during the protein-limited rainy season compared with those conceived in the dry harvest season in Gambia (Waterland et al., 2010). Differences in DNA methylation were associated with periconceptional maternal plasma concentrations of key micronutrients involved in $C_1$ metabolism, suggesting that the changes in DNA methylation found in this population may be linked not to the negative energy balance observed in mothers during the rainy season, but rather to the limited dietary levels of methyl donors and co-factors required for $C_1$ metabolism.

A number of studies have also reported associations between maternal intake and/or status of $C_1$ donors and cofactors with DNA methylation levels in the offspring. However, variations in the effect size, direction of effect, and genes differentially methylated are observed in these studies. For instance, periconceptional folic acid has been both positively (Steegers-Theunissen et al., 2009) and negatively (Pauwels et al., 2017) associated with methylation at the IGF2 locus in offspring. Conversely, studies have also reported no effect of periconceptional folic acid exposure (Haggarty et al., 2012) on DNA methylation. There are also examples of maternal macronutrient intake influencing DNA methylation in the offspring. A prenatal diet high in fat and sugar was positively associated with offspring IGF2 methylation in blood (Rijlaarsdam et al., 2017), and maternal carbohydrate intake during the second trimester was negatively associated with methylation of retinoid X receptor α at birth (Godfrey et al., 2011). Furthermore, increased protein intake in pregnancy was positively associated with GR methylation in the adult offspring (Drake et al., 2012). Data from recent randomized trials have reported that the epigenetic impact of a dysglycemia prenatal maternal environment is modified by lifestyle intervention in pregnancy (Antoun et al., 2020) and that vitamin D supplementation in pregnancy altered the methylation of a CpG site previously linked with offspring bone development (Harvey et al., 2014; Curtis et al., 2019).

## 10.2.7 Mechanisms by which maternal nutrition modifies the epigenome and modulates long-term health

A primary mechanism by which nutrition has been considered to modulate the epigenome is through one-carbon ($C_1$) metabolism (Anderson et al., 2012). Methyl groups for all biological methylation reactions, which includes both DNA and histone methylation, are mainly supplied from dietary methyl donors and cofactors via $C_1$ metabolism. Within the $C_1$, pathway S-adenosylmethionine (SAM) functions as a primary methyl donor regulating methyl group transfer to a number of substrates, which include nucleic acids and histone proteins resulting in DNA and histone methylation respectively. After methyl group transfer, S-adenosylmethionine is then converted to S-adenosylhomocysteine, which is converted to homocysteine. Homocysteine is either recycled to methionine by the enzyme betaine homocysteine methyltransferase, which uses betaine or choline, or via a folate-dependent remethylation pathway, where 5-methyltetrahydrofolate is reduced to 5,10-methylenetetrahydrofolate by 5,10-methylenetetrahydrofolate reductase. The methyl group is subsequently used by methionine synthase to convert homocysteine back to methionine using vitamin $B_{12}$ as a cofactor. Many studies have demonstrated the effects of imbalances in dietary methyl donors on the epigenome, such as folate, a water-soluble vitamin (B9) of which deficiency has been implicated in modified disease risk (Mahajan et al., 2019). Furthermore, the effects of synthetic methyl donors such as folic acid, fortified in staple foods in many countries in order to reduce folate deficiency associated neural tube defects, has been shown to modulate offspring DNA methylation when supplemented during pregnancy, and is also implicated as a potential modifier of long term disease risk (Richmond et al., 2018).

Although $C_1$ metabolism pathways have been the predominant pathways implicated in methyl supply and transfer reactions, modulation of the epigenome may not, however, be limited to $C_1$ donors and cofactors. For example, many transcription factors which recruit epigenetic writers are regulated by nutritional factors, and indeed many of the readers, writers, and erasers of the epigenetic code themselves are regulated at least in part by the concentration of specific metabolic substrates or cofactors. For instance, the PPAR family of nuclear receptors, which play a key role in lipid metabolism, are activated by polyunsaturated fatty acids (Kliewer et al., 1994), while the lysine-specific histone demethylase 1A, which demethylates lysine 4 of histone 3, uses the reduction of the cofactor FAD to $FADH_2$. Thus, variations in dietary intake in terms of either individual components or total energy are likely to influence the epigenome.

## 10.2.8 The effect of paternal nutrition as a modifier of offspring health

Until recently, studies have focused predominately on understanding the effects of maternal nutrition on the fetal epigenome and the health of the offspring; however, research has now begun to investigate how paternal environment or exposures may contribute to developmental programming prior to and at the time of conception (Fleming et al., 2018). It was shown many years ago that paternal nutritional intake is of critical importance and can modulate long-term effects on offspring health. For example, studies in Sweden showed that the paternal grandfather's nutritional intake in pre-puberty was associated with the risk of diabetes and CVD in male but not female grandchildren (Pembrey et al., 2006; Kaati et al., 2002). Furthermore, experimental studies in rodents have identified that variations in paternal diet induce phenotypic changes in the offspring linked to modified disease risk. For example, offspring from males exposed to dietary restriction demonstrated reduced birth weight and impaired glucose tolerance (Jimenez-Chillaron et al., 2009), while feeding male rats a PR diet prior to mating led to elevated hepatic expression of genes involved in lipid and cholesterol biosynthesis and a decrease in cholesterol esters, relative to the offspring of males fed a control diet. Further studies have also reported that chronic HF feeding in Sprague–Dawley fathers led to increased body weight, adiposity, and impaired glucose tolerance and insulin sensitivity in the offspring (Ng et al., 2014) (Fig. 10.3).

### 10.2.9 Epigenetic mechanisms by which paternal diet may influence the offspring's long-term health

Lifestyle and environmental factors such as nutrition (Carone et al., 2010; Ng et al., 2014) have been shown to alter semen composition and sperm quality parameters such as motility. Such exposures are thought to leave an imprint on the sperm epigenome and transcriptome that may be transmitted to the zygote during conception resulting in phenotypic changes in the offspring (Bedi et al., 2019; Siddeek et al., 2018; Donkin and Barrès, 2018). To understand the mechanisms of paternal transmission, experimental studies have begun to examine

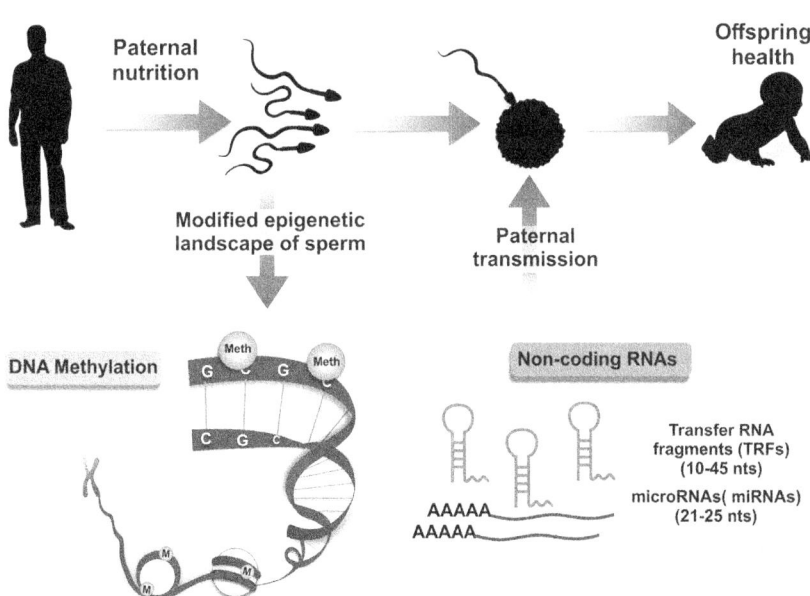

**FIG. 10.3** Shows a graphical summary of how paternal nutrition is proposed to modulate paternal transmission and offspring health. Changes in paternal nutrition prior to and around the time of conception have been shown to alter the epigenetic and transcriptomic landscape of sperm, in particular levels of DNA methylation and sncRNA expression. Changes in sncRNAs, namely miRNAs and tRFs cleaved from tRNAs, have been shown to be sensitive to dietary intake, and in experimental animal models confer information at conception which modulates disease phenotype.

the effect of paternal diet on epigenetic modifiers, namely DNA methylation, histone modifications, and/or the ncRNA content of sperm. For example, Watkins et al. (2018) reported that sperm from male mice fed a PR diet for 8 weeks showed hypomethylation at 972 loci compared to controls, although Carone et al. reported that cytosine methylation patterns are highly correlated in sperm from control, low protein or energy-restricted fathers, suggesting the sperm epigenome may be refractory to differences in diet. The different effects on the sperm methylome between these two studies may reflect the different diets given, exposure time to such diets, and the methods used to assess DNA methylation changes.

Paternal HF diets have also been associated with changes in the sperm methylome and histone profiles. Donkin and Barres reported differential methylation of 18 regions in the sperm genome of males fed a HF diet and their offspring, including CpGs within the solute carrier family 3 amino acid transporter heavy chain member 2, and within transforming growth factor β regulator 4 and major facilitator superfamily domain containing 7 (Donkin and Barrès, 2018). Furthermore, using a high-fat diet (HFD)-induced obesity mouse model, Terashima et al., reported differential histone H3-occupancy at genes involved in the regulation of embryogenesis and differential H3K4me1-enrichment at transcription regulatory genes in sperm from HFD fathers compared to control mice. Such findings suggest that dietary exposure can modulate histone composition at regulatory genes implicated in key processes such as embryogenesis and sperm regulation which are critical to development (Terashima et al., 2015). Nutritional intake has also been linked with changes in the sperm transcriptome. For example, *Let-7* miRNA, which regulates lipid and glucose metabolism, has been shown to be down-regulated in spermatozoa after exposure of males to a low-protein diet (Sharma et al., 2016); expression of Let-7 was also differentially expressed in spermatozoa of rats fed a HF diet as well as in their offspring (de Castro Barbosa et al., 2016).

While paternal diet can clearly modulate the sperm transcriptome affecting miRNA expression and DNA methylation; recent studies have identified tRNA derived fragments (tRFs), a class of tsRNAs, as potential mediators by which information on the father's environment is transmitted to the offspring. Chen et al. demonstrated that feeding a HF diet to male mice over a 6-month period substantially altered the composition of tRFs within the sperm; injection of tRFs isolated from sperm from males fed a HF diet into control zygotes resulted in altered expression of metabolic genes in the early embryo and metabolic disorders in the offspring, akin to those seen after natural mating of the high-fat fed fathers to control dams (Chen et al., 2016). In humans, a study by Natt et al. demonstrated that sperm are acutely sensitive to nutrient flux, both in terms of sperm motility and changes in sperm tsRNAs. Over the course of a 2-week diet intervention, in which participants were first introduced to a healthy diet followed by a diet rich in sugar, sperm motility increased and stabilized at high levels. Furthermore, tsRNAs were up-regulated after eating a high-sugar diet for just 1 week (Nätt et al., 2019). In addition, we have shown that a 6 week dietary intervention containing vitamin D and omega −3 fatty acids modulates the sperm non-coding transcriptome, with changes in tRFs, miRNAs, and piRNAs. Moreover, the predicted targets of the altered ncRNAs included genes involved in fatty acid metabolism and vitamin D response (Vaz et al., 2021). The rapid response to a dietary intervention on tRFs in human sperm is attuned with the paternal intergenerational metabolic responses found in model organisms (Carone et al., 2010). More importantly, these studies suggest diet-sensitive mechanisms between sperm quality and the biogenesis of tsRNAs, which provide novel insights into the interplay between nutrition and male reproductive health. Such studies also provide evidence that variations in paternal diet alter the sperm transcriptome and that sncRNAs capture the epigenetic imprint of this change. Furthermore, the changes seen in human sncRNA profiles in response to paternal exposures mirror those previously observed in experimental rodent models that have been shown to induce persistent changes to the health of the offspring. This suggests that similar mechanisms also occur in humans, and paternal diet may also be a key determinant of the future health of the child.

## 10.3 Contribution of perinatal epigenetic marks to later phenotype epigenetic biomarkers and future health

There is increasing evidence that epigenetic changes, particularly during early life, play critical roles in determining future disease susceptibility. The detection of such epigenetic marks in early life may therefore provide valuable 'disease biomarkers', quantifiable biological parameters which serve as indices for current or predicted disease risk to identify individuals at increased risk of later disease (Oses et al., 2019). However, in humans there is limited tissue availability; easily accessible tissues include cord, cord blood, placenta, buccal, and blood, but whether methylation changes in these tissues adequately reflect methylation in more metabolically relevant cell types is uncertain. Such methylation changes even in peripheral tissue may nonetheless act as markers of a particular early life exposure and may be useful to detect individuals at increased risk of metabolic disease. Consistent with this paradigm, our studies have shown that DNA methylation changes measured in the umbilical cord at birth predicted adiposity in later childhood. We found that the methylation of a CpG site in the promoter region of the nuclear retinoic acid receptor RXR-alpha was strongly related to childhood adiposity in both boys and girls in two independent cohorts, explaining >25% of the variance in childhood fat mass (Godfrey et al., 2011), while methylation of specific CpG loci in the promoter of peroxisome proliferator-activated receptor gamma coactivator 1-alpha (Clarke-Harris et al., 2014), at 5 years of age-predicted adiposity year-on-year from 8 to 14 years, strongly supporting the hypothesis that developmentally induced epigenetic marks may be valuable predictors of later adiposity even in peripheral tissues.

Genome-wide methylome analysis has also identified CpG loci within solute carrier family 6 member 4, a serotonin transporter linked with energy balance and appetite, in umbilical cord correlated with % and total fat mass from birth to 4 and 6 years., and with triceps skinfold thickness at birth, 6 and 12 mo and 2, 3, and 6 years (Lillycrop et al., 2019). Methylation of the same CpG locus in cord blood was also associated with triceps skinfold thickness from birth to 6 years. and predicted obesity in adipose tissue during adulthood. We have also identified novel associations between the level of CpG methylation at birth within the promoter of the lncRNA ANRIL and adiposity in children aged 6-years, in birth tissues from ethnically diverse neonates, in peripheral blood from adolescents, and in adipose tissue from adults (Lillycrop et al., 2017). As DNA methylation is influenced by both the environment and genotype (Teh et al., 2014), the detection of perinatal epigenetic biomarkers may potentially provide more powerful biomarkers than genotype and environmental exposures alone, allowing the integration of environmental signals with genetic profiles. This would provide a more complete profile of disease risk, how imbalances in the supply of specific nutrients may influence inter-individual disease susceptibility (García-Giménez et al., 2017; Amenyah et al., 2020), and response to preventative and intervention strategies (García-Giménez et al., 2017). However, it remains to be determined whether these methylation changes are causally involved in the development and progression of NCDs or whether they are simply markers or a consequence of the change in phenotype. Direct experimental proof of a causal role for such methylation changes remains elusive because of the technical difficulty in methylating specific CpG sites. However, the recent studies demonstrating a role for ncRNAs in mediating the effect of paternal environment on the offspring's phenotype, suggest a role for epigenetic processes in the causal pathway by which early life environment affects later health, with perhaps DNA methylation changes consolidating transcriptional changes induced by ncRNAs in response to the environment.

## 10.4 Conclusion

Non-communicable diseases, which include obesity, T2D, and CVD, are becoming increasingly prevalent globally. This has led agencies worldwide to now advocate for taking a life course approach to disease prevention from preconception through to adulthood and old age. Primary prevention of NCDs therefore not only requires an intrinsic understanding of the underlying environmental, lifestyle, and societal influences that may affect such disease risks, but also of the cellular and molecular mechanisms underpinning the programmed memory of early developmental exposures and whether specific early biological detection and reversal strategies are achievable in order to mitigate risk. Substantial evidence now shows that early-life nutrition of both mother and father is a key determinant of future disease risk, and that the underlying mechanism by which alterations in early-life nutrition can induce phenotypic changes in offspring involves the altered epigenetic regulation of genes.

Compelling evidence suggests that such epigenetic processes (DNA methylation, histone modifications, and ncRNAs) not only can function independently but are also interconnected, forming an epigenetic network that works in concert to modulate gene expression in response to environmental exposures such as changes in nutritional intakes. The central role of epigenetic processes as mechanisms by which both paternal and maternal diet can influence the health of the offspring provides an opportunity for intervention aimed at reversing the adverse effects of the early-life environment, as epigenetic processes, although stable, have been shown to be reversible. Experimental evidence is accruing that endocrine or nutritional interventions during early postnatal life can reverse epigenetic and phenotypic changes induced, for example, by an unbalanced maternal diet during pregnancy (Hoile et al., 2012). Furthermore, changes in paternal diet during the period prior to conception may alter epigenetic marks in sperm prior to conception leading to improved sperm health, increased conception rates, enhanced embryo development, and future offspring health. Thus, elucidation of such epigenetic mechanisms may permit perinatal identification of individuals at risk of later NCD and facilitate a new generation of early intervention strategies to mitigate such risk. Thus, a deeper understanding of molecular signaling pathways activated by bioactive food components and such effects on epigenetic process and gene regulation is required. Such findings have important implications for public health policy and the engagement of the current generation in discussions about healthy nutritional intake and its implications on long-term health of the next generation.

## 10.5 Future trends and research

Research to date has clearly demonstrated that environmental exposures and our lifestyle choices such as nutritional intake can modulate the epigenetic landscape of cells, leading to changes in gene expression and metabolism, affecting susceptibility to NCDs in later life. The detection of such epigenetic changes may provide potential predictive biomarkers of disease risk and allow the identification of novel targets for therapeutic interventions. With the development of a new generation of robust high-throughput sequencing technologies together with the decreasing cost of such approaches, this is paving the way for personalized epigenetic screening and research on the development of tailored nutritional interventions to ameliorate the risk of NCD in later life. Furthermore, this research demonstrates that both the mothers and father's diet can influence the health of the child, reinforcing the message of many public health campaigns that early life nutrition is critical to reduce the burden of disease in the next generation.

## Sources of additional information

Burdge, G., Lillycrop, K., 2016 Nutrition, Epigenetics and Health. World Scientific Publishing, Singapore, 225 pp.

Burton, M. A., Lillycrop, K. A., 2019. Nutritional modulation of the epigenome and its implication for future health. Proc. Nutr. Soc. 78, 305–312.

Donkin, I., Barrès, R., 2018. Sperm epigenetics and influence of environmental factors. Mol. Metab. 14, 1–11.

Fleming, T. P., Watkins, A. J., Velazquez, M. A., Mathers, J. C., Prentice, A. M., Stephenson, J., Barker, M., Saffery, R., Yajnik, C. S., Eckert, J. J., Hanson, M. A., Forrester, T., Gluckman, P. D., Godfrey, K. M., 2018. Origins of lifetime health around the time of conception: causes and consequences. Lancet 391, 1842–1852.

Koletzko, B., Godfrey, K. M., Poston, L., Szajewska, H., Van Goudoever, J. B., De Waard, M., Brands, B., Grivell, R. M., Deussen, A. R., Dodd, J. M., Patro-Golab, B., Zalewski, B. M., 2019. Nutrition during pregnancy, lactation and early childhood and its implications for maternal and long-term child health: the early nutrition project recommendations. Ann. Nutr. Metab. 74, 93–106.

Leroy, J. L., Frongillo, E. A., Dewan, P., Black, M. M., Waterland, R. A. 2020. Can children catch up from the consequences of undernourishment? evidence from child linear growth, developmental epigenetics, and brain and neurocognitive development. Adv. Nutr. 11, 1032–1041.

Low, F. M., Gluckman, P. D., Hanson, M. A., 2020. Maternal and child health: is making 'healthy choices' an oxymoron? Glob. Health Promot. 1757975920967351.

Patro-Gołąb, B., Zalewski, B. M., Kołodziej, M., Kouwenhoven, S., Poston, L., Godfrey, K. M., Koletzko, B., Van Goudoever, J. B., Szajewska, H. 2016. Nutritional interventions or exposures in infants and children aged up to 3 years and their effects on subsequent risk of overweight, obesity and body fat: a systematic review of systematic reviews. Obes Rev., 17, 1245–1257.

# References

Amenyah, S.D., Ward, M., Strain, J.J., McNulty, H., Hughes, C.F., Dollin, C., Walsh, C.P., Lees-Murdock, D.J., 2020. Nutritional epigenomics and age-related disease. Curr. Dev. Nutr. 4, nzaa097.

Anderson, O.S., Sant, K.E., Dolinoy, D.C., 2012. Nutrition and epigenetics: an interplay of dietary methyl donors, one-carbon metabolism and DNA methylation. J. Nutr. Biochem. 23, 853–859.

Antoun, E., Kitaba, N.T., Titcombe, P., Dalrymple, K.V., Garratt, E.S., Barton, S.J., Murray, R., Seed, P.T., Holbrook, J.D., Kobor, M.S., Lin, D.T.S., MacIsaac, J.L., Burdge, G.C., White, S.L., Poston, L., Godfrey, K.M., Lillycrop, K.A., Consortium, U., 2020. Maternal dysglycaemia, changes in the infant's epigenome modified with a diet and physical activity intervention in pregnancy: secondary analysis of a randomised control trial. PLoS Med. 17, e1003229.

Atlasi, Y., Stunnenberg, H.G., 2017. The interplay of epigenetic marks during stem cell differentiation and development. Nat. Rev. Genet. 18, 643–658.

Bannister, A.J., Kouzarides, T., 2011. Regulation of chromatin by histone modifications. Cell Res. 21, 381–395.

Barker, D.J., Osmond, C., 1988. Low birth weight and hypertension. BMJ 297, 134–135.

Barker, D.J.P., Osmond, C., Winter, P.D., Margetts, B., Simmonds, S.J., 1989. Weight in infancy and death from ischaemic heart disease. Lancet 334, 577–580.

Barker, D.J.P., Hales, C.N., Fall, C.H.D., Osmond, C., Phipps, K., Clark, P.M.S., 1993. Type 2 (non-insulin-dependent) diabetes mellitus, hypertension and hyperlipidaemia (syndrome X): relation to reduced fetal growth. Diabetologia 36, 62–67.

Bateson, P., Barker, D., Clutton-Brock, T., Deb, D., D'udine, B., Foley, R.A., Gluckman, P., Godfrey, K., Kirkwood, T., Lahr, M.M., McNamara, J., Metcalfe, N.B., Monaghan, P., Spencer, H.G., Sultan, S.E., 2004. Developmental plasticity and human health. Nature 430, 419–421.

Bedi, Y., Chang, R.C., Gibbs, R., Clement, T.M., Golding, M.C., 2019. Alterations in sperm-inherited noncoding RNAs associate with late-term fetal growth restriction induced by preconception paternal alcohol use. Reprod. Toxicol. 87, 11–20.

Bertram, C.E., Hanson, M.A., 2001. Animal models and programming of the metabolic syndrome: type 2 diabetes. Br. Med. Bull. 60, 103–121.

Bird, A., Macleod, D., 2004. Reading the DNA methylation signal. Cold Spring Harb. Symp. Quant. Biol. 69, 113–118.

Blin, G., Liand, M., Mauduit, C., Chehade, H., Benahmed, M., Simeoni, U., Siddeek, B., 2020. Maternal exposure to high-fat diet induces long-term derepressive chromatin marks in the heart. Nutrients 12, 181.

Burdge, G.C., Lillycrop, K.A., 2010. Nutrition, epigenetics, and developmental plasticity: implications for understanding human disease. Annu. Rev. Nutr. 30, 315–339.

Burdge, G.C., Lillycrop, K.A., Phillips, E.S., Slater-Jefferies, J.L., Jackson, A.A., Hanson, M.A., 2009. Folic acid supplementation during the juvenile-pubertal period in rats modifies the phenotype and epigenotype induced by prenatal nutrition. J. Nutr. 139, 1054–1060.

Burns, S.P., Desai, M., Cohen, R.D., Hales, C.N., Iles, R.A., Germain, J.P., Going, T.C., Bailey, R.A., 1997. Gluconeogenesis, glucose handling, and structural changes in livers of the adult offspring of rats partially deprived of protein during pregnancy and lactation. J. Clin. Invest. 100, 1768–1774.

Carone, B.R., Fauquier, L., Habib, N., Shea, J.M., Hart, C.E., Li, R., Bock, C., Li, C., Gu, H., Zamore, P.D., 2010. Paternally induced transgenerational environmental reprogramming of metabolic gene expression in mammals. Cell 143, 1084–1096.

Chen, Q., Yan, M., Cao, Z., Li, X., Zhang, Y., Shi, J., Feng, G.-H., Peng, H., Zhang, X., Zhang, Y., Qian, J., Duan, E., Zhai, Q., Zhou, Q., 2016. Sperm tsRNAs contribute to intergenerational inheritance of an acquired metabolic disorder. Science 351, 397–400.

Clarke-Harris, R., Wilkin, T.J., Hosking, J., Pinkney, J., Jeffery, A.N., Metcalf, B.S., Godfrey, K.M., Voss, L.D., Lillycrop, K.A., Burdge, G.C., 2014. PGC1α promoter methylation in blood at 5–7 years predicts adiposity from 9 to 14 years (EarlyBird 50). Diabetes 63, 2528–2537.

Cleal, J.K., Poore, K.R., Boullin, J.P., Khan, O., Chau, R., Hambidge, O., Torrens, C., Newman, J.P., Poston, L., Noakes, D.E., Hanson, M.A., Green, L.R., 2007. Mismatched pre- and postnatal nutrition leads to cardiovascular dysfunction and altered renal function in adulthood. Proc. Natl. Acad. Sci. 104, 9529–9533.

Crozier, S.R., Inskip, H.M., Godfrey, K.M., Cooper, C., Harvey, N.C., Cole, Z.A., Robinson, S.M., Group, S. W. S. S. S, 2010. Weight gain in pregnancy and childhood body composition: findings from the Southampton Women's survey. Am. J. Clin. Nutr. 91, 1745–1751.

Curtis, E.M., Krstic, N., Cook, E., D'angelo, S., Crozier, S.R., Moon, R.J., Murray, R., Garratt, E., Costello, P., Cleal, J., Ashley, B., Bishop, N.J., Kennedy, S., Papageorghiou, A.T., Schoenmakers, I., Fraser, R., Gandhi, S.V., Prentice, A., Javaid, M.K., Inskip, H.M., Godfrey, K.M., Bell, C.G., Lillycrop, K.A., Cooper, C., Harvey, N.C., 2019. Gestational vitamin D supplementation leads to reduced perinatal RXRA DNA methylation: results from the Mavidos trial. J. Bone Miner. Res. 34, 231–240.

De Castro Barbosa, T., Ingerslev, L.R., Alm, P.S., Versteyhe, S., Massart, J., Rasmussen, M., Donkin, I., Sjögren, R., Mudry, J.M., Vetterli, L., Gupta, S., Krook, A., Zierath, J.R., Barrès, R., 2016. High-fat diet reprograms the epigenome of rat spermatozoa and transgenerationally affects metabolism of the offspring. Mol. Metab. 5, 184–197.

Donkin, I., Barrès, R., 2018. Sperm epigenetics and influence of environmental factors. Mol. Metab. 14, 1–11.

Drake, A.J., McPherson, R.C., Godfrey, K.M., Cooper, C., Lillycrop, K.A., Hanson, M.A., Meehan, R.R., Seckl, J.R., Reynolds, R.M., 2012. An unbalanced maternal diet in pregnancy associates with offspring epigenetic changes in genes controlling glucocorticoid action and foetal growth. Clin. Endocrinol. 77, 808–815.

Fall, C.H.D., 2013. Fetal programming and the risk of noncommunicable disease. Indian J. Pediatr. 80 (Suppl 1), S13–S20.

Ferguson-Smith, A.C., 2011. Genomic imprinting: the emergence of an epigenetic paradigm. Nat. Rev. Genet. 12, 565–575.

Fleming, T.P., Watkins, A.J., Velazquez, M.A., Mathers, J.C., Prentice, A.M., Stephenson, J., Barker, M., Saffery, R., Yajnik, C.S., Eckert, J.J., Hanson, M.A., Forrester, T., Gluckman, P.D., Godfrey, K.M., 2018. Origins of lifetime health around the time of conception: causes and consequences. Lancet 391, 1842–1852.

Forsdahl, A., 1977. Are poor living conditions in childhood and adolescence an important risk factor for arteriosclerotic heart disease? Br. J. Prev. Soc. Med. 31, 91–95.

García-Giménez, J.L., Seco-Cervera, M., Tollefsbol, T.O., Romá-Mateo, C., Peiró-Chova, L., Lapunzina, P., Pallardó, F.V., 2017. Epigenetic biomarkers: current strategies and future challenges for their use in the clinical laboratory. Crit. Rev. Clin. Lab. Sci. 54, 529–550.

Gluckman, P.D., Hanson, M.A., Spencer, H.G., 2005. Predictive adaptive responses and human evolution. Trends Ecol. Evol. 20, 527–533.

Gluckman, P.D., Lillycrop, K.A., Vickers, M.H., Pleasants, A.B., Phillips, E.S., Beedle, A.S., Burdge, G.C., Hanson, M.A., 2007. Metabolic plasticity during mammalian development is directionally dependent on early nutritional status. Proc. Natl. Acad. Sci. 104, 12796.

Godfrey, K.M., Barker, D.J., 2001. Fetal programming and adult health. Public Health Nutr. 4, 611–624.

Godfrey, K.M., Lillycrop, K.A., Burdge, G.C., Gluckman, P.D., Hanson, M.A., 2007. Epigenetic mechanisms and the mismatch concept of the developmental origins of health and disease. Pediatr. Res. 61, 5–10.

Godfrey, K.M., Sheppard, A., Gluckman, P.D., Lillycrop, K.A., Burdge, G.C., Mclean, C., Rodford, J., Slater-Jefferies, J.L., Garratt, E., Crozier, S.R., Emerald, B.S., Gale, C.R., Inskip, H.M., Cooper, C., Hanson, M.A., 2011. Epigenetic gene promoter methylation at birth is associated with child's later adiposity. Diabetes 60, 1528–1534.

Godfrey, K.M., Reynolds, R.M., Prescott, S.L., Nyirenda, M., Jaddoe, V.W.V., Eriksson, J.G., Broekman, B.F.P., 2017. Influence of maternal obesity on the long-term health of offspring. Lancet Diabetes Endocrinol. 5, 53–64.

Haggarty, P., Hoad, G., Campbell, D.M., Horgan, G.W., Piyathilake, C., McNeill, G., 2012. Folate in pregnancy and imprinted gene and repeat element methylation in the offspring. Am. J. Clin. Nutr. 97, 94–99.

Hales, C.N., Barker, D.J., Clark, P.M., Cox, L.J., Fall, C., Osmond, C., Winter, P.D., 1991. Fetal and infant growth and impaired glucose tolerance at age 64. Br. Med. J. 303, 1019–1022.

Hanson, M.A., Gluckman, P.D., 2014. Early developmental conditioning of later health and disease: physiology or pathophysiology? Physiol. Rev. 94, 1027–1076.

Hanson, M., Godfrey, K.M., Lillycrop, K.A., Burdge, G.C., Gluckman, P.D., 2011. Developmental plasticity and developmental origins of non-communicable disease: theoretical considerations and epigenetic mechanisms. Prog. Biophys. Mol. Biol. 106, 272–280.

Harvey, N.C., Sheppard, A., Godfrey, K.M., Mclean, C., Garratt, E., Ntani, G., Davies, L., Murray, R., Inskip, H.M., Gluckman, P.D., Hanson, M.A., Lillycrop, K.A., Cooper, C., 2014. Childhood bone mineral content is associated with methylation status of the RXRA promoter at birth. J. Bone Miner. Res. 29, 600–607.

Hawkins, P.G., Santoso, S., Adams, C., Anest, V., Morris, K.V., 2009. Promoter targeted small RNAs induce long-term transcriptional gene silencing in human cells. Nucleic Acids Res. 37, 2984–2995.

Heijmans, B.T., Tobi, E.W., Stein, A.D., Putter, H., Blauw, G.J., Susser, E.S., Slagboom, P.E., Lumey, L.H., 2008. Persistent epigenetic differences associated with prenatal exposure to famine in humans. Proc. Natl. Acad. Sci. 105, 17046–17049.

Heindel, J.J., Vandenberg, L.N., 2015. Developmental origins of health and disease: a paradigm for understanding disease cause and prevention. Curr. Opin. Pediatr. 27, 248–253.

Hoile, S.P., Lillycrop, K.A., Grenfell, L.R., Hanson, M.A., Burdge, G.C., 2012. Increasing the folic acid content of maternal or post-weaning diets induces differential changes in phosphoenolpyruvate carboxykinase mRNA expression and promoter methylation in rats. Br. J. Nutr. 108, 852–857.

Hoile, S.P., Irvine, N.A., Kelsall, C.J., Sibbons, C., Feunteun, A., Collister, A., Torrens, C., Calder, P.C., Hanson, M.A., Lillycrop, K.A., Burdge, G.C., 2013. Maternal fat intake in rats alters 20:4n-6 and 22:6n-3 status and the epigenetic regulation of Fads2 in offspring liver. J. Nutr. Biochem. 24, 1213–1220.

Jimenez-Chillaron, J.C., Isganaitis, E., Charalambous, M., Gesta, S., Pentinat-Pelegrin, T., Faucette, R.R., Otis, J.P., Chow, A., Diaz, R., Ferguson-Smith, A., Patti, M.-E., 2009. Intergenerational transmission of glucose intolerance and obesity by in utero undernutrition in mice. Diabetes 58, 460–468.

Kaati, G., Bygren, L.O., Edvinsson, S., 2002. Cardiovascular and diabetes mortality determined by nutrition during parents' and grandparents' slow growth period. Eur. J. Hum. Genet. 10, 682–688.

Kelly, T.K., De Carvalho, D.D., Jones, P.A., 2010. Epigenetic modifications as therapeutic targets. Nat. Biotechnol. 28, 1069–1078.

Kelsall, C.J., Hoile, S.P., Irvine, N.A., Masoodi, M., Torrens, C., Lillycrop, K.A., Calder, P.C., Clough, G.F., Hanson, M.A., Burdge, G.C., 2012. Vascular dysfunction induced in offspring by maternal dietary fat involves altered arterial polyunsaturated fatty acid biosynthesis. PLoS One 7, e34492.

Kim, D.H., Sætrom, P., Snøve, O., Rossi, J.J., 2008. MicroRNA-directed transcriptional gene silencing in mammalian cells. Proc. Natl. Acad. Sci. 105, 16230–16235.

Kliewer, S.A., Forman, B.M., Blumberg, B., Ong, E.S., Borgmeyer, U., Mangelsdorf, D.J., Umesono, K., Evans, R.M., 1994. Differential expression and activation of a family of murine peroxisome proliferator-activated receptors. Proc. Natl. Acad. Sci. 91, 7355.

Krek, A., Grün, D., Poy, M.N., Wolf, R., Rosenberg, L., Epstein, E.J., Macmenamin, P., Da Piedade, I., Gunsalus, K.C., Stoffel, M., Rajewsky, N., 2005. Combinatorial microRNA target predictions. Nat. Genet. 37, 495–500.

Langley, S.C., Seakins, M., Grimble, R.F., Jackson, A.A., 1994. The acute phase response of adult rats is altered by in utero exposure to maternal low protein diets. J. Nutr. 124, 1588–1596.

Lillycrop, K.A., Slater-Jefferies, J.L., Hanson, M.A., Godfrey, K.M., Jackson, A.A., Burdge, G.C., 2007. Induction of altered epigenetic regulation of the hepatic glucocorticoid receptor in the offspring of rats fed a protein-restricted diet during pregnancy suggests that reduced DNA methyltransferase-1 expression is involved in impaired DNA methylation and changes in histone modifications. Br. J. Nutr. 97, 1064–1073.

Lillycrop, K.A., Phillips, E.S., Torrens, C., Hanson, M.A., Jackson, A.A., Burdge, G.C., 2008. Feeding pregnant rats a protein-restricted diet persistently alters the methylation of specific cytosines in the hepatic PPARα promoter of the offspring. Br. J. Nutr. 100, 278–282.

Lillycrop, K., Murray, R., Cheong, C., Teh, A.L., Clarke-Harris, R., Barton, S., Costello, P., Garratt, E., Cook, E., Titcombe, P., Shunmuganathan, B., Liew, S.J., Chua, Y.C., Lin, X., Wu, Y., Burdge, G.C., Cooper, C., Inskip, H.M., Karnani, N., Hopkins, J.C., Childs, C.E., Chavez, C.P., Calder, P.C., Yap, F., Lee, Y.S., Chong, Y.S., Melton, P.E., Beilin, L., Huang, R.C., Gluckman, P.D., Harvey, N., Hanson, M.A., Holbrook, J.D., Godfrey, K.M., 2017. ANRIL promoter DNA methylation: a perinatal marker for later adiposity. EBioMedicine 19, 60–72.

Lillycrop, K.A., Garratt, E.S., Titcombe, P., Melton, P.E., Murray, R.J.S., Barton, S.J., Clarke-Harris, R., Costello, P.M., Holbrook, J.D., Hopkins, J.C., Childs, C.E., Paras-Chavez, C., Calder, P.C., Mori, T.A., Beilin, L., Burdge, G.C., Gluckman, P.D., Inskip, H.M., Harvey, N.C., Hanson, M.A., Huang, R.-C., Cooper, C., Godfrey, K.M., Epigen, C., 2019. Differential SLC6A4 methylation: a predictive epigenetic marker of adiposity from birth to adulthood. Int. J. Obes. 43, 974–988.

Mahajan, A., Sapehia, D., Thakur, S., Mohanraj, P.S., Bagga, R., Kaur, J., 2019. Effect of imbalance in folate and vitamin B12 in maternal/parental diet on global methylation and regulatory miRNAs. Sci. Rep. 9, 17602.

Marco, A., Kisliouk, T., Weller, A., Meiri, N., 2013. High fat diet induces hypermethylation of the hypothalamic Pomc promoter and obesity in post-weaning rats. Psychoneuroendocrinology 38, 2844–2853.

Mathers, C.D., Loncar, D., 2006. Projections of global mortality and burden of disease from 2002 to 2030. PLoS Med. 3, e442.

Maute, R.L., Schneider, C., Sumazin, P., Holmes, A., Califano, A., Basso, K., Dalla-Favera, R., 2013. tRNA-derived microRNA modulates proliferation and the DNA damage response and is down-regulated in B cell lymphoma. Proc. Natl. Acad. Sci. U. S. A. 110, 1404–1409.

Miller, J.L., Grant, P.A., 2013. The role of DNA methylation and histone modifications in transcriptional regulation in humans. Subcell. Biochem. 61, 289–317.

Moosavi, A., Motevalizadeh Ardekani, A., 2016. Role of epigenetics in biology and human diseases. Iran. Biomed. J. 20, 246–258.

Morris, K.V., Chan, S.W.-L., Jacobsen, S.E., Looney, D.J., 2004. Small interfering RNA-induced transcriptional gene silencing in human cells. Science 305, 1289–1292.

Nätt, D., Kugelberg, U., Casas, E., Nedstrand, E., Zalavary, S., Henriksson, P., Nijm, C., Jäderquist, J., Sandborg, J., Flinke, E., Ramesh, R., Örkenby, L., Appelkvist, F., Lingg, T., Guzzi, N., Bellodi, C., Löf, M., Vavouri, T., Öst, A., 2019. Human sperm displays rapid responses to diet. PLoS Biol. 17, e3000559.

Ng, S.F., Lin, R.C.Y., Maloney, C.A., Youngson, N.A., Owens, J.A., Morris, M.J., 2014. Paternal high-fat diet consumption induces common changes in the transcriptomes of retroperitoneal adipose and pancreatic islet tissues in female rat offspring. FASEB J. 28, 1830–1841.

Ong, K.K., 2006. Size at birth, postnatal growth and risk of obesity. Horm. Res. Paediatr. 65 (suppl 3), 65–69.

Oses, M., Margareto Sanchez, J., Portillo, M.P., Aguilera, C.M., Labayen, I., 2019. Circulating miRNAs as biomarkers of obesity and obesity-associated comorbidities in children and adolescents: a systematic review. Nutrients 11, 2890.

O'Tierney, P.F., Barker, D.J.P., Osmond, C., Kajantie, E., Eriksson, J.G., 2009. Duration of breast-feeding and adiposity in adult life. J. Nutr. 139 (2), 422S–425S. https://doi.org/10.3945/jn.108.097089.

Painter, R.C., Roseboom, T.J., Bleker, O.P., 2005. Prenatal exposure to the Dutch famine and disease in later life: an overview. Reprod. Toxicol. 20, 345–352.

Patel, N., Pasupathy, D., Poston, L., 2015. Determining the consequences of maternal obesity for offspring health. Exp. Physiol. 100, 1421–1428.

Pauwels, S., Ghosh, M., Duca, R.C., Bekaert, B., Freson, K., Huybrechts, I., Langie, S.A.S., Koppen, G., Devlieger, R., Godderis, L., 2017. Maternal intake of methyl-group donors affects Dna methylation of metabolic genes in infants. Clin. Epigenetics 9, 16.

Pembrey, M.E., Bygren, L.O., Kaati, G., Edvinsson, S., Northstone, K., Sjöström, M., Golding, J., The, A.S.T., 2006. Sex-specific, male-line transgenerational responses in humans. Eur. J. Hum. Genet. 14, 159–166.

Pettitt, D.J., Jovanovic, L., 2001. Birth weight as a predictor of type 2 diabetes mellitus: the U-shaped curve. Curr. Diab. Rep. 1, 78–81.

Plagemann, A., Harder, T., Brunn, M., Harder, A., Roepke, K., Wittrock-Staar, M., Ziska, T., Schellong, K., Rodekamp, E., Melchior, K., Dudenhausen, J.W., 2009. Hypothalamic proopiomelanocortin promoter methylation becomes altered by early overfeeding: an epigenetic model of obesity and the metabolic syndrome. J. Physiol. 587, 4963–4976.

Rakyan, V.K., Blewitt, M.E., Druker, R., Preis, J.I., Whitelaw, E., 2002. Metastable epialleles in mammals. Trends Genet. 18, 348–351.

Richmond, R.C., Sharp, G.C., Herbert, G., Atkinson, C., Taylor, C., Bhattacharya, S., Campbell, D., Hall, M., Kazmi, N., Gaunt, T., McArdle, W., Ring, S., Davey Smith, G., Ness, A., Relton, C.L., 2018. The long-term impact of folic acid in pregnancy on offspring DNA methylation: follow-up of the Aberdeen folic acid supplementation trial (AFAST). Int. J. Epidemiol. 47, 928–937.

Rijlaarsdam, J., Cecil, C.A.M., Walton, E., Mesirow, M.S.C., Relton, C.L., Gaunt, T.R., McArdle, W., Barker, E.D., 2017. Prenatal unhealthy diet, insulin-like growth factor 2 gene (IGF2) methylation, and attention deficit hyperactivity disorder symptoms in youth with early-onset conduct problems. J. Child Psychol. Psychiatry 58, 19–27.

Robinson, S.M., Marriott, L.D., Crozier, S.R., Harvey, N.C., Gale, C.R., Inskip, H.M., Baird, J., Law, C.M., Godfrey, K.M., Cooper, C., 2009. Variations in infant feeding practice are associated with body composition in childhood: a prospective cohort study. J. Clin. Endocrinol. Metab. 94, 2799–2805.

Robinson, S.M., Crozier, S.R., Harvey, N.C., Barton, B.D., Law, C.M., Godfrey, K.M., Cooper, C., Inskip, H.M., 2015. Modifiable early-life risk factors for childhood adiposity and overweight: an analysis of their combined impact and potential for prevention. Am. J. Clin. Nutr. 101, 368–375.

Roseboom, T., De Rooij, S., Painter, R., 2006. The Dutch famine and its long-term consequences for adult health. Early Hum. Dev. 82, 485–491.

Samuelsson, A.-M., Matthews, P.A., Argenton, M., Christie, M.R., McConnell, J.M., Jansen, E.H.J.M., Piersma, A.H., Ozanne, S.E., Twinn, D.F., Remacle, C., Rowlerson, A., Poston, L., Taylor, P.D., 2008. Diet-induced obesity in female mice leads to offspring hyperphagia, adiposity, hypertension, and insulin resistance. Hypertension 51, 383–392.

Sandovici, I., Smith, N.H., Nitert, M.D., Ackers-Johnson, M., Uribe-Lewis, S., Ito, Y., Jones, R.H., Marquez, V.E., Cairns, W., Tadayyon, M., O'neill, L.P., Murrell, A., Ling, C., Constancia, M., Ozanne, S.E., 2011. Maternal diet and aging alter the epigenetic control of a promoter-enhancer interaction at the Hnf4a gene in rat pancreatic islets. Proc. Natl. Acad. Sci. U. S. A. 108, 5449–5454.

Schimmel, P., 2018. The emerging complexity of the tRNA world: mammalian tRNAs beyond protein synthesis. Nat. Rev. Mol. Cell Biol. 19, 45–58.

Sharma, U., Conine, C.C., Shea, J.M., Boskovic, A., Derr, A.G., Bing, X.Y., Belleannee, C., Kucukural, A., Serra, R.W., Sun, F., Song, L., Carone, B.R., Ricci, E.P., Li, X.Z., Fauquier, L., Moore, M.J., Sullivan, R., Mello, C.C., Garber, M., Rando, O.J., 2016. Biogenesis and function of tRNA fragments during sperm maturation and fertilization in mammals. Science 351, 391–396.

Siddeek, B., Mauduit, C., Simeoni, U., Benahmed, M., 2018. Sperm epigenome as a marker of environmental exposure and lifestyle, at the origin of diseases inheritance. Mutat. Res. Rev. Mutat. Res. 778, 38–44.

Siddeek, B., Mauduit, C., Chehade, H., Blin, G., Liand, M., Chindamo, M., Benahmed, M., Simeoni, U., 2019. Long-term impact of maternal high-fat diet on offspring cardiac health: role of micro-RNA biogenesis. Cell Death Dis. 5, 71.

Steegers-Theunissen, R.P., Obermann-Borst, S.A., Kremer, D., Lindemans, J., Siebel, C., Steegers, E.A., Slagboom, P.E., Heijmans, B.T., 2009. Periconceptional maternal folic acid use of 400 μg per day is related to increased methylation of the IGF2 gene in the very young child. PLoS One 4, e7845.

Teh, A.L., Pan, H., Chen, L., Ong, M.L., Dogra, S., Wong, J., MacIsaac, J.L., Mah, S.M., McEwen, L.M., Saw, S.M., Godfrey, K.M., Chong, Y.S., Kwek, K., Kwoh, C.K., Soh, S.E., Chong, M.F., Barton, S., Karnani, N., Cheong, C.Y., Buschdorf, J.P., Stünkel, W., Kobor, M.S., Meaney, M.J., Gluckman, P.D., Holbrook, J.D., 2014. The effect of genotype and in utero environment on interindividual variation in neonate DNA methylomes. Genome Res. 24, 1064–1074.

Terashima, M., Barbour, S., Ren, J., Yu, W., Han, Y., Muegge, K., 2015. Effect of high fat diet on paternal sperm histone distribution and male offspring liver gene expression. Epigenetics 10, 861–871.

Tessarz, P., Kouzarides, T., 2014. Histone core modifications regulating nucleosome structure and dynamics. Nat. Rev. Mol. Cell Biol. 15, 703–708.

Titcombe, P., Murray, R., Hewitt, M., Antoun, E., Cooper, C., Inskip, H.M., Holbrook, J.D., Godfrey, K.M., Lillycrop, K., Hanson, M., Barton, S.J., 2021. Human non-CpG methylation patterns display both tissue-specific and interindividual differences suggestive of underlying function. Epigenetics, 1–12.

Tobi, E.W., Lumey, L.H., Talens, R.P., Kremer, D., Putter, H., Stein, A.D., Slagboom, P.E., Heijmans, B.T., 2009. DNA methylation differences after exposure to prenatal famine are common and timing- and sex-specific. Hum. Mol. Genet. 18, 4046–4053.

Torrens, C., Poston, L., Hanson, M.A., 2008. Transmission of raised blood pressure and endothelial dysfunction to the F2 generation induced by maternal protein restriction in the F0, in the absence of dietary challenge in the F1 generation. Br. J. Nutr. 100, 760–766.

Turner, B.M., 2000. Histone acetylation and an epigenetic code. BioEssays 22, 836–845.

Vaz, C., Kermack, A.J., Burton, M., Tan, P.F., Huan, J., Yoo, T.P.X., Donnelly, K., Wellstead, S.J., Fisk, H.L., Houghton, F.D., Lewis, S., Chong, Y.S., Gluckman, P.D., Cheong, Y., Macklon, N.S., Calder, P.C., Dutta, A., Godfrey, K.M., Kumar, P., Lillycrop, K.A., Karnani, N., 2021. Short-Term Diet Intervention Alters the Small Non-coding RNA (sncRNA) Landscape of Human Sperm. BioRxiv. 2021.07.08.451257.

Voerman, E., Santos, S., Patro Golab, B., Amiano, P., Ballester, F., Barros, H., Bergström, A., Charles, M.-A., Chatzi, L., Chevrier, C., Chrousos, G.P., Corpeleijn, E., Costet, N., Crozier, S., Devereux, G., Eggesbø, M., Ekström, S., Fantini, M.P., Farchi, S., Forastiere, F., Georgiu, V., Godfrey, K.M., Gori, D., Grote, V., Hanke, W., Hertz-Picciotto, I., Heude, B., Hryhorczuk, D., Huang, R.-C., Inskip, H., Iszatt, N., Karvonen, A.M., Kenny, L.C., Koletzko, B., Küpers, L.K., Lagström, H., Lehmann, I., Magnus, P., Majewska, R., Mäkelä, J., Manios, Y., McAuliffe, F.M., McDonald, S.W., Mehegan, J., Mommers, M., Morgen, C.S., Mori, T.A., Moschonis, G., Murray, D., Chaoimh, C.N., Nohr, E.A., Nybo Andersen, A.-M., Oken, E., Oostvogels, A.J.J.M., Pac, A., Papadopoulou, E., Pekkanen, J., Pizzi, C., Polanska, K., Porta, D., Richiardi, L., Rifas-Shiman, S.L., Ronfani, L., Santos, A.C., Standl, M., Stoltenberg, C., Thiering, E., Thijs, C., Torrent, M., Tough, S.C., Trnovec, T., Turner, S., Van Rossem, L., Von Berg, A., Vrijheid, M., Vrijkotte, T.G.M., West, J., Wijga, A., Wright, J., Zvinchuk, O., Sørensen, T.I.A., Lawlor, D.A., Gaillard, R., Jaddoe, V.W.V., 2019. Maternal body mass index, gestational weight gain, and the risk of overweight and obesity across childhood: an individual participant data meta-analysis. PLoS Med. 16, e1002744.

Vucetic, Z., Kimmel, J., Totoki, K., Hollenbeck, E., Reyes, T.M., 2010. Maternal high-fat diet alters methylation and gene expression of dopamine and opioid-related genes. Endocrinology 151, 4756–4764.

Waterland, R.A., Kellermayer, R., Laritsky, E., Rayco-Solon, P., Harris, R.A., Travisano, M., Zhang, W., Torskaya, M.S., Zhang, J., Shen, L., Manary, M.J., Prentice, A.M., 2010. Season of conception in rural Gambia affects DNA methylation at putative human metastable Epialleles. PLoS Genet. 6, e1001252.

Watkins, A.J., Dias, I., Tsuro, H., Allen, D., Emes, R.D., Moreton, J., Wilson, R., Ingram, R.J.M., Sinclair, K.D., 2018. Paternal diet programs offspring health through sperm- and seminal plasma-specific pathways in mice. Proc. Natl. Acad. Sci. 115, 10064–10069.

Wolff, G.L., Kodell, R.L., Moore, S.R., Cooney, C.A., 1998. Maternal epigenetics and methyl supplements affect agouti gene expression in Avy/a mice. FASEB J. 12, 949–957.

Yadav, D.K., Shrestha, S., Lillycrop, K.A., Joglekar, C.V., Pan, H., Holbrook, J.D., Fall, C.H., Yajnik, C.S., Chandak, G.R., 2018. Vitamin B(12) supplementation influences methylation of genes associated with type 2 diabetes and its intermediate traits. Epigenomics 10, 71–90.

Yang, A.Y., Kim, H., Li, W., Kong, A.-N.T., 2016. Natural compound-derived epigenetic regulators targeting epigenetic readers, writers and erasers. Curr. Top. Med. Chem. 16, 697–713.

Zampetaki, A., Albrecht, A., Steinhofel, K., 2018. Long non-coding RNA structure and function: is there a link? Front. Physiol. 9, 1201.

Zhang, Y., Kutateladze, T.G., 2018. Diet and the epigenome. Nat. Commun. 9, 3375.

Zhang, J., Zhang, F., Didelot, X., Bruce, K.D., Cagampang, F.R., Vatish, M., Hanson, M., Lehnert, H., Ceriello, A., Byrne, C.D., 2009. Maternal high fat diet during pregnancy and lactation alters hepatic expression of insulin like growth factor-2 and key microRNAs in the adult offspring. BMC Genomics 10, 478.

Zheng, J., Xiao, X., Zhang, Q., Wang, T., Yu, M., Xu, J., 2017. Maternal low-protein diet modulates glucose metabolism and hepatic microRNAs expression in the early life of offspring†. Nutrients 9, 205.

# PART II

# Early nutrition and development of non-communicable diseases

# Early life nutrition and its effect on the development of obesity and type-2 diabetes

*Mark H. Vickers*

Liggins Institute, University of Auckland, Auckland, New Zealand

## LEARNING OBJECTIVES

- To understand factors influencing the relationship between early life nutrition and subsequent development of obesity and type 2 diabetes.

- To identify evidence from human observational studies and animal research models that demonstrate developmental programming of obesity and type 2 diabetes in offspring.

- To describe how altered maternal nutrition, including under- and overnutrition, and

- emerging evidence for paternal effects contribute to transgenerational impacts related to obesity and type 2 diabetes.

- To recognize potential mechanisms by which early nutrition and epigenetics can result in lifelong changes in metabolic processes involved in the development of obesity and type 2 diabetes.

## 11.1 Introduction

Despite intensive research and public policy efforts, the prevalence of obesity and related cardiometabolic disorders including type 2 diabetes mellitus (T2DM) continues to rise rapidly globally and presents a growing health and economic burden (Blüher, 2019; Chatterjee et al., 2017). Once seen as a problem in developed countries, rates of obesity and related noncommunicable diseases including T2DM are rising rapidly in developing and transitioning economies, particularly in urban settings with changes in lifestyle including nutrition transitions. The number of people with T2DM was estimated to have increased from 171 million in 2000 to 415 million in 2015 with the incidence projected to rise to 642 million adults by 2040 (Guariguata et al., 2014; Zheng et al., 2018). With regard to obesity, the worldwide prevalence has almost tripled between 1975 and 2016 (Marousez et al., 2019). Of increasing concern are the rising rates of childhood and adolescent overweight/obesity (Lascar et al., 2018; Weihrauch-Blüher and Wiegand, 2018), with overweight and obesity in children and adolescents rising from 4% in 1975 to over 18% in 2016 (WHO, 2018) with T2DM rates increasing in parallel to the increased rates of pediatric obesity. Although in part, the increasing prevalence arises due to increased rates of obesity in those with a genetic predisposition, studies examining the genetic contribution to obesity have demonstrated that of the variants characterized to date, the estimated genetic contribution to T2DM is less than 10%, suggesting that additional environmental factors and gene–environment interactions contribute to disease risk (Morris et al., 2012; Lango et al., 2008; McCarthy and Zeggini, 2009; Jackson et al., 2020). As such, obesity and T2DM risk can arise from a complex interaction between genetic susceptibility and exposure to a suboptimal nutritional environment and, as stated by Bray, "Genes load the gun, the environment pulls the trigger." In this context, data derived from epidemiological studies and experimental animal models have highlighted a relationship between early life development (i.e., periconceptual, fetal, and infancy, also commonly referred to as the "First 1000 Days") and later predisposition to a range of cardiometabolic disorders including obesity and T2DM. The term "developmental programming" is used to describe these associations under the developmental origins of health and disease (DOHaD) framework. The mechanistic processes underpinning such early life programming and the relative roles of genes versus environment and the interactions therein are yet to be fully defined. It has been proposed that, in response to a suboptimal environment in utero, the fetus makes physiological adaptations during development to optimize the chances for survival in the immediate environment. Such adaptations may include the resetting of homeostatic set points for cardiometabolic processes and altered growth trajectory resulting in an altered birth phenotype. The "thrifty phenotype" (Hales and Barker, 2001) and "predictive adaptive response" (PARs) hypotheses propose that the extent of the "mismatch" between the prenatal and postnatal environments may represent a key determinant (and potential trigger) for later disease risk. Thus, while adaptive changes in physiology in early development may be beneficial for short-term survival in utero and early infancy, they may become maladaptive over time and result in adverse health outcomes in later life when offspring are exposed to, for example, obesogenic diets, catch-up growth, and other environmental triggers. The role of the maternal diet in the programming of later obesity and T2DM risk has been well established with fetal malnutrition and/or rapid postnatal growth, as well as a maternal obesogenic environment, all associated with an increased propensity for offspring to develop obesity and T2DM. Further complicating mechanistic insights, there are clear evidence of sex-specific effects as well as an emerging body of evidence for the role of paternal factors influencing obesity and T2DM risk in progeny (Paternal Origins of Health and Disease) (Ng et al., 2014, 2010; Soubry, 2018; Magnus et al., 2018; Hur et al., 2017). In addition, evidence suggests transgenerational transmission of disease risk thus mediating a perpetuating cycle of disease across generations (Berends and Ozanne, 2012; Catalano, 2003).

## 11.2 Developmental programming of obesity and T2DM

### 11.2.1 Evidence from human observations

The early work of David Barker highlighted a clear association between born of low birth weight (LBW) and later risk for obesity, T2DM, hypertension, and disorders of lipid metabolism. Following these observations, studies of famine exposure were used to examine the impact of altered maternal nutrition and the effect of suboptimal nutrition in utero on birth outcomes and later disease outcomes. Of these, the most widely reported is that of the Dutch Hunger Winter (also known as the Dutch Famine) of 1944–45. In these studies, the timing of famine exposure was observed to be a major driver of later offspring outcomes. As an example, whereas exposure to famine during early pregnancy was linked to a greater later risk for the development of hypertension in adulthood, maternal exposure to famine in late pregnancy resulted in an increased risk for adiposity and impaired glucose tolerance in adults. Further, exposure to famine in late pregnancy predisposed offspring to a greater degree of glucose intolerance than during early or mid-pregnancy. Obesity rates were higher in male offspring exposed in the first half of pregnancy and lower in males exposed in the last trimester of pregnancy as compared to non-exposed males. These observations thus suggested that while exposure of the fetus to a substrate-limited environment at most stages of development leads to metabolic disorders in adulthood, the precise mechanisms and degree of severity of dysregulation can vary with the timing/duration of exposure. Studies in adults born during the Great Chinese Famine (1959–61) reported that famine-exposed offspring were more likely to be overweight and have T2DM as compared to those born post-famine (Li and Lumey, 2017). Of note, interactions between the effects of the famine with a transgenerational risk of developing T2DM have been proposed as a key factor contributing to the current epidemic of T2DM in China (Zimmet et al., 2018). Of interest, a more recent example of adverse maternal exposures, the Quebec Ice Storm (1998), further highlighted the link between increased prenatal stress and alterations in metabolic pathways involved in energy metabolism in offspring thus predisposing to later insulin resistance (IR) and obesity (Paxman et al., 2018; Liu et al., 2016).

In populations such as those in India which were historically undernourished, rapid urbanization has resulted in individuals born of LBW being increasingly exposed to obesogenic Western-style diets with the rates of obesity and T2DM reaching epidemic levels (Gulati and Misra, 2014; Misra et al., 2011). In India, babies born of LBW commonly exhibit relatively increased visceral adiposity (the so-called thin-fat phenotype (D'angelo et al., 2015)), and their increased risk for T2DM in later life is reflected in higher leptin and insulin and reduced adiponectin concentrations in cord blood (Yajnik, 2014). This is supported in other studies of LBW babies where, despite a lower body mass index, they show a disproportionate abdominal fat mass in adulthood. In a multi-ethnic cohort of around 3000 women, LBW was directly predictive of a higher risk for development of T2DM in later life with the associations between LBW (< 2.72 kg) and later T2DM risk primarily driven by IR but further explained by systolic blood pressure and circulating concentrations of sex hormone-binding globulin and E-selectin (Song et al., 2015). Although there remains a debate whether rapid catch-up growth in the early postnatal period is indeed beneficial or not, most human and experimental evidence to date suggest that such "catch-up" growth is linked to adverse metabolic outcomes in adulthood. As an example, it has been shown that children born small for gestational age

(SGA) who then have catch-up growth have increased circulating leptin concentrations which were correlated significantly with markers of insulin sensitivity.

Early research in the area of developmental programming focused on LBW as a proxy for a perturbed in-utero environment. However, although fetal growth restriction has been demonstrated to impact the long-term risk of increased adiposity in offspring, it needs to be noted that the link between weight at birth and disease risk in later life is not a linear relationship and represents a "U" shaped response curve. As such, those babies born large for gestational age (macrosomic) may also be at an increased risk of developing obesity and T2DM, associations supported by studies examining the long-term outcomes of maternal diabetes or gestational diabetes (GDM) on offspring. Further, even though some obese mothers are not clinically diagnosed with GDM, they may still have cardiometabolic risk factors that impact the growth of the fetus and later health outcomes. This has also been explored under the "fetal insulin hypothesis" and the "fuel-mediated hypothesis" (Shapiro et al., 2015). Under the "fetal insulin hypothesis," genetically determined IR leads to an impairment of insulin-mediated fetal growth as well as IR in adulthood. Under the "fuel mediated hypothesis," it is proposed that metabolic phenotypes in overweight/obese pregnant women, characterized by increased IR and increased circulating fuels, lead to fetal "overnutrition" and subsequent increase of adiposity in offspring. It needs to be noted that, although maternal obesity is often associated with macrosomia and large birth weight arising from GDM in particular, obese pregnancies can also be characterized by intrauterine growth restriction (IUGR) (Radulescu et al., 2013; Ornoy, 2011). This may be due to placental insufficiency with impaired placental structure and function resulting in altered nutrient transport as has been shown previously in the rat (Mark et al., 2011).

In developed societies and those societies that have transitioned or are transitioning to "Western" style diets and lifestyle habits, consumption of poor quality diets high in fats and sugar is generally excessive with maternal overweight/obesity becoming a common complication of pregnancy. Maternal obesity is well established to be associated with a number of complications of pregnancy including fetal and neonatal mortality and lactational insufficiency and remains the most significant predictor of obesity in childhood and later development of the metabolic syndrome. These effects lead to a cycle of disease, as those offspring of obese mothers are themselves predisposed to T2DM and obesity, leading to intergenerational effects via the so-called vicious cycle of obesity and cardiometabolic disorders (Catalano, 2003).

## 11.2.2 Evidence from experimental animal models

Extensive work across a range of experimental animal models have provided extensive empirical data to support the DOHaD framework and have been key to understanding the mechanisms underpinning the link between altered early life nutrition and later risk for development of obesity and T2DM. Although data from epidemiological studies suggest that programming can occur within the normal birth weight ranges, early animal models were primarily focused on inducing significant IUGR given that insults impacting on the normal growth of the fetus were likely those that lead to aberrant developmental programming. Experimental approaches of altered maternal nutrition across a wide range of model species have been utilized to induce IUGR. In the rodent, obesity and cardiometabolic disorders have been induced in offspring using moderate (50%–70% of ad-libitum) or severe (30% of ad-libitum) global maternal undernutrition, a low protein (LP) diet (typically 8% vs 20% protein) (Ma et al., 2018), and maternal micronutrient deficiencies (Tomat et al., 2011; Vanhees et al., 2014). In this context, however, it is not *essential* to induce IUGR to lead to developmental programming, but provides surrogate evidence for aberrant in utero development.

Epidemiological observations and evidence derived from animal models clearly demonstrates that IUGR is associated with an increased risk for a range of adult metabolic disorders, implying that nutrient deprivation in early life is a strong programming stimulus. However, in many developed and transitioning societies, maternal and postnatal caloric intake can be excessive. As such, a range of pre-clinical models of excess maternal caloric intake have been developed using either single fat "open source" diets or a cafeteria diet-style approach. Both dietary approaches have some limitations, for example, the nutritional component of a cafeteria diet is relatively uncontrolled (Moore, 1987), while a single fat source diet is not reflective of a complex Western-style human diet (Sampey et al., 2011). However, experimental models using both ends of the maternal dietary range have clearly shown that programming of obesity and T2DM risk represents a "U-shaped" curve with increased rates of obesity and T2DM in adults who were exposed to either suboptimal or excessive levels of maternal nutrition. It also needs to be noted that models of "overnutrition" may indeed reflect models of malnutrition (the so-called double burden of malnutrition (Wells et al., 2020)) due to deficiencies in key vitamins and minerals and may in part reflect the similar phenotypic outcomes seen across disparate nutritional models.

### 11.2.2.1 *Maternal undernutrition*

Undernutrition can be achieved through restriction of the maternal diet during the periconceptional period and during pregnancy and/or lactation. Two dietary approaches in experimental models have been widely used, which are global undernutrition or isocaloric LP diets (Vickers et al., 2000; Howie et al., 2012; Desai et al., 2005).

Global dietary restriction during pregnancy and/or lactation is a commonly used approach to examine the impact of nutritional programming of obesity and T2DM with a number of rodent models developed and characterized utilizing global maternal undernutrition at different levels/developmental stages. In the rat, pregnant mothers fed at 30% of ad-libitum intake throughout pregnancy (i.e., a "severe" level of undernutrition) have birthweights and placental weights that are typically 25%–30% lower than the offspring of ad-libitum fed mothers. These offspring exhibit increased fat mass, IR, elevated blood pressure, hyperleptinemia, reduced voluntary locomotor activity, and appetite dysregulation in adulthood, these effects will be amplified when they are exposed to a post-weaning high fat (HF) diet. When the level of undernutrition in the mother is reduced to a moderate level (50% of controls), offspring still display increased fat mass and metabolic disturbances in adulthood. Of note, if catch-up growth in offspring in the pre-weaning period is prevented by continuation of the dietary restriction of the mother throughout lactation, offspring are conferred protection against the later development of obesity and related metabolic disorders (Howie et al., 2012). This is similar to reports in the LP model (detailed below), whereby extending the period of exposure to the LP diet into lactation can prevent the development of the metabolic phenotype, further suggesting that rapid catch-up growth can potentially have deleterious effects in offspring in the long term.

The LP model in the rodent involves feeding of a diet containing 8%–9% (w/w) protein (casein), approximately half the protein content but equivalent in energy of a standard control diet containing 18%–20% protein. LP-fed mothers have offspring that have birthweights typically 15%–20% lower than offspring of control-fed mothers. Feeding the LP diet through the period of lactation further exacerbates the differences in body weight and leads to persistent growth reductions. If LP offspring are cross-fostered to mothers fed a standard diet, they demonstrate rapid catch-up growth, which as detailed earlier may predispose to an increased risk for later disease (Singhal, 2017). The LP diet model has provided utility in highlighting a range of potential mechanistic processes that may be involved in the development and progression of obesity and T2DM. In particular, protein supply during pregnancy has been widely demonstrated to play a major role in the development of pancreatic β-cells with offspring of LP dams exhibiting reduced proliferation of neonatal β-cells, islet size, and vasculature in addition to glucose intolerance in adulthood (Fernandez-Twinn and Ozanne, 2010; Snoeck et al., 1990). However, it needs to be recognized that since LP models utilize an isocaloric diet approach, LP diets are typically characterized by relative increases in fat and carbohydrate intake, thus ascribing the observed deleterious effects in offspring directly to protein deficiency per se can be difficult.

Although programming effects associated with altered maternal macronutrient intake have been well described, micronutrient restriction has not been as widely investigated. Even in developed countries, where a balanced diet is accessible, micronutrient inadequacies remain common due to intake of generally high fat: high sugar and low-quality diets with suboptimal intake particularly of iron, vitamin D, folate, iodine, vitamin B12, and docosahexaenoic acid (Cetin et al., 2019). Restriction of specific micronutrients during pregnancy has been associated with the nutritional programming of a number of cardiometabolic abnormalities in offspring. As an example, maternal anemia in the rat results in several characteristics of the metabolic syndrome (Gambling et al., 2002), with the timing of iron supplementation to the mother key in ameliorating the in utero effects of maternal anemia and later outcomes in offspring. These data are supported by evidence from clinical studies where maternal iron supplementation results in a reduced incidence of LBW and a higher average birth weight. In the rat, maternal diets either high or low in salt result in altered renal development and increases in systolic blood pressure in adult male offspring with work by Segovia et al. also showing that maternal HF and high salt diets lead to differential and sex-specific programming effects on metabolism in offspring (Segovia et al., 2018; Reynolds et al., 2015c).

Vitamin D status in woman in the second trimester has also been associated with an elevated risk for offspring being born SGA (Gernand et al., 2014). With the well-established effects of vitamin D on glucose homeostasis and IR, it is therefore unsurprising that vitamin D deficiency in some populations parallels increases in T2DM prevalence (G and Gupta, 2014; Van Belle et al., 2013). There remains limited evidence as to whether supplementation with vitamin D during pregnancy and lactation improves fetal and infant growth and developmental outcomes in populations characterized by high rates of vitamin D deficiency. In a recent study by Roth et al. in a population with widespread prenatal vitamin D deficiency and fetal and infant growth restriction, supplementation with vitamin D from mid-pregnancy until birth or until 6 months postnatally did not significantly improve fetal or infant growth (Roth et al., 2018). However, a meta-analysis on the effect of vitamin D supplementation during pregnancy showed associations with increased birth weight and birth length although acknowledged that larger, better-designed randomized control trials were required to reach a definitive conclusion (Pérez-López et al., 2015).

In the rat, magnesium restriction during pregnancy and the early neonatal period can predispose offspring to glucose intolerance and IR. Chronic maternal chromium restriction in the rat results in a significant increase in body weight and adiposity, particularly visceral adiposity, in both male and female offspring. Further work by Zhang et al. has also shown that chromium restriction during pregnancy in the mouse alters methylation patterns in genes associated with insulin signaling in the liver of adult male offspring (Zhang et al., 2017). A maternal diet deficient in calcium increases IR and blood pressure in adult rat offspring (Takaya et al., 2018; Bergel and Belizán, 2002). A 50% vitamin restriction during pregnancy can predispose female and male rat offspring to IR and increased risk for obesity when fed a post-weaning obesogenic diet. Given the outcomes of experimental models and observations in human cohorts to date, it is clear that the impact of altered micronutrient status on early nutrition programming requires greater understanding to further address the limited awareness that remains around the potential long-term health outcomes micronutrient deficiencies during pregnancy and/or lactation on offspring health (Cetin et al., 2019).

### 11.2.2.2 Maternal obesity

Given the significant increases in overweight/obesity in women of reproductive age (18–44), there has been an increase in focus on experimental models of maternal obesity and GDM. A number of models utilizing maternal obesogenic exposures, primarily in the rodent, have demonstrated a consistent phenotype of growth and cardiometabolic disorders in offspring, although, as with undernutrition, the severity of effects can differ with the timing/duration of the nutritional exposure and the composition of the diets used. As detailed earlier, although maternal obesity is often associated with macrosomia and large birth weights arising from GDM, obese pregnancies can also lead to an increased risk for IUGR (Radulescu et al., 2013; Ornoy, 2011). This may be a consequence of placental insufficiency with impaired placental structure and function resulting in altered placental transport of nutrients as has been shown previously in the rat (Mark et al., 2011). IR, impaired glucose-stimulated insulin secretion, and altered β-cell mass have been reported in offspring of dams fed an obesogenic diet (HF or cafeteria-style diet) throughout gestation (Taylor et al., 2005; Cerf et al., 2005). Even a moderate maternal obesogenic diet can result in increased body weights, adiposity, impaired glucose tolerance, hyperinsulinemia, and alterations in central regulators of appetite regulation in offspring which are independent of the level of post-weaning diet. It is also of interest that a lifetime exposure to a HF diet (i.e., from weaning) produced a phenotype in offspring that was similar to that of HF nutrition restricted to pregnancy and lactation alone, thus suggesting that the postnatal sequelae of maternal HF nutrition can occur independently of the dietary environment preconception (Howie et al., 2009). In ovine models, maternal obesity (150% of National Research Council dietary recommendations) has been shown to impact on pancreatic β-cell development in the fetus with alterations in β-cell maturation rates potentially contributing to premature β-cell function loss and increased risk for obesity and related metabolic disorders (Zhang et al., 2011). As mentioned earlier, a caveat for models using "overnutrition" is that in many cases, obesity is reflected in key micronutrient deficiencies, thus the phenotypic similarities observed in offspring from mothers either undernourished or "overnourished" may arise as a result of reduced/suboptimal placental/lactational nutrient transport in those offspring of "overnourished" dams, i.e., "obesity malnutrition" (Via, 2012).

## 11.3  Role of epigenetics in programming of obesity and T2DM

Although the mechanistic processes underpinning developmental programming of obesity and T2DM remain unclear, epigenetic processes have emerged as playing a key role (Ong and Ozanne, 2015). Certain nutrients act as key substrates for epigenetic modifications and therefore alterations in the nutritional environment in early life can impact on epigenetic patterns due to alterations in the activity of the enzymes that are involved in the addition/removal of epigenetic marks or variations in substrate availability. An example of this is S-adenosylmethionine that has a key role as a methyl donor substrate for a number of biological and biochemical processes (Chiang et al., 1996). During early life development, the epigenome is labile and therefore can be adaptive in response to environmental stressors, including an altered nutritional environment (Jang and Serra, 2014). At a mechanistic level, human studies examining changes in the epigenome with disease risk remain limited and largely associative, although there is evidence for inheritance of tissue-specific DNA methylation patterns (Silva and White, 1988). To date, most evidence has been derived from experimental models as human studies are limited by a range of factors, including the availability of accurate methods to quantify nutritional components in the one-carbon cycle and ability to assess tissue-specific effects. Gene promoter methylation at birth has been associated with alterations in fat mass in children at 9 years of age, thus suggesting that a major component of metabolic disease risk has a prenatal developmental basis (Godfrey et al., 2011). Further, a recent trial providing omega-3 polyunsaturated fatty acids to pregnant women reported differences in methylation in some DNA regions in offspring as compared to the unsupplemented group, although the functional consequences of these changes have yet to be determined (Van Dijk et al., 2016). In the Dutch Famine cohort, relative hypomethylation of the imprinted insulin-like growth factor (IGF)-2 gene adult was seen in offspring exposed to famine prenatally as compared to unexposed siblings. The association was specific for exposure during the preconceptional period, further reinforcing that the very early developmental window is a critical period for establishing and maintaining epigenetic marks (Heijmans et al., 2008; Tobi et al., 2009). Further work in this cohort utilizing genome-scale analysis in whole blood identified differential patterns of methylation in regions linked to birthweight and cholesterol metabolism (Tobi et al., 2014). Establishment of these methylation signatures appeared to be dependent on specific exposure to famine during pregnancy as they did not overlap with tissue-specific differentially methylated regions that have been previously described in adults. The impact of altered maternal nutrition on the epigenome in offspring has also been shown in the Kiang West Longitudinal Population Study in The Gambia. In this region, characterized by marked seasonal fluctuations in maternal nutritional intake, i.e., a wet "hungry" season, and reduced energy intakes, DNA methylation at metastable epialleles (MEs) was increased in those individuals who were conceived during the nutritionally challenged rainy season, and provides the first evidence of a persistent effect of the periconceptional environment on human epigenotype (Waterland et al., 2010). Further work in this cohort revealed that naturally occurring seasonal variations in food availability had marked effects on methyl-donor biomarker status (including folate, choline, and betaine) resulting in persistent and systemic epigenetic changes at human MEs (Dominguez-Salas et al., 2013, 2014).

In experimental animal models, it has now been clearly shown that nutritional challenges during pregnancy and/or lactation can result in changes in promoter methylation and thus either directly or indirectly affect gene expression and impact across a range of physiologic processes (Gicquel et al., 2008; Jirtle and Skinner, 2007; Pham et al., 2003; Bogdarina et al., 2007; Weaver et al., 2004; Dudley et al., 2011). Although maternal macronutrient status is clearly implicated as a mediator of developmental programming (McMillen et al., 2008), micronutrient levels during pregnancy are of interest given their requirement for one-carbon metabolism with an imbalance in these nutrients (including folate, choline, and vitamin B12 (Gicquel et al., 2008, MacLennan et al., 2004, Vanhees et al., 2014)) impacting on DNA methylation patterns. As an example, increased maternal vitamin B12 concentrations are associated with decreased global DNA methylation in newborn infants while increased circulating B12 concentrations in newborns are associated with a reduction in the methylation of the IGF binding protein-3 gene, a key mediator of fetal growth (McKay et al., 2012). It has also been suggested that other factors such as magnesium, zinc, and chromium can induce epigenetic modifications by reducing or increasing the methylation level at the promoter region of some genes (Cetin et al., 2019). A maternal LP diet results in aberrant changes in DNA methylation in key genes in offspring which can be reversed via maternal dietary supplementation with cofactors (Lillycrop et al., 2005; Cho et al., 2013). In the rat, for example, altered gene expression and promoter methylation have been shown for the hepatic peroxisome proliferator-activated receptor and the glucocorticoid receptor (GR) (Lillycrop et al., 2005, 2007), influencing lipid and carbohydrate metabolism (Burdge et al., 2007). A maternal LP diet results in hypomethylation and increased gene expression of PPAR-$\alpha$ and GR in offspring that is normalized to that of controls following maternal supplementation with folate (Lillycrop et al., 2005).

In addition to maternal dietary restriction, it has now been well established that a maternal obesogenic diet and early life "overnutrition" can both elicit similar epigenetic changes in offspring, that is, the "U"-shaped response curve. For example, an obesogenic diet during lactation can lead to epigenetic modifications in key genes in skeletal muscle involved in the insulin signaling pathway and manifest as IR in later life (Liu et al., 2013). In the mouse, maternal obesity has been shown to induce epigenetic modifications that facilitate and enhance adipocyte differentiation, thereby programming for adiposity and metabolic disorders in later life (Yang et al., 2013). Hypermethylation of the proopiomelanocortin (POMC) gene has been shown in female offspring in the setting of a maternal obesogenic diet and corresponded with increased body weight and decreased POMC transcription (Marco et al., 2014). Of note, these effects appeared to be permanent in nature and could not be reprogrammed by feeding of a standard diet post-weaning.

In the context of parental obesity, it has been shown that infants born to obese parents have altered DNA methylation patterns at imprinted genes (Soubry et al., 2015) with paternal obesity associated with hypomethylation of IGF-2 in newborn infants (Soubry et al., 2013). Maternal obesity and GDM have been shown to be associated with tissue-specific alterations in leptin promoter methylation in a sex-specific manner and may therefore have implications for later metabolic health of offspring (Lesseur et al., 2013, 2014). In the rat, a chronic paternal HF diet leads to programmed changes in $\beta$-cell function in female offspring and induces glucose intolerance and changes in the transcriptome of the pancreas and adipose tissue (Ng et al., 2014, 2010). These effects of paternal metabolic status are also associated with hypomethylation of the IL13ra2 gene (Ng et al., 2010). Of note, the significant and independent association between paternal obesity and the methylation status of offspring suggests the developing sperm is highly susceptible to environmental insults. Of note, a potential limitation of observations to date is that many studies are performed utilizing whole tissues and mixed cell populations thus changes in methylation observed may be due to tissue or cell population heterogeneity (Marousez et al., 2019). Further, many reports to date have only described small changes in methylation (1%–10%) (Breton et al., 2017; Leenen et al., 2016), thus these differences could arise to variations in cell populations with the same tissue although the functional consequences of such small absolute changes cannot be discounted.

Research on epigenetic mechanisms in the setting of programming have primarily focused on alterations in DNA methylation arising due to altered nutritional exposures (Delage and Dashwood, 2008). However, a number of studies have now highlighted the role of nutritional manipulations on other epigenetic processes including altered histone structure and function and micro RNAs (miRNAs). Methylation of either DNA or histone proteins requires availability of methyl donors from dietary folate and the presence of vitamins B12, B6, methionine, choline, and a range of methyltransferases (Wolffe, 1998; Callinan and Feinberg, 2006; Tosh et al., 2010). Histone methylation can impact on gene expression, either repressing or promoting gene expression, depending on the location. As an example, a rat model that utilized maternal hyperglycemia to induce adult cardiovascular disease reported changes in H3Me3K36 of the IGF-1 gene in the liver (Zinkhan et al., 2012). A further study using uteroplacental insufficiency to induce IUGR in the rat has also reported a decrease in histone 3 trimethylation of lysine 36 of the IGF-1 gene (H3Me3K36) (Fu et al., 2009). Taken together, these data suggest that H3Me3K36 of the IGF-1 gene is sensitive to prenatal glucose concentrations, with resultant changes in expression of IGF-1 and progression toward IR in adulthood (Zinkhan et al., 2012). Work in sheep models of IUGR have also reported histone modifications associated with the hypothalamic POMC promoter which could predispose the offspring to altered glucose homeostasis, appetite regulation, and energy expenditure later in life (Stevens et al., 2011).

miRNAs are small molecules (21–24 nucleotides in length) that bind to the 3' untranslated regions of mRNA and either sequester mRNA for degradation or prevents translation via interference with the translation machinery. The expression of certain miRNAs is controlled by DNA methylation and chromatin modifications. Conversely, miRNAs can mediate the machinery that regulates methylation and the expression of proteins involved in the modification of histones, a key post-translational process that plays a key role in gene expression. Work on miRNAs and long non-coding RNAs (lncRNAs) in the setting of developmental programming has revealed a complex network of reciprocal interactions. miRNAs can control expression of genes at a post-transcriptional level, thereby representing an important class of regulatory molecules as well as being directly connected to the "epigenetic machinery" through a regulatory loop (Iorio et al., 2010). In addition, lncRNAs can bind mRNAs and exert opposing roles in transcript stabilization/destabilization. Recent work by Saeedi Borujeni et al. has reviewed the roles of these systems in the pathogenesis of T2DM and β-cell dysfunction (Saeedi Borujeni et al., 2019).

Alterations in miRNAs have been implicated in the programming of both adipogenesis and IR. Maternal periconceptional undernutrition in the sheep results in altered expression of miRNAs in offspring which may play a role in the progression toward development of IR in adulthood (Lie et al., 2014). In the rat maternal LP model, the imprinted miR-483 is programmed in adipose tissue in offspring leading to a reduction in adipose tissue expandability resulting in ectopic lipid deposition which is known to contribute to the progression of NAFLD and IR (Ferland-McCollough et al., 2012). Of interest, adipose tissue from humans born with LBW reveals similar changes in miR-483, suggesting conservation of this programming mechanism (Ferland-McCollough et al., 2012).

A maternal LP diet has also been reported to alter miRNA profiles and expression of mechanistic target of rapamycin (mTOR) in offspring influencing glucose homeostasis and insulin secretion with the glucose intolerance observed in adult offspring a result of an insulin secretory defect as opposed to a programmed reduction in β-cell mass (Alejandro et al., 2014). Islets of LP offspring exhibited reduced expression of mTOR and increased expression of a subset of miRNAs and blockade of these miRNAs normalized mTOR and insulin secretion. A specific set of miRNAs has been shown to play a key role in pancreatic β-cell differentiation and is essential for the maintenance of normal insulin secretion and for compensatory β-cell mass expansion in response to IR (Guay et al., 2011; Nesca et al., 2013). A number of studies have now reported altered profiles of miRNAs in the pancreatic islets of experimental models of diabetes and in isolated islets from patients with T2DM. However, a number of the changes in miRNA expression observed in the islets of diabetic patients were not detected in animal models of diabetes and vice versa which may reflect fundamental differences in the experimental approaches (Guay and Regazzi, 2014). Nutritional modulation of miRNAs may also underlie the increased susceptibility to T2DM in offspring. As an example, a maternal HF diet can lead to alterations in miRNAs in the liver concomitant with changes in gene expression including IGF-2 which is known to be important for survival of pancreatic β-cells (Zhang et al., 2009). A maternal HF diet can also lead to an increase in miR-126, resulting in a reduction in its primary target, IRS-1, in adipose tissue of offspring. Given the programmed phenotype was maintained in vitro, it was suggested that this mechanism was cell autonomous and may drive the progression toward IR in later life (Fernandez-Twinn et al., 2014).

It is important to note that the phenotypic effects of epigenetic modifications during development arising due to nutritional programming may not manifest until later in life, particularly where they impact on genes that modulate responses to later environmental insults, such as a post-weaning dietary challenge with an obesogenic diet, i.e., a "second hit" or "trigger."

## 11.4 Role of the gut microbiome in the development of obesity and T2DM

There is increasing interest in the role of the gut microbiome in the initiation and progression of cardiometabolic diseases with the suggestion that alterations in the gut flora may lead to changes in energy harvested from the diet. As a result, there is increasing interest in the potential use of microbiota in clinical applications for understanding and treating obesity and T2DM (Gurung et al., 2020). Early postnatal nutrition may represent a key determinant of adult health by impacting on the development of the gut microbiome and thus provides a key window for intervention for at-risk individuals. During the neonatal period, early colonizers play an important role in health of the host because they are involved in nutritional, physiologic, and immunologic functions (Nauta et al., 2013). Alterations in the composition of the gut microbiota has been proposed as an early diagnostic markers for the development of T2DM in high-risk patients (Hartstra et al., 2015). Disruption of the gut microbial community in newborns of obese mothers has been shown to contribute to an increased risk of childhood obesity (Soderborg and Friedman, 2018), and alterations in early gut microbiota composition and function appear to be associated with aberrant programming of later immune function and overall health status. Ley et al. reported that the obese leptin-deficient *ob/ob* mice had a 50% decrease in the abundance of Bacteriodetes and a relative increase in Firmicutes as compared to their lean control group (Ley et al., 2005). Given that the composition of the gut microbiota can differ between obese and lean individuals (Ley et al., 2006; Turnbaugh et al., 2006), transplantation of gut flora from lean subjects to those with metabolic syndrome demonstrated improvements in insulin sensitivity (Kootte et al., 2012; Vrieze et al., 2012). In this context, the use of probiotics to restore intestinal microbiota balance may have efficacy in preventing the development of chronic immune-mediated diseases (Canani et al., 2011). In the piglet, probiotic supplementation during the sucking period has been demonstrated to improve intestinal health via beneficial effects on immune function and conferring protection against pathogenic challenges in neonates born following IUGR (Hu et al., 2017). Further, supplementation with synbiotics (a mixture of probiotics and prebiotics) can confer protection against adipose accumulation in the setting of a HF dietary challenge in mice (Mischke et al., 2018). The important role of the gut microbiota in potential mediation of programming-related outcomes is further supported by reports that exposure to antibiotics during critical periods of early development can result in an increased obesity risk via effects on the developing gut microbiota (Azad et al., 2017).

While mechanistic studies in experimental animal models support a causal role for alterations in the microbiota and risk for metabolic disorders, the majority of outcomes reported in human studies are associative and thus hinder cause-effect inferences (Allin et al., 2015). Further, different studies have reported different taxa to be associated with T2DM (Gurung et al., 2020) with a recent study reporting that different microbial populations were found to be associated with the same metabolic outcomes across different geographical areas (He et al., 2018). From an epigenetic perspective, a recent study has shown that the gut microbiota is able to drive distinct methylome and transcriptome changes during postnatal development (Pan et al., 2018), but more work is required to establish the link between infant gut microbiota and epigenetic reprogramming. Of interest, in addition to potential programming effects on the gut microbiome, it has also been shown that a maternal HF diet can result in sex-specific changes in gene expression of taste receptors and inflammatory markers in the gut that may impact on glucose sensing pathways (Reynolds et al., 2015b).

## 11.5 Transgenerational effects

Human evidence and those derived from experimental animal models has shown that developmental programming represents a transgenerational phenomenon and seen as a form of epigenetic inheritance, via either parental line. There is evidence for both somatic and germline inheritance of epigenetic modifications that may underpin phenotypic changes that span further generations (Aiken and Ozanne, 2014). In particular, given the rising prevalence of maternal overweight/obesity, there is increasing interest in the detrimental impact of a maternal obesogenic environment on the risk of disease beyond the F1 generation. Of note, both ends of the range of maternal nutritional intakes appear to elicit similar transgenerational effects with both maternal obesity and maternal undernutrition resulting in transmission of disease traits related to the risk of developing obesity and T2DM. As detailed earlier, whether the mechanisms are similar and that a maternal obesogenic dietary environment also reflects a form of malnutrition arising due to vitamin/mineral deficiencies remains poorly defined.

A number of studies in programming models have reported transmission to the F2 lineage. However, transmission to the F3 or subsequent generation (a true marker of transgenerational transmission as it represents the first generation not exposed to the initial pregnancy perturbation) has been less defined with some studies suggesting a resolution of the offspring phenotype by the F3 generation. In a meta-analysis by Aiken and Ozanne, of the studies carried through to F3, over half failed to show any effect (Aiken and Ozanne, 2014). Human evidence remains limited although studies have demonstrated that parents who were born of LBW also had babies with a LBW transmitted via both the maternal (Qian et al., 2017) or paternal (Jaquet et al., 2005) lineages, and in a British 1958 birth cohort study, this growth restriction was subsequently passed onto the F3 generation via the maternal line (Emanuel et al., 1992).

There is also increasing evidence for the impact of the health status of the father in transgenerational inheritance (Fullston et al., 2013; Hur et al., 2017). In the work of Fulston et al., paternal obesity in mice was shown to initiate metabolic disturbances through to the F2 offspring albeit with only partial phenotype transmission to the F2 generation. Paternal obesity modulated germ methylation status and sperm microRNA content which can initiate the transmission of disease risk to future generations. Studies in sperm from F1 offspring have suggested a role for altered expression of IGF-2 and H19 in transmission of phenotypic traits to F2 offspring (Ding et al., 2012). However, not all studies reporting a paternal line transmission have reported epigenetic alterations in the F1 sperm (Drake et al., 2011). In a study by Radford et al., there was no evidence that maternal nutritional restriction resulted in epigenetic reprogramming of imprinting control regions in the germline thus, suggesting that mechanisms other than direct germline transmission may be responsible (Radford et al., 2012).

Although transmission of a phenotype across generations is often viewed as a form of epigenetic inheritance, evidence to date also highlights the role of non-genomic components and interactions between the in-utero environment and the developing fetus in transmission of disease traits. These include altered maternal adaptations to pregnancy, a suboptimal reproductive tract environment, or other societal factors. In addition, females who were born SGA and/or have a reduced nephron number (a common observation in programming models) are at an increased risk for pregnancy complications, which can influence the growth and development of the next generation (Briffa et al., 2020). As such, programming effects could potentially be transmitted through the maternal line de novo beyond the F2 generation as a consequence of development in a suboptimal intrauterine tract and not necessarily through directly transmitted epigenetic mechanisms (Aiken and Ozanne, 2014).

## 11.6 Critical developmental windows and strategies for intervention

It is clear that maternal health status and nutritional environment are key determinants in influencing fetal and infant development with numerous studies supporting the notion that a number of risk factors for the development of metabolic disorders may be modifiable by dietary or other therapeutic interventions during critical and sensitive windows of early life development (Aaltonen et al., 2011; Laitinen et al., 2009; Luoto et al., 2010).

Work in animal models has shown that nutritional and pharmacologic interventions may have efficacy in ameliorating or reversing the adverse growth and cardiometabolic impacts associated with adverse nutritional programming (Vickers and Sloboda, 2012b). One of the earliest reported potential treatment modality was in a rat model using maternal taurine supplementation to LP mothers. In pre-diabetic and diabetic states, taurine concentrations are reduced with maintenance of physiological concentrations of taurine important for normal β-cell function and insulin action. In offspring of LP-fed dams, β-cell mass was reduced at birth and metabolic dysregulation persisted into adulthood despite provision of a standard diet after birth or after weaning. However, supplementation of LP dams with taurine (via the drinking water) lead to a restoration of insulin release of insulin from LP fetal pancreatic islets, demonstrating the important role of taurine in the development and maintenance of normal β-cell function in the developing fetus. Further, it has recently been shown that taurine supplementation to pregnant mothers in the setting of a maternal obesogenic diet can partially prevent programming events in rat offspring in later life (Li et al., 2013, 2015). Work with other amino acids such as arginine, citrulline, and cysteine have also reported beneficial effects of supplementation on programming-related outcomes (Hsu and Tain, 2020). As an example, arginine supplementation during pregnancy in animal models has been shown to have protective effects against IUGR, although wider reprogramming effects have not been fully examined (Lassala et al., 2010).

Leptin, an adipokine produced primarily by adipocytes, has been widely investigated as a potential mediator of developmental programming (Vickers and Sloboda, 2012a), thus representing a key target for intervention strategies. It has been proposed that altered leptin action during critical developmental windows can lead to a "hardwiring" of obesity and related metabolic disorders. Leptin acts centrally to regulate food intake by regulating the activity of neurons in the arcuate nucleus (ARH). Neural projection pathways from the ARH are disrupted in leptin-deficient *ob/ob* mice with neonatal leptin treatment normalizing the development of ARH projections. In humans, children born SGA are hypoleptinemic with significantly reduced cord blood leptin concentrations but go on to develop hyperleptinemia, obesity, and IR in adult life. It is therefore clear from animal data and clinical observations that alterations in the early life environment that impact on leptin concentrations may have long-term consequences for the formation and function of circuits involved in the regulation of food intake, energy expenditure, and body weight. Moreover, leptin interacts in a feedback loop with insulin (adipoinsular axis)—insulin is adipogenic, increases body fat mass, and stimulates the production and secretion of leptin. Conversely, leptin suppresses insulin secretion via both central actions and direct actions on pancreatic β-cells (Kieffer and Habener, 2000). As circulating leptin concentrations are directly proportional to adiposity, an increase in fat mass increases circulating leptin concentrations, thereby curtailing insulin production and further increasing fat mass. Defects in the adipoinsular axis, as has been shown in offspring following maternal undernutrition (Vickers et al., 2001b), results in hyperinsulinemia, hyperleptinemia, and compensatory leptin production by pancreatic δ-cells in an attempt to reduce the hypersecretion of insulin and the progression to adipogenic diabetes.

In the rat, leptin treatment to female neonates born following maternal undernutrition prevented the development of diet-induced obesity and associated cardiometabolic disorders in adulthood. Specifically, leptin administration resulted in a normalization of body weight, fat mass, caloric intake, voluntary locomotor activity and fasting glucose, insulin, leptin, and c-peptide concentrations; suggesting that the effects observed were not restricted to a central mechanism. Moreover, the effects of leptin treatment were specific to animals born of LBW, with leptin having no effect in female offspring born to normally nourished mothers. The observations of leptin efficacy in the rat as a potential intervention strategy have been replicated in a piglet model of growth restriction. IUGR in piglets was characterized by altered distribution of the leptin receptor within the hypothalamic regions involved in metabolic regulation with leptin administration partially reversing the IUGR phenotype. The translation of findings across animal models itself offers promise for defining the role of leptin and potential as a modifiable risk factor during this critical window of development. It has been proposed that the period of developmental plasticity is still open during the timing of treatment and normalizing of leptin concentrations reverses the cuing effects of fetal undernutrition. Next remains the question of the leptin surge that occurs in neonates—while the leptin surge has been well characterized in rodents and other model species such as the sheep (Smith et al., 2018), the absence or presence of a leptin surge in humans remains uncertain and would likely reflect a late gestation phenomenon. Although alterations in maternal nutrition can alter the profile of the leptin surge with regard to timing and/or duration, results have not been consistent across experimental paradigms. Yura et al. reported that the neonatal leptin surge occurred prematurely in the mouse following moderate maternal undernutrition, whereas offspring of LP-fed mothers display a delayed leptin surge. Further work in the rat showed that maternal undernutrition significantly reduced the leptin surge in neonates and altered the development of the POMC neurons in the ARH of male neonates. In the sheep, reduced maternal nutrition during early- to mid-gestation eliminates the neonatal leptin surge and appears to be mediated by cortisol concentrations in the newborn lambs (Smith et al., 2018). To date, only a few studies have investigated the leptin surge in maternal obesogenic models. In rat neonates, exposure to a maternal HF diet has been shown to result in a prolonged and amplified leptin surge. Similar to that of undernutrition in the sheep, maternal obesity has also been shown to eliminate the plasma leptin peak in neonatal lambs (Long et al., 2011), further suggesting a "U"-shaped response to different programming stimuli. Further, in the sheep model of maternal overnutrition/obesity, transgenerational impacts on the leptin surge have been reported with lambs in the F2 generation failing to exhibit the early postnatal leptin peak compared to controls (Shasa et al., 2015). Interestingly, treatment of neonatal offspring of obese rat dams with a leptin antagonist partially prevented the development of growth and metabolic disorders in offspring (Beltrand et al., 2012).

Work in rodents has shown that both growth hormone (GH) and IGF-I can normalize several aspects of the cardiometabolic phenotype in offspring following developmental programming. Utilizing a model of IUGR induced via maternal global undernutrition, offspring were fed either a chow or HF diet postnatally. These offspring had increased fat mass and were obese, hyperphagic, hyperinsulinemic, and hyperleptinemic with elevated blood pressure as a result of the maternal diet; the effects of which were exacerbated when exposed to a HF diet post-weaning. Treatment of adult offspring with GH led to a reduction in fat mass and a normalization of systolic blood pressure. However, hyperinsulinemia was worsened in adults as a result of the diabetogenic effects of GH administration. GH treatment during the neonatal period to offspring of undernourished mothers has recently been shown to be efficacious in ameliorating metabolic and cardiovascular disorders in adult offspring (Gray et al., 2013, 2014; Reynolds et al., 2013) and negated the diabetogenic effects associated with adult GH treatment. Treatment with IGF-I in adult female rat offspring of mothers undernourished during pregnancy led to a normalization of fat mass, caloric intake, and fasting plasma insulin and leptin concentrations. In the sheep, intrauterine therapy in the setting of fetal growth restriction with intra-amniotic IGF-1 improved fetal growth and altered markers of perinatal growth and metabolism in a sex-specific manner with effects that persist into young adulthood (Spiroski et al., 2020). Collectively, these studies highlight the role of the GH-IGF axis in cardiometabolic disturbances arising via developmental programming although the long-term outcomes of such treatment approaches targeting this axis are not known. In SGA children, GH administration has been shown to normalize systolic blood pressure, effects that persisted throughout the 6 year duration of treatment. However, clinical data, albeit limited, have suggested that GH treatment to SGA children may enhance later T2DM risk but this may reflect an acceleration of the disorder in predisposed individuals (Cutfield et al., 2000).

Using a rat model of HF feeding, Reynolds et al. has shown that maternal supplementation with conjugated linoleic acid can reverse some programming effects including normalization of the inflammatory phenotype in mothers and normalization of insulin sensitivity, lipid profiles, and inflammatory markers in offspring (Segovia et al., 2017; Reynolds et al., 2015a). Further work in this model using fish oil supplementation during pregnancy also demonstrated normalization of insulin sensitivity in adult male offspring, although here was no effect on body composition (Albert et al., 2017). The use of dietary polyphenols has gained some attention as a strategy for preventing IUGR given its role in increasing circulating antioxidant capacity and improving markers of oxidative stress and glucose homeostasis across the feto-placental unit (Ly et al., 2015). As an example, experimental evidence across a range of animal models suggests a role for the polyphenol resveratrol in reversing features of the metabolic syndrome in offspring, particularly attenuation of obesity and IR (Tain and Hsu, 2018). In the context of maternal obesity, these effects may be mediated via protective effects on the fetal brain. However, translation to the human may be difficult given that the metabolism of resveratrol differs between humans and other species (Wang and Sang, 2018). A dietary intervention in the preconceptional period (changing from an obesogenic diet to a normal control diet) has been shown to partially reverse metabolic programming in male offspring. Of note, in addition to dietary and supplement-based approaches, it has also been shown that exercise can potentially ameliorate programming effects. In the rat, exercise in the setting of maternal obesity can have beneficial effects on both mother and offspring across a range of markers of metabolic health and oxidative stress including triglycerides, cholesterol, leptin, and corticosterone (Vega et al., 2015). Exercise during normal pregnancy in the rat has been demonstrated to enhance insulin sensitivity and glucose homeostasis in female offspring (Carter et al., 2013) and promote physical activity in adult offspring (Eclarinal et al., 2016). It has also been shown in human studies that maternal gestational weight gain can provide an important biological predictor of offspring physical activity. Moreover, these effects were sex-specific and provide support for the sex-dependent early developmental programming influence of maternal weight gain on activity in offspring (Wasenius et al., 2017). However, the effects of exercise in the setting of programming models has yet to be well characterized.

As regards, GDM and primary prevention, a number of clinical studies have been conducted utilizing a range nutritional manipulations and lifestyle modifications, although only a limited number of trials to date have shown a reduction in the proportion of women with GDM (Simmons, 2015). Nutritional supplements such as probiotics and myo-inositol may have some efficacy for primary prevention—a recent meta-analysis by Zheng et al. reported that myo-inositol supplementation reduced GDM rates although noted that further evaluation in large-scale controlled trials was required (Zheng et al., 2015). In experimental models, it has been shown that leptin treatment can prevent spontaneous GDM in the *db/db* mouse model of leptin receptor deficiency (Yamashita et al., 2001), but this model is limited as regards translation to the human where leptin receptor deficiency is not an important contributor to T2DM (Wang et al., 2014). Other animal studies have also reported efficacy of agents such as resveratrol (Yao et al., 2015) and PPAR agonists (Arck et al., 2010), but these are as avenues for treatment, not primary GDM prevention, and some safety issues remain to be resolved before any clinical translation can be considered.

Although a number of different experimental paradigms in animal models have now shown that targeted interventions can reverse or ameliorate metabolic disorders arising due to developmental programming, translation to the human setting remains difficult as first need to identify those at risk or programmed disorders. Further, some interventions, including leptin and GH, have sex-specific effects and may also predispose offspring of healthy pregnancies to later metabolic disorders. An example of this is neonatal leptin treatment with leptin administration to male neonates of control pregnancies eliciting adverse metabolic response including increased diet-induced weight gain, hyperinsulinemia, and increased total body adiposity compared to controls (Vickers et al., 2008). This is further highlighted by early work showing that the response to leptin treatment, as an example, is directionally dependent upon prior maternal nutritional status suggesting that the response to one cue can be determined by previous exposure to another, for example, undernutrition (Gluckman et al., 2007b). Some human trials support the initial findings from animal studies, particularly around micronutrient supplementation. For example, supplementation with folic acid and iron during pregnancy has been shown to result in increased birthweights, but this response was modified by maternal nutritional status, with infants born to women with improved short-term nutrition having a greater birthweight response. Whether these observations have an epigenetic basis as has been reported for the animal models is not clear although alterations in H19 methylation is a potential mechanism by which folic acid risks and/or benefits are conferred in utero. Other interventions have yet to be translated from preclinical models. In the clinic, for example, concentrations of taurine are reduced in both pre-diabetic and diabetic states with physiological concentrations of taurine in the circulation known to be important for maintenance of β-cell function. Animal studies have shown that taurine supplementation of the mother during pregnancy can partially reverse the cardiometabolic disorders that arise in offspring in the setting of both maternal obesity and LP diet exposure. However, translation of these findings and restoration of taurine levels in at-risk patients with pre-diabetes/diabetes has yet to be fully explored. A number of interventions (e.g., leptin, GH, taurine, and methyl donors) during key periods of developmental plasticity elicit similar reversal effects in offspring across a range of experimental paradigms highlighting the importance of early developmental windows as the optimal target for intervention strategies.

## 11.7  Summary

Data derived from epidemiological cohorts, clinical studies, and extensive work in experimental animal models have clearly shown that the propensity to develop obesity and related cardiometabolic disorders including T2DM in adulthood is increased when development during early life has been adversely affected. The disease etiology is not based on genetic defects but on alterations in gene expression as a consequence of predictive (mal) adaptation to environmental changes during early life development. However, there is little known about the interaction between the pre- and postnatal nutritional environments on either exacerbation or resolution of the programming phenotype depending on the degree and severity of nutritional match/mismatch, for example, regulation of catch-up growth. Thus, further mechanistic studies examining the thrifty phenotype/PARS hypothesis are required in conjunction with transgenerational work through to F3 to further the DOHaD paradigm and development of potential DOHaD "circuit breakers."

The molecular mechanisms underpinning nutritional programming of disease susceptibility are only recently beginning to be investigated with epigenetic profiling becoming a key tool for DOHaD research. DNA methylation and histone modifications are the two most epigenetic mechanisms studied to date which remain largely associative in nature. Dietary intake and availability of methyl donors and cofactors during critical windows of development will alter patterns of DNA methylation. Thus, early methyl donor malnutrition could effectively lead to premature epigenetic aging, thereby conferring an enhanced susceptibility to diseases such as obesity and T2DM in later life. However, there is now emerging data on the role of miRNAs with evidence that maternal diet-induced changes in miRNAs may underlie pancreatic β-cell dysfunction in offspring (Alejandro et al., 2014). A limitation of epigenetic profiling to date is that most studies have utilized a candidate approach, whereas more global approaches are required and a move toward genome-wide screening of methylation patterns using the high throughput platforms now available (Marousez et al., 2019). An example of a more global approach is the recent work by Kupers et al., where a meta-analysis of epigenome-wide association studies in neonates has revealed widespread differential DNA methylation patterns associated with birthweight outcomes although a causal link has yet to be confirmed (Küpers et al., 2019).

Although there has been extensive work focusing on early life nutrition and later T2DM risk, how the fetal nutrient environment induces lasting changes in the structure or function of the pancreatic β-cell remains largely unknown (Alejandro et al., 2014). The consistency of finding across a range of epidemiological studies and experimental models highlights the necessity to gain a better understanding of the mechanisms by which obesity and T2DM risk is programmed via early life exposures, including the interaction between the prenatal and postnatal environment in exacerbating disease risk. By understanding mechanisms, intervention strategies become feasible and thus offer the chance to reduce disease risk in current and future generations.

## 11.8  Future trends and research

Alterations in the nutritional environment during early development can exert lasting adverse effects on the health of offspring. These effects are consistent across a range of experimental models and human cohorts and may be transmitted across generations. Animal models have been key in understanding some of the potential mechanisms involved and gene–environment interactions including the so-called second hit, such as a postnatal obesogenic nutritional environment compounding the effects of early life programming. Experimental models have also highlighted critical developmental windows that offer opportunities for intervention and amelioration of risk for programmed disorders via a range of early nutritional and pharmacologic treatment strategies to both mother and offspring.

There remains a need for further additional longitudinal human studies, supported by ongoing data from animal models, to build the evidence for a casual role of epigenetic effects in mediating the effects of developmental programming. Effective research translation, communication and uptake of the preclinical observations into the clinic are important next steps. At present, there is a critical unmet need for basic, translational, and human intervention studies targeting pathways that connect the nutritional environment, microbiota, and metabolism in mothers with obesity and their infants and present new challenges for disease prevention in the next generation (Friedman, 2018). With strategies aimed at reversal of programming this can be difficult as safety remains the primary consideration—some studies have shown that interventions are only efficacious in those at risk of programmed disorders with the same intervention potentially eliciting adverse outcomes when utilized in the setting of a "control" early life environment. As programming represents a continuum rather than a defined subset of phenotypes, identifying those at risk can therefore be difficult outside of broader surrogate markers of a perturbed in utero environment such as altered birth weight. This is further compounded by the known sex-specific effects on programming outcomes detailed in animal models and ideally, all studies should address outcomes in both males and females as will provide further mechanistic insight. Translation to a clinic may rely on the establishment of effective early life biomarkers to identify those at a later risk. In this context, epigenetic marks, although to date largely associative in nature, may still offer utility as early predictive biomarkers of later disease risk. In addition, more attention to the role of paternal factors in the transmission of disease traits is required, particularly as regards programmed glucose intolerance, and this will undoubtedly increase as an area of focus in the next phase of DOHaD research.

## Sources of additional information

Gyllenhammer LE, Sonja Entringer S, Buss C, Wadhwa PD. Developmental programming of mitochondrial biology: a conceptual framework and review. 2020;287(1926):20192713.
Friedman JE. Developmental Programming of Obesity and Diabetes in Mouse, Monkey, and Man in 2018: Where Are We Headed? Diabetes 2018;67(11):2137–2151.
Dearden L, Bouret SG, Ozanne SE. Nutritional and developmental programming effects of insulin. J Neuroendocrinol. 2021;e12933.
Bianco-Miotto T, Craig JM, Gasser YP, van Dijk SJ, Ozanne SE. Epigenetics and DOHaD: from basics to birth and beyond. J Dev Orig Health Dis. 2017;8(5):513–519.
Vickers MH, Sloboda DM. Strategies for reversing the effects of metabolic disorders induced as a consequence of developmental programming. Front Physiol. 2012; 2;3:242.
Fernandez-Twinn DS, Hjort L, Novakovic B, Ozanne SE, Saffery R. Intrauterine programming of obesity and type 2 diabetes. Diabetologia. 2019;62(10):1789–1801.

Nicholas LM, Morrison JL, Rattanatray L, Zhang S, Ozanne SE, McMillen IC. The early origins of obesity and IR: timing, programming and mechanisms. Int J Obes (Lond). 2016;40(2):229–38.

# References

Aaltonen, J., Ojala, T., Laitinen, K., Poussa, T., Ozanne, S., Isolauri, E., 2011. Impact of maternal diet during pregnancy and breastfeeding on infant metabolic programming: a prospective randomized controlled study. Eur. J. Clin. Nutr. 65, 10–19.

Aiken, C.E., Ozanne, S.E., 2014. Transgenerational developmental programming. Hum. Reprod. Update 20, 63–75.

Albert, B.B., Vickers, M.H., Gray, C., Reynolds, C.M., Segovia, S.A., Derraik, J.G.B., Garg, M.L., Cameron-Smith, D., Hofman, P.L., Cutfield, W.S., 2017. Fish oil supplementation to rats fed high-fat diet during pregnancy prevents development of impaired insulin sensitivity in male adult offspring. Sci. Rep. 7, 5595.

Alejandro, E.U., Gregg, B., Wallen, T., Kumusoglu, D., Meister, D., Chen, A., Merrins, M.J., Satin, L.S., Liu, M., Arvan, P., Bernal-Mizrachi, E., 2014. Maternal diet-induced microRNAs and mTOR underlie beta cell dysfunction in offspring. J. Clin. Invest. 124, 4395–4410.

Allin, K.H., Nielsen, T., Pedersen, O., 2015. Mechanisms in endocrinology: gut microbiota in patients with type 2 diabetes mellitus. Eur. J. Endocrinol. 172, R167–R177.

Arck, P., Toth, B., Pestka, A., Jeschke, U., 2010. Nuclear receptors of the peroxisome proliferator-activated receptor (PPAR) family in gestational diabetes: from animal models to clinical trials. Biol. Reprod. 83, 168–176.

Azad, M.B., Moossavi, S., Owora, A., Sepehri, S., 2017. Early-life antibiotic exposure, gut microbiota development, and predisposition to obesity. Nestle Nutr. Inst. Workshop Ser. 88, 67–79.

Beltrand, J., Sloboda, D.M., Connor, K.L., Truong, M., Vickers, M.H., 2012. The effect of neonatal leptin antagonism in male rat offspring is dependent upon the interaction between prior maternal nutritional status and post-weaning diet. J. Nutr. Metab. 2012, 296935.

Berends, L.M., Ozanne, S.E., 2012. Early determinants of type-2 diabetes. Best Pract. Res. Clin. Endocrinol. Metab. 26, 569–580.

Bergel, E., Belizán, J.M., 2002. A deficient maternal calcium intake during pregnancy increases blood pressure of the offspring in adult rats. BJOG 109, 540–545.

Blüher, M., 2019. Obesity: global epidemiology and pathogenesis. Nat. Rev. Endocrinol. 15, 288–298.

Bogdarina, I., Welham, S., King, P.J., Burns, S.P., Clark, A.J., 2007. Epigenetic modification of the renin-angiotensin system in the fetal programming of hypertension. Circ. Res. 100, 520–526.

Breton, C.V., Marsit, C.J., Faustman, E., Nadeau, K., Goodrich, J.M., Dolinoy, D.C., Herbstman, J., Holland, N., Lasalle, J.M., Schmidt, R., Yousefi, P., Perera, F., Joubert, B.R., Wiemels, J., Taylor, M., Yang, I.V., Chen, R., Hew, K.M., Freeland, D.M., Miller, R., Murphy, S.K., 2017. Small-magnitude effect sizes in epigenetic end points are important in children's environmental health studies: the Children's environmental health and disease prevention research Center's epigenetics working group. Environ. Health Perspect. 125, 511–526.

Briffa, J.F., Wlodek, M.E., Moritz, K.M., 2020. Transgenerational programming of nephron deficits and hypertension. Semin. Cell Dev. Biol. 103, 94–103.

Burdge, G.C., Lillycrop, K.A., Jackson, A.A., Gluckman, P.D., Hanson, M.A., 2007. The nature of the growth pattern and of the metabolic response to fasting in the rat are dependent upon the dietary protein and folic acid intakes of their pregnant dams and post-weaning fat consumption. Br. J. Nutr. 99, 540–549.

Callinan, P.A., Feinberg, A.P., 2006. The emerging science of epigenomics. Hum. Mol. Genet. 15, R95–101.

Canani, R.B., Costanzo, M.D., Leone, L., Bedogni, G., Brambilla, P., Cianfarani, S., Nobili, V., Pietrobelli, A., Agostoni, C., 2011. Epigenetic mechanisms elicited by nutrition in early life. Nutr. Res. Rev. 24, 198–205.

Carter, L.G., Qi, N.R., De Cabo, R., Pearson, K.J., 2013. Maternal exercise improves insulin sensitivity in mature rat offspring. Med. Sci. Sports Exerc. 45, 832–840.

Catalano, P.M., 2003. Obesity and pregnancy—the propagation of a viscous cycle? J. Clin. Endocrinol. Metab. 88, 3505–3506.

Cerf, M.E., Williams, K., Nkomo, X.I., Muller, C.J., Du Toit, D.F., Louw, J., Wolfe-Coote, S.A., 2005. Islet cell response in the neonatal rat after exposure to a high-fat diet during pregnancy. Am. J. Phys. Regul. Integr. Comp. Phys. 288, R1122–R1128.

Cetin, I., Bühling, K., Demir, C., Kortam, A., Prescott, S.L., Yamashiro, Y., Yarmolinskaya, M., Koletzko, B., 2019. Impact of micronutrient status during pregnancy on early nutrition programming. Ann. Nutr. Metab. 74, 269–278.

Chatterjee, S., Khunti, K., Davies, M.J., 2017. Type 2 diabetes. Lancet 389, 2239–2251.

Chiang, P.K., Gordon, R.K., Tal, J., Zeng, G.C., Doctor, B.P., Pardhasaradhi, K., McCann, P.P., 1996. S-adenosylmethionine and methylation. FASEB J. 10, 471–480.

Cho, C.E., Sanchez-Hernandez, D., Reza-Lopez, S.A., Huot, P.S., Kim, Y.I., Anderson, G.H., 2013. High folate gestational and post-weaning diets alter hypothalamic feeding pathways by DNA methylation in Wistar rat offspring. Epigenetics 8, 710–719.

Cutfield, W.S., Wilton, P., Bennmarker, H., Albertsson-Wikland, K., Chatelain, P., Ranke, M.B., Price, D.A., 2000. Incidence of diabetes mellitus and impaired glucose tolerance in children and adolescents receiving growth-hormone treatment. Lancet 355, 610–613.

D'angelo, S., Yajnik, C.S., Kumaran, K., Joglekar, C., Lubree, H., Crozier, S.R., Godfrey, K.M., Robinson, S.M., Fall, C.H., Inskip, H.M., 2015. Body size and body composition: a comparison of children in India and the UK through infancy and early childhood. J. Epidemiol. Community Health 69, 1147–1153.

Delage, B., Dashwood, R.H., 2008. Dietary manipulation of histone structure and function. Annu. Rev. Nutr. 28, 347–366.

Desai, M., Gayle, D., Babu, J., Ross, M.G., 2005. Programmed obesity in intrauterine growth-restricted newborns: modulation by newborn nutrition. Am. J. Phys. Regul. Integr. Comp. Phys. 288, R91–R96.

Ding, G.L., Wang, F.F., Shu, J., Tian, S., Jiang, Y., Zhang, D., Wang, N., Luo, Q., Zhang, Y., Jin, F., Leung, P.C., Sheng, J.Z., Huang, H.F., 2012. Transgenerational glucose intolerance with Igf2/H19 epigenetic alterations in mouse islet induced by intrauterine hyperglycemia. Diabetes 61, 1133–1142.

Dominguez-Salas, P., Moore, S.E., Cole, D., Da Costa, K.A., Cox, S.E., Dyer, R.A., Fulford, A.J., Innis, S.M., Waterland, R.A., Zeisel, S.H., Prentice, A.M., Hennig, B.J., 2013. DNA methylation potential: dietary intake and blood concentrations of one-carbon metabolites and cofactors in rural African women. Am. J. Clin. Nutr. 97, 1217–1227.

Dominguez-Salas, P., Moore, S.E., Baker, M.S., Bergen, A.W., Cox, S.E., Dyer, R.A., Fulford, A.J., Guan, Y., Laritsky, E., Silver, M.J., Swan, G.E., Zeisel, S.H., Innis, S.M., Waterland, R.A., Prentice, A.M., Hennig, B.J., 2014. Maternal nutrition at conception modulates DNA methylation of human metastable epialleles. Nat. Commun. 5, 3746.

Drake, A.J., Liu, L., Kerrigan, D., Meehan, R.R., Seckl, J.R., 2011. Multigenerational programming in the glucocorticoid programmed rat is associated with generation-specific and parent of origin effects. Epigenetics 6, 1334–1343.

Dudley, K.J., Sloboda, D.M., Connor, K.L., Beltrand, J., Vickers, M.H., 2011. Offspring of mothers fed a high fat diet display hepatic cell cycle inhibition and associated changes in gene expression and DNA methylation. PLoS One 6, e21662.

Eclarinal, J.D., Zhu, S., Baker, M.S., Piyarathna, D.B., Coarfa, C., Fiorotto, M.L., Waterland, R.A., 2016. Maternal exercise during pregnancy promotes physical activity in adult offspring. FASEB J. 30, 2541–2548.

Emanuel, I., Filakti, H., Alberman, E., Evans, S.J., 1992. Intergenerational studies of human birthweight from the 1958 birth cohort. 1. Evidence for a multigenerational effect. Br. J. Obstet. Gynaecol. 99, 67–74.

Ferland-McCollough, D., Fernandez-Twinn, D.S., Cannell, I.G., David, H., Warner, M., Vaag, A.A., Bork-Jensen, J., Brøns, C., Gant, T.W., Willis, A.E., Siddle, K., Bushell, M., Ozanne, S.E., 2012. Programming of adipose tissue miR-483-3p and GDF-3 expression by maternal diet in type 2 diabetes. Cell Death Differ. 19, 1003–1012.

Fernandez-Twinn, D.S., Ozanne, S.E., 2010. Early life nutrition and metabolic programming. Ann. N. Y. Acad. Sci. 1212, 78–96.

Fernandez-Twinn, D.S., Alfaradhi, M.Z., Martin-Gronert, M.S., Duque-Guimaraes, D.E., Piekarz, A., Ferland-McCollough, D., Bushell, M., Ozanne, S.E., 2014. Downregulation of IRS-1 in adipose tissue of offspring of obese mice is programmed cell-autonomously through post-transcriptional mechanisms. Mol Metab 3, 325–333.

Friedman, J.E., 2018. Developmental programming of obesity and diabetes in mouse, monkey, and man in 2018: where are we headed? Diabetes 67, 2137–2151.

Fu, Q., Yu, X., Callaway, C.W., Lane, R.H., McKnight, R.A., 2009. Epigenetics: intrauterine growth retardation (IUGR) modifies the histone code along the rat hepatic IGF-1 gene. FASEB J. 23, 2438–2449.

Fullston, T., Ohlsson Teague, E.M., Palmer, N.O., Deblasio, M.J., Mitchell, M., Corbett, M., Print, C.G., Owens, J.A., Lane, M., 2013. Paternal obesity initiates metabolic disturbances in two generations of mice with incomplete penetrance to the F2 generation and alters the transcriptional profile of testis and sperm microRNA content. FASEB J. 27, 4226–4243.

G, R., Gupta, A., 2014. Vitamin D deficiency in India: prevalence, causalities and interventions. Nutrients 6, 729–775.

Gambling, L., Charania, Z., Hannah, L., Antipatis, C., Lea, R.G., McArdle, H.J., 2002. Effect of iron deficiency on placental cytokine expression and fetal growth in the pregnant rat. Biol. Reprod. 66, 516–523.

Gernand, A.D., Simhan, H.N., Caritis, S., Bodnar, L.M., 2014. Maternal vitamin D status and small-for-gestational-age offspring in women at high risk for preeclampsia. Obstet. Gynecol. 123, 40–48.

II. Early nutrition and development of non-communicable diseases

Gicquel, C., El-Osta, A., Le Bouc, Y., 2008. Epigenetic regulation and fetal programming. Best Pract. Res. Clin. Endocrinol. Metab. 22, 1–16.

Gluckman, P.D., Lillycrop, K.A., Vickers, M.H., Pleasants, A.B., Phillips, E.S., Beedle, A.S., Burdge, G.C., Hanson, M.A., 2007b. Metabolic plasticity during mammalian development is directionally dependent on early nutritional status. Proc. Natl. Acad. Sci. U. S. A. 104, 12796–12800.

Godfrey, K.M., Sheppard, A., Gluckman, P.D., Lillycrop, K.A., Burdge, G.C., Mclean, C., Rodford, J., Slater-Jefferies, J.L., Garratt, E., Crozier, S.R., Emerald, B.S., Gale, C.R., Inskip, H.M., Cooper, C., Hanson, M.A., 2011. Epigenetic gene promoter methylation at birth is associated with child's later adiposity. Diabetes 60, 1528–1534.

Gray, C., Li, M., Reynolds, C.M., Vickers, M.H., 2013. Pre-weaning growth hormone treatment reverses hypertension and endothelial dysfunction in adult male offspring of mothers undernourished during pregnancy. PLoS One 8, e53505.

Gray, C., Li, M., Reynolds, C.M., Vickers, M.H., 2014. Let-7 miRNA profiles are associated with the reversal of left ventricular hypertrophy and hypertension in adult male offspring from mothers undernourished during pregnancy following pre-weaning growth hormone treatment. Endocrinology 155, 4808–4817.

Guariguata, L., Whiting, D.R., Hambleton, I., Beagley, J., Linnenkamp, U., Shaw, J.E., 2014. Global estimates of diabetes prevalence for 2013 and projections for 2035. Diabetes Res. Clin. Pract. 103, 137–149.

Guay, C., Regazzi, R., 2014. Role of islet microRNAs in diabetes: which model for which question? Diabetologia 58, 456–463.

Guay, C., Roggli, E., Nesca, V., Jacovetti, C., Regazzi, R., 2011. Diabetes mellitus, a microRNA-related disease? Transl. Res. 157, 253–264.

Gulati, S., Misra, A., 2014. Sugar intake, obesity, and diabetes in India. Nutrients 6, 5955–5974.

Gurung, M., Li, Z., You, H., Rodrigues, R., Jump, D.B., Morgun, A., Shulzhenko, N., 2020. Role of gut microbiota in type 2 diabetes pathophysiology. EBioMedicine 51, 102590.

Hales, C.N., Barker, D.J., 2001. The thrifty phenotype hypothesis. Br. Med. Bull. 60, 5–20.

Hartstra, A.V., Bouter, K.E., Backhed, F., Nieuwdorp, M., 2015. Insights into the role of the microbiome in obesity and type 2 diabetes. Diabetes Care 38, 159–165.

He, Y., Wu, W., Zheng, H.M., Li, P., McDonald, D., Sheng, H.F., Chen, M.X., Chen, Z.H., Ji, G.Y., Zheng, Z.D., Mujagond, P., Chen, X.J., Rong, Z.H., Chen, P., Lyu, L.Y., Wang, X., Wu, C.B., Yu, N., Xu, Y.J., Yin, J., Raes, J., Knight, R., Ma, W.J., Zhou, H.W., 2018. Regional variation limits applications of healthy gut microbiome reference ranges and disease models. Nat. Med. 24, 1532–1535.

Heijmans, B.T., Tobi, E.W., Stein, A.D., Putter, H., Blauw, G.J., Susser, E.S., Slagboom, P.E., Lumey, L.H., 2008. Persistent epigenetic differences associated with prenatal exposure to famine in humans. Proc. Natl. Acad. Sci. U. S. A. 105, 17046–17049.

Howie, G.J., Sloboda, D.M., Kamal, T., Vickers, M.H., 2009. Maternal nutritional history predicts obesity in adult offspring independent of postnatal diet. J. Physiol. 587, 905–915.

Howie, G.J., Sloboda, D.M., Vickers, M.H., 2012. Maternal undernutrition during critical windows of development results in differential and sex-specific effects on postnatal adiposity and related metabolic profiles in adult rat offspring. Br. J. Nutr. 108, 298–307.

Hsu, C.N., Tain, Y.L., 2020. Amino acids and developmental origins of hypertension. Nutrients 12, 1763.

Hu, L., Peng, X., Chen, H., Yan, C., Liu, Y., Xu, Q., Fang, Z., Lin, Y., Xu, S., Feng, B., Li, J., Wu, D., Che, L., 2017. Effects of intrauterine growth retardation and Bacillus subtilis PB6 supplementation on growth performance, intestinal development and immune function of piglets during the suckling period. Eur. J. Nutr. 56, 1753–1765.

Hur, S.S.J., Cropley, J.E., Suter, C.M., 2017. Paternal epigenetic programming: evolving metabolic disease risk. J. Mol. Endocrinol. 58, R159–R168.

Iorio, M.V., Piovan, C., Croce, C.M., 2010. Interplay between microRNAs and the epigenetic machinery: an intricate network. Biochim. Biophys. Acta 1799, 694–701.

Jackson, S.E., Llewellyn, C.H., Smith, L., 2020. The obesity epidemic—nature via nurture: a narrative review of high-income countries. SAGE Open Med. 8. 2050312120918265.

Jang, H., Serra, C., 2014. Nutrition, epigenetics, and diseases. Clin. Nutr. Res. 3, 1–8.

Jaquet, D., Swaminathan, S., Alexander, G.R., Czernichow, P., Collin, D., Salihu, H.M., Kirby, R.S., Lévy-Marchal, C., 2005. Significant paternal contribution to the risk of small for gestational age. BJOG 112, 153–159.

Jirtle, R.L., Skinner, M.K., 2007. Environmental epigenomics and disease susceptibility. Nat. Rev. Genet. 8, 253–262.

Kieffer, T.J., Habener, J.F., 2000. The adipoinsular axis: effects of leptin on pancreatic beta-cells. Am. J. Physiol. Endocrinol. Metab. 278, E1–E14.

Kootte, R.S., Vrieze, A., Holleman, F., Dallinga-Thie, G.M., Zoetendal, E.G., De Vos, W.M., Groen, A.K., Hoekstra, J.B., Stroes, E.S., Nieuwdorp, M., 2012. The therapeutic potential of manipulating gut microbiota in obesity and type 2 diabetes mellitus. Diabetes Obes. Metab. 14, 112–120.

Küpers, L.K., Monnereau, C., Sharp, G.C., Yousefi, P., Salas, L.A., Ghantous, A., et al., 2019. Meta-analysis of epigenome-wide association studies in neonates reveals widespread differential DNA methylation associated with birthweight. Nat. Commun. 10, 1893.

Laitinen, K., Poussa, T., Isolauri, E., 2009. Probiotics and dietary counselling contribute to glucose regulation during and after pregnancy: a randomised controlled trial. Br. J. Nutr. 101, 1679–1687.

Lango, H., Palmer, C.N., Morris, A.D., Zeggini, E., Hattersley, A.T., McCarthy, M.I., Frayling, T.M., Weedon, M.N., 2008. Assessing the combined impact of 18 common genetic variants of modest effect sizes on type 2 diabetes risk. Diabetes 57, 3129–3135.

Lascar, N., Brown, J., Pattison, H., Barnett, A.H., Bailey, C.J., Bellary, S., 2018. Type 2 diabetes in adolescents and young adults. Lancet Diabetes Endocrinol. 6, 69–80.

Lassala, A., Bazer, F.W., Cudd, T.A., Datta, S., Keisler, D.H., Satterfield, M.C., Spencer, T.E., Wu, G., 2010. Parenteral administration of L-arginine prevents fetal growth restriction in undernourished ewes. J. Nutr. 140, 1242–1248.

Leenen, F.A., Muller, C.P., Turner, J.D., 2016. DNA methylation: conducting the orchestra from exposure to phenotype? Clin. Epigenetics 8, 92.

Lesseur, C., Armstrong, D.A., Paquette, A.G., Koestler, D.C., Padbury, J.F., Marsit, C.J., 2013. Tissue-specific leptin promoter DNA methylation is associated with maternal and infant perinatal factors. Mol. Cell. Endocrinol. 381, 160–167.

Lesseur, C., Armstrong, D.A., Paquette, A.G., Li, Z., Padbury, J.F., Marsit, C.J., 2014. Maternal obesity and gestational diabetes are associated with placental leptin DNA methylation. Am. J. Obstet. Gynecol. 211 (654), e1–e9.

Ley, R.E., Backhed, F., Turnbaugh, P., Lozupone, C.A., Knight, R.D., Gordon, J.I., 2005. Obesity alters gut microbial ecology. Proc. Natl. Acad. Sci. U. S. A. 102, 11070–11075.

Ley, R.E., Turnbaugh, P.J., Klein, S., Gordon, J.I., 2006. Microbial ecology: human gut microbes associated with obesity. Nature 444, 1022–1023.

Li, C., Lumey, L.H., 2017. Exposure to the Chinese famine of 1959-61 in early life and long-term health conditions: a systematic review and meta-analysis. Int. J. Epidemiol. 46, 1157–1170.

Li, M., Reynolds, C.M., Sloboda, D.M., Gray, C., Vickers, M.H., 2013. Effects of taurine supplementation on hepatic markers of inflammation and lipid metabolism in mothers and offspring in the setting of maternal obesity. PLoS One 8, e76961.

Li, M., Reynolds, C.M., Sloboda, D.M., Gray, C., Vickers, M.H., 2015. Maternal taurine supplementation attenuates maternal fructose-induced metabolic and inflammatory dysregulation and partially reverses adverse metabolic programming in offspring. J. Nutr. Biochem. 26, 267–276.

Lie, S., Morrison, J.L., Williams-Wyss, O., Suter, C.M., Humphreys, D.T., Ozanne, S.E., Zhang, S., MacLaughlin, S.M., Kleemann, D.O., Walker, S.K., Roberts, C.T., McMillen, I.C., 2014. Periconceptional undernutrition programs changes in insulin-signaling molecules and microRNAs in skeletal muscle in singleton and twin fetal sheep. Biol. Reprod. 90, 5.

Lillycrop, K.A., Phillips, E.S., Jackson, A.A., Hanson, M.A., Burdge, G.C., 2005. Dietary protein restriction of pregnant rats induces and folic acid supplementation prevents epigenetic modification of hepatic gene expression in the offspring. J. Nutr. 135, 1382–1386.

Lillycrop, K.A., Slater-Jefferies, J.L., Hanson, M.A., Godfrey, K.M., Jackson, A.A., Burdge, G.C., 2007. Induction of altered epigenetic regulation of the hepatic glucocorticoid receptor in the offspring of rats fed a protein-restricted diet during pregnancy suggests that reduced DNA methyltransferase-1 expression is involved in impaired DNA methylation and changes in histone modifications. Br. J. Nutr. 97, 1064–1073.

Liu, H.W., Mahmood, S., Srinivasan, M., Smiraglia, D.J., Patel, M.S., 2013. Developmental programming in skeletal muscle in response to overnourishment in the immediate postnatal life in rats. J. Nutr. Biochem. 24, 1859–1869.

Liu, G.T., Dancause, K.N., Elgbeili, G., Laplante, D.P., King, S., 2016. Disaster-related prenatal maternal stress explains increasing amounts of variance in body composition through childhood and adolescence: project ice storm. Environ. Res. 150, 1–7.

Long, N.M., Ford, S.P., Nathanielsz, P.W., 2011. Maternal obesity eliminates the neonatal lamb plasma leptin peak. J. Physiol. 589, 1455–1462.

Luoto, R., Kalliomaki, M., Laitinen, K., Isolauri, E., 2010. The impact of perinatal probiotic intervention on the development of overweight and obesity: follow-up study from birth to 10 years. Int. J. Obes. 34, 1531–1537.

Ly, C., Yockell-Lelièvre, J., Ferraro, Z.M., Arnason, J.T., Ferrier, J., Gruslin, A., 2015. The effects of dietary polyphenols on reproductive health and early development. Hum. Reprod. Update 21, 228–248.

Ma, D., Ozanne, S.E., Guest, P.C., 2018. Generation of the maternal low-protein rat model for studies of metabolic disorders. Methods Mol. Biol. 1735, 201–206.

MacLennan, N.K., James, S.J., Melnyk, S., Piroozi, A., Jernigan, S., Hsu, J.L., Janke, S.M., Pham, T.D., Lane, R.H., 2004. Uteroplacental insufficiency alters DNA methylation, one-carbon metabolism, and histone acetylation in IUGR rats. Physiol. Genomics 18, 43–50.

Magnus, M.C., Olsen, S.F., Granstrom, C., Lund-Blix, N.A., Svensson, J., Johannesen, J., Fraser, A., Skrivarhaug, T., Joner, G., Njølstad, P.R., Størdal, K., Stene, L.C., 2018. Paternal and maternal obesity but not gestational weight gain is associated with type 1 diabetes. Int. J. Epidemiol. 47, 417–426.

Marco, A., Kisliouk, T., Tabachnik, T., Meiri, N., Weller, A., 2014. Overweight and CpG methylation of the Pomc promoter in offspring of high-fat-diet-fed dams are not "reprogrammed" by regular chow diet in rats. FASEB J. 28, 4148–4157.

Mark, P.J., Sisala, C., Connor, K., Patel, R., Lewis, J.L., Vickers, M.H., Waddell, B.J., Sloboda, D.M., 2011. A maternal high-fat diet in rat pregnancy reduces growth of the fetus and the placental junctional zone, but not placental labyrinth zone growth. J. Dev. Orig. Health Dis. 2, 63–70.

Marousez, L., Lesage, J., Eberlé, D., 2019. Epigenetics: linking early postnatal nutrition to obesity programming? Nutrients 11, 2966.

McCarthy, M.I., Zeggini, E., 2009. Genome-wide association studies in type 2 diabetes. Curr. Diab. Rep. 9, 164–171.

McKay, J.A., Groom, A., Potter, C., Coneyworth, L.J., Ford, D., Mathers, J.C., Relton, C.L., 2012. Genetic and non-genetic influences during pregnancy on infant global and site specific DNA methylation: role for folate gene variants and vitamin B12. PLoS One 7, e33290.

McMillen, I.C., MacLaughlin, S.M., Muhlhausler, B.S., Gentili, S., Duffield, J.L., Morrison, J.L., 2008. Developmental origins of adult health and disease: the role of periconceptional and foetal nutrition. Basic Clin. Pharmacol. Toxicol. 102, 82–89.

Mischke, M., Arora, T., Tims, S., Engels, E., Sommer, N., Van Limpt, K., Baars, A., Oozeer, R., Oosting, A., Bäckhed, F., Knol, J., 2018. Specific synbiotics in early life protect against diet-induced obesity in adult mice. Diabetes Obes. Metab. 20, 1408–1418.

Misra, A., Singhal, N., Sivakumar, B., Bhagat, N., Jaiswal, A., Khurana, L., 2011. Nutrition transition in India: secular trends in dietary intake and their relationship to diet-related non-communicable diseases. J. Diabetes 3, 278–292.

Moore, B.J., 1987. The cafeteria diet-an inappropriate tool for studies of thermogenesis. J. Nutr. 117, 227–231.

Morris, A.P., Voight, B.F., Teslovich, T.M., Ferreira, T., Segre, A.V., Steinthorsdottir, V., et al., 2012. Large-scale association analysis provides insights into the genetic architecture and pathophysiology of type 2 diabetes. Nat. Genet. 44, 981–990.

Nauta, A.J., Ben Amor, K., Knol, J., Garssen, J., Van Der Beek, E.M., 2013. Relevance of pre- and postnatal nutrition to development and interplay between the microbiota and metabolic and immune systems. Am. J. Clin. Nutr. 98, 586S–593S.

Nesca, V., Guay, C., Jacovetti, C., Menoud, V., Peyot, M.L., Laybutt, D.R., Prentki, M., Regazzi, R., 2013. Identification of particular groups of microRNAs that positively or negatively impact on beta cell function in obese models of type 2 diabetes. Diabetologia 56, 2203–2212.

Ng, S.F., Lin, R.C., Laybutt, D.R., Barres, R., Owens, J.A., Morris, M.J., 2010. Chronic high-fat diet in fathers programs beta-cell dysfunction in female rat offspring. Nature 467, 963–966.

Ng, S.F., Lin, R.C., Maloney, C.A., Youngson, N.A., Owens, J.A., Morris, M.J., 2014. Paternal high-fat diet consumption induces common changes in the transcriptomes of retroperitoneal adipose and pancreatic islet tissues in female rat offspring. FASEB J. 28, 1830–1841.

Ong, T.P., Ozanne, S.E., 2015. Developmental programming of type 2 diabetes: early nutrition and epigenetic mechanisms. Curr. Opin. Clin. Nutr. Metab. Care 18, 354–360.

Ornoy, A., 2011. Prenatal origin of obesity and their complications: gestational diabetes, maternal overweight and the paradoxical effects of fetal growth restriction and macrosomia. Reprod. Toxicol. 32, 205–212.

Pan, W.H., Sommer, F., Falk-Paulsen, M., Ulas, T., Best, P., Fazio, A., et al., 2018. Exposure to the gut microbiota drives distinct methylome and transcriptome changes in intestinal epithelial cells during postnatal development. Genome Med. 10, 27.

Paxman, E.J., Boora, N.S., Kiss, D., Laplante, D.P., King, S., Montina, T., Metz, G.A.S., 2018. Prenatal maternal stress from a natural disaster alters urinary metabolomic profiles in project ice storm participants. Sci. Rep. 8, 12932.

Pérez-López, F.R., Pasupuleti, V., Mezones-Holguin, E., Benites-Zapata, V.A., Thota, P., Deshpande, A., Hernandez, A.V., 2015. Effect of vitamin D supplementation during pregnancy on maternal and neonatal outcomes: a systematic review and meta-analysis of randomized controlled trials. Fertil. Steril. 103, 1278–1288.e4.

Pham, T.D., MacLennan, N.K., Chiu, C.T., Laksana, G.S., Hsu, J.L., Lane, R.H., 2003. Uteroplacental insufficiency increases apoptosis and alters p53 gene methylation in the full-term IUGR rat kidney. Am. J. Phys. Regul. Integr. Comp. Phys. 285, R962–R970.

Qian, M., Chou, S.Y., Gimenez, L., Liu, J.T., 2017. The intergenerational transmission of low birth weight and intrauterine growth restriction: a large cross-generational cohort study in Taiwan. Matern. Child Health J. 21, 1512–1521.

Radford, E.J., Isganaitis, E., Jimenez-Chillaron, J., Schroeder, J., Molla, M., Andrews, S., Didier, N., Charalambous, M., McEwen, K., Marazzi, G., Sassoon, D., Patti, M.E., Ferguson-Smith, A.C., 2012. An unbiased assessment of the role of imprinted genes in an intergenerational model of developmental programming. PLoS Genet. 8, e1002605.

Radulescu, L., Munteanu, O., Popa, F., Cirstoiu, M., 2013. The implications and consequences of maternal obesity on fetal intrauterine growth restriction. J. Med. Life 6, 292–298.

Reynolds, C.M., Li, M., Gray, C., Vickers, M.H., 2013. Pre-weaning growth hormone treatment ameliorates adipose tissue insulin resistance and inflammation in adult male offspring following maternal undernutrition. Endocrinology 154, 2676–2686.

Reynolds, C.M., Segovia, S.A., Zhang, X.D., Gray, C., Vickers, M.H., 2015a. Conjugated linoleic acid supplementation during pregnancy and lactation reduces maternal high-fat-diet-induced programming of early-onset puberty and hyperlipidemia in female rat offspring. Biol. Reprod. 92, 40.

Reynolds, C.M., Segovia, S.A., Zhang, X.D., Gray, C., Vickers, M.H., 2015b. Maternal high-fat diet-induced programming of gut taste receptor and inflammatory gene expression in rat offspring is ameliorated by CLA supplementation. Phys. Rep. 3, e12588.

Reynolds, C.M., Vickers, M.H., Harrison, C.J., Segovia, S.A., Gray, C., 2015c. Maternal high fat and/or salt consumption induces sex-specific inflammatory and nutrient transport in the rat placenta. Phys. Rep. 3, e12399.

Roth, D.E., Morris, S.K., Zlotkin, S., Gernand, A.D., Ahmed, T., Shanta, S.S., et al., 2018. Vitamin D supplementation in pregnancy and lactation and infant growth. N. Engl. J. Med. 379, 535–546.

Saeedi Borujeni, M.J., Esfandiary, E., Baradaran, A., Valiani, A., Ghanadian, M., Codoñer-Franch, P., Basirat, R., Alonso-Iglesias, E., Mirzaei, H., Yazdani, A., 2019. Molecular aspects of pancreatic β-cell dysfunction: oxidative stress, microRNA, and long noncoding RNA. J. Cell. Physiol. 234, 8411–8425.

Sampey, B.P., Vanhoose, A.M., Winfield, H.M., Freemerman, A.J., Muehlbauer, M.J., Fueger, P.T., Newgard, C.B., Makowski, L., 2011. Cafeteria diet is a robust model of human metabolic syndrome with liver and adipose inflammation: comparison to high-fat diet. Obesity (Silver Spring) 19, 1109–1117.

Segovia, S.A., Vickers, M.H., Gray, C., Zhang, X.D., Reynolds, C.M., 2017. Conjugated linoleic acid supplementation improves maternal high fat diet-induced programming of metabolic dysfunction in adult male rat offspring. Sci. Rep. 7, 6663.

Segovia, S.A., Vickers, M.H., Harrison, C.J., Patel, R., Gray, C., Reynolds, C.M., 2018. Maternal high-fat and high-salt diets have differential programming effects on metabolism in adult male rat offspring. Front. Nutr. 5, 1.

Shapiro, A.L., Schmiege, S.J., Brinton, J.T., Glueck, D., Crume, T.L., Friedman, J.E., Dabelea, D., 2015. Testing the fuel-mediated hypothesis: maternal insulin resistance and glucose mediate the association between maternal and neonatal adiposity, the healthy start study. Diabetologia 58, 937–941.

Shasa, D.R., Odhiambo, J.F., Long, N.M., Tuersunjiang, N., Nathanielsz, P.W., Ford, S.P., 2015. Multigenerational impact of maternal overnutrition/obesity in the sheep on the neonatal leptin surge in granddaughters. Int. J. Obes. 39, 695–701.

Silva, A.J., White, R., 1988. Inheritance of allelic blueprints for methylation patterns. Cell 54, 145–152.

Simmons, D., 2015. Prevention of gestational diabetes mellitus: where are we now? Diabetes Obes. Metab. 17, 824–834.

Singhal, A., 2017. Long-term adverse effects of early growth acceleration or catch-up growth. Ann. Nutr. Metab. 70, 236–240.

Smith, A.M., Pankey, C.L., Odhiambo, J.F., Ghnenis, A.B., Nathanielsz, P.W., Ford, S.P., 2018. Rapid communication: reduced maternal nutrition during early- to mid-gestation elevates newborn lamb plasma cortisol concentrations and eliminates the neonatal leptin surge. J. Anim. Sci. 96, 2640–2645.

Snoeck, A., Remacle, C., Reusens, B., Hoet, J.J., 1990. Effect of a low protein diet during pregnancy on the fetal rat endocrine pancreas. Biol. Neonate 57, 107–118.

Soderborg, T.K., Friedman, J.E., 2018. Imbalance in gut microbes from babies born to obese mothers increases gut permeability and myeloid cell adaptations that provoke obesity and NAFLD. Microb. Cell 6, 102–104.

II. Early nutrition and development of non-communicable diseases

Song, Y., Huang, Y., Song, Y., Hevener, A.L., Ryckman, K.K., Qi, L., Leblanc, E.S., Kazlauskaite, R., Brennan, K.M., Liu, S., 2015. Birthweight, mediating biomarkers and the development of type 2 diabetes later in life: a prospective study of multi-ethnic women. Diabetologia 58, 1220–1230.

Soubry, A., 2018. POHaD: why we should study future fathers. Environ. Epigenet. 4, dvy007.

Soubry, A., Murphy, S.K., Wang, F., Huang, Z., Vidal, A.C., Fuemmeler, B.F., Kurtzberg, J., Murtha, A., Jirtle, R.L., Schildkraut, J.M., Hoyo, C., 2015. Newborns of obese parents have altered DNA methylation patterns at imprinted genes. Int. J. Obes. 39, 650–657.

Soubry, A., Schildkraut, J.M., Murtha, A., Wang, F., Huang, Z., Bernal, A., Kurtzberg, J., Jirtle, R.L., Murphy, S.K., Hoyo, C., 2013. Paternal obesity is associated with IGF2 hypomethylation in newborns: results from a newborn epigenetics study (NEST) cohort. BMC Med. 11, 29.

Spiroski, A.M., Oliver, M.H., Jaquiery, A.L., Gunn, T.D., Harding, J.E., Bloomfield, F.H., 2020. Effects of intrauterine insulin-like growth factor-1 therapy for fetal growth restriction on adult metabolism and body composition are sex specific. Am. J. Physiol. Endocrinol. Metab. 318, E568–E578.

Stevens, A., Begum, G., White, A., 2011. Epigenetic changes in the hypothalamic pro-opiomelanocortin gene: a mechanism linking maternal undernutrition to obesity in the offspring? Eur. J. Pharmacol. 660, 194–201.

Tain, Y.L., Hsu, C.N., 2018. Developmental programming of the metabolic syndrome: can we reprogram with resveratrol? Int. J. Mol. Sci. 19, 584.

Takaya, J., Yamanouchi, S., Kino, J., Tanabe, Y., Kaneko, K., 2018. A calcium-deficient diet in dams during gestation increases insulin resistance in male offspring. Nutrients 10, 1745.

Taylor, P.D., McConnell, J., Khan, I.Y., Holemans, K., Lawrence, K.M., Asare-Anane, H., Persaud, S.J., Jones, P.M., Petrie, L., Hanson, M.A., Poston, L., 2005. Impaired glucose homeostasis and mitochondrial abnormalities in offspring of rats fed a fat-rich diet in pregnancy. Am. J. Phys. Regul. Integr. Comp. Phys. 288, R134–R139.

Tobi, E.W., Goeman, J.J., Monajemi, R., Gu, H., Putter, H., Zhang, Y., Slieker, R.C., Stok, A.P., Thijssen, P.E., Müller, F., Van Zwet, E.W., Bock, C., Meissner, A., Lumey, L.H., Eline Slagboom, P., Heijmans, B.T., 2014. DNA methylation signatures link prenatal famine exposure to growth and metabolism. Nat. Commun. 5, 5592.

Tobi, E.W., Lumey, L.H., Talens, R.P., Kremer, D., Putter, H., Stein, A.D., Slagboom, P.E., Heijmans, B.T., 2009. DNA methylation differences after exposure to prenatal famine are common and timing- and sex-specific. Hum. Mol. Genet. 18, 4046–4053.

Tomat, A.L., Costa Mde, L., Arranz, C.T., 2011. Zinc restriction during different periods of life: influence in renal and cardiovascular diseases. Nutrition 27, 392–398.

Tosh, D.N., Fu, Q., Callaway, C.W., McKnight, R.A., McMillen, I.C., Ross, M.G., Lane, R.H., Desai, M., 2010. Epigenetics of programmed obesity: alteration in IUGR rat hepatic IGF1 mRNA expression and histone structure in rapid vs. delayed postnatal catch-up growth. Am. J. Physiol. Gastrointest. Liver Physiol. 299, G1023–G1029.

Turnbaugh, P.J., Ley, R.E., Mahowald, M.A., Magrini, V., Mardis, E.R., Gordon, J.I., 2006. An obesity-associated gut microbiome with increased capacity for energy harvest. Nature 444, 1027–1031.

Van Belle, T.L., Gysemans, C., Mathieu, C., 2013. Vitamin D and diabetes: the odd couple. Trends Endocrinol. Metab. 24, 561–568.

Van Dijk, S.J., Zhou, J., Peters, T.J., Buckley, M., Sutcliffe, B., Oytam, Y., Gibson, R.A., McPhee, A., Yelland, L.N., Makrides, M., Molloy, P.L., Muhlhausler, B.S., 2016. Effect of prenatal DHA supplementation on the infant epigenome: results from a randomized controlled trial. Clin. Epigenetics 8, 114.

Vanhees, K., Vonhogen, I.G., Van Schooten, F.J., Godschalk, R.W., 2014. You are what you eat, and so are your children: the impact of micronutrients on the epigenetic programming of offspring. Cell. Mol. Life Sci. 71, 271–285.

Vega, C.C., Reyes-Castro, L.A., Bautista, C.J., Larrea, F., Nathanielsz, P.W., Zambrano, E., 2015. Exercise in obese female rats has beneficial effects on maternal and male and female offspring metabolism. Int. J. Obes. 39, 712–719.

Via, M., 2012. The malnutrition of obesity: micronutrient deficiencies that promote diabetes. ISRN Endocrinol. 2012, 103472.

Vickers, M.H., Breier, B.H., Cutfield, W.S., Hofman, P.L., Gluckman, P.D., 2000. Fetal origins of hyperphagia, obesity, and hypertension and postnatal amplification by hypercaloric nutrition. Am. J. Physiol. Endocrinol. Metab. 279, E83–E87.

Vickers, M.H., Gluckman, P.D., Coveny, A.H., Hofman, P.L., Cutfield, W.S., Gertler, A., Breier, B.H., Harris, M., 2008. The effect of neonatal leptin treatment on postnatal weight gain in male rats is dependent on maternal nutritional status during pregnancy. Endocrinology 149, 8.

Vickers, M.H., Reddy, S., Ikenasio, B.A., Breier, B.H., 2001b. Dysregulation of the adipoinsular axis—a mechanism for the pathogenesis of hyperleptinemia and adipogenic diabetes induced by fetal programming. J. Endocrinol. 170, 323–332.

Vickers, M.H., Sloboda, D.M., 2012a. Leptin as mediator of the effects of developmental programming. Best Pract. Res. Clin. Endocrinol. Metab. 26, 677–687.

Vickers, M.H., Sloboda, D.M., 2012b. Strategies for reversing the effects of metabolic disorders induced as a consequence of developmental programming. Front. Physiol. 3, 242.

Vrieze, A., Van Nood, E., Holleman, F., Salojarvi, J., Kootte, R.S., Bartelsman, J.F., et al., 2012. Transfer of intestinal microbiota from lean donors increases insulin sensitivity in individuals with metabolic syndrome. Gastroenterology 143, 913–916.e7.

Wang, B., Chandrasekera, P.C., Pippin, J.J., 2014. Leptin- and leptin receptor-deficient rodent models: relevance for human type 2 diabetes. Curr. Diabetes Rev. 10, 131–145.

Wang, P., Sang, S., 2018. Metabolism and pharmacokinetics of resveratrol and pterostilbene. Biofactors 44, 16–25.

Wasenius, N.S., Grattan, K.P., Harvey, A.L.J., Barrowman, N., Goldfield, G.S., Adamo, K.B., 2017. Maternal gestational weight gain and objectively measured physical activity among offspring. PLoS One 12, e0180249.

Waterland, R.A., Kellermayer, R., Laritsky, E., Rayco-Solon, P., Harris, R.A., Travisano, M., Zhang, W., Torskaya, M.S., Zhang, J., Shen, L., Manary, M.J., Prentice, A.M., 2010. Season of conception in rural Gambia affects DNA methylation at putative human metastable epialleles. PLoS Genet. 6, e1001252.

Weaver, I.C., Cervoni, N., Champagne, F.A., D'alessio, A.C., Sharma, S., Seckl, J.R., Dymov, S., Szyf, M., Meaney, M.J., 2004. Epigenetic programming by maternal behavior. Nat. Neurosci. 7, 847–854.

Weihrauch-Blüher, S., Wiegand, S., 2018. Risk factors and implications of childhood obesity. Curr. Obes. Rep. 7, 254–259.

Wells, J.C., Sawaya, A.L., Wibaek, R., Mwangome, M., Poullas, M.S., Yajnik, C.S., Demaio, A., 2020. The double burden of malnutrition: aetiological pathways and consequences for health. Lancet 395, 75–88.

Wolffe, A.P., 1998. Packaging principle: how DNA methylation and histone acetylation control the transcriptional activity of chromatin. J. Exp. Zool. 282, 239–244.

World Health Organisation, 2018. Obesity and Overweight. World Health Organisation, Geneva, Switzerland.

Yajnik, C.S., 2014. Transmission of obesity-adiposity and related disorders from the mother to the baby. Ann. Nutr. Metab. 64, 8–17.

Yamashita, H., Shao, J., Ishizuka, T., Klepcyk, P.J., Muhlenkamp, P., Qiao, L., Hoggard, N., Friedman, J.E., 2001. Leptin administration prevents spontaneous gestational diabetes in heterozygous Lepr(db/+) mice: effects on placental leptin and fetal growth. Endocrinology 142, 2888–2897.

Yang, Q.Y., Liang, J.F., Rogers, C.J., Zhao, J.X., Zhu, M.J., Du, M., 2013. Maternal obesity induces epigenetic modifications to facilitate Zfp423 expression and enhance adipogenic differentiation in fetal mice. Diabetes 62, 3727–3735.

Yao, L., Wan, J., Li, H., Ding, J., Wang, Y., Wang, X., Li, M., 2015. Resveratrol relieves gestational diabetes mellitus in mice through activating AMPK. Reprod. Biol. Endocrinol. 13, 118.

Zhang, J., Zhang, F., Didelot, X., Bruce, K.D., Cagampang, F.R., Vatish, M., Hanson, M., Lehnert, H., Ceriello, A., Byrne, C.D., 2009. Maternal high fat diet during pregnancy and lactation alters hepatic expression of insulin like growth factor-2 and key microRNAs in the adult offspring. BMC Genomics 10, 478.

Zhang, L., Long, N.M., Hein, S.M., Ma, Y., Nathanielsz, P.W., Ford, S.P., 2011. Maternal obesity in ewes results in reduced fetal pancreatic beta-cell numbers in late gestation and decreased circulating insulin concentration at term. Domest. Anim. Endocrinol. 40, 30–39.

Zhang, Q., Sun, X., Xiao, X., Zheng, J., Li, M., Yu, M., Ping, F., Wang, Z., Qi, C., Wang, T., Wang, X., 2017. Dietary chromium restriction of pregnant mice changes the methylation status of hepatic genes involved with insulin signaling in adult male offspring. PLoS One 12, e0169889.

Zheng, X., Liu, Z., Zhang, Y., Lin, Y., Song, J., Zheng, L., Lin, S., 2015. Relationship between myo-inositol supplementary and gestational diabetes mellitus: a meta-analysis. Medicine (Baltimore) 94, e1604.

Zheng, Y., Ley, S.H., Hu, F.B., 2018. Global aetiology and epidemiology of type 2 diabetes mellitus and its complications. Nat. Rev. Endocrinol. 14, 88–98.

Zimmet, P., Shi, Z., El-Osta, A., Ji, L., 2018. Epidemic T2DM, early development and epigenetics: implications of the Chinese famine. Nat. Rev. Endocrinol. 14, 738–746.

Zinkhan, E.K., Fu, Q., Wang, Y., Yu, X., Callaway, C.W., Segar, J.L., Scholz, T.D., McKnight, R.A., Joss-Moore, L., Lane, R.H., 2012. Maternal hyperglycemia disrupts histone 3 lysine 36 trimethylation of the IGF-1 gene. J. Nutr. Metab. 2012, 930364.

# Early nutrition and development of cardiovascular disease

*Tricia L. Hart[a], Kristina S. Petersen[a,b],*
*and Penny M. Kris-Etherton[a]*

[a]Penn State University, University Park, PA, United States [b]Texas Tech University, Lubbock, TX, United States

## CHAPTER LEARNING OBJECTIVES

(1) Understand the importance of a heart healthy diet throughout childhood and adolescence

(2) Describe components of a heart healthy diet

(3) Discuss evidence for CVD risk reduction with recommended dietary patterns

## 12.1 Introduction

Cardiovascular disease (CVD) is the leading cause of death globally accounting for 17.9 million deaths in 2019, or 32% of all deaths (Roth et al., 2017; World Health Organization, 2021). Coronary heart disease (CHD) is the most prevalent type of CVD and accounted for the largest increase in cause-specific deaths globally between 2000 and 2019 (by more than 2 million) (World Health Organization, 2020). CVD is a chronic disease that results from accruing exposure to risk factors, including poor diet quality, throughout the life span.

Dietary risk factors are the number one contributor to CVD mortality in adults accounting for approximately 72% of all CVD-related deaths (GBD, 2015). Dietary behaviors in childhood, however, strongly influence CVD risk in adulthood (Daniels et al., 2019). Most children are born with ideal cardiovascular health, which the American Heart Association (AHA) defines as the simultaneous presence of four favorable health behaviors (related to smoking, body mass index (BMI), physical activity, and healthy diet status) and three favorable health factors (total cholesterol, blood pressure (BP), and fasting blood glucose levels; Table 12.1) (Steinberger et al., 2016). However, throughout early childhood the number of children with

TABLE 12.1    Traditional cardiovascular disease risk factor definitions and prevalence in children.

| Risk factor | Definition | Definition ages[a] | Children meeting recommendation |
|---|---|---|---|
| (1) Overweight/obesity | BMI-for-age values ≥ 85th percentile of the 2000 Centers for Disease Control and Prevention CDC growth charts | 2–5 years | 86.1% |
| | | 6–11 years | 81.6% |
| | | 12–19 years | 79.4% |
| (2) Blood pressure | > 90th percentile of blood pressure | 8–12 years | 94.7% |
| | | 13–17 years | 95.6% |
| (3) Dyslipidemia | Fasting TG > 150 mg/dL LDL-C > 130 mg/dL HDL-C < 35 mg/dL TC > 170 mg/dL | 6–19 years | 51.4% |
| | | 12–19 years | 46.8% |
| (4) Fasting plasma glucose | Fasting blood glucose > 100 mg/dL | 12–19 years | 86.2% |

[a] Data are not available for other ages.
Data from Lloyd-Jones, D.M., Hong, Y., Labarthe, D., Mozaffarian, D., Appel, L.J., Van Horn, L., et al., 2010. Defining and setting national goals for cardiovascular health promotion and disease reduction: the American Heart Association's strategic Impact Goal through 2020 and beyond. Circulation 121(4), 586–613. https://doi.org/10.1161/CIRCULATIONAHA.109.192703; Data from Virani, S.S., Alonso, A., Aparicio, H.J., Benjamin, E.J., Bittencourt, M.S., Callaway, C.W., et al., 2021. Heart Disease and Stroke Statistics-2021 update: a report from the American Heart Association. Circulation 143(8), e254–e743. https://doi.org/10.1161/CIR.0000000000000950.

ideal cardiovascular health declines. Currently, less than 1% of children have an ideal diet based on the AHA definition (meeting recommendations for fruits and vegetables, whole grains, fish, sodium, sweets/sugar sweetened beverages) (Virani et al., 2021). Thus, management of dietary risk factors in childhood is critical to CVD risk reduction throughout life (Bowen et al., 2018; Steinberger et al., 2016).

A healthy dietary pattern in early life promotes cardiovascular health through life and decreases the risk of premature death and disability from CVD. This chapter will summarize the role of early nutrition (age 2 through age 19 years) in the prevention of modifiable CVD risk factors in childhood as well as adult-onset CVD. Specifically, the prevalence of poor diet quality in early life and the impact this has on CVD risk factors will be reviewed. In addition, dietary recommendations for CVD risk reduction in early life and strategies for implementation will be described. Optimal early life nutrition decreases CVD risk factors and, consequently, CVD risk throughout the life span. Thus, childhood and adolescence are critical windows of opportunity to establish healthy dietary behaviors to promote life-long cardiovascular health.

## 12.2  Importance of CVD risk reduction in childhood

CVD risk factors may develop early in life and affect cardiovascular health throughout the lifespan. Some CVD risk factors are non-modifiable (age, sex, genetics), although many CVD risk factors are modifiable, e.g., poor diet quality, physical inactivity, tobacco product use or exposure, overweight/obesity, high BP, dyslipidemia and elevated fasting plasma glucose (Table 12.1). A healthy lifestyle, including a healthy diet, can attenuate CVD risk in those at high CVD risk due to the presence of non-modifiable risk factors. In a prospective cohort study of adults (ages 44–80 years) at high genetic risk for coronary events (91% higher based on the top quintile of polygenic scores from DNA), compared to the lowest genetic risk, the risk of coronary events was reduced by 46% when at least three of four healthy life-style behaviors (not smoking, BMI < 30 kg/m$^2$, physical activity at least one time per week and a healthy eating pattern) were implemented versus fewer than three (Khera et al., 2016; Niinikoski et al., 2009).

Childhood obesity, hypertension, dyslipidemia, and hyperglycemia increase CVD risk in adulthood. The AHA reported that adolescents with overweight or obesity had two- to three-fold higher risk of CVD mortality compared to their normal weight counterparts and that a graded relationship exists between high BP in adolescence and CVD events decades later (de Ferranti et al., 2019). Further evidence from a prospective study showed that children ages 6–18 years with overweight or obesity (≥ 85th CDC 2000 age-gender specific percentile) had increased risk of CVD (OR 3.03, CI 95% 1.18–7.73) 26 years later compared to those without overweight or obesity. Similarly, children with high triglycerides (≥ 110 mg/dL; OR 5.85, CI 95% 2.33–14.7), high BP (≥ 90th age-height specific percentile; OR 3.02, CI 95% 0.92–9.89) or high fasting plasma glucose (≥ 110 mg/dL; 3.09, CI 95% 0.68–14.0) had significantly increased risk of CVD in adulthood compared to children without these risk factors (Morrison et al., 2012).

Onset of CVD risk factors is increasingly common in childhood (Table 12.1). Currently, 40% of US children have overweight and 19% have obesity (Fryar et al., 2020; Virani et al., 2021). Obesity prevalence differs by ethnicity with the obesity prevalence of Hispanic children being the highest at 25.6%, and lowest among non-Hispanic Asian children at 8.7% (Centers for Disease Control and Prevention, 2021). The percentage of children affected by obesity has more than tripled since 1970 (Fryar et al., 2020). Of further concern is the increase in obesity by age. In 2017–18, 13.4% of children ages 2–5 years had obesity, 20.3% of children ages 6–11 years had obesity, and 21.2% of children ages 12–19 years had obesity (Centers for Disease Control and Prevention, 2021). The CDC reports that 6.1% of the pediatric population has severe obesity (Fryar et al., 2020). During the past 18 years, there have been significant increases in obesity severity following the adult model of class I, II, and III obesity independent of age, race, and sex (Skinner et al., 2018).

Approximately 210,000 Americans younger than 20 years are estimated to have diagnosed diabetes, about 0.25% of that population (Centers for Disease Control and Prevention, 2020). From 2002 to 2015, the prevalence of type 2 diabetes in children younger than 20 years increased by 4.8% across all ages, genders, and races except for whites (Center for Disease Control and Prevention, 2020; Divers et al., 2020). The greatest increase in type 2 diabetes prevalence was seen in non-Hispanic blacks (Centers for Disease Control and Prevention, 2020).

Hypertension and dyslipidemia can begin in childhood. Approximately 4.9% of children ages 8–17 years have BPs greater than the 95th percentile and 13.3% have systolic or diastolic BP in the 90th percentile (Virani et al., 2021). Between the ages of 6 and 19 years, total cholesterol has trended downwards from 1999 to 2016; however, even with the improvement, only 51.4% of children have ideal cholesterol and lipid levels (see Table 12.1) (Perak et al., 2019).

Dietary intake strongly influences obesity, hypertension, dyslipidemia, and hyperglycemia development in childhood and adulthood. Given the significant effect diet has on CVD risk factors, a key component of primordial prevention is a healthy diet. The 2020–25 Dietary Guidelines for Americans recommend consuming a healthy eating pattern at every life stage with an emphasis on nutrient-dense foods. A healthy eating pattern meets food group and nutrient recommendations and limits added sugar, sodium, and saturated fat. Current recommendations are that saturated fat and added sugar each is limited to less than 10% of total energy; sodium recommendations are based on age. Healthy eating patterns should be individualized to align with food preferences, cultural preferences, and budgetary constraints (U.S. Department of Health and Human Services and U.S. Department of Agriculture, 2020).

## 12.3 Childhood nutrition and CVD risk factors

In the United States, the majority of children do not meet dietary recommendations, with over 99% not having a healthy diet score (Virani et al., 2021). The Healthy Eating Index-2015 was developed to assess adherence to the 2015–20 Dietary Guidelines for Americans. Table 12.2 presents the Healthy Eating Index-2015 scores as well as the percentage of children exceeding saturated fat, sodium, and added sugar recommendations.

Throughout childhood diet quality declines. In adolescents (ages 14–18 years), the Healthy Eating Index-2015 is 10 points lower than in children aged 2–4 years. The majority of children in all age groups exceed saturated fat, sodium, and added sugar recommendations (see Table 12.2). Interestingly, fewer adolescents consumed excess sugar and saturated fat than younger age groups. There is also a difference between genders in sodium intake as 97% of males compared to 77% of females exceed the recommended 2300 mg of sodium, which likely reflects energy intake since sodium tracks with calories (U.S. Department of Health and Human Services and U.S. Department of Agriculture, 2020). The discrepancy between recommendations and consumption throughout childhood widens with age with a concomitant increased risk of developing major CVD risk factors. See Table 12.3 for average current intakes of children versus recommendations.

## 12.4 Early nutrition and CVD risk

Current childhood dietary intake patterns are characterized as suboptimal because of low intake of fruits, vegetables, and whole grains, and high intake of added sugars,

TABLE 12.2   Healthy eating index scores for children ages 2–18 years.

| Age | Healthy eating index[a] | Children exceeding saturated fat recommendations | Children exceeding sodium recommendations | Children exceeding sugar recommendations |
|-----|-----|-----|-----|-----|
| 2–4 | 61 | 87% | 96% | 59% |
| 5–8 | 55 | 83% | 97% | 79% |
| 9–13 | 52 | 87% | 96% | 78% |
| 14–18 | 51 | 82% | 87% | 74% |

[a] *Maximum score 100.*
*Data from U.S. Department of Agriculture and U.S. Department of Health and Human Services. Dietary Guidelines for Americans, 2020–2025, ninth ed.*

TABLE 12.3 Current dietary intake of children.

| Food group | Daily amount of food from each group | | | | | |
| | Ages 2–5 | | Ages 6–11 | | Ages 12–19 | |
| | M | F | M | F | M | F |
| --- | --- | --- | --- | --- | --- | --- |
| Total vegetables (cup eq/day) | 0.70 (1–2) | 0.66 (1–1½) | 0.85 (1½–3½) | 0.90 (1½–3) | 1.06 (2–4) | 0.96 (1½–3) |
| Total fruits (cup eq/day) | 1.23 (1–1½) | 1.19 (1–1½) | 0.93 (1–2) | 0.91 (1–2) | 0.87 (1½–2½) | 0.88 (1½–2) |
| Total grains (oz. eq/day) | 5.34 (3–5) | 4.53 (3–5) | 7.42 (4–9) | 6.85 (4–7) | 8.18 (5–10) | 6.44 (5–8) |
| Total dairy (cup eq/day) | 1.98 (2–2½) | 1.90 (2–2½) | 2.09 (2½–3) | 1.91 (2½–3) | 2.16 (3–3½) | 1.60 (3–3½) |
| Total protein foods (oz. eq/day) | 3.13 (2–5) | 2.91 (2–4) | 4.19 (3–6½) | 3.77 (3–6) | 5.58 (5–7) | 4.01 (4–6½) |

Recommendations are denoted in parentheses.
Data from U.S. Department of Agriculture and U.S. Department of Health and Human Services. Dietary Guidelines for Americans, 2020–2025, ninth ed.; Data from U.S. Department of Agriculture, Agricultural Research Service, 2018. Nutrient Intakes from Food and Beverages: Mean Amounts Consumed per Individual, by Gender and Age. In: What We Eat in America, NHANES 2015–2016.

saturated fat, and sodium. Better diet quality is consistently associated with lower risk of CVD risk factors and CVD risk (Dietary Guidelines Advisory Committee, 2020). In the following sections, the relationship between these dietary factors and CVD risk will be summarized.

## 12.4.1 Dietary patterns and CVD risk

Numerous studies have shown that a heart-healthy diet in childhood is associated with fewer CVD risk factors. A prospective analysis of children ages 7–15 years found that poorer diet quality (i.e., high energy density, high fat, and low fiber diets) was associated with a 13% increase in likelihood of being in the highest quintile for fat mass per one standard deviation increase (through age 15) (Ambrosini et al., 2012). In Korean children (ages 6–15 years), intake of fruits and vegetables less than once per day was associated with a 21% increase (6 years later) in the risk of having two or more CVD risk factors (i.e., waist circumference > 90th%, elevated BP, low HDL-C, high TG, high fasting blood glucose) (Seo et al., 2018). A prospective cohort study evaluated the relationship between adherence to the DASH diet and Metabolic Syndrome in children (ages 6–18 years) and found that those in the highest quintile for adherence had a decreased risk of hypertension (OR 0.30, 95% CI 0.10–0.88), high fasting plasma glucose (OR 0.40, 95% CI 0.15–0.99), and abdominal obesity (OR 0.35, 95% CI 0.14–0.89) compared to the lowest quintile (Asghari et al., 2016). Children younger than 20 years with type 1 diabetes were assessed at baseline, 1 year and 5 years to evaluate Mediterranean Diet adherence in relation to lipids, BP, and obesity. Results indicated that an increase of one standard deviation in adherence correlated with a 0.4 mg/dL lower total cholesterol, 3.4 mg/dL lower LDL-C, and 3.9 mg/dL lower non-HDL cholesterol at baseline. Throughout follow-up, a one standard deviation improvement in Mediterranean Diet adherence was associated with a 1.8 mg/dL lower total cholesterol, 1.6 mg/dL lower LDL-C, and 1.8 mg/dL lower non-HDL-C (Zhong et al., 2016).

Prospective cohort studies demonstrate that diet quality in childhood is associated with CVD risk factor burden in adults. In the Cardiovascular Risk in Young Finns Study, fruit and vegetable consumption during childhood (ages 3–18 years) and adulthood was inversely related to pulse wave velocity, a measure of arterial stiffness that increases likelihood of CVD complications. Notably, consistently higher intake of fruits and vegetables from childhood through adulthood (over 27 years) was associated with lower (better) pulse wave velocity when compared to individuals with consistently low consumption (Aatola et al., 2010). In the same cohort, intake of a traditional (lower nutrient) diet pattern, determined by a principal component analysis, during childhood (ages 3–18 years) was associated with higher LDL-cholesterol and total cholesterol in adulthood (ages 24–29 years). In women ages 24–39 years, intake of a traditional diet from age 9 was associated with higher insulin levels and higher systolic BP. Also of importance, across three follow-ups from childhood through adulthood, dietary patterns remained consistent within subjects (Mikkila et al., 2007). Thus, healthy dietary practices in early life are associated with decreased risk of CVD in adults.

## 12.4.2 Energy intake

While genetics, age, sex, and environmental factors influence obesity, a primary contributor is excess calorie intake relative to energy expenditure (Sahoo et al., 2015). In adults, studies have shown reducing caloric intake decreases body weight, waist circumference, triglycerides, LDL-C, and improves insulin sensitivity (Garcia-Prieto and Fernandez-Alfonso, 2016; Kraus et al., 2019). Similar findings have been observed in children. A systematic review of 16 studies reported unhealthy dietary patterns (assessed via cluster, factor, and/or principal component analysis) were associated with increased odds of obesity in children and adolescents [OR1.02 (95% CI, 0.91–1.15) to 3.55 (95% CI, 1.80–7.03)]. Potentially obesogenic foods (fatty cheeses, sugary drinks, processed foods, fast food, candies, snacks, cakes, animal products, whole milk, and refined grains) increased the likelihood of being overweight, while healthier foods (low intakes s of sugar and fat and high intakes of fruits, vegetables, whole grains, fish, nuts, legumes, and yogurt) were not associated with obesity (Liberali et al., 2020). When 14 behavioral factors in 199 studies were analyzed in relation to childhood overweight/obesity drinking sugar-sweetened beverages 4 or more times per week (OR 1.24, 95% CI, 1.07–1.43) increased the risk of obesity (Poorolajal et al., 2020).

The Academy of Nutrition and Dietetics' (AND) Evidence Analysis Library recommends a hypocaloric diet, between 900 and 1200 calories, with medical monitoring and registered dietitian supervision in children ages 6–12 and no lower than 1200 calories in children ages 13 through 18 years to improve weight status. The evidence supporting both caloric restriction strategies to improve weight status was classified as strong (Academy of Nutrition and Dietetics, 2007). When children with obesity between 8 and 18 years of age consumed a reduced calorie diet (500 kcal less per day) under the supervision of a dietitian for 6 months, those consuming fewer calories lost an average of 5.7 kg, decreased BMI by an average of 3.3 kg/m$^2$, and reduced fat mass by 5.1 kg. No differences were observed in blood lipid levels or BP, but fasting insulin decreased (Partsalaki et al., 2012). Calorie reduction in children with obesity may lead to favorable cardiovascular health outcomes. A systemic review suggests that energy density plays an integral role in calorie intake. Both children (ages 3 to 5 years) and adults were more likely to eat similar quantities (weight) of food, rather than consistent caloric intake suggesting consuming high water content, low energy density foods may aid in the regulation of intake, avoiding excess calories, and weight gain (Rolls, 2017). The American Psychological Association and the AND support this recommendation by encouraging fruit and vegetable consumption and improving diet quality rather than extreme energy restriction. The AND suggests a multifaceted approach through nutrition, physical activity, and behavioral counseling with parental/caregiver involvement being critical in children between ages 2 through 5 years (Hoelscher et al., 2013).

### 12.4.3 Saturated fat

Saturated fat in children 2–19 years should be limited to less than 10% of total energy intake (and trans fat should be avoided) to prevent elevated LDL-C and total cholesterol levels (Te Morenga and Montez, 2017). In a meta-analysis of randomized control trials and prospective cohort studies intake of low saturated fat diets in children and adolescents between the ages of 2–18 years significantly lowered total cholesterol (− 2.88 mg/dL) and LDL-C (− 2.34 mg/dL) as well as diastolic BP (− 1.45 mmHg) compared to higher saturated fat containing diets. As saturated fat does not inherently increase BP, this decrease may be attributable to the reduction in calories or improvement in diet quality. There were no adverse effects on growth or development in groups that reduced saturated fat intake (Te Morenga and Montez, 2017). In support of limiting saturated fat intake, the Special Turku Coronary Risk Factor Intervention Project (STRIP) provided education from infancy through age 20 years focused on replacing saturated fat with unsaturated fat, and also reducing salt intake and incorporating whole grains and fruits and vegetables, and was effective in reducing saturated fat intake, and increasing mono- and polyunsaturated fat, fiber, and potassium intake compared to the control group, that did not receive counseling (Oranta et al., 2013). After 15–20 years, the intervention group had a 41% reduction in risk of Metabolic Syndrome (Nupponen et al., 2015). Furthermore, in the experimental group boys had lower very-low-density-lipoprotein cholesterol and intermediate-density-lipoprotein cholesterol, and triglycerides and LDL-C was lower in girls when compared to the group that did not receive education (Niinikoski et al., 2012). Children in the intervention group had 1 mmHg lower systolic and diastolic BP, which was measured yearly from age 7 to 15 (Niinikoski et al., 2009). Replacing saturated fat with poly- and mono-unsaturated fatty acids and fiber-rich, whole grain carbohydrates, has the greatest impact on decreasing total cholesterol and LDL-C (Briggs et al., 2017; Te Morenga and Montez, 2017). The disagreement about reducing dietary saturated fat to reduce CVD risk has been clearly refuted (Kris-Etherton and Krauss, 2020; U.S. Department of Health and Human Services and U.S. Department of Agriculture, 2020). The 2020 Dietary Guidelines Advisory Committee (DGAC) concluded that strong evidence shows that diets lower in saturated fatty acids and cholesterol lead to lower levels of total blood and LDL-C (Dietary Guidelines Advisory Committee, 2020). Since so many children are exceeding saturated fat recommendations, this is an important dietary target because of the relationship with CVD risk, and early CVD events via a sustained increase in LDL-C for many years.

## 12.4.4 Added sugar

Limiting added sugars to less than 10% of calories per day is recommended by the 2020–25 Dietary Guidelines for Americans for all age groups. Adherence to the Dietary Guidelines for Americans inherently limits the contribution of calories from added sugars (U.S. Department of Health and Human Services and U.S. Department of Agriculture, 2020). About 24% (or 266 kcal) of added sugars consumed in children older than 1 year come from sugar-sweetened beverages (U.S. Department of Health and Human Services and U.S. Department of Agriculture, 2020). Sugar-sweetened beverages provide a substantial number of calories with no nutritive qualities (Vos et al., 2017). Sugar-sweetened beverages should be limited as high intake is associated with obesity among children of all ages (Vos et al., 2017). Further, in a study of 1987 children (average age of 8.3 years), a 7 ounce increase in daily sugar-sweetened beverage intake was associated with a 0.2% increase in BMI and increased odds of obesity (OR 1.22, 95% CI 1.04, 1.44) (Muckelbauer et al., 2016).

Reducing intake of added sugars may lower BP in children. A recent meta-analysis of 14 studies reported that children and adolescents with the highest intake of sugar sweetened beverages had higher systolic BP (pooled estimate weighted mean difference 1.67 mmHg; 95% CI) than those with the lowest consumption of sugar-sweetened beverages (Farhangi et al., 2020). However, more evidence is needed to support the link between added sugars and BP. The 2020 DGAC concluded that there is limited evidence that high consumption of sugar sweetened beverages is associated with increased cardiovascular mortality and insufficient evidence for the relationship between added sugar consumption and risk of CVD in children. The 2020 DGAC reported that excess consumption of added sugars may add to unhealthy weight gain and obesity and contribute to an unhealthy diet pattern (Dietary Guidelines Advisory Committee, 2020). Thus, reducing added sugar intake and achieving current dietary recommendations may decrease cardiovascular risk factors in children.

## 12.4.5 Salt

It is well established that salt intake increases BP, a major CVD risk factor. Moderate strength evidence shows higher salt intake increases the risk of cardiovascular events in adults. Similarly, reducing salt intake reduces the incidence of hypertension (National Academies of Sciences, Engineering, and Medicine, 2019). A meta-analysis of randomized controlled studies showed that decreasing salt consumption by 2.0–2.3 g per day decreased cardiovascular events by 20% in normotensive and hypertensive adults (He and MacGregor, 2011). Salt has similar hypertensive effects in children (He and MacGregor, 2011). A meta-analysis of 14 experimental studies reported that salt reduction interventions reduce systolic BP by 0.06 mmHg and diastolic BP by 1.2 mmHg in children from birth to 18 years. Each additional gram of salt consumed in childhood and adolescence was associated with a 0.8 mmHg increase in systolic BP and 0.7 mmHg increase in diastolic pressure. These results were more pronounced in children with overweight (Leyvraz et al., 2018). Salt reduction decreases the risk of hypertension and CVD in adults and also reduces the likelihood of childhood hypertension (Lava et al., 2015). The AHA recommends reducing intake of packaged and heavily processed foods and decreasing table salt use, to reduce salt intake and prevent hypertension. Achieving current salt recommendations in childhood will help prevent hypertension and arterial stiffness and decrease early onset CVD in adulthood.

## 12.4.6 Fiber

Fiber is another component of a healthy diet that has been shown to decrease CVD risk (Funtikova et al., 2015; McRae, 2017). High intakes of soluble, gel-forming fiber decrease LDL-C and total cholesterol by decreasing absorption of cholesterol (McRae, 2017). The 2020 DGAC reports that higher intakes of fiber reduce the risk of coronary heart disease (Dietary Guidelines Advisory Committee, 2020). A review of diet quality and health in children and adolescents reported that children with none of the criteria for Metabolic Syndrome had a higher soluble fiber intake than children with Metabolic Syndrome. Children with high fiber intake also had lower insulin resistance and a lower waist circumference (Funtikova et al., 2015). In a longitudinal cohort study over 24 years, individuals (ages 13–36 years) who consumed more fiber in the form of fruits, vegetables, and whole grains had less carotid artery stiffness at older ages (36 years) (van de Laar et al., 2012). In addition, consumption of vegetables was shown to have an inverse relationship to hyperglycemia, perhaps related, in part, to dietary fiber (Villegas et al., 2008). Meeting dietary fiber recommendations in childhood by achieving food-based recommendations for fruits, vegetables, whole grains, legumes, and other fiber containing foods is important for health and decreasing CVD risk factors early in life to prevent CVD later in life.

## 12.4.7 Micronutrients

A healthy dietary pattern meets recommendations for all micronutrients, including potassium and magnesium. Micronutrients are important for maintaining ideal cardiovascular health. For example, associations between high BP and sodium intake were stronger in children who did not meet recommendations for potassium (Leyvraz et al., 2018). Increasing potassium and decreasing sodium will benefit cardiovascular health in childhood. Low levels of magnesium, which can result from poor diet quality has been associated with high BP. Analysis of nearly 4000 healthy children ages 6–15 years showed a positive relationship between hypomagnesemia ($< 1.8 \, mg/dL$) and hypertension and magnesium intake has a significant negative relationship for both systolic ($r = -0.201$) and diastolic ($r = -0.206$) BP (Guerrero-Romero et al., 2016).

## 12.5 Dietary recommendations for children

The 2020–25 Dietary Guidelines for Americans recommends three healthy dietary patterns that can be enjoyed at any stage of life (The Healthy US-Style Dietary Pattern, The Healthy Mediterranean-Style Dietary Pattern and the Healthy Vegetarian-Style Dietary Pattern). The Healthy US-Style Dietary Pattern for children ages 2–8, 9–13, and 14–18 is summarized in Table 12.4. Meeting these food group recommendations will ensure adequate nutrient intake for growth and development and minimize risk of developing CVD risk factors. When following these food-based guidelines, a small number of calories remain and can be used for added sugars and saturated fat, as well as for more of the recommended foods.

## 12.6 Implementation of dietary recommendations in childhood

Given the importance of early nutrition on long-term cardiovascular health and the high prevalence of poor dietary practices in US children and adolescents, significant changes are

TABLE 12.4  DGA 2020–25 healthy US-style dietary pattern for children ages 2 through 18.

| Food group or subgroup | Daily amount of food from each group | | |
| --- | --- | --- | --- |
| | Ages 2–8 | Ages 9–13 | Ages 14–18 |
| | 1400 kcal level pattern | 1800 kcal level pattern | 2600 kcal level pattern |
| Vegetables (cup eq/day) | 1½ | 2½ | 3½ |
| | Vegetable subgroups in weekly amounts | | |
| Dark-green vegetables (cup eq/week) | 1 | 1½ | 2½ |
| Red and orange vegetables (cup eq/week) | 3 | 5½ | 7 |
| Beans, peas, lentils (cup eq/week) | ½ | 1½ | 2½ |
| Starchy vegetables (cup eq/week) | 3½ | 5 | 7 |
| Other vegetables (cup eq/week) | 2½ | 4 | 5½ |
| Fruit (cup eq/day) | 1½ | 1½ | 2 |
| Grains (oz. eq/day) | 5 | 6 | 9 |
| Whole grains (oz. eq/day) | 2½ | 3 | 4½ |
| Refined grains (oz. eq/day) | 2½ | 3 | 4½ |
| Dairy (cup eq/day) | 2½ | 3 | 3 |
| Protein foods (oz. eq/day) | 4 | 5 | 6½ |
| | Protein food sub-groups in weekly amounts | | |
| Meats, poultry, eggs (oz. eq/week) | 19 | 23 | 31 |
| Seafood (oz. eq/week) | 6 | 8 | 10 |
| Nuts, seeds, soy products (oz. eq/week) | 3 | 4 | 5 |
| Oils (g/day) | 17 | 24 | 34 |
| Limit on calories for other uses (kcal/day) | 90 | 140 | 350 |
| Limit on calories for other uses (% kcal/day) | 6 | 8 | 13 |

*Data from U.S. Department of Agriculture and U.S. Department of Health and Human Services. Dietary Guidelines for Americans, 2020–2025, ninth ed.*

required to improve cardiovascular health throughout life. Healthy eating habits that are learned and implemented early in life have lifelong impacts on cardiovascular health. Starting good nutrition practices as early as possible is one of the best strategies for decreasing CVD risk in early adulthood, as well as later. In order to implement dietary recommendations, family, caregivers, and healthcare providers play a crucial role in impacting the dietary habits of children and adolescents and, as a result, risk factors for CVD.

Since families and caregivers have a very significant impact on dietary behaviors of children, interventions should be targeted at children as well as their caregivers. The caregiver environment has been associated with children's self-regulation of eating. For example, an indulgent feeding style in parents correlates with higher adiposity and lower self-regulation in children. Research supports allowing the child to start and stop eating autonomously that is guided by satiety, while also providing healthy foods. Setting times to eat and encouraging healthy options supports children's autonomy and self-regulation (Wood et al., 2020). Specific strategies should be utilized to create an environment that offers healthy foods rather than focuses on the amount or what is eaten. This allows children to decide when they are hungry. Helpful strategies include responding to verbal and non-verbal cues regarding food choices, providing structure for mealtimes and selective food availability (Wood et al., 2020). Since young children are reliant on caregivers for food, setting an example of good dietary habits can shape a child's eating behavior. Children's habits typically are similar to those of the household. Therefore, providing nutrient dense, heart-healthy foods, while restricting foods that are nutrient-poor and energy-dense, establishes healthy eating behaviors (U.S. Department of Health and Human Services and U.S. Department of Agriculture, 2020).

A healthcare provider, preferably a registered dietitian, can assist in setting specific nutrition goals throughout childhood and adolescence. Health professionals can recommend simple strategies to improve a child's diet. Realistic goals may include replacing one processed snack a day for a child's favorite fruit or vegetable to increase fiber and decrease sodium, substituting whole fat milk with 2% milk to decrease saturated fat, or replacing a sugar sweetened beverage with water to reduce calories and added sugar intake.

While younger children present a variety of challenges including aversions to certain foods, adolescents often present a different set of barriers to healthy food choices. As age increases, the overall role of the caregiver decreases, including their influence on dietary intake. Teenagers are no longer solely reliant on the caregiver for food as peer influences and autonomy increase (U.S. Department of Health and Human Services and U.S. Department of Agriculture, 2020). Goals and strategies to continue CVD preventive care through healthy dietary practices during adolescence are likely to vary from childhood. Including teenagers in meal planning, grocery shopping, and cooking allows the caregiver to maintain some control and empowers the child to begin making heart-healthy choices. Continuing to provide healthier options in the home should remain a priority as this offers the adolescent convenient access to these foods (U.S. Department of Health and Human Services and U.S. Department of Agriculture, 2020). Lastly, nutrition education can be an effective strategy for prevention in this age group. As reported in the STRIP study, education about a healthy diet had significant impacts on cardiovascular health both in childhood and early adulthood (Nupponen et al., 2015).

Another important step after prevention is screening and monitoring CVD risk factors throughout childhood and adolescence. This is often overlooked as evidenced by the only 3.2% of children (ages 20 years and under) who received lipid tests (Force et al., 2016). Screening to diagnose medical risks requires information about fasting blood glucose, lipid panels, BP, and weight. Children should also be screened for lifestyle behaviors (i.e., dietary habits, physical activity, smoking) that are associated with risk of CVD. Screening for dyslipidemia before 20 years of age may improve lipid markers and reduce premature CVD (Force et al., 2016). Diagnosing and treating hypertension in children could reduce target organ damage as well. Children with uncontrolled hypertension had significantly higher levels of left ventricular hypertrophy than those who had treated hypertension (Seeman et al., 2012). Because maintaining ideal cardiovascular health reduces CVD risk, if behavioral therapy and diet modifications alone do not treat major controllable CVD risk factors (i.e., hyperglycemia, hypertension, dyslipidemia), pharmacological intervention should be considered (Barlow and Expert, 2007).

With the development of CVD risk factors or CVD, implementation of dietary interventions that address the causes of CVD risk factors in the form of medical nutrition therapy is recommended. Implementing a healthy diet (including the Dietary Guidelines food-based and nutrient recommendations) early in life is a recommended preventive strategy. Nutrition therapies often focus on the components previously discussed (i.e., saturated fat, added sugar, salt, fiber) to attenuate risk factors. Research has investigated the DASH diet, Mediterranean diet, and vegetarian diet to mitigate risk factors in children.

The Dietary Approach to Stop Hypertension (DASH) diet emphasizes vegetables, fruits, whole grains, fat-free/low-fat dairy, low-fat meats, vegetable oils, and nuts while limiting saturated fat, sodium, and added sugar (Steinberg et al., 2017). In a randomized controlled study, children ages 11–17 years either received general healthy eating education, or DASH diet education. After 10 weeks, the DASH diet group showed a significant improvement in systolic BP, LDL-C, HDL-C, total cholesterol, triglycerides, and fasting blood glucose, when compared to the healthy diet education group (Mahdavi et al., 2021). Because of the cardiovascular benefits of increasing fiber, potassium, calcium, magnesium, and other nutrients while decreasing saturated fat, sodium and added sugar, the DASH diet reduces CVD risk factors, and prevents the development of CVD in early life.

The Mediterranean Diet features vegetables, fruits, extra-virgin olive oil, nuts, legumes, and whole grains, while limiting added sugar and red meat and has been shown to be effective for CVD risk reduction in children and adults (Salas-Salvado et al., 2018). This dietary pattern is high in dietary fiber, mono-, and polyunsaturated fatty acids (Becerra-Tomas et al., 2020). Pre-pubertal hypercholesterolemic children received education on the Mediterranean Diet over 12 months resulting in a decrease of total cholesterol and LDL-C compared to baseline measurements (Giannini et al., 2014). While further clinical trial research is needed investigating the effect of a Mediterranean diet on CVD risk in children, this study provides compelling evidence that adherence to a healthy dietary pattern is associated with cardiovascular health benefits in early life.

Vegetarian diets typically are low in saturated fat and cholesterol because of the elimination of some or all animal products. There are a variety of ways to implement vegetarian diets. All avoid meat and most avoid seafood including lacto vegetarians (consume dairy), ovo vegetarians (eat eggs), lacto-ovo vegetarians (eat eggs and milk), pescatarians (consume seafood), and vegans - eat no animal products. Few studies have evaluated the effect of different types of vegetarian diets on CVD risk factors in children (Schurmann et al., 2017). In children ages 9–18 with obesity and elevated cholesterol levels, following a vegan diet and limiting added fat for 4 weeks decreased BMI z-score (− 0.14), systolic BP by 6.43 mmHg, weight by 3.05 kg, total cholesterol by 22.5 mg/dL, LDL-C by 13.14 mg/dL, and insulin by 5.42 uU/mL compared to baseline (Macknin et al., 2015). A systematic review of 16 studies investigating vegetarian diets in children from birth to 18 years found that nutritional inadequacies especially in children younger than 4 years may result from following this diet. During early life the following nutrient deficiencies may result from restricting animal products: protein, calcium, vitamin D, vitamin B12, iron, and iodine. The need for these nutrients is relatively high in children, putting them at greater risk for one or more nutrient deficiencies when eliminating certain foods (Schurmann et al., 2017). Eliminating meat and animal products from a child's diet requires careful planning to assure that all nutrient needs are met including iron. An omnivorous diet that emphasizes plant-based foods is one recommended strategy to meet nutrient needs in childhood.

Dietary interventions can be implemented to optimize health during this important time for growth and development in children, as well as reducing risk for CVD later in life. Diets that support heart health are high in fruits, vegetables, whole grains, lean protein foods, low-fat dairy or alternatives, legumes, nuts and seeds, liquid vegetable oils and are low in saturated fat, sodium and added sugars. Increasing fiber and nutrient density also decreases CVD risk. Given that there is much evidence that supports the cardiovascular benefits of a healthy dietary pattern in children, efforts are needed to improve the current diets of children with the goal being to achieve a healthy dietary pattern for all children. Practitioners should work with caregivers and children to identify realistic diet changes. Evaluating individual factors such as food accessibility, food preferences, and intake patterns can aid in tailoring recommended dietary changes for primordial prevention of CVD.

## 12.7 Conclusions

Good nutrition early in life is important for decreasing CVD risk throughout life. Benefits of good nutrition range from creating healthy eating habits to preventing early onset adult CVD morbidity and mortality. There is convincing evidence that poor nutrition during childhood increases the risk of premature CVD in adulthood. Limiting excess calories, sodium and added sugar, replacing saturated fat with unsaturated fat and fiber, and increasing dietary fiber in a healthy eating pattern decreases CVD risk. Because of the significant gaps between current dietary recommendations and intakes at all life stages, including children, there is a pressing need to improve diet quality. Caregivers play a central role in implementing heart-healthy dietary practices and teaching children about good nutrition principles. Nutrition education for children and caregivers will benefit many health outcomes, including CVD, throughout life. In addition, screening and monitoring of behavioral risks and CVD risk factors by health professionals can encourage early intervention with strong and consistent messages about the benefits of a heart-healthy diet. Through preventive measures and dietary interventions in children and adolescents, CVD risk can be reduced significantly.

## 12.8 Research needs

Strong and consistent evidence supports our understanding of the benefits of a healthy dietary pattern in childhood on CVD risk. However, challenges remain in achieving an optimal dietary pattern in children. Given this, clinical trials are needed to evaluate interventions that elicit dietary changes that are sustained in children. In addition, follow-up assessments of CVD risk throughout adulthood will provide important information about the long-term benefits of healthy diets starting in childhood. Evaluating adherence issues to heart-healthy diets throughout life stages (childhood, adolescence, adulthood) and cardiovascular outcomes will provide additional insight into the type of intervention strategies (e.g., type of intervention, intensity, duration, timing, etc.) that work best. Great strides have been made in identifying heart-healthy diets for the primordial prevention of CVD. Identification and effective implementation of interventions that promote healthy dietary practices in children will be a major step forward for reducing CVD.

## Sources of additional information

**(1)** https://www.heart.org/
**(2)** https://www.dietaryguidelines.gov/
**(3)** https://www.nutrition.org/

## References

Aatola, H., Koivistoinen, T., Hutri-Kahonen, N., Juonala, M., Mikkila, V., Lehtimaki, T., Kahonen, M., 2010. Lifetime fruit and vegetable consumption and arterial pulse wave velocity in adulthood: the cardiovascular risk in Young Finns study. Circulation 122 (24), 2521–2528. https://doi.org/10.1161/CIRCULATIONAHA.110.969279.

Academy of Nutrition and Dietetics, 2007. Pediatric Weight Management: Executive Summary of Recommendations. (Retrieved from).

Ambrosini, G.L., Emmett, P.M., Northstone, K., Howe, L.D., Tilling, K., Jebb, S.A., 2012. Identification of a dietary pattern prospectively associated with increased adiposity during childhood and adolescence. Int. J. Obes. 36 (10), 1299–1305. https://doi.org/10.1038/ijo.2012.127.

Asghari, G., Yuzbashian, E., Mirmiran, P., Hooshmand, F., Najafi, R., Azizi, F., 2016. Dietary approaches to stop hypertension (DASH) dietary pattern is associated with reduced incidence of metabolic syndrome in children and adolescents. J. Pediatr. 174, 178–184.e171. https://doi.org/10.1016/j.jpeds.2016.03.077.

Barlow, S.E., Expert, C., 2007. Expert committee recommendations regarding the prevention, assessment, and treatment of child and adolescent overweight and obesity: summary report. Pediatrics 120 (Suppl. 4), S164–S192. https://doi.org/10.1542/peds.2007-2329C.

Becerra-Tomas, N., Blanco Mejia, S., Viguiliouk, E., Khan, T., Kendall, C.W.C., Kahleova, H., Salas-Salvado, J., 2020. Mediterranean diet, cardiovascular disease and mortality in diabetes: a systematic review and meta-analysis of prospective cohort studies and randomized clinical trials. Crit. Rev. Food Sci. Nutr. 60 (7), 1207–1227. https://doi.org/10.1080/10408398.2019.1565281.

Bowen, K.J., Sullivan, V.K., Kris-Etherton, P.M., Petersen, K.S., 2018. Nutrition and cardiovascular disease-an update. Curr. Atheroscler. Rep. 20 (2), 8. https://doi.org/10.1007/s11883-018-0704-3.

Briggs, M.A., Petersen, K.S., Kris-Etherton, P.M., 2017. Saturated fatty acids and cardiovascular disease: replacements for saturated fat to reduce cardiovascular risk. Healthcare (Basel) 5 (2). https://doi.org/10.3390/healthcare5020029.

Center for Disease Control and Prevention, 2020. Rates of New Diagnosed Cases of Type 1 and Type 2 Diabetes Continue to Rise Among Children, Teens. Retrieved from https://www.cdc.gov/diabetes/research/reports/children-diabetes-rates-rise.html.

Centers for Disease Control and Prevention, 2020. National diabetes statistics report. Atlanta, GA.

Centers for Disease Control and Prevention, 2021. Obesity and Overweight. Retrieved from https://www.cdc.gov/nchs/fastats/obesity-overweight.htm.

Daniels, S.R., Pratt, C.A., Hollister, E.B., Labarthe, D., Cohen, D.A., Walker, J.R., Young, M.E., 2019. Promoting cardiovascular health in early childhood and transitions in childhood through adolescence: a workshop report. J. Pediatr. 209, 240–251.e241. https://doi.org/10.1016/j.jpeds.2019.01.042.

de Ferranti, S.D., Steinberger, J., Ameduri, R., Baker, A., Gooding, H., Kelly, A.S., Zaidi, A.N., 2019. Cardiovascular risk reduction in high-risk pediatric patients: a scientific statement from the American Heart Association. Circulation 139 (13), e603–e634. https://doi.org/10.1161/CIR.0000000000000618.

Dietary Guidelines Advisory Committee, 2020. Scientific report of the 2020 dietary guidelines advisory committee: advisory report to the secretary of agriculture and the secretary of health and human services. Retrieved from Washington, DC.

Divers, J., Mayer-Davis, E.J., Lawrence, J.M., Isom, S., Dabelea, D., Dolan, L., Wagenknecht, L.E., 2020. Trends in incidence of type 1 and type 2 diabetes among youths—selected counties and Indian reservations, United States, 2002-2015. MMWR Morb. Mortal. Wkly Rep. 69 (6), 161–165. https://doi.org/10.15585/mmwr.mm6906a3.

Farhangi, M.A., Nikniaz, L., Khodarahmi, M., 2020. Sugar-sweetened beverages increases the risk of hypertension among children and adolescence: a systematic review and dose-response meta-analysis. J. Transl. Med. 18 (1), 344. https://doi.org/10.1186/s12967-020-02511-9.

Force, U.S.P.S.T., Bibbins-Domingo, K., Grossman, D.C., Curry, S.J., Davidson, K.W., Epling Jr., J.W., Siu, A.L., 2016. Screening for lipid disorders in children and adolescents: US preventive services task force recommendation statement. JAMA 316 (6), 625–633. https://doi.org/10.1001/jama.2016.9852.

Fryar, C.D., Carroll, M.D., Affu, J., 2020. Prevalence of Overweight, Obesity, and Severe Obesity Among Children and Adolescents Aged 2–19 Years: United States, 1963–1965 Through 2017–2018. NCHS Health E-Stats.

Funtikova, A.N., Navarro, E., Bawaked, R.A., Fito, M., Schroder, H., 2015. Impact of diet on cardiometabolic health in children and adolescents. Nutr. J. 14, 118. https://doi.org/10.1186/s12937-015-0107-z.

Garcia-Prieto, C.F., Fernandez-Alfonso, M.S., 2016. Caloric restriction as a strategy to improve vascular dysfunction in metabolic disorders. Nutrients 8 (6). https://doi.org/10.3390/nu8060370.

GBD, 2015. Global, regional, and national age–sex specific all-cause and cause-specific mortality for 240 causes of death, 1990–2013: a systematic analysis for the global burden of disease study 2013. Lancet 385, 117–171. https://doi.org/10.1016/S0140-6736(14)61682-2.

Giannini, C., Diesse, L., D'Adamo, E., Chiavaroli, V., de Giorgis, T., Di Iorio, C., Mohn, A., 2014. Influence of the Mediterranean diet on carotid intima-media thickness in hypercholesterolaemic children: a 12-month intervention study. Nutr. Metab. Cardiovasc. Dis. 24 (1), 75–82. https://doi.org/10.1016/j.numecd.2013.04.005.

Guerrero-Romero, F., Rodriguez-Moran, M., Hernandez-Ronquillo, G., Gomez-Diaz, R., Pizano-Zarate, M.L., Wacher, N.H., Network of Childhood Obesity of the Mexican Social Security, I, 2016. Low serum magnesium levels and its association with high blood pressure in children. J. Pediatr. 168, 93–98.e91. https://doi.org/10.1016/j.jpeds.2015.09.050.

He, F.J., MacGregor, G.A., 2011. Salt reduction lowers cardiovascular risk: meta-analysis of outcome trials. Lancet 378 (9789), 380–382. https://doi.org/10.1016/S0140-6736(11)61174-4.

Hoelscher, D.M., Kirk, S., Ritchie, L., Cunningham-Sabo, L., Academy Positions, C., 2013. Position of the academy of nutrition and dietetics: interventions for the prevention and treatment of pediatric overweight and obesity. J. Acad. Nutr. Diet. 113 (10), 1375–1394. https://doi.org/10.1016/j.jand.2013.08.004.

Khera, A.V., Emdin, C.A., Drake, I., Natarajan, P., Bick, A.G., Cook, N.R., Kathiresan, S., 2016. Genetic risk, adherence to a healthy lifestyle, and coronary disease. N. Engl. J. Med. 375 (24), 2349–2358. https://doi.org/10.1056/NEJMoa1605086.

Kraus, W.E., Bhapkar, M., Huffman, K.M., Pieper, C.F., Krupa Das, S., Redman, L.M., Investigators, C, 2019. 2 years of calorie restriction and cardiometabolic risk (CALERIE): exploratory outcomes of a multicentre, phase 2, randomised controlled trial. Lancet Diabetes Endocrinol. 7 (9), 673–683. https://doi.org/10.1016/S2213-8587(19)30151-2.

Kris-Etherton, P.M., Krauss, R.M., 2020. Public health guidelines should recommend reducing saturated fat consumption as much as possible: YES. Am. J. Clin. Nutr. 112 (1), 13–18. https://doi.org/10.1093/ajcn/nqaa110.

Lava, S.A., Bianchetti, M.G., Simonetti, G.D., 2015. Salt intake in children and its consequences on blood pressure. Pediatr. Nephrol. 30 (9), 1389–1396. https://doi.org/10.1007/s00467-014-2931-3.

Leyvraz, M., Chatelan, A., da Costa, B.R., Taffe, P., Paradis, G., Bovet, P., Chiolero, A., 2018. Sodium intake and blood pressure in children and adolescents: a systematic review and meta-analysis of experimental and observational studies. Int. J. Epidemiol. 47 (6), 1796–1810. https://doi.org/10.1093/ije/dyy121.

Liberali, R., Kupek, E., Assis, M.A.A., 2020. Dietary patterns and childhood obesity risk: a systematic review. Child. Obes. 16 (2), 70–85. https://doi.org/10.1089/chi.2019.0059.

Macknin, M., Kong, T., Weier, A., Worley, S., Tang, A.S., Alkhouri, N., Golubic, M., 2015. Plant-based, no-added-fat or American Heart Association diets: impact on cardiovascular risk in obese children with hypercholesterolemia and their parents. J. Pediatr. 166 (4), 953–959.e951-953. https://doi.org/10.1016/j.jpeds.2014.12.058.

Mahdavi, A., Mohammadi, H., Foshati, S., Shokri-Mashhadi, N., Clark, C.C.T., Moafi, A., Rouhani, M.H., 2021. Effects of the dietary approach to stop hypertension (DASH) diet on blood pressure, blood glucose, and lipid profile in adolescents with hemophilia: a randomized clinical trial. Food Sci. Nutr. 9 (1), 145–153. https://doi.org/10.1002/fsn3.1972.

McRae, M.P., 2017. Dietary fiber is beneficial for the prevention of cardiovascular disease: an umbrella review of meta-analyses. J. Chiropr. Med. 16 (4), 289–299. https://doi.org/10.1016/j.jcm.2017.05.005.

Mikkila, V., Rasanen, L., Raitakari, O.T., Marniemi, J., Pietinen, P., Ronnemaa, T., Viikari, J., 2007. Major dietary patterns and cardiovascular risk factors from childhood to adulthood. The cardiovascular risk in Young Finns study. Br. J. Nutr. 98 (1), 218–225. https://doi.org/10.1017/S0007114507691831.

Morrison, J.A., Glueck, C.J., Wang, P., 2012. Childhood risk factors predict cardiovascular disease, impaired fasting glucose plus type 2 diabetes mellitus, and high blood pressure 26 years later at a mean age of 38 years: the Princeton-lipid research clinics follow-up study. Metabolism 61 (4), 531–541. https://doi.org/10.1016/j.metabol.2011.08.010.

Muckelbauer, R., Gortmaker, S.L., Libuda, L., Kersting, M., Clausen, K., Adelberger, B., Muller-Nordhorn, J., 2016. Changes in water and sugar-containing beverage consumption and body weight outcomes in children. Br. J. Nutr. 115 (11), 2057–2066. https://doi.org/10.1017/S0007114516001136.

National Academies of Sciences, Engineering, and Medicine, 2019. In: Oria, M., Harrison, M., Stallings, V.A. (Eds.), Dietary Reference Intakes for Sodium and Potassium. National Academies of Sciences, Engineering, and Medicine, Washington, DC.

Niinikoski, H., Jula, A., Viikari, J., Ronnemaa, T., Heino, P., Lagstrom, H., Simell, O., 2009. Blood pressure is lower in children and adolescents with a low-saturated-fat diet since infancy: the special turku coronary risk factor intervention project. Hypertension 53 (6), 918–924. https://doi.org/10.1161/HYPERTENSIONAHA.109.130146.

Niinikoski, H., Pahkala, K., Ala-Korpela, M., Viikari, J., Ronnemaa, T., Lagstrom, H., Raitakari, O.T., 2012. Effect of repeated dietary counseling on serum lipoproteins from infancy to adulthood. Pediatrics 129 (3), e704–e713. https://doi.org/10.1542/peds.2011-1503.

Nupponen, M., Pahkala, K., Juonala, M., Magnussen, C.G., Niinikoski, H., Ronnemaa, T., Raitakari, O.T., 2015. Metabolic syndrome from adolescence to early adulthood: effect of infancy-onset dietary counseling of low saturated fat: the special Turku coronary risk factor intervention project (STRIP). Circulation 131 (7), 605–613. https://doi.org/10.1161/CIRCULATIONAHA.114.010532.

Oranta, O., Pahkala, K., Ruottinen, S., Niinikoski, H., Lagstrom, H., Viikari, J.S., Raitakari, O.T., 2013. Infancy-onset dietary counseling of low-saturated-fat diet improves insulin sensitivity in healthy adolescents 15-20 years of age: the special Turku coronary risk factor intervention project (STRIP) study. Diabetes Care 36 (10), 2952–2959. https://doi.org/10.2337/dc13-0361.

Partsalaki, I., Karvela, A., Spiliotis, B.E., 2012. Metabolic impact of a ketogenic diet compared to a hypocaloric diet in obese children and adolescents. J. Pediatr. Endocrinol. Metab. 25 (7–8), 697–704. https://doi.org/10.1515/jpem-2012-0131.

Perak, A.M., Ning, H., Kit, B.K., de Ferranti, S.D., Van Horn, L.V., Wilkins, J.T., Lloyd-Jones, D.M., 2019. Trends in levels of lipids and apolipoprotein B in US youths aged 6 to 19 years, 1999-2016. JAMA 321 (19), 1895–1905. https://doi.org/10.1001/jama.2019.4984.

Poorolajal, J., Sahraei, F., Mohamdadi, Y., Doosti-Irani, A., Moradi, L., 2020. Behavioral factors influencing childhood obesity: a systematic review and meta-analysis. Obes. Res. Clin. Pract. 14 (2), 109–118. https://doi.org/10.1016/j.orcp.2020.03.002.

Rolls, B.J., 2017. Dietary energy density: applying behavioural science to weight management. Nutr. Bull. 42 (3), 246–253. https://doi.org/10.1111/nbu.12280.

Roth, G.A., Johnson, C., Abajobir, A., Abd-Allah, F., Abera, S.F., Abyu, G., Murray, C., 2017. Global, regional, and national burden of cardiovascular diseases for 10 causes, 1990 to 2015. J. Am. Coll. Cardiol. 70 (1), 1–25. https://doi.org/10.1016/j.jacc.2017.04.052.

Sahoo, K., Sahoo, B., Choudhury, A.K., Sofi, N.Y., Kumar, R., Bhadoria, A.S., 2015. Childhood obesity: causes and consequences. J. Family Med. Prim. Care 4 (2), 187–192. https://doi.org/10.4103/2249-4863.154628.

Salas-Salvado, J., Becerra-Tomas, N., Garcia-Gavilan, J.F., Bullo, M., Barrubes, L., 2018. Mediterranean diet and cardiovascular disease prevention: what do we know? Prog. Cardiovasc. Dis. 61 (1), 62–67. https://doi.org/10.1016/j.pcad.2018.04.006.

Schurmann, S., Kersting, M., Alexy, U., 2017. Vegetarian diets in children: a systematic review. Eur. J. Nutr. 56 (5), 1797–1817. https://doi.org/10.1007/s00394-017-1416-0.

Seeman, T., Dostalek, L., Gilik, J., 2012. Control of hypertension in treated children and its association with target organ damage. Am. J. Hypertens. 25 (3), 389–395. https://doi.org/10.1038/ajh.2011.218.

Seo, Y.G., Choi, M.K., Kang, J.H., Lee, H.J., Jang, H.B., Park, S.I., Park, K.H., 2018. Cardiovascular disease risk factor clustering in children and adolescents: a prospective cohort study. Arch. Dis. Child. 103 (10), 968–973. https://doi.org/10.1136/archdischild-2017-313226.

Skinner, A.C., Ravanbakht, S.N., Skelton, J.A., Perrin, E.M., Armstrong, S.C., 2018. Prevalence of obesity and severe obesity in US children, 1999-2016. Pediatrics 141 (3). https://doi.org/10.1542/peds.2017-3459.

Steinberg, D., Bennett, G.G., Svetkey, L., 2017. The DASH diet, 20 years later. JAMA 317 (15), 1529–1530. https://doi.org/10.1001/jama.2017.1628.

Steinberger, J., Daniels, S.R., Hagberg, N., Isasi, C.R., Kelly, A.S., Lloyd-Jones, D., Stroke, C., 2016. Cardiovascular health promotion in children: challenges and opportunities for 2020 and beyond: a scientific statement from the American Heart Association. Circulation 134 (12), e236–e255. https://doi.org/10.1161/CIR.0000000000000441.

Te Morenga, L., Montez, J.M., 2017. Health effects of saturated and trans-fatty acid intake in children and adolescents: systematic review and meta-analysis. PLoS One 12 (11). https://doi.org/10.1371/journal.pone.0186672, e0186672.

U.S. Department of Health and Human Services and U.S. Department of Agriculture, 2020. Dietary Guidelines for Americans. Retrieved from https://www.dietaryguidelines.gov/sites/default/files/2020-12/Dietary_Guidelines_for_Americans_2020-2025.pdf.

van de Laar, R.J., Stehouwer, C.D., van Bussel, B.C., te Velde, S.J., Prins, M.H., Twisk, J.W., Ferreira, I., 2012. Lower lifetime dietary fiber intake is associated with carotid artery stiffness: the Amsterdam growth and health longitudinal study. Am. J. Clin. Nutr. 96 (1), 14–23. https://doi.org/10.3945/ajcn.111.024703.

Villegas, R., Shu, X.O., Gao, Y.T., Yang, G., Elasy, T., Li, H., Zheng, W., 2008. Vegetable but not fruit consumption reduces the risk of type 2 diabetes in Chinese women. J. Nutr. 138 (3), 574–580. https://doi.org/10.1093/jn/138.3.574.

Virani, S.S., Alonso, A., Aparicio, H.J., Benjamin, E.J., Bittencourt, M.S., Callaway, C.W., Stroke Statistics, S, 2021. Heart disease and stroke statistics-2021 update: a report from the American Heart Association. Circulation 143 (8), e254–e743. https://doi.org/10.1161/CIR.0000000000000950.

Vos, M.B., Kaar, J.L., Welsh, J.A., Van Horn, L.V., Feig, D.I., Anderson, C.A.M., Council on, H., 2017. Added sugars and cardiovascular disease risk in children: a scientific statement from the American Heart Association. Circulation 135 (19), e1017–e1034. https://doi.org/10.1161/CIR.0000000000000439.

Wood, A.C., Blissett, J.M., Brunstrom, J.M., Carnell, S., Faith, M.S., Fisher, J.O., Stroke, C., 2020. Caregiver influences on eating behaviors in young children: a scientific statement from the American Heart Association. J. Am. Heart Assoc. 9 (10). https://doi.org/10.1161/JAHA.119.014520, e014520.

World Health Organization, 2020. The Top Ten Causes of Death. Retrieved from https://www.who.int/news-room/fact-sheets/detail/the-top-10-causes-of-death.

World Health Organization, 2021. Cardiovascular Diseases. Retrieved from https://www.who.int/news-room/fact-sheets/detail/cardiovascular-diseases-(cvds.

Zhong, V.W., Lamichhane, A.P., Crandell, J.L., Couch, S.C., Liese, A.D., The, N.S., Mayer-Davis, E.J., 2016. Association of adherence to a Mediterranean diet with glycemic control and cardiovascular risk factors in youth with type I diabetes: the SEARCH nutrition ancillary study. Eur. J. Clin. Nutr. 70 (7), 802–807. https://doi.org/10.1038/ejcn.2016.8.

# Early nutrition and the development of allergic diseases

*Edward G.A. Iglesia[a], David M. Fleischer[b], and Elissa M. Abrams[c]*

[a]Vanderbilt University Medical Center, Nashville, TN, United States [b]Children's Hospital of Colorado, University of Colorado School of Medicine, Aurora, CO, United States [c]University of Manitoba, Winnipeg, MB, Canada

## CHAPTER LEARNING OBJECTIVES

1. Identify the role of pre-natal exposures in the prevention of allergic disease

2. Review the role of early childhood exposures, including early food

3. introduction, in the prevention of allergic disease

4. Describe ongoing controversies in the role of early food introduction in the prevention of allergic disease

## 13.1 Introduction

Often first appearing in infancy and early childhood, asthma, atopic dermatitis, food allergy, and allergic rhinitis are some of the most common chronic childhood conditions, impacting directly up to 10% of children and indirectly up to 50% of the population according to some estimates (Soller et al., 2012; Pawankar et al., 2013; Gupta et al., 2018; Clarke et al., 2020). In absolute global estimates, 300 million people suffer from asthma, and 200–250 million people have a food allergy (Pawankar et al., 2013). Many allergies, including some food allergies such as peanut and tree nuts, are rarely outgrown (Fleischer, 2007; Boyce et al., 2011). Additionally, allergic conditions and in particular food allergy, have a profound ongoing impact on day-to-day quality of life (Couratier et al., 2020; DunnGalvin et al., 2020; Nowak-Wegrzyn et al., 2021) and exert a substantial economic burden (Pawankar et al., 2013; Gupta et al., 2013). Given the rise of allergic disease prevalence in primarily Westernized and urban

*Early Nutrition and Long-Term Health*
https://doi.org/10.1016/B978-0-12-824389-3.00016-7

327

centers over a relatively short time frame over the past century, much attention has been given to environmental exposures as potential inciting factors, especially in potentially genetically susceptible individuals (Pawankar et al., 2013). As some of these factors (e.g., indoor/outdoor environment) are potentially modifiable and possibly scalable on a population level, there has been a heightened interest toward the prevention of allergic diseases by intervening in early life. The maternal and infant diets present opportunities to impact immune development and potentially prevent allergic sensitization and/or clinical allergic disease.

The goal of this chapter is to review pre-natal and post-natal nutritional factors that may influence the development of allergic disease in childhood. It will cover maternal and infant nutrition, including maternal diet, breastfeeding, use of pre- and probiotics, dietary diversity, hydrolyzed formula, age of food introduction, polyunsaturated fatty acids, and vitamin D. The majority of the studies cited are observational, with the exception of a few randomized controlled studies on early food introduction. There are limitations in drawing significant conclusions with many of the interventions discussed, due to the nature of the studies to date.

With respect to breastfeeding studies, several challenges exist in conducting observational and interventional studies in human milk exposures and related health outcomes (Matheson et al., 2012; Blyuss et al., 2019). Given that human milk is the desired normative standard for its optimal caloric and nutrient density for infants, as well as for its known and purported maternal and infant health benefits, it is unethical to assign a mother-infant dyad to a non-human milk arm. As study designs are typically limited to observational studies, it is difficult to draw causal inferences between breastfeeding and health outcomes of interest. A particular causal inference problem that is also present in other nutrition research studies (whether interventional or strictly observational) is the issue of reverse causality. Reverse causality can occur when an outcome of interest is instead the cause of the studied exposure, rather than the exposure causing the outcome. For example, mothers of infants who develop eczema may continue to breastfeed longer than mothers of infants who do not develop eczema. Without accounting for this, a biased result may conclude that breastfeeding increases the risk of eczema, where in fact the opposite may be true (Bigman, 2020).

Other traditional threats to internal validity inherent to observational studies that are particularly salient in breastfeeding studies, but also are seen in other nutritional studies, include firstly measurement error, as quantifying the dose (i.e., amount, frequency, pattern, and duration) of exposure is challenging. For example, exposures may be categorized as exclusive breastfeeding, partial breastfeeding, or never breastfeeding; or by duration (e.g., less than 2 months vs 2 months or longer; or as a continuous variable). However, breastfeeding and weaning behaviors are generally dynamic and may not be neatly categorized. Additionally, quantification of these exposures may be subject to recall bias. Classifying atopic outcomes also presents various measurement challenges, as outcome definitions vary by natural history (e.g., infant wheeze vs asthma) and whether a diagnosis is ascertained by a standardized instrument (e.g., spirometry or oral food challenge) or patient-report, clinician report, or surrogate markers (e.g., markers of allergic sensitization).

In addition, confounding is a concern as the proclivity to develop an atopic state is influenced by a multitude of hypothesized factors—including genetics, various environmental exposures, infectious challenges, alterations in the human microbiome, dietary patterns, among other factors. By definition, observational studies are subject to residual confounding that may affect the effect size of any intervention on atopic outcomes.

Finally, sufficient sample size and power are a challenge. In part due to the various confounders mentioned above, the aforementioned measurement challenges, and relative infrequency of atopic conditions with respect to study design, large samples are required to detect modest effect sizes and to properly and statistically account for a priori confounders.

Despite these limitations, there has been a surge in evidence in allergy prevention, both in the pre-natal and early post-natal course, that will be reviewed in depth below.

## 13.2 Maternal diet during lactation and pregnancy

Barker's "fetal origins hypothesis" solidified the concept of intrauterine nutrition and its influence on the development of chronic disease (Barker and Martyn, 1992). Extending this principle to allergic diseases, there has been broad interest in identifying immunomodulatory mechanisms of specific nutrients and other maternal dietary approaches to atopic prevention in the perinatal period. This section will focus on maternal exposures, including vitamin D, long-chain polyunsaturated fatty acids, dietary antigens, and pre/probiotics (Fig. 13.1).

### 13.2.1 Vitamin D

Vitamin D is a fat-soluble micronutrient well-known for its central role in calcium homeostasis and bone health. The discovery of vitamin D receptor expression on immune cells has drawn attention to vitamin D's potential regulatory role in inflammation and immune pathways, principally through its physiologically active metabolite $1,25(OH)_2D_3$ (Aranow, 2011). Both the innate and adaptive immune systems have been shown to be involved in vitamin D's immunomodulatory mechanisms (Mora et al., 2008). For example, in antigen-presenting dendritic cells, vitamin D suppresses interleukin (IL)-12 production, a key cytokine that promotes $T_H1$ responses, and upregulates production of IL-10, a key cytokine that promotes immune tolerance. As another example, among effector and memory T cells, vitamin D has been shown to inhibit T-cell proliferation, T-cell expression of IL-2 and interferon (IFN)-$\gamma$, and CD8-mediated cytotoxicity (Jeffery et al., 2009). Vitamin D's involvement in promoting the development of allergy is supported by a number of basic, clinical, and epidemiologic studies (Reinholz et al., 2012).

Despite mechanistic and epidemiologic support for vitamin D's role in atopy development, evidence for vitamin D supplementation during pregnancy has been mixed. A 2020 systematic review and meta-analysis to investigate the association of various maternal diet factors with allergic outcomes included 17 randomized control trials and 78 observational studies (Venter et al., 2020a). Among randomized control trials, pre-natal vitamin D supplementation was associated with reduced risk of wheeze (OR 0.72 [95% CI 0.56, 0.92]). There were two notable trials that contributed to the summary estimate. The Vitamin D Antenatal Asthma Reduction Trial (VDAART) randomly assigned 881 women between 10 and 18 weeks gestational age to vitamin D3 4400 IU daily vs vitamin D3 400 mg IU daily (Litonjua et al., 2016). Among the 806 children at age 3 years, there was a 20% risk reduction for asthma or recurrent wheeze in children born to mothers who supplemented with 4400 IU of vitamin D3 vs children born to mothers who supplemented with 400 IU (hazard ratio [HR] 0.8 [95% CI 0.6, 1.0]). Follow-up at 6 years did not find an association with increased pre-natal vitamin

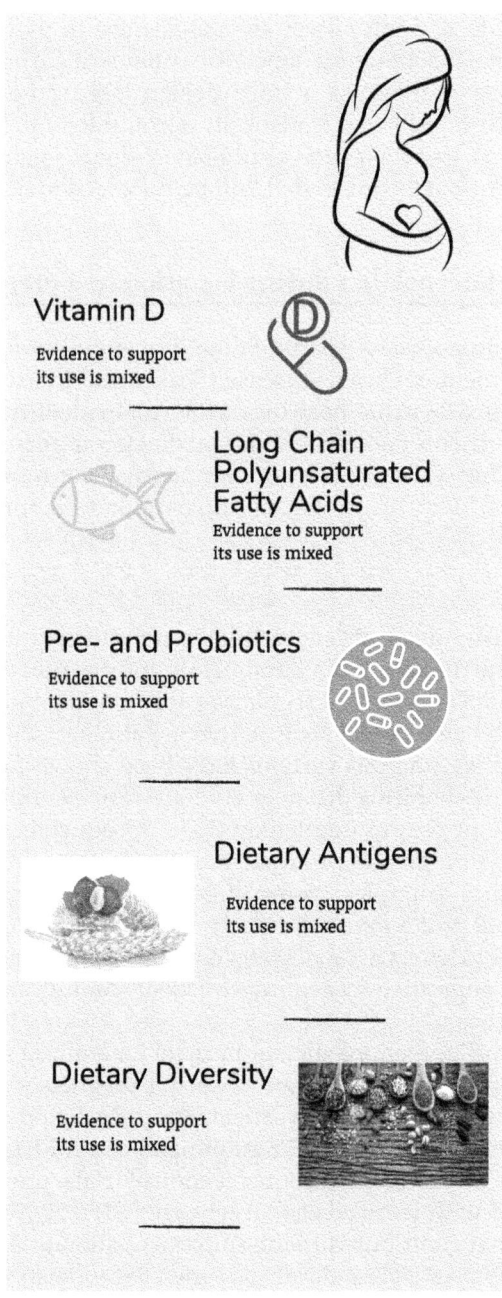

**FIG. 13.1**    Pre-natal exposures and influence on allergic outcomes. *Credit: Elissa M. Abrams, MD, MPH.*

D supplementation with asthma or recurrent wheeze. The Copenhagen Prospective Studies on Asthma in Childhood (COPSAC) randomly assigned 623 women at 23 weeks gestation to vitamin D3 2800 IU daily vs 400 IU daily (Chawes et al., 2016). Among 581 children born, higher vitamin D supplementation did not confer a significant risk reduction in the primary outcome of persistent wheeze at 3 years of age (HR 0.76 [95% CI 0.52, 1.12]), in the secondary outcome of asthma (OR 0.83 [95% CI 0.50, 1.36]), nor in the yearly prevalence of persistent wheeze/asthma through age 6 years (OR 0.87 [95% CI 0.59, 1.28]). Despite the trials not meeting their primary outcome, consistency in the direction of effect support a possible protective role of pre-natal vitamin D supplementation against childhood wheeze/asthma, especially in mothers who might be vitamin D insufficient at baseline (Litonjua, 2017). A secondary analysis of the VDAART trial found a protective effect in offspring born to mothers in the 4400 IU daily arm and an initial 25-hydroxyvitamin D level greater than 30 ng/mL vs offspring born to mothers in the 400 IU daily arm and an initial vitamin D level less than 20 mg/mL (aOR 0.42 [95% CI 0.19, 0.91]) (Litonjua et al., 2016). This systematic review identified no association between vitamin D supplementation and other allergic outcomes, including atopic dermatitis or food allergy.

Overall, while evidence continues to emerge regarding maternal vitamin D supplementation and its potential protective effect against allergic disease, in particular asthma/wheeze, there are no formal recommendations to proactively supplement high doses of vitamin D during pregnancy or lactation for the purposes of allergy prevention. Current allergy professional organizations do not suggest using vitamin D in pregnant women or lactating mothers (Yepes-Nunez et al., 2016; Greer et al., 2019; Fleischer et al., 2021; Halken et al., 2021), though a determination to do so is subject to shared-decision making. The Dietary Guidelines for Americans 2020–25 recommended daily allowance (RDA) of vitamin D is 600 IU daily for pregnant and lactating women, regardless of age, trimester, or postpartum period and irrespective of role in allergy prevention (US Department of Agriculture and US Department of Health and Human Services, 2020).

## 13.2.2 Long-chain polyunsaturated fatty acids

Dietary long-chain polyunsaturated acids (PUFAs) are essential nutrients that participate in cellular homeostasis, including membrane protein function, membrane fluidity, and regulation of cell signaling and gene expression (Das, 2006). Divided into two principal families, dietary n-6 PUFA (omega-6; linoleic acid) is found in vegetable oils (e.g., corn, sunflower, soybean) and related derived products (e.g., margarine), while dietary n-3 PUFA (omega-3, alpha-linoleic acid) is present in fatty/oily fish, fish oil, and nuts. The concomitant rise in n-6 PUFA consumption in the Western diet during the latter half of the 20th century with the increased prevalence of atopic and other inflammatory conditions helped generate the hypothesis that an imbalance between n-6 PUFAs and n-3 PUFAs might be causally related to the development of allergic disease.

N-6 PUFAs promote pro-inflammatory responses principally via its metabolism to arachidonic acid, which promotes the synthesis of numerous eicosanoids via the enzyme actions of cyclooxygenases and lipoxygenases (Calder et al., 2010). Eicosanoids, such as prostaglandins, leukotrienes, and thromboxanes, are important pro-inflammatory mediators, including those involved in both the immediate and late-phase allergic responses (e.g., $PG_2$, $PG2_a$, thromboxane $A_2$, $LTE_4$).

The consumption of n-3 PUFAs counterbalances n-6 PUFAs by competitively incorporating them into inflammatory cell membranes, effectively displacing arachidonic acid to an extent (Calder et al., 2010). Consequentially, the decreased availability of arachidonic acid substrate results in decreased inflammatory cell synthesis of arachidonic acid-derived eicosanoid mediators. Thus, the overall balance of n-3 and n-6 PUFAs is important in curbing inflammatory responses and achieving an anti-inflammatory state via n-3 PUFA supplementation.

Though supported by strong biologic plausibility and ecologic patterns, data from both observational and interventional studies have been mixed with regards to n-3 PUFA supplementation as an effective strategy against the development of atopic disease. A 2011 systematic review that included five observational studies found a protective effect of maternal fish consumption during pregnancy on allergic outcomes in offspring (decrease in childhood atopy between 25% and 95%), though one study of maternal fish consumption during lactation did not identify an effect (Kremmyda et al., 2011). A 2015 Cochrane review included eight randomized trials to investigate maternal pre-natal and/or post-natal n-3 PUFA supplementation as a preventive strategy for childhood allergy development in offspring (Gunaratne et al., 2015). While the authors concluded overall that the evidence was limited to support n-3 PUFA supplementation in pregnancy and/or lactation to prevent childhood allergic diseases, their results show that n-3 PUFA supplementation reduced medically diagnosed IgE allergy in children 12–36 months of age (RR 0.66 [95% CI 0.44, 0.98]). However, this effect was not seen for medically diagnosed IgE allergy beyond 36 months of age (RR 0.86 [95% CI 0.71, 1.11]) or any allergy (medically diagnosed IgE-mediated and/or parental report) at either age 12–36 months or greater than age 36 months. In secondary analyses, the authors found reductions in children 12 months or younger favoring n-3 PUFA supplementation for medically diagnosed IgE-mediated food allergies and IgE-mediated atopic dermatitis, as well as reductions in egg sensitization to egg and sensitization to any allergen in children between 12 and 36 months of age. Overall, there were no differences in childhood allergic disease among women who supplemented with n-3 PUFA vs those who did not.

Subsequent systematic reviews also identified a protective effect of n-3 PUFA supplementation in pregnancy and/or lactation against egg sensitization in offspring at 1 year of age, but otherwise have found inconsistent results of n-3 PUFA supplementation effects on offspring allergic outcomes (Best et al., 2016; Garcia-Larsen et al., 2018). A 2020 systematic review observed a non-statistically significant association between increased pre-natal n-3 PUFA supplementation and decreased asthma/wheeze (OR 0.70 [95% CI 0.45, 1.08]) and allergic rhinitis (OR 0.76 [95% CI 0.56, 1.04]) (Venter et al., 2020a).

As a result, in conclusion, there is no firm evidence at this time (despite a strong biologic plausibility) that maternal polyunsaturated fatty acid supplementation plays a role in allergy prevention.

### 13.2.3 Pre- and probiotics

The intestinal microbiome plays an important role in immune homeostasis and is a vital component of the local immunologic milieu in promoting oral tolerance (Penders et al., 2007; Prescott and Bjorksten, 2007; Chistiakov et al., 2014). Immune-protective effects of the intestinal microbiome include production of IgA, induction of tolerogenic dendritic cells and regulatory T cells, with subsequent production of pro-tolerogenic cytokines (e.g., IL-10 and transforming growth factor [TGF]-β). A study in a pathogen-free murine model demonstrated that the presence of an adequate intestinal microbiome is required for full immune function and the development of oral tolerance (Sudo et al., 1997). In the same model, appropriately regulated susceptibility to $T_H2$ responses was necessary for oral tolerance induction and was restored with normal intestinal microbiota (i.e., *Bifidobacterium infantis*) that was introduced early in the neonatal stage.

This basic mechanistic framework underlies the "old friends" hypothesis, which supposes the rise in allergic disease is a result of reduced early childhood microbial exposure, resulting in corresponding alterations in co-evolved commensal microbial flora needed for tolerogenic immune responses (Rook and Brunet, 2005). The "old friends" hypothesis builds upon the classic "hygiene hypothesis," which posits that the skewing from a $T_H1$ to a $T_H2$ phenotype occurs in the absence of sufficient microbial antigen-stimulation (Strachan, 1989). In this framework, the population growth in allergic and autoimmune disease is a consequence of a decreased burden of viral, bacterial, and parasitic infections in the Western world (Okada et al., 2010). Regardless of which hypothesis is invoked, the post-industrial environmental and "westernized" lifestyle changes that began in the 20th century (i.e., changes in diet, food manufacturing, physical activity, family and community structures), along with public health and clinical advances against communicable disease, are felt to be among the distal causes of the present-day preponderance of immune-related conditions (Thorburn et al., 2014). Observational studies in different countries have documented a notably lower prevalence of allergic diseases in groups living in traditional farming communities than those from the general population who are presumed to be living a "modern" lifestyle (Gerrard et al., 1976; Von Mutius et al., 1994; Martina et al., 2016).

Prebiotic and probiotic supplementation to prevent allergy is proposed to occur via influences on neonatal and infant immune development, though precise mechanisms are not fully understood (West et al., 2015). Prebiotics are non-digestible oligosaccharides that selectively stimulate the growth and activity of health-promoting commensal microbiota (bifidobacteria and lactobacilli species). Additionally, anti-inflammatory short-chain fatty acids are produced via microbial fermentation of prebiotics (Wong et al., 2006). These are naturally present in human milk, cereals, vegetables, or can be manufactured. Probiotics are proposed to positively influence intestinal flora composition, act as an immunomodulator toward a $T_H1$ phenotype, and/or interact with other luminal and mucosal products generated from microbes, the host, or food (Michail, 2009; Sestito et al., 2020).

Overall, the body of clinical evidence to date to support the use of pre- or probiotics for allergy prevention is not definitive. Studies using prebiotics in pregnant or lactating women for the purpose of allergy prevention are lacking (Cuello-Garcia et al., 2017, 2016). Regarding probiotics, a 2015 systematic review identified 29 randomized trials assessing the effects of probiotics administered to pregnant women, lactating women, and/or infants (Cuello-Garcia et al., 2015). The risk of atopic dermatitis was reduced when probiotics were used by mothers during their third trimester of pregnancy (RR 0.71 [95% CI 0.60, 0.84]) and during lactation (RR 0.57 [95% CI 0.47, 0.69]) compared to mothers taking placebo; however, the level of certainty in the evidence was low due to risk of bias, imprecision, and indirect causality. A 2015 review by the World Allergy Organization found similar conclusions among eight trials (RR 0.72 [95% CI 0.61, 0.85]), and subsequently issued a conditional recommendation to recommend probiotic supplementation to women who are pregnant and/or lactating whose offspring is at high risk of allergy development (Fiocchi et al., 2015). A 2019 systematic review of 28 studies focused on probiotics and offspring atopic dermatitis development found that only a combined pre-natal and post-natal probiotic supplementation approach was protective against atopic dermatitis (OR 0.69 [95% CI 0.58, 0.82]) (Li et al., 2019). These systematic reviews have not demonstrated a significant effect of probiotic supplementation in pregnant or lactating mothers on allergic outcomes other than atopic dermatitis.

Limitations to the literature to date include varying intervals of probiotic supplementation, different microorganisms in the probiotic products used, varying dose, and varying definitions of allergic outcomes. Systematic reviews which include different probiotic bacteria may not be appropriate or reflective of the effect of one specific genus or strain, as different bacteria would be expected to behave differently. At this time, there is insufficient evidence to recommend the addition of pre- or probiotics in general to mothers during pregnancy or breastfeeding to prevent allergic diseases or food allergy.

### 13.2.4 Dietary antigens

Dietary and inhalant antigens, including those derived from milk, egg, and birch pollen, have been noted to have transplacental transfer (Szepfalusi et al., 2000). Dietary antigens are also known to be passed into human breast milk (Kilshaw and Cant, 1984; Vadas et al., 2001). These routes of exposure to the fetus and/or infant have provided the basis for investigation into a purposeful exclusion or consumption of allergenic foods in the maternal diet, during pregnancy or lactation, for prevention of allergic sensitization and clinical allergy. Possible explanatory mechanisms of dietary antigen consumption during lactation have been gleaned from clinical studies. For example, in one study, lower levels of milk-specific IgA, IgG,1, and IgG4 antibodies in infants of mothers avoiding cow's milk was associated with infant cow's milk allergy (Jarvinen et al., 2014). Another study of maternal egg consumption during lactation on egg protein levels in breast milk, infant serum IgG4 specific to egg ovalbumin (a hen's egg component protein) at 6 months of age was positively correlated with high-egg ingestion by mothers (Metcalfe et al., 2016). These are relevant as IgG4 is thought to be a 'protective' antibody that is a surrogate of oral tolerance. Additionally, cord blood IgA positively correlated with maternal consumption of milk during pregnancy in the Finnish Type I Diabetes Prediction and Prevention Prospective Cohort Study (Nwaru et al., 2013). In this study, the highest quartile intake of cow's milk during pregnancy was associated with lower odds of offspring cow's milk allergy (OR 0.30, [95% CI 013, 0.68]).

However, clinical evidence to date is not conclusive of a protective effect of maternal manipulation of diet with allergenic foods. Three systematic reviews from 2014 (Kramer and Kakuma, 2014; De Silva et al., 2014; Netting et al., 2014), including one Cochrane review synthesizing evidence from five trials (952 participants), (Kramer and Kakuma, 2014) did not identify a protective effect of maternal dietary antigen avoidance on offspring allergic outcomes, either while pregnant or during lactation. This was the case for both infants at risk for atopy and infants at standard risk. Overall, avoidance diets are not recommended given insufficient evidence for efficacy and evidence of harm in restricting important macro- and micronutrients required to maintain optimal nutrition for mother and fetus/infant.

### 13.2.5 Diet diversity

Defined as the variety of different food or food groups eaten over a given time period, diet diversity has drawn increased attention in recent years as a practical intervention to optimizing health given its approach to whole foods and due to the difficulty of focusing on isolated nutrients (Venter et al., 2020b). While precise mechanisms are not yet understood, several hypotheses have been proposed by which diet diversity can promote tolerance, namely, (1) support of increased gut microbial diversity, which may in turn promote pro-tolerogenic immune adaptations; (2) incorporation of increased nutrient intake, including those that are proposed to be associated with allergy prevention (i.e., n3-PUFAs and prebiotics); (3) incorporation of increased exposure to dietary antigens and promotion of tolerance through early allergen exposure via the gut (Venter et al., 2020b).

To date, there are no published studies on the formal role of diet diversity in pregnancy or lactation and allergy outcomes in offspring. There have been, however, studies examining the association of diet indices (i.e., formally defined dietary patterns) used in pregnancy with subsequent atopic disease in offspring (D'auria et al., 2020). Two birth cohort studies found no association between the Healthy Eating Index (HEI) with allergic outcomes during childhood in offspring (Lange et al., 2010; Moonesinghe et al., 2016), while one Irish cohort found that higher HEI-2015 scores were associated with lower risk of asthma (OR 0.77 [95% CI 0.64,0.93]) (Chen et al., 2020). The same Irish cohort found an association between Diet Inflammatory Index (DII) scores during pregnancy and asthma outcomes in offspring over a 10-year period. A US-based cohort also showed an association between DII scores in pregnancy with wheeze, but not asthma at age 7.5 years (Hanson et al., 2020). Among five cohorts that examined the association between the Mediterranean diet index and offspring allergic outcomes, four studies did not find an association (Lange et al., 2010; Chatzi et al., 2008, 2013; Castro-Rodriguez et al., 2016; Hanson et al., 2020). One study found an association between Mediterranean diet score with childhood persistent wheeze, atopic wheeze, and overall atopic, while another study found an association between Mediterranean diet scores and relevant spirometry parameters.

## 13.3 Infant diet—Breastfeeding

### 13.3.1 Breastfeeding

Leading health authorities recognize that human breast milk (HBM), ideally fed exclusively, is the optimal source of infant nutrition in early life (Organization, 2017; Section on, 2012, American College of et al., 2016). Numerous positive infant and child health outcomes are attributed to HBM feeding (Victora et al., 2016; Ip et al., 2007). As the effects of HBM against pathogens are mediated via its various immunomodulatory properties, there has also been interest in HBM's influence on other immune-mediated disease, including atopic conditions, with some studies published as early as the 1930s attempting to delineate an effect (Grulee and Sanford, 1936).

Human breast milk contains numerous immunologically active components that participate in the developing immune systems of infants (Jarvinen et al., 2019; Andreas et al., 2015; Ballard and Morrow, 2013). Roles of HBM include host defense against pathogens, regulation of inflammatory/immunomodulatory pathways, and promotion of immune tolerance. Numerous identified innate and acquired immune components include various leukocytes, immunoglobulins, cytokines, growth factors, hormones, mucins, among other substances. Additionally, macronutrients such as long-chain polyunsaturated fatty acids, human milk oligosaccharides, lactoferrin, and dietary antigens are present in HBM and have been implicated in protective mechanisms against atopic disease. However, to date, the literature is mixed regarding the role of HBM in the prevention of atopic disease (Fig. 13.2).

## 13.3.2 Breastfeeding and atopic dermatitis

A 2001 systematic review and meta-analysis supported a protective effect of breastfeeding during the first 3 months of life and subsequent atopic dermatitis (AD) (Gdalevich et al., 2001). Using a fixed-effect model to summarize results across 18 prospective studies from developed countries, the study's authors report a summary odds ratio (OR) was 0.68 (95% CI 0.52, 0.88). When stratified by a family history of atopy, the OR was 0.58 (95% CI 0.41, 0.92) for a positive family history vs a non-statistically significant association for breastfed infants without a family history of atopy (OR 0.84 [95% 0.59, 1.19]). These results are cited by a 2007 Agency for Healthcare Research Quality evidence report for the US Depart of Health and Human Services Office on Women's Health are often used as the basis for public health messaging on the protective effect of breastfeeding and AD (Ip et al., 2007).

However, several updated systematic reviews and meta-analyses incorporating newer studies present evidence that is less supportive of a protective effect of breastfeeding on AD. In a 2009 systematic review and meta-analysis of 21 studies, the authors did not find a significant protective effect of exclusive breastfeeding for 3 months' duration against AD vs partial breastfeeding or conventional infant formula (OR 0.89, [95% CI 0.76, 1.04]) (Yang et al., 2009). Furthermore, as part of a sensitivity analysis whereby a controversial study was excluded in comparing exclusive breastfeeding to conventional formula only, the summary OR was 0.94 (95% CI 0.81, 1.08). An updated 2015 systematic review and meta-analysis performed pooled analyses that examined breastfeeding exposures of (a) "more vs less breastfeeding"; (b) breastfeeding for at least 3–4 months, with eczema outcomes; (c) before 2 years of age; and (d) after 2 years of age (Lodge et al., 2015). In pooling six cohort studies, the authors found a protective effect of exclusive breastfeeding for at least 3–4 months against the risk of eczema up to 2 years of age (re OR 0.74 95% CI 0.57, 0.97). Conversely, the authors did not identify an association between the exposure of more vs. less breastfeeding and eczema outcomes at 2 years of age, nor on breastfeeding exposures and eczema outcomes after 2 years of age, thus raising the question of breastfeeding as potentially protective against a specific infantile eczema phenotype. In both of the 2009 and 2015 meta-analyses, family history of atopy was not found to be an effect modifier, and heterogeneity among studies was high.

Most recently, the United States Department of Agriculture (USDA) commissioned a systematic review in 2019 in order to inform the evidence base for the 2020–25 Dietary Guidelines for Americans (Gungor et al., 2019). Key questions examined breastfeeding exposures of (a) never vs ever feeding human milk and (b) shorter vs longer durations of any human milk feedings, with allergic outcomes (food allergies, allergic rhinitis, atopic dermatitis, and asthma) in (c) childhood and (d) birth through 24 months. Among studies that examined the association of the never vs ever feeding human milk exposures and atopic dermatitis, the study authors found inconclusive evidence among 16 articles and the outcome of eczema in the birth through the 24-month period. Among eight prospective cohort studies and one nested case-control study, the authors identified only one study to have a statistically significant association between ever feeding human milk and atopic dermatitis, though half of the

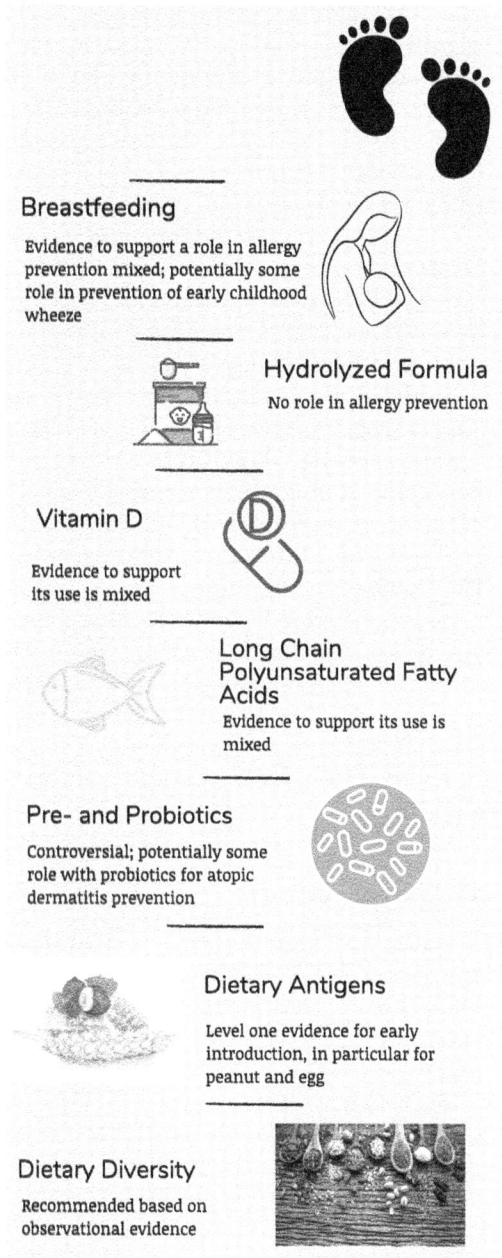

**Breastfeeding**

Evidence to support a role in allergy prevention mixed; potentially some role in prevention of early childhood wheeze

**Hydrolyzed Formula**

No role in allergy prevention

**Vitamin D**

Evidence to support its use is mixed

**Long Chain Polyunsaturated Fatty Acids**

Evidence to support its use is mixed

**Pre- and Probiotics**

Controversial; potentially some role with probiotics for atopic dermatitis prevention

**Dietary Antigens**

Level one evidence for early introduction, in particular for peanut and egg

**Dietary Diversity**

Recommended based on observational evidence

**FIG. 13.2** Post-natal exposures and influence on allergic outcomes. *Credit: Elissa M. Abrams, MD, MPH.*

study sample was noted to be born small for gestational age (Purvis et al., 2005). The other eight studies reported non-significant associations and were inconsistent in direction.

Regarding the exposure of shorter vs longer duration of any human milk feeding, the authors deemed that eight included articles presented inconclusive evidence on an association with atopic dermatitis from birth to 24 months. When looking at this exposure and the outcome of atopic dermatitis in childhood, the authors included a large cluster randomized controlled trial (RCT) conducted by Kramer et al. (Promotion of Breastfeeding Intervention Trial [PROBIT]) (Kramer et al., 2007). In this trial, 17,046 healthy mothers of full-term infants in Belarus were followed for 12 months. Study sites were randomized to a health promotion intervention to increase duration and exclusivity of human milk feeding who elected to breastfeed, or to a control intervention of usual infant feeding practices and policies. Kramer et al. did not find an association between intervention arm and ever having eczema by 6.5 years of age as measured by a standardized physician-assessment of eczema (ISAAC instrument). The systematic review authors note that most of the other six prospective cohort studies reported non-significant associations between any duration of human milk feeding and atopic dermatitis and childhood. Bergmann et al. found a seemingly paradoxical association of any duration human milk feeding with increased risk of atopic dermatitis through 7 years of age (OR 1.029 [95% CI 1.002, 1.057]) in the Multicentre Allergy Study, though this and related findings were limited to select analyses in their report (Bergmann et al., 2000).

The authors of the USDA systematic review concluded that there was limited evidence on the association of breastfeeding exposures on AD outcomes (Gungor et al., 2019), thus breastfeeding is not included as a protective factor against AD in the updated Dietary Guidelines for Americans (Services.). This differs from other recommendations that affirm that breastfeeding for the first 3–4 months decreases the risk of eczema in the first 2 years of life (Greer et al., 2019).

Overall, the literature to date does not strongly support a role for breastfeeding as a protective factor against atopic dermatitis.

### 13.3.3 Breastfeeding and allergic rhinitis

The evidence on the role of breastfeeding in the prevention of allergic rhinitis is sparse, with significant methodologic limitations. A 2002 meta-analysis of 6 prospective studies noted a borderline protective effect of exclusive breastfeeding for the first 3 months of life against the development of allergic rhinitis (summary OR 0.74 [95%CI 0.54, 1.01]) (Mimouni Bloch et al., 2002). The Lodge et al. meta-analysis (based on 5 cohorts and 11 cross-sectional studies) noted that more vs less breastfeeding was associated with a non-significant protective effect for allergic rhinitis (OR 0.92 [95%CI 0.84, 1.01]) (Lodge et al., 2015). Studies to date have noted a range of results, from increased risk of allergic rhinitis with breastfeeding, no protective role, or decreased risk (Kramer et al., 2007; Matheson et al., 2007; Codispoti et al., 2010). Both a 2019 American Academy of Pediatrics Clinical Report and the 2019 USDA-commissioned systematic review concluded there is currently insufficient evidence to demonstrate an association between breastfeeding and the development of allergic rhinitis throughout the lifespan (Greer et al., 2019; Gungor et al., 2019). Limitations of the evidence to date include largely observational studies, lack of long-term follow-up for many of these studies, varying definitions of allergic rhinitis, and minimal data from low to middle-income countries. Longer-term studies would be beneficial as seasonal allergies can change and develop even into adolescence.

## 13.3.4 Breastfeeding and food allergy

The data on breastfeeding as a food allergy prevention strategy are mixed. Some studies demonstrate a reduced risk of food allergy with breastfeeding, while others demonstrate no association between breastfeeding duration and food allergy (Van Odijk et al., 2003). For example, the Copenhagen Prospective Study on Asthma in Childhood (COPSAC) found no significant association between duration of exclusive breastfeeding and development of sensitization in the first 6 years of life (OR 0.96 [95% CI 0.84, 1.10]) at 6 years of age) (Jelding-Dannemand et al., 2015). Both the 2019 AAP Clinical Report and the 2019 USDA-commissioned systematic review suggest that no conclusions can be made about the role of breastfeeding in preventing or delaying any specific food allergy (Greer et al., 2019; Gungor et al., 2019). Similarly, the North American consensus guideline notes no association between exclusive breastfeeding and the primary prevention of any specific food allergy (Fleischer et al., 2021).

## 13.3.5 Breastfeeding and asthma

The evidence on the role of exclusive breastfeeding in asthma prevention is changing rapidly. In the last decade, there have been more than 50 studies examining the relationship between asthma and breastfeeding (Greer et al., 2019). The picture, as a result, is complicated by divergent data and heterogeneity in the literature. A 2014 systematic review noted that the index of heterogeneity between studies on asthma prevention and exclusive breastfeeding vary between 71% and 91% (Dogaru et al., 2014).

Despite the limitations, the evidence is relatively consistent in demonstrating a protective effect against early childhood wheeze with breastfeeding in the first few months of life. A study of 3296 infants in a Canadian birth cohort noted that the risk of probable asthma at 3 years of age was significantly increased in infants who were not exclusively breastfed for the first 3 months of life (Klopp et al., 2017). Compared with those exclusively fed at the breast, those who received some expressed breastmilk had a 43% increased odds of asthma, and those who received only formula had a 70% increased odds, even after adjustment for maternal atopy, ethnicity, mode of birth, infant sex, gestational age, and daycare attendance. Similarly, the Copenhagen Study on Asthma in Childhood (COPSAC) birth cohort of 411 infants noted that increased duration of exclusive breastfeeding reduced the risk of wheezy episodes in multivariate analysis (RR 0.67; 95%CI:0.48–0.96) (Giwercman et al., 2010).

There is also some evidence that prolonged duration of breastfeeding is protective. In the Canadian cohort, among infants at risk of asthma, exclusive breastfeeding for 6 months of age reduced wheezing episodes in infancy by 62% (aRR0.38; 95%CI 0.20–0.71) compared to no breastfeeding and by 37% compared with partial breastfeeding (supplemented with formula or complementary foods) (aRR 0.63; 95%CI 0.43–0.93). (Azad et al., 2017) A 2014 systematic review and meta-analysis of 117 studies noted that more vs less breastfeeding was associated with a 22% reduced risk of "asthma ever" (OR 0.78 [95%CI 0.74, 0.84]) and a 24% reduced risk of "recent asthma" (OR 0.76 [95% CI 0.67, 0.86]) (Dogaru et al., 2014). When stratified by age, the strongest protective effect was seen in the first 2 years of life but did persist until 7 years of age or more. The Lodge et al. systematic review also noted a longer-term protective effect. In the 29 studies that looked at more vs less breastfeeding duration, more breastfeeding was associated with a reduced risk of asthma into school age (5–18 years; OR 0.90; 95% CI:0.84–0.97), particularly in medium to low-income countries (Lodge et al., 2015). The 2019 USDA-commissioned systematic review included 17 studies examining "never" vs "ever" being fed human milk and asthma in childhood, as well as 20 studies examining the duration of any human milk feeding and asthma in childhood (Gungor et al., 2019). With the exception of one study, all studies demonstrated that no exposure, or shorter duration of exposure, of breast-milk was associated with a higher risk of childhood asthma. The 2019 AAP Clinical Report also recommends exclusive breastfeeding months as protective against wheezing early in life, citing similar evidence that suggests that part of the protective effect is related to duration and not exclusivity of breastfeeding (Greer et al., 2019). The guideline also notes that longer duration of breastfeeding may protect against asthma after 5 years of age.

In summary, there is moderate evidence that any and longer duration of HBM feeding is associated with a decreased risk of childhood wheeze and asthma. Evidence is unclear regarding the role of exclusive HBM in atopic dermatitis prevention. Limited evidence does not suggest a link between HBM consumption and other atopic diseases such as food allergies and allergic rhinitis. Studies are limited by their observational, non-randomized designs, acknowledging that randomized, controlled trials would be difficult and unethical to conduct as breastfeeding is the preferred means of infant feeding due to its many other benefits to mother and infant.

## 13.4 Infant diet—Hydrolyzed formula and supplementation

### 13.4.1 Hydrolyzed formula

Infant formula simulates the caloric density and nutrient content of human milk and provides a suitable substitute in situations where human milk use is contraindicated, insufficient, or not desired. Infant formula is derived from a variety of alternative protein sources, most commonly cow's milk. However, infants with a food protein hypersensitivity (e.g., IgE-mediated cow's milk allergy or non-IgE-mediated food protein enterocolitis) do not tolerate standard infant formulas derived from whole, intact protein. In these cases, extensively hydrolyzed formulas, or crystalline amino-acid-based formulas (also referred to as hypoallergenic formulas in the US), are recommended. Hydrolyzed formulas are classified by the degree of hydrolysis and subsequent peptide size: partially hydrolyzed (<5 kDa, range 3–10 kDa), extensively hydrolyzed (<3 kDa). Due to various proprietary hydrolysis methods, there may also be qualitative changes to peptide composition that influence allergenicity in addition to peptide size and protein source. Hydrolyzed formulas may be derived from two general cow's milk protein fractions: whey or casein. In addition, the term 'hypoallergenic' differs from region to region, due to regulation.

Antigen uptake and presentation leading to oral tolerance in the gastrointestinal immune system underlies potential mechanisms for the role of hydrolyzed formula in prevention of allergic sensitization and allergic disease. The lamina propria, which contains populations of effector T cells, antibody-secreting plasma cells, and CD103+ dendritic cells, plays an important role in promotion of oral tolerance (Pabst and Mowat, 2012; Chistiakov et al., 2014). The lamina propria acquires soluble antigens that have diffused via tight junctions or through epithelial transcellular routes. Gut-associated lymphoid tissue (GALT), composed of Peyer's patches, isolated lymphoid follicles, gut-draining mesenteric lymph nodes, plays a smaller role in induction of oral tolerance, primarily facilitating transport of luminal particulate antigens and microbiota via M-cell-mediated transcytosis (Pabst and Mowat, 2012). Within this mechanistic framework, the decreased molecular weight of smaller hydrolyzed peptides, with their associated decreased allergenicity, is hypothesized to promote oral tolerance without sensitization (Cabana, 2017).

Despite the utility of hydrolyzed formula in treating cow's milk-mediated allergies and the hypothesized mechanistic basis for prevention of sensitization, evidence from clinical studies to date has not been consistent in supporting the use of hydrolyzed formulas over standard intact cow's milk formulas in preventing allergic disease. Data from Cochrane systematic reviews and meta-analyses from the 2000s initially underpinned professional society recommendations for use of hydrolyzed formula, as a category, to prevent or delay atopic dermatitis in high-risk infants who are unable to breastfeed (Fleischer et al., 2013; Greer et al., 2008; Osborn and Sinn, 2006, 2003). Among the included studies was a notable large intervention trial (German Infant Nutritional Intervention-Program [GINI]) that randomized 2252 term infants with a family history of atopy to one of three hydrolyzed formulas (partially or extensively hydrolyzed whey formula, extensively hydrolyzed casein formula) or cow's milk formula as a substitute for the first 4 months of life when breastfeeding was insufficient. Compared with those who used cow's milk formula, infant atopic dermatitis incidence was reduced among those using an extensively hydrolyzed casein-based formula (OR 0.42 [95% CI 0.22, 0.79]) or partially hydrolyzed formula (OR 0.56 [95% CI 0.32, 0.99]) (von Berg et al., 2003). An extensively hydrolyzed whey-based formula had no impact on infant atopic dermatitis (OR 0.81 [95% CI 0.48, 1.4]). Similar results were found in subsequent follow-ups at 3, 6, 10, and 20 years of age, with greater effect sizes in the extensively hydrolyzed casein, and partially hydrolyzed whey-based groups, but not in the extensively hydrolyzed whey formula group (von Berg et al., 2007, 2008; Rzehak et al., 2011; Gappa et al., 2020).

However, a 2016 systematic review and meta-analysis of 37 intervention trials (28 randomized control trials; greater than 19,000 participants) examined allergic outcomes between infants treated with any hydrolyzed cow's milk formula vs non-hydrolyzed cow's milk formula or human milk (Boyle et al., 2016). The odds of developing atopic dermatitis between 0 and 4 years among the hydrolyzed formula group were no better than those in the standard infant formula group: partially hydrolyzed formula (OR 0.84 [95% CI 0.67, 1.07], extensively hydrolyzed casein-based formula (OR 0.55 [95% CI, 0.28, 1.09]), and extensively hydrolyzed whey-based formula (OR 1.12, [95% CI 0.88, 1.42]). Synthesized evidence also did find support for prevention of atopic dermatitis from 5 to 14 years, recurrent wheeze from 0 to 14 years, allergic rhinitis 0–14 years, food allergy, or allergic sensitization. An updated 2018 Cochrane review and meta-analysis and a 2019 systematic review similarly found no substantial evidence to support use of hydrolyzed formula of any duration over cow's milk formula to prevent allergic disease in infants who are unable to exclusively breastfeed, although a limitation of systematic reviews is the inclusion of multiple different hydrolyzed formulas which may not be reflective of the effect of one specific type of hydrolysate (Osborn et al., 2018; Vandenplas et al., 2019). In a recent population-based cohort study of 11,720 infants in France, the use of partially hydrolyzed formula vs non-hydrolyzed formula increased the odds of wheezing at 1 year of age in at-risk infants (OR 1.68 [95% CI 1.24, 2.28]), and in food allergy at 2 years of age in both standard-risk infants (OR 3.78 [95% CI 1.52, 9.41]) and at-risk infants (OR 2.31 [95% CI 1.36, 3.94]) (Davisse-Paturet et al., 2019).

As a result of inconsistent and conflicting evidence, updated guidelines do not recommend the use of hydrolyzed formulas in general as a means to prevent allergic disease.

### 13.4.2 Vitamin D

In the 2018 systematic review of vitamin D supplementation and primary prevention of allergic diseases, there were no randomized control trials that assessed allergic outcomes in infants (Yepes-Nunez et al., 2018). Three observational studies examined infant outcomes, but results were inconsistent with very low certainty in the evidence (Hypponen et al., 2004; Bener et al., 2012; Anderson et al., 2015). One cohort study showing an increased relative risk of allergic rhinitis among infants who regularly supplemented vitamin D with infants who did not supplement or supplemented irregularly (RR 1.95 [95% CI 1.15, 1.49]) and a RR of 1.33 (95% CI, 1.00, 1.79) of asthma/wheeze in the same comparator groups (Hypponen et al., 2004). Another cohort study had no impact of infant vitamin D supplementation of childhood wheezing (OR 1.00 [95% CI 0.81, 1.23]) (Anderson et al., 2015), and a case-control demonstrated a reduced risk of food allergy development at 1 year of age (RR 0.49 [95% CI 0.27, 0.88]) (Bener et al., 2012). No randomized control trial or observational study addressed vitamin D supplementation and allergic outcomes in childhood.

Current allergy professional organizations do not specifically recommend for or against high dose vitamin D supplementation to infants for the purposes of allergy prevention (Yepes-Nunez et al., 2016; Fleischer et al., 2021; Halken et al., 2021).

### 13.4.3 Long-chain polyunsaturated fatty acids

A 2016 Cochrane review identified 17 randomized and quasi-RCTs that compared the use of PUFA with no PUFA in infants for the primary prevention of allergy, with nine studies included in the meta-analysis (2704 infants) (Schindler et al., 2016). Overall, the authors found no evidence that infant PUFA supplementation impacted infant or childhood allergy (RR 0.96 [95% CI 0.73, 1.26]), asthma (RR 1.04 [95% CI 0.80, 1.35]), atopic dermatitis (RR 0.93 [95% CI 0.82, 1.06]), or food allergy (RR 0.81 [95% CI 0.56, 1.19]). Data were insufficient to estimate an effect on allergic rhinitis. The quality of the evidence was very low.

*Pre- and Probiotics.* A 2015 World Allergy Organization (WAO) review identified 18 randomized trials that included non-exclusively breastfed infants (term infancy to 3 years of age) and addressed the use of prebiotics vs no prebiotics for allergy prevention (Cuello-Garcia et al., 2015). Prebiotic supplementation in the first year of life reduced the risk of asthma or recurrent wheeze (RR 0.37 [95% CI 0.17, 0.80]), had a RR of 0.28 (95% CI 0.08, 1.00) for food allergy, and a RR of 0.57 (95% CI 0.30, 1.08) for atopic dermatitis. This led to a conditional recommendation for prebiotic supplementation in not-exclusively breastfed infants, both at high and low risk for development of allergy. Among 22 RCTs in a 2017 systematic review and meta-analysis, prebiotic supplementation in the infant period, compared to placebo: had the following estimates on allergic outcomes: atopic dermatitis (RR 0.68 [95% CI 0.40, 1.15]), wheeze/asthma (RR 0.37 [95% CI 0.17, 0.80]), and food allergy (RR 0.28 [95% CI 0.08, 1.00])

(Cuello-Garcia et al., 2017). Overall certainty in the results of both reviews was very low due to serious risk of bias and imprecise estimates of the original studies.

A 2015 systematic review identified 29 randomized trials that addressed the use of probiotics in the infant period for allergy prevention. Compared to no probiotic use, administration of probiotics to infants reduced the risk of atopic dermatitis (RR 0.80 [95% CI 0.68, 0.94]) (Cuello-Garcia et al., 2015). Certainty in the evidence was low, and there was no evidence to support an effect of probiotics on other allergic conditions. The limitations of this systematic review, as identified by the authors, includes the paucity of direct evidence, the likelihood of bias in primary studies, and the imprecision of the estimated pooled effects. A 2015 WAO systematic review focused on probiotics for the prevention of allergies identified 23 randomized trials conducted in infants (Fiocchi et al., 2015). Infant probiotic supplementation decreased the risk of atopic dermatitis compared to placebo (RR 0.81 [95% CI 0.70, 0.94]). No differences were identified outcomes of wheeze/asthma, food allergy, allergic rhinitis, or "any allergy." While certainty in the evidence was low, authors of a conditional recommendation judged a net benefit to probiotic supplementation in infants at high risk for developing allergies. Overall, the WAO is the only professional society that has issued recommendations regarding the use of pre- and probiotics for the primary prevention of allergic disease (Fiocchi et al., 2015).

## 13.5 Infant diet—Timing of complementary food introduction

*Egg and Peanut.* Beginning in approximately 2008, observational studies began to emerge suggesting that introduction of potentially allergenic foods, in particular egg and peanut, before the age of 6 months may be associated with a decreased risk of developing a food allergy. In 2008, a clinically validated questionnaire determined the prevalence of peanut allergy among Jewish schoolchildren in the United Kingdom to be approximately 10-fold higher than those in Israel (Du Toit et al., 2008). The main difference noted between these populations was that peanut was introduced earlier, eaten more frequently, and eaten in larger amounts in Israel than in the United Kingdom. In 2010, a large Australian population-based cross-sectional study (HealthNuts) reported that compared to general-population infants introduced to egg at 4–6 months of age, later introduction was associated with a higher risk of egg allergy, even among children considered at lower risk for egg allergy (Koplin et al., 2010). This study also noted that the type of egg introduced influenced the development of egg allergy—first exposure to cooked egg reduced the risk of egg allergy compared to first exposure as egg in baked goods.

While observational studies can show an association but not demonstrate causation, this trend toward early introduction for egg and peanut as a means of allergy prevention has since been supported by several key RCTs over the past few years.

The most significant 'leap' forward in the field of allergy prevention was the LEAP (Learning Early About Peanut) study, a RCT of 640 infants in the United Kingdom considered at high risk of peanut allergy due to either severe eczema and/or egg allergy (Du Toit et al., 2015). These infants were randomized to either early and ongoing peanut ingestion (starting at 4–11 months of age with ongoing peanut ingestion of at least 6 g of peanut protein per week, distributed in three or more servings, until 5 years of age) or avoidance (until 5 years of age). Results revealed an 80% reduction in peanut allergy with early peanut ingestion. The LEAP study found a preventative effect in both peanut skin-test negative and peanut skin-test positive infants, supporting early peanut introduction as a means of both primary and secondary prevention. The LEAP study also demonstrated that early peanut ingestion in high-risk infants is safe; only 2.2% of infants randomly assigned to early peanut introduction had a reaction, and none required epinephrine.

There have been five RCTs examining early egg introduction as a means of egg allergy prevention. The studies have discrepant results, perhaps because the form of egg ingested (cooked in one study; pasteurized raw egg powder in four studies) varied. The only RCT to examine early cooked egg ingestion, PETIT, found that randomization of infants with eczema to heated egg powder at 6 months of life was associated with a significantly lower rate of egg allergy than egg avoidance until 12 months of age (Natsume et al., 2017). This trial was so successful it was halted prematurely.

In contrast, four RCTs examining early pasteurized raw egg ingestion failed to show a preventative effect against egg allergy, revealed a high rate of adverse events, or both (Wei-Liang Tan et al., 2017; Palmer et al., 2013, 2017; Bellach et al., 2017). The Beating Egg Allergy (BEAT) study of 319 infants with a family history of atopy randomized to ingestion of egg starting at 4 months of age, or avoidance of egg until 8 months of age, with outcome of egg allergy at a year of age (Wei-Liang Tan et al., 2017). While this study demonstrated a significant reduction in egg sensitization with early egg ingestion, there was no effect on the proportion of infants with probable egg allergy. No serious adverse events occurred during the study, no significant difference in reaction rates between the groups, and no epinephrine was required. The Solids Timing for Allergy Research randomized infants with moderate-to-severe eczema to daily raw whole egg powder ingestion from 4 to 8 months of age, or avoidance until 8 months of age, with outcome based on development of egg allergy at a year of age (Palmer et al., 2013). There was a lower (but not significant) proportion of infants in the early egg ingestion group with egg allergy compared to the delayed egg ingestion group. However, 31% of those infants randomized to early introduction of egg had an allergic reaction and halted ongoing ingestion. The Starting Time of Egg Protein randomized 820 non-eczematous infants with a family history of atopy to early introduction of pasteurized raw egg powder at 4–6 months of age or avoidance until 10 months and found a non-significant trend toward reduced risk of egg allergy but significantly decreased egg sensitization in the early introduction group (Palmer et al., 2017). There was a higher rate of allergic reactions in the early introduction group. Data from the Hen's Egg Allergy Prevention (HEAP) study are the most potentially concerning. In this trial of 406 general population infants, early pasteurized raw egg powder introduction at 4–6 months of age vs placebo was not associated with any difference in the rate of development of egg allergy or egg sensitization at 1 year of age (Bellach et al., 2017). However, among 23 children with baseline egg sensitization who were excluded from randomization but then challenged to egg separately, 11/17 had anaphylaxis upon this initial introduction.

A 2016 meta-analysis and systematic review of timing of allergenic food introduction during the first year of life and reported allergic disease or sensitization noted moderate certainty evidence (2 trials; 1550 participants) that early peanut introduction between 4 and 11 months of age was associated with a reduced risk of peanut allergy (Ierodiakonou et al., 2016). Absolute risk reduction for a population with a 2.5% incidence of peanut allergy was 18 cases per 1000 population. There was also moderate certainty evidence from five trials (1915 participants) that early egg introduction at 4–6 months of age was associated with reduced egg allergy. Absolute risk reduction for a population with a 5.4% incidence of egg allergy was 24 cases per 1000 population.

## 13.5.1 Cow's milk

There have been three observational studies demonstrating an association between very early (within the first few months of life) cow's milk ingestion (in the form of cow's milk formula) and risk of cow's milk allergy, in predominantly general population infants. In 2010, a prospective study of the feeding history of over 13,000 Israeli infants found that regular exposure to cow's milk formula starting in the first 14 days of life was associated with an almost 20-fold lower risk of cow's milk allergy compared with later exposure (Katz et al., 2010). A case-control study of children with cow's milk allergy, compared to general population and egg-allergic controls, noted that delaying cow's milk introduction for more than a month after birth, or feeding it irregularly, was associated with a higher rate of cow's milk allergy (Onizawa et al., 2016). The HealthNuts study also found that early ingestion of cow's milk formula within the first 3 months of life reduced the risk of cow's milk allergy at a year of age (Peters et al., 2019).

Similar to egg and peanut, there is now an RCT examining the benefit of early cow's milk ingestion in the prevention of cow's milk allergy. The Strategy for Prevention of Milk Allergy by Daily Ingestion of Infant Formula in Early Infancy (SPADE) study randomized 504 general population infants to daily cow's milk formula supplementation with ongoing breastfeeding or cow's milk formula avoidance (soy supplementation if required) between 1 and 2 months of age and found a significant reduction in cow's milk allergy in the cow's milk ingestion compared to the cow's milk avoidance groups (Sakihara et al., 2021). A dose-response relationship was observed, with none of the infants who consumed at least 70 mL of cow's milk formula per week between 1 and 2 months of age developing cow's milk allergy.

Another recent RCT, the Atopy Induced by Breastfeeding or Cow's Milk Formula (ABC) study, suggests that regularity of ingestion may be as important as early exposure (Urashima et al., 2019). This study randomized 330 newborns with a family history of atopy to breastfeeding with or without amino acid-based elemental formula (BF/EF) for at least the first 3 days of life or breastfeeding supplemented with cow's milk formula (BF/CMF) from the first day of life to 5 months of age. It demonstrated a significantly reduced risk of cow's milk allergy at 2 years of age among the BF/EF group than the BF/CMF group, suggesting that infants who are fed cow's milk formula for a very brief, and not ongoing, period of time after birth may have an increased risk of cow's milk allergy compared to use of elemental formula. It is important to note that several of the observational studies supporting a role of early cow's milk ingestion in the prevention of cow's milk allergy have also included, as part of the study design, ongoing regular cow's milk ingestion, raising the possibility that it is the ongoing regular ingestion instead of early exposure that could be protective (Katz et al., 2010; Onizawa et al., 2016; Abrams and Sicherer, 2021).

## 13.5.2 Multiple allergens

There has only been one randomized study examining the early introduction of multiple allergenic foods (cow's milk first for all children, then randomly ordered introduction of egg, wheat, sesame, peanut, and finned fish) the Enquiring About Tolerance (EAT) study (Perkin et al., 2016). The EAT study randomized 1303 general-population infants to either early (3 months) ingestion of these allergens or standard (6 months) ingestion. This study showed no significant difference in the rates of allergy development between groups in the intention to treat analysis, although there were significant reductions in the rates of egg and peanut allergy in the adjusted per protocol analysis. This study had significant issues with protocol adherence, with only 42.8% of families in the early introduction group adhering to the diet. While this raises the issue of possible reverse causality, poor protocol adherence may have contributed to insufficient power to have detected what otherwise would have been a meaningful difference between groups on a population level (Iglesia and Kim, 2020).

### 13.5.3 Other allergens (wheat, tree nuts, shellfish, finned fish, seeds)

To date, there are no RCTs nor definitive observational studies demonstrating a clear benefit with early ingestion of other common allergens. However, it is thought that the mechanism of sensitization is likely similar for common allergens (Fleischer et al., 2013).

### 13.5.4 Guideline recommendations on age of introduction of allergenic foods

Following the release of the LEAP study, the National Institute of Allergy and Infectious Diseases (NIAID) released addendum guidelines for the prevention of peanut allergy in the United States recommending that infants with severe eczema, egg allergy, or both have peanut introduced into the diet at 4–6 months of age (Togias et al., 2017). For infants with mild to moderate eczema, the recommendation was at-home peanut introduction at around 6 months of age, and for infants without atopic risk factors, the recommendation was introduction in accordance with parental preference and cultural norms. More recently, a consensus approach to the primary prevention of food allergy endorsed by the American Academy of Allergy, Asthma and Immunology (AAAAI), the American College of Allergy, Asthma and Immunology (ACAAI), and the Canadian Society of Allergy and Clinical Immunology (CSACI) has been released (Fleischer et al., 2021). This consensus statement recommends peanut and egg introduction at around 6 months of life, though not before 4 months of life, in all infants irrespective of baseline risk. For other food allergens, the recommendation is not to deliberately delay their introduction once complementary feeding has commenced, as there are no data showing harm in introducing other allergens within the first year of life, but also no data suggesting a specific benefit.

## 13.6 Ongoing controversies regarding early allergen introduction

### 13.6.1 Safety of early allergen ingestion

Studies have demonstrated early peanut ingestion to be safe, with very low rates of anaphylaxis. In the LEAP study, only 2.2% of infants assigned to the early peanut ingestion group had a positive oral food challenge, and none required epinephrine (Du Toit et al.,

2015). In the HealthNuts cohort, among infants who were introduced to peanut at home within the first year of life, reactions were rare (2.4% [95% CI 1.7%, 3.4%]; irrespective of baseline risk) and only one infant (0.08%) met criteria for anaphylaxis due to wheeze although this same infant later tolerated peanut at 14 months of age (Koplin et al., 2016). A follow-up general population cross-sectional study nearly one decade later using an identical sampling frame (EarlyNuts) found a non-statistically difference in the rate of peanut reactions (4.0% [95% CI 2.7%, 5.8%]; $P = 0.054$) in a sample highly adherent to updated Australian infant feeding guidelines to introduce peanut before 12 months of age (9 in 10 infants) (Netting et al., 2017; Soriano et al., 2019). Even among cohorts of only high-risk infants, such as those with baseline high positive skin prick tests to peanut, severe reactions are rare (Abrams et al., 2020b; Volertas et al., 2020; Lin et al., 2020). While some of the egg RCTs demonstrated a high rate of reactions, this was only seen in the studies that utilized pasteurized raw egg powder as a means of egg introduction, something that would lack feasibility in the real world. Those studies that utilized cooked or baked egg have also demonstrated early egg introduction to be safe (Koplin et al., 2010). In general, infant anaphylaxis tends to be milder than in older children (Abrams et al., 2020b). In particular, respiratory symptoms are less likely in infant allergic reactions than they are in older children (Samady et al., 2018; Ko et al., 2020). Mortality on first ingestion of an allergen in infancy has never been described in the literature (Abrams et al., 2020b).

## 13.6.2 Amount and frequency of ingestion

SPADE suggests at least 10 mL of cow's milk per day is required. The LEAP and EAT studies suggested that ingestion of 2 g/week of egg and peanut protein was sufficient to prevent egg or peanut allergy. However, the absolute amount required for tolerance is unclear. The recommended frequency of allergenic solid food ingestion remains unknown, although all RCTs completed thus far required regular ingestion (typically several times a week) as a part of the protocol (Du Toit et al., 2015; Perkin et al., 2016; Katz et al., 2010; Onizawa et al., 2016). It has also been suggested in the cow's milk studies that irregularity of exposure can increase the risk of cow's milk allergy (Katz et al., 2010; Onizawa et al., 2016; Peters et al., 2019). While the exact frequency of ingestion is unclear, ongoing ingestion on a regular basis appears important.

## 13.6.3 Risk of non-IgE mediated food allergy with early ingestion

A theoretical harm related to early introduction may be an increased risk of non-IgE mediated food allergies, such as food protein-induced enterocolitis syndrome (FPIES) (Nowak-Wegrzyn et al., 2017; Leonard et al., 2018). Guidelines around the prevention of FPIES recommend that higher-risk foods for FPIES, such as grains, be introduced later (Leonard et al., 2018). Allergy prevention guidelines to date do not specifically tend to address this issue. However, as IgE-mediated food allergy is more prevalent and generally more difficult to outgrow, the potential risk of developing IgE-mediated allergy to foods such as peanut or egg is likely to be a greater concern to stakeholders than the potential theoretical benefit of delayed introduction in the prevention of FPIES.

## 13.6.4 Population- or risk-based introduction if early (and how to define risk)

There is no international consensus on the definition of an infant at high risk for food allergy development (Fleischer et al., 2021). The NIAID defines an infant at high risk of peanut allergy as having severe eczema and/or egg allergy, largely in keeping with the LEAP study inclusion criteria (Togias et al., 2017). The North American consensus guidance has a stratified approach to risk, categorizing infants at highest risk of food allergy development as those with severe eczema, and infants at some increased risk as those with a history of mild to moderate eczema, a family history of atopy in one or both parents, or a known food allergy (Fleischer et al., 2021).

It is important to recognize that food allergy can develop in infants who have no risk factors (Fleischer et al., 2021). There is a consistent association between the presence of eczema in infancy and the development of food allergy ((Tsakok et al., 2016; Du Toit et al., 2016; Abrams, 2021), although this risk factor is neither necessary nor sufficient for food allergy development (Abrams, 2021). Other risk factors, such as a family history of atopy, are less consistently associated with the development of food allergy (Fleischer et al., 2021; Abrams, 2021). For example, a particular interest has been whether a sibling of a peanut-allergic child is at increased risk of peanut allergy. While observational studies have demonstrated a higher rate, more recent literature has not supported an increased risk and has suggested that previously noted higher rates of peanut allergy in siblings are not due to inherent genetic susceptibility but to delayed peanut ingestion in infancy (Hourihane et al., 1996; Liem et al., 2008; Gupta et al., 2016; Shaker et al., 2019; Abrams et al., 2018; Keet et al., 2021a). The intervention of early ingestion of allergens has been shown to be effective in the general population of infants, and no study to date has ever demonstrated early allergen ingestion to be detrimental in infants, irrespective of whether or not they are higher risk (Du Toit et al., 2015; Perkin et al., 2016; Katz et al., 2010; Abrams et al., 2020b).

## 13.6.5 Pre-emptive screening

The NIAID guideline recommends that infants at high risk for peanut allergy (due to egg allergy and/or severe eczema) be strongly considered for pre-emptive testing prior to peanut introduction (Togias et al., 2017). This is in contrast to multiple other international guidelines, including the North American consensus statement, which discourage pre-emptive testing in any infant, irrespective of risk (Abrams et al., 2019a; Immunology, 2018; Netting et al., 2017; Nutrition, 2018; Fleischer et al., 2021). Arguments in favor of a pre-emptive screening approach include that peanut screening tests are sensitive, that a subset of infants can be identified as higher risk, and that there is often parental hesitancy to introduce peanut without screening (Abrams et al., 2020a; Greenhawt et al., 2020; Keet et al., 2021a,b). However, while screening tests are sensitive, they lack specificity, and many infants with positive allergy testing are, in fact, clinically tolerant to the food being screened (Fleischer et al., 2011; Abrams et al., 2020a; Greenhawt et al., 2020). Pre-emptive screening may also lack feasibility at a populational level due to the high prevalence of egg allergy and eczema within the population (Silverberg et al., 2021; Abrams et al., 2020a; Greenhawt and Shaker, 2019; Shaker et al., 2018; Koplin et al., 2016). The HealthNuts study demonstrated that screening all infants with early-onset eczema and/or egg allergy would require screening 16% of the population, of whom 29% would require follow up because of positive testing, and still miss 23.4% of all peanut allergy cases (Koplin et al., 2016). Pre-emptive screening prior to peanut introduction has been demonstrated to be poorly cost-effective (Greenhawt and Shaker, 2019; Shaker et al., 2018). In addition, there is a risk of a 'screening creep' in which infants at lower risk are screened (Turner and Campbell, 2017), as well as a risk that the resource limitations associated with a screening approach could inadvertently increase the risk of peanut allergy by delaying peanut introduction (Abrams et al., 2019b).

## 13.7 Infant diet diversity

In addition to the emergence of an evidence base for infant allergenic food introduction as a protective factor against food allergy, the role of infant diet diversity (the number of food groups an infant ingests) is also being explored as a potentially modifiable risk factor in influencing atopic development (D'auria et al., 2020; Fleischer et al., 2021). A 2020 systematic review conducted by a European Academy of Allergy and Clinical Immunology Taskforce on Diet and Immunomodulation investigated the association between diet diversity and allergy outcomes (Venter et al., 2020b). Regarding allergic sensitization to foods and environmental aeroallergens, one multi-country study in Europe (Prospective Birth Cohort Study Against Allergy Study in Rural Environments [PASTURE]) found that low diet diversity in the infant period (first 6–12 months of life) was associated with increased risk of sensitization to food allergens at ages 4.5 and 6 years, but not to environmental aeroallergens, though this association was attenuated when accounting for reverse causality (Roduit et al., 2014). One German study found that high diet diversity was associated with lower odds of aeroallergen sensitization only (Markevych et al., 2017), while the Finnish Type I Diabetes Prediction and Prevention Prospective Cohort Study found that low diet diversity was associated with increased risk of both food and aeroallergen sensitization at age 5 years (Nwaru et al., 2013). Regarding the association of infant diet diversity and food allergy, the PASTURE study was the only study included in the systematic review and found that increased diet diversity in the first year of life was associated with reduced risk of a clinician-diagnosis of food allergy up to 6 years (Roduit et al., 2014). Recently, an additional birth cohort study reported an association between increased diet diversity in the first year of life (as measured by four different measures) and reduced odds of developing food allergy up to 10 years of age (OR 0.69, [95% CI 0.5, 0.9]) (Venter et al., 2020c). The effect of increased infant diet diversity on atopic dermatitis is unclear, with some studies showing protective benefit,[refs], some studies showing no association, and some studies showing increased risk (Venter et al., 2019). The 2020 systematic review included both the PASTURE and Finnish cohort studies in examining asthma and allergic rhinitis outcomes. In both studies, there was an association between increased diet diversity in the first year of life and reduction of asthma cases up to 5–6 years of life. Lower diet diversity at 6–12 months was associated with the development of allergic rhinitis in the PASTURE study, while there was no effect in the Finnish cohort (Markevych et al., 2017; Nwaru et al., 2013).

Overall, while no RCT has assessed the efficacy of a diet diversity strategy to prevent food allergy or other allergic outcomes, the North American consensus emphasizes the balance of observational evidence suggesting a food allergy prevention benefit with the absence of known harm (Fleischer et al., 2021). A diverse infant diet has practical concordance with intentional incorporation of allergenic foods to support food allergy prevention (D'auria et al., 2020). Furthermore, a diverse infant diet may support other nutritional outcomes and may conform with normative infant feeding practices, depending on cultural and familial preferences.

## 13.8 Conclusion

While there is much interest in modification of pre-natal exposures, and a solid basis for the pathophysiologic influence of intrauterine nutrition on the development of chronic disease, to date, there is no consistent evidence for any specific modification of maternal diet during pregnancy or lactation and the prevention of allergic disease. Specifically, it remains unclear whether vitamin D supplementation, polyunsaturated fatty acid ingestion, pre- and probiotic supplementation, nor diversity of maternal diet influences childhood allergy development.

While breastfeeding is uniformly recommended for multiple benefits to both mother and child, the data regarding its influence on the development of allergic disease, with the exception of early childhood wheeze, is mixed. Hydrolyzed formulas in general are not recommended as a means of allergy prevention in mothers who cannot or choose not to breastfeed. The role of infant vitamin D supplementation, polyunsaturated fatty acid ingestion, and pre- and probiotic supplementation remains unclear.

There is level one evidence that ingestion of egg and peanut shortly after complementary feeding begins (e.g., around 6 months of age), in particular for infants at high risk, has a role in prevention of egg and peanut allergy, respectively. However, there remain controversies regarding frequency, duration, and amount of ingestion. Pre-emptive screening prior to introduction of allergens in an infant's diet, in general, is not recommended. While there have been no level one studies on dietary diversity, observational data does support a benefit to infant dietary diversity in allergic disease prevention, in particular for food allergy, and no harm to this approach has been seen.

## 13.9 Future trends and research

Further research into the roles of some specific interventions in food allergy prevention—such as vitamin supplementation, polyunsaturated fatty acid ingestion, pre- and probiotic supplementation—is required. In addition, studies examining the role of maternal dietary interventions are required before any firm conclusions can be drawn. The data on breastfeeding as a means of allergy prevention remain mixed, although this intervention is difficult to capture, and randomization is unethical. With respect to early food introduction, several areas of uncertainty remain. The optimal amount of allergenic solid required to promote tolerance is unclear, as is the duration of ingestion required to maintain tolerance. There is lack of evidence concerning early introduction of some specific allergenic foods (such as shellfish, sesame, finned fish, and grains) although some could argue that at this stage randomized trials with other allergens could be considered unethical as the evidence of benefit has been so firmly established for some allergens.

## Sources of additional information

Greer, F. R., Sicherer, S. H., Burks, A. W., American Academy Of Pediatrics Committee On, N., American Academy Of Pediatrics Section On, A. & Immunology 2008. Effects of early nutritional interventions on the development of atopic disease in infants and children: the role of maternal dietary restriction, breastfeeding, timing of introduction of complementary foods, and hydrolyzed formulas. *Pediatrics,* 121**,** 183–91.

Fleischer, D. M., Chan, E. S., Venter, C., Spergel, J. M., Abrams, E. M., Stukus, D., Groetch, M., Shaker, M. & Greenhawt, M. 2021. A Consensus Approach to the Primary Prevention of Food Allergy Through Nutrition: Guidance from the American Academy of Allergy, Asthma, and Immunology; American College of Allergy, Asthma, and Immunology; and the Canadian Society for Allergy and Clinical Immunology. *J Allergy Clin Immunol Pract,* 9**,** 22–43 e4.

U.S. Department of Agriculture and U.S. Department of Health and Human Services. Dietary Guidelines for Americans, 2020-2025. 9th Edition. December 2020. Available at DietaryGuidelines.gov.

Gungor, D., Nadaud, P., Lapergola, C. C., Dreibelbis, C., Wong, Y. P., Terry, N., Abrams, S. A., Beker, L., Jacobovits, T., Jarvinen, K. M., Nommsen-Rivers, L. A., O'brien, K. O., Oken, E., Perez-Escamilla, R., Ziegler, E. E. & Spahn, J. M. 2019. Infant milk-feeding practices and food allergies, allergic rhinitis, atopic dermatitis, and asthma throughout the life span: a systematic review. *Am J Clin Nutr,* 109**,** 772S–799S.

Halken, S., Muraro, A., De Silva, D., Khaleva, E., Angier, E., Arasi, S., Arshad, H., Bahnson, H. T., Beyer, K., Boyle, R., Du Toit, G., Ebisawa, M., Eigenmann, P., Grimshaw, K., Hoest, A., Jones, C., Lack, G., Nadeau, K., O'mahony, L., Szajewska, H., Venter, C., Verhasselt, V., Wong, G. W. K., Roberts, G., European Academy Of, A., Clinical Immunology Food, A. & Anaphylaxis Guidelines, G. 2021. EAACI guideline: Preventing the development of food allergy in infants and young children (2020 update). *Pediatr Allergy Immunol.*

Togias, A., Cooper, S. F., Acebal, M. L., Assa'ad, A., Baker, J. R., Jr., Beck, L. A., Block, J., Byrd-Bredbenner, C., Chan, E. S., Eichenfield, L. F., Fleischer, D. M., Fuchs, G. J., 3rd, Furuta, G. T., Greenhawt, M. J., Gupta, R. S., Habich, M., Jones, S. M., Keaton, K., Muraro, A., Plaut, M., Rosenwasser, L. J., Rotrosen, D., Sampson, H. A., Schneider, L. C., Sicherer, S. H., Sidbury, R., Spergel, J., Stukus, D. R., Venter, C. & Boyce, J. A. 2017. Addendum guidelines for the prevention of peanut allergy in the United States: Report of the National Institute of Allergy and Infectious Diseases-sponsored expert panel. *J Allergy Clin Immunol,* 139**,** 29–44.

Venter, C., Greenhawt, M., Meyer, R. W., Agostoni, C., Reese, I., Du Toit, G., Feeney, M., Maslin, K., Nwaru, B. I., Roduit, C., Untersmayr, E., Vlieg-Boerstra, B., Pali-Scholl, I., Roberts, G. C., Smith, P., Akdis, C. A., Agache, I., Ben-Adallah, M., Bischoff, S., Frei, R., Garn, H., Grimshaw, K., Hoffmann-Sommergruber, K., Lunjani, N., Muraro, A., Poulsen, L. K., Renz, H., Sokolowska, M., Stanton, C. & O'mahony, L. 2020b. EAACI position paper on diet diversity in pregnancy, infancy and childhood: Novel concepts and implications for studies in allergy and asthma. *Allergy,* 75**,** 497–523.

Venter, C., Meyer, R. W., Nwaru, B. I., Roduit, C., Untersmayr, E., Adel-Patient, K., Agache, I., Agostoni, C., Akdis, C. A., Bischoff, S. C., Du Toit, G., Feeney, M., Frei, R.,

Garn, H., Greenhawt, M., Hoffmann-Sommergruber, K., Lunjani, N., Maslin, K., Mills, C., Muraro, A., Pali-Scholl, I., Poulson, L. K., Reese, I., Renz, H., Roberts, G. C., Smith, P., Smolinska, S., Sokolowska, M., Stanton, C., Vlieg-Boerstra, B. & O'mahony, L. 2019. EAACI position paper: Influence of dietary fatty acids on asthma, food allergy, and atopic dermatitis. *Allergy*, 74, 1429–1444.

Yepes-Nunez, J. J., Fiocchi, A., Pawankar, R., Cuello-Garcia, C. A., Zhang, Y., Morgano, G. P., Ahn, K., Al-Hammadi, S., Agarwal, A., Gandhi, S., Beyer, K., Burks, W., Canonica, G. W., Ebisawa, M., Kamenwa, R., Lee, B. W., Li, H., Prescott, S., Riva, J. J., Rosenwasser, L., Sampson, H., Spigler, M., Terracciano, L., Vereda, A., Waserman, S., Schunemann, H. J. & Brozek, J. L. 2016. World Allergy Organization-McMaster University Guidelines for Allergic Disease Prevention (GLAD-P): Vitamin D. *World Allergy Organ J*, 9, 17.

Cuello-Garcia, C. A., Fiocchi, A., Pawankar, R., Yepes-Nunez, J. J., Morgano, G. P., Zhang, Y., Ahn, K., Al-Hammadi, S., Agarwal, A., Gandhi, S., Beyer, K., Burks, W., Canonica, G. W., Ebisawa, M., Kamenwa, R., Lee, B. W., Li, H., Prescott, S., Riva, J. J., Rosenwasser, L., Sampson, H., Spigler, M., Terracciano, L., Vereda, A., Waserman, S., Schunemann, H. J. & Brozek, J. L. 2016. World Allergy Organization-McMaster University Guidelines for Allergic Disease Prevention (GLAD-P): Prebiotics. *World Allergy Organ J*, 9, 10.

Fiocchi, A., Pawankar, R., Cuello-Garcia, C., Ahn, K., Al-Hammadi, S., Agarwal, A., Beyer, K., Burks, W., Canonica, G. W., Ebisawa, M., Gandhi, S., Kamenwa, R., Lee, B. W., Li, H., Prescott, S., Riva, J. J., Rosenwasser, L., Sampson, H., Spigler, M., Terracciano, L., Vereda-Ortiz, A., Waserman, S., Yepes-Nunez, J. J., Brozek, J. L. & Schunemann, H. J. 2015. World Allergy Organization-McMaster University Guidelines for Allergic Disease Prevention (GLAD-P): Probiotics. *World Allergy Organ J*, 8, 4.

# References

Abrams, E.M., 2021. Removing risk stratification in food allergy prevention guidelines. Can. J. Public Health 112, 289–291.

Abrams, E.M., Sicherer, S.H., 2021. Cow's milk allergy prevention. Ann. Allergy Asthma Immunol. 127, 36–41.

Abrams, E.M., Chan, E.S., Sicherer, S.H., 2018. Should younger siblings of peanut allergic children be screened for peanut allergy? J Allergy Clin Immunol Pract 6, 414–418.

Abrams, E.M., Hildebrand, K., Blair, B., Chan, E.S., 2019a. Timing of introduction of allergenic solids for infants at high risk. Paediatr. Child Health 24, 56–57.

Abrams, E.M., Singer, A.G., Chan, E.S., 2019b. Pre-emptive screening for peanut allergy before peanut ingestion in infants is not standard of care. CMAJ 191, E1169–E1170.

Abrams, E.M., Brough, H.A., Keet, C., Shaker, M.S., Venter, C., Greenhawt, M., 2020a. Pros and cons of pre-emptive screening programmes before peanut introduction in infancy. Lancet Child Adolesc. Health 4, 526–535.

Abrams, E.M., Primeau, M.N., Kim, H., Gerdts, J., Chan, E.S., 2020b. Increasing awareness of the low risk of severe reaction at infant peanut introduction: implications during COVID-19 and beyond. J. Allergy Clin. Immunol. Pract. 8, 3259–3260.

American College Of, O., Gynecologists' Committee On Obstetric, P, Breastfeeding Expert Work, G, 2016. Committee opinion no. 658: optimizing support for breastfeeding as part of obstetric practice. Obstet. Gynecol. 127, e86–e92.

Anderson, L.N., Chen, Y., Omand, J.A., Birken, C.S., Parkin, P.C., To, T., Maguire, J.L., Collaboration, T.A.K., 2015. Vitamin D exposure during pregnancy, but not early childhood, is associated with risk of childhood wheezing. J. Dev. Orig. Health Dis. 6, 308–316.

Andreas, N.J., Kampmann, B., Mehring Le-Doare, K., 2015. Human breast milk: a review on its composition and bioactivity. Early Hum. Dev. 91, 629–635.

Aranow, C., 2011. Vitamin D and the immune system. J. Investig. Med. 59, 881–886.

Azad, M.B., Vehling, L., Lu, Z., Dai, D., Subbarao, P., Becker, A.B., Mandhane, P.J., Turvey, S.E., Lefebvre, D.L., Sears, M.R., Investigators, C.S., 2017. Breastfeeding, maternal asthma and wheezing in the first year of life: a longitudinal birth cohort study. Eur. Respir. J. 49.

Ballard, O., Morrow, A.L., 2013. Human milk composition: nutrients and bioactive factors. Pediatr. Clin. N. Am. 60, 49–74.

Barker, D.J., Martyn, C.N., 1992. The maternal and fetal origins of cardiovascular disease. J. Epidemiol. Community Health 46, 8–11.

Bellach, J., Schwarz, V., Ahrens, B., Trendelenburg, V., Aksunger, O., Kalb, B., Niggemann, B., Keil, T., Beyer, K., 2017. Randomized placebo-controlled trial of hen's egg consumption for primary prevention in infants. J. Allergy Clin. Immunol. 139, 1591–1599.e2.

Bener, A., Ehlayel, M.S., Tulic, M.K., Hamid, Q., 2012. Vitamin D deficiency as a strong predictor of asthma in children. Int. Arch. Allergy Immunol. 157, 168–175.

Bergmann, R.L., Edenharter, G., Bergmann, K.E., Lau, S., Wahn, U., 2000. Socioeconomic status is a risk factor for allergy in parents but not in their children. Clin. Exp. Allergy 30, 1740–1745.

Best, K.P., Gold, M., Kennedy, D., Martin, J., Makrides, M., 2016. Omega-3 long-chain PUFA intake during pregnancy and allergic disease outcomes in the offspring: a systematic review and meta-analysis of observational studies and randomized controlled trials. Am. J. Clin. Nutr. 103, 128–143.

Bigman, G., 2020. The relationship of breastfeeding and infant eczema: the role of reverse causation. Breastfeed. Med. 15, 114–116.

Blyuss, O., Cheung, K.Y., Chen, J., Parr, C., Petrou, L., Komarova, A., Kokina, M., Luzan, P., Pasko, E., Eremeeva, A., Peshko, D., Eliseev, V.I., Pedersen, S.A., Azad, M.B., Jarvinen, K.M., Peroni, D.G., Verhasselt, V., Boyle, R.J., Warner, J.O., Simpson, M.R., Munblit, D., 2019. Statistical approaches in the studies assessing associations between human milk immune composition and allergic diseases: a scoping review. Nutrients 11.

Boyce, J.A., Assa'A, A., Burks, A.W., Jones, S.M., Sampson, H.A., Wood, R.A., Plaut, M., Cooper, S.F., Fenton, M.J., Arshad, S.H., Bahna, S.L., Beck, L.A., Byrd-Bredbenner, C., Camargo Jr., C.A., Eichenfield, L., Furuta, G.T., Hanifin, J.M., Jones, C., Kraft, M., Levy, B.D., Lieberman, P., Luccioli, S., McCall, K.M., Schneider, L.C., Simon, R.A., Simons, F.E., Teach, S.J., Yawn, B.P., Schwaninger, J.M., Panel, N. I.-S. E, 2011. Guidelines for the diagnosis and management of food allergy in the United States: summary of the NIAID-sponsored expert panel report. Nutrition 27, 253–267.

Boyle, R.J., Ierodiakonou, D., Khan, T., Chivinge, J., Robinson, Z., Geohegan, N., Jarrold, K., Afxentiou, T., Reeves, T., Cunha, S., Trivella, M., Garcia-Larsen, V., Leonardi-Bee, J., 2016. Hydrolysed formula and risk of allergic or autoimmune disease: systematic review and meta-analysis. BMJ 352, i974.

Cabana, M.D., 2017. The role of hydrolyzed formula in allergy prevention. Ann. Nutr. Metab. 70 (Suppl. 2), 38–45.

Calder, P.C., Kremmyda, L.S., Vlachava, M., Noakes, P.S., Miles, E.A., 2010. Is there a role for fatty acids in early life programming of the immune system? Proc. Nutr. Soc. 69, 373–380.

Castro-Rodriguez, J.A., Ramirez-Hernandez, M., Padilla, O., Pacheco-Gonzalez, R.M., Perez-Fernandez, V., Garcia-Marcos, L., 2016. Effect of foods and Mediterranean diet during pregnancy and first years of life on wheezing, rhinitis and dermatitis in preschoolers. Allergol Immunopathol (Madr) 44, 400–409.

Chatzi, L., Torrent, M., Romieu, I., Garcia-Esteban, R., Ferrer, C., Vioque, J., Kogevinas, M., Sunyer, J., 2008. Mediterranean diet in pregnancy is protective for wheeze and atopy in childhood. Thorax 63, 507–513.

Chatzi, L., Garcia, R., Roumeliotaki, T., Basterrechea, M., Begiristain, H., Iniguez, C., Vioque, J., Kogevinas, M., Sunyer, J., Group, I. S, Group, R. S, 2013. Mediterranean diet adherence during pregnancy and risk of wheeze and eczema in the first year of life: INMA (Spain) and RHEA (Greece) mother-child cohort studies. Br. J. Nutr. 110, 2058–2068.

Chawes, B.L., Bonnelykke, K., Stokholm, J., Vissing, N.H., Bjarnadottir, E., Schoos, A.M., Wolsk, H.M., Pedersen, T.M., Vinding, R.K., Thorsteinsdottir, S., Arianto, L., Hallas, H.W., Heickendorff, L., Brix, S., Rasmussen, M.A., Bisgaard, H., 2016. Effect of vitamin D3 supplementation during pregnancy on risk of persistent wheeze in the offspring: a randomized clinical trial. JAMA 315, 353–361.

Chen, L.W., Lyons, B., Navarro, P., Shivappa, N., Mehegan, J., Murrin, C.M., Hebert, J.R., Kelleher, C.C., Phillips, C.M., 2020. Maternal dietary inflammatory potential and quality are associated with offspring asthma risk over 10-year follow-up: the lifeways cross-generation cohort study. Am. J. Clin. Nutr. 111, 440–447.

Chistiakov, D.A., Bobryshev, Y.V., Kozarov, E., Sobenin, I.A., Orekhov, A.N., 2014. Intestinal mucosal tolerance and impact of gut microbiota to mucosal tolerance. Front. Microbiol. 5, 781.

Clarke, A.E., Elliott, S.J., St Pierre, Y., Soller, L., La Vieille, S., Ben-Shoshan, M., 2020. Temporal trends in prevalence of food allergy in Canada. J Allergy Clin Immunol Pract 8, 1428–1430.e5.

II. Early nutrition and development of non-communicable diseases

Codispoti, C.D., Levin, L., Lemasters, G.K., Ryan, P., Reponen, T., Villareal, M., Burkle, J., Stanforth, S., Lockey, J.E., Khurana Hershey, G.K., Bernstein, D.I., 2010. Breast-feeding, aeroallergen sensitization, and environmental exposures during infancy are determinants of childhood allergic rhinitis. J. Allergy Clin. Immunol. 125, 1054–1060.e1.

Couratier, P., Montagne, R., Acaster, S., Gallop, K., Patel, R., Vereda, A., Pouessel, G., 2020. Allergy to peanuts imPacting emotions and life (APPEAL): the impact of peanut allergy on children, adolescents, adults and caregivers in France. Allergy Asthma Clin. Immunol. 16, 86.

Cuello-Garcia, C.A., Brozek, J.L., Fiocchi, A., Pawankar, R., Yepes-Nunez, J.J., Terracciano, L., Gandhi, S., Agarwal, A., Zhang, Y., Schunemann, H.J., 2015. Probiotics for the prevention of allergy: a systematic review and meta-analysis of randomized controlled trials. J. Allergy Clin. Immunol. 136, 952–961.

Cuello-Garcia, C.A., Fiocchi, A., Pawankar, R., Yepes-Nunez, J.J., Morgano, G.P., Zhang, Y., Ahn, K., Al-Hammadi, S., Agarwal, A., Gandhi, S., Beyer, K., Burks, W., Canonica, G.W., Ebisawa, M., Kamenwa, R., Lee, B.W., Li, H., Prescott, S., Riva, J.J., Rosenwasser, L., Sampson, H., Spigler, M., Terracciano, L., Vereda, A., Waserman, S., Schunemann, H.J., Brozek, J.L., 2016. World Allergy Organization-McMaster University Guidelines for allergic disease prevention (GLAD-P): prebiotics. World Allergy Organ. J. 9, 10.

Cuello-Garcia, C., Fiocchi, A., Pawankar, R., Yepes-Nunez, J.J., Morgano, G.P., Zhang, Y., Agarwal, A., Gandhi, S., Terracciano, L., Schunemann, H.J., Brozek, J.L., 2017. Prebiotics for the prevention of allergies: a systematic review and meta-analysis of randomized controlled trials. Clin. Exp. Allergy 47, 1468–1477.

Das, U.N., 2006. Essential fatty acids: biochemistry, physiology and pathology. Biotechnol. J. 1, 420–439.

D'auria, E., Peroni, D.G., Sartorio, M.U.A., Verduci, E., Zuccotti, G.V., Venter, C., 2020. The role of diet diversity and diet indices on allergy outcomes. Front. Pediatr. 8, 545.

Davisse-Paturet, C., Raherison, C., Adel-Patient, K., Divaret-Chauveau, A., Bois, C., Dufourg, M.N., Lioret, S., Charles, M.A., De Lauzon-Guillain, B., 2019. Use of partially hydrolysed formula in infancy and incidence of eczema, respiratory symptoms or food allergies in toddlers from the ELFE cohort. Pediatr. Allergy Immunol. 30, 614–623.

De Silva, D., Geromi, M., Halken, S., Host, A., Panesar, S.S., Muraro, A., Werfel, T., Hoffmann-Sommergruber, K., Roberts, G., Cardona, V., Dubois, A.E., Poulsen, L.K., Van Ree, R., Vlieg-Boerstra, B., Agache, I., Grimshaw, K., O'mahony, L., Venter, C., Arshad, S.H., Sheikh, A., Allergy, E.F., Anaphylaxis Guidelines, G., 2014. Primary prevention of food allergy in children and adults: systematic review. Allergy 69, 581–589.

Dogaru, C.M., Nyffenegger, D., Pescatore, A.M., Spycher, B.D., Kuehni, C.E., 2014. Breastfeeding and childhood asthma: systematic review and meta-analysis. Am. J. Epidemiol. 179, 1153–1167.

Du Toit, G., Katz, Y., Sasieni, P., Mesher, D., Maleki, S.J., Fisher, H.R., Fox, A.T., Turcanu, V., Amir, T., Zadik-Mnuhin, G., Cohen, A., Livne, I., Lack, G., 2008. Early consumption of peanuts in infancy is associated with a low prevalence of peanut allergy. J. Allergy Clin. Immunol. 122, 984–991.

Du Toit, G., Roberts, G., Sayre, P.H., Bahnson, H.T., Radulovic, S., Santos, A.F., Brough, H.A., Phippard, D., Basting, M., Feeney, M., Turcanu, V., Sever, M.L., Gomez Lorenzo, M., Plaut, M., Lack, G., Team, L. S, 2015. Randomized trial of peanut consumption in infants at risk for peanut allergy. N. Engl. J. Med. 372, 803–813.

Du Toit, G., Tsakok, T., Lack, S., Lack, G., 2016. Prevention of food allergy. J. Allergy Clin. Immunol. 137, 998–1010.

Dunngalvin, A., Gallop, K., Acaster, S., Timmermans, F., Regent, L., Schnadt, S., Podesta, M., Sanchez, A., Ryan, R., Couratier, P., Feeney, M., Hjorth, B., Fisher, H.R., Blumchen, K., Vereda, A., Fernandez-Rivas, M., 2020. APPEAL-2: a pan-European qualitative study to explore the burden of peanut-allergic children, teenagers and their caregivers. Clin. Exp. Allergy 50, 1238–1248.

Fiocchi, A., Pawankar, R., Cuello-Garcia, C., Ahn, K., Al-Hammadi, S., Agarwal, A., Beyer, K., Burks, W., Canonica, G.W., Ebisawa, M., Gandhi, S., Kamenwa, R., Lee, B.W., Li, H., Prescott, S., Riva, J.J., Rosenwasser, L., Sampson, H., Spigler, M., Terracciano, L., Vereda-Ortiz, A., Waserman, S., Yepes-Nunez, J.J., Brozek, J.L., Schunemann, H.J., 2015. World Allergy Organization-McMaster University guidelines for allergic disease prevention (GLAD-P): probiotics. World Allergy Organ. J. 8, 4.

Fleischer, D.M., 2007. The natural history of peanut and tree nut allergy. Curr. Allergy Asthma Rep. 7, 175–181.

Fleischer, D.M., Bock, S.A., Spears, G.C., Wilson, C.G., Miyazawa, N.K., Gleason, M.C., Gyorkos, E.A., Murphy, J.R., Atkins, D., Leung, D.Y., 2011. Oral food challenges in children with a diagnosis of food allergy. J. Pediatr. 158, 578–583.e1.

Fleischer, D.M., Spergel, J.M., Assa'ad, A.H., Pongracic, J.A., 2013. Primary prevention of allergic disease through nutritional interventions. J. Allergy Clin. Immunol. Pract. 1, 29–36.

Fleischer, D.M., Chan, E.S., Venter, C., Spergel, J.M., Abrams, E.M., Stukus, D., Groetch, M., Shaker, M., Greenhawt, M., 2021. A consensus approach to the primary prevention of food allergy through nutrition: guidance from the American academy of allergy, asthma, and immunology; American college of allergy, asthma, and immunology; and the Canadian society for allergy and clinical immunology. J. Allergy Clin. Immunol. Pract. 9, 22–43.e4.

Gappa, M., Filipiak-Pittroff, B., Libuda, L., Von Berg, A., Koletzko, S., Bauer, C.P., Heinrich, J., Schikowski, T., Berdel, D., Standl, M., 2020. Long-term effects of hydrolyzed formulae on atopic diseases in the GINI study. Allergy 76, 1903–1907.

Garcia-Larsen, V., Ierodiakonou, D., Jarrold, K., Cunha, S., Chivinge, J., Robinson, Z., Geoghegan, N., Ruparelia, A., Devani, P., Trivella, M., Leonardi-Bee, J., Boyle, R.J., 2018. Diet during pregnancy and infancy and risk of allergic or autoimmune disease: a systematic review and meta-analysis. PLoS Med. 15, e1002507.

Gdalevich, M., Mimouni, D., David, M., Mimouni, M., 2001. Breast-feeding and the onset of atopic dermatitis in childhood: a systematic review and meta-analysis of prospective studies. J. Am. Acad. Dermatol. 45, 520–527.

Gerrard, J.W., Geddes, C.A., Reggin, P.L., Gerrard, C.D., Horne, S., 1976. Serum IgE levels in white and metis communities in Saskatchewan. Ann. Allergy 37, 91–100.

Giwercman, C., Halkjaer, L.B., Jensen, S.M., Bonnelykke, K., Lauritzen, L., Bisgaard, H., 2010. Increased risk of eczema but reduced risk of early wheezy disorder from exclusive breast-feeding in high-risk infants. J. Allergy Clin. Immunol. 125, 866–871.

Greenhawt, M., Shaker, M., 2019. Determining levers of cost-effectiveness for screening infants at high risk for peanut sensitization before early peanut introduction. JAMA Netw. Open 2, e1918041.

Greenhawt, M., Shaker, M., Wang, J., Oppenheimer, J.J., Sicherer, S., Keet, C., Swaggart, K., Rank, M., Portnoy, J.M., Bernstein, J., Chu, D.K., Dinakar, C., Golden, D., Horner, C., Lang, D.M., Lang, E.S., Khan, D.A., Lieberman, J., Stukus, D., Wallace, D., 2020. Peanut allergy diagnosis: a 2020 practice parameter update, systematic review, and GRADE analysis. J. Allergy Clin. Immunol. 146, 1302–1334.

Greer, F.R., Sicherer, S.H., Burks, A.W., American Academy of Pediatrics Committee on, N., American Academy of Pediatrics Section on, A. & Immunology, 2008. Effects of early nutritional interventions on the development of atopic disease in infants and children: the role of maternal dietary restriction, breastfeeding, timing of introduction of complementary foods, and hydrolyzed formulas. Pediatrics 121, 183–191.

Greer, F.R., Sicherer, S.H., Burks, A.W., Committee On, N., Section On, A. & Immunology, 2019. The effects of early nutritional interventions on the development of atopic disease in infants and children: the role of maternal dietary restriction, breastfeeding, hydrolyzed formulas, and timing of introduction of allergenic complementary foods. Pediatrics 143.

Grulee, C.G., Sanford, H.N., 1936. The influence of breast and artificial feeding on infantile eczema. J. Pediatr. 9, 223–225.

Gunaratne, A.W., Makrides, M., Collins, C.T., 2015. Maternal prenatal and/or postnatal n-3 long chain polyunsaturated fatty acids (LCPUFA) supplementation for preventing allergies in early childhood. Cochrane Database Syst. Rev., CD010085.

Gungor, D., Nadaud, P., Lapergola, C.C., Dreibelbis, C., Wong, Y.P., Terry, N., Abrams, S.A., Beker, L., Jacobovits, T., Jarvinen, K.M., Nommsen-Rivers, L.A., O'brien, K.O., Oken, E., Perez-Escamilla, R., Ziegler, E.E., Spahn, J.M., 2019. Infant milk-feeding practices and food allergies, allergic rhinitis, atopic dermatitis, and asthma throughout the life span: a systematic review. Am. J. Clin. Nutr. 109, 772S–799S.

Gupta, R., Holdford, D., Bilaver, L., Dyer, A., Holl, J.L., Meltzer, D., 2013. The economic impact of childhood food allergy in the United States. JAMA Pediatr. 167, 1026–1031.

Gupta, R.S., Walkner, M.M., Greenhawt, M., Lau, C.H., Caruso, D., Wang, X., Pongracic, J.A., Smith, B., 2016. Food Allergy sensitization and presentation in siblings of food allergic children. Cochrane Database Syst. Rev. 4, 956–962.

Gupta, R.S., Warren, C.M., Smith, B.M., Blumenstock, J.A., Jiang, J., Davis, M.M., Nadeau, K.C., 2018. The public health impact of parent-reported childhood food allergies in the United States. Pediatrics 142.

Halken, S., Muraro, A., De Silva, D., Khaleva, E., Angier, E., Arasi, S., Arshad, H., Bahnson, H.T., Beyer, K., Boyle, R., Du Toit, G., Ebisawa, M., Eigenmann, P., Grimshaw, K., Hoest, A., Jones, C., Lack, G., Nadeau, K., O'mahony, L., Szajewska, H., Venter, C., Verhasselt, V., Wong, G.W.K., Roberts, G., European Academy Of, A., Clinical Immunology Food, A. & Anaphylaxis Guidelines, G, 2021. EAACI guideline: preventing the development of food allergy in infants and young children (2020 update). Pediatr. Allergy Immunol. 32, 843–858.

Hanson, C., Rifas-Shiman, S.L., Shivappa, N., Wirth, M.D., Hebert, J.R., Gold, D., Camargo Jr., C.A., Sen, S., Sordillo, J.E., Oken, E., Litonjua, A.A., 2020. Associations of prenatal dietary inflammatory potential with childhood respiratory outcomes in project viva. J Allergy Clin Immunol Pract 8, 945–952.e4.

Hourihane, J.O., Dean, T.P., Warner, J.O., 1996. Peanut allergy in relation to heredity, maternal diet, and other atopic diseases: results of a questionnaire survey, skin prick testing, and food challenges. BMJ 313, 518–521.

Hypponen, E., Sovio, U., Wjst, M., Patel, S., Pekkanen, J., Hartikainen, A.L., Jarvelinb, M.R., 2004. Infant vitamin d supplementation and allergic conditions in adulthood: Northern Finland birth cohort 1966. Ann. N. Y. Acad. Sci. 1037, 84–95.

II.  Early nutrition and development of non-communicable diseases

Ierodiakonou, D., Garcia-Larsen, V., Logan, A., Groome, A., Cunha, S., Chivinge, J., Robinson, Z., Geoghegan, N., Jarrold, K., Reeves, T., Tagiyeva-Milne, N., Nurmatov, U., Trivella, M., Leonardi-Bee, J., Boyle, R.J., 2016. Timing of allergenic food introduction to the infant diet and risk of allergic or autoimmune disease: a systematic review and meta-analysis. JAMA 316, 1181–1192.

Iglesia, E.G.A., Kim, E.H., 2020. Low-risk infants may still benefit from allergenic food consumption. J. Allergy Clin. Immunol. 145, 1305.

Immunology, F. A. S. G. O. T. B. D. A. A. P. A. G. O. T. B. S. F. A. C, 2018. Preventing Food Allergy in Higher Risk Infants: Guidance for Healthcare Professionals.

Ip, S., Chung, M., Raman, G., Chew, P., Magula, N., Devine, D., Trikalinos, T., Lau, J., 2007. Breastfeeding and maternal and infant health outcomes in developed countries. Evid. Rep. Technol. Assess., 1–186.

Jarvinen, K.M., Westfall, J.E., Seppo, M.S., James, A.K., Tsuang, A.J., Feustel, P.J., Sampson, H.A., Berin, C., 2014. Role of maternal elimination diets and human milk IgA in the development of cow's milk allergy in the infants. Clin. Exp. Allergy 44, 69–78.

Jarvinen, K.M., Martin, H., Oyoshi, M.K., 2019. Immunomodulatory effects of breast milk on food allergy. Ann. Allergy Asthma Immunol. 123, 133–143.

Jeffery, L.E., Burke, F., Mura, M., Zheng, Y., Qureshi, O.S., Hewison, M., Walker, L.S., Lammas, D.A., Raza, K., Sansom, D.M., 2009. 1,25-Dihydroxyvitamin D3 and IL-2 combine to inhibit T cell production of inflammatory cytokines and promote development of regulatory T cells expressing CTLA-4 and FoxP3. J. Immunol. 183, 5458–5467.

Jelding-Dannemand, E., Malby Schoos, A.M., Bisgaard, H., 2015. Breast-feeding does not protect against allergic sensitization in early childhood and allergy-associated disease at age 7 years. J. Allergy Clin. Immunol. 136, 1302–8e1-13.

Katz, Y., Rajuan, N., Goldberg, M.R., Eisenberg, E., Heyman, E., Cohen, A., Leshno, M., 2010. Early exposure to cow's milk protein is protective against IgE-mediated cow's milk protein allergy. J. Allergy Clin. Immunol. 126, 77–82.e1.

Keet, C., Pistiner, M., Plesa, M., Szelag, D., Shreffler, W., Wood, R., Dunlop, J., Peng, R., Dantzer, J., Togias, A., 2021a. Age and eczema severity, but not family history, are major risk factors for peanut allergy in infancy. J. Allergy Clin. Immunol. 147, 984–991.e5.

Keet, C., Plesa, M., Szelag, D., Shreffler, W., Wood, R., Dunlop, J., Peng, R., Dantzer, J., Hamilton, R.G., Togias, A., Pistiner, M., 2021b. Ara h 2-specific IgE is superior to whole peanut extract-based serology or skin prick test for diagnosis of peanut allergy in infancy. J. Allergy Clin. Immunol. 147, 977–983.e2.

Kilshaw, P.J., Cant, A.J., 1984. The passage of maternal dietary proteins into human breast milk. Int. Arch. Allergy Appl. Immunol. 75, 8–15.

Klopp, A., Vehling, L., Becker, A.B., Subbarao, P., Mandhane, P.J., Turvey, S.E., Lefebvre, D.L., Sears, M.R., Investigators, C.S., Azad, M.B., 2017. Modes of infant feeding and the risk of childhood asthma: a prospective birth cohort study. J. Pediatr. 190, 192–199.e2.

Ko, J., Zhu, S., Alabaster, A., Wang, J., Sax, D.R., 2020. Prehospital treatment and emergency department outcomes in young children with food allergy. J. Allergy Clin. Immunol. Pract. 8, 2302–2309.e2.

Koplin, J.J., Osborne, N.J., Wake, M., Martin, P.E., Gurrin, L.C., Robinson, M.N., Tey, D., Slaa, M., Thiele, L., Miles, L., Anderson, D., Tan, T., Dang, T.D., Hill, D.J., Lowe, A.J., Matheson, M.C., Ponsonby, A.L., Tang, M.L., Dharmage, S.C., Allen, K.J., 2010. Can early introduction of egg prevent egg allergy in infants? A population-based study. J. Allergy Clin. Immunol. 126, 807–813.

Koplin, J.J., Peters, R.L., Dharmage, S.C., Gurrin, L., Tang, M.L.K., Ponsonby, A.L., Matheson, M., Togias, A., Lack, G., Allen, K.J., Healthnuts Study, I, 2016. Understanding the feasibility and implications of implementing early peanut introduction for prevention of peanut allergy. J. Allergy Clin. Immunol. 138, 1131–1141.e2.

Kramer, M.S., Kakuma, R., 2014. Maternal dietary antigen avoidance during pregnancy or lactation, or both, for preventing or treating atopic disease in the child. Evid. Based Child Health 9, 447–483.

Kramer, M.S., Matush, L., Vanilovich, I., Platt, R., Bogdanovich, N., Sevkovskaya, Z., Dzikovich, I., Shishko, G., Mazer, B., Promotion Of Breastfeeding Intervention Trial Study, G, 2007. Effect of prolonged and exclusive breast feeding on risk of allergy and asthma: cluster randomised trial. BMJ 335, 815.

Kremmyda, L.S., Vlachava, M., Noakes, P.S., Diaper, N.D., Miles, E.A., Calder, P.C., 2011. Atopy risk in infants and children in relation to early exposure to fish, oily fish, or long-chain omega-3 fatty acids: a systematic review. Clin. Rev. Allergy Immunol. 41, 36–66.

Lange, N.E., Rifas-Shiman, S.L., Camargo Jr., C.A., Gold, D.R., Gillman, M.W., Litonjua, A.A., 2010. Maternal dietary pattern during pregnancy is not associated with recurrent wheeze in children. J. Allergy Clin. Immunol. 126, 250–255. 255 e1-4.

Leonard, S.A., Pecora, V., Fiocchi, A.G., Nowak-Wegrzyn, A., 2018. Food protein-induced enterocolitis syndrome: a review of the new guidelines. World Allergy Organ J. 11, 4.

Li, L., Han, Z., Niu, X., Zhang, G., Jia, Y., Zhang, S., He, C., 2019. Probiotic supplementation for prevention of atopic dermatitis in infants and children: a systematic review and meta-analysis. Am. J. Clin. Dermatol. 20, 367–377.

Liem, J.J., Huq, S., Kozyrskyj, A.L., Becker, A.B., 2008. Should younger siblings of peanut-allergic children be assessed by an allergist before being fed peanut? Allergy Asthma Clin. Immunol. 4, 144–149.

Lin, A., Uygungil, B., Robbins, K., Ackerman, O., Sharma, H., 2020. Low-dose peanut challenges can facilitate infant peanut introduction regardless of skin prick test size. Ann. Allergy Asthma Immunol. 125, 97–99.

Litonjua, A.A., 2017. Vitamin D levels, asthma, and lung function: time to act on deficiency? J. Allergy Clin. Immunol. Pract. 5, 797–798.

Litonjua, A.A., Carey, V.J., Laranjo, N., Harshfield, B.J., Mcelrath, T.F., O'connor, G.T., Sandel, M., Iverson Jr., R.E., Lee-Paritz, A., Strunk, R.C., Bacharier, L.B., Macones, G.A., Zeiger, R.S., Schatz, M., Hollis, B.W., Hornsby, E., Hawrylowicz, C., Wu, A.C., Weiss, S.T., 2016. Effect of prenatal supplementation with vitamin D on asthma or recurrent wheezing in offspring by age 3 years: the VDAART randomized clinical trial. JAMA 315, 362–370.

Lodge, C.J., Tan, D.J., Lau, M.X., Dai, X., Tham, R., Lowe, A.J., Bowatte, G., Allen, K.J., Dharmage, S.C., 2015. Breastfeeding and asthma and allergies: a systematic review and meta-analysis. Acta Paediatr. 104, 38–53.

Markevych, I., Standl, M., Lehmann, I., Von Berg, A., Heinrich, J., 2017. Food diversity during the first year of life and allergic diseases until 15 years. J. Allergy Clin. Immunol. 140, 1751–1754.e4.

Martina, C., Looney, R.J., Marcus, C., Allen, M., Stahlhut, R., 2016. Prevalence of allergic disease in old order mennonites in New York. Ann. Allergy Asthma Immunol. 117, 562–563.e1.

Matheson, M.C., Erbas, B., Balasuriya, A., Jenkins, M.A., Wharton, C.L., Tang, M.L., Abramson, M.J., Walters, E.H., Hopper, J.L., Dharmage, S.C., 2007. Breast-feeding and atopic disease: a cohort study from childhood to middle age. J. Allergy Clin. Immunol. 120, 1051–1057.

Matheson, M.C., Allen, K.J., Tang, M.L., 2012. Understanding the evidence for and against the role of breastfeeding in allergy prevention. Clin. Exp. Allergy 42, 827–851.

Metcalfe, J.R., Marsh, J.A., D'vaz, N., Geddes, D.T., Lai, C.T., Prescott, S.L., Palmer, D.J., 2016. Effects of maternal dietary egg intake during early lactation on human milk ovalbumin concentration: a randomized controlled trial. Clin. Exp. Allergy 46, 1605–1613.

Michail, S., 2009. The role of probiotics in allergic diseases. Allergy Asthma Clin. Immunol. 5, 5.

Mimouni Bloch, A., Mimouni, D., Mimouni, M., Gdalevich, M., 2002. Does breastfeeding protect against allergic rhinitis during childhood? A meta-analysis of prospective studies. Acta Paediatr. 91, 275–279.

Moonesinghe, H., Patil, V.K., Dean, T., Arshad, S.H., Glasbey, G., Grundy, J., Venter, C., 2016. Association between healthy eating in pregnancy and allergic status of the offspring in childhood. Ann. Allergy Asthma Immunol. 116, 163–165.

Mora, J.R., Iwata, M., Von Andrian, U.H., 2008. Vitamin effects on the immune system: vitamins A and D take centre stage. Nat. Rev. Immunol. 8, 685–698.

Natsume, O., Kabashima, S., Nakazato, J., Yamamoto-Hanada, K., Narita, M., Kondo, M., Saito, M., Kishino, A., Takimoto, T., Inoue, E., Tang, J., Kido, H., Wong, G.W., Matsumoto, K., Saito, H., Ohya, Y., Team, P. S, 2017. Two-step egg introduction for prevention of egg allergy in high-risk infants with eczema (PETIT): a randomised, double-blind, placebo-controlled trial. Lancet 389, 276–286.

Netting, M.J., Middleton, P.F., Makrides, M., 2014. Does maternal diet during pregnancy and lactation affect outcomes in offspring? A systematic review of food-based approaches. Nutrition 30, 1225–1241.

Netting, M.J., Campbell, D.E., Koplin, J.J., Beck, K.M., Mcwilliam, V., Dharmage, S.C., Tang, M.L.K., Ponsonby, A.L., Prescott, S.L., Vale, S., Loh, R.K.S., Makrides, M., Allen, K.J., Centre For, F., Allergy Research, T. A. S. O. C. I., Allergy, T. N. A. S, The Australian Infant Feeding Summit Consensus, G, 2017. An Australian consensus on infant feeding guidelines to prevent food allergy: outcomes from the Australian infant feeding summit. J. Allergy Clin. Immunol. Pract. 5, 1617–1624.

Nowak-Wegrzyn, A., Chehade, M., Groetch, M.E., Spergel, J.M., Wood, R.A., Allen, K., Atkins, D., Bahna, S., Barad, A.V., Berin, C., Brown Whitehorn, T., Burks, A.W., Caubet, J.C., Cianferoni, A., Conte, M., Davis, C., Fiocchi, A., Grimshaw, K., Gupta, R., Hofmeister, B., Hwang, J.B., Katz, Y., Konstantinou, G.N., Leonard, S.A., Lightdale, J., McGhee, S., Mehr, S., Sopo, S.M., Monti, G., Muraro, A., Noel, S.K., Nomura, I., Noone, S., Sampson, H.A., Schultz, F., Sicherer, S.H., Thompson, C.C., Turner, P.J., Venter, C., Westcott-Chavez, A.A., Greenhawt, M., 2017. International consensus guidelines for the diagnosis and management of food protein-induced enterocolitis syndrome: executive summary-workgroup report of the adverse reactions to foods committee, American academy of allergy, asthma & immunology. J. Allergy Clin. Immunol. 139, 1111–1126.e4.

II. Early nutrition and development of non-communicable diseases

Nowak-Wegrzyn, A., Hass, S.L., Donelson, S.M., Robison, D., Cameron, A., Etschmaier, M., Duhig, A., McCann, W.A., 2021. The peanut allergy burden study: impact on the quality of life of patients and caregivers. World Allergy Organ. J. 14, 100512.

Nutrition, S. A. C. O, 2018. Feeding in the First Year of Life. Public Health England.

Nwaru, B.I., Takkinen, H.M., Niemela, O., Kaila, M., Erkkola, M., Ahonen, S., Tuomi, H., Haapala, A.M., Kenward, M.G., Pekkanen, J., Lahesmaa, R., Kere, J., Simell, O., Veijola, R., Ilonen, J., Hyoty, H., Knip, M., Virtanen, S.M., 2013. Introduction of complementary foods in infancy and atopic sensitization at the age of 5 years: timing and food diversity in a Finnish birth cohort. Allergy 68, 507–516.

Okada, H., Kuhn, C., Feillet, H., Bach, J.F., 2010. The 'hygiene hypothesis' for autoimmune and allergic diseases: an update. Clin. Exp. Immunol. 160, 1–9.

Onizawa, Y., Noguchi, E., Okada, M., Sumazaki, R., Hayashi, D., 2016. The association of the delayed introduction of cow's milk with IgE-mediated Cow's Milk allergies. J. Allergy Clin. Immunol. Pract. 4, 481–488.e2.

Organization, W. H, 2017. Guideline: Protecting, Promoting and Supporting Breastfeeding in Facilities Providing Maternity and Newborn Services. Geneva.

Osborn, D.A., Sinn, J., 2003. Formulas containing hydrolysed protein for prevention of allergy and food intolerance in infants. Cochrane Database Syst. Rev., CD003664.

Osborn, D.A., Sinn, J., 2006. Formulas containing hydrolysed protein for prevention of allergy and food intolerance in infants. Cochrane Database Syst. Rev., CD003664.

Osborn, D.A., Sinn, J.K., Jones, L.J., 2018. Infant formulas containing hydrolysed protein for prevention of allergic disease. Cochrane Database Syst. Rev. 10, CD003664.

Pabst, O., Mowat, A.M., 2012. Oral tolerance to food protein. Mucosal Immunol. 5, 232–239.

Palmer, D.J., Metcalfe, J., Makrides, M., Gold, M.S., Quinn, P., West, C.E., Loh, R., Prescott, S.L., 2013. Early regular egg exposure in infants with eczema: a randomized controlled trial. J. Allergy Clin. Immunol. 132, 387–392.e1.

Palmer, D.J., Sullivan, T.R., Gold, M.S., Prescott, S.L., Makrides, M., 2017. Randomized controlled trial of early regular egg intake to prevent egg allergy. J. Allergy Clin. Immunol. 139, 1600–1607.e2.

Pawankar, R., Canonica, G.W., Holgate, S.T., Lockey, R.F., Blaiss, M.S., 2013. World allergy organization (WAO) white book on allergy: update 2013. World Allergy Organization, Milwaukee, WI.

Penders, J., Stobberingh, E.E., Van Den Brandt, P.A., Thijs, C., 2007. The role of the intestinal microbiota in the development of atopic disorders. Allergy 62, 1223–1236.

Perkin, M.R., Logan, K., Tseng, A., Raji, B., Ayis, S., Peacock, J., Brough, H., Marrs, T., Radulovic, S., Craven, J., Flohr, C., Lack, G., Team, E. A. T. S, 2016. Randomized trial of introduction of allergenic foods in breast-fed infants. N. Engl. J. Med. 374, 1733–1743.

Peters, R.L., Koplin, J.J., Dharmage, S.C., Tang, M.L.K., Mcwilliam, V.L., Gurrin, L.C., Neeland, M.R., Lowe, A.J., Ponsonby, A.L., Allen, K.J., 2019. Early exposure to cow's milk protein is associated with a reduced risk of cow's milk allergic outcomes. J. Allergy Clin. Immunol. Pract. 7, 462–470.e1.

Prescott, S.L., Bjorksten, B., 2007. Probiotics for the prevention or treatment of allergic diseases. J. Allergy Clin. Immunol. 120, 255–262.

Purvis, D.J., Thompson, J.M., Clark, P.M., Robinson, E., Black, P.N., Wild, C.J., Mitchell, E.A., 2005. Risk factors for atopic dermatitis in New Zealand children at 3.5 years of age. Br. J. Dermatol. 152, 742–749.

Reinholz, M., Ruzicka, T., Schauber, J., 2012. Vitamin D and its role in allergic disease. Clin. Exp. Allergy 42, 817–826.

Roduit, C., Frei, R., Depner, M., Schaub, B., Loss, G., Genuneit, J., Pfefferle, P., Hyvarinen, A., Karvonen, A.M., Riedler, J., Dalphin, J.C., Pekkanen, J., Von Mutius, E., Braun-Fahrlander, C., Lauener, R., Group, P. S, 2014. Increased food diversity in the first year of life is inversely associated with allergic diseases. J. Allergy Clin. Immunol. 133, 1056–1064.

Rook, G.A., Brunet, L.R., 2005. Microbes, immunoregulation, and the gut. Gut 54, 317–320.

Rzehak, P., Sausenthaler, S., Koletzko, S., Reinhardt, D., Von Berg, A., Kramer, U., Berdel, D., Bollrath, C., Grubl, A., Bauer, C.P., Wichmann, H.E., Heinrich, J., Group, G. I.-P. S, 2011. Long-term effects of hydrolyzed protein infant formulas on growth—extended follow-up to 10 y of age: results from the German infant nutritional intervention (GINI) study. Am. J. Clin. Nutr. 94, 1803S–1807S.

Sakihara, T., Otsuji, K., Arakaki, Y., Hamada, K., Sugiura, S., Ito, K., 2021. Randomized trial of early infant formula introduction to prevent cow's milk allergy. J. Allergy Clin. Immunol. 147, 224–232.e8.

Samady, W., Trainor, J., Smith, B., Gupta, R., 2018. Food-induced anaphylaxis in infants and children. Ann. Allergy Asthma Immunol. 121, 360–365.

Schindler, T., Sinn, J.K., Osborn, D.A., 2016. Polyunsaturated fatty acid supplementation in infancy for the prevention of allergy. Cochrane Database Syst. Rev. 10, CD010112.

II. Early nutrition and development of non-communicable diseases

Section On, B., 2012. Breastfeeding and the use of human milk. Pediatrics 129, e827–e841.

Sestito, S., D'auria, E., Baldassarre, M.E., Salvatore, S., Tallarico, V., Stefanelli, E., Tarsitano, F., Concolino, D., Pensabene, L., 2020. The role of prebiotics and probiotics in prevention of allergic diseases in infants. Front. Pediatr. 8, 583946.

Shaker, M., Stukus, D., Chan, E.S., Fleischer, D.M., Spergel, J.M., Greenhawt, M., 2018. "To screen or not to screen": comparing the health and economic benefits of early peanut introduction strategies in five countries. Allergy 73, 1707–1714.

Shaker, M.S., Iglesia, E., Greenhawt, M., 2019. The health and economic benefits of approaches for peanut introduction in infants with a peanut allergic sibling. Allergy 74, 2251–2254.

Silverberg, J.I., Barbarot, S., Gadkari, A., Simpson, E.L., Weidinger, S., Mina-Osorio, P., Rossi, A.B., Brignoli, L., Saba, G., Guillemin, I., Fenton, M.C., Auziere, S., Eckert, L., 2021. Atopic dermatitis in the pediatric population: a cross-sectional, international epidemiologic study. Ann. Allergy Asthma Immunol. 126, 417–428.e2.

Soller, L., Ben-Shoshan, M., Harrington, D.W., Fragapane, J., Joseph, L., St Pierre, Y., Godefroy, S.B., La Vieille, S., Elliott, S.J., Clarke, A.E., 2012. Overall prevalence of self-reported food allergy in Canada. J. Allergy Clin. Immunol. 130, 986–988.

Soriano, V.X., Peters, R.L., Ponsonby, A.L., Dharmage, S.C., Perrett, K.P., Field, M.J., Knox, A., Tey, D., Odoi, S., Gell, G., Camesella Perez, B., Allen, K.J., Gurrin, L.C., Koplin, J.J., 2019. Earlier ingestion of peanut after changes to infant feeding guidelines: the EarlyNuts study. J. Allergy Clin. Immunol. 144, 1327–1335.e5.

Strachan, D.P., 1989. Hay fever, hygiene, and household size. BMJ 299, 1259–1260.

Sudo, N., Sawamura, S., Tanaka, K., Aiba, Y., Kubo, C., Koga, Y., 1997. The requirement of intestinal bacterial flora for the development of an IgE production system fully susceptible to oral tolerance induction. J. Immunol. 159, 1739–1745.

Szepfalusi, Z., Loibichler, C., Pichler, J., Reisenberger, K., Ebner, C., Urbanek, R., 2000. Direct evidence for transplacental allergen transfer. Pediatr. Res. 48, 404–407.

Thorburn, A.N., Macia, L., Mackay, C.R., 2014. Diet, metabolites, and "western-lifestyle" inflammatory diseases. Immunity 40, 833–842.

Togias, A., Cooper, S.F., Acebal, M.L., Assa'ad, A., Baker Jr., J.R., Beck, L.A., Block, J., Byrd-Bredbenner, C., Chan, E.S., Eichenfield, L.F., Fleischer, D.M., Fuchs 3rd, G.J., Furuta, G.T., Greenhawt, M.J., Gupta, R.S., Habich, M., Jones, S.M., Keaton, K., Muraro, A., Plaut, M., Rosenwasser, L.J., Rotrosen, D., Sampson, H.A., Schneider, L.C., Sicherer, S.H., Sidbury, R., Spergel, J., Stukus, D.R., Venter, C., Boyce, J.A., 2017. Addendum guidelines for the prevention of peanut allergy in the United States: report of the National Institute of Allergy and Infectious Diseases-sponsored expert panel. J. Allergy Clin. Immunol. 139, 29–44.

Tsakok, T., Marrs, T., Mohsin, M., Baron, S., Du Toit, G., Till, S., Flohr, C., 2016. Does atopic dermatitis cause food allergy? A systematic review. J. Allergy Clin. Immunol. 137, 1071–1078.

Turner, P.J., Campbell, D.E., 2017. Implementing primary prevention for peanut allergy at a population level. JAMA 317, 1111–1112.

Urashima, M., Mezawa, H., Okuyama, M., Urashima, T., Hirano, D., Gocho, N., Tachimoto, H., 2019. Primary prevention of cow's milk sensitization and food allergy by avoiding supplementation with cow's milk formula at birth: a randomized clinical trial. JAMA Pediatr. 173, 1137–1145.

US Department of Agriculture, US Department of Health and Human Services, 2020. Dietary Guidelines for Americans, 2020–2025, ninth ed. US Department of Agriculture. December. Available at: DietaryGuidelines.gov.

Vadas, P., Wai, Y., Burks, W., Perelman, B., 2001. Detection of peanut allergens in breast milk of lactating women. JAMA 285, 1746–1748.

Van Odijk, J., Kull, I., Borres, M.P., Brandtzaeg, P., Edberg, U., Hanson, L.A., Host, A., Kuitunen, M., Olsen, S.F., Skerfving, S., Sundell, J., Wille, S., 2003. Breastfeeding and allergic disease: a multidisciplinary review of the literature (1966-2001) on the mode of early feeding in infancy and its impact on later atopic manifestations. Allergy 58, 833–843.

Vandenplas, Y., Latiff, A.H.A., Fleischer, D.M., Gutierrez-Castrellon, P., Miqdady, M.S., Smith, P.K., Von Berg, A., Greenhawt, M.J., 2019. Partially hydrolyzed formula in non-exclusively breastfed infants: a systematic review and expert consensus. Nutrition 57, 268–274.

Venter, C., Meyer, R.W., Nwaru, B.I., Roduit, C., Untersmayr, E., Adel-Patient, K., Agache, I., Agostoni, C., Akdis, C.A., Bischoff, S.C., Du Toit, G., Feeney, M., Frei, R., Garn, H., Greenhawt, M., Hoffmann-Sommergruber, K., Lunjani, N., Maslin, K., Mills, C., Muraro, A., Pali-Scholl, I., Poulson, L.K., Reese, I., Renz, H., Roberts, G.C., Smith, P., Smolinska, S., Sokolowska, M., Stanton, C., Vlieg-Boerstra, B., O'Mahony, L., 2019. EAACI position paper: influence of dietary fatty acids on asthma, food allergy, and atopic dermatitis. Allergy 74, 1429–1444.

Venter, C., Agostoni, C., Arshad, S.H., Ben-Abdallah, M., Du Toit, G., Fleischer, D.M., Greenhawt, M., Glueck, D.H., Groetch, M., Lunjani, N., Maslin, K., Maiorella, A., Meyer, R., Antonella, M., Netting, M.J., Ibeabughichi Nwaru, B., Palmer, D.J., Palumbo, M.P., Roberts, G., Roduit, C., Smith, P., Untersmayr, E., Vanderlinden, L.A., O'mahony, L., 2020a. Dietary factors during pregnancy and atopic outcomes in childhood: a systematic review from the European academy of allergy and clinical immunology. Pediatr. Allergy Immunol. 31, 889–912.

Venter, C., Greenhawt, M., Meyer, R.W., Agostoni, C., Reese, I., Du Toit, G., Feeney, M., Maslin, K., Nwaru, B.I., Roduit, C., Untersmayr, E., Vlieg-Boerstra, B., Pali-Scholl, I., Roberts, G.C., Smith, P., Akdis, C.A., Agache, I., Ben-Adallah, M., Bischoff, S., Frei, R., Garn, H., Grimshaw, K., Hoffmann-Sommergruber, K., Lunjani, N., Muraro, A., Poulsen, L.K., Renz, H., Sokolowska, M., Stanton, C., O'mahony, L., 2020b. EAACI position paper on diet diversity in pregnancy, infancy and childhood: novel concepts and implications for studies in allergy and asthma. Allergy 75, 497–523.

Venter, C., Maslin, K., Holloway, J.W., Silveira, L.J., Fleischer, D.M., Dean, T., Arshad, S.H., 2020c. Different measures of diet diversity during infancy and the association with childhood food allergy in a UK birth cohort study. J Allergy Clin Immunol Pract 8, 2017–2026.

Victora, C.G., Bahl, R., Barros, A.J., Franca, G.V., Horton, S., Krasevec, J., Murch, S., Sankar, M.J., Walker, N., Rollins, N.C., Lancet Breastfeeding Series, G, 2016. Breastfeeding in the 21st century: epidemiology, mechanisms, and lifelong effect. Lancet 387, 475–490.

Volertas, S., Coury, M., Sanders, G., Mcmorris, M., Gupta, M., 2020. Real-life infant peanut allergy testing in the post-NIAID peanut guideline world. J. Allergy Clin. Immunol. Pract. 8, 1091–1093.e2.

von Berg, A., Koletzko, S., Grübl, A., Filipiak-Pittroff, B., Wichmann, H.-E., Bauer, C.P., Reinhardt, D., Berdel, D., German Infant Nutritional Intervention Study Group, 2003. The effect of hydrolyzed cow's milk formula for allergy prevention in the first year of life: the German Infant Nutritional Intervention Study, a randomized double-blind trial. J. Allergy Clin. Immunol. 111 (3), 533–540. https://doi.org/10.1067/mai.2003.101.

Von Berg, A., Koletzko, S., Filipiak-Pittroff, B., Laubereau, B., Grubl, A., Wichmann, H.E., Bauer, C.P., Reinhardt, D., Berdel, D., German Infant Nutritional Intervention Study, G, 2007. Certain hydrolyzed formulas reduce the incidence of atopic dermatitis but not that of asthma: three-year results of the German infant nutritional intervention study. J. Allergy Clin. Immunol. 119, 718–725.

Von Berg, A., Filipiak-Pittroff, B., Kramer, U., Link, E., Bollrath, C., Brockow, I., Koletzko, S., Grubl, A., Heinrich, J., Wichmann, H.E., Bauer, C.P., Reinhardt, D., Berdel, D., Group, G. I. S, 2008. Preventive effect of hydrolyzed infant formulas persists until age 6 years: long-term results from the German infant nutritional intervention study (GINI). J. Allergy Clin. Immunol. 121, 1442–1447.

Von Mutius, E., Martinez, F.D., Fritzsch, C., Nicolai, T., Roell, G., Thiemann, H.H., 1994. Prevalence of asthma and atopy in two areas of West and East Germany. Am. J. Respir. Crit. Care Med. 149, 358–364.

Wei-Liang Tan, J., Valerio, C., Barnes, E.H., Turner, P.J., Van Asperen, P.A., Kakakios, A.M., Campbell, D.E., Beating Egg Allergy Trial Study, G, 2017. A randomized trial of egg introduction from 4 months of age in infants at risk for egg allergy. J. Allergy Clin. Immunol. 139, 1621–1628.e8.

West, C.E., Jenmalm, M.C., Prescott, S.L., 2015. The gut microbiota and its role in the development of allergic disease: a wider perspective. Clin. Exp. Allergy 45, 43–53.

Wong, J.M., De Souza, R., Kendall, C.W., Emam, A., Jenkins, D.J., 2006. Colonic health: fermentation and short chain fatty acids. J. Clin. Gastroenterol. 40, 235–243.

Yang, Y.W., Tsai, C.L., Lu, C.Y., 2009. Exclusive breastfeeding and incident atopic dermatitis in childhood: a systematic review and meta-analysis of prospective cohort studies. Br. J. Dermatol. 161, 373–383.

Yepes-Nunez, J.J., Fiocchi, A., Pawankar, R., Cuello-Garcia, C.A., Zhang, Y., Morgano, G.P., Ahn, K., Al-Hammadi, S., Agarwal, A., Gandhi, S., Beyer, K., Burks, W., Canonica, G.W., Ebisawa, M., Kamenwa, R., Lee, B.W., Li, H., Prescott, S., Riva, J.J., Rosenwasser, L., Sampson, H., Spigler, M., Terracciano, L., Vereda, A., Waserman, S., Schunemann, H.J., Brozek, J.L., 2016. World allergy Organization-McMaster University guidelines for allergic disease prevention (GLAD-P): vitamin D. World Allergy Organ. J. 9, 17.

Yepes-Nunez, J.J., Brozek, J.L., Fiocchi, A., Pawankar, R., Cuello-Garcia, C., Zhang, Y., Morgano, G.P., Agarwal, A., Gandhi, S., Terracciano, L., Schunemann, H.J., 2018. Vitamin D supplementation in primary allergy prevention: systematic review of randomized and non-randomized studies. Allergy 73, 37–49.

# 14

# Early nutrition and its effect on the development of celiac disease

*Carlo Catassi and Elena Lionetti*

Department of Pediatrics, Marche Polytechnic University, Ancona, Italy

## LEARNING OBJECTIVES

1. To improve knowledge on celiac disease epidemiology and pathogenesis, with particular attention to the possible role of environmental factors on celiac disease pathogenesis.

2. To learn major results of randomized controlled trials and longitudinal cohort studies performed so far on the role of early infant nutrition on celiac disease development.

3. To improve knowledge on the role of intestinal microbiota on celiac disease development.

## 14.1 Celiac disease

### 14.1.1 Definition

Celiac disease is a systemic immune-mediated disorder caused by the ingestion of gluten-containing grains (wheat, rye, and barley) in genetically susceptible persons (Fasano and Catassi, 2012).

### 14.1.2 Epidemiology

Celiac disease is one of the most common lifelong disorders, affecting approximately 1%–2% of the population worldwide (Singh et al., 2018). The prevalence of celiac disease has increased in developed countries over recent decades (Lionetti et al., 2015). The total prevalence of celiac disease has doubled during the last decades in Finland (1.05% in 1978–80 and 1.99% in 2000–01) (Lohi et al., 2007) and in Italy (0.8% in 1993–95 and 1.5% in 2015–16) (Gatti et al.,

2020), an increase that cannot simply be attributed to a better detection rate. The frequency of celiac disease autoimmunity doubled between 1974 (1 in every 501 subjects) and 1989 (1 in every 219 subjects) in a sample of the US population. This trend apparently continued in the following years (1 in 105 subjects in the year 2001) followed by a stabilization in recent years (0.7%–0.8% in 2008–14) (Catassi et al., 2010; Choung et al., 2017). These findings point to the role of one or more possible environmental triggers, other than gluten, that could be involved in celiac disease pathogenesis.

### 14.1.3 Pathogenesis

The development of celiac disease is determined by both environmental and genetic factors. A familial aggregation is found in 5%–15% of celiac disease patients and a striking 83%–86% concordance rate was observed among monozygotic twin pairs (Wolters and Wijmenga, 2008). The genetic determinants that confer susceptibility to the disease are however not yet fully understood. The most important genetic factor identified so far is the human leukocyte antigen (HLA) locus. The HLA-DQ2 (DQA1*0501-DQB1*0201) haplotype is expressed in the majority of affected patients (90%), the DQ8 haplotype (DQA1*0301-DQB1*0302) is expressed in 5%, and 5% carry at least one of the two DQ2 alleles (usually the DQB1*0201) (Abadie et al., 2011). An increased risk of celiac disease has been observed among persons who carry two DQB1*02 alleles (Liu et al., 2014; Lionetti et al., 2014). The ability of these alleles in conferring individual susceptibility to celiac disease is related to their peculiar capacity to bind negatively charged peptides such as gliadin peptides deamidated by the anti-transglutaminase. The HLA-antigen link results in the activation of T lymphocytes, whose secretion products play a key role in causing mucosal lesions (Liu et al., 2014). The associations found in non-HLA genome wide linkage and association studies are much weaker. This might be because a large number of non-HLA genes (about 40) contribute to the pathogenesis of celiac disease. Hence, the contribution of a single predisposing non-HLA gene might be quite modest (Wolters and Wijmenga, 2008).

Gluten is the environmental factor required to trigger the disease, but other factors may be involved in a model of a complex multifactorial disease (Lionetti and Catassi, 2011). According to the "hygiene hypothesis," the cleaner environment found nowadays in developed countries led to lower frequency of early childhood infections and differences in the spectrum of microorganisms populating the gut. These changes could modify the immune response being responsible for higher risk of different autoimmune disorders like celiac disease (Bach, 2002). However, the rising prevalence of adult-onset celiac disease that was observed in the US study can hardly be explained by hygienic changes occurring in childhood. The reasons for these changes are still unclear, but have to do with the environmental components of celiac disease, since genetic changes are too slow to drive these phenomena (Lionetti et al., 2015).

It has been recently hypothesized that all the following environmental factors are possibly involved in the switches of the tolerance–intolerance immune balance: the amount and the quality of ingested gluten, the type and duration of wheat dough fermentation, early infant feeding, the spectrum of intestinal microorganisms and how they change over time, intestinal infections, and vaccination schedule (Lindfors et al., 2019). However, more research is needed to determine whether and how these factors can cause loss of gluten tolerance.

## 14.1.4 Treatment and prevention

The only available treatment consists in dietary exclusion of grains containing gluten. New pharmacological treatments are currently under scrutiny. In order to achieve the ambitious goal of celiac disease prevention, recent randomized controlled trials and longitudinal cohort studies have been performed to clarify the role of early nutrition on later development of celiac disease.

## 14.2 Early nutrition and the risk of celiac disease

## 14.2.1 Timing of gluten introduction

The introduction of gluten at 6 months of age is a long-standing practice, at least in Western countries, however the optimal time of introduction of gluten in the diet of the child had never been rigorously tested. Investigations following the "epidemic" of celiac disease that occurred in Sweden during the 1980s and 90s showed that the introduction of a small amount of gluten during breastfeeding between 4 and 6 months of age was associated with a reduced risk of the disease. These data provided the basis for the hypothesis of the so-called window of tolerance, according to which there would be a window of time, between 4 and 7 months of age, during which the introduction of gluten could facilitate the induction of tolerance (Ivarsson et al., 2000, 2013). The concept of the "window of tolerance" gained popularity and a US study reported that children at genetic risk for type 1 diabetes exposed to gluten between 4 and 6 months of age had a reduced risk of celiac disease than those exposed to gluten before 4 and after 7 months of age; however, it is worth noting that the number of patients in this study with a diagnosis of celiac disease confirmed by intestinal biopsy was very small (Norris et al., 2005). Later, the Norwegian Mother and Child Cohort Study (MoBa), a large population-based study including 324 cases with celiac disease and 81,843 healthy controls, reported that only the delayed (> 6 months), but not the early introduction of gluten (< 4 months) was associated with an increased risk of celiac disease (Størdal et al., 2013; Lund-Blix et al., 2019), although with a border-line significance. The main limitation of these case–control studies was the lack of an intervention arm.

In 2014, two randomized controlled trials, aimed to clarify the relationship between timing of gluten introduction in the infant diet and the risk of celiac disease, were finally published (Lionetti et al., 2014; Vriezinga et al., 2014). The Risk of Celiac Disease and Age at Gluten Introduction (CELIPREV) trial is a multicenter, prospective intervention trial comparing early (6 months) and delayed (12 months) introduction of gluten in infants with a familial risk of celiac disease, followed from birth to 10 years of age (Lionetti et al., 2014). Infants who had a family risk of celiac disease (i.e., infants who had at least one first-degree relative affected with celiac disease) were recruited in 20 centers in Italy between 2003 and 2008. Infants were randomly assigned to one of the two groups: those in group A were introduced to gluten-containing foods (pasta, semolina, and biscuits) at 6 months of age, and those in group B at 12 months of age. The main objective of this study was to compare the prevalence of celiac disease according to the time of gluten introduction at 5 years of age. The percentage of children with celiac disease at 5 years of age was the same in group A and in group B (16% and 16%, $P = 0.78$); at 10 years there was still no significant difference between the two groups (hazard ratio at 10 years: 0.9; 95% confidence interval: 0.6–1.4; $P = 0.79$). However, the average age at which celiac disease developed was 26 months in group A and 34 months in group B ($P = 0.01$). Worth noting, in children with higher-risk HLA genotype (characterized by homozygosis for HLA-DQ2), the prevalence of celiac disease was higher in group A than in group B at all ages, although the difference was not statistically significant ($P = 0.51$), probably to the small number of children with this genotype. During the follow-up, complications related to celiac disease (i.e., autoimmune thyroid diseases, type 1 diabetes) did not develop in any child of the two groups. Therefore, the CELIPREV study showed that postponing the introduction of gluten at 12 months of age has no effect on the risk of developing the disease in the long term and does not reduce or increase the risk of disease. However, delaying the introduction of gluten had two potentially positive consequences: (1) to delay the development of the disease; and (2) to reduce the frequency of celiac disease in babies with a double copy of the HLA-DQ2 gene. Although this last effect did not reach the statistical significance, it is worthy of further investigations.

The other European multi-center project Prevent Celiac Disease (PREVENT-CD) trial is a randomized, double-blind, placebo-controlled dietary intervention study aimed to compare the introduction of small quantities of gliadin (100 mg/daily) from 16 to 24 weeks of age vs placebo, followed by standard gluten consumption in infants with a familial risk of celiac disease, followed from birth to at least 3 years of age (Vriezinga et al., 2014). The results of this trial demonstrated that the introduction of small amounts of gluten during the "supposed" window of tolerance does not reduce the risk of the disease. The cumulative incidence of celiac disease among children at 3 years of age was indeed similar in the gluten group and the placebo group (5.9 and 4.5%, respectively, hazard ratio at 3 years: 1.23; 95% confidence interval, 0.79–1.91, $P = 0.47$).

Therefore, the results of both the CELIPREV and the PREVENT-CD studies showed that the timing of introduction of gluten does not modify the risk of developing celiac disease, at least in subjects with a family history of disease.

After these interventional trials, two large observational cohort studies drew the same conclusions. The Generation R study found that the introduction of gluten from the age of 6 months onward, compared to earlier exposure, was not significantly associated with celiac disease (Jansen et al., 2014); the Environmental Determinants of Diabetes in the Young (TEDDY), a prospective observational birth cohort study designed to identify environmental triggers of type 1 diabetes and celiac disease, including six clinical centers in Finland, Germany, Sweden, and the United States, compared first exposure to gluten occurring < 17 weeks, between 17 and 26 weeks, or > 17 weeks. No difference was found in the risk of developing celiac disease between the three groups differing in age of exposure (Andrén Aronsson et al., 2016).

At variance with these studies, a recent randomized controlled trial suggests the validity of the "window of tolerance" hypothesis, due to the finding of a protective role of early high-dose consumption of gluten on celiac disease development. The Enquiring About Tolerance (EAT) Study was an open-label randomized clinical trial (Logan et al., 2020). A total of 1004 children from the general population in England and Wales were recruited and followed up. Infants were randomized to consume 6 allergenic foods (peanut, sesame, hen's egg, cow's milk, cod fish, and wheat) in addition to breast milk from age 4 months (early introduction group) or to avoid allergenic foods and follow UK infant feeding recommendations of exclusive breastfeeding until approximately age 6 months (standard introduction group). Of note, the mean quantity of gluten consumed between ages 4 and 6 months was 0.49 g/week in the standard intervention group and 2.66 g/week in the early intervention group ($P < 0.001$). Seven of 516 children from the standard intervention group (1.4%) had a diagnosis of CD confirmed vs none of the 488 children in the early intervention group ($P = 0.02$, risk difference between the groups using the bootstrap, 1.4%; 95% confidence interval, 0.6%–2.6%).

Table 14.1 summarizes the characteristics of randomized controlled trials on timing of gluten introduction and the risk of celiac disease. Overall, the discordant results of early intervention studies do not consent to draw conclusions about timing of the first gluten introduction.

## 14.2.2 Quantity of gluten

Table 14.2 shows the main results of available studies on the amount of gluten and the risk of celiac disease. The effect of the quantity of gluten at the time of weaning and in the first years of life on the risk of celiac disease is still a debated issue. Data from two recent longitudinal cohort studies and one population study suggest that large amounts of gluten may increase the risk of celiac disease. In detail, the Diabetes Autoimmunity Study in the Young (DAISY), conducted in Denver, followed children genetically at risk for type 1 diabetes and celiac disease (Lund-Blix et al., 2019). Gluten intake from age 1 year throughout childhood was assessed via repeated food-frequency questionnaires. Overall, 31,766 newborns were screened, of which 2547 (8%) were included in the study, and 1243 had analyzable data on gluten (3.3% of the screened number). Children in the highest quartile of gluten consumption between the ages of 1 and 2 years had a twofold greater hazard of celiac disease (hazard ratio 1.96; 95% confidence interval, 0.90–4.24; $P = 0.09$) than those in the lowest quartile. The incidence of celiac disease increased with the cumulative gluten intake throughout childhood (per 1 g, hazard ratio 1.01; 95% confidence interval 1.00–1.01; $P = 0.04$). Almost simultaneously, Andrén-Aronsson published the results of the TEDDY study (Andrén Aronsson et al., 2019). Overall, 424,788 newborn infants were screened for HLA, and 21,589 were eligible for screening but only 40% ($n = 8676$) agreed to participate. Of these, even fewer ($n = 6757$) were screened for CD annually. Gluten intake was estimated from 3-day food records collected at ages 6, 9, and 12 months and biannually thereafter until the age of 5 years. The researchers' main finding was that each additional gram of gluten consumption per day was associated with a 50% increased risk of celiac disease at the age of 3 years (hazard ratio 1.50; 95% confidence interval, 1.35–1.66). Finally, in the MoBa study 113,000 children were initially enrolled; of them, 67,608 were included in the study and followed up for a mean of 11.5 years (Lund-Blix et al., 2019). Information regarding celiac disease diagnosis was obtained from the Norwegian Patient Register 2008–16. Gluten intake at age 18 months was estimated from a prospectively collected parental questionnaire. This study found that for each gram of extra gluten intake per day, the risk of celiac disease increased by 3% (95% confidence interval, 1.01–1.05). Taken together, these studies suggest that one extra small slice of bread (2 g of gluten) per day seems to be linked to a 20%–50% increased risk of celiac disease.

## 14.2.3 Quality of gluten

There are no data on any correlation between the type of gluten introduced at weaning (e.g., from different gluten-containing cereals) and subsequent celiac disease development

**TABLE 14.1** Characteristics of randomized controlled trials on timing of gluten introduction and risk celiac disease.

| Author | Study name | Study design | Setting | Objective | Participants | Methods | Prevalence of CD | Effect |
|---|---|---|---|---|---|---|---|---|
| Lionetti (2014) | Celi-PREV | RCT | Italy | To compare 6 vs 12 months' introduction of gluten on CD risk | 553 infants HLA-DQ2/-DQ8 positive | Randomization to gluten at 6 or 12 months | 16.8% at 10 years | CD HR 0.9 (0.6–1.4) |
| Vriezinga et al. (2014) | PREVENT-CD | RCT | Croatia, Germany, Hungary, Italy, The Netherlands, Poland, Spain | To compare the introduction of 200 mg of vital gluten at 4 months vs 6 months' introduction on CD risk | 994 infants HLA-DQ2/-DQ8 positive. | Randomization to 200 mg of vital gluten at 4 months or to gluten at 6 months | 12.1% at 5 years | CD HR 1.23 (0.79–1.91) |
| Logan et al. (2020) | EAT | RCT | England and Wales | To determine whether early introduction of high-dose gluten lowers the prevalence of CD at age 3 years | 1004 infants from the general population | Randomization to high-dose gluten at 4 months or to standard gluten at 6 months (mean weekly gluten consumption: 4 g/week vs 0.9 g/week at age 6 months) | 0.7% at 3 years | CD RD 1.4% (0.6%–2.6%) |

**TABLE 14.2** Characteristics of studies on amount of gluten and risk celiac disease.

| Author | Study name | Study design | Setting | Objective | Methods | Participants | Prevalence of CD | Effect |
|---|---|---|---|---|---|---|---|---|
| Vriezinga et al. (2014) | PREVENT-CD | RCT | Croatia, Germany, Hungary, Italy, The Netherlands, Poland, Spain | To compare the introduction of 200mg of vital gluten at 4months vs 6months' introduction on CD risk | Randomization to 200mg of vital gluten at 4months or to gluten at 6months | 994 infants HLA-DQ2/-DQ8 positive | 12.1% at 5years | CD HR per extra-gram of gluten intake per day: 1.2 (0.98–1.3) |
| Andrén Aronsson et al. (2019) | Teddy | Prospective cohort study | Finland, Germany, Sweden, United States | To investigate if the amount of gluten intake is associated with celiac disease risk | Estimates of gluten intake from 3-day food records collected at ages 6, 9, and 12months and biannually thereafter until the age of 5years | 6605 infants HLA-DQ2/-DQ8 positive. | 7% at 9years | CD HR per extra-gram of gluten intake per day: 1.5 (1.35–1.66) |
| (Mårild et al., 2019) | DAISY | Prospective cohort study | United States | To determine the association between the amount of gluten intake in childhood and later CD | Annual estimates of gluten intake (g/day) between ages 1 and 2 from food-frequency questionnaires | 1243 infants HLA-DQ2/-DQ8 positive | 4.5% at 13years | CD HR per extra-gram of gluten intake per day: 1.04 (0.98–1.10). Third tertile vs first tertile of gluten intake: HR 1.96 (0.9–4.24) |
| Lund-Blix et al. (2019) | MoBa | Prospective nationwide-cohort study | Norway | To determine whether the amount of gluten intake at age 18months predicted later risk of CD | Estimates of gluten intake at 18months from a parental questionnaire | 67,608 infants from the general population | 1.1% at 11.5years | CD RR per extra-gram of gluten intake per day: 1.03 (1.01–1.05). Fourth quartile vs first quartile of gluten intake: RR 1.27 (1.04–1.55) |
| Logan et al. (2020) | EAT | RCT | England and Wales | To determine whether early introduction of high-dose gluten lowers the prevalence of CD at age 3years | Randomization to high-dose of gluten at 4 or to standard gluten at 6months | 1004 infants from the general population | 0.7% at 3years | CD RD 1.4% (0.6%–2.6%) |

CD: celiac disease; HR: hazard ratio; RCT: randomized controlled trial; RD: risk difference; RR: relative risk.

from randomized controlled trials. Only one observational study evaluated this relationship, showing that the type of gluten-containing cereal given was not an independent risk factor for developing celiac disease (Ivarsson et al., 2002).

### 14.2.4 Breastfeeding and infant formula

A protective role of breastfeeding against celiac disease has long been perceived, mostly based on some retrospective studies (Ivarsson et al., 2002; Peters et al., 2001; Greco et al., 1988; Auricchio et al., 1983) and a systematic review of the literature (Akobeng et al., 2006) and a meta-analysis that summarized those results (Szajewska et al., 2012). The previously reported Norwegian investigation had instead shown that breastfeeding does not exert any protective effect against the development of celiac disease; the average duration of breastfeeding was, indeed, even longer in children with celiac disease (10.4 months) compared with controls (9.9 months) and the risk of disease was significantly higher in babies that had been breastfed for more than 12 months (Størdal et al., 2013).

The CELIPREV study contributed to clarify this important aspect of child nutrition. In the cohort of infants at familial risk of celiac disease, it was not observed any protective effect of breastfeeding on the development of celiac disease: the average duration of breastfeeding was similar for children that developed celiac disease and for those that did not develop celiac disease (5.6 and 5.8 months, respectively); there was no significant difference in the percentage of children that developed celiac disease among children breastfed and in those never breastfed, and among those breastfed for more or less than 6 months; finally, there was no significant difference in the percentage of children that developed celiac disease among children that introduced gluten during breastfeeding and in those that introduced gluten without breastfeeding (Lionetti et al., 2014). The same results were reported by the PREVENT-CD study (Vriezinga et al., 2014). Therefore, although there are many good reasons to recommend prolonged breastfeeding of newborns, prospective studies have not confirmed any protective effect against celiac disease.

Two studies have subsequently analyzed the characteristics of powdered formulas and their relationship with the development of celiac disease. Hyytinen et al. analyzed whether there was a difference in genetically predisposed subjects in taking conventional artificial formula or extensively hydrolyzed formula during the first 6–8 months of life, finding no differences in the risk of celiac disease (Hyytinen et al., 2017). Segerstad et al. evaluated the risk of developing celiac disease in relation to artificial feeding in genetically predisposed subjects. They analyzed the amounts of powdered milk that infants ingested and observed that there were no differences in the development of the disease depending on the amount of powdered milk, although the follow-up was only 2 years, thus losing the diagnosis of those subjects who developed the disease years later (Segerstad et al., 2018).

### 14.2.5 HLA genotype

Both CELIPREV and PREVENT-CD showed that the risk of celiac disease was far higher among children with high-risk HLA (double copy of HLA-DQ2) than among those with a standard-risk HLA, confirming that predisposing HLA gene dosing is, at our knowledge, the most influential variable in increasing the risk to develop celiac disease (Lionetti et al., 2014; Vriezinga et al., 2014; Liu et al., 2014).

## 14.2.6 Intestinal microbiota

There is now accumulating evidence that gut microbiota plays an important role in the regulation of intestinal immune responses and in the maintenance of intestinal homeostasis. Most observational studies in children and adults have shown intestinal dysbiosis (i.e., altered gut microbiota composition or function) in celiac disease patients, untreated and treated with the gluten-free diet, compared to healthy controls (Cenit et al., 2015; Verdu et al., 2015; Cheng et al., 2013; Sánchez et al., 2013; Sellitto et al., 2012; Di Cagno et al., 2011; Collado et al., 2008). Recently, Zafeiropoulou et al. explored the gut microbiota and metabolome of patients with untreated celiac disease at onset, and healthy controls and found that 11 distinctive operational taxonomic units (OTUs) composed a microbe signature specific to celiac disease with high diagnostic probability; in detail, they identified two OTUs most characterizing celiac disease: OTU_53 Clostridium sensu stricto 1 and OTU_143 *Ruminococcus* (Zafeiropoulou et al., 2020). However, it still remains unclear whether the changes in the microbiota are a cause or a secondary consequence of celiac disease development.

Dysbiosis may be the result of both genetic and environmental factors. Specific host-genetic makeup could promote the colonization of pathobionts and reduce symbionts, thus leading to dysbiosis (Cenit et al., 2015). The genotype of infants at family risk of developing celiac disease, carrying the HLA-DQ2 haplotypes, has indeed been shown to influence the early gut microbiota composition, suggesting that a specific disease-biased host genotype may select for the first gut colonizers and could contribute to determining disease risk (Olivares et al., 2015). Recent studies also showed a significant association of celiac disease with homozygosity for a nonsense mutation in the fucosyltransferase 2 non-secretor status, which has been shown to be a major determinant for the gut microbial spectrum (Parmar et al., 2012). The non-secretor individuals were demonstrated to have an altered mucosa-associated microbiota in their intestinal tract, characterized by reduced diversity, richness, and abundance of *Bifidobacterium* spp., a bacterial genus that may play an important role in autoimmune disease risk (Wacklin et al., 2011, 2014b). Besides host genetics, environmental factors could also influence microbiota composition; indeed, the milk-feeding type (breast milk vs formula), the amount of gluten in the diet, the mode of delivery, antibiotics, and other drugs are also well-known environmental factors exerting a profound impact on the microbiota composition, potentially modifying its functional role in health and disease (Cenit et al., 2015; Martín-Masot et al., 2020). Interestingly, Sanz et al. analyzed samples from a sub-set of mothers ($n = 49$) included in the Prevent-CD project, whose children did or did not develop celiac disease and found that certain microbial species were more abundant in milk samples from mothers whose children developed celiac disease compared to those that remained healthy. These included increases in facultative methylotrophs such as *Methylobacterium komagatae* and *Methylocapsa palsarum* as well as in species such as *Bacteroides vulgatus*, that consumes fucosylated-oligosaccharides present in human milk, and other breast-abscess associated species. Theoretically, these microbiota components could be vertically transmitted from mothers-to-infants during breastfeeding, thereby influencing celiac disease risk (Benítez-Páez et al., 2020).

Intestinal dysbiosis might contribute to the pathophysiology of celiac disease by either providing proteolytic activities that influence the generation of toxic and immunogenic peptides from gluten and mediating host–microbe interactions, which could influence the intestinal barrier and immune function (e.g., via regulation of the cytokine network of proinflammatory and anti-inflammatory factors) (Cenit et al., 2015). Animal models, including germ-free and gnotobiotic models, will be of critical value to study whether the composition of the gut microbiota influences the loss of tolerance to gluten in genetically susceptible hosts and the mechanisms through which microbes can influence host responses to gluten. These types of studies will be helpful in determining causality, but their direct translational value might be limited due to the associated limitations with animal models of celiac disease. Thus, clinical studies will be needed to provide translational value of basic studies. Prospective studies in healthy infants at family risk of celiac disease are underway to decipher the co-evolution of the gut microbiome and the host genome in response to environmental factors and the possible causal relationships with celiac disease onset.

## 14.3 Conclusions

Initially suspected as major risk factors, both breastfeeding duration and age at gluten introduction were deemed less important or perhaps even irrelevant by two randomized clinical trials published in 2014 that failed to find an effect on the risk of celiac disease. Based on these results, a revision of the recommendations of the European Society of Gastroenterology, Hepatology and Pediatric Nutrition (ESPGHAN) on weaning (Committee on et al., 2008), which recommended the introduction of gluten from 4 to 7 months of age, during the "window of tolerance," and to introduce gluten while the infant is still being breastfed, in order to reduce the risk of celiac disease has been recently published (Szajewska et al., 2016). Since then attention has shifted, and some evidence emerged on the possible role of the quantity of gluten on the risk of celiac disease. The idea that nutrition in the first years of life is not the only factor for the development of the disease is gaining ground in the recent years, but it may concur with other risk factors (in particular infections in the first years of life) to the development of CD.

## 14.4 Future trends and research

Further studies are needed to determine whether nutrition in early infancy together with other environmental factors, such as infections, the composition of the intestinal microbiota, the metabolic profile, the vaccination program, the use of antibiotics or other drugs, and the intrauterine and perinatal exposures, actually influence the balance between the tolerance and abnormal immune response to gluten.

## Sources of additional information

1. www.espghan.org/guidelines/gastroenterology/
2. www.early-nutrition.org/
3. http://www.nejm.org/doi/full/10.1056/NEJMoa1400697

4. Marild, K., Ye, W., Lebwohl, B., Green, P.H., Blaser, M.J., Card, T., Ludvigsson, J.F., 2013. Antibiotic exposure and the development of coeliac disease: a nationwide case-control study. BMC Gastroenterol. 13, 109.

5. Meji, T.G., Budding, A.E., Grasman, M.E., Kneepkens, C.M., Savelkoul, P.H., Mearin, M.L., 2013. Composition and diversity of the duodenal mucosa-associated microbiome in children with untreated coeliac disease. Scand. J. Gastroenterol. 48, 530–536.

6. Norris, J.M., Barriga, K., Klingensmith, G., Hoffman, M., Eisenbarth, G.S., Erwlich, H.A., Rewers, M., 2003. Timing of initial cereal exposure in infancy and risk of islet autoimmunity. JAMA 290, 1713–1720.

7. Wacklin, P., Laurikka, P., Lindfors, K., Collin, P., Salmi, T., Lahdeaho, M.-L., Saavalainen, P., Maki, M., Matto, J., Kurppa, K., et al., 2014a. Altered duodenal microbiota composition in celiac disease patients suffering from persistent symptoms on a long-term gluten-free diet. Am. J. Gastroenterol. 109, 1933–1941.

# References

Abadie, V., Sollid, L.M., Barreiro, L.B., Jabri, B., 2011. Integration of genetic and immunological insights into a model of celiac disease pathogenesis. Annu. Rev. Immunol. 29, 493–525.

Akobeng, A.K., Ramanan, A.V., Buchan, I., Heller, R.F., 2006. Effect of breast feeding on risk of coeliac disease: a systematic review and meta-analysis of observational studies. Arch. Dis. Child. 91, 39–43.

Andrén Aronsson, C., Lee, H.S., Hård Af Segerstad, E.M., Uusitalo, U., Yang, J., Koletzko, S., Liu, E., Kurppa, K., Bingley, P.J., Toppari, J., Ziegler, A.G., She, J.X., Hagopian, W.A., Rewers, M., Akolkar, B., Krischer, J.P., Virtanen, S.M., Norris, J.M., Agardh, D., TEDDY Study Group, 2019. Association of gluten intake during the first 5 years of life with incidence of celiac disease autoimmunity and celiac disease among children at increased risk. JAMA 13 (322), 514–523.

Andrén Aronsson, C., Lee, H.S., Koletzko, S., et al., for the TEDDY Study Group, 2016. Effects of gluten intake on risk of celiac disease: a case-control study on a Swedish birth cohort. Clin. Gastroenterol. Hepatol. 14, 403–409.

Auricchio, S., Follo, D., de Ritis, G., Giunta, A., Marzorati, D., Prampolini, L., Ansaldi, N., Levi, P., Dall'Olio, D., Bossi, A., 1983. Does breast feeding protect against the development of clinical symptoms of celiac disease in children? J. Pediatr. Gastroenterol. Nutr. 2, 428–433.

Bach, J.F., 2002. The effect of infections on susceptibility to autoimmune and allergic diseases. N. Engl. J. Med. 347, 911–920.

Benítez-Páez, A, Olivares, M, Szajewska, H, Pieścik-Lech, M, Polanco, I, Castillejo, G, Nuñez, M, Ribes-Koninckx, C, Korponay-Szabó, IR, Koletzko, S, Meijer, CR, Mearin, ML, Sanz, Y, 2020. Breast-milk microbiota linked to celiac disease development in children: a pilot study from the prevent CD cohort. Front. Microbiol. 11, 1335.

Catassi, C., Kryszak, D., Bhatti, B., Sturgeon, C., Helzlsouer, K., Clipp, S.L., Gelfond, D., Puppa, E., Sferruzza, A., Fasano, A., 2010. Natural history of celiac disease autoimmunity in a USA cohort followed since 1974. Ann. Med. 42, 530–538.

Cenit, M.C., Olivares, M., Codoñer-Franch, P., Sanz, Y., 2015. Intestinal microbiota and celiac disease: cause, consequence or co-evolution? Nutrients 7, 6900–6923.

Cheng, J., Kalliomäki, M., Heilig, H.G., Palva, A., Lähteenoja, H., de Vos, W.M., Salojärvi, J., Satokari, R., 2013. Duodenal microbiota composition and mucosal homeostasis in pediatric celiac disease. BMC Gastroenterol. 13, 113.

Choung, R.S., Larson, S.A., Khaleghi, S., Rubio-Tapia, A., Ovsyannikova, I.G., King, K.S., Larson, J.J., Lahr, B.D., Poland, G.A., Camilleri, M.J., Murray, J.A., 2017. Prevalence and morbidity of undiagnosed celiac disease from a community-based study. Gastroenterology 152, 830–839.

Collado, M.C., Donat, E., Ribes-Koninckx, C., Calabuig, M., Sanz, Y., 2008. Imbalances in faecal and duodenal bifidobacterium species composition in active and non-active coeliac disease. BMC Microbiol. 8, 232.

Di Cagno, R., de Angelis, M., de Pasquale, I., Ndagijimana, M., Vernocchi, P., Ricciuti, P., Gagliardi, F., Laghi, L., Crecchio, C., Guerzoni, M.E., et al., 2011. Duodenal and faecal microbiota of celiac children: molecular, phenotype and metabolome characterization. BMC Microbiol. 11, 219.

ESPGHAN, Committee, on Nutrition, Agostoni, C., Decsi, T., Fewtrell, M., Goulet, O., Kolacek, S., Koletzko, B., Michaelsen, K.F., Moreno, L., Puntis, J., Rigo, J., Shamir, R., Szajewska, H., Turck, D., van Goudoever, J., 2008. Complementary feeding: a commentary by the ESPGHAN committee on nutrition. J. Pediatr. Gastroenterol. Nutr. 46, 99–110.

Fasano, A., Catassi, C., 2012. Celiac disease. N. Engl. J. Med. 367, 2419–2426.

Gatti, S., Lionetti, E., Balanzoni, L., Verma, A.K., Galeazzi, T., Gesuita, R., Scattolo, N., Cinquetti, M., Fasano, A., Catassi, C., 2020. Increased prevalence of celiac disease in school-age children in Italy. Clin. Gastroenterol. Hepatol. 18, 596–603.

Greco, L., Auricchio, S., Mayer, M., Grimaldi, M., 1988. Case control study on nutritional risk factors in celiac disease. J. Pediatr. Gastroenterol. Nutr. 7, 395–399.

Hyytinen, M.M., Savilahti, E., Virtanen, S.M., Härkönen, T., Ilonen, J., Luopajärvi, K., Uibo, R., Vaarala, O., Åkerblom, H.K., Knip, M., 2017. Avoidance of cow's milk-based formula for at-risk infants does not reduce development of celiac disease: a randomized controlled trial. Gastroenterology 153, 961–970.

Ivarsson, A., Persson, L.A., Nyström, L., Ascher, H., Cavell, B., Danielsson, L., Dannaeus, A., Lindberg, T., Lindquist, B., Stenhammar, L., Hernell, O., 2000. Epidemic of coeliac disease in Swedish children. Acta Paediatr. 89, 165–171.

Ivarsson, A., Hernell, O., Stenlund, H., Persson, L.A., 2002. Breast-feeding protects against celiac disease. Am. J. Clin. Nutr. 75, 914–921.

Ivarsson, A., Myléus, A., Norström, F., van der Pals, M., Rosén, A., Högberg, L., Danielsson, L., Halvarsson, B., Hammarroth, S., Hernell, O., Karlsson, E., Stenhammar, L., Webb, C., Sandström, O., Carlsson, A., 2013. Prevalence of childhood celiac disease and changes in infant feeding. Pediatrics 131, 687–694.

Jansen, M.A.E., Tromp, I.I.M., Kiefte-de Jong, J.C., et al., 2014. Infant feeding and anti-tissue transglutaminase antibody concentrations in the Generation RStudy. Am. J. Clin. Nutr. 100, 1095–1101.

Lindfors, K., Ciacci, C., Kurppa, K., Lundin, K.E.A., Makharia, G.K., Mearin, M.L., Murray, J.A., Verdu, E.F., Kaukinen, K., 2019. Coeliac disease. Nat. Rev. Dis. Primers 5, 3.

Lionetti, E., Catassi, C., 2011. New clues in celiac disease epidemiology, pathogenesis, clinical manifestations, and treatment. Int. Rev. Immunol. 30, 219–231.

Lionetti, E., Castellaneta, S., Francavilla, R., Pulvirenti, A., Tonutti, E., Amarri, S., Barbato, M., Barbera, C., Barera, G., Bellantoni, A., Castellano, E., Guariso, G., Limongelli, M.G., Pellegrino, S., Polloni, C., Ughi, C., Zuin, G., Fasano, A., Catassi, C., 2014. SIGENP (Italian Society of Pediatric Gastroenterology, hepatology, and nutrition) working group on weaning and celiac disease risk. Introduction of gluten, HLA status, and the risk of celiac disease in children. N. Engl. J. Med. 371, 1295–1303.

Lionetti, E., Gatti, S., Pulvirenti, A., Catassi, C., 2015. Celiac disease from a global perspective. Best Pract. Res. Clin. Gastroenterol. 29, 365–379.

Liu, E., Lee, H.S., Aronsson, C.A., Hagopian, W.A., Koletzko, S., Rewers, M.J., Eisenbarth, G.S., Bingley, P.J., Bonifacio, E., Simell, V., Agardh, D., 2014. TEDDY study group. Risk of pediatric celiac disease according to HLA haplotype and country. N. Engl. J. Med. 371, 42–49.

Logan, K., Perkin, M.R., Marrs, T., Radulovic, S., Craven, J., Flohr, C., Bahnson, H.T., Lack, G., 2020. Early gluten introduction and celiac disease in the EAT study: a prespecified analysis of the EAT randomized clinical trial. JAMA Pediatr. 174, 1041–1047.

Lohi, S., Mustalahti, K., Kaukinen, K., Laurila, K., Collin, P., Rissanen, H., Lohi, O., Bravi, E., Gasparin, M., Reunanen, A., Mäki, M., 2007. Increasing prevalence of coeliac disease over time. Aliment. Pharmacol. Ther. 26, 1217–1225.

Lund-Blix, N.A., Marild, K., Tapia, G., Norris, J.M., Stene, L.C., Størdal, K., 2019. Gluten intake in early child- hood and risk of celiac disease in childhood: a nationwide cohort study. Am. J. Gastroenterol. 114, 1299–1306.

Mårild, K., Dong, F., Lund-Blix, N.A., Seifert, J., Barón, A.E., Waugh, K.C., Taki, I., Størdal, K., Tapia, G., Stene, L.C., Johnson, R.K., Liu, E., Rewers, M.J., Norris, J.M., 2019. Gluten intake and risk of celiac disease: long-term follow-up of an at-risk birth cohort. Am. J. Gastroenterol. 114, 1307–1314.

Martín-Masot, R., Diaz-Castro, J., Moreno-Fernandez, J., Navas-López, V.M., Nestares, T., 2020. The role of early programming and early nutrition on the development and progression of celiac disease: a review. Nutrients 12 (11), 3427.

Norris, J.M., Barriga, K., Hoffenberg, E.J., Taki, I., Miao, D., Haas, J.E., Emery, L.M., Sokol, R.J., Erlich, H.A., Eisenbarth, G.S., Rewers, M., 2005. Risk of celiac disease autoimmunity and timing of gluten introduction in the diet of infants at increased risk of disease. JAMA 293, 2343–2451.

Olivares, M., Neef, A., Castillejo, G., Palma, G.D., Varea, V., Capilla, A., Palau, F., Nova, E., Marcos, A., Polanco, I., et al., 2015. The HLA-DQ2 genotype selects for early intestinal microbiota composition in infants at high risk of developing coeliac disease. Gut 64, 406–417.

Parmar, A.S., Alakulppi, N., Paavola-Sakki, P., Kurppa, K., Halme, L., Färkkilä, M., Turunen, U., Lappalainen, M., Kontula, K., Kaukinen, K., et al., 2012. Association study of FUT2 (rs601338) with celiac disease and inflammatory bowel disease in the Finnish population. Tissue Antigens 80, 488–493.

Peters, U., Schneeweiss, S., Trautwein, E.A., Erbersdobler, H.F., 2001. A case-control study of the effect of infant feeding on celiac disease. Ann. Nutr. Metab. 45, 135–142.

Sánchez, E., Donat, E., Ribes-Koninckx, C., Fernández-Murga, M.L., Sanz, Y., 2013. Duodenalmucosal bacteria associated with celiac disease in children. Appl. Environ. Microbiol. 79, 5472–5479.

Segerstad, E.M.H.A., Lee, H., Aronsson, C.A., Yang, J., Uusitalo, U., Sjöholm, I., Rayner, M., Kurppa, K., Virtanen, S.M., Norris, J.M., 2018. Daily intake of milk powder and risk of celiac disease in early childhood: a nested case-control study. Nutrients 10, 550.

Sellitto, M., Bai, G., Serena, G., Fricke, W.F., Sturgeon, C., Gajer, P., White, J.R., Koenig, S.S., Sakamoto, J., Boothe, D., et al., 2012. Proof of concept of microbiome-metabolome analysis and delayed gluten exposure on celiac disease autoimmunity in genetically at-risk infants. PLoS One 7, e33387.

Singh, P., Arora, A., Strand, T.A., Leffler, D.A., Catassi, C., Green, P.H., Kelly, C.P., Ahuja, V., Makharia, G.K., 2018. Global prevalence of celiac disease: systematic review and meta-analysis. Clin. Gastroenterol. Hepatol. 16, 823–836.

Størdal, K., White, R.A., Eggesbø, M., 2013. Early feeding and risk of celiac disease in a prospective birth cohort. Pediatrics 132, 1202–1209.

Szajewska, H., Chmielewska, A., Pieścik-Lech, M., Ivarsson, A., Kolacek, S., Koletzko, S., Mearin, M.L., Shamir, R., Auricchio, R., Troncone, R., 2012. PREVENTceliac disease study group. Systematic review: early infant feeding and the prevention of coeliac disease. Aliment. Pharmacol. Ther. 36, 607–618.

Szajewska, H., Shamir, R., Mearin, L., Ribes-Koninckx, C., Catassi, C., Domellof, M., Fewtrell, M.S., Husby, S., Papadopoulou, A., Vandenplas, Y., Castillejo, G., Kolacek, S., Koletzko, S., Korponay-Szabo, I.R., Kionetti, E., Polanco, I., Troncone, R., 2016. Gluten introduction and the risk of coeliac disease: a position paper by the European Society for Paediatric Gastroenterology. Hepatology and nutrition. J. Pediatr. Gastroenterol. Nutr. 62, 507–513.

Verdu, E.F., Galipeau, H.J., Jabri, B., 2015. Novel players in coeliac disease pathogenesis: role of the gut microbiota. Nat. Rev. Gastroenterol. Hepatol. 12, 497–506.

Vriezinga, S.L., Auricchio, R., Bravi, E., Castillejo, G., Chmielewska, A., Crespo Escobar, P., Kolac̆ek, S., Koletzko, S., Korponay-Szabo, I.R., Mummert, E., Polanco, I., Putter, H., Ribes Koninckx, C., Shamir, R., Szajewska, H., Werkstetter, K., Greco, L., Gyimesi, J., Hartman, C., Hogen Esch, C., Hopman, E., Ivarsson, A., Koltai, T., Koning, F., Martinez-Ojinaga, E., te Marvelde, C., Pavic, A., Romanos, J., Stoopman, E., Villanacci, V., Wijmenga, C., Troncone, R., Mearin, M.L., 2014. Randomized feeding intervention in infants at high risk for celiac disease. N. Engl. J. Med. 371, 1304–1315.

Wacklin, P., Mäkivuokko, H., Alakulppi, N., Nikkilä, J., Tenkanen, H., Räbinä, J., Partanen, J., Aranko, K., Mättö, J., 2011. Secretor genotype (FUT2 gene) is strongly associated with the composition of bifidobacteria in the human intestine. PLoS One 6, e20113.

Wacklin, P., Tuimala, J., Nikkilä, J., Sebastian, T., Mäkivuokko, H., Alakulppi, N., Laine, P., Rajilic-Stojanovic, M., Paulin, L., de Vos, W.M., et al., 2014b. Faecal microbiota composition in adults is associated with the FUT2 gene determining the secretor status. PLoS One 14, e94863.

Wolters, V.M., Wijmenga, C., 2008. Genetic background of celiac disease and its clinical implications. Am. J. Gastroenterol. 103, 190–195.

Zafeiropoulou, K., Nichols, B., Mackinder, M., Biskou, O., Rizou, E., Karanikolou, A., Clark, C., Buchanan, E., Cardigan, T., Duncan, H., Wands, D., Russell, J., Hansen, R., Russell, R.K., McGrogan, P., Edwards, C.A., Ijaz, U.Z., Gerasimidis, K., 2020. Alterations in intestinal microbiota of children with celiac disease at the time of diagnosis and on a gluten-free diet. Gastroenterology 159, 2039–2051.

# Early nutrition and its effect on the development of functional gastrointestinal disorders

*Silvia Salvatore[a] and Yvan Vandenplas[b]*

[a]Pediatric Department, Hospital "F. Del Ponte," University of Insubria, Varese, Italy
[b]Vrije Universiteit Brussel, UZ Brussel, KidZ Health Castle, Brussels, Belgium

## LEARNING OBJECTIVES

[3–5 learning objectives for academic use of chapter]
Review the information supporting the following key messages:

- Functional gastrointestinal disorders (FGIDs) in infants are toddlers are frequent as ~50% of infants can present with at least one FGID.

- About half of infants in the general population present with more than one FGID.

- FGIDs have short and long-term negative consequences on health and quality of life.

- The gastrointestinal microbiota composition plays a significant role in the pathogenesis of certain FGIDs.

- Dietary interventions, including restoring a balanced gastrointestinal microbiota, have shown safety and varying degrees of efficacy for the prevention and management of FGIDs in infants and toddlers

## 15.1 Introduction

Functional gastrointestinal (GI) symptoms are accompaniments to physiological development or arise from maladaptive behavioral responses to internal or external stimuli (Shamir et al., 2013). The Rome IV consensus proposes definitions and diagnostic criteria for FGIDs but does not include management recommendations (Benninga et al., 2016).

During infancy, according to a systematic review, FGIDs such as regurgitation, infantile colic, and constipation occur in almost half of the infants. Each of these FGIDs is reported to occur in 10%–25% (Vandenplas et al., 2015a). Their prevalence shows geographical differences. FGIDs are commonly discussed separately. However, a highly variable number of infants presents with a combination of FGIDs: 4.2% according to data from The Netherlands, Belgium, and Italy (Steutel et al., 2020), 35% according to data from Turkey (Beser et al., 2021) 50% according to data from Africa (Bellaiche et al., 2020)and 75% according to data from France (Bellaiche et al., 2018). Up to 15% of infants may present simultaneously three or more FGIDs (Bellaiche et al., 2018).

FGIDs are a cause of parental stress and anxiety. As a consequence, FGIDs during infancy are a major reason for parents to consult healthcare providers (HCPs), as they are searching for a remedy to decrease these manifestations that impact quality of life.

Recent and growing evidence indicates that the gastrointestinal microbiota of the infant can play a major role in the pathogenesis of FGIDs in childhood. Studies have suggested that gut bacteria can impact neurological outcomes–altering behavior and potentially affecting the onset and/or severity of nervous system disorders (Sampson and Mazmanian, 2015). Germ-free mice display alterations in stress-responsivity, central neurochemistry, and behavior indicative of a reduction in anxiety in comparison to conventional mice (Cryan and O'Mahony, 2011). Steenbergen et al. showed evidence that the intake of probiotics may help reduce negative thoughts associated with sad mood (Steenbergen et al., 2015). A review by Mohajeri et al. provided evidence for communication between the GI microbiome and brain function in adults: probiotics were shown to have an influence on cognitive function and mood (Mohajeri et al., 2018). The precocious neural maturation in stressed infants is prevented by a non-invasive probiotic treatment in infant rats (Cowan et al., 2019). Sialic acid and sialylated oligosaccharide supplementation during lactation improve learning and memory in rats (Oliveros et al., 2018). In infants, the gastrointestinal microbiota composition at the age of 1 year was shown to be associated with cognitive function at the age of 2 years (Carlson et al., 2018).

## 15.2 FGIDS and consequences

Traditionally, FGIDs during infancy are considered to be benign as they are transient and self-limiting conditions. But FGIDs often frustrate parents and caregivers, impair parental-child interaction and behavior (Salvatore et al., 2018a, b, c). The occurrence of FGIDs, especially infant colic and crying, has been associated with a shorter duration of breastfeeding (Hazard Ratio=2.4, 95% CI 1.4 to 4.2; $P=0.001$) (Howard et al., 2006). Multiple vs single FGIDs are even more likely to be associated with: shorter duration of breastfeeding, but also with lower weight gain, increased drug prescriptions, slower recovery, decreased quality of life (Bellaiche et al., 2018).

Infants presenting with infantile colic have a two to five times higher risk to present with other FGIDs as well (Vandenplas et al., 2017a, b). Families with colicky infants had more distress 3 years later (Rautava et al., 1995). A prospective follow-up study suggested that early bouts of unsoothable crying represent an early manifestation of abdominal pain-related FGIDs at the age of 13 years (Pärtty et al., 2013). Children with abdominal pain-related FGIDs at 7.9 years of age had a two to five times higher prevalence of GI distress during the first 3 months of life (Indrio et al., 2015).

According to Savino et al., infants with severe colic are at increased risk to present at the age of 10 years more frequently with allergic, gastrointestinal, and behavioral disease (Savino et al., 2005a, b). Data suggest that functional GI symptoms, such as infantile colic, may be associated with multiple disorders, such as recurrent abdominal pain, migraine, allergic manifestations, sleep disturbances, and maladaptive behavior, and also aggressiveness later in life (Sillanpää and Saarinen, 2015). A number of studies reported an increased risk of emotional, behavioral, and cognitive disturbances, reduced joy, and selective eating during childhood in ex-colicky children compared to non-colic matches (Canivet et al., 2000; Neu and Robinson, 2003; Santos et al., 2015; Rao et al., 2004; Lemcke et al., 2016).

Infants spilling more than 90 days during the first 2 years of life are more likely to have GER symptoms at 9 years of age (Martin et al., 2002). The majority of infants presenting with constipation will improve over time, but some of them remain at increased risk for relapse (Pijpers et al., 2010).

In summary: the standard statement "that FGIDs in infants are benign since they are transient" is challenged by many data from the literature that report a relationship between early life FGIDs and long-term consequences during child- and adulthood. However, there are no data that evaluated if an early intervention does change the natural evolution and association with other FGIDs later in life. Studies evaluating the long-term effect of early intervention are a research priority.

## 15.3 Infants (0–12 months)

### 15.3.1 Breastfeeding

None of the FGIDs in infants are a reason to stop breastfeeding (Vandenplas et al., 2016).

Constipation is much more frequent in formula-fed than in breastfed infants, as it occurs in 1% of exclusively breastfed infants and in almost 10% of formula-fed infants (Tunc et al., 2008). While breastfed infants generally produce soft stools ranging in frequency from 1 per 7 days to 7 stools per day, extremes of up to 12 times a day or once in 3–4 weeks are reported (Vandenplas et al., 2016). It is not clear if regurgitation occurs more frequently in formula-fed than in breastfed infants. While some authors report the same frequency in formula and breastfed infants, others report a higher incidence in formula-fed infants (Hegar et al., 2009; Miyazawa et al., 2002; Martin et al., 2002; Osatakul et al., 2002).

Exclusively breastfed infants have a significantly lower incidence and severity of irritability and colic episodes, and longer nocturnal sleep than formula-fed infants (Cohen Engler et al., 2012). This could be partially related to the content of melatonin in breast milk. Indeed, melatonin has a hypnotic and relaxing effect on the smooth muscle of the GI tract, and is secreted during the night in adults but not in infants (Cohen Engler et al., 2012). The enterochromaffin cells of the GI tract secrete 400 times as much melatonin as the pineal gland (Werbach, 2008). Although melatonin has not been used in the treatment of GER-disease, there are indications that melatonin reduces GER (Brzozowska et al., 2014).

In summary: overall, there are indications that breastfed infants develop less frequently FGIDs than formula-fed ones. The role of the duration of exclusive breastfeeding on the development of FGIDs in older children, adolescents, and adults is not known. However, the exact role of breastfeeding is difficult to substantiate, since studies comparing breast- to formula feeding cannot be randomized, and numerous confounding variables are known to intervene.

## 15.3.2 Formula feeding

### 15.3.2.1 Regurgitation

Regurgitation can be a consequence of inappropriate formula preparation, feeding technique, and most of all of overfeeding. Therefore, the management of regurgitation starts with the reassurance of parents and nutritional management by adapting the frequency and volume of feeds (Rosen et al., 2018). Thickened formula or anti-regurgitation (AR) formula decreases regurgitation (Rosen et al., 2018; Salvatore et al., 2018a, b, c). Commercialized AR-formulas (contain different thickening agents: processed rice, corn or potato starch, guar gum, or locust bean gum. Because of the absence of comparative trials, there are insufficient data to recommend one thickener over another (Salvatore et al., 2018a, b, c). If commercial AR formula is not available, a thickening product can be used. Locust bean gum does not increase the caloric density, but may cause bloating (Meunier et al., 2014). A large study in over 2500 infants showed that locust bean gum-thickened formula decreases infant regurgitation, is well tolerated, and improves quality of life of the infants and parents (Tounian et al., 2020). In the past, insufficient attention may have been given to the fact that improvement of regurgitation with thickened formula is observed within the first week, often even more rapid. Bean gum does not change stool composition and frequency (Tounian et al., 2020). Cereals increase caloric intake, possibly inducing excessive weight gain and altering the fat and protein-energy ratio. Home thickening" of a regular formula increases the osmolarity, which may increase the number of transient lower esophageal sphincter relaxations (Vandenplas et al., 2009) and may delay gastric emptying time, and thus have negative effects.

In an infant with persistent and recurrent regurgitation, unresponsive to thickened formula, especially when associated with other manifestations of allergic disease, such as atopic dermatitis and/or wheezing, cow's milk allergy (CMA) should be suspected (Vandenplas et al., 2016). The cow milk-related symptom score (CoMiSS) may help to recognize infants with cow's milk-related manifestations (Vandenplas et al., 2015b). Extensive cow's milk-based hydrolysates are recommended in the management of CMA, but rice hydrolysates may be considered as well. A thickened extensive hydrolysate has the advantage to treat CMA and regurgitation, but does as a consequence, not allow to differentiate between both the conditions (Vandenplas and De Greef, 2014). The gastric emptying of a protein hydrolysate is faster than that of intact protein, which may decrease regurgitation (Vandenplas et al., 2016): improvement of GER with a hydrolysate may be due to faster gastric emptying and is not a proof of allergy.

Limited literature suggests that specific probiotics (*Lactobacillus reuteri* DSM 17938) and prebiotics prevent regurgitation and may fasten gastric emptying (Indrio et al., 2014; Savino et al., 2005a, b).

There is no indication for drug treatment in "happy spitters," while alginate may be useful in the management of troublesome regurgitation (Savino et al., 2005a, b; Tighe et al., 2014). Proton pump inhibitors do not decrease infant regurgitation. This drug class does also not decrease crying, distress, or irritability in infants who do not suffer acid GER-disease

Stepwise approach for infants with persistent (≥1 week) regurgitation and distress

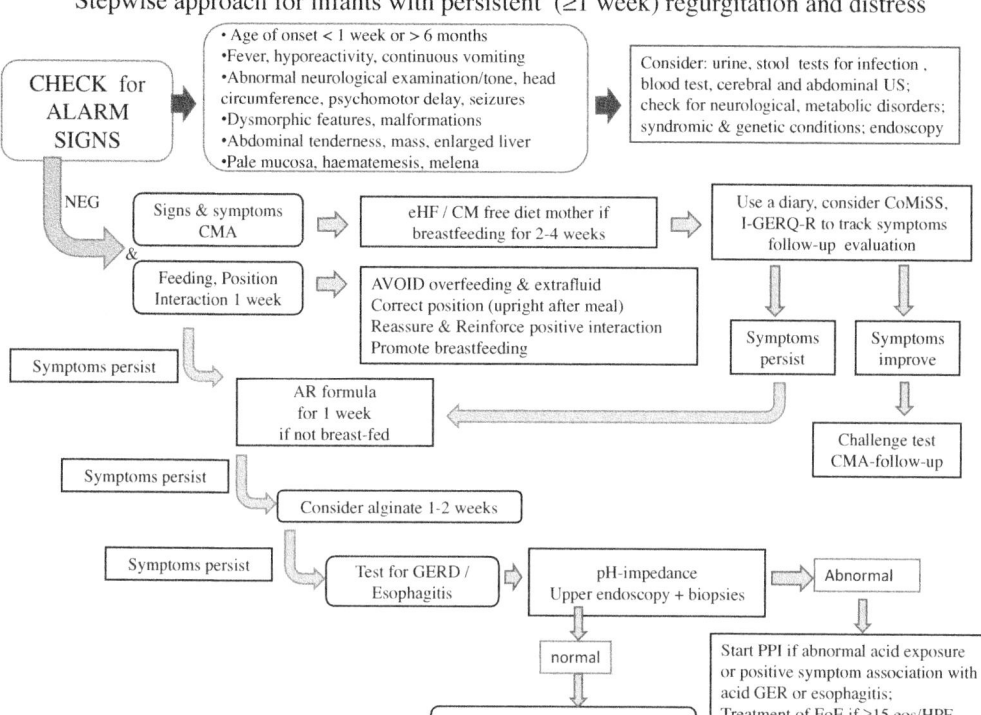

**FIG. 15.1** Algorithm for the approach of troublesome infant regurgitation. *AR*: anti-regurgitation; *CMA*: cow's milk allergy; *CoMiSS*: cow's milk related symptom score; *eHF*: extensively hydrolyzed formula; *EoE*: eosinophilic esophagitis; *Eos*: eosinophils; *GERD*: gastro-esophageal reflux disease; *HPF*: high power field; *I-GERQ-R*: infant gastro-esophageal reflux questionnaire—revised; *NEG*: negative; *PPI*: proton pump inhibitor; *US*: ultrasound.

(Gieruszczak-Białek et al., 2015). Moreover, proton pump inhibitors cause dysbiosis resulting in small intestinal bacterial overgrowth and increasing the risk for respiratory and gastrointestinal tract infections (Levy et al., 2020) (Fig. 15.1).

In summary, AR-formula does what it has to do: decrease regurgitation, and as a consequence, reassure parents, and improve quality of life of the family. There are no data to support that management of troublesome regurgitation in infants has an impact on the risk of developing FGIDs later in life.

### 15.3.2.2 Constipation

Traditionally, stool composition is described using the Bristol stool scale, which was developed for adults and is inappropriate to describe stool consistency in non-toilet trained children. The Brussels Infants and Toddlers Stool Scale (BITSS) has been developed to better describe stool consistency in non-toilet trained children (Huysentruyt et al., 2019). A digital tool was developed to describe stool consistency more objectively (Ludwig et al., 2021).

Hard stools are frequent in infants fed formula containing palm oil, which is rich in palmitic acid that is found mainly at the Sn-1 and Sn-3 positions (with Sn being an abbreviation for stereospecific numbering). In mother's milk, palmitic acid is mainly in the Sn-2 position (Lasekan et al., 2017). The Sn-1 and Sn-3 positions can be broken down by lipase, and displaced palmitic acid favors the formation of calcium soaps, responsible for the hard stools. Whereas palmitic acid in the Sn-2 position is not broken down by lipase, remains intact, and thus does not form calcium soaps since it does not bind with calcium ions.

In children with food-related chronic constipation, an increase in both rectal mast cell density and spatial interactions between mast cells and nerve fibers correlates with anal motor abnormalities was described (Borrelli et al., 2009).

Constipation is in some infants related to the intake of cow's milk protein because of allergy (seldom) or the formation of calcium soaps (frequent). The first step in the management of functional constipation is parental education and reassurance (Vandenplas et al., 2016; Tabbers et al., 2011, 2014). Different nutritional options have been proposed, but dietary changes were reported to resolve constipation less effectively than laxatives (Tabbers et al., 2014; Salvatore, 2007). Both milk of magnesia and polyethylene glycol are efficient and safe in infants and toddlers (Tabbers et al., 2014). Polyethylene glycol is registered in most countries from the age of 6 months onwards and is at least equally effective as lactulose and has fewer adverse effects of gassiness and bloating (Tabbers et al., 2014). Juices containing sorbitol, such as prune, pear, and apple juices, decrease constipation but induce a risk for unbalanced nutrition (Tabbers et al., 2014). Glycerine suppositories can be helpful if acute relief by rectal emptying is needed (Tabbers et al., 2014). Evidence does not support the use of mineral oil (risk of lipoid pneumonia due to aspiration) or enemas (e.g., phosphate) in young infants (Tabbers et al., 2014).

## 15.4 Hydrolysates can soften the stools

Manipulation of the GI microbiome in constipated infants has been poorly studied. *L. reuteri* DSM 17938 has been reported to increase stool frequency in a study in healthy infants (Indrio et al., 2014). Another study showed that *L. reuteri* DSM 17938 increases bowel movements in constipated infants, without difference in consistency and crying episodes (Coccorullo et al., 2010). Some "anti-constipation formulae" have a high content of magnesium, although within regulatory limits (Tabbers et al., 2014). Infant formula with high magnesium levels was shown to increase stool frequency, reduce stool consistency, and defecation related pain (Benninga et al., 2019). A formula with a partial whey hydrolysate supplemented with the same *L. reuteri* and high levels of magnesium was shown to reduce constipation from 18.8% to 6.5% within a time frame of 3 days (Vandenplas et al., 2021). An underpowered study performed with a partial hydrolysate, a prebiotic, and beta-palmitate (palmitic acid enriched at the Sn-2 position) showed a trend for a softer stool consistency (Bongers et al., 2007). Supplementation of infant formula with prebiotics (in particular a specific combination of fructo- and galacto-oligosaccharides) and synbiotics has been shown to increase stool frequency and soften stool consistency (Vlieger et al., 2009; Moro et al., 2003). Only 3.2% of infants fed a formula with synbiotics (*Bifidobacterium lactis* and fructo-oligosaccharides) presented with constipation, which is a lower incidence than that reported in the literature in formula-fed infants (Vandenplas et al., 2017b) (Fig. 15.2).

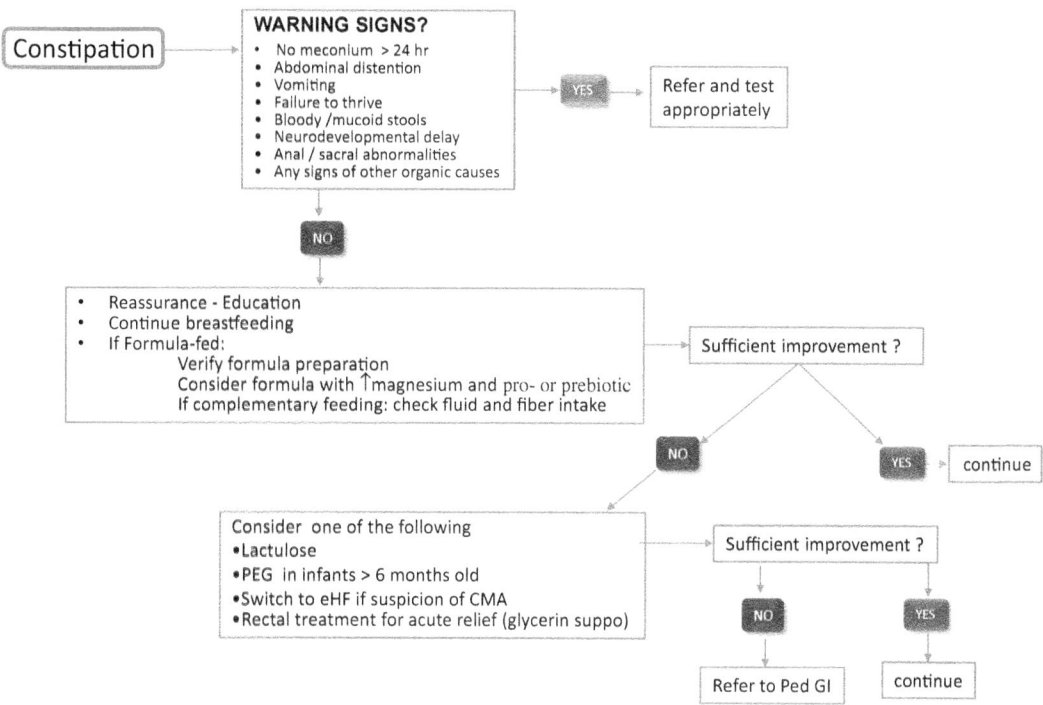

FIG. 15.2   Algorithm for the approach of infant constipation. *CMA*: cow's milk allergy; *eHF*: extensively hydrolyzed formula; *PEG*: polyethylene glycol; *Ped GI*: pediatric gastroenterologist.

In summary, several infant formulas with adapted protein and lipid composition, with high magnesium content, and with "biotics" have been shown to increase stool frequency and decrease stool consistency. The impact on the persistence of constipation later in life or the development of other FGIDs has not been studied.

## 15.4.1 Infantile colic

The cardinal manifestation of infantile colic is excessive, persistent, unconsolable, or unsoothable loud crying, especially in the late afternoon. During each episode the child appears irritable, distressed, and fussy, flexes the hip joints, becomes red-faced, and has episodes of borborygmi. In the absence of warning signs (Vandenplas et al., 2016), caregivers should be reassured and supported (Salvatore et al., 2018a, b, c). Parents may misinterpret crying and distress in infants, and should be educated on the recognition of signs of hunger and fatigue, and instructed on offering structure and regularity. Since infantile colic is a multi-factorial condition, it is unlikely that a single intervention will significantly reduce infantile colic in an unselected population. Selection of patients is likely to be a major bias in these studies.

Infants with colic vs non-colicky infants have slower colonization, lower diversity, and stability of their GI microbiome (de Weerth et al., 2013). Colicky infants have fewer butyrate-producing species and more proteobacteria, including species producing gas and inflammation, decreased levels of lactobacilli and bifidobacteria, including species with anti-inflammatory effects (de Weerth et al., 2013). Infantile colic is associated with increased levels of fecal calprotectin and low-grade systemic inflammation (Pärtty and Kalliomäki, 2017; Savino et al., 2018).

Preparations containing fennel oil appear to some extent effective for reducing colic (Harb et al., 2016). Limited literature suggests that a transient low lactase activity can trigger excessive crying (Hall et al., 2012; Kanabar et al., 2001). After some initial enthusiasm about the role of administration of lactase, negative results suggest a minor role of lactase in infantile colic (Hall et al., 2012). The evidence for maternal dietary manipulation, lactase, sucrose, glucose, and simethicone is weak (Harb et al., 2016). The NICE guidelines propose a two-week trial of lactase drops in breastfed and formula-fed infants, although the evidence for this recommendation is limited. A preventive trial with a formula containing a stable lactase and postbiotics as the result of a fermentation process indicated a decreased incidence of infant crying at the age of 4 weeks (Vandenplas et al., 2014b).

Low-quality studies report a reduction in crying time with soy formula (Vandenplas et al., 2016; Hall et al., 2012). In selected formula-fed infants, there is some evidence that an extensively hydrolyzed protein formula reduces infantile colic (Vandenplas et al., 2016). A partially hydrolyzed protein formula has also been shown to be beneficial (Vandenplas et al., 2014a). Most of these formulae are lactose-reduced or lactose-free and contain prebiotics or probiotics, which all may contribute to a reduction of crying time (Hall et al., 2012; Vandenplas et al., 2014a).

A double-blind, placebo-controlled trial with a partial hydrolysate, with beta-palmitate and a specific prebiotic mixture of galacto- and fructooligosaccharides showed a significant decrease of infantile colic within 1 week of intervention (Savino et al., 2006). A partial whey hydrolysate, synbiotic, and reduced lactose significantly reduced the duration of crying and improved quality of life of the parents and infants (Xinias et al., 2017). Infants with colic treated with *L. reuteri* for 30 days had a significantly decreased crying time and an increased FOXP3 concentration, resulting in a decreased RORγ/FOXP3 ratio (Savino et al., 2018). The probiotic treatment also reduced fecal calprotectin (Savino et al., 2018). Given the safety profile and the data suggesting evidence of *L. reuteri* DSM 17938, this therapeutic option should be proposed to caregivers. Data on other probiotics, either positive or negative, are too limited to allow reliable conclusions (Szajewska and Dryl, 2016). The same probiotic strain was shown to significantly prevent the onset of infantile colic in formula and breastfed infants (Indrio et al., 2014). *L. rhamnosus* GG in infants treated in tandem with behavioral support and a cow's milk elimination diet did not provide additional treatment effect for diary-verified colic crying, although parental report of crying suggested the probiotic intervention was effective (Pärtty et al., 2015).

According to a network meta-analysis, *L. reuteri* DSM 17938 and dietary adaptations are the only evidence-based interventions to reduce infantile colic (Gutiérrez-Castrellón et al., 2017). However, although infants with infantile colic have a GI dysbiosis, it should be considered that colic vanishes around the age of 4 months, also without administration of pre- or probiotics. The question that arises is if, around the age of 3–5 months, there is a significant change in GI microbiota in colicky infants (Fig. 15.3).

In summary: there is no standard recommended treatment for infantile colic. Accumulating evidence favors to consider formula with "biotics" since trials some probiotics such as

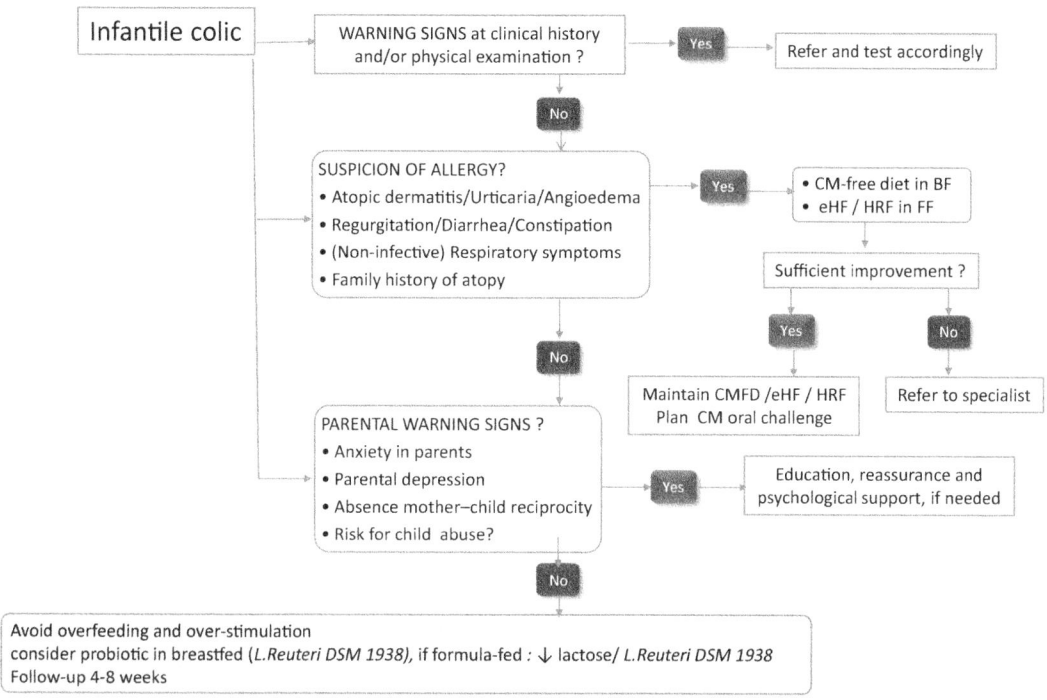

**FIG. 15.3** Proposes a practical approach to colicky infants. *BF*: breastfeeding; *CM*: cow's milk; *CMFD*: cow's milk free diet; *eHF*: extensively hydorlyzed formula; *FF*: formula fed; *L. reuteri*: *Limosilactobacillus reuteri*; *HRF*: hydrolyzed rice formula.

*L. reuteri* DSM 17938, but also with prebiotics, synbiotics, and postbiotics. Limited evidence suggests that lactase or lactose reduction may be beneficial as well. However, there are no data that effective reduction of infant distress and crying has an impact on the development of FGIDs later in life. More data on the natural evolution of babies with infantile colic and the long-term effects of various interventions are a research priority (Salvatore et al., 2020).

## 15.5 Between 1 and 4 years

Early-life events constitute an additional risk factor for the development of irritable bowel syndrome (IBS) and other FGIDs. Toddlers with FGIDs have a lower quality of life, increased medical and mental health visits, and increased hospital stays compared to age-matched controls (Rouster et al., 2016). GI inflammation and infection, allergy, trauma, and stress have been associated with visceral hyperalgesia and various GI symptoms in children (Saps et al., 2008, 2011; Pensabene et al., 2018, 2015; Chogle et al., 2014; Di Nardo et al., 2018; Tan et al., 2017).

However, data in toddlers are very limited since almost no study restricts the assessment to this age group and often incorporates subjects aged 0–12 months in the total prevalence of FGIDs. Both American and European data showed that functional constipation is the most frequent FGID in toddlers, without any difference in age, sex, or race, whereas infantile colic and regurgitation do no longer occur at this age (van Tilburg et al., 2015). When a sub-group analysis is performed, regurgitation progressively disappeared while the rate of constipation increased with age, from 4.7% to 9.4% and 29% in subjects < 1 year and 1–3 years, cyclic vomiting syndrome from 0% to 3.4% to 10% and functional diarrhea passed from 2.4% to 6.4% (van Tilburg et al., 2015; Rouster et al., 2016). A recent cross-sectional study in European infants and toddlers confirmed that constipation was more frequent in the group aged 13–48 months compared to infants (9.7% vs 3%). At least one FGID was found in 11.3% of toddlers, multiple FGIDs in 0.3%, cyclic vomiting in 1.5%, and functional diarrhea in 0.6% of subjects (Steutel et al., 2020).

IBS is a common disorder in older children characterized by abdominal pain associated with a change in stool consistency or frequency, including low-grade inflammation and intestinal microbiota changes (Guandalini et al., 2015). In a large Swedish cohort study, several perinatal and familial factors, such as cesarean section, low birth weight (< 2500 g), being second in birth order, young maternal age (< 20 years), maternal marital status (divorced/widowed), maternal education, parental history of IBS, of anxiety, and of depression significantly increased the risk of IBS later in life (Waehrens et al., 2018). In another population, a shorter period of breastfeeding was significantly associated with IBS (5.6 months vs 8.1 months, $P = 0.009$) in adult life (Koloski et al., 2015). A systematic review of 27 studies highlighted parental IBS, substance abuse, parental punishment, and rejection as parental risk factors for the development of IBS; low birth weight as a perinatal risk factor; and crowded living conditions in low-income families, childhood anxiety, depression, or child abuse as childhood risk factors (Low et al., 2020). Male sex (Waehrens et al., 2018), parental emotional warmth, and advanced maternal age (≥ 35 years) were found as protective factors for IBS (Waehrens et al., 2018; Low et al., 2020). However, IBS is difficult to diagnose in toddlers, and is not reported in the studies evaluating the prevalence of FGIDS in this age group. The most accepted framework to explain IBS is a biopsychosocial model, which conceptualizes chronic pain as a dysregulation of the gut-brain homeostasis with peripheral and central factors mutually influencing each other (Chogle et al., 2014). Environmental factors and maladaptive coping predispose children to develop IBS with greater disability and more frequent medical consultations (Chogle et al., 2014). The contribution of heredity and social learning on the development of IBS was first assessed in a study on US 6060 twin pairs (Levy et al., 2001). Concordance for IBS was significantly greater ($P = 0.030$) in monozygotic (17.2%) than in dizygotic (8.4%) twins. However, having a mother or a father with IBS were stronger independent predictors of irritable bowel status ($P < 0.001$) than having a twin with IBS. A child was more likely to suffer from hard stools if the parent also reported hard stools, but a similar association was not found with loose stools (van Tilburg et al., 2015).

Many (adult) studies showed significant changes in intestinal microbiota in IBS, with reduced Lactobacillus, Bifidobacterium, and *Faecalibacterium prausnitzii*, particularly in diarrhea-predominant IBS (Liu et al., 2017). Dysbiosis leading to abnormal intestinal fermentation and motility, altered bile acid metabolism, mucosal immunity, and pain perception has been suggested as a possible pathogenic mechanism in IBS. In a small group of American school-aged children, the microbiota of the 22 IBS subjects was characterized by greater percentages of *Haemophilus* and taxa of the genus *Veillonella*, whereas there were corresponding reductions in *Eubacterium* and *Anaerovorax*. Additionally, individual taxa belonging to the genera *Akkermansia* and *Parabacteroides*, and a member of the family *Ruminococcaceae* were found in children with an increased number of abdominal pain episodes (Saulnier et al., 2011). However, there are no data analyzing the GI microbiota composition in toddlers and its impact on the later development of IBS or other FGIDs. Few and disappointing data are available for prebiotic supplementation (Guandalini et al., 2015). There is insufficient evidence to recommend any therapeutic intervention in pediatric IBS, including manipulation of the gastrointestinal tract microbiome, despite the evidence that dysbiosis seems to be an associated pathophysiologic factor (Levy et al., 2021).

Microbiota composition is strongly influenced by different diet components, starting from breast milk feeding in infancy and long-term intake of carbohydrates and fibers (Oluwagbemigun et al., 2021). Dietary habits of toddlers show geographical and ethnic differences, but all parents should be instructed and encouraged to implement children's healthy eating habits since early life and to facilitate their child's participation in appropriate family meals (Foterek et al., 2016).

A nutritional analysis of 200 (13–24 month-old) and 173 (25–36 month-old) young children in Belgium showed that median energy intake was 15%–20% above the recommended daily intake (RDI) of 79–82 kcal/kg/day in almost 75% of the subjects (Huysentruyt et al., 2016). Except for one child, protein intake was above the RDI in all children, and in 78% of the included population, this was above the upper tolerable limit of 15% of total energy intake (Huysentruyt et al., 2016; Agostoni et al., 2008). The median fat intake increased with age but was slightly below the RDI. Water and carbohydrate intake were in accordance with the RDI, whereas fiber intake was below the RDI of 15 g/day for 93% of the oldest and 83% of the middle age group. Milk represented the most important source of energy and macronutrients in the first 24 months of life (Huysentruyt et al., 2016). After this age, cakes and sweets gain importance in providing energy, protein, and fat (Huysentruyt et al., 2016; Walton, 2012; Fox et al., 2006).

The mean energy intake was similar in a Belgian and Finnish study, and higher in a Dutch cohort (Huysentruyt et al., 2016; Kyttala et al., 2010; Ocké et al., 2008). Noteworthy, the RDIs for energy and protein have decreased with time, lowering by 20%–25% in 20 years (FOA/WHO/UNU, 1985, 2004; FOA/WHO/UNU, 1985; FOA/WHO/UNU, 2002). In contrast to frequent high energy and protein intake, Belgian and Dutch toddlers showed a fat intake 5%–20% below the RDI (Ocké et al., 2008), whereas it was higher in Italy (Sette et al., 2011) and reached 40% of energy intake in Greece (Manios et al., 2008). Low fiber intake is frequent in all European countries, varying between 7.6 and 13 g/day (Kyttala et al., 2010; Ocké et al., 2008; Manios et al., 2008; Sette et al., 2011; Walton et al., 2017; Huybrechts and De Henauw, 2007).

Data collecting from nationally representative dietary surveys across the world found total sugars (glucose, fructose, lactose, sucrose, and maltose), as a percentage of energy, were highest in the infant (< 4 years), with mean values ranging from 20.0% to 38.4%, and decreased over the lifespan to 13.5%–24.6% in adults (Newens and Walton, 2016). Gastrointestinal symptoms attributed to carbohydrate malabsorption often determine a diet with limited lactose and Fermentable Oligosaccharides, Disaccharides, Monosaccharides, and Polyols (FODMAP).

Fermentable oligosaccharides, disaccharides, monosaccharides, and polyols ("FODMAP") are short-chain carbohydrates that are poorly absorbed in the small intestine and are prone to absorb water and to be fermented in the colon. FODMAPS include short-chain oligosaccharide polymers of fructose (fructans) and galactooligosaccharides (GOS, stachyose, raffinose), disaccharides (lactose), monosaccharides (fructose), and sugar alcohols (polyols), such as sorbitol, mannitol, xylitol, and maltitol. Most FODMAPs are naturally present in food and the human diet, but the polyols may be added artificially in commercially prepared foods and beverages. FODMAPs may cause digestive discomfort in some infants, children, and adults.

The impact of this intervention on FGIDs in children is very limited (Turco et al., 2018). In children, only two small studies (in 33 and 8 children, aged 7–17 years) from the same group, one RCT lasting only 48 h (Chumpitazi et al., 2015) and one open-label study lasting 1 week (Chumpitazi et al., 2014) reported positive results of low FODMAP diet. Responders were enriched at baseline in taxa with known greater saccharolytic metabolic capacity (e.g., Bacteroides, Ruminococcaceae, *Faecalibacterium prausnitzii*) and three Kyoto Encyclopedia of Genes and Genomes orthologues, of which two relate to carbohydrate metabolism (Chumpitazi et al., 2015). However, a more recent RCT in 27 children with functional abdominal pain concluded that a low FODMAP diet for 4 weeks did not reduce symptoms (Boradyn et al., 2020). One RCT showed exacerbation of symptoms with fructans in children with IBS; no effect was found for the lactose-free diet, whilst fructose-restricted diets were effective in 5/6 studies (Pensabene et al., 2019). However, starting lactose and/or FODMAP restriction in early life may promote a different intestinal colonization, a limited production of short-chain fatty acids, selective appetite, food aversions, eating disorders as well as an imbalanced nutrient intake that may compromise growth and development (Bhesania and Cresci, 2017). A typical Western diet, high in saturated fat, simple sugars, emulsifiers, and processed foods, and low in fibers has been suggested to alter microbiota composition, favor intestinal inflammatory response, and Crohn's disease (Chassaing et al., 2017; Hou et al., 2011). In contrast, the Mediterranean diet is rich in fresh fruits, vegetables, whole grains, olive oil, omega-3 fatty acids (fish), nuts, and legumes, with reduced consumption of red meat and saturated fat. Interestingly, in a prospective analysis of gastrointestinal symptoms, Italian adolescent and young adults (aged 17–24 years) who had lower Mediterranean diet adherence scores reported a higher incidence of IBS and functional dyspepsia, particularly among females, compared to the other aged group subjects with better adherence to the diet (Zito et al., 2016).

There is a lack of prospective data collection to analyze if feeding during early life has an impact on FGIDs in childhood and adulthood. However, both genetic, environmental, and dietary factors may be related to the association of constipation in parents and their children (van Tilburg et al., 2015).

Several studies have been conducted to evaluate the effect of specific strains of probiotics on modifying intestinal microbiota and relieving FGIDs in children. A report from the Rome foundation group included 32 RCTs evaluating the efficacy of probiotics in IBS, most of which showed an overall modest improvement in symptoms, with the patients most benefiting from probiotics being those with predominant diarrhea and those having a post-infectious IBS (Guandalini et al., 2015). A review focusing only on children with FGIDs concluded that probiotics are more effective than placebo in the treatment of patients with abdominal pain-related FGIDs, although without effect on constipation (Guandalini et al., 2015). *L. rhamnosus* GG was shown to significantly reduce the frequency and severity of abdominal pain in children with IBS; this effect is sustained during 8 weeks follow-up and may be secondary to improvement of the gut barrier (Francavilla et al., 2010). VSL#3 has been studied in an older group of children (4–18 years old, and was shown to be significantly superior to placebo, although the latter was in as many as half of the patients (Guandalini et al., 2010). Four pediatric studies assessed the effect of *L. reuteri* DSM17938 on functional abdominal pain and IBS and found a significant reduction of intensity (Romano et al., 2014; Weizman et al., 2016; Maragkoudaki et al., 2017; Jadresin et al., 2017) and frequency of symptoms (Weizman et al., 2016; Maragkoudaki et al., 2017; Jadresin et al., 2017). In one study (Romano et al., 2014), the frequency was unchanged, and in another trial (Eftekhari et al., 2015) no significant difference with the placebo group was noted.

Hence, there is moderate evidence for *L. reuteri* DSM 17938 and *L.GG* and limited evidence (based on one study each) for the beneficial effect of mixed probiotics and a three-strain bifidobacteria mix in abdominal pain FGIDs, particularly in the IBS sub-group of children, but neither in functional dyspepsia nor in constipation (Salvatore et al., 2018a, b, c).

Noteworthy, all the above studies were performed in school-aged children. Whether early intervention with specific strains of probiotics in younger children may modify the natural history of FGIDs is unknown. An open, prospective cohort study on 220 young children with CMA in the first year of life compared to 110 healthy controls found a higher prevalence of FGIDs at 4–6 years in the allergic subjects compared to the control group. Of interest, the group treated with extensive casein hydrolyzed formula supplemented with L. *GG* had fewer FGIDs compared to the ones fed with the same hydrolyzed formula without the probiotic (Nocerino et al., 2019).

In summary: data on the incidence of FGIDs in toddlers are scarce. As a consequence, it is not possible to propose age-related recommendations. It is very likely that constipation is frequent in this age group. Treatment with polyethylene glycol and behavioral recommendations including toilet training can be proposed as there are some data suggesting efficacy and because these are devoid of risk for adverse effects.

## 15.6 Conclusions

There is evidence that food intake is a major interfering factor in the development of FGIDs in infants and toddlers. Breastfeeding should always be promoted in infants, including those with FGIDs because of its multiple benefits, including nutritional and immunological factors. If human milk is not possible, the choice of different formulas should be based on characteristic components and evidence of efficacy for the occurring disorders. Because many infants present with more than one FGID, a dietary intervention that tackles the different FGIDs makes sense.

A balanced diet and appropriate dietetic and microbiota interventions may also alleviate FGIDs in toddlers, although data are so far very limited.

## 15.7 Future trends and research

More data are needed on the prevalence of FGIDs in toddlers. Long-term follow-up studies in infants with FGIDS are a priority in research, as it is not clear if early intervention has an impact on long-term health. Since early life FGIDs are a risk factor for FGIDs later in life, information on the long-term effect of early intervention would be of major interest.

Considering the high prevalence of FGIDs in infants, prevention would of course be preferable to treatment. The role of macronutrients (protein, carbohydrates, and lipids) will be investigated. Are partial hydrolysates better tolerated than intact protein? Does a reduced lactose content have negative consequences, and does it decrease colic? What about the benefits of a palm-oil-free formula? What is the role of the GI microbiome in the prevention of FGIDs? It can be concluded that much more research is needed on the prevention of FGIDS in infants and toddlers.

Data on the long-term effects of effective management of FGIDs are also a priority for research. Since the literature suggests an association between FGIDs during infancy and toddlerhood and later in life, another question is if prevention of FGIDs in infants and young children would reduce FGIDs in adults?

## Sources of additional information

Hyams, J.S., Di Lorenzo, C., Saps, M., Shulman, R.J., Staiano, A., van Tilburg, M., 2016. Functional disorders: children and adolescents. Gastroenterology.

Benninga, M.A., Faure, C., Hyman, P.E., et al., 2016. Childhood functional gastrointestinal disorders: neonate/toddler. Gastroenterology.

Gensollen, T., Iyer, S.S., Kasper, D.L., Blumberg, R.S., 2016. How colonization by microbiota in early life shapes the immune system. Science 352 (6285), 539–544.

Logan, A.C., Jacka, F.N., Craig, J.M., Prescott, S.L., 2016. The microbiome and mental health: looking back, moving forward with lessons from allergic diseases. Clin. Psychopharmacol. Neurosci. 14, 131–147.

Zhang, C., Yin, A., Li, H., Wang, R., Wu, G., Shen, J., Zhang, M., Wang, L., Hou, Y., Ouyang, H., Zhang, Y., Zheng, Y., Wang, J., Lv, X., Wang, Y., Zhang, F., Zeng, B., Li, W., Yan, F., Zhao, Y., Pang, X., Zhang, X., Fu, H., Chen, F., Zhao, N., Hamaker, B.R., Bridgewater, L.C., Weinkove, D., Clement, K., Dore, J., Holmes, E., Xiao, H., Zhao, G., Yang, S., Bork, P., Nichol- son, J.K., Wei, H., Tang, H., Zhang, X., Zhao, L., 2015. Dietary modulation of gut microbiota contributes to alleviation of both genetic and simple obesity in children. EBioMedicine 2, 968–984.

Tabbers, M.M., Chmielewska, A., Roseboom, M.G., Crastes, N., Perrin, C., Reitsma, J.B., Norbruis, O., Szajewska, H., Benninga, M.A., 2011. Fermented milk containing Bifidobacterium lactis DN-173 010 in childhood constipation: a randomized, double-blind, controlled trial. Pediatrics 127 (6), e1392–e1399. https://doi.org/10.1542/peds.2010-2590.

## References

Agostoni, C., Decsi, T., Fewtrell, M., Goulet, O., Kolacek, S., Koletzko, B., Michaelsen, K.F., Moreno, L., Puntis, J., Rigo, J., Shamir, R., Szajewska, H., Turck, D., van Goudoever, J., 2008. Complementary feeding: a commentary by the ESPGHAN Committee on nutrition. J. Pediatr. Gastroenterol. Nutr. 46, 99–110.

Bellaiche, M., Oozeer, R., Gerardi-Temporel, G., Faure, C., Vandenplas, Y., 2018. Multiple functional gastrointestinal disorders are frequent in formula-fed infants and decrease their quality of life. Acta Paediatr. 107 (7), 1276–1282. https://doi.org/10.1111/apa.14348.

Bellaiche, M., Ategbo, S., Krumholz, F., Ludwig, T., Miqdady, M., Abkari, A., Vandenplas, Y., 2020. A large-scale study to describe the prevalence, characteristics and management of functional gastrointestinal disorders in African infants. Acta Paediatr. 109, 2366–2373. https://doi.org/10.1111/apa.15248.

Benninga, M.A., Faure, C., Hyman, P.E., St James Roberts, I., Schechter, N.L., Nurko, S., 2016. Childhood functional gastrointestinal disorders: neonate/toddler. Gastroenterology 150 (6), 1443–1455.e2. https://doi.org/10.1053/j.gastro.2016.02.016.

Benninga, M.A., MENA Infant Constipation Study Group, Benninga MA, V.Y., et al., 2019. The magnesium-rich formula for functional constipation in infants: a randomized comparator-controlled study. Pediatr. Gastroenterol. Hepatol. Nutr. 22, 270–281.

Beser, O.F., Cokugras, F.C., Dogan, G., Akgun, O., Elevli, M., Yilmazbas, P., et al., 2021. The frequency of and factors affecting functional gastrointestinal disorders in infants that presented to tertiary care hospitals. Eur. J. Pediatr. 180, 2443–2452. https://doi.org/10.1007/s00431-021-04059-2.

Bhesania, N., Cresci, G.A.M., 2017. A nutritional approach for managing irritable bowel syndrome. Curr. Opin. Pediatr. 29 (5), 584–591. https://doi.org/10.1097/MOP.0000000000000536.

Bongers, M.E., de Lorijn, F., Reitsma, J.B., Groeneweg, M., Taminiau, J.A., Benninga, M.A., 2007. The clinical effect of a new infant formula in term infants with constipation: a double-blind, randomized cross-over trial. Nutr. J. 6, 8.

Boradyn, K.M., Przybyłowicz, K.E., Jarocka-Cyrta, E., 2020. Low FODMAP diet is not effective in children with functional abdominal pain: a randomized controlled trial. Ann Nutr Metab. 76 (5), 334–344.

Borrelli, O., Barbara, G., Di Nardo, G., Cremon, C., Lucarelli, S., Frediani, T., et al., 2009. Neuro- immune interaction and anorectal motility in children with food allergy-related chronic constipation. Am. J. Gastroenterol. 104, 454–463.

Brzozowska, I., Strzalka, M., Drozdowicz, D., Konturek, S.J., Brzozowski, T., 2014. Mechanisms of esophageal protection, gastroprotection and ulcer healing by melatonin. Implications for the therapeutic use of melatonin in gastro esophageal reflux disease (GERD) and peptic ulcer disease. Curr. Pharm. Des. 20, 4807–4815. https://doi.org/10.2174/1381612819666131119110258.

Canivet, C., Jakobsson, I., Hagander, B., 2000. Infantile colic. Follow-up at four years of age: still more "emotional". Acta Paediatr. 89, 13–17. https://doi.org/10.1080/080352500750028988.

Carlson, A.L., Xia, K., Azcarate-Peril, M.A., Goldman, B.D., Ahn, M., Styner, M.A., Thompson, A.L., Geng, X., Gilmore, J.H., Knickmeyer, R.C., 2018. Infant gut microbiome associated with cognitive development. Biol. Psychiatry 83, 148–159. https://doi.org/10.1016/j.biopsych.2017.06.021.

Chassaing, B., Van de Wiele, T., De Bodt, J., et al., 2017. Dietary emulsifiers directly alter human microbiota composition and gene epression ex vivo potentiating intestinal inflammation. Gut 0, 1–14.

Chogle, A., Mintjens, S., Saps, M., 2014. Pediatric IBS: an overview on pathophysiology, diagnosis, and treatment. Pediatr. Ann. 43, e76–e82.

Chumpitazi, B.P., Hollister, E.B., Oezguen, N., Tsai, C.M., McMeans, A.R., Luna, R.A., et al., 2014. Gut microbiota influences low fermentable substrate diet efficacy in children with irritable bowel syndrome. Gut Microbes 5 (2), 165–175.

Chumpitazi, B.P., Cope, J.L., Hollister, E.B., Tsai, C.M., McMeans, A.R., Luna, R.A., Versalovic, J., Shulman, R.J., 2015. Randomised clinical trial: gut microbiome biomarkers are associated with clinical response to a low FODMAP diet in children with irritable bowel syndrome. Aliment. Pharmacol. Ther. 42, 418–427.

Coccorullo, P., Strisciuglio, C., Martinelli, M., Miele, E., Greco, L., Staiano, A., 2010. Lactobacillus reuteri (DSM 17938) in infants with functional chronic constipation: a double-blind, random- ized, placebo-controlled study. J. Pediatr. 157, 598–602.

Cohen Engler, A., Hadash, A., Shehadeh, N., Pillar, G., 2012. Breastfeeding may improve nocturnal sleep and reduce infantile colic: potential role of breast milk melatonin. Eur. J. Pediatr. 171, 729–732.

Cowan, C.S.M., Stylianakis, A.A., Richardson, R., 2019. Early-life stress, microbiota, and brain development: probiotics reverse the effects of maternal separation on neural circuits underpinning fear expression and extinction in infant rats. Dev. Cogn. Neurosci. 37. https://doi.org/10.1016/j.dcn.2019.100627, 100627 (Epub 2019 Apr 3).

Cryan, J.F., O'Mahony, S.M., 2011. The microbiome-gut-brain axis: from bowel to behavior. Neurogastroenterol. Motil. 23, 187–192. https://doi.org/10.1111/j.1365-2982.2010.01664.x.

de Weerth, C., Fuentes, S., Puylaert, P., de Vos, W.M., 2013. Intestinal microbiota of infants with colic: development and specific signatures pediatrics. 131 (2), e550–e558. https://doi.org/10.1542/peds.2012-1449 (Epub 2013 Jan 14).

Di Nardo, G., Cremon, C., et al., 2018. Allergic Proctocolitis is a risk factor for functional gastrointestinal disorders in children. J. Pediatr. 195, 128–133.e1.

Eftekhari, K., Vahedi, Z., Kamali Aghdam, M., Diaz, D.N., 2015. A randomized double-blind placebo-controlled trial of Lactobacillus reuteri for chronic functional abdominal pain in children. Iran. J. Pediatr. 25 (6), e2616.

FOA/WHO/UNU (Food and Agriculture Organization of the United States/World Health Organization/ United Nations University), 2002. Protein and Amino Acid Requirements in Human Nutrition: A Report of a Joint FAO/ WHO/UNU Expert Consultation. WHO Technical Report Series. WHO, Geneva.

FOA/WHO/UNU (Food and Agriculture Organization of the United States/World Health Organization/United Nations University), 1985. Energy and Protein Requirements: Report of a Joint FAO/ WHO/UNU Expert Consultation. WHO Technical Report Series. FOA/WHO/UNU, Rome.

FOA/WHO/UNU (Food and Agriculture Organization of the United States/World Health Organization/United Nations University), 2004. Human Energy Requirements: Report of a Joint FAO/ WHO/UNU Expert Consultation. Food and Nutrition Technical Report Series. FOA/WHO/UNU, Rome.

Foterek, K., Hilbig, A., Kersting, M., Alexy, U., 2016. Age and time trends in the diet of young children: results of the DONALD study. Eur. J. Nutr. 55 (2), 611–620.

Fox, M.K., Reidy, K., Novak, T., Ziegler, P., 2006. Sources of energy and nutrients in the diets of infants and toddlers. J. Am. Diet. Assoc. 106 (1 Suppl. 1), S28–S42.

Francavilla, R., Miniello, V., Magistà, A.M., De Canio, A., Bucci, N., Gagliardi, F., Lionetti, E., Castellaneta, S., Polimeno, L., Peccarisi, L., Indrio, F., Cavallo, L., 2010. A randomized con- trolled trial of *Lactobacillus* GG in children with functional abdominal pain. Pediatrics 126, e1445–e1452.

Gieruszczak-Białek, D., Konarska, Z., Skórka, A., Vandenplas, Y., Szajewska, 2015. No effect of proton pump inhibitors on crying and irritability in infants: systematic review of randomized controlled trials. J. Pediatr. 166, 767–770. e3.

Guandalini, S., Magazzù, G., Chiaro, A., La Balestra, V., Di Nardo, G., Gopalan, S., Sibal, A., Romano, C., Canani, R.B., Lionetti, P., Setty, M., 2010. VSL#3 improves symptoms in children with irritable bowel syndrome: a multicenter, randomized, placebo-controlled, double-blind, crossover study. J. Pediatr. Gastroenterol. Nutr. 51, 24–30.

Guandalini, S., Cernat, E., Moscoso, D., 2015. Prebiotics and probiotics in irritable bowel syndrome and inflamma- tory bowel disease in children. Benef. Microbes 6, 209–217.

Gutiérrez-Castrellón, P., Indrio, F., Bolio-Galvis, A., Jiménez-Gutiérrez, C., Jimenez-Escobar, I., López-Velázquez, G., 2017. Efficacy of Lactobacillus reuteri DSM 17938 for infantile colic: systematic review with network meta- analysis. Medicine (Baltimore) 96 (51), e9375.

Hall, B., Chesters, J., Robinson, A., 2012. Infantile colic: a systematic review of medical and con- ventional therapies. J. Paediatr. Child Health 48, 128–137.

Harb, T., Matsuyama, M., David, M., Hill, R., 2016. Infant Colic—what works: a systematic review of interventions for breastfed infants. J. Pediatr. Gastroenterol. Nutr. 62 (5), 668–686.

Hegar, B., Dewanti, N.R., Kadim, M., Alatas, S., Firmansyah, A., Vandenplas, Y., 2009. Natural evolution of regurgi- tation in healthy infants. Acta Paediatr. 98, 1189–1193.

Hou, J.K., Abraham, B., El-Serag, H., 2011. Dietary intake and risk of developing inflammatory bowel disease: a sys- tematic review of the literature. Am. J. Gastroenterol. 106 (4), 563–573.

Howard, C.R., Lanphear, N., Lanphear, B.P., Eberly, S., Lawrence, R.A., 2006. Parental responses to infant crying and colic: the effect on breastfeeding duration. Breastfeed. Med. 1 (3), 146–155.

Huybrechts, I., De Henauw, S., 2007. Energy and nutrient intakes by pre-school children in Flanders-Belgium. Br. J. Nutr. 98, 600–610.

Huysentruyt, K., Laire, D., Van Avondt, T., De Schepper, J., Vandenplas, Y., 2016. Energy and mac- ronutrient intakes and adherence to dietary guidelines of infants and toddlers in Belgium. Eur. J. Nutr. 55 (4), 1595–1604.

Huysentruyt, K., Koppen, I., Benninga, M., Cattaert, T., Cheng, J., De Geyter, C., Faure, C., Gottrand, F., Hegar, B., Hojsak, I., Miqdady, M., Osatakul, S., Ribes-Koninckx, C., Salvatore, S., Saps, M., Shamir, R., Staiano, A., Szajewska, H., Vieira, M., Vandenplas, Y., 2019. BITSS working group. The Brussels infant and toddler stool scale: a study on Interobserver reliability. J. Pediatr. Gastroenterol. Nutr. 68, 207–213.

Indrio, F., Di Mauro, A., Riezzo, G., Civardi, E., Intini, C., Corvaglia, L., Ballardini, E., Bisceglia, M., Cinquetti, M., Brazzoduro, E., Del Vecchio, A., Tafuri, S., 2014. Prophylactic use of a probiotic in the prevention of colic, regurgi- tation, and functional constipation: a randomized clinical trial. JAMA Pediatr. 168, 228–233.

Indrio, F., Di Mauro, A., Riezzo, G., Cavallo, L., Francavilla, R., 2015. Infantile colic, regurgitation, and constipation: an early traumatic insult in the development of functional gastrointestinal disorders in children? Eur. J. Pediatr. 174 (6), 841–842. https://doi.org/10.1007/s00431-014-2467-3.

Jadresin, O., Hojsak, I., Misak, Z., Kekez, A.J., Trbojevic, T., Ivkovic, L., Kolacek, S., 2017. Lactobacillus reuteri DSM 17938 in the treatment of functional abdominal pain in children: RCT study. J. Pediatr. Gastroenterol. Nutr. 64 (6), 925–929.

Kanabar, D., Randhawa, M., Clayton, P., 2001. Improvement of symptoms in infant colic following reduction of lactose load with lactase. J. Hum. Nutr. Diet. 14, 359–363.

Koloski, N.A., Jones, M., Weltman, M., et al., 2015. Identification of early environmental risk factors for irritable bowel syndrome and dyspepsia. Neurogastroenterol. Motil. 27, 1317–1325.

Kyttala, P., Erkkola, M., Kronberg-Kippila, C., Tapanainen, H., Veijola, R., Simell, O., Knip, M., Virtanen, S.M., 2010. Food consumption and nutrient intake in Finnish 1–6-year-old children. Public Health Nutr. 13 (6a), 947–956.

Lasekan, J.B., Hustead, D.S., Masor, M., Murray, R., 2017. Impact of palm olein in infant formulas on stool consistency and frequency: a meta-analysis of randomized clinical trials. Food Nutr. Res. 61 (1), 1330104. https://doi.org/10.1080/16546628.2017.1330104.

Lemcke, S., Parner, E.T., Bjerrum, M., Thomsen, P.H., Lauritsen, M.B., 2016. Early development in children that are later diagnosed with disorders of attention and activity: a longitudinal study in the Danish National Birth Cohort. Eur. Child Adolesc. Psychiatry 25 (10), 1055–1066. https://doi.org/10.1007/s00787-016-0825-6 (Epub 2016 Feb 9).

Levy, R.L., Jones, K.R., Whitehead, W.E., Feld, S.I., Talley, N.J., Corey, L.A., 2001. Irritable bowel syndrome in twins: heredity and social learning both contribute to etiology. Gastroenterology 121 (4), 799–804.

Levy, E.I., Hoang, D.M., Vandenplas, Y., 2020. The effects of proton pump inhibitors on the microbiome in young children. Acta Paediatr. 109, 1531–1538. https://doi.org/10.1111/apa.15213.

Levy, E.I., De Geyter, C., Ouald Chaib, A., Aman, B.A., Hegar, B., Vandenplas, Y., 2021. How to manage irritable bowel syndrome in children. Acta Paediatr. (in press).

Liu, H.N., Wu, H., Chen, Y.Z., Chen, Y.J., Shen, X.Z., Liu, T.T., 2017. Altered molecular signature of intestinal microbiota in irritable bowel syndrome patients compared with healthy controls: a systematic review and meta-analysis. Dig. Liver Dis. 49 (4), 331–337.

Low, E.X.S., Mandhari, M.N.K.A., Herndon, C.C., Loo, E.X.L., Tham, E.H., Siah, K.T.H., 2020. Parental, perinatal, and childhood risk factors for development of irritable bowel syndrome: a systematic review. J Neurogastroenterol Motil. 26 (4), 437–446. https://doi.org/10.5056/jnm20109.

Ludwig, T., Oukid, I., Wong, J., Ting, S., Huysentruyt, K., Roy, P., Foussat, A.C., Vandenplas, Y., 2021. J. Pediatr. Gastroenterol. Nutr. 72 (2), 255–261.

Manios, Y., Grammatikaki, E., Papoutsou, S., Liarigkovinos, T., Kondaki, K., Moschonis, G., 2008. Nutrient intakes of toddlers and preschoolers in Greece: the GENESIS study. J. Am. Diet. Assoc. 108, 357–361.

Maragkoudaki, M., Chouliaras, G., Orel, R., Horvath, A., Szajewska, H., Pappadopoulou, A., 2017. Lactobacillus reuteri DSM 17938 and a placebo both significantly reduced symptoms in children with functional abdominal pain. Acta Paediatr. 106 (11), 1857–1862.

Martin, A.J., Pratt, N., Kennedy, J.D., Ryan, P., Ruffin, R.E., Miles, H., et al., 2002. Natural history and familial relationships of infant spilling to 9 years of age. Pediatrics 109, 1061–1067.

Meunier, L., Garthoff, J.A., Schaafsma, A., Krul, L., Schrijver, J., van Goudoever, J.B., 2014. Locust bean gum safety in neonates and young infants: an integrated review of the toxicologi- cal database and clinical evidence. Regul. Toxicol. Pharmacol. 70, 155–169.

Miyazawa, R., Tomomasa, T., Kaneko, H., Tachibana, A., Ogawa, T., Morikawa, A., 2002. Prevalence of gastroesophagealgastro-esophageal reflux-related symptoms in Japanese infants. Pediatr. Int. 44, 513–516.

Mohajeri, M.H., La Fata, G., Steinert, R.E., Weber, P., 2018. Relationship between the gut microbiome and brain function. Nutr. Rev. 76, 481–496. https://doi.org/10.1093/nutrit/nuy009.

Moro, G., Mosca, F., Miniello, V., Fanaro, S., Jelinek, J., Stahl, B., Boehm, G. (Eds.), 2003. Effects of a new mixture of prebiotics on faecal flora and stools in term infants. Acta Paediatr. 91 (Suppl. 441), 77–79.

Neu, M., Robinson, J.A., 2003. Infants with colic: their childhood characteristics. J. Pediatr. Nurs. 18 (1), 12–20. https://doi.org/10.1053/jpdn.2003.3.

Newens, K.J., Walton, J., 2016. A review of sugar consumption from nationally representative dietary surveys across the world. J. Hum. Nutr. Diet. 29 (2), 225–240. https://doi.org/10.1111/jhn.12338.

Nocerino, R., Di Costanzo, M., Bedogni, G., Cosenza, L., Maddalena, Y., Di Scala, C., Della Gatta, G., Carucci, L., Voto, L., Coppola, S., Iannicelli, A.M., Berni, C.R., 2019. Dietary treatment with extensively hydrolyzed casein formula containing the probiotic Lactobacillus rhamnosus GG prevents the occurrence of functional gastrointestinal disorders in children with cow's milk allergy. J. Pediatr. 213, 137–142. e2Ocké.

Ocké, M.C., van Rossum, C.T.M., Fransen, H.P., Buurma, E.M., de Boer, E.J., Brants, H.A.M., Niekerk, E.M., van der Laan, J.D., Drijvers, J.J.M.M., Ghameshlou, Z., 2008. Dutch National Food Consumption Survey: Young Children 2005/2006. National Institute for Public Health and the Environment.

Oliveros, E., Vázquez, E., Barranco, A., Ramírez, M., Gruart, A., Delgado-García, J.M., Buck, R., Rueda, R., Martín, M.J., 2018. Sialic acid and Sialylated oligosaccharide supplementation during lactation improves learning and memory in rats. Nutrients 10, 1519. https://doi.org/10.3390/nu10101519.

Oluwagbemigun, K., O'Donovan, A.N., Berding, K., Lyons, K., Alexy, U., Schmid, M., Clarke, G., Stanton, C., Cryan, J., Nöthlings, U., 2021. Long-term dietary intake from infancy to late adolescence is associated with gut microbiota composition in young adulthood. Am. J. Clin. Nutr. 113 (3), 647–656.

Osatakul, S., Sriplung, H., Puetpaiboon, A., Junjana, C.O., Chamnongpakdi, S., 2002. Prevalence and natural course of gastroesophageal reflux symptoms: a 1-year cohort study in Thai infants. J. Pediatr. Gastroenterol. Nutr. 34, 63–67.

Pärtty, A., Kalliomäki, M., 2017. Infant colic is still a mysterious disorder of the microbiota-gut-brain axis. Acta Paediatr. 106 (4), 528–529. https://doi.org/10.1111/apa.13754.

Pärtty, A., Kalliomaki, M., Salminen, S., Isolauri, E., 2013. Infant distress and development of functional gastrointestinal disorders in childhood: is there a connection? JAMA Pediatr. 167 (10), 977–978. https://doi.org/10.1001/jamapediatrics.2013.99.

Pärtty, A., Lehtonen, L., Kalliomäki, M., Salminen, S., Isolauri, E., 2015. Probiotic Lactobacillus rhamnosus GG therapy and microbiological programming in infantile colic: a randomized, controlled trial. Pediatr. Res. 78, 470–475.

Pensabene, L., Talarico, V., Concolino, D., Ciliberto, D., Campanozzi, A., Gentile, T., Rutigliano, V., Salvatore, S., Staiano, A., Di Lorenzo, C., 2015. Post-infectious functional gastrointestinal disorders study Group of Italian Society for pediatric gastroenterology, hepatology and nutrition. Postinfectious functional gastrointestinal disorders in children: a multicenter prospective study. J. Pediatr. 166 (4), 903–907.

Pensabene, L., Salvatore, S., D'Auria, E., Parisi, F., Concolino, D., Borrelli, O., Thapar, N., Staiano, A., Vandenplas, Y., Saps, M., 2018. Cow's milk protein allergy in infancy: a risk factor for functional gastrointestinal disorders in children? Nutrients 10 (11). https://doi.org/10.3390/nu10111716. pii: E1716.

Pensabene, L., Salvatore, S., Turco, R., Tarsitano, F., Concolino, D., Baldassarre, M.E., Borrelli, O., Thapar, N., Vandenplas, Y., Staiano, A., Saps, M., 2019. Low FODMAPs diet for functional abdominal pain disorders in children: critical review of current knowledge. J. Pediatr. 95 (6), 642–656.

Pijpers, M.A.M., Bongers, M.E.J., Benninga, M.A., Berger, M.Y., 2010. Functional constipation in children: a systematic review on prognosis and predictive factors. J. Pediatr. Gastroenterol. Nutr. 50 (3), 256–268. https://doi.org/10.1097/MPG.0b013e3181afcdc3.

Rao, M.R., Brenner, R.A., Schisterman, E.F., Vik, T., Mills, J.M., 2004. Long term cognitive development in children with prolonged crying. Arch. Dis. Child. 89 (11), 989–992. https://doi.org/10.1136/adc.2003.039198.

Rautava, P., Lehtonen, L., Helenius, H., Sillanpää, M., 1995. Infantile colic: child and family three years later. Pediatrics 96 (1 Pt 1), 43–47.

Romano, C., Ferrau, V., Cavataio, F., Iacono, G., Spina, M., Lionetti, E., Comisi, F., Famiani, A., Comito, D., 2014. Lactobacillus reuteri in children with functional abdominal pain (FAP). J. Paediatr. Child Health 50, E68–E71.

Rosen, R., Vandenplas, Y., Singendonk, M., Cabana, M., DiLorenzo, C., Gottrand, F., Gupta, S., Langendam, M., Staiano, A., Thapar, N., Tipnis, N., Tabbers, M., 2018. Pediatric gastroesophageal reflux clinical practice guidelines: joint recommendations of the north American Society for pediatric gastroenterology, hepatology, and nutrition and the European Society for pediatric gastroenterology, hepatology, and nutrition. J. Pediatr. Gastroenterol. Nutr. 66 (3), 516–554. https://doi.org/10.1097/MPG.0000000000001889.

Rouster, A.S., Karpinski, A.C., Silver, D., Monagas, J., Hyman, P.E., 2016. Functional gastrointestinal disorders dominate pediatric gastroenterology outpatient practice. J. Pediatr. Gastroenterol. Nutr. 62 (6), 847–851.

Salvatore, S., 2007. Nutritional options for infant constipation. Nutrition 23 (7–8), 615–616.

Salvatore, S., Abkari, A., Cai, W., Catto-Smith, A., Cruchet, S., Gottrand, F., Hegar, B., Lifschitz, C., Ludwig, T., Shah, N., Staiano, A., Szajewska, H., Treepongkaruna, S., Vandenplas, Y., 2018a. Review shows that parental reassurance and nutritional advice help to optimise the management of functional gastrointestinal disorders in infants. Acta Paediatr. 107 (9), 1512–1520.

Salvatore, S., Pensabene, L., Borrelli, O., Saps, M., Thapar, N., Concolino, D., Staiano, A., Vandenplas, Y., 2018b. Mind the gut: probiotics in paediatric neurogastroenterology. Benef. Microbes. 9 (6), 883–898.

Salvatore, S., Savino, F., Singendonk, M., Tabbers, M., Benninga, M.A., Staiano, A., Vandenplas, Y., 2018c. Thickened infant formula: what to know? Nutrition 49, 51–56. https://doi.org/10.1016/j.nut.2017.10.010 (Epub 2018 Feb 26).

Salvatore, S., Pagliarin, F., Huysentruyt, K., Bosco, A., Fumagalli, L., Van De Maele, K., Agosti, M., Vandenplas, Y., 2020. Distress in infants and young children: Don't blame acid reflux. J. Pediatr. Gastroenterol. Nutr. 71 (4), 465–469. https://doi.org/10.1097/MPG.0000000000002841.

Sampson, T.R., Mazmanian, S.K., 2015. Control of brain development, function, and behavior by the microbiome. Cell Host Microbe 17 (5), 565–576. https://doi.org/10.1016/j.chom.2015.04.011.

Santos, I.S., Matijasevich, A., Capilheira, M.F., Anselmi, L., Barros, F.C., 2015. Excessive crying at 3 months of age and behavioural problems at 4 years age: a prospective cohort study. J. Epidemiol. Community Health 69 (7), 654–659. https://doi.org/10.1136/jech-2014-204568.

Saps, M., Pensabene, L., Di Martino, L., et al., 2008. Post-infectious functional gastrointestinal disorders in children. J. Pediatr. 152, 812–816.

Saps, M., Lu, P., Bonilla, S., 2011. Cow's-milk allergy is a risk factor for the development of FGIDs in children. J. Pediatr. Gastroenterol. Nutr. 52, 166–169.

Savino, F., Garro, M., Montanari, P., Galliano, I., Bergallo, M., 2018. Crying time and RORγ/FOXP3 expression in *Lactobacillus reuteri* DSM17938-treated infants with colic: a randomized trial. J. Pediatr. 192, 171–177.e1. https://doi.org/10.1016/j.jpeds.2017.08.062.

Savino, F., Maccario, S., Castagno, E., Cresi, F., Cavallo, F., Dalmasso, P., Fanaro, S., Oggero, R., Silvestro, L., 2005a. Advances in the management of digestive problems during the first months of life. Acta Paediatr. 94 (Suppl. 449), 120–124.

Saulnier, D.M., Riehle, K., Mistretta, T.A., Diaz, M.A., Mandal, D., Raza, S., Weidler, E.M., Qin, X., Coarfa, C., Milosavljevic, A., Petrosino, J.F., Highlander, S., Gibbs, R., Lynch, S.V., Shulman, R.J., Versalovic, J., 2011. Gastrointestinal microbiome signatures of pediatric patients with irritable bowel syndrome. Gastroenterology 141 (5), 1782–1791. https://doi.org/10.1053/j.gastro.2011.06.072.

Savino, F., Castagno, E., Bretto, R., Brondello, C., Palumeri, E., Oggero, R., 2005b. A prospective 10-year study on children who had severe infantile colic. Acta Paediatr. Suppl. 94 (449), 129–132. https://doi.org/10.1111/j.1651-2227.2005.tb02169.x.

Savino, F., Palumeri, E., Castagno, E., Cresi, F., Dalmasso, P., Cavallo, F., 2006. Reduction of cry- ing episodes owing to infantile colic: a randomized controlled study on the efficacy of a new infant formula. Eur. J. Clin. Nutr. 60, 1304–1310.

Sette, S., Le Donne, C., Piccinelli, R., Arcella, D., Turrini, A., Leclercq, C., 2011. The third Italian national food consumption survey, INRAN-SCAI 2005-06–part 1: nutrient intakes in Italy. Nutr. Metab. Cardiovasc. Dis. 21, 922–932.

Shamir, R., St James-Roberts, I., Di Lorenzo, C., et al., 2013. Infant crying, colic, and gastrointes- tinal discomfort in early childhood: a review of the evidence and most plausible mechanisms. J. Pediatr. Gastroenterol. Nutr. 57 (Suppl. 1), S1–S45.

Sillanpää, M., Saarinen, M., 2015. Infantile colic associated with childhood migraine: a prospective cohort study. Cephalalgia 35, 1246–1251.

Steenbergen, L., Sellaro, R., van Hemert, S., Bosch, J.A., Colzato, L.S., 2015. A randomized controlled trial to test the effect of multispecies probiotics on cognitive reactivity to sad mood. Brain Behav. Immun. 48, 258–264. https://doi.org/10.1016/j.bbi.2015.04.003 (Epub 2015 Apr 7).

Steutel, N.F., Zeevenhooven, J., Scarpato, E., Vandenplas, Y., Tabbers, M.M., Staiano, A., Benninga, M.A., 2020. Prevalence of functional gastrointestinal disorders in European infants and toddlers. J. Pediatr. 221, 107–114.

Szajewska, H., Dryl, D., 2016. Probiotics for the management of infantile colic. J. Pediatr. Gastroenterol. Nutr. 63 (Suppl 1), S22–S24. https://doi.org/10.1097/MPG.0000000000001220.

Tabbers, M.M., Boluyt, N., Berger, M.Y., Benninga, M.A., 2011. Nonpharmacologic treatments for childhood constipation: systematic review. Pediatrics 128 (4), 753–761. https://doi.org/10.1542/peds.2011-0179.

Tabbers, M.M., DiLorenzo, C., Berger, M.Y., Faure, C., Langendam, M.W., Nurko, S., Staiano, A., Vandenplas, Y., Benninga, M.A., 2014. European society for pediatric gastroenterology, hepatology, and nutrition; north american society for pediatric gastroenterology. Evaluation and treatment of functional constipation in infants and children: evidence-based recommendations from ESPGHAN and NASPGHAN. J. Pediatr. Gastroenterol. Nutr. 8, 265–281.

Tan, T.K., Chen, A.C., Lin, C.L., Shen, T.C., Li, T.C., Wei, C.C., 2017. Preschoolers with allergic diseases have an in- creased risk of irritable bowel syndrome when reaching school age. J. Pediatr. Gastroenterol. Nutr. 64 (1), 26–30.

Tighe, M., Afzal, N.A., Bevan, A., Hayen, A., Munro, A., Beattie, R.M., 2014. Pharmacological treatment of children with gastro-oesophageal reflux. Cochrane Database Syst. Rev. 11. https://doi.org/10.1002/14651858.CD008550.pub2, CD008550.

Tounian, P., Meunier, L., Speijers, G., Oozeer, R., Vandenplas, Y., 2020. Effectiveness and tolerance of a locust bean gum-thickened formula: a real-life study. Pediatr. Gastroenterol. Hepatol. Nutr. 23 (6), 511–520. https://doi.org/10.5223/pghn.2020.23.6.511 (Epub 2020 Nov 5).

Tunc, V.T., Camurdan, A.D., Ilhan, M.N., Sahin, F., Beyazova, U., 2008. Factors associated with defecation patterns in 0–24-month-old children. Eur. J. Pediatr. 167, 1357–1362.

Turco, R., Salvatore, S., Miele, E., Romano, C., Marseglia, G.L., Staiano, A., 2018. Does a low FODMAPs diet reduce symptoms of functional abdominal pain disorders? A systematic review in adult and paediatric population, on behalf of Italian Society of Pediatrics. Ital. J. Pediatr. 44 (1), 53.

van Tilburg, M.A., Hyman, P.E., Walker, L., Rouster, A., Palsson, O.S., Kim, S.M., Whitehead, W.E., 2015. Prevalence of functional gastrointestinal disorders in infants and toddlers. J. Pediatr. 166, 684–689.

Vandenplas, Y., De Greef, E., 2014. ALLAR study group. Extensive protein hydrolysate formula effectively reduces regurgitation in infants with positive and negative challenge tests for cow's milk allergy. Acta Paediatr. 103, e243–e250.

Vandenplas, Y., Rudolph, C.D., Di Lorenzo, C., Hassall, E., Liptak, G., Mazur, L., Sondheimer, J., Staiano, A., Thomson, M., Veereman-Wauters, G., Wenzl, T.G., 2009. Pediatric gastroesopha- geal reflux clinical practice guidelines: joint recommendations of the North American society for pediatric gastroenterology, hepatology and nutrition (NASPGHAN) and the European society for pediatric gastroenterology, hepatology and nutrition (ESPGHAN). J. Pediatr. Gastroenterol. Nutr. 49, 498–547.

Vandenplas, Y., Cruchet, S., Faure, C., Lee, H., Di Lorenzo, C., Staiano, A., 2014a. When should we use partially hydrolysed formulae for frequent gastrointestinal symptoms and allergy prevention? Acta Paediatr. 103, 689–695.

Vandenplas, Y., Ludwig, T., Bouritius, H., 2014b. The combination of scGOS/lcFOS with ferment- ed infant formula reduces the incidence of colic in 4 week old infants. Arch. Dis. Child. 99 (Suppl. 2), A91–A92.

Vandenplas, Y., Abkari, A., Bellaiche, M., Benninga, M., Chouraqui, J.P., Çokura, F., Harb, T., Hegar, B., Lifschitz, C., Ludwig, T., Miqdady, M., de Morais, M.B., Osatakul, S., Salvatore, S., Shamir, R., Staiano, A., Szajewska, H., Thapar, N., 2015a. Prevalence and health outcomes of functional gastrointestinal symptoms in infants from birth to 12 months of age. J. Pediatr. Gastroenterol. Nutr. 61, 531–537.

Vandenplas, Y., Dupont, C., Eigenmann, P., Host, A., Kuitunen, M., Ribes-Koninckx, C., Shah, N., Shamir, R., Staiano, A., Szajewska, H., Von Berg, A., 2015b. A workshop report on the development of the Cow's milk-related symptom score awareness tool for young children. Acta Paediatr. 104, 334–339.

Vandenplas, Y., Benninga, M., Broekaert, I., Falconer, J., Gottrand, F., Guarino, A., Lifschitz, C., Lionetti, P., Orel, R., Papadopoulou, A., Ribes-Koninckx, C., Ruemmele, F.M., Salvatore, S., Shamir, R., Schäppi, M., Staiano, A., Szajewska, H., Thapar, N., Wilschanski, M., 2016. Functional gastrointestinal disorder algorithms focus on early recognition, parental reassurance and nutritional strategies. Acta Paediatr. 105 (3), 244–252.

Vandenplas, Y., Ludwig, T., Bouritius, H., Alliet, P., Forde, D., Peeters, S., Huet, F., Hourihane, J., 2017a. Randomised controlled trial demonstrates that fermented infant formula with short-chain galacto-oligosaccharides and long-chain fructo-oligosaccharides reduces the incidence of infantile colic. Acta Paediatr. 106 (7), 1150–1158. https://doi.org/10.1111/apa.13844 (Epub 2017 Apr 19).

Vandenplas, Y., Analitis, A., Tziouvara, C., Kountzoglou, A., Drakou, A., Tsouvalas, M., Mavroudi, A., Xinias, I., 2017b. Safety of a new Synbiotic starter formula. Pediatr. Gastroenterol. Hepatol. Nutr. 20 (3), 167–177. https://doi.org/10.5223/pghn.2017.20.3.167 (Epub 2017 Sep 26).

Vandenplas, Y., Gerlier, L., Caekelbergh, K., Nan-Study-Group, Possner, M., 2021. An observational real-life study with a new infant formula in infants with functional gastrointestinal disorders. Nutrients 13, 336. https://doi.org/10.3390/nu13103336.

Vlieger, A.M., Robroch, A., van Buuren, S., Kiers, J., Rijkers, G., Benninga, M.A., te Biesebeke, R., 2009. Tolerance and safety of *Lactobacillus paracasei* ssp. paracasei in combination with *Bifidobacterium animalis* ssp. lactis in a prebiotic-containing infant formula: a randomised controlled trial. Br. J. Nutr. 102, 869–875.

Waehrens, R., Li, X., Sundquist, J., Sundquist, K., Zöller, B., 2018. Perinatal and familial risk factors for irritable bowel syndrome in a Swedish national cohort. Scand. J. Gastroenterol. 53 (5), 559–564.

Walton, J.E., 2012. National Pre-School Nutrition Survey-Summary Report. Available from www. iuna.net.

Walton, J., Kehoe, L., McNulty, B.A., Nugent, A.P., Flynn, A., 2017. Nutrient intakes and compliance with nutrient recommendations in children aged 1–4 years in Ireland. J. Hum. Nutr. Diet. 30 (5), 665–676. https://doi.org/10.1111/jhn.12452.

Weizman, Z., Abu-Abed, J., Binsztok, M., 2016. Lactobacillus reuteri DSM17938 for the management of functional abdominal pain in childhood: a randomized, double-blind, placebo-controlled trial. J. Pediatr. 174, 160–164.

Werbach, M.R., 2008. Melatonin for the treatment of gastroesophageal reflux disease. Altern. Ther. Health Med. 14, 54–58.

Xinias, I., Analitis, A., Mavroudi, A., Roilides, I., Lykogeorgou, M., Delivoria, V., Milingos, V., Mylonopoulou, M., Vandenplas, Y., 2017. Innovative dietary intervention answers to baby colic. Pediatr. Gastroenterol. Hepatol. Nutr. 20 (2), 100–106.

Zito, F.P., Polese, B., Vozzella, L., et al., 2016. Good adherence to Mediterranean diet can prevent gastrointestinal symptoms: a survey from southern Italy. World J Gastrointest Pharmacol Ther. 7 (4), 564–571.

# PART III

# Promoting long-term health: Taking action in the first 1000 days

# 16

# Prenatal nutrition and nutrition in pregnancy: Effects on long-term growth and development

*Zohra S. Lassi[a], Zahra A. Padhani[b], Rehana A. Salam[b], and Zulfiqar A. Bhutta[c,d]*

[a]Robinson Research Institute, University of Adelaide, Adelaide, SA, Australia [b]Division of Women and Child Health, Aga Khan University, Karachi, Pakistan [c]Centre for Global Child Health, The Hospital for Sick Children, Toronto, ON, Canada [d]Institute of Global Health and Development, Aga Khan University, Karachi, Pakistan

## LEARNING OBJECTIVES

1. To understand the epidemiology of malnutrition particularly in girls/women.

2. To learn nutritional pathways before and during pregnancy on growth and developmental outcomes of the child.

3. To study the existing evidence on the long-term effects of pre-conception and maternal nutrition from animal and human studies.

4. To study the beneficial effects of pre-conception and maternal nutrition interventions on long-term health and development outcomes of a child.

## 16.1 Background

Pregnancy is a state of high nutritional demand, and provision of optimal micro and macronutrients are important for both mother and the growing fetus (Abu-Saad and Fraser, 2010; Ramakrishnan et al., 2014). Malnutrition, before and during pregnancy, has been associated with poor maternal, neonatal, and child health outcomes (MNCH) that include anemia, preeclampsia, obstructed labor, intrauterine growth restriction (IUGR), cesarean birth, preterm

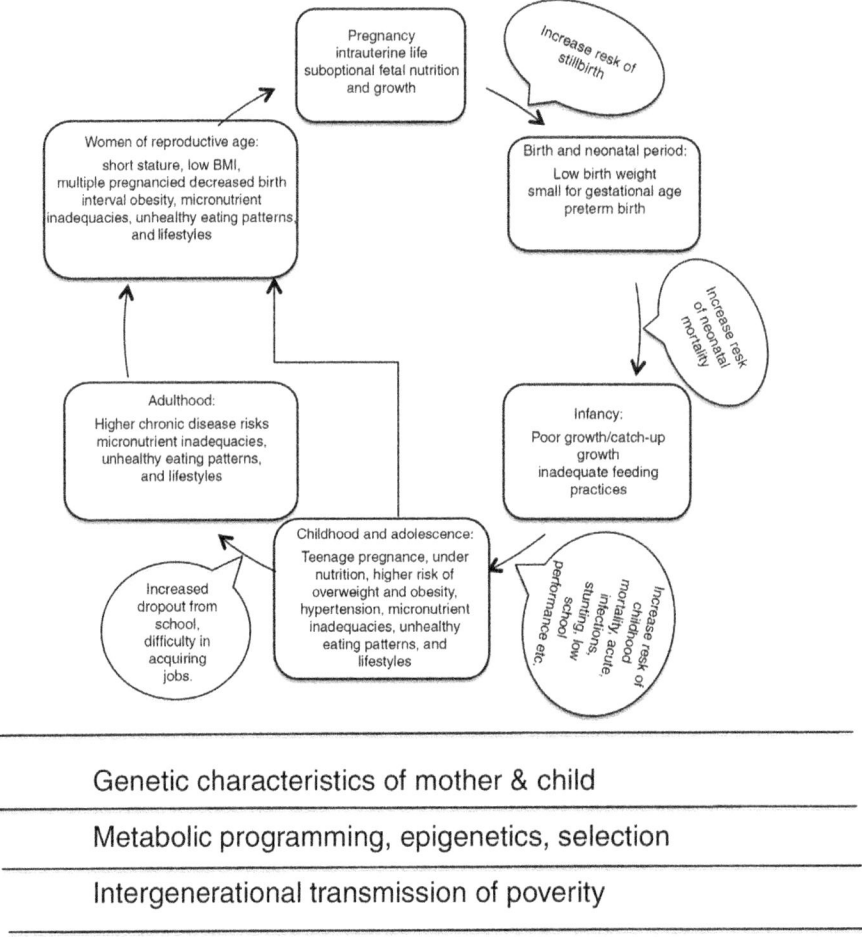

**FIG. 16.1** Conceptual framework: intergenerational relationship of maternal and child nutrition. *Credit: Modified from Martorell, R., Zongrone, A., 2012. Intergenerational influences on child growth and undernutrition. Paediatr. Perinat. Epidemiol. 26 (Suppl. 1), 302–314.*

birth, stillbirth, low birth weight (LBW), macrosomia, neonatal hypothermia, neonatal and maternal mortality, and child stunted growth (Fig. 16.1) (Ronnenberg et al., 2003; Subramanian et al., 2009; Ahmed et al., 2012; Black et al., 2013; Christian et al., 2015; Zerfu et al., 2016).

Newborns who are born to mothers with malnutrition or those who are born with LBW are at increased risk of complications after birth but also the risk for long-term health conditions in later life (Kimani-Murage et al., 2015; Salam et al., 2014; Victora et al., 2008). The Barker Hypothesis on the developmental origin of health and diseases demonstrates that the fetus experiences epigenetic modifications that impact gene expression and influence disease development in later life (Barker and Thornburg, 2013). Fetal exposure to under- and over-nutrition can lead to changes in fetal metabolic pathways which increase the risk of long-term adverse health outcomes such as diabetes mellitus, obesity, hypertension, and neurocognitive dysfunction.

Various nutrition interventions have been evaluated for women of reproductive age (WRA), including pregnant women, to optimize the nutritional status of mothers and their effects on maternal, birth, and neonatal outcomes. For example, folic acid supplementation during peri-conception has shown to reduce the risk of neural tube defects (NTD) in babies (Lassi et al., 2020a), likewise, balanced energy protein (BEP) supplementation during pregnancy has shown to reduce the risk of babies born small for gestational age (SGA) (Lassi et al., 2020a). Other pre-conception and maternal nutritional interventions include multiple micronutrient (MMN) supplementation, lipid-based nutrient supplements (LNS) and food distribution programs, etc. However, the effect of these interventions in terms of growth during early childhood and non-communicable disease during adulthood is not well established in the literature.

This chapter will focus on the effects of nutrition before conception (pre-conception) and during pregnancy on long-term growth and developmental outcomes. We will first describe the epidemiology of maternal malnutrition, followed by the evidence on maternal nutrition interventions on long-term effects for offspring from animal and human studies. In this chapter, the terms 'long-term' is used interchangeably with 'intergenerational effects' and mainly describes adverse outcomes associated with maternal malnutrition for offspring during childhood or adulthood.

## 16.2 Epidemiology

Global epidemiological transition across various countries has documented the co-existence of under- and over-nutrition. Globally about 462 million adults are underweight while 1.9 billion are overweight or obese (WHO, 2020). About 12% of the underweight population globally are women, with a high prevalence in Africa and Asia (Black et al., 2013). In addition, the global prevalence of anemia among non-pregnant women is 38.2% while that among pregnant women is 29.4% (WHO, 2015). Many underweight women are also stunted or wasted, which are the known risk factors for obstetric complications such as obstructed labor, and in severe cases, injury or death of mothers and their babies (Elder and Ransom, 2003).

Adolescent girls aged 10–19 years are susceptible to malnutrition because they are growing faster than at any other time after their first year of life and, therefore, require more nutrients to support the growth and development to meet the increased body demands (Elder and Ransom, 2003). Currently, about 1.2 billion adolescents make up to 16% of the world's population, of which half are living in Asia alone (UNICEF, 2019). Today, more than 340 million children and adolescents aged 5–19 years are either overweight or obese (WHO, 2020), and about 8.4% of girls are underweight ((NCD-RisC), 2017). Inadequate nutrition and teenage pregnancy are the leading contributing factors to many of the predominant causes of adolescent deaths (Black et al., 2013; Elder and Ransom, 2003). Adolescents who become pregnant and are stunted or underweight are most likely to experience obstructed labor and other obstetric complications. A recent systematic review reported that teenage pregnancy and shorter inter-pregnancy intervals are the leading cause of adverse pregnancy and neonatal outcomes (Lassi et al., 2020a). The existing evidence also suggests that the bodies of the still-growing adolescent mother and her baby may compete for nutrients, raising the risk of LBW, pre-term birth, and early death (Ganchimeg et al., 2014; Marvin-Dowle et al., 2018).

## 16.3 Evidence from animal studies

Animal studies demonstrate that restriction on maternal nutritional intake during pregnancy can affect fetal growth and reduce birth weight (Kind et al., 2006). Previous animal studies have reported that in utero exposure to undernutrition can lead to permeant growth impairments despite subsequent improvement in nutritional status after birth (Plagemann et al., 1999). However, recent evidence on mice, rats, sheep, and guinea pigs has reported that in utero undernutrition is mainly affected by placental nutrient transport, uterine and umbilical blood flows, and placental and fetal metabolism rate (Muhlhausler et al., 2006). This may also vary by nature, duration, time, and severity of nutrition insult. Early nutrition restriction not only affects fetal growth but also impairs the growth and development of specific organs which increases the risk of diseases in later life. Maternal nutrient restriction impairs fetal nephrogenesis in mice, rats, and sheep (Harding et al., 2010). It reduces angiogenesis and increases peripheral vascular resistance, which contributes to the development of hypertension in offspring (Khorram et al., 2007). Similarly, maternal low protein diet in rats reduces cardiomyocyte proliferation in the heart and increases cardiomyocyte apoptosis leading to cardiac dysfunction in post-natal life (Cheema et al., 2005). Moreover, maternal protein restriction during pregnancy alters the fat distribution and food intake, impairs glucose tolerance and cardiac function which results in the development of hypertension in the offspring (Hoppe et al., 2004). Changes in balanced dietary protein also increase the risk of disease in later life. Micronutrient deficiency (i.e., calcium, iron, and zinc, etc.) in the maternal diet has shown fetal growth retardation in rats which have been demonstrated to be associated with increased blood pressure in adulthood (Taylor and Poston, 2007; Woodall et al., 1996).

Apart from undernutrition, overfeeding has also demonstrated adverse long-term health consequences in animals. Exposure to a high-fat diet (HFD) in rats during gestation has been reported to result in impaired endothelial function, glucose tolerance, metabolism, and may lead to increased body weight and fat mass, reduced insulin sensitivity, increased blood glucose, and hypertension in offspring (Sebert et al., 2009). Studies on sheep have shown that over nourishment in pregnancy may result in increased adiposity, placental growth restriction, pre-term birth, and LBW (Wallace et al., 1996, 2004, 2006). The sensitive window for these effects is not known, but animal models suggest that the most vulnerable period is during pregnancy. Most of these studies are observational in design, therefore, further studies are needed to establish an exact mechanism by which maternal under- and over-nutrition adversely affect the offspring. Whether such effects are evident in human subjects is a critical question for public health policy and future nutrition research (Lanigan and Singhal, 2009).

## 16.4 Evidence from human studies

### 16.4.1 Effect of pre-conception nutritional status

Pre-pregnancy nutritional status has a profound effect on a child's linear growth in the first 1000 days of birth (Young et al., 2018). Pre-pregnancy nutrition affects birth outcomes by influencing embryonic and placental development, epigenetic effects, and the distribution of nutrients to mother and fetus (King, 2016). Women with weight <43 kg, height <150 cm, and body mass index (BMI) <17.5 or <18 kg/m$^2$ have an increased risk of having a child with stunted growth at 2 years of age (Young et al., 2018). A review reported an increased risk of pre-term birth and SGA among women with low pre-conception BMI (<18.5 kg/m$^2$) (Dean et al., 2013). Conversely, pre-conceptional obesity has also found to be associated with neonatal and infant mortality, stillbirths, miscarriages, cesarean section, neonatal intensive care unit (NICU) admission, pre-term birth, NTDs, cleft palate, decreased 5-min APGAR scores in the infant, macrosomia, and babies born large for gestational age (LGA) (Hemond et al., 2016; Shin et al., 2016). Additionally, it is also associated with long-term adverse outcomes such as cardiovascular diseases, metabolic syndrome, asthma, and obesity in adulthood (Hemond et al., 2016; Thanoon et al., 2015; Papachatzi et al., 2013).

## 16.4.2 Effect of overweight and obesity

Women who enter pregnancy as overweight/obese are at higher risk of adverse maternal and child health outcomes including gestational diabetes mellitus (GDM), gestational hypertension, depressive disorders, pre-eclampsia, cesarean section, macrosomia, congenital anomalies, and delivery of a LGA baby (Catalano and Demouzon, 2015; Fleming et al., 2018; Gluckman and Hanson, 2008; Poston et al., 2016; Yang et al., 2019; Rozowski and Parodi, 2008; Reiss et al., 2015; Lindam et al., 2016; Cedergren, 2004; Ebbeling et al., 2002). Evidence suggests that overweight and obese women have high rates of miscarriages (especially in the first trimester) compared to the women with normal weight (Rittenberg et al., 2011; Metwally et al., 2008). A study revealed that overweight females do not have a greater embryo euploidy rate in the first trimester miscarriages (Landres et al., 2010), however, some studies concluded that the increased risk of miscarriages in overweight women is independent of embryonic aneuploidy (Metwally et al., 2008; Bellver et al., 2011), and this can be because of some existing conditions in obese women which includes insulin resistance or polycystic ovary syndrome (PCOS), which, is also associated with a higher occurrence of pregnancy loss in women (Barton et al., 2014). The risk of stillbirths, fetal death, neonatal, and infant death also increases among mothers with high BMI (Aune et al., 2014). Obese mothers are also at risk of having a fetus with NTD (Odds ratio (OR) 1.87; 95% confidence interval (CI) 1.62–2.15), spina bifida (OR 2.24; 95% CI 1.86–2.69), cardiovascular anomalies (OR 1.30; 95% CI 1.12–1.51), cleft lip and palate (OR 1.20; 95% CI 1.03–1.40), cleft palate (OR, 1.23; 95% CI, 1.03–1.47), septal anomalies (OR 1.20; 95% CI 1.09–1.31), hydrocephaly (OR 1.68; 95% CI 1.19–2.36), anorectal atresia (OR 1.48; 95% CI 1.12–1.97), and limb reduction anomalies (OR 1.34; 95% CI 1.03–1.73) (Stothard et al., 2009). These risks appear to increase with the increase in maternal BMI (Stothard et al., 2009). A meta-analysis of observational studies also found an association between maternal obesity with increased risk in asthma/wheeze (OR 1.35 95% CI 1.08–1.68) (Forno et al., 2014).

Multiple studies suggested that greater gestational weight gain (GWG) and higher pre-conception BMI are associated with a higher BMI in adolescents and adults (Laitinen et al., 2012; Hochner et al., 2012; Tequeanes et al., 2009; Reynolds et al., 2010; Schack-Nielsen et al., 2010; Hrolfsdottir et al., 2015; Rooney et al., 2011; Mamun et al., 2009). A study of 2432 Australians found that greater maternal GWG was associated with a higher BMI (on average 0.3 kg/m$^2$ (95% CI 0.1–0.4 kg/m$^2$) higher for each 0.1 kg/week greater GWG) in the offspring at the age

21 years (Mamun et al., 2009). Similarly, a study among 6000 Dutch mother-offspring dyads showed that early-pregnancy weight gain was associated with an adverse cardio-metabolic profile (OR 1.20 95% CI 1.07–1.35) in childhood (Gaillard et al., 2015). Maternal obesity is also implicated in the rising burden of asthma and allergic diseases (Godfrey et al., 2017). A meta-analysis of 14 studies including 108,321 mother–child pairs reported that maternal overweight and obesity were associated with increased risk of childhood asthma or wheeze (OR 1.31, 95%CI 1.16–1.49) (Forno et al., 2014). Danish National Birth Cohort's follow-up reported that maternal obesity did not increase the risk of eczema, sensitization (largely assessed to aeroallergens), or hay fever (Harpsøe et al., 2013). These results are consistent with evidence that allergic diseases result from both tissue-specific effects and systemic immune dysregulation during critical stages of development (Godfrey et al., 2017).

### 16.4.3 Effect of gestational diabetes mellitus (GDM)

Diabetes Mellitus Type 2 (T2DM) is a chronic disease caused by insulin resistance in the body (Kadayifci et al., 2019). Women with GDM are at risk of developing T2DM postpregnancy, and fetuses of mothers with T2DM and GDM are at high risk of having glucose intolerance (Noctor and Dunne, 2015). Early-life exposure to GDM, malnutrition, IUGR, HFD, protein restriction, bisphenol, taurine deficiency, alcohol, and excessive weight gain during pregnancy contribute to beta-cell dysfunction, decreased beta-cell mass, pancreatic islet abnormalities, and impaired insulin sensitivity that increases the risk of T2DM in fetus later life (Kadayifci et al., 2019; Nielsen et al., 2014). Women with GDM are also at higher risk of having gestational pre-eclampsia, hypertension, and cesarean birth (Bulletins–Obstetrics, 2013). However, the underlying mechanism relating to adverse pregnancy outcomes and maternal obesity lacks enough evidence in the literature (Valsamakis et al., 2015; Yang et al., 2019).

Environmental, epigenetic, and genetic modifications also play a major role in the development of T2DM in adulthood. The epigenetic modifications interact with maternal diet, genetic alterations, and intrauterine environment. Hereditary factors such as the heritability of epigenetic changes, sex, maternal nutrition, and family history of disease regulate the genetic process which may link to the development of the T2DM in the child (Table 16.1) (Kadayifci et al., 2019; Nielsen et al., 2014). Studies also report that maternal obesity (Retnakaran and Shah, 2016), GDM (Retnakaran and Shah, 2016), and pre-term birth (before 35 weeks of gestation) (Kajantie et al., 2010) contribute to the development of T2DM in later life; however, the mechanism is still unknown (Kadayifci et al., 2019).

Metabolic status during pregnancy affects the fetal environment and the early programming of T2DM during critical developmental stages (Cardin et al., 2007). Luo, et al. conducted a prospective pregnancy cohort study to test the effect of impaired glucose tolerance during pregnancy on fetal insulin sensitivity and beta-cell function (Luo et al., 2010). The study reported that glucose intolerance during pregnancy may result in fetal insulin sensitivity impairment but not beta-cell function and predispose progeny to increase risks of T2DM (Choi et al., 2011). Studies suggest that dysfunction of the insulin-like growth factor 1 receptor (IGF-1R) gene is associated with postnatal growth and LBW (Choi et al., 2011).

**TABLE 16.1** Summary of studies reporting specific target genetic modifications in fetal and early life programming.

| Studies | Gene of interest | Genetic and epigenetic regulations | Physiological outcome |
|---------|------------------|-----------------------------------|----------------------|
| Guarente (2006) and Liang et al. (2009) | SIRT1 | Nutrient-sensing histone deacetylase | Associated with the risk of metabolic syndrome including T2DM |
| Mazaki-Tovi et al. (2010) | RBP4 | Retinol binding protein is responsible for adipokine mediating systemic insulin sensitivity | GDM resulted in higher levels of RBP4 in which related to fetal growth |
| Cooper et al. (2012) | IGR2R, GTPL2–2 | 2 methylated regions examined in cord blood showed DNA methylation alteration | IGR2R in girls and GTPL2–2 in boys were reduced after micronutrient supplementation |
| Valtat et al. (2013) | PGC-1α | Coregulator of glucocorticoids receptor and Pdx1 promoter region | Overexpression during the fetal period impaired glucose tolerance and altered β-cell function |
| Vuguin et al. (2013) | GLUT 4 | Not mentioned in the study | Deletion of GLUT4 led to hypertension and increased serum cytokines |
| Berends et al. (2013) | IRS-1, p110β, and Akt-2 | Prenatal protein restriction resulted in reduced mRNA expression of these insulin-signaling genes | No differences are shown in blood glucose and insulin levels |
| Um et al. (2015) | S6K1 | Downstream effector in the mTOR complex 1 signaling pathway | Deficiency yielded an intrauterine growth restriction phenotype |
| Baier et al. (2015) | ABCC8 | Encodes for a sub-unit of ATP-sensitive potassium channels | Variation in the ABCC8 gene showed higher birth weights and an increased risk of diabetes |

*Kadayifci, F.Z., Haggard, S., Jeon, S., Ranard, K., Tao, D., Pan, Y.-X., 2019. Early-life programming of type 2 diabetes mellitus: Understanding the association between epigenetics/genetics and environmental factors. Curr. Genom. 20 (6), 453–463.*

## 16.5 Evidence from nutrition interventions studies among human

Several nutrition interventions have shown to have a positive impact on maternal and infant outcomes (Keats et al., 2020); however, the long-term effects of these interventions are not well studied. In this section, we will present the most recent data on the long-term effects of nutrition interventions given during the pre-conception period and/or during pregnancy (Table 16.2).

TABLE 16.2 Effect of nutrition intervention on maternal and birth outcomes and long-term effect for offspring.

| Nutrition intervention | Population | Effect on maternal and birth outcomes | Long term effects for offspring |
|---|---|---|---|
| Multiple micronutrient supplementation | Pre-conception (specifically adolescents) | **Significant effects:** reduction in anemia prevalence: (relative risk [RR]: 0.69; 95% confidence interval [CI]: 0.62–0.76), improved birthweight: (standard mean difference:0.25; 95% CI: 0.08–0.41), decreased low birth weight (RR: 0.70; 95% CI: 0.57–0.84), and pre-term birth (RR: 0.73; 95% CI: 0.57–0.95) (Salam et al., 2016) | No intervention study reported data for long-term outcomes for offspring for MMN supplementation at pre-conception |
| | During pregnancy | Significant effects: Child serum/plasma retinol concentration (average MD 0.06 umol/L, 95% CI 0.02–0.09) (Oh et al., 2020) | Maternal supplementation showed a 16% reduction in the risk of diarrhea among children ages 6 months to under-five when compared to IFA (average RR 0.84; 95% CI 0.76–0.92). No improvement in the risk of child wasting (average RR 1.02, 95% CI 0.88–1.18), stunting (average RR 0.99, 95% CI 0.92–1.07), and child underweight status (average RR 0.95, 95% CI 0.84–1.07) was observed (Oh et al., 2020) |
| Iron-folic acid (IFA) supplementation | Women of reproductive age (WRA), including adolescents | Significant effects: Reduction in incidence of neural tube defects (RR = 0.53; 95% CI = 0.41–0.77), and improvement in rate of anemia (RR = 0.66, 95% CI = 0.53–0.81) (Lassi et al., 2020a) | No intervention study reported data for long-term outcomes for offspring for folic acid supplementation |
| | During pregnancy | **Significant effects: Reduction in the risk of maternal anemia by 47% (average RR 0.53, 95% CI 0.43–0.65), and LBW (average RR 0.88, 95% CI 0.78–0.99). It did not affect perinatal mortality** It improved maternal hemoglobin concentration (average MD 7.80 g/L, 95% CI 4.08–11.52) and maternal serum/plasma ferritin concentrations (average MD 25.30 µg/L, 95% CI 9.74–40.8) (Oh et al., 2020) | |

| | | | |
|---|---|---|---|
| Long-chain fatty acids | During pregnancy | Significant effects: reduced risk of pre-eclampsia (RR 0.84, 95% CI 0.69–1.01), early pre-term birth <34 weeks (RR 0.58, 95% CI 0.44–0.77), pre-term birth <37 weeks (RR 0.89, 95% CI 0.81–0.97), perinatal death (RR 0.75, 95% CI 0.54–1.03), LBW babies (RR 0.90, 95% CI 0.82–0.99) (Middleton et al., 2018) <br><br> It may have a possible increase in large-for-gestational-age (LGA) babies (RR 1.15, 95% CI 0.97–1.36). It may have little or no difference on small-for-gestational-age or intrauterine growth restriction (RR 1.01, 95% CI 0.90–1.13) (Middleton et al., 2018) | No impact on BMI of pre-school (<5 years) (standardized mean difference (SMD) 0.07, 95% CI −0.22, 0.36), school-aged children (6–12 years) (SMD=0.12, 95% CI=−0.06, 0.30) (Stratakis et al., 2014) and on children of 19 years old (MD 0, 95% CI −0.83 to 0.83) (Middleton et al., 2018) |
| Vitamin D Supplementation | During pregnancy | Significant effects: reduced risks of SGA infant (RR 0.72, 95% CI 0.52–0.99) (Bi et al., 2018) | Vitamin D supplementation during pregnancy has found reduced risks of wheeze/asthma in offspring (odds ratio 0.72, 95% CI 0.56–0.92)(Venter et al., 2020). Insignificant effects on eczema/atopic dermatitis and food allergies were also noted (Venter et al., 2020). There was no increase in risks of fetal or neonatal mortality or congenital abnormality (Bi et al., 2018) |
| Calcium supplementation | During pregnancy | Significant effects: in LMICs, studies that provided only calcium to mothers showed a greater reduction in the risk of pre-eclampsia/eclampsia (average RR 0.30, 95% CI 0.17–0.52) (according to a posthoc analysis) (Oh et al., 2020) In HICs, High-dose calcium supplementation (≥1 g/day) showed reduction in risk of high blood pressure (BP) (RR 0.65, 95% CI 0.53–0.81), pre-term births (RR 0.45, 95% CI 0.31–0.65). The composite outcome of maternal death or serious morbidity showed reduction (RR 0.80, 95% CI 0.65–0.97) (Hofmeyr et al., 2018) | One study reported a 27% reduction in the risk of developing at least one decayed, missing, or filled surfaces (DMFT) (RR: 0.73, CI 95%: [0.62: 0.87]) (Bergel et al., 2010) Another study showed a statistically significant reduction of −1.92 mmHg (95% CI −3.14 to −0.71) in offspring (1–9 years) systolic blood pressure (Bergel and Barros, 2007) |
| Iodine Supplementation | Women in the pre-conception, pregnancy, or post-partum period | Significant effects: decrease in adverse effects of postpartum hyperthyroidism by 68% (average RR 0.32; 95% CI 0.11–0.91) (Harding et al., 2017) No effect on pre-term birth (average RR 0.71; 95% CI 0.30–1.66) and LBW (average RR 0.56; 95% CI 0.26–1.23) (Harding et al., 2017) | One study reported a higher mean intelligence quotient (IQ) scores among children who were provided with iodine compared to the placebo group(85.6±13.9 compared with 74.4±14.8, respectively; P=0.002) psychological age retardation was lower (15.5±11.6% compared with 26.6±14.1%, respectively; P<0.0001). No differences between groups were reported for the growth rate, skinfold thicknesses, and post-natal bone maturation up to 5 y of age (Zhou et al., 2013) |

Continued

**TABLE 16.2** Effect of nutrition intervention on maternal and birth outcomes and long-term effect for offspring.—cont'd

| Nutrition intervention | Population | Effect on maternal and birth outcomes | Long term effects for offspring |
|---|---|---|---|
| Zinc supplementation | During pregnancy | No impact on pre-eclampsia/eclampsia (average RR 1.01, 95% CI 0.53–1.93) LBW (average RR 1.08, 95% CI 0.94–1.25), pre-term birth (average RR 0.97, 95% CI 0.80–1.17, and SGA babies (average RR 1.05, 9% CI 0.97–1.13) (Oh et al., 2020) | No intervention study reported data for long-term outcomes for offspring for zinc supplementation during pregnancy |
| Balanced energy-protein (BEP) supplementation | During pregnancy | Significant effects: reduction in stillbirths (RR 0.39, 95% CI 0.19–0.80), 40% reduction in the incidence of low birth weight (LBW) births (birth weight <2500 g) (RR 0.60; 95% CI 0.41–0.86), significant increases in birth weight (MD 107.28, 95% CI 68.51–146.04), 9% significant decrease in the incidence of small-for-gestational-age (SGA) births (RR 0.71; 95% CI 0.54–0.94), reduction in perinatal mortality (RR 0.50; 95% CI 0.30–0.84). The evidence reports no impact of BEP supplementation on the birth length and pre-term birth (Lassi et al., 2020b). | No intervention study reported data for long-term outcomes for offspring for BEP supplementation during pregnancy |
| LNS supplementation | At pre-conception | A multi-country trial reported reduction small-for-gestational-age (RR: 0.78; 95% CI: 0.70, 0.88) (Hambidge et al., 2019) | A multi-country trial reported reduction in stunting (RR: 0.69; 95% CI: 0.49, 0.98) (Hambidge et al., 2019) |
| | During pregnancy | No effect on miscarriage (average RR 1.12, 95% CI 0.69–1.80), perinatal mortality (average RR 1.01, 95% CI 0.65–1.65), pre-term birth (average RR 1.15, 95% CI 0.93), LBW (average RR 0.92, 95% CI 0.75–1.13), and on SGA babies (average RR 0.96; 95% CI 0.86–1.07) (Oh et al., 2020) | No intervention study reported data for long-term outcomes for offspring for LNS supplementation during pregnancy |
| Food distribution programs | During pregnancy | Significant effects: improvement in mean birth weight by 46 g (MD 46.00 g, 95% CI 45.10–46.90), and in birth length by 0.20 cm (MD 0.20 cm, 95% CI 0.20–0.20). There was no effect of FDP on miscarriage, maternal mortality, perinatal mortality, neonatal mortality, infant mortality, pre-term birth, LBW, SGA, head circumference, and underweight babies (Lassi et al., 2020b) | Reduction in stunting by 18% (RR 0.82, 95% CI 0.71–0.94), and wasting by 13% (RR 0.87, 95% CI 0.78–0.97) (Lassi et al., 2020b) |

## 16.5.1 Pre-conception care

Pre-conception care is recognized as an important tool for maternal and child health care which involves optimization of nutritional status prior to conception (Dean et al., 2013). Pre-conception care interventions involve lifestyle modification including nutrition (MMN and iron and folic acid supplementation) and physical activity (Lassi et al., 2020a). Adequate intake of folic acid before conception and until the first trimester of pregnancy has shown to reduce NTDs (Gernand et al., 2016), however, a cohort study with a sample of 85,000 children born in 2002 and 2008 showed an inverse relation between periconceptional folic acid supplementation and pregnancy outcomes (Surén et al., 2013). The study reported the development of autism spectrum disorders (ASD) with an adjusted odds ratio of 0.61 for a group of mothers who were supplemented with folic acid from 4 weeks before to 8 weeks after conception (Surén et al., 2013). A systematic review of five studies also demonstrated an increase in the risk of ASD in children born to mothers who were obese (Li et al., 2016), and an inverse association between higher pre-conception BMI and lower serum folate concentrations (Shin et al., 2016). The high risk of ASD has shown to be associated with BMI independent of GWG (Ling et al., 2015).

## 16.5.2 Multiple micronutrient supplementation

MMN supplements contain three or more micronutrients and WHO endorses antenatal supplementation of MMN (Organization, 2020). Micronutrients are vital during pregnancy for metabolic activities that support tissue growth, development, and functioning of the fetus (Gernand et al., 2016). Micronutrient deficiencies result in adverse health outcomes affecting both mother and baby, which is often aggravated due to increased nutritional demand (Black et al., 2013). One of the reasons for micronutrient deficiency could be short inter-pregnancy intervals and repeated pregnancies (Darnton-Hill and Mkparu, 2015). Evidence from the recent reviews on MMN supplementation during the pre-conception period has shown improvements in fetal survival rate, and reductions in anemia prevalence rates (Ahmed et al., 2010; Salam et al., 2016; Sri, 2015). MMN supplementation has also shown improvements in birth weight and reduction in the rates of LBW, and pre-term births among pregnant adolescents (Salam et al., 2016).

MMN supplementation during pregnancy has shown a significant reduction in the risk of LBW and SGA babies (Keats et al., 2019), however, there is no effect on the rates of perinatal mortality, neonatal mortality, and stillbirths (Keats et al., 2019; Smith et al., 2017; Christian et al., 2005; Haider et al., 2011; Ronsmans et al., 2009). Evidence on MMN supplementation to mothers in low- and middle-income countries (LMICs) has reported a reduction in the risk of delivering LBW babies, stillbirths, and SGA babies (Oh et al., 2020). It has shown to reduce the risk of diarrhea among children aged 6 months to under 5 years of age; however, no improvements were observed in the rates of maternal mortality, perinatal mortality, maternal anemia, iron deficiency anemia, and child growth outcomes (such as stunting, wasting, and underweight) (Oh et al., 2020).

## 16.5.3 Iron-folic acid (IFA) supplementation

WHO currently recommends 400 µg folic acid and 30–60 mg of iron daily for all women throughout pregnancy (WHO, 2016). IFA supplementation during pregnancy reduces the risk of LBW babies and the prevalence of anemia, and iron deficiency anemia at term (Oh et al., 2020; Cantor et al., 2015). There is no strong evidence that iron supplementation in non-anemic pregnant women improves maternal or child clinical outcomes. Iron is found to be important for fetal brain development and it has been proposed that treatment of iron deficiency before the development of anemia may benefit in improving neurodevelopmental outcomes (Garner, 2020).

Periconceptional folic acid supplementation to WRA including adolescents from preconception until the first trimester of pregnancy has shown a reduction in the risk of anemia and NTDs (Lassi et al., 2020a). However, studies have not studied the long-term outcomes.

### 16.5.4 Long-chain fatty acids

Long-chain polyunsaturated fatty acids (LCPUFA), such as arachidonic acid (AA) and docosahexaenoic acid (DHA) are important components of the human brain that increase during the third trimester of pregnancy and early infancy (Koletzko et al., 2015; Verfuerden et al., 2020). Human breast milk also contains AA and DHA and their fatty acid precursors, that is why breastfeeding is more encouraged than infant formula. DHA and AA are considered essential because the human body cannot synthesize them.

Reviews evaluating omega-3 LCPUFA interventions (supplements and food) during pregnancy found that it reduces the risk of pre-eclampsia, early pre-term birth, pre-term birth, perinatal death, and LBW (Middleton et al., 2018). It was also found to have a possible increase in LGA babies and had no impact on SGA births. Omega-3 LCPUFA interventions showed no difference in cognition, intelligence quotient, vision, other neurodevelopment and growth outcomes, language, and behavior of the child (Middleton et al., 2018). LCPUFA supplementation during pregnancy also had no impact on BMI among pre-school children (<5 years), school-aged children (6–12 years) (Stratakis et al., 2014), and among the 19-years-old age group (Middleton et al., 2018).

### 16.5.5 Vitamin D supplementation during pregnancy

Institute of Medicine (IoM) 2010 suggests a recommended dietary allowance of 600 international units of vitamin D for all WRA, including pregnant and lactating women (Medicine, 2010). Vitamin D supplementation during pregnancy has shown to reduce the risk of maternal pre-eclampsia (Hollis and Wagner, 2017), SGA infants (Bi et al., 2018), wheeze/asthma (Venter et al., 2020; Litonjua et al., 2016), and autism in offspring (Cannell, 2017); while the evidence from LMICs has shown reductions in the risk of pre-term births (Oh et al., 2020).

### 16.5.6 Calcium supplementation during pregnancy

In populations with low dietary calcium intake, WHO recommends daily oral calcium supplementation of 1.5–2.0 g for pregnant women to prevent pre-eclampsia (WHO, 2018). Any dose of calcium supplementation among healthy pregnant women with low calcium intake has shown to improve the risk of maternal pre-eclampsia/eclampsia in LMICs (Oh et al., 2020). High dose (≥1 g/day) of calcium supplementation in high-income countries (HICs) has shown to reduce the risk of pre-eclampsia, high blood pressure, maternal deaths or serious morbidity, pre-term births, and reduced risk of LBW among women at risk of hypertensive disorder during pregnancy (Hofmeyr et al., 2018). Maternal dietary calcium supplementation has also shown a reduction in the offspring's (1–9 years) systolic BP (Jamshidi and Kelishadi, 2015; Belizán et al., 1997; Bergel and Barros, 2007).

A randomized control trial conducted in one of the hospitals of Rosario, Argentina included a random sample of 195 children of 12-year-old from a follow-up study of 614 women who were randomized during pregnancy to calcium supplementation or placebo group (Bergel et al., 2010). This follow-up study showed improvement in dental caries in children among women who were supplemented with calcium during pregnancy (Bergel et al., 2010).

## 16.5.7 Iodine supplementation

Iodine is an essential nutrient for the biosynthesis of thyroid hormones, which are responsible for regulating growth, development, and metabolism (Harding et al., 2017). Iodine supplementation among WRA has shown a decrease in the likelihood of post-partum hyperthyroidism but did not affect LBW and pre-term birth (Harding et al., 2017). Iodine supplementation in regions of severe iodine deficiency during pre-conception and pregnancy has reported a reduction in risk of cretinism, but no improvements were observed in childhood growth, gross development, intelligence, or pregnancy outcomes, although there was an improvement in some motor functions (Zhou et al., 2013).

## 16.5.8 Zinc supplementation during pregnancy

Zinc is essential for many biological functions such as protein synthesis, cell division, and nucleic acid metabolism (King, 2006). Zinc deficiency can lead to poor birth outcomes and compromised infant development (King, 2006). In LMICs, zinc supplementation during pregnancy has shown no effect in the reduction of risk of pre-eclampsia/eclampsia, pre-term birth, LBW, and SGA babies (Oh et al., 2020). Moreover, the literature lacks evidence on the long-term effects of zinc supplementation at pre-conception and during pregnancy.

## 16.5.9 Balanced energy-protein supplementation

Undernourished women are at high risk of delivering LBW babies, thus providing them with BEP has shown to promote GWG and improve pregnancy outcomes (WHO, 2019). BEP supplementation is defined as a food supplement where proteins provide less than 25% of the total energy content (Imdad and Bhutta, 2012). Previous evidence shows that BEP supplementation during pregnancy reduces the incidence of LBW, SGA babies, stillbirths, and increases birth weight (Imdad and Bhutta, 2012; Ota et al., 2015; Kramer and Kakuma, 2003). The recent evidence on BEP supplementation during pregnancy in LMICs also reports a reduction in incidences of stillbirths, LBW, and SGA births (Lassi et al., 2020b). However, the evidence reports no impact of BEP supplementation on the birth length and pre-term birth (Lassi et al., 2020b). The literature lacks evidence on the effect of BEP on maternal anemia, iron deficiency anemia, maternal mortality, pre-eclampsia, placental abruption, overweight, obesity, congenital anomalies, macrosomia, and child stunting, wasting, and underweight.

### 16.5.10 Lipid-based nutrient supplements (LNS)

Lipid-based nutrient supplements (LNS) include MMN fortified semisolid pastes usually prepared from groundnut paste, vegetable oil, sugar, milk, and different concentrations of micronutrients depending on the type of product and the specific nutritional conditions in the target population. The existing evidence on the impact of LNS pre-conception and during pregnancy is limited; however, a recent review reported no improvements on the rates of LBW, SGA babies, pre-term birth, miscarriage, perinatal mortality, and neonatal mortality when supplemented during pregnancy (Oh et al., 2020; Das et al., 2018). A recent multi-country trial on the small-quantity lipid-nutrient supplement (SQ-LNS) at pre-conception on underweight women reported no difference in mean newborn length-for-age Z-scores (LAZ), but it showed a reduction in rates of stunting and SGA (Hambidge et al., 2019).

### 16.5.11 Food distribution programs

Food distribution programs are defined as the direct provision of food to pregnant women. Eligible food distribution programs could be locally or internationally led and may or may not include elements of nutrition education.

General food distribution programs during pregnancy have shown a reduction in the risk of LBW, SGA births, and improved birth weight and birth length (Lassi et al., 2020b). Besides, it was noted that newborns born to mothers provided food had a lower risk of stunting and wasting in infancy (Lassi et al., 2020b).

## 16.6 Future trends and research

There is an increasing acknowledgment of the double and triple burden of malnutrition (Davis et al., 2020; Singh et al., 2007). In most cases, under-nutrition, over-nutrition, and other micronutrient deficiencies share the common causes, and interventions targeting the first 1000 days of life are beneficial (Naja et al., 2016). Poor nutrition in early life has long-term adverse consequences including short stature, delayed cognition, less schooling, and reduced work capacity and income (Victora et al., 2008; Ramakrishnan et al., 1999). Therefore, avoidance of pregnancy early in life, healthy body composition at the time of conception, optimal weight gain during pregnancy, adequate micronutrient stores during pregnancy, early and exclusive breastfeeding for the first 6 months, appropriate complementary feeding during infancy, healthy diet, and physical activity may promote growth and developmental outcomes. Future research should focus on the efficacy, delivery, and feasibility of these interventions. There is also an increasing concern on the linkage of maternal malnutrition and the growing burden of cardiovascular and other non-communicable diseases in adults; however, evidence of maternal nutrition on long-term health outcomes is limited, thus no robust conclusion can be drawn at this stage. Therefore, further research to understand the maternal nutrition pathways to the development of chronic disease during adulthood should be conducted.

## 16.7 Conclusion

Maternal nutrition plays an important role in fetal growth, infant health, and survival as well as long-term child health and development. Animal and human-based studies do suggest that poor maternal nutrition intake (either before or during pregnancy) has adverse consequences on neonatal, infant, and child health outcomes. However, intervention studies with long-term follow are limited and therefore, further nutritional intervention studies with long-term follow-ups are needed to understand the relationship between maternal nutrition and risks of developing adverse long-term outcomes during childhood and adulthood.

## Sources of additional information

Garner, C. D. Post, T. W. 2017. *Nutrition in pregnancy.* Waltham (MA): Wolters Kluwer.
UNICEF. 2019. *Adolescent demographics* [Online]. United Nations International Children's Emergency Fund. Available: https://data.unicef.org/topic/adolescents/demographics/ [Accessed February 12, 2021].
WHO. 2019. *Balanced energy and protein supplementation during pregnancy* [Online]. World Health Organization. Available: https://www.who.int/elena/titles/energy_protein_pregnancy/en/#:~:text=Current%20evidence%20indicates%20that%20balanced,especially%20among%20undernourished%20pregnant%20women. [Accessed February 9, 2021]. Last update 11 Feb, 2019.
WHO. 2020. *Malnurition* [Online]. World Health Organization (WHO). Available: https://www.who.int/news-room/fact-sheets/detail/malnutrition [Accessed February 3, 2021]. WHO. Last update June 9, 2021.

## References

(NCD-RISC), N. R. F. C, 2017. Worldwide trends in body-mass index, underweight, overweight, and obesity from 1975 to 2016: a pooled analysis of 2416 population-based measurement studies in 128·9 million children, adolescents, and adults. Lancet 390, 2627–2642.

Abu-Saad, K., Fraser, D., 2010. Maternal nutrition and birth outcomes. Epidemiol. Rev. 32, 5–25.

Ahmed, F., Khan, M.R., Akhtaruzzaman, M., Karim, R., Williams, G., Torlesse, H., Darnton-Hill, I., Dalmiya, N., Banu, C.P., Nahar, B., 2010. Long-term intermittent multiple micronutrient supplementation enhances hemoglobin and micronutrient status more than iron+ folic acid supplementation in Bangladeshi rural adolescent girls with nutritional anemia. J. Nutr. 140, 1879–1886.

Ahmed, T., Hossain, M., Sanin, K.I., 2012. Global burden of maternal and child undernutrition and micronutrient deficiencies. Ann. Nutr. Metab. 61 (Suppl 1), 8–17.

Aune, D., Saugstad, O.D., Henriksen, T., Tonstad, S., 2014. Maternal body mass index and the risk of fetal death, stillbirth, and infant death: a systematic review and meta-analysis. JAMA 311, 1536–1546.

Baier, L.J., Muller, Y.L., Remedi, M.S., Traurig, M., Piaggi, P., Wiessner, G., Huang, K., Stacy, A., Kobes, S., Krakoff, J., 2015. ABCC8 R1420H loss-of-function variant in a southwest American Indian community: association with increased birth weight and doubled risk of type 2 diabetes. Diabetes 64, 4322–4332.

Barker, D.J., Thornburg, K.L., 2013. The obstetric origins of health for a lifetime. Clin. Obstet. Gynecol. 56, 511–519.

Barton, J.R., Sibai, A.J., Istwan, N.B., Rhea, D.J., Desch, C.N., Sibai, B.M., 2014. Spontaneously conceived pregnancy after 40: influence of age and obesity on outcome. Am. J. Perinatol. 31, 795–798.

Belizán, J.M., Villar, J., Bergel, E., Del Pino, A., Di Fulvio, S., Galliano, S.V., Kattan, C., 1997. Long term effect of calcium supplementation during pregnancy on the blood pressure of offspring: follow up of a randomised controlled trial. BMJ 315, 281–285.

Bellver, J., Cruz, F., Martínez, M.C., Ferro, J., Ramírez, J.F., Pellicer, A., Garrido, N., 2011. Female overweight is not associated with a higher embryo euploidy rate in first trimester miscarriages karyotyped by hysteroembryoscopy. Fertil. Steril. 96 (931–933), e1.

Berends, L., Fernandez-Twinn, D., Martin-Gronert, M., Cripps, R., Ozanne, S., 2013. Catch-up growth following intra-uterine growth-restriction programmes an insulin-resistant phenotype in adipose tissue. Int. J. Obes. 37, 1051–1057.

Bergel, E., Barros, A.J., 2007. Effect of maternal calcium intake during pregnancy on children's blood pressure: a systematic review of the literature. BMC Pediatr. 7, 1–9.

Bergel, E., Gibbons, L., Rasines, M.G., Luetich, A., Belizán, J.M., 2010. Maternal calcium supplementation during pregnancy and dental caries of children at 12 years of age: follow-up of a randomized controlled trial. Acta Obstet. Gynecol. Scand. 89, 1396–1402.

Bi, W.G., Nuyt, A.M., Weiler, H., Leduc, L., Santamaria, C., Wei, S.Q., 2018. Association between vitamin D supplementation during pregnancy and offspring growth, morbidity, and mortality: a systematic review and meta-analysis. JAMA Pediatr. 172, 635–645.

Black, R.E., Victora, C.G., Walker, S.P., Bhutta, Z.A., Christian, P., De Onis, M., Ezzati, M., Grantham-McGregor, S., Katz, J., Martorell, R., Uauy, R., 2013. Maternal and child undernutrition and overweight in low-income and middle-income countries. Lancet 382, 427–451.

Bulletins-Obstetrics, C. O. P, 2013. Practice bulletin no. 137: gestational diabetes mellitus. Obstet. Gynecol. 122, 406–416.

Cannell, J.J., 2017. Vitamin D and autism, what's new? Rev. Endocr. Metab. Disord. 18, 183–193.

Cantor, A.G., Bougatsos, C., Dana, T., Blazina, I., McDonagh, M., 2015. Routine iron supplementation and screening for iron deficiency anemia in pregnancy: a systematic review for the US preventive services task force. Ann. Intern. Med. 162, 566–576.

Cardin, S., Libby, E., Pelletier, P., Le Bouter, S., Shiroshita-Takeshita, A., Le Meur, N., Léger, J., Demolombe, S., Ponton, A., Glass, L., 2007. Contrasting gene expression profiles in two canine models of atrial fibrillation. Circ. Res. 100, 425–433.

Catalano, P., Demouzon, S., 2015. Maternal obesity and metabolic risk to the offspring: why lifestyle interventions may have not achieved the desired outcomes. Int. J. Obes. 39, 642–649.

Cedergren, M.I., 2004. Maternal morbid obesity and the risk of adverse pregnancy outcome. Obstet. Gynecol. 103, 219–224.

Cheema, K.K., Dent, M.R., Saini, H.K., Aroutiounova, N., Tappia, P.S., 2005. Prenatal exposure to maternal undernutrition induces adult cardiac dysfunction. Br. J. Nutr. 93, 471–477.

Choi, J.-H., Kang, M., Kim, G.-H., Hong, M., Jin, H.Y., Lee, B.-H., Park, J.-Y., Lee, S.-M., Seo, E.-J., Yoo, H.-W., 2011. Clinical and functional characteristics of a novel heterozygous mutation of the IGF1R gene and IGF1R haploinsufficiency due to terminal 15q26. 2-> qter deletion in patients with intrauterine growth retardation and postnatal catch-up growth failure. J. Clin. Endocrinol. Metab. 96, E130–E134.

Christian, P., Osrin, D., Manandhar, D.S., Khatry, S.K., Anthony, M.D.L., West, K.P., 2005. Antenatal micronutrient supplements in Nepal. Lancet 366, 711–712.

Christian, P., Mullany, L.C., Hurley, K., Katz, J., Black, R., 2015. Erratum to "Nutrition and maternal, neonatal, and child health"[Semin Perinatol 39 (5)(2015) 361–372]. Semin. Perinatol. 39, 505.

Cooper, W.N., Khulan, B., Owens, S., Elks, C.E., Seidel, V., Prentice, A.M., Belteki, G., Ong, K.K., Affara, N.A., Constância, M., 2012. DNA methylation profiling at imprinted loci after periconceptional micronutrient supplementation in humans: results of a pilot randomized controlled trial. FASEB J. 26, 1782–1790.

Darnton-Hill, I., Mkparu, U.C., 2015. Micronutrients in pregnancy in low-and middle-income countries. Nutrients 7, 1744–1768.

Das, J.K., Hoodbhoy, Z., Salam, R.A., Bhutta, A.Z., Valenzuela-Rubio, N.G., Prinzo, Z.W., Bhutta, Z.A., 2018. Lipid-based nutrient supplements for maternal, birth, and infant developmental outcomes. Cochrane Database Syst. Rev. 8, CD012610.

Davis, J.N., Oaks, B.M., Engle-Stone, R., 2020. The double burden of malnutrition: a systematic review of operational definitions. Curr. Dev. Nutr. 4, nzaa127.

Dean, S.V., Imam, A.M., Lassi, Z.S., Bhutta, Z.A., 2013. Importance of intervening in the preconception period to impact pregnancy outcomes. Nestle Nutr. Inst. Workshop Ser. 74, 63–73. Maternal and child nutrition: the first 1,000 days.

Ebbeling, C.B., Pawlak, D.B., Ludwig, D.S., 2002. Childhood obesity: public-health crisis, common sense cure. Lancet 360, 473–482.

Elder, L., Ransom, E., 2003. Nutrition of Women and Adolescent Girls: Why It Matters. Population Reference Bureau. (Online). Available from: https://www.prb.org/nutritionofwomenandadolescentgirlswhyitmatters/. (Accessed 12 February 2021).

Fleming, T.P., Watkins, A.J., Velazquez, M.A., Mathers, J.C., Prentice, A.M., Stephenson, J., Barker, M., Saffery, R., Yajnik, C.S., Eckert, J.J., 2018. Origins of lifetime health around the time of conception: causes and consequences. Lancet 391, 1842–1852.

Forno, E., Young, O.M., Kumar, R., Simhan, H., Celedón, J.C., 2014. Maternal obesity in pregnancy, gestational weight gain, and risk of childhood asthma. Pediatrics 134, e535–e546.

Gaillard, R., Steegers, E., Franco, O., Hofman, A., Jaddoe, V., 2015. Maternal weight gain in different periods of pregnancy and childhood cardio-metabolic outcomes. The generation R study. Int. J. Obes. 39, 677–685.

Ganchimeg, T., Ota, E., Morisaki, N., Laopaiboon, M., Lumbiganon, P., Zhang, J., Yamdamsuren, B., Temmerman, M., Say, L., Tunçalp, Ö., 2014. Pregnancy and childbirth outcomes among adolescent mothers: a World Health Organization multicountry study. BJOG Int. J. Obstet. Gynaecol. 121, 40–48.

Garner, C.D., 2020. Nutrition in Pregnancy. (Online). Available from: https://www.uptodate.com/contents/nutrition-in-pregnancy#H717781762. (Accessed 9 February 2021).

Gernand, A.D., Schulze, K.J., Stewart, C.P., West, K.P., Christian, P., 2016. Micronutrient deficiencies in pregnancy worldwide: health effects and prevention. Nat. Rev. Endocrinol. 12, 274–289.

Gluckman, P., Hanson, M., 2008. Developmental and epigenetic pathways to obesity: an evolutionary-developmental perspective. Int. J. Obes. 32, S62–S71.

Godfrey, K.M., Reynolds, R.M., Prescott, S.L., Nyirenda, M., Jaddoe, V.W., Eriksson, J.G., Broekman, B.F., 2017. Influence of maternal obesity on the long-term health of offspring. Lancet Diabetes Endocrinol. 5, 53–64.

Guarente, L., 2006. Sirtuins as potential targets for metabolic syndrome. Nature 444, 868–874.

Haider, B.A., Yakoob, M.Y., Bhutta, Z.A., 2011. Effect of multiple micronutrient supplementation during pregnancy on maternal and birth outcomes. BMC Public Health 11, 1–9.

Hambidge, K.M., Westcott, J.E., Garces, A., Figueroa, L., Goudar, S.S., Dhaded, S.M., Pasha, O., Ali, S.A., Tshefu, A., Lokangaka, A., Derman, R.J., Goldenberg, R.L., Bose, C.L., Bauserman, M., Koso-Thomas, M., Thorsten, V.R., Sridhar, A., Stolka, K., Das, A., McClure, E.M., Krebs, N.F., Women First Preconception Trial Study, G, 2019. A multicountry randomized controlled trial of comprehensive maternal nutrition supplementation initiated before conception: the women first trial. Am. J. Clin. Nutr. 109, 457–469.

Harding, J.E., Derraik, J.G., Bloomfield, F.H., 2010. Maternal undernutrition and endocrine development. Expert. Rev. Endocrinol. Metab. 5, 297–312.

Harding, K.B., Peña-Rosas, J.P., Webster, A.C., Yap, C.M., Payne, B.A., Ota, E., De-Regil, L.M., 2017. Iodine supplementation for women during the preconception, pregnancy and postpartum period. Cochrane Database Syst. Rev. 3, CD011761.

Harpsøe, M.C., Basit, S., Bager, P., Wohlfahrt, J., Benn, C.S., Nøhr, E.A., Linneberg, A., Jess, T., 2013. Maternal obesity, gestational weight gain, and risk of asthma and atopic disease in offspring: a study within the Danish National Birth Cohort. J. Allergy Clin. Immunol. 131, 1033–1040.

Hemond, J., Robbins, R.B., Young, P.C., 2016. The effects of maternal obesity on neonates, infants, children, adolescents, and adults. Clin. Obstet. Gynecol. 59, 216–227.

Hochner, H., Friedlander, Y., Calderon-Margalit, R., Meiner, V., Sagy, Y., Avgil-Tsadok, M., Burger, A., Savitsky, B., Siscovick, D.S., Manor, O., 2012. Associations of maternal prepregnancy body mass index and gestational weight gain with adult offspring cardiometabolic risk factors: the Jerusalem perinatal family follow-up study. Circulation 125, 1381–1389.

Hofmeyr, G.J., Lawrie, T.A., Atallah, A.N., Torloni, M.R., 2018. Calcium supplementation during pregnancy for preventing hypertensive disorders and related problems. Cochrane Database Syst. Rev. 10, CD001059.

Hollis, B.W., Wagner, C.L., 2017. Vitamin D supplementation during pregnancy: improvements in birth outcomes and complications through direct genomic alteration. Mol. Cell. Endocrinol. 453, 113–130.

Hoppe, C., Rovenna Udam, T., Lauritzen, L., Mølgaard, C., Juul, A., Fleischer Michaelsen, K., 2004. Animal protein intake, serum insulin-like growth factor I, and growth in healthy 2.5-y-old Danish children. Am. J. Clin. Nutr. 80, 447–452.

Hrolfsdottir, L., Rytter, D., Olsen, S., Bech, B., Maslova, E., Henriksen, T., Halldorsson, T., 2015. Gestational weight gain in normal weight women and offspring cardio-metabolic risk factors at 20 years of age. Int. J. Obes. 39, 671–676.

Imdad, A., Bhutta, Z.A., 2012. Maternal nutrition and birth outcomes: effect of balanced protein-energy supplementation. Paediatr. Perinat. Epidemiol. 26, 178–190.

Jamshidi, F., Kelishadi, R., 2015. A systematic review on the effects of maternal calcium supplementation on offspring's blood pressure. J. Res. Med. Sci. 20, 994.

Kadayifci, F.Z., Haggard, S., Jeon, S., Ranard, K., Tao, D., Pan, Y.-X., 2019. Early-life programming of type 2 diabetes mellitus: understanding the association between epigenetics/genetics and environmental factors. Curr. Genomics 20, 453–463.

Kajantie, E., Osmond, C., Barker, D.J., Eriksson, J.G., 2010. Preterm birth—a risk factor for type 2 diabetes?: the Helsinki birth cohort study. Diabetes Care 33, 2623–2625.

Keats, E.C., Haider, B.A., Tam, E., Bhutta, Z.A., 2019. Multiple-micronutrient supplementation for women during pregnancy. Cochrane Database Syst. Rev. 3, CD004905.

Keats, E.C., Das, J.K., Salam, R.A., Lassi, Z.S., Imdad, A., Black, R.E., Bhutta, Z., 2020. What Works for Maternal and Child Undernutrition: A Review of the Evidence. Available from SSRN 3541130.

Khorram, O., Khorram, N., Momeni, M., Han, G., Halem, J., Desai, M., Ross, M.G., 2007. Maternal undernutrition inhibits angiogenesis in the offspring: a potential mechanism of programmed hypertension. Am. J. Phys. Regul. Integr. Comp. Phys. 293, R745–R753.

Kimani-Murage, E.W., Muthuri, S.K., Oti, S.O., Mutua, M.K., Van De Vijver, S., Kyobutungi, C., 2015. Evidence of a double burden of malnutrition in urban poor settings in Nairobi, Kenya. PLoS One 10, e0129943.

Kind, K.L., Moore, V.M., Davies, M.J., 2006. Diet around conception and during pregnancy–effects on fetal and neonatal outcomes. Reprod. BioMed. Online 12, 532–541.

King, J., 2006. Zinc. In: Shils, M.E., Shike, M. (Eds.), Modern Nutrition in Health and Disease. Lippincott Williams & Wilkins, Philadelphia, PA.

King, J.C., 2016. A summary of pathways or mechanisms linking preconception maternal nutrition with birth outcomes. J. Nutr. 146, 1437S–1444S.

Koletzko, B., Bhatia, J., Bhutta, Z.A., Cooper, P., Makrides, M., Uauy, R., Wang, W., 2015. Pediatric Nutrition in Practice. Karger Medical and Scientific Publishers.

Kramer, M.S., Kakuma, R., 2003. Energy and protein intake in pregnancy. Cochrane Database Syst. Rev. (4), CD000032.

Laitinen, J., Jääskeläinen, A., Hartikainen, A.L., Sovio, U., Vääräsmäki, M., Pouta, A., Kaakinen, M., Järvelin, M.R., 2012. Maternal weight gain during the first half of pregnancy and offspring obesity at 16 years: a prospective cohort study. BJOG Int. J. Obstet. Gynaecol. 119, 716–723.

Landres, I.V., Milki, A.A., Lathi, R.B., 2010. Karyotype of miscarriages in relation to maternal weight. Hum. Reprod. 25, 1123–1126.

Lanigan, J., Singhal, A., 2009. Early nutrition and long-term health: a practical approach: symposium on 'early nutrition and later disease: current concepts, research and implications'. Proc. Nutr. Soc. 68, 422–429.

Lassi, Z.S., Kedzior, S., Tariq, W., Jadoon, Y., Das, J.K., Bhutta, Z.A., 2020a. Effects of preconception care and periconception interventions on maternal nutritional status and birth outcomes in low and middle income countries: a systematic review. Nutrients 12, 606.

Lassi, Z.S., Padhani, Z.A., Rabbani, A., Rind, F., Salam, R., Das, J.K., Bhutta, Z.A., 2020b. Impact of dietary interventions during pregnancy on maternal, neonatal and child outcomes in low- and middle-income countries. Nutrients 12 (2), 531.

Li, Y.-M., Ou, J.-J., Liu, L., Zhang, D., Zhao, J.-P., Tang, S.-Y., 2016. Association between maternal obesity and autism spectrum disorder in offspring: a meta-analysis. J. Autism Dev. Disord. 46, 95–102.

Liang, F., Kume, S., Koya, D., 2009. SIRT1 and insulin resistance. Nat. Rev. Endocrinol. 5, 367.

Lindam, A., Johansson, S., Stephansson, O., Wikström, A.-K., Cnattingius, S., 2016. High maternal body mass index in early pregnancy and risks of stillbirth and infant mortality—a population-based sibling study in Sweden. Am. J. Epidemiol. 184, 98–105.

Ling, Z., Wang, J., Li, X., Zhong, Y., Qin, Y., Xie, S., Yang, S., Zhang, J., 2015. Association between mothers' body mass index before pregnancy or weight gain during pregnancy and autism in children. Zhonghua Liu Xing Bing Xue Za Zhi 36, 949–952.

Litonjua, A.A., Carey, V.J., Laranjo, N., Harshfield, B.J., McElrath, T.F., O'connor, G.T., Sandel, M., Iverson, R.E., Lee-Paritz, A., Strunk, R.C., 2016. Effect of prenatal supplementation with vitamin D on asthma or recurrent wheezing in offspring by age 3 years: the VDAART randomized clinical trial. JAMA 315, 362–370.

Luo, Z.-C., Delvin, E., Fraser, W.D., Audibert, F., Deal, C.I., Julien, P., Girard, I., Shear, R., Levy, E., Nuyt, A.-M., 2010. Maternal glucose tolerance in pregnancy affects fetal insulin sensitivity. Diabetes Care 33, 2055–2061.

Mamun, A.A., O'Callaghan, M., Callaway, L., Williams, G., Najman, J., Lawlor, D.A., 2009. Associations of gestational weight gain with offspring body mass index and blood pressure at 21 years of age: evidence from a birth cohort study. Circulation 119 (13), 1720–1727.

Marvin-Dowle, K., Kilner, K., Burley, V.J., Soltani, H., 2018. Impact of adolescent age on maternal and neonatal outcomes in the born in Bradford cohort. BMJ Open 8, e016258.

Mazaki-Tovi, S., Romero, R., Vaisbuch, E., Kusanovic, J.P., Chaiworapongsa, T., Kim, S.K., Mittal, P., Dong, Z., Pacora, P., Yeo, L., 2010. Retinol-binding protein 4: a novel adipokine implicated in the genesis of LGA in the absence of gestational diabetes mellitus. J. Perinat. Med. 38, 147–155.

Medicine, I.O., 2010. Report at a Glance, Report Brief: Dietary Reference Intakes for Calcium and Vitamin D.

Metwally, M., Ong, K.J., Ledger, W.L., Li, T.C., 2008. Does high body mass index increase the risk of miscarriage after spontaneous and assisted conception? A meta-analysis of the evidence. Fertil. Steril. 90, 714–726.

Middleton, P., Gomersall, J.C., Gould, J.F., Shepherd, E., Olsen, S.F., Makrides, M., 2018. Omega-3 fatty acid addition during pregnancy. Cochrane Database Syst. Rev. 11, CD003402.

Muhlhausler, B.S., Adam, C.L., Findlay, P., Duffield, J., McMillen, I., Muhlhausler, B., Adam, C., Findlay, P., Duffield, J., McMillen, I., 2006. Increased maternal nutrition alters development of the appetite-regulating network in the brain. FASEB J. 20, E556–E565.

Naja, F., Nasreddine, L., Yunis, K., Clinton, M., Nassar, A., Jarrar, S.F., Moghames, P., Ghazeeri, G., Rahman, S., Al-Chetachi, W., 2016. Study protocol: mother and infant nutritional assessment (MINA) cohort study in Qatar and Lebanon. BMC Pregnancy Childbirth 16, 1–11.

Nielsen, J.H., Haase, T.N., Jaksch, C., Nalla, A., Søstrup, B., Nalla, A.A., Larsen, L., Rasmussen, M., Dalgaard, L.T., Gaarn, L.W., 2014. Impact of fetal and neonatal environment on beta cell function and development of diabetes. Acta Obstet. Gynecol. Scand. 93, 1109–1122.

Noctor, E., Dunne, F.P., 2015. Type 2 diabetes after gestational diabetes: the influence of changing diagnostic criteria. World J. Diabetes 6, 234.

Oh, C., Keats, E.C., Bhutta, Z.A., 2020. Vitamin and mineral supplementation during pregnancy on maternal, birth, child health and development outcomes in low- and middle-income countries: a systematic review. Nutrients 12 (2), 491.

Organization, W. H, 2020. WHO Antenatal Care Recommendations for a Positive Pregnancy Experience: Nutritional Interventions Update: Vitamin D Supplements during Pregnancy.

Ota, E., Hori, H., Mori, R., Tobe-Gai, R., Farrar, D., 2015. Antenatal dietary education and supplementation to increase energy and protein intake. Cochrane Database Syst. Rev. (6), CD000032.

Papachatzi, E., Dimitriou, G., Dimitropoulos, K., Vantarakis, A., 2013. Pre-pregnancy obesity: maternal, neonatal and childhood outcomes. J. Neonatal-Perinatal Med. 6, 203–216.

Plagemann, A., Harder, T., Melchior, K., Rake, A., Rohde, W., Dörner, G., 1999. Elevation of hypothalamic neuropeptide Y-neurons in adult offspring of diabetic mother rats. Neuroreport 10, 3211–3216.

Poston, L., Caleyachetty, R., Cnattingius, S., Corvalán, C., Uauy, R., Herring, S., Gillman, M.W., 2016. Preconceptional and maternal obesity: epidemiology and health consequences. Lancet Diabetes Endocrinol. 4, 1025–1036.

Ramakrishnan, U., Martorell, R., Schroeder, D.G., Flores, R., 1999. Role of intergenerational effects on linear growth. J. Nutr. 129, 544S–549S.

Ramakrishnan, U., Imhoff-Kunsch, B., Martorell, R., 2014. Maternal nutrition interventions to improve maternal, newborn, and child health outcomes. Nestle Nutr. Inst. Workshop Ser. 78, 71–80.

Reiss, K., Breckenkamp, J., Borde, T., Brenne, S., David, M., Razum, O., 2015. Contribution of overweight and obesity to adverse pregnancy outcomes among immigrant and non-immigrant women in Berlin, Germany. Eur. J. Pub. Health 25, 839–844.

Retnakaran, R., Shah, B., 2016. Sex of the baby and future maternal risk of type 2 diabetes in women who had gestational diabetes. Diabet. Med. 33, 956–960.

Reynolds, R., Osmond, C., Phillips, D., Godfrey, K., 2010. Maternal BMI, parity, and pregnancy weight gain: influences on offspring adiposity in young adulthood. J. Clin. Endocrinol. Metab. 95, 5365–5369.

Rittenberg, V., Seshadri, S., Sunkara, S.K., Sobaleva, S., Oteng-Ntim, E., El-Toukhy, T., 2011. Effect of body mass index on IVF treatment outcome: an updated systematic review and meta-analysis. Reprod. BioMed. Online 23, 421–439.

Ronnenberg, A.G., Wang, X., Xing, H., Chen, C., Chen, D., Guang, W., Guang, A., Wang, L., Ryan, L., Xu, X., 2003. Low preconception body mass index is associated with birth outcome in a prospective cohort of Chinese women. J. Nutr. 133, 3449–3455.

Ronsmans, C., Fisher, D.J., Osmond, C., Margetts, B.M., Fall, C.H.D., 2009. Multiple micronutrient supplementation during pregnancy in low-income countries: a meta-analysis of effects on stillbirths and on early and late neonatal mortality. Food Nutr. Bull. 30, S547–S555.

Rooney, B.L., Mathiason, M.A., Schauberger, C.W., 2011. Predictors of obesity in childhood, adolescence, and adulthood in a birth cohort. Matern. Child Health J. 15, 1166–1175.

Rozowski, J., Parodi, C.G., 2008. Implications of the nutrition transition in the nutritional status on pregnant women. In: Lammi-Keefe, C.J., Couch, S.C., Philipson, E.H. (Eds.), Handbook of Nutrition and Pregnancy. Humana Press, Totowa, NJ.

Salam, R.A., Das, J.K., Bhutta, Z.A., 2014. Impact of intrauterine growth restriction on long-term health. Curr. Opin. Clin. Nutr. Metab. Care 17 (3), 249–254.

Salam, R.A., Hooda, M., Das, J.K., Arshad, A., Lassi, Z.S., Middleton, P., Bhutta, Z.A., 2016. Interventions to improve adolescent nutrition: a systematic review and meta-analysis. J. Adolesc. Health 59, S29–S39.

Schack-Nielsen, L., Michaelsen, K., Gamborg, M., Mortensen, E., Sørensen, T., 2010. Gestational weight gain in relation to offspring body mass index and obesity from infancy through adulthood. Int. J. Obes. 34, 67–74.

Sebert, S., Hyatt, M., Chan, L., Patel, N., Bell, R., Keisler, D., Stephenson, T., Budge, H., Symonds, M., Gardner, D., 2009. Maternal nutrient restriction between early and midgestation and its impact upon appetite regulation after juvenile obesity. Endocrinology 150, 634–641.

Shin, D., Lee, K.W., Song, W.O., 2016. Pre-pregnancy weight status is associated with diet quality and nutritional biomarkers during pregnancy. Nutrients 8, 162.

Singh, R.B., Pella, D., Mechirova, V., Kartikey, K., Demeester, F., Tomar, R.S., Beegom, R., Mehta, A.S., Gupta, S.B., De, A.K., 2007. Prevalence of obesity, physical inactivity and undernutrition, a triple burden of diseases during transition in a developing economy. The Five City study Group. Acta Cardiol. 62, 119–127.

Smith, E.R., Shankar, A.H., Wu, L.S., Aboud, S., Adu-Afarwuah, S., Ali, H., Agustina, R., Arifeen, S., Ashorn, P., Bhutta, Z.A., 2017. Modifiers of the effect of maternal multiple micronutrient supplementation on stillbirth, birth outcomes, and infant mortality: a meta-analysis of individual patient data from 17 randomised trials in low-income and middle-income countries. Lancet Glob. Health 5, e1090–e1100.

Sri, S., 2015. Micronutrients supplementation during preconception period improves fetal survival and cord blood insulin-like growth factor 1. Asian J. Clin. Nutr. 7, 33–44.

Stothard, K.J., Tennant, P.W., Bell, R., Rankin, J., 2009. Maternal overweight and obesity and the risk of congenital anomalies: a systematic review and meta-analysis. JAMA 301, 636–650.

Stratakis, N., Gielen, M., Chatzi, L., Zeegers, M.P., 2014. Effect of maternal n-3 long-chain polyunsaturated fatty acid supplementation during pregnancy and/or lactation on adiposity in childhood: a systematic review and meta-analysis of randomized controlled trials. Eur. J. Clin. Nutr. 68, 1277–1287.

Subramanian, S., Ackerson, L.K., Smith, G.D., John, N.A., 2009. Association of maternal height with child mortality, anthropometric failure, and anemia in India. JAMA 301, 1691–1701.

Surén, P., Roth, C., Bresnahan, M., Haugen, M., Hornig, M., Hirtz, D., Lie, K.K., Lipkin, W.I., Magnus, P., Reichborn-Kjennerud, T., 2013. Association between maternal use of folic acid supplements and risk of autism spectrum disorders in children. JAMA 309, 570–577.

Taylor, P., Poston, L., 2007. Developmental programming of obesity in mammals. Exp. Physiol. 92, 287–298.

Tequeanes, A.L.L., Gigante, D.P., Assunção, M.C.F., Chica, D.A.G., Horta, B.L., 2009. Maternal anthropometry is associated with the body mass index and waist: height ratio of offspring at 23 years of age. J. Nutr. 139, 750–754.

Thanoon, O., Gharaibeh, A., Mahmood, T., 2015. The implications of obesity on pregnancy outcome. Obstet. Gynaecol. Reprod. Med. 25, 102–105.

Um, S.H., Sticker-Jantscheff, M., Chau, G.C., Vintersten, K., Mueller, M., Gangloff, Y.-G., Adams, R.H., Spetz, J.-F., Elghazi, L., Pfluger, P.T., 2015. S6K1 controls pancreatic β cell size independently of intrauterine growth restriction. J. Clin. Invest. 125, 2736–2747.

UNICEF, 2019. Adolescent Demographics. United Nations International Children's Emergency Fund. (Online). Available from: https://data.unicef.org/topic/adolescents/demographics/. (Accessed 12 February 2021).

Valsamakis, G., Kyriazi, E.L., Mouslech, Z., Siristatidis, C., Mastorakos, G., 2015. Effect of maternal obesity on pregnancy outcomes and long-term metabolic consequences. Hormones 14, 345–357.

Valtat, B., Riveline, J.-P., Zhang, P., Singh-Estivalet, A., Armanet, M., Venteclef, N., Besseiche, A., Kelly, D.P., Tronche, F., Ferré, P., 2013. Fetal Pgc-1α overexpression programs adult pancreatic β-cell dysfunction. Diabetes 62, 1206–1216.

Venter, C., Agostoni, C., Arshad, S.H., Ben-Abdallah, M., Du Toit, G., Fleischer, D.M., Greenhawt, M., Glueck, D.H., Groetch, M., Lunjani, N., 2020. Dietary factors during pregnancy and atopic outcomes in childhood: a systematic review from the European academy of allergy and clinical immunology. Pediatr. Allergy Immunol. 31, 889–912.

Verfuerden, M.L., Dib, S., Jerrim, J., Fewtrell, M., Gilbert, R.E., 2020. Effect of long-chain polyunsaturated fatty acids in infant formula on long-term cognitive function in childhood: a systematic review and meta-analysis of randomised controlled trials. PLoS One 15, e0241800.

Victora, C.G., Adair, L., Fall, C., Hallal, P.C., Martorell, R., Richter, L., Sachdev, H.S., Maternal & Child Undernutrition Study, G, 2008. Maternal and child undernutrition: consequences for adult health and human capital. Lancet 371, 340–357.

Vuguin, P.M., Hartil, K., Kruse, M., Kaur, H., Lin, C.-L.V., Fiallo, A., Glenn, A.S., Patel, A., Williams, L., Seki, Y., 2013. Shared effects of genetic and intrauterine and perinatal environment on the development of metabolic syndrome. PLoS One 8, e63021.

Wallace, J., Aitken, R., Cheyne, M., 1996. Nutrient partitioning and fetal growth in rapidly growing adolescent ewes. Reproduction 107, 183–190.

Wallace, J.M., Aitken, R.P., Milne, J.S., Hay Jr., W.W., 2004. Nutritionally mediated placental growth restriction in the growing adolescent: consequences for the fetus. Biol. Reprod. 71, 1055–1062.

Wallace, J.M., Milne, J.S., Redmer, D.A., Aitken, R.P., 2006. Effect of diet composition on pregnancy outcome in overnourished rapidly growing adolescent sheep. Br. J. Nutr. 96, 1060–1068.

WHO, 2015. The Global Prevalence of Anaemia in 2011. World Health Organization. (Online). Available from: https://apps.who.int/iris/bitstream/handle/10665/177094/9789241564960_eng.pdf?sequence=1. (Accessed 12 February 2021).

WHO, 2016. WHO Recommendations on Antenatal Care for a Positive Pregnancy Experience. World Health Organization, Geneva.

WHO, 2018. WHO Recommendation: Calcium Supplementation during Pregnancy for Prevention of Pre-Eclampsia and its Complications. World Health Organization.

WHO, 2019. Balanced Energy and Protein Supplementation during Pregnancy. World Health Organization. (Online). Available from: https://www.who.int/elena/titles/energy_protein_pregnancy/en/#:~:text=Current%20evidence%20indicates%20that%20balanced,especially%20among%20undernourished%20pregnant%20women. (Accessed 9 February 2021).

WHO, 2020. Malnurition. World Health Organization (WHO). (Online). Available from: https://www.who.int/news-room/fact-sheets/detail/malnutrition. (Accessed 3 February 2021).

Woodall, S., Johnston, B., Breier, B., Gluckman, P., 1996. Chronic maternal undernutrition in the rat leads to delayed postnatal growth and elevated blood pressure of offspring. Pediatr. Res. 40, 438–443.

Yang, Z., Phung, H., Freebairn, L., Sexton, R., Raulli, A., Kelly, P., 2019. Contribution of maternal overweight and obesity to the occurrence of adverse pregnancy outcomes. Aust. N. Z. J. Obstet. Gynaecol. 59, 367–374.

Young, M.F., Nguyen, P.H., Gonzalez Casanova, I., Addo, O.Y., Tran, L.M., Nguyen, S., Martorell, R., Ramakrishnan, U., 2018. Role of maternal preconception nutrition on offspring growth and risk of stunting across the first 1000 days in Vietnam: a prospective cohort study. PLoS One 13, e0203201.

Zerfu, T.A., Umeta, M., Baye, K., 2016. Dietary diversity during pregnancy is associated with reduced risk of maternal anemia, preterm delivery, and low birth weight in a prospective cohort study in rural Ethiopia. Am. J. Clin. Nutr. 103, 1482–1488.

Zhou, S.J., Anderson, A.J., Gibson, R.A., Makrides, M., 2013. Effect of iodine supplementation in pregnancy on child development and other clinical outcomes: a systematic review of randomized controlled trials. Am. J. Clin. Nutr. 98, 1241–1254.

# Addressing nutritional needs in preterm infants to promote long-term health

Monique van de Lagemaat[a,b,*], Charlotte A. Ruys[a,b,*], Harrie N. Lafeber[a,b,†], Johannes B. van Goudoever[a,b], and Chris H.P. van den Akker[a,b]

[a]Department of Pediatrics and Neonatology, Amsterdam UMC, location Vrije Universiteit Amsterdam and location University of Amsterdam, Emma Children's Hospital, Amsterdam, The Netherlands [b]Amsterdam Reproduction and Development (AR&D), Amsterdam, The Netherlands

## CHAPTER LEARNING OBJECTIVES

- To learn about the long-term cardiometabolic and neurodevelopmental consequences in preterm infants, especially in those experiencing extra-uterine growth restriction
- To learn about the need to start parenteral nutrition shortly after birth with rapid replacement by enteral nutrition aiming to mimic intra-uterine growth rates
- To learn about the pivotal role of human milk and the need for multinutrient fortification
- To learn about nutrition after discharge with a role for human milk or nutrient-enriched formula if human milk is unavailable.

* Authors contributed equally.

† Harrie N. Lafeber has sadly passed away during the writing of this chapter. He had an extraordinary critical intellect and a highly productive career in neonatal nutrition and physiology. Harrie was recognized for his remarkable work on growth restriction, bone mineralization, and postdischarge formula and served within the Committee on Nutrition of ESPGHAN.

## 17.1  Introduction

About 10% of all neonates are born preterm, i.e., before completing 37 weeks of pregnancy (Blencowe et al., 2012). Most of them are moderately preterm, but approximately 2% of all neonates are born very preterm, i.e., before completing 32 weeks of pregnancy (Blencowe et al., 2012). Consequently, worldwide, an estimated 15 million infants are born prematurely every year, and this number is rising each year (Blencowe et al., 2012). Preterm infants are overall immature at birth, leaving them at a high risk of acute and chronic morbidity or even death. During the last decades, improvements in medical and nursing care have led to a considerable increase in survival chances for preterm infants (Stoll et al., 2015). However, many preterm infants face problems in later life, and the occurrence of these problems has remained unchanged or has even increased over time (Stoll et al., 2015; Costeloe et al., 2012; Twilhaar et al., 2018b). As a result, the focus of perinatal interventions has shifted more and more to enhance long-term health and quality of life. Long-term health in those born preterm may be modulated by growth and nutrition in early life. This chapter will review and discuss the nutritional needs of preterm infants and how they may influence their long-term health.

## 17.2  Prematurity and long-term consequences

Many of the causes that result in detrimental effects arising from preterm birth can probably never be prevented completely. Apart from direct complications of neonatal disease, adverse outcomes may also be related to the very different physical environment once the infant is born prematurely, while optimal development should take place in the womb. For example, neonates are exposed to higher oxygen levels, gravity, different thermoregulation, and an environment full of microbes. Examples of improved neonatal care include the reduction of the fraction of inspired oxygen exposure during the resuscitation, which decreases oxidative stress with subsequently long-term benefits in preterm infants who have reduced antioxidant capacities (Lara-Canton et al., 2020; Rantakari et al., 2021). Another intervention to reduce morbidity is strict infection prevention, since preterm infants are prone to sepsis because of an immature immune system. Additionally, psycho-emotional stress reduction programs for both parents (Westrup et al., 2004) and their infants may ameliorate outcomes (Bracht et al., 2013; van Veenendaal et al., 2019, 2020) as stress is known to influence brain development (de Kloet et al., 2005) possibly through epigenetic changes (Lucassen et al., 2013).

Severe illness during the first few weeks of life may have a negative impact on later quality of life. These morbidities include, for example, necrotizing enterocolitis (NEC), sepsis, bronchopulmonary dysplasia (BPD), retinopathy of prematurity, periventricular leukomalacia, and intracranial hemorrhages. With or without these major morbidities, preterm-born children are at risk for neurodevelopmental problems as well as cardiometabolic diseases in later life, as described in the following paragraphs.

During the intrauterine third trimester, rapid fetal brain growth and development take place (Cormack et al., 2019). Unfortunately, very preterm infants often show delayed cortical maturation at term equivalent age (Vinall et al., 2013) and have an increased risk of white matter injury (Cormack et al., 2019). Especially serious infections in the neonatal period have been associated with white matter damage, which is still apparent in the brains of school-aged children (de Kieviet et al., 2012; van Vliet et al., 2013; Matei et al., 2020). Systematic reviews and meta-analyses show that those born very preterm have their intelligence quotient score reduced by 0.86 SD (Twilhaar et al., 2018b). Overall, 20%–45% of very preterm infants have suboptimal neurodevelopment, including cognitive, motor, and behavioral problems in childhood and adolescence compared to those born at term (Martinez-Jimenez et al., 2020; Guellec et al., 2016; Fenton et al., 2021; Sammallahti et al., 2014; Cormack et al., 2019; Franz et al., 2018; Agrawal et al., 2018; Twilhaar et al., 2018a). Furthermore, it must be noted that not only those infants suffering from major morbidities in the direct postnatal phase (Serenius et al., 2013; Vliegenthart et al., 2019; Matei et al., 2020), but also preterm infants without severe complications during hospitalization have poorer performance in specific neurocognitive skills than term-born children at school-age or young adulthood (Kallankari et al., 2015). In particular, preterm infants who experience extra-uterine growth restriction (EUGR) are at risk of impaired neurodevelopment, including autism and attention-deficit hyperactivity disorder in later life (Kuzniewicz et al., 2014; Wong et al., 2014; Keir et al., 2014; Lampi et al., 2012), whereas those with more rapid postnatal growth have a more favorable outcome (Ruys et al., 2019; Sammallahti et al., 2014; Cormack et al., 2019; Taine et al., 2018; Frondas-Chauty et al., 2018; Simon et al., 2017; Guellec et al., 2016).

Not only are neurocognitive effects noted, but many other organ systems are affected in early life with later consequences. Those born preterm show features of increased glucocorticoid bioactivity and metabolic syndrome, including raised blood pressure, increased fat mass, dyslipidemia, insulin resistance, and diabetes mellitus type 2 (Lawlor et al., 2006; Hofman et al., 2004; Sipola-Leppanen and Kajantie, 2015; Parkinson et al., 2013; Mathai et al., 2013; Ueda et al., 2014; Markopoulou et al., 2019; Chiavaroli et al., 2021). Young adults born preterm or with very low birth weight (VLBW), despite having a relatively normal body mass index, exhibit decreased lean mass, increased fat content, and centralization of fat distribution (Euser et al., 2005; Thomas et al., 2011). It has been hypothesized that the link between metabolic syndrome and prematurity is partly explained by infant adiposity that is related to infant nutrition, and subsequently tracks into childhood and adulthood, predisposing those born preterm to metabolic syndrome (Singh et al., 2008; Kerkhof et al., 2012). However, many of the previously cited studies included infants born several decades ago, in a time when less attention was paid to early nutrition and capabilities, and knowledge was less available to support growth resembling intrauterine rates. It therefore remains speculative whether neonates born nowadays, who have a greater chance of long-term survival, and who are on average less growth-restricted around discharge than before, are still at higher risk for long-term metabolic complications as described previously.

Although current literature is focused mostly on the very preterm population, the possible long-term effects of moderate to late preterm birth (i.e., after 32–36 weeks of pregnancy) are increasingly gaining attention. A higher risk for both cardiometabolic disease and neurodevelopmental delay has been described (Kajantie et al., 2019; Sharma et al., 2021). Although individual risks may only marginally be increased, at a population level substantial burden is to be expected because of the large number of infants born at these gestational ages.

## 17.3 Feeding the preterm infant: Nutritional needs and feeding practices

### 17.3.1 General aspects

Early nutritional management plays an important role in neonatology through its impact on somatic growth, including bone growth (Meneghelli et al., 2016; Ryan and Kovacs, 2020), as well as promoting the development of the gastrointestinal tract (prevention of intestinal atrophy), the immune system (van Belkum et al., 2020) and the brain, despite inconsistent findings with regard to the latter (Hortensius et al., 2019; Lin et al., 2019). Especially in VLBW (birth weight $\leq 1500\,g$) and extremely low birth weight (ELBW; birth weight $\leq 1000\,g$) infants, poor nutrition and impaired growth are associated with adverse long-term consequences. However, due to feeding intolerance and the perceived risk of NEC, providing enteral nutrition to preterm infants remains a major challenge. Although the incidence and severity of so-called extra-uterine growth failure have decreased over the last decades, it is still too common (Stevens et al., 2018; Hiltunen et al., 2018; Martinez-Jimenez et al., 2020). In a recent report from 11 European countries, infants had lost 1.2 standard deviations on average at discharge when compared to their birth weight standard deviation (El Rafei et al., 2021). In fact, 14% lost more than two standard deviations when compared to their birth $z$-score. On the other hand, there are also some reports, typically from single centers, that show that this fall in the growth percentile can be prevented in the majority of preterm infants by paying meticulous attention to nutrition and growth (Andrews et al., 2019). In addition, among very preterm or VLBW infants, final height at adult age was reduced by 0.5 standard deviations (SD) compared to population-specific-reference data (Euser et al., 2008).

The overall goal of feeding preterm and VLBW infants, for example, stated by the European Society for Pediatric Gastroenterology Hepatology and Nutrition (ESPGHAN), is to mimic intrauterine growth rate (15–20 g/kg/day) and body composition, and to achieve long-term functional outcomes comparable to term-born infants (Agostoni et al., 2010). With regard to postnatal nutrition, energy, and all individual macronutrients, as well as micronutrients, including trace elements and vitamins, are equally important. These substrates can all be delivered via parenteral nutrition, but are preferably provided with enteral nutrition, thereby reducing the need for indwelling catheters and consequently lowering the risk of infections.

However, preterm infants frequently have a reduced initial tolerance to enteral nutrition. Besides, proper coordination of sucking and swallowing only starts around 32–34 weeks postconceptional age, so, until that time, enteral nutrition is provided through an orogastric or nasogastric tube. In preterm infants, reduced gut maturation and diminished gut peristalsis are likely to contribute to reduced tolerance of enteral nutrition, sometimes leading to abdominal distention, voluminous residuals, or vomiting. A more severe complication, although not solely due to feeding intolerance, is NEC. Therefore, many interventions have been tried in an attempt to increase tolerance to enteral nutrition. Currently, it is well-known that very and even extremely preterm infants can tolerate small amounts of milk immediately after birth, so that initial fasting or providing minimal enteral feeding for several days should no longer be common practice (Morgan et al., 2013, 2014). Further rapid advancements of daily enteral intakes are, however, a continuing matter of debate. Generally, preterm infants can tolerate daily increases in enteral volumes of at least 15–20 mL/kg/day and possibly higher (Walsh et al., 2020; Oddie et al., 2017), so that most preterm infants are on full enteral nutrition between 7 and 10 days after birth, and parenteral nutrition can be fully stopped. More rapid advancements have the advantage of lower dependency on parenteral nutrition and invasive catheters, which could be cost-efficient and possibly reduce infection rates, although the latter has not been shown consistently. A recent large randomized controlled trial (RCT) aimed to increase daily enteral volumes with 30 mL/kg versus 18 mL/kg from day 4 of life onwards, but showed that in real life, the high rates were far from being realized (Dorling et al., 2019). Nonetheless, time on parenteral nutrition was reduced in the faster group, and NEC rates were unaltered. In the long-term, a yet unexplained higher incidence of cerebral palsy was seen in the faster increment group. A biological explanation is not apparent, so this adverse outcome might have been found by chance. Another recent very large case-control study ($n = 12{,}387$) suggested, however, that slower feeding increments were slightly protective in reducing NEC incidence (Masoli et al., 2021). Other measures which could possibly influence feeding tolerance include providing either intermittent bolus or continuous feedings (Rovekamp-Abels et al., 2015; Razak, 2020; Wang et al., 2020), and even abdominal massage (Tekgunduz et al., 2014) and olfactory stimuli (Muelbert et al., 2019b) have been or are being tried, although evidence for specific interventions remains limited.

Certain probiotic strains have been shown to be efficacious in improving feeding tolerance and reducing NEC rates (van den Akker et al., 2018, 2020; Beghetti et al., 2021; Sharif et al., 2020; Pell et al., 2019; Underwood, 2019). Studies on the addition of other bioactive factors, such as lactoferrin, hormones, enzymes, or high dose vitamins, to nutrition for preterm infants are limited, and firm conclusions cannot yet be drawn (Mank et al., 2020; Pammi and Suresh, 2020; Buhrer et al., 2020).

## 17.3.2 Parenteral nutrition

Prior to the year ~ 2005, it was common to withhold parenteral nutrition in the first days after birth, as it was assumed that preterm infants would not be able to tolerate parenteral nutrition. In those first days after birth, only intravenous glucose with some calcium was provided. However, the current consensus is that, similar to a fetus who receives nutrients through the umbilical cord while in utero, a preterm infant should be able to metabolize nutrients provided via parenteral nutrition after birth. Key differences, however, include the fact that there no longer is a placenta to excrete metabolic waste components. Furthermore, defining fetal nutrient uptake from the placenta remains elusive (van den Akker and van Goudoever, 2010, 2016; Hay Jr., 2018).

Nonetheless, several RCTs, as well as observational studies, have shown beneficial effects of starting parenteral nutrition, including amino acids, lipids, and all micronutrients directly after birth (Leenders et al., 2018; Moon and Rao, 2021; Osborn et al., 2018; Moyses et al., 2013). Most of these beneficial effects have only been shown on short-term outcomes, i.e., improved nitrogen balances and various other biochemical indices as well as shorter duration of time to regain birth weight. While these may all be important, long-term functional outcomes remain sparsely studied, and convincing beneficial clinical effects are lacking (Bellagamba et al., 2016; Blanco et al., 2012; Roelants et al., 2018; van den Akker et al., 2014; Blakstad et al., 2015; Strommen et al., 2015; Vlaardingerbroek et al., 2012). The small increments made when increasing parenteral nutrition in combination with a lack of power (i.e., a limited number of studied infants) may be held responsible, although a true lack of long-term functional effects of using higher amounts of parenteral nutrition may be possible as well.

Nonetheless, immediate commencement of full parenteral nutrition, that includes all macro- and micronutrients, shortly after birth, is considered safe and well tolerated and is now the recommendation from several international guidelines for very preterm infants (Mihatsch et al., 2018). Evidence on how to feed moderately preterm infants (i.e., born between 32 and 37 weeks of pregnancy) is much less clear (Lapillonne et al., 2019; Muelbert et al., 2019a), as RCTs are even more limited. Currently, the DIAMOND trial on nutrition is enrolling >500 moderately preterm infants and will hopefully provide some true experimental evidence to guide clinicians (Bloomfield et al., 2018).

Adverse effects of high parenteral nutritional intakes are, however, also possible, as has been reported in adults, children, and term infants who are admitted to an intensive care unit. Recently, large RCTs in these patient groups indicated that intravenous delivery of high amounts of nutrients proved detrimental in the acute phase of critical illness (Fivez et al., 2016; Casaer et al., 2011), although others did not find these adverse effects (Alsharif et al., 2020). Specifically intravenous amino acids have been shown to sort adverse effects, including higher risk of a new infection and longer ICU admission, in patients during critical illness (Gunst et al., 2018; Vanhorebeek et al., 2017), as excess amino acids may suppress autophagy processes, which are vital in recovery and serve as a cleanup mechanism in cells (Chun and Kim, 2018). Noteworthy, in a large pediatric RCT on withholding full parenteral nutrition during critical illness (Fivez et al., 2016), the subgroup of term-born infants who were younger than 1 month of age showed the largest benefits, which consisted of fewer nosocomial infections (van Puffelen et al., 2018). Long-term neurocognitive outcomes were also apparent, and were most prominent in those between 1 month and 1 year of age (Verlinden et al., 2021). Unfortunately, preterm infants were not included in this trial, and it remains speculative how to extrapolate these results to preterm infants if they suffer acute critical illness in addition to their prematurity (Moon and Rao, 2021). Preterm infants have limited body reserves, and experience the largest growth and developmental rates in their lives. Thus, current common practice in many neonatal intensive care units is to always provide full dose parenteral nutrition in addition to enteral nutrition as tolerated, although this is still debated during critical illness (Moon et al., 2020; Moltu et al., 2021; Westin et al., 2020). ESPGHAN very recently published its nutritional recommendations for unstable and critically ill preterm infants during, for example, sepsis or surgery (Moltu et al., 2021). They advise limiting parenteral intakes of energy and macronutrients during the early and late acute phases of critically ill preterm infants. Still, to date, the evidence is inconclusive to support firm recommendations on optimal composition and timing of parenteral nutrition in unstable and critically ill preterm infants (Moltu et al., 2021; Moon and Rao, 2021; van Goudoever and van den Akker, 2021).

### 17.3.3 Enteral nutrition

After preterm birth, establishing adequate enteral administration of nutrients is pivotal, as adequate growth is best achieved with optimal enteral nutrition. Lack of enteral nutrition causes gut atrophy in animal models, with an increased risk of bacterial translocation. This could help explain increased sepsis rates during parenteral nutrition associated with microbial migration along indwelling catheters. Moreover, early establishment of enteral nutrition will also minimize other complications caused by prolonged parenteral nutrition as well, such as metabolic derangements, cholestasis, and central venous catheter-related complications including thrombosis, sepsis, and catheter malfunction (Corpeleijn et al., 2011). Generally, preterm infants will require parenteral nutrition during the first 1 or 2 weeks of life, while enteral nutrition is gradually increased, as explained above.

To achieve the enteral nutrition goals in preterm infants at different ages, there are several options. These include the infant's own mother's milk and donor milk, which require multinutrient fortification to meet the high nutrient requirements. Alternatively, preterm formula or nutrient-enriched formula can be given, as discussed below.

### 17.3.3.1 Mother's own milk and donor milk

Given the well-known short- and long-term benefits of mother's own milk, leading health authorities such as the World Health Organization (WHO), ESPGHAN, and the American Academy of Pediatrics (AAP) strongly recommend it as the preferred source of enteral nutrition for all newborn infants, particularly for those born preterm (Boquien, 2018). Yet, it remains impossible to obtain direct experimental evidence from RCTs that compare mother's own milk versus (preterm) formula, as randomization between these is both impossible and unethical (Brown et al., 2019; Granger et al., 2021). Nevertheless, it has been shown in cohort studies that preterm infants that are fed mother's own milk tolerate full enteral feeding earlier, compared to those that are formula-fed, and have a lower incidence of several neonatal morbidities, including NEC and BPD (Villamor-Martinez et al., 2019; Miller et al., 2018; Huang et al., 2019; Altobelli et al., 2020; Zhang et al., 2020). Additionally, there appears to be an independent beneficial positive effect on long-term neurodevelopmental outcome (Lechner and Vohr, 2017; Belfort et al., 2016; Gibertoni et al., 2015; Koo et al., 2014), despite slower in-hospital growth compared to formula-fed infants, often termed the "breastfeeding paradox" (Roze et al., 2012; Cerasani et al., 2020). Human milk is full of bioactive factors (Bardanzellu et al., 2020; Gila-Diaz et al., 2019). These include antimicrobial molecules such as immunoglobulins, cytokines, and lactoferrin. Also, numerous growth factors like epithelial growth factor or insulin-like growth factors 1 and 2 are naturally present in human milk and are thought to stimulate maturation of the premature gut (Walsh and McGuire, 2019; Granger et al., 2021). Improved neurodevelopment in those fed human milk could also be due to other functional building blocks like long-chain polyunsaturated fatty acids (e.g., docosahexaenoic acid; DHA) or larger lipid classes like sphingomyelin and cholesterol (Boquien, 2018). Independently, however, a clear long-term benefit of supplementing preterm infants with DHA has not been proven (Collins et al., 2015; Wang et al., 2016).

When mother's own milk is unavailable, pasteurized donor (human) milk is recommended as the first alternative, as this might replicate some of the beneficial effects of mother's own milk (Nutrition et al., 2013). Limited available data suggest that donor milk is associated with improved feeding tolerance and a decreased risk of NEC when compared to preterm formula feeding, whereas rates of infection and mortality rates are not affected (Quigley et al., 2019; Silano et al., 2019). In meta-analyses that assessed both cohort and randomized studies, it appeared that donor milk-fed infants had lower BPD rates in the cohort studies, though this was not confirmed in the RCTs (Miller et al., 2018; Villamor-Martinez et al., 2018). Long-term follow-up after donor milk was assessed in only one RCT, suggesting that at 18 months' corrected age outcome scores were similar when compared to formula-fed infants (O'Connor et al., 2016).

There are several reasons why pasteurized donor milk is not as beneficial as mother's own milk. For example, donor milk is often provided by women who gave birth to term infants several months before, and thus contains a lower protein content (Gidrewicz and Fenton, 2014). In addition, almost all donor milk banks pasteurize donated milk to avoid transmission of pathogens, mainly bacteria, cytomegalovirus, and human immunodeficiency virus. Both the processing and heating of donor milk lower the quantity and quality of macronutrients and bioactive substances. For example, the classical Holder pasteurization method (which maintains milk temperature above 62.5°C for 30 min) will partially or completely inactivate many bioactive factors, including immunological components, growth hormones, and digestive enzymes such as bile-salt stimulated lipase, further impairing enteral fat uptake (Hard et al., 2019; Colaizy, 2021).

Regardless of whether mother's own milk or donor milk is given to preterm infants, with the goal of mimicking intrauterine growth rates, its nutrient content is too low, particularly regarding protein, energy, calcium, and phosphate. Unfortified human milk is known to result in poor postnatal growth and metabolic bone deficiency of prematurity, and can be improved by supplementing a multinutrient fortifier to match the nutritional requirements of preterm infants. Unfortunately, the underlying experimental and beneficial clinical evidence regarding optimal multinutrient fortification is still not very strong (Agostoni et al., 2010; Thanigainathan and Abiramalatha, 2020; Brown et al., 2020; van den Akker et al., 2021), especially with regard to long-term benefits (Modi, 2021; Gao et al., 2020). Nonetheless, ESPGHAN (Moro et al., 2015), the European Milk Bank Association (EMBA) (Arslanoglu et al., 2019), and the AAP (Section On, 2012) recommend that a multinutrient fortifier be added to human milk for preterm infants. Moreover, from the available evidence, no adverse effects of fortification, such as NEC, were seen, which seems reassuring (Brown et al., 2020).

In most of the multinutrient fortifiers, the protein source is bovine milk origin. However, there is also a fortifier available that is produced from donor human milk. Evaluation of the clinical advantage of a so-called "human milk only" diet, however, requires further large high-quality trials (Premkumar et al., 2019). Currently, only one RCT in infants where mother's own milk was not available, compared a standard multinutrient fortifier from bovine origin with a human milk-based fortifier (O'Connor et al., 2018). In this trial ($n = 125$), there were no differences in feeding intolerance as the primary outcome, nor were there differences in NEC stage $\geq 2$, sepsis, or death, although there was less severe retinopathy of prematurity in the intervention group as a secondary outcome. A downside of human milk derived fortifiers is that they are liquid and replace 30% of the volume of own mother's milk intake. Furthermore, the costs of this type of fortifier are very high, and there is a range of societal, ethical, and logistical issues that might preclude widespread rollout of this type of product (Prouse, 2021; Cohen, 2019). Therefore, well-designed, large-scale independent trials will be needed before this approach can be recommended.

### 17.3.3.2 Postdischarge nutrition

When approaching term equivalent age and from hospital discharge onwards, preterm infants are likely to drink directly from the breast, and this makes fortification less practical. Yet, many infants have suboptimal growth outcomes around discharge, as discussed above. Despite the fact that sound evidence is lacking, it may still be advisable to continue fortification of human milk as long as practically possible if growth is less than optimal (Young et al., 2013; McCormick et al., 2021).

In case infants are not fully breastfed around discharge, nutrient-enriched postdischarge formulas are available. However, compelling evidence of an effect on growth and neuro-development of preterm infants is lacking until now (Lapillonne et al., 2013; Young et al., 2016; Ruys et al., 2017, 2019, 2021). Although not unequivocally, some studies demonstrate that nutrient-enriched formulas tend to improve growth and body composition during the first 6 months (Teller et al., 2016). It is suggested that these possible benefits are associated with a higher protein-to-energy ratio in these nutrient-enriched formulas (Teller et al., 2016). However, these possible effects on growth and body composition do not persist into childhood (Ruys et al., 2017) and no positive effects on later neurodevelopment have been demonstrated (Teller et al., 2016; Ruys et al., 2019; Young et al., 2016). Nonetheless, nutrient-enriched for-mulas are still recommended for preterm infants up to 3 months corrected age (i.e., 3 months after term equivalent age), unless growth is accelerating above desired levels. Thereafter, it is recommended to switch to a standard term formula (Ruys et al., 2021; Agostoni et al., 2010). With respect to the use of a protein-enriched formula beyond 3 months corrected age, caution is warranted, since excessive protein intake during the first 2 years of life has been shown to predispose to later adiposity (Michaelsen and Greer, 2014). Continuation of protein-enriched formula after 3 months corrected age should be guided by critically evaluating the infant's growth pattern.

Regarding moderate-late preterm infants, hardly any evidence is currently available on what type of enteral feeding regimen should be used both before and after discharge from the hospital (Lapillonne et al., 2013; Asadi et al., 2019). Ongoing and future studies may give more insight into the specific needs for this large group of preterm infants (Bloomfield et al., 2018; Kakaroukas et al., 2021).

## 17.4 Conclusions

During the first weeks to months of their lives, preterm infants face the most rapid growth and developmental phase of their lives. Adverse complications, including growth restriction during that period, have been shown to have long-lasting detrimental effects that last into adulthood. Those effects are notable on all body systems, altering growth and body com-position, and can lead to cardiovascular disease and poor neurodevelopmental outcomes. The overall aim of neonatology is to mimic the outcomes of healthy term-born neonates. Nutrition, especially fortified mother's own milk, has proven to play a pivotal role in ame-liorating these outcomes, not only by directly enhancing growth, but also by decreasing the incidence of adverse neonatal complications and stimulating brain development.

## 17.5 Future trends and research

First, despite moderate and late preterm infants (i.e., those born between 32 and 37 weeks of pregnancy) outnumber those born very preterm, evidence how to optimally feed the former remains less clear (Lapillonne et al., 2019). This holds true not only during the period of hospitalization, but also thereafter. Currently, the DIAMOND trial on nutrition is enrolling moderate-late preterm infants for a nutritional intervention during hospital admission (98). Furthermore, the LEGO trial (Dutch Trial Registry NL4979, www.trialregister.nl) is currently being conducted and investigates a nutritional intervention in moderate-late preterm infants after hospital discharge. Future research should also focus on the risk of cardiometabolic disease and impaired neurodevelopmental outcome in moderate-late preterm infants.

Second, recently, ESPGHAN published recommendations to limit parenteral intakes of energy and macronutrients during early and late acute phases of critically ill preterm infants (Moltu et al., 2021). However, as evidence remains inconclusive to support firm recommendations on optimal composition and timing of parenteral nutrition in unstable and critically ill preterm infants, future studies should focus on this.

## Sources of additional information

Mihatsch, W. A., Braegger, C., Bronsky, J., Cai, W., Campoy, C., Carnielli, V., Darmaun, D., Desci, T., Domellof, M., Embleton, N., Fewtrell, M., Mis, N. F., Franz, A., Goulet, O., Hartman, C., Susan, H., Hojsak, I., Iacobelli, S., Jochum, F., Joosten, K., Kolacek, S., Koletzko, B., Ksiazyk, J., Lapillonne, A., Lohner, S., Mesotten, D., Mihalyi, K., Mimouni, F., Molgaard, C., Moltu, S. J., Nomayo, A., Picaud, J. C., Prell, C., Puntis, J., Riskin, A., de Pipaon, M. S., Senterre, T., Shamir, R., Simchowitz, V., Szitanyi, P., Tabbers, M. M., van den Akker, C. H. B., van Goudoever, J. B., van Kempen, A., Verbruggen, S., Wu, J. & Yan, W. 2018. ESPGHAN/ESPEN/ESPR/CSPEN guidelines on pediatric parenteral nutrition. Clin Nutr, 37, 2303–2305.
Moltu, S. J., Bronsky, J., Embleton, N., Gerasimidis, K., Indrio, F., Koglmeier, J., de Koning, B., Lapillonne, A., Norsa, L., Verduci, E., Domellof, M. & Espghan Committee On Nutrition 2021. Nutritional Management of the Critically Ill Neonate: A Position Paper of the ESPGHAN Committee on Nutrition. J Pediatr Gastroenterol Nutr, 73, 274–289.
Lapillonne, A., Bronsky, J., Campoy, C., Embleton, N., Fewtrell, M., Fidler Mis, N., Gerasimidis, K., Hojsak, I., Hulst, J., Indrio, F., Molgaard, C., Moltu, S. J., Verduci, E., Domellof, M. & Espghan COMMITTEE On Nutrition 2019. Feeding the Late and Moderately Preterm Infant: A Position Paper of the European Society for Pediatric Gastroenterology, Hepatology and Nutrition Committee on Nutrition. J Pediatr Gastroenterol Nutr, 69, 259–270.
Buhrer, C., Fischer, H. S. & Wellmann, S. 2020. Nutritional interventions to reduce rates of infection, necrotizing enterocolitis and mortality in very preterm infants. Pediatr Res, 87, 371–377.
Ruys, C. A., van de Lagemaat, M., Rotteveel, J., Finken, M. J. J. & Lafeber, H. N. 2021. Improving long-term health outcomes of preterm infants: how to implement the findings of nutritional intervention studies into daily clinical practice. Eur J Pediatr, 180, 1665–1673.
Arslanoglu, S., Boquien, C. Y., King, C., Lamireau, D., Tonetto, P., Barnett, D., Bertino, E., Gaya, A., Gebauer, C., Grovslien, A., Moro, G. E., Weaver, G., Wesolowska, A. M. & Picaud, J. C. 2019. Fortification of Human Milk for Preterm Infants: Update and

Recommendations of the European Milk Bank Association (EMBA) Working Group on Human Milk Fortification. Front Pediatr, 7, 76.

Fenton, T. R., Griffin, I. J., Groh-Wargo, S., Gura, K., Martin, C. R., Taylor, S. N., Rozga, M. & Moloney, L. 2021. Very Low Birthweight Preterm Infants: A 2020 Evidence Analysis Center Evidence-Based Nutrition Practice Guideline. J Acad Nutr Diet.

# References

Agostoni, C., Buonocore, G., Carnielli, V.P., de Curtis, M., Darmaun, D., Decsi, T., Domellof, M., Embleton, N.D., Fusch, C., Genzel-Boroviczeny, O., Goulet, O., Kalhan, S.C., Kolacek, S., Koletzko, B., Lapillonne, A., Mihatsch, W., Moreno, L., Neu, J., Poindexter, B., Puntis, J., Putet, G., Rigo, J., Riskin, A., Salle, B., Sauer, P., Shamir, R., Szajewska, H., Thureen, P., Turck, D., van Goudoever, J.B., Ziegler, E.E., Espghan Committee On Nutrition, 2010. Enteral nutrient supply for preterm infants: commentary from the European Society of Paediatric Gastroenterology, Hepatology and Nutrition Committee on Nutrition. J. Pediatr. Gastroenterol. Nutr. 50, 85–91.

Agrawal, S., Rao, S.C., Bulsara, M.K., Patole, S.K., 2018. Prevalence of autism spectrum disorder in preterm infants: a meta-analysis. Pediatrics 142, e20180134.

Alsharif, D.J., Alsharif, F.J., Aljuraiban, G.S., Abulmeaty, M.M.A., 2020. Effect of supplemental parenteral nutrition versus enteral nutrition alone on clinical outcomes in critically ill adult patients: a systematic review and meta-analysis of randomized controlled trials. Nutrients 12, 2968.

Altobelli, E., Angeletti, P.M., Verrotti, A., Petrocelli, R., 2020. The impact of human milk on necrotizing enterocolitis: a systematic review and meta-analysis. Nutrients 12, 1322.

Andrews, E.T., Ashton, J.J., Pearson, F., Beattie, R.M., Johnson, M.J., 2019. Early postnatal growth failure in preterm infants is not inevitable. Arch. Dis. Child. Fetal Neonatal Ed. 104, F235–F241.

Arslanoglu, S., Boquien, C.Y., King, C., Lamireau, D., Tonetto, P., Barnett, D., Bertino, E., Gaya, A., Gebauer, C., Grovslien, A., Moro, G.E., Weaver, G., Wesolowska, A.M., Picaud, J.C., 2019. Fortification of human milk for preterm infants: update and recommendations of the European Milk Bank Association (EMBA) working group on human milk fortification. Front. Pediatr. 7, 76.

Asadi, S., Bloomfield, F.H., Harding, J.E., 2019. Nutrition in late preterm infants. Semin. Perinatol. 43, 151160.

Bardanzellu, F., Peroni, D.G., Fanos, V., 2020. Human breast milk: bioactive components, from stem cells to health outcomes. Curr. Nutr. Rep. 9, 1–13.

Beghetti, I., Panizza, D., Lenzi, J., Gori, D., Martini, S., Corvaglia, L., Aceti, A., 2021. Probiotics for preventing necrotizing enterocolitis in preterm infants: a network meta-analysis. Nutrients 13, 192.

Belfort, M.B., Anderson, P.J., Nowak, V.A., Lee, K.J., Molesworth, C., Thompson, D.K., Doyle, L.W., Inder, T.E., 2016. Breast milk feeding, brain development, and neurocognitive outcomes: a 7-year longitudinal study in infants born at less than 30 Weeks' gestation. J. Pediatr. 177, 133–139.e1.

Bellagamba, M.P., Carmenati, E., D'ascenzo, R., Malatesta, M., Spagnoli, C., Biagetti, C., Burattini, I., Carnielli, V.P., 2016. One extra gram of protein to preterm infants from birth to 1800 g: a single-blinded randomized clinical trial. J. Pediatr. Gastroenterol. Nutr. 62, 879–884.

Blakstad, E.W., Strommen, K., Moltu, S.J., Wattam-Bell, J., Nordheim, T., Almaas, A.N., Gronn, M., Ronnestad, A.E., Braekke, K., Iversen, P.O., von Hofsten, C., Veierod, M.B., Westerberg, A.C., Drevon, C.A., Nakstad, B., 2015. Improved visual perception in very low birth weight infants on enhanced nutrient supply. Neonatology 108, 30–37.

Blanco, C.L., Gong, A.K., Schoolfield, J., Green, B.K., Daniels, W., Liechty, E.A., Ramamurthy, R., 2012. Impact of early and high amino acid supplementation on Elbw infants at 2 years. J. Pediatr. Gastroenterol. Nutr. 54, 601–607.

Blencowe, H., Cousens, S., Oestergaard, M.Z., Chou, D., Moller, A.B., Narwal, R., Adler, A., Vera Garcia, C., Rohde, S., Say, L., Lawn, J.E., 2012. National, regional, and worldwide estimates of preterm birth rates in the year 2010 with time trends since 1990 for selected countries: a systematic analysis and implications. Lancet 379, 2162–2172.

Bloomfield, F.H., Harding, J.E., Meyer, M.P., Alsweiler, J.M., Jiang, Y., Wall, C.R., Alexander, T., Group, D. S, 2018. The DIAMOND trial – dIfferent approaches to MOderate & late preterm Nutrition: determinants of feed tolerance, body composition and development: protocol of a randomised trial. BMC Pediatr. 18, 220.

Boquien, C.Y., 2018. Human Milk: an ideal food for nutrition of preterm newborn. Front. Pediatr. 6, 295.

Bracht, M., O'Leary, L., Lee, S.K., O'brien, K., 2013. Implementing family-integrated care in the NICU: a parent education and support program. Adv. Neonatal Care 13, 115–126.

Brown, J.V.E., Walsh, V., McGuire, W., 2019. Formula versus maternal breast milk for feeding preterm or low birth weight infants. Cochrane Database Syst. Rev. 8, CD002972.

Brown, J.V.E., Lin, L., Embleton, N.D., Harding, J.E., McGuire, W., 2020. Multi-nutrient fortification of human milk for preterm infants. Cochrane Database Syst. Rev. 2020, CD000343.

Buhrer, C., Fischer, H.S., Wellmann, S., 2020. Nutritional interventions to reduce rates of infection, necrotizing enterocolitis and mortality in very preterm infants. Pediatr. Res. 87, 371–377.

Casaer, M.P., Mesotten, D., Hermans, G., Wouters, P.J., Schetz, M., Meyfroidt, G., van Cromphaut, S., Ingels, C., Meersseman, P., Muller, J., Vlasselaers, D., Debaveye, Y., Desmet, L., Dubois, J., van Assche, A., Vanderheyden, S., Wilmer, A., van den Berghe, G., 2011. Early versus late parenteral nutrition in critically ill adults. N. Engl. J. Med. 365, 506–517.

Cerasani, J., Ceroni, F., de Cosmi, V., Mazzocchi, A., Morniroli, D., Roggero, P., Mosca, F., Agostoni, C., Gianni, M.L., 2020. Human milk feeding and preterm Infants' growth and body composition: a literature review. Nutrients 12, 1155.

Chiavaroli, V., Derraik, J.G.B., Jayasinghe, T.N., Rodrigues, R.O., Biggs, J.B., Battin, M., Hofman, P.L., O'sullivan, J.M., Cutfield, W.S., 2021. Lower insulin sensitivity remains a feature of children born very preterm. Pediatr. Diabetes 22, 161–167.

Chun, Y., Kim, J., 2018. Autophagy: an essential degradation program for cellular homeostasis and life. Cell 7, 278.

Cohen, M., 2019. Should human milk be regulated? UC Irvine Law Rev. 9, 557–634.

Colaizy, T.T., 2021. Effects of milk banking procedures on nutritional and bioactive components of donor human milk. Semin. Perinatol. 45, 151382.

Collins, C.T., Gibson, R.A., Anderson, P.J., McPhee, A.J., Sullivan, T.R., Gould, J.F., Ryan, P., Doyle, L.W., Davis, P.G., McMichael, J.E., French, N.P., Colditz, P.B., Simmer, K., Morris, S.A., Makrides, M., 2015. Neurodevelopmental outcomes at 7 years' corrected age in preterm infants who were fed high-dose docosahexaenoic acid to term equivalent: a follow-up of a randomised controlled trial. BMJ Open 5, e007314.

Cormack, B.E., Harding, J.E., Miller, S.P., Bloomfield, F.H., 2019. The influence of early nutrition on brain growth and neurodevelopment in extremely preterm babies: a narrative review. Nutrients 11, 2029.

Corpeleijn, W.E., Vermeulen, M.J., van den Akker, C.H., van Goudoever, J.B., 2011. Feeding very-low-birth-weight infants: our aspirations versus the reality in practice. Ann. Nutr. Metab. 58 (Suppl. 1), 20–29.

Costeloe, K.L., Hennessy, E.M., Haider, S., Stacey, F., Marlow, N., Draper, E.S., 2012. Short term outcomes after extreme preterm birth in England: comparison of two birth cohorts in 1995 and 2006 (the EPICure studies). BMJ 345, e7976.

de Kieviet, J.F., Oosterlaan, J., Vermeulen, R.J., Pouwels, P.J., Lafeber, H.N., van Elburg, R.M., 2012. Effects of glutamine on brain development in very preterm children at school age. Pediatrics 130, e1121–e1127.

de Kloet, E.R., Sibug, R.M., Helmerhorst, F.M., Schmidt, M.V., 2005. Stress, genes and the mechanism of programming the brain for later life. Neurosci. Biobehav. Rev. 29, 271–281.

Dorling, J., Abbott, J., Berrington, J., Bosiak, B., Bowler, U., Boyle, E., Embleton, N., Hewer, O., Johnson, S., Juszczak, E., Leaf, A., Linsell, L., McCormick, K., McGuire, W., Omar, O., Partlett, C., Patel, M., Roberts, T., Stenson, B., Townend, J., Group, S. I, 2019. Controlled trial of two incremental milk-feeding rates in preterm infants. N. Engl. J. Med. 381, 1434–1443.

El Rafei, R., Jarreau, P.H., Norman, M., Maier, R.F., Barros, H., Reempts, P.V., Pedersen, P., Cuttini, M., Zeitlin, J., Group, E. R, 2021. Variation in very preterm extrauterine growth in a European multicountry cohort. Arch. Dis. Child. Fetal Neonatal Ed. 106, 316–323.

Euser, A.M., Finken, M.J., Keijzer-Veen, M.G., Hille, E.T., Wit, J.M., Dekker, F.W., Dutch, P.-C.S.G., 2005. Associations between prenatal and infancy weight gain and BMI, fat mass, and fat distribution in young adulthood: a prospective cohort study in males and females born very preterm. Am. J. Clin. Nutr. 81, 480–487.

Euser, A.M., de Wit, C.C., Finken, M.J., Rijken, M., Wit, J.M., 2008. Growth of preterm born children. Horm. Res. 70, 319–328.

Fenton, T.R., Groh-Wargo, S., Gura, K., Martin, C.R., Taylor, S.N., Griffin, I.J., Rozga, M., Moloney, L., 2021. Effect of enteral protein amount on growth and health outcomes in very-low-birth-weight preterm infants: phase II of the pre-B project and an evidence analysis center systematic review. J. Acad. Nutr. Diet. 121, 2287–2300.e12.

Fivez, T., Kerklaan, D., Mesotten, D., Verbruggen, S., Wouters, P.J., Vanhorebeek, I., Debaveye, Y., Vlasselaers, D., Desmet, L., Casaer, M.P., Garcia Guerra, G., Hanot, J., Joffe, A., Tibboel, D., Joosten, K., van den Berghe, G., 2016. Early versus late parenteral nutrition in critically ill children. N. Engl. J. Med. 374, 1111–1122.

Franz, A.P., Bolat, G.U., Bolat, H., Matijasevich, A., Santos, I.S., Silveira, R.C., Procianoy, R.S., Rohde, L.A., Moreira-Maia, C.R., 2018. Attention-deficit/hyperactivity disorder and very preterm/very low birth weight: a meta-analysis. Pediatrics 141, e20171645.

Frondas-Chauty, A., Simon, L., Flamant, C., Hanf, M., Darmaun, D., Roze, J.C., 2018. Deficit of fat free mass in very preterm infants at discharge is associated with neurological impairment at age 2 years. J. Pediatr. 196, 301–304.

Gao, C., Miller, J., Collins, C.T., Rumbold, A.R., 2020. Comparison of different protein concentrations of human milk fortifier for promoting growth and neurological development in preterm infants. Cochrane Database Syst. Rev. 11, CD007090.

Gibertoni, D., Corvaglia, L., Vandini, S., Rucci, P., Savini, S., Alessandroni, R., Sansavini, A., Fantini, M.P., Faldella, G., 2015. Positive effect of human milk feeding during NICU hospitalization on 24 month neurodevelopment of very low birth weight infants: an Italian cohort study. PLoS One 10, e0116552.

Gidrewicz, D.A., Fenton, T.R., 2014. A systematic review and meta-analysis of the nutrient content of preterm and term breast milk. BMC Pediatr. 14, 216.

Gila-Diaz, A., Arribas, S.M., Algara, A., Martin-Cabrejas, M.A., Lopez De Pablo, A.L., Saenz De Pipaon, M., Ramiro-Cortijo, D., 2019. A review of bioactive factors in human breastmilk: a focus on prematurity. Nutrients 11, 1307.

Granger, C.L., Embleton, N.D., Palmer, J.M., Lamb, C.A., Berrington, J.E., Stewart, C.J., 2021. Maternal breastmilk, infant gut microbiome and the impact on preterm infant health. Acta Paediatr. 110, 450–457.

Guellec, I., Lapillonne, A., Marret, S., Picaud, J.C., Mitanchez, D., Charkaluk, M.L., Fresson, J., Arnaud, C., Flamant, C., Cambonie, G., Kaminski, M., Roze, J.C., Ancel, P.Y., Etude Epidemiologique Sur Les Petits Ages Gestationnels Study, G, 2016. Effect of intra- and extrauterine growth on long-term neurologic outcomes of very preterm infants. J. Pediatr. 175, 93–99.e1.

Gunst, J., Vanhorebeek, I., Thiessen, S.E., van den Berghe, G., 2018. Amino acid supplements in critically ill patients. Pharmacol. Res. 130, 127–131.

Hard, A.L., Nilsson, A.K., Lund, A.M., Hansen-Pupp, I., Smith, L.E.H., Hellstrom, A., 2019. Review shows that donor milk does not promote the growth and development of preterm infants as well as maternal milk. Acta Paediatr. 108, 998–1007.

Hay Jr., W.W., 2018. Nutritional support strategies for the preterm infant in the neonatal intensive care unit. Pediatr. Gastroenterol. Hepatol. Nutr. 21, 234–247.

Hiltunen, H., Loyttyniemi, E., Isolauri, E., Rautava, S., 2018. Early nutrition and growth until the corrected age of 2 years in extremely preterm infants. Neonatology 113, 100–107.

Hofman, P.L., Regan, F., Jackson, W.E., Jefferies, C., Knight, D.B., Robinson, E.M., Cutfield, W.S., 2004. Premature birth and later insulin resistance. N. Engl. J. Med. 351, 2179–2186.

Hortensius, L.M., van Elburg, R.M., Nijboer, C.H., Benders, M., de Theije, C.G.M., 2019. Postnatal nutrition to improve brain development in the preterm infant: a systematic review from bench to bedside. Front. Physiol. 10, 961.

Huang, J., Zhang, L., Tang, J., Shi, J., Qu, Y., Xiong, T., Mu, D., 2019. Human milk as a protective factor for bronchopulmonary dysplasia: a systematic review and meta-analysis. Arch. Dis. Child. Fetal Neonatal Ed. 104, F128–F136.

Kajantie, E., Strang-Karlsson, S., Evensen, K.A.I., Haaramo, P., 2019. Adult outcomes of being born late preterm or early term – what do we know? Semin. Fetal Neonatal Med. 24, 66–83.

Kakaroukas, A., Abrahamse-Berkeveld, M., Berrington, J.E., McNally, R.J.Q., Stewart, C.J., Embleton, N.D., van Elburg, R.M., 2021. An observational cohort study and nested randomized controlled trial on nutrition and growth outcomes in moderate and late preterm infants (FLAMINGO). Front. Nutr. 8, 561419.

Kallankari, H., Kaukola, T., Olsen, P., Ojaniemi, M., Hallman, M., 2015. Very preterm birth and foetal growth restriction are associated with specific cognitive deficits in children attending mainstream school. Acta Paediatr. 104, 84–90.

Keir, A., McPhee, A., Wilkinson, D., 2014. Beyond the borderline: outcomes for inborn infants born at </=500 grams. J. Paediatr. Child Health 50, 146–152.

Kerkhof, G.F., Willemsen, R.H., Leunissen, R.W., Breukhoven, P.E., Hokken-Koelega, A.C., 2012. Health profile of young adults born preterm: negative effects of rapid weight gain in early life. J. Clin. Endocrinol. Metab. 97, 4498–4506.

Koo, W., Tank, S., Martin, S., Shi, R., 2014. Human milk and neurodevelopment in children with very low birth weight: a systematic review. Nutr. J. 13, 94.

Kuzniewicz, M.W., Wi, S., Qian, Y., Walsh, E.M., Armstrong, M.A., Croen, L.A., 2014. Prevalence and neonatal factors associated with autism spectrum disorders in preterm infants. J. Pediatr. 164, 20–25.

Lampi, K.M., Lehtonen, L., Tran, P.L., Suominen, A., Lehti, V., Banerjee, P.N., Gissler, M., Brown, A.S., Sourander, A., 2012. Risk of autism spectrum disorders in low birth weight and small for gestational age infants. J. Pediatr. 161, 830–836.

Lapillonne, A., O'Connor, D.L., Wang, D., Rigo, J., 2013. Nutritional recommendations for the late-preterm infant and the preterm infant after hospital discharge. J. Pediatr. 162, S90–100.

Lapillonne, A., Bronsky, J., Campoy, C., Embleton, N., Fewtrell, M., Fidler Mis, N., Gerasimidis, K., Hojsak, I., Hulst, J., Indrio, F., Molgaard, C., Moltu, S.J., Verduci, E., Domellof, M., Espghan Committee On Nutrition, 2019. Feeding the late and moderately preterm infant: a position paper of the European Society for Paediatric Gastroenterology, hepatology and nutrition committee on nutrition. J. Pediatr. Gastroenterol. Nutr. 69, 259–270.

Lara-Canton, I., Solaz, A., Parra-Llorca, A., Garcia-Robles, A., Millan, I., Torres-Cuevas, I., Vento, M., 2020. Oxygen supplementation during preterm stabilization and the relevance of the first 5 min after birth. Front. Pediatr. 8, 12.

Lawlor, D.A., Davey Smith, G., Clark, H., Leon, D.A., 2006. The associations of birthweight, gestational age and childhood BMI with type 2 diabetes: findings from the Aberdeen children of the 1950s cohort. Diabetologia 49, 2614–2617.

Lechner, B.E., Vohr, B.R., 2017. Neurodevelopmental outcomes of preterm infants fed human milk: a systematic review. Clin. Perinatol. 44, 69–83.

Leenders, E., de Waard, M., van Goudoever, J.B., 2018. Low- versus high-dose and early versus late parenteral amino-acid administration in very-low-birth-weight infants: a systematic review and meta-analysis. Neonatology 113, 187–205.

Lin, L., Amissah, E., Gamble, G.D., Crowther, C.A., Harding, J.E., 2019. Impact of macronutrient supplements for children born preterm or small for gestational age on developmental and metabolic outcomes: a systematic review and meta-analysis. PLoS Med. 16, e1002952.

Lucassen, P.J., Naninck, E.F., van Goudoever, J.B., Fitzsimons, C., Joels, M., Korosi, A., 2013. Perinatal programming of adult hippocampal structure and function; emerging roles of stress, nutrition and epigenetics. Trends Neurosci. 36, 621–631.

Mank, E., Naninck, E.F.G., Limpens, J., van Toledo, L., van Goudoever, J.B., van den Akker, C.H.P., 2020. Enteral bioactive factor supplementation in preterm infants: a systematic review. Nutrients 12, 2916.

Markopoulou, P., Papanikolaou, E., Analytis, A., Zoumakis, E., Siahanidou, T., 2019. Preterm birth as a risk factor for metabolic syndrome and cardiovascular disease in adult life: a systematic review and meta-analysis. J. Pediatr. 210, 69–80.e5.

Martinez-Jimenez, M.D., Gomez-Garcia, F.J., Gil-Campos, M., Perez-Navero, J.L., 2020. Comorbidities in childhood associated with extrauterine growth restriction in preterm infants: a scoping review. Eur. J. Pediatr. 179, 1255–1265.

Masoli, D., Dominguez, A., Tapia, J.L., Uauy, R., Fabres, J., Network, N.C., 2021. Enteral feeding and necrotizing enterocolitis: does time of first feeds and rate of advancement matter? J. Pediatr. Gastroenterol. Nutr. 72, 763–768.

Matei, A., Montalva, L., Goodbaum, A., Lauriti, G., Zani, A., 2020. Neurodevelopmental impairment in necrotising enterocolitis survivors: systematic review and meta-analysis. Arch. Dis. Child. Fetal Neonatal Ed. 105, 432–439.

Mathai, S., Derraik, J.G., Cutfield, W.S., Dalziel, S.R., Harding, J.E., Biggs, J., Jefferies, C., Hofman, P.L., 2013. Increased adiposity in adults born preterm and their children. PLoS One 8, e81840.

McCormick, K., King, C., Clarke, S., Jarvis, C., Johnson, M., Parretti, H.M., Greene, N., Males, J., 2021. The role of breast milk fortifier in the post-discharge nutrition of preterm infants. Br. J. Hosp. Med. (Lond.) 82, 42–48.

Meneghelli, M., Pasinato, A., Salvadori, S., Gaio, P., Fantinato, M., Vanzo, V., de Terlizzi, F., Verlato, G., 2016. Bone status in preterm infant: influences of different nutritional regimens and possible markers of bone disease. J. Perinatol. 36, 394–400.

Michaelsen, K.F., Greer, F.R., 2014. Protein needs early in life and long-term health. Am. J. Clin. Nutr. 99, 718S–722S.

Mihatsch, W.A., Braegger, C., Bronsky, J., Cai, W., Campoy, C., Carnielli, V., Darmaun, D., Desci, T., Domellof, M., Embleton, N., Fewtrell, M., Mis, N.F., Franz, A., Goulet, O., Hartman, C., Susan, H., Hojsak, I., Iacobelli, S., Jochum, F., Joosten, K., Kolacek, S., Koletzko, B., Ksiazyk, J., Lapillonne, A., Lohner, S., Mesotten, D., Mihalyi, K., Mimouni, F., Molgaard, C., Moltu, S.J., Nomayo, A., Picaud, J.C., Prell, C., Puntis, J., Riskin, A., de Pipaon, M.S., Senterre, T., Shamir, R., Simchowitz, V., Szitanyi, P., Tabbers, M.M., van den Akker, C.H.B., van Goudoever, J.B., van Kempen, A., Verbruggen, S., Wu, J., Yan, W., 2018. ESPGHAN/ESPEN/ESPR/CSPEN guidelines on pediatric parenteral nutrition. Clin. Nutr. 37, 2303–2305.

Miller, J., Tonkin, E., Damarell, R.A., McPhee, A.J., Suganuma, M., Suganuma, H., Middleton, P.F., Makrides, M., Collins, C.T., 2018. A systematic review and meta-analysis of human milk feeding and morbidity in very low birth weight infants. Nutrients 10, 707.

Modi, N., 2021. The implications of routine milk fortification for the short and long-term health of preterm babies. Semin. Fetal Neonatal Med. 26, 101216.

Moltu, S.J., Bronsky, J., Embleton, N., Gerasimidis, K., Indrio, F., Koglmeier, J., de Koning, B., Lapillonne, A., Norsa, L., Verduci, E., Domellof, M., Espghan Committee On Nutrition, 2021. Nutritional Management of the Critically ill neonate: a position paper of the ESPGHAN Committee on Nutrition. J. Pediatr. Gastroenterol. Nutr. 73, 274–289.

Moon, K., Rao, S.C., 2021. Early or delayed parenteral nutrition for infants: what evidence is available? Curr. Opin. Clin. Nutr. Metab. Care 24, 281–286.

Moon, K., Athalye-Jape, G.K., Rao, U., Rao, S.C., 2020. Early versus late parenteral nutrition for critically ill term and late preterm infants. Cochrane Database Syst. Rev. 4, CD013141.

Morgan, J., Bombell, S., McGuire, W., 2013. Early trophic feeding versus enteral fasting for very preterm or very low birth weight infants. Cochrane Database Syst. Rev. (3), CD000504.

Morgan, J., Young, L., McGuire, W., 2014. Delayed introduction of progressive enteral feeds to prevent necrotising enterocolitis in very low birth weight infants. Cochrane Database Syst. Rev. 2014, CD001970.

Moro, G.E., Arslanoglu, S., Bertino, E., Corvaglia, L., Montirosso, R., Picaud, J.C., Polberger, S., Schanler, R.J., Steel, C., van Goudoever, J., Ziegler, E.E., American Academy of, Pediatrics, European Society For Pediatric Gastroenterology, Hepatology & Nutrition, 2015. XII. Human milk in feeding premature infants: consensus statement. J. Pediatr. Gastroenterol. Nutr. 61 (suppl 1). S16-9.

Moyses, H.E., Johnson, M.J., Leaf, A.A., Cornelius, V.R., 2013. Early parenteral nutrition and growth outcomes in preterm infants: a systematic review and meta-analysis. Am. J. Clin. Nutr. 97, 816–826.

Muelbert, M., Harding, J.E., Bloomfield, F.H., 2019a. Nutritional policies for late preterm and early term infants – can we do better? Semin. Fetal Neonatal Med. 24, 43–47.

Muelbert, M., Lin, L., Bloomfield, F.H., Harding, J.E., 2019b. Exposure to the smell and taste of milk to accelerate feeding in preterm infants. Cochrane Database Syst. Rev. 7, CD013038.

Nutrition, E.C.O., Arslanoglu, S., Corpeleijn, W., Moro, G., Braegger, C., Campoy, C., Colomb, V., Decsi, T., Domellof, M., Fewtrell, M., Hojsak, I., Mihatsch, W., Molgaard, C., Shamir, R., Turck, D., van Goudoever, J., 2013. Donor human milk for preterm infants: current evidence and research directions. J. Pediatr. Gastroenterol. Nutr. 57, 535–542.

O'Connor, D.L., Gibbins, S., Kiss, A., Bando, N., Brennan-Donnan, J., Ng, E., Campbell, D.M., Vaz, S., Fusch, C., Asztalos, E., Church, P., Kelly, E., Ly, L., Daneman, A., Unger, S., Group, G. T. A. D. F, 2016. Effect of supplemental donor human milk compared with preterm formula on neurodevelopment of very low-birth-weight infants at 18 months: a randomized clinical trial. JAMA 316, 1897–1905.

O'Connor, D.L., Kiss, A., Tomlinson, C., Bando, N., Bayliss, A., Campbell, D.M., Daneman, A., Francis, J., Kotsopoulos, K., Shah, P.S., Vaz, S., Williams, B., Unger, S., Optimo, M.F.G., 2018. Nutrient enrichment of human milk with human and bovine milk-based fortifiers for infants born weighing <1250 g: a randomized clinical trial. Am. J. Clin. Nutr. 108, 108–116.

Oddie, S.J., Young, L., McGuire, W., 2017. Slow advancement of enteral feed volumes to prevent necrotising enterocolitis in very low birth weight infants. Cochrane Database Syst. Rev. 8, CD001241.

Osborn, D.A., Schindler, T., Jones, L.J., Sinn, J.K., Bolisetty, S., 2018. Higher versus lower amino acid intake in parenteral nutrition for newborn infants. Cochrane Database Syst. Rev. 3, CD005949.

Pammi, M., Suresh, G., 2020. Enteral lactoferrin supplementation for prevention of sepsis and necrotizing enterocolitis in preterm infants. Cochrane Database Syst. Rev. 3, CD007137.

Parkinson, J.R., Hyde, M.J., Gale, C., Santhakumaran, S., Modi, N., 2013. Preterm birth and the metabolic syndrome in adult life: a systematic review and meta-analysis. Pediatrics 131, e1240-63.

Pell, L.G., Loutet, M.G., Roth, D.E., Sherman, P.M., 2019. Arguments against routine administration of probiotics for NEC prevention. Curr. Opin. Pediatr. 31, 195–201.

Premkumar, M.H., Pammi, M., Suresh, G., 2019. Human milk-derived fortifier versus bovine milk-derived fortifier for prevention of mortality and morbidity in preterm neonates. Cochrane Database Syst. Rev. 2019, CD013145.

Prouse, C., 2021. Mining liquid gold: the lively, contested terrain of human milk valuations. Environ. Plan. A 53, 958–976.

Quigley, M., Embleton, N.D., McGuire, W., 2019. Formula versus donor breast milk for feeding preterm or low birth weight infants. Cochrane Database Syst. Rev. 7, CD002971.

Rantakari, K., Rinta-Koski, O.P., Metsaranta, M., Hollmen, J., Sarkka, S., Rahkonen, P., Lano, A., Lauronen, L., Nevalainen, P., Leskinen, M.J., Andersson, S., 2021. Early oxygen levels contribute to brain injury in extremely preterm infants. Pediatr. Res. 90, 131–139.

Razak, A., 2020. Two-hourly versus three-hourly feeding in very low-birth-weight infants: a systematic review and meta-analysis. Am. J. Perinatol. 37, 898–906.

Roelants, J.A., Vlaardingerbroek, H., van den Akker, C.H.P., de Jonge, R.C.J., van Goudoever, J.B., Vermeulen, M.J., 2018. Two-year follow-up of a randomized controlled nutrition intervention trial in very low-birth-weight infants. JPEN J. Parenter. Enteral Nutr. 42, 122–131.

Rovekamp-Abels, L.W., Hogewind-Schoonenboom, J.E., de Wijs-Meijler, D.P., Maduro, M.D., Jansen-Van Der Weide, M.C., van Goudoever, J.B., Hulst, J.M., 2015. Intermittent bolus or semicontinuous feeding for preterm infants? J. Pediatr. Gastroenterol. Nutr. 61, 659–664.

Roze, J.C., Darmaun, D., Boquien, C.Y., Flamant, C., Picaud, J.C., Savagner, C., Claris, O., Lapillonne, A., Mitanchez, D., Branger, B., Simeoni, U., Kaminski, M., Ancel, P.Y., 2012. The apparent breastfeeding paradox in very preterm infants: relationship between breast feeding, early weight gain and neurodevelopment based on results from two cohorts, epipage and lift. BMJ Open 2, e000834.

Ruys, C.A., van de Lagemaat, M., Finken, M.J., Lafeber, H.N., 2017. Follow-up of a randomized trial on postdischarge nutrition in preterm-born children at age 8 y. Am. J. Clin. Nutr. 106, 549–558.

Ruys, C.A., Broring, T., van Schie, P.E.M., van de Lagemaat, M., Rotteveel, J., Finken, M.J.J., Oostrom, K.J., Lafeber, H.N., 2019. Neurodevelopment of children born very preterm and/or with a very low birth weight: 8-year follow-up of a nutritional RCT. Clin. Nutr. ESPEN 30, 190–198.

Ruys, C.A., van de Lagemaat, M., Rotteveel, J., Finken, M.J.J., Lafeber, H.N., 2021. Improving long-term health outcomes of preterm infants: how to implement the findings of nutritional intervention studies into daily clinical practice. Eur. J. Pediatr. 180, 1665–1673.

Ryan, B.A., Kovacs, C.S., 2020. Calciotropic and phosphotropic hormones in fetal and neonatal bone development. Semin. Fetal Neonatal Med. 25, 101062.

Sammallahti, S., Pyhala, R., Lahti, M., Lahti, J., Pesonen, A.K., Heinonen, K., Hovi, P., Eriksson, J.G., Strang-Karlsson, S., Andersson, S., Jarvenpaa, A.L., Kajantie, E., Raikkonen, K., 2014. Infant growth after preterm birth and neurocognitive abilities in young adulthood. J. Pediatr. 165, 1109–1115.e3.

Section On, B., 2012. Breastfeeding and the use of human milk. Pediatrics 129, e827-41.

Serenius, F., Kallen, K., Blennow, M., Ewald, U., Fellman, V., Holmstrom, G., Lindberg, E., Lundqvist, P., Marsal, K., Norman, M., Olhager, E., Stigson, L., Stjernqvist, K., Vollmer, B., Stromberg, B., Group, E, 2013. Neurodevelopmental outcome in extremely preterm infants at 2.5 years after active perinatal care in Sweden. JAMA 309, 1810–1820.

Sharif, S., Meader, N., Oddie, S.J., Rojas-Reyes, M.X., McGuire, W., 2020. Probiotics to prevent necrotising enterocolitis in very preterm or very low birth weight infants. Cochrane Database Syst. Rev. 10, CD005496.

Sharma, D., Padmavathi, I.V., Tabatabaii, S.A., Farahbakhsh, N., 2021. Late preterm: a new high risk group in neonatology. J. Matern. Fetal Neonatal Med. 34, 2717–2730.

Silano, M., Milani, G.P., Fattore, G., Agostoni, C., 2019. Donor human milk and risk of surgical necrotizing enterocolitis: a meta-analysis. Clin. Nutr. 38, 1061–1066.

Simon, L., Nusinovici, S., Flamant, C., Cariou, B., Rouger, V., Gascoin, G., Darmaun, D., Roze, J.C., Hanf, M., 2017. Post-term growth and cognitive development at 5 years of age in preterm children: evidence from a prospective population-based cohort. PLoS One 12, e0174645.

Singh, A.S., Mulder, C., Twisk, J.W., van Mechelen, W., Chinapaw, M.J., 2008. Tracking of childhood overweight into adulthood: a systematic review of the literature. Obes. Rev. 9, 474–488.

Sipola-Leppanen, M., Kajantie, E., 2015. Should we assess cardiovascular risk in young adults born preterm? Curr. Opin. Lipidol. 26, 282–287.

Stevens, T.P., Shields, E., Campbell, D., Combs, A., Horgan, M., La Gamma, E.F., Xiong, K., Kacica, M., 2018. Statewide initiative to reduce postnatal growth restriction among infants <31 weeks of gestation. J. Pediatr. 197, 82–89.e2.

Stoll, B.J., Hansen, N.I., Bell, E.F., Walsh, M.C., Carlo, W.A., Shankaran, S., Laptook, A.R., Sanchez, P.J., van Meurs, K.P., Wyckoff, M., Das, A., Hale, E.C., Ball, M.B., Newman, N.S., Schibler, K., Poindexter, B.B., Kennedy, K.A., Cotten, C.M., Watterberg, K.L., D'angio, C.T., Demauro, S.B., Truog, W.E., Devaskar, U., Higgins, R.D., Eunice Kennedy Shriver National Institute Of Child, H, Human Development Neonatal Research, N, 2015. Trends in care practices, morbidity, and mortality of extremely preterm neonates, 1993-2012. JAMA 314, 1039–1051.

Strommen, K., Blakstad, E.W., Moltu, S.J., Almaas, A.N., Westerberg, A.C., Amlien, I.K., Ronnestad, A.E., Nakstad, B., Drevon, C.A., Bjornerud, A., Courivaud, F., Hol, P.K., Veierod, M.B., Fjell, A.M., Walhovd, K.B., Iversen, P.O., 2015. Enhanced nutrient supply to very low birth weight infants is associated with improved white matter maturation and head growth. Neonatology 107, 68–75.

Taine, M., Charles, M.A., Beltrand, J., Roze, J.C., Leger, J., Botton, J., Heude, B., 2018. Early postnatal growth and neurodevelopment in children born moderately preterm or small for gestational age at term: a systematic review. Paediatr. Perinat. Epidemiol. 32, 268–280.

Tekgunduz, K.S., Gurol, A., Apay, S.E., Caner, I., 2014. Effect of abdomen massage for prevention of feeding intolerance in preterm infants. Ital. J. Pediatr. 40, 89.

Teller, I.C., Embleton, N.D., Griffin, I.J., van Elburg, R.M., 2016. Post-discharge formula feeding in preterm infants: a systematic review mapping evidence about the role of macronutrient enrichment. Clin. Nutr. 35, 791–801.

Thanigainathan, S., Abiramalatha, T., 2020. Early fortification of human milk versus late fortification to promote growth in preterm infants. Cochrane Database Syst. Rev. 7, CD013392.

Thomas, E.L., Parkinson, J.R., Hyde, M.J., Yap, I.K., Holmes, E., Dore, C.J., Bell, J.D., Modi, N., 2011. Aberrant adiposity and ectopic lipid deposition characterize the adult phenotype of the preterm infant. Pediatr. Res. 70, 507–512.

Twilhaar, E.S., de Kieviet, J.F., Aarnoudse-Moens, C.S., van Elburg, R.M., Oosterlaan, J., 2018a. Academic performance of children born preterm: a meta-analysis and meta-regression. Arch. Dis. Child. Fetal Neonatal Ed. 103, F322–F330.

Twilhaar, E.S., Wade, R.M., de Kieviet, J.F., van Goudoever, J.B., van Elburg, R.M., Oosterlaan, J., 2018b. Cognitive outcomes of children born extremely or very preterm since the 1990s and associated risk factors: a meta-analysis and Meta-regression. JAMA Pediatr. 172, 361–367.

Ueda, P., Cnattingius, S., Stephansson, O., Ingelsson, E., Ludvigsson, J.F., Bonamy, A.K., 2014. Cerebrovascular and ischemic heart disease in young adults born preterm: a population-based Swedish cohort study. Eur. J. Epidemiol. 29, 253–260.

Underwood, M.A., 2019. Arguments for routine administration of probiotics for NEC prevention. Curr. Opin. Pediatr. 31, 188–194.

van Belkum, M., Mendoza Alvarez, L., Neu, J., 2020. Preterm neonatal immunology at the intestinal interface. Cell. Mol. Life Sci. 77, 1209–1227.

van den Akker, C.H., van Goudoever, J.B., 2010. Recent advances in our understanding of protein and amino acid metabolism in the human fetus. Curr. Opin. Clin. Nutr. Metab. Care 13, 75–80.

van den Akker, C.H., van Goudoever, J.B., 2016. Defining protein requirements of preterm infants by using metabolic studies in fetuses and preterm infants. Nestle Nutr. Inst. Workshop Ser. 86, 139–149.

van den Akker, C.H., Te Braake, F.W., Weisglas-Kuperus, N., van Goudoever, J.B., 2014. Observational outcome results following a randomized controlled trial of early amino acid administration in preterm infants. J. Pediatr. Gastroenterol. Nutr. 59, 714–719.

van den Akker, C.H.P., van Goudoever, J.B., Szajewska, H., Embleton, N.D., Hojsak, I., Reid, D., Shamir, R., Espghan Working Group For Probiotics And Prebiotics & Committee On Nutrition, 2018. Probiotics for preterm infants: a strain-specific systematic review and network meta-analysis. J. Pediatr. Gastroenterol. Nutr. 67, 103–122.

van den Akker, C.H.P., van Goudoever, J.B., Shamir, R., Domellof, M., Embleton, N.D., Hojsak, I., Lapillonne, A., Mihatsch, W.A., Berni Canani, R., Bronsky, J., Campoy, C., Fewtrell, M.S., Fidler Mis, N., Guarino, A., Hulst, J.M., Indrio, F., Kolacek, S., Orel, R., Vandenplas, Y., Weizman, Z., Szajewska, H., 2020. Probiotics and preterm infants: a position paper by the European Society for Paediatric Gastroenterology Hepatology and Nutrition Committee on Nutrition and the European Society for Paediatric Gastroenterology Hepatology and Nutrition Working Group for probiotics and prebiotics. J. Pediatr. Gastroenterol. Nutr. 70, 664–680.

van den Akker, C.H.P., Embleton, N.D., Vermeulen, M.J., van Goudoever, J.B., 2021. Meeting protein and energy requirements of preterm infants receiving human milk. Nestle Nutr. Inst. Workshop Ser. 96, 72–85. E Pub 2022 May 10. https://doi.org/10.1159/000519397. 35537430.

van Goudoever, J.B., van den Akker, C.H.P., 2021. Parenteral Nutrition for critically ill term and preterm neonates: a commentary on the 2021 European Society for paediatric gastroenterology, hepatology and nutrition position paper. J. Pediatr. Gastroenterol. Nutr. 73, 137–138.

van Puffelen, E., Vanhorebeek, I., Joosten, K.F.M., Wouters, P.J., van den Berghe, G., Verbruggen, S., 2018. Early versus late parenteral nutrition in critically ill, term neonates: a preplanned secondary subgroup analysis of the PEPaNIC multicentre, randomised controlled trial. Lancet Child Adolesc. Health 2, 505–515.

van Veenendaal, N.R., Heideman, W.H., Limpens, J., van der Lee, J.H., van Goudoever, J.B., van Kempen, A., van der Schoor, S.R.D., van Veenendaal, N.R., van der Schoor, S.R.D., Heideman, W.H., Rijnhart, J.J.M., Heymans, M.W., Twisk, J.W.R., van Goudoever, J.B., van Kempen, A., 2019. Hospitalising preterm infants in single family rooms versus open bay units: a systematic review and meta-analysis. Lancet Child Adolesc. Health 3, 147–157.

van Veenendaal, N.R., van der Schoor, S.R.D., Heideman, W.H., Rijnhart, J.J.M., Heymans, M.W., Twisk, J.W.R., van Goudoever, J.B., van Kempen, A., 2020. Family integrated care in single family rooms for preterm infants and late-onset sepsis: a retrospective study and mediation analysis. Pediatr. Res. 88, 593–600.

van Vliet, E.O., de Kieviet, J.F., Oosterlaan, J., van Elburg, R.M., 2013. Perinatal infections and neurodevelopmental outcome in very preterm and very low-birth-weight infants: a meta-analysis. JAMA Pediatr. 167, 662–668.

Vanhorebeek, I., Verbruggen, S., Casaer, M.P., Gunst, J., Wouters, P.J., Hanot, J., Guerra, G.G., Vlasselaers, D., Joosten, K., van den Berghe, G., 2017. Effect of early supplemental parenteral nutrition in the paediatric ICU: a preplanned observational study of post-randomisation treatments in the PEPanic trial. Lancet Respir. Med. 5, 475–483.

Verlinden, I., Dulfer, K., Vanhorebeek, I., Guiza, F., Hordijk, J.A., Wouters, P.J., Guerra, G.G., Joosten, K.F., Verbruggen, S.C., van den Berghe, G., 2021. Role of age of critically ill children at time of exposure to early or late parenteral nutrition in determining the impact hereof on long-term neurocognitive development: a secondary analysis of the PEPaNIC-RCT. Clin. Nutr. 40, 1005–1012.

Villamor-Martinez, E., Pierro, M., Cavallaro, G., Mosca, F., Kramer, B.W., Villamor, E., 2018. Donor human milk protects against bronchopulmonary dysplasia: a systematic review and meta-analysis. Nutrients 10, 238.

Villamor-Martinez, E., Pierro, M., Cavallaro, G., Mosca, F., Villamor, E., 2019. Mother's own milk and bronchopulmonary dysplasia: a systematic review and meta-analysis. Front. Pediatr. 7, 224.

Vinall, J., Grunau, R.E., Brant, R., Chau, V., Poskitt, K.J., Synnes, A.R., Miller, S.P., 2013. Slower postnatal growth is associated with delayed cerebral cortical maturation in preterm newborns. Sci. Transl. Med. 5, 168ra8.

Vlaardingerbroek, H., Veldhorst, M.A., Spronk, S., van den Akker, C.H., van Goudoever, J.B., 2012. Parenteral lipid administration to very-low-birth-weight infants–early introduction of lipids and use of new lipid emulsions: a systematic review and meta-analysis. Am. J. Clin. Nutr. 96, 255–268.

Vliegenthart, R.J.S., van Kaam, A.H., Aarnoudse-Moens, C.S.H., van Wassenaer, A.G., Onland, W., 2019. Duration of mechanical ventilation and neurodevelopment in preterm infants. Arch. Dis. Child. Fetal Neonatal Ed. 104, F631–F635.

Walsh, V., McGuire, W., 2019. Immunonutrition for preterm infants. Neonatology 115, 398–405.

Walsh, V., Brown, J.V.E., Copperthwaite, B.R., Oddie, S.J., McGuire, W., 2020. Early full enteral feeding for preterm or low birth weight infants. Cochrane Database Syst. Rev. 12, CD013542.

Wang, Q., Cui, Q., Yan, C., 2016. The effect of supplementation of long-chain polyunsaturated fatty acids during lactation on neurodevelopmental outcomes of preterm infant from infancy to school age: a systematic review and meta-analysis. Pediatr. Neurol. 59, 54–61.e1.

Wang, Y., Zhu, W., Luo, B.R., 2020. Continuous feeding versus intermittent bolus feeding for premature infants with low birth weight: a meta-analysis of randomized controlled trials. Eur. J. Clin. Nutr. 74, 775–783.

Westin, V., Vanpée, M., Norman, M., Stoltz Sjöström, E., 2020. Perioperative nutrition in extremely preterm infants undergoing surgery for patent ductus arteriosus. Clin. Nutr. Exp. 33, 60–71.

Westrup, B., Bohm, B., Lagercrantz, H., Stjernqvist, K., 2004. Preschool outcome in children born very prematurely and cared for according to the newborn individualized developmental care and assessment program (NIDCAP). Acta Paediatr. 93, 498–507.

Wong, H.S., Huertas-Ceballos, A., Cowan, F.M., Modi, N., Medicines For Neonates Investigator, G, 2014. Evaluation of early childhood social-communication difficulties in children born preterm using the quantitative checklist for autism in toddlers. J. Pediatr. 164, 26–33.e1.

Young, L., Embleton, N.D., McCormick, F.M., McGuire, W., 2013. Multinutrient fortification of human breast milk for preterm infants following hospital discharge. Cochrane Database Syst. Rev. 2013, CD004866.

Young, L., Embleton, N.D., McGuire, W., 2016. Nutrient-enriched formula versus standard formula for preterm infants following hospital discharge. Cochrane Database Syst. Rev. 12, CD004696.

Zhang, B., Xiu, W., Dai, Y., Yang, C., 2020. Protective effects of different doses of human milk on neonatal necrotizing enterocolitis. Medicine (Baltimore) 99, e22166.

# 18

# Early nutrition, the development of obesity, and its long term consequences

## Jose M. Saavedra

Johns Hopkins University, School of Medicine, Baltimore, MD, United States

## LEARNING OBJECTIVES

- To review the current global burden of childhood obesity, and examine early life growth and nutrition as major determinants of obesity risk and other long-term health consequences.

- Review the prenatal and postnatal diet and behavior-related modifiable factors in

a child's immediate environment that are associated with increased risk of obesity in childhood and later life.

- Discuss approaches to address the global problem of obesity, with a focus on modifiable factors related to obesity in early life.

## 18.1 Introduction

Despite some progress in certain parts of the world, obesity is the largest and fastest grow-ing epidemic of modern times. By estimates from the World Health Organization (WHO), the worldwide prevalence of obesity nearly tripled between 1975 and 2016. In 2016 more than 1.9 billion adults were overweight, and 650 million were obese. More alarmingly, the problem has increasingly affected the younger and the more disadvantaged populations (UNICEF et al., 2021; WHO, 2016a, 2021).

Although the prevalence of overweight and obesity in children has been lower than that of adults, over the last decades, the rate of increase in childhood obesity in many countries has been greater than the rate of increase in adult obesity. From 1975 to 2016, the global prevalence of overweight or obese 5–19-year-olds increased more than fourfold from 4% to

18% globally (WHO, 2021). In the same time period, the prevalence of obesity alone rose from 0.7% to 5.6% in girls, and from 0.9% to 7.8% in boys, an eightfold increase overall. The global age-standardized BMI for children and adolescents rose from 17.2 to 18.6 in girls and 16.8 to 18.5 for boys (NCD Risk Factor Collaboration, 2017). In round terms, from 2000 to 2016, the proportion of overweight 5- to 19-year-old children rose from 1 in 10 to almost 1 in 5 (United Nations Children's Fund UNICEF, 2019). Given these trends, a 2017 estimate suggests that this year, 2022, the world will have swung to having more obese than moderate and severely underweight children and adolescents (NCD Risk Factor Collaboration, 2017).

For children 2–4 years of age, between 1980 and 2015, the global prevalence of obesity almost doubled, from 3.9% to 7.2% in boys and 3.7% to 6.4% in girls (Di Cesare et al., 2019). The recent Joint Child Malnutrition Estimates from UNICEF, WHO, and the World Bank indicate that from 2000 to 2020 (before the start of the COVID-19 pandemic), global obesity rates for children under 5 increased only slightly, from 5.4% to 5.7% or 33.3 to 38.9 million children (UNICEF et al., 2021; WHO, 2021), with the fastest growing prevalence in Asia and Africa. The Brookings Institution estimates that by 2030, 90 million children aged 2 to 4 years, equal to 22% of the world's total, will be overweight (Kharas et al., 2018).

However, these global numbers and trends are very unevenly distributed between more and less vulnerable populations. In high come countries like the United States and Europe over the last decade, the prevalence of obesity appears to have leveled off or slightly decreased in 2–5-year-olds (Ogden et al., 2014) and in young children (Buoncristiano et al., 2021). In low- and middle-income countries, however, it continues to rise. Today, most countries with the largest number of undernourished children also have the greatest numbers of overweight and obesity. In 2020, 75% of all overweight children under 5 years lived in Asia and Africa. And independent of the country, most children with overweight and obesity are from the most socioeconomically disadvantaged families (UNICEF et al., 2021).

It is not uncommon to find undernutrition and obesity co-existing within the same country, the same community, and the same household. In more developed regions, weight and BMI tend to be associated with lower SES and minorities. In the United States, for example, among 2–5-year-old children, 16.7% of Hispanic boys and girls were obese, compared with a population average of 8.4%, and 8.8% of infants 0–2 years of age were > 97.7 percentile of weight/length WHO growth charts, compared to 5.5% of white (non-Hispanic) infants (Ogden et al., 2014). In some environments, unhealthy infant feeding practices in early infancy appear to be the primary mechanism mediating the relationship between SES and early childhood obesity (Taveras et al., 2010b; Gibbs and Forste, 2014). In 2020, 94% of all stunted children, and 97% of all children affected by wasting, under 5 years of age, lived in Asia and Africa (UNICEF et al., 2021). Thus, most low- and middle-income countries confront the "double burden" of poor nutrition and related disease.

The global state of nutrition and health has been dramatically disrupted by the emergence of the SARS-CoV-2 virus leading to the COVID-19 pandemic we are currently enduring. Since its beginning, it became abundantly clear that it would affect child nutrition and long-lasting global health. On the one hand, COVID-19 has deeply affected agricultural production and all aspects of the food supply, as well as altering global, local, and family economies. These have similarly had a more profound effect on low-income groups. The World Food Program estimated that the number of people facing acute food insecurity doubled to 265 million in 2020 (World Food Program (WFP), 2020) and will further worsen in 2022. This, coupled with severe losses in the coverage of nutrition services for vulnerable groups (UNICEF et al., 2021), is leading to major increases in child undernutrition and mortality, particularly for children in low-income countries (UNICEF et al., 2021; Headey et al., 2020).

On the other hand, the pandemic has also adversely affected the quality of children's diets, particularly in middle- and high-income countries, and in these, especially among vulnerable groups. Early surveys in Europe show significant adverse changes, including increased intake of less nutrient-dense foods, increased snacking, and increased inactivity (Zemrani et al., 2021), associated with changes in schooling, quarantines, and lockdowns. The SARS-CoV-2 virus has fortunately had a lesser infectious impact on children; however, the pandemic's severe and profound social and economic fall-out will have acute and long-term nutrition consequences (Crowder et al., 2021). The pandemic may exacerbate both under and overnutrition and further exacerbate present inequities. Its effects on the trends and projections related to children's nutrition will need to be reassessed and dealt with in the years to come.

Obesity starts early in the life cycle. It is well documented that the growth patterns in infancy are critical determinants of obesity in late childhood and later life. Infant adiposity or increased BMI, as early as 2 weeks of age (Winter et al., 2010) through 24 months of age (Stettler and Iotova, 2010; Moss and Yeaton, 2012), has been associated with a significantly increased risk of overweight in toddler or preschool age years. Children who were obese at 9 months or 24 months were three times more likely to retain an obese weight at age 4 years, compared to nonobese children measured during their first 2 years of life (Moss and Yeaton, 2012). The majority of children who are obese by 3 years of age remain obese into adolescence. Overweight 5-year-olds were four times as likely as normal-weight children to become obese adolescents (Cunningham et al., 2014). In turn, these early changes strongly correlate with adult overweight (De Kroon et al., 2010). Thus, the growth trajectory of children likely to become obese is greatly determined by weight in infancy and early childhood. Any serious attempts to curb this epidemic demand focus and actions to prevent the development of overweight and obesity in the first 2 years of life (Deal et al., 2020).

Overweight and obesity in infancy correlates with childhood obesity, which is associated with breathing difficulties, increased risk of fractures, hypertension, early markers of cardiovascular disease, insulin resistance, and psychological effects. Furthermore, obesity in early life heralds and correlates not only with adolescent and adult obesity, but with the risk of development of noncommunicable diseases (NCDs) and their attendant complications. These include cardiovascular diseases (heart disease and stroke), diabetes, musculoskeletal disorders (especially osteoarthritis), and some cancers (including endometrial, breast, ovarian, prostate, liver, gallbladder, kidney, and colon). Today, most of the world's population live in countries where overweight and obesity kill more people than underweight (WHO, 2021).

Obesity is a present and growing problem worldwide. The epidemic transcends geographical, ethnic, and socioeconomic boundaries, affecting all population groups. Obesity in infancy is a major predictor of later obesity and its short- and long-term-associated health complications. Current trends in obesity prevalence also widen disparities in health and its social and economic consequences. The enormous healthcare costs of NCDs, many, if not most of which have their origins in infancy, are being passed on to future generations, threatening health and the development and economic growth of nations. The need for action is clear.

## 18.2 Addressing the problem

The fundamental underlying cause of obesity and overweight is ultimately a mismatch between energy consumed and energy expended. Globally, there has been an increased intake of energy and a decrease in physical inactivity, with increasingly sedentary work and lifestyle behaviors, changing modes of transportation, and increasing urbanization. Managing the epidemic of obesity will require decreasing this mismatch, starting very early in life.

The genetic contribution to obesity as a phenotypic expression of this energy intake-expenditure imbalance has been increasingly investigated, and estimates have varied. Twin studies demonstrate that environmental factors significantly affect genetic expression and BMI in childhood, and this influence varies with age and sex (Silventoinen et al., 2016). Adult BMI-associated single-nucleotide genetic polymorphisms have been found to exert their effect between birth and 5 years of age. Genetic predisposition can thus explain differences in the development of obesity but not enough to trigger obesity. Dietary interventions and proper lifestyle changes can decrease obesity development in genetically predisposed children (Mărginean et al., 2018). Thus, overweight and obesity are largely preventable, and early intervention seems critical.

In early life, the imbalance between intake and expenditure is mediated by diet and feeding behaviors as well as activity-related behaviors of parents and caregivers toward the infant. This dynamic is also affected by broader mediators in the family (e.g., socioeconomic status, parental education, and occupation), and in the larger community and society (adequacy of social networks and support, employment, physical environments, and social advantages or disadvantages), which can foster obesogenic behaviors and obesity among children (Gibbs and Forste, 2014; Iguacel et al., 2021).

Addressing these factors requires supportive policies in multiple sectors, including health, education, agriculture, transport, urban and environmental planning, and food processing, distribution, and marketing. Thus, identifying solutions to curb the epidemic needs to assess, consider and address these multiple factors in a holistic and comprehensive approach. No single approach will be successful, nor can this be addressed without clear, transparent, and determined multisectoral involvement of government, NGOs, the private sector, communities, families, and individuals.

At a global level, the WHO is currently implementing a process to update guiding principles on complementary feeding (WHO, 2019). In 2016, the World Health Assembly welcomed the report of the Commission on Ending Childhood Obesity and its six specific recommendations (WHO, 2016b). See Table 18.1.

Two recommendations (#1 and 2) tackle the environment and norms to modify the "obesogenic" environment, including reduction of "unhealthy foods" and sweetened beverages, adding that there is a broader need for addressing political and commercial factors (e.g., trade agreements, fiscal and agricultural policies and food systems, availability of healthy foods, infrastructure, and opportunities for physical activity in the neighborhood, etc.) One recommendation (#6) addresses the management and treatment of obesity and related disorders, and three recommendations (#3–5) are focused on reducing the risk of obesity in the life course: one focuses on implementing programs to foster adequate school, health nutrition, and activity environments for school-aged children, and two focus on the topic of this chapter, the potential effect of nutritional and behavioral interventions during preconception and pregnancy, and in infancy and early childhood.

**TABLE 18.1** Recommendations from the report of the commission on ending childhood obesity.

Tackle the obesogenic environment and norms

1. Reduce the intake of unhealthy foods and sugar-sweetened beverages by children and adolescents.

2. Implement comprehensive programs that promote physical activity and reduce sedentary behaviors in children and adolescents.

Reduce the risk of obesity by addressing critical elements in the life-course

3. Integrate and strengthen guidance for noncommunicable disease prevention with current guidance for preconception and antenatal care, to reduce the risk of childhood obesity.

4. Provide guidance on and support for healthy diet, sleep, and physical activity in early childhood to ensure children grow appropriately and develop healthy habits.

5. Implement comprehensive programs that promote healthy school environments, health and nutrition literacy, and physical activity among school-age children and adolescents.

Treat children who are obese to improve their current and future health roles and responsibilities

6. Provide family-based, multicomponent lifestyle weight management services for children, and young people who are obese.

*Adapted from World Health Organization, 2016. WHO Report of the Commission on Ending Childhood Obesity. http://apps.who.int/iris/bitstream/10665/204176/1/9789241510066_eng.pdf.*

On the bright side, gestation and the first 2 years of life shape metabolic, immunologic, sensory, behavioral, developmental, and growth parameters for the rest of a person's life. This gives us a unique window of opportunity, which, if well utilized, can provide the greatest return on the investment of our efforts in combating the epidemic.

While nutrition-related factors associated with obesity can be addressed at multiple levels—family, communal, and societal—this chapter will refer to "modifiable factors," defined as *prenatal conditions and practices, and postnatal dietary and feeding-related behavioral practices, that can be addressed by parents and direct caregivers, in the immediate child's environment, in their first two years of life.* The evidence for these is discussed below, noting that the focus is on otherwise healthy mothers and children born at term.

## 18.3 Modifiable factors in preconception and pregnancy

There is a significant level of evidence to show that the following factors can independently increase the likelihood of obesity during infancy and childhood: maternal undernutrition (whether global or nutrient-specific), maternal overweight or obesity, excess pregnancy weight gain, maternal hyperglycemia (including gestational diabetes), and smoking or exposure to alcohol and toxins (Dattilo et al., 2012; Weng et al., 2012; Woo Baidal et al., 2016). In addition, evidence has mounted pointing to antibiotic use during pregnancy or perinatally, as well as mode of birth (cesarean section versus vaginal delivery) as independent risk factors for overweight and obesity in children, likely mediated by alterations in maternal and infant microbiota (Mueller et al., 2015a).

Table 18.2 summarizes the prenatal modifiable factors and behaviors associated with overweight or obesity in children discussed below, and potential actions for preventive interventions.

TABLE 18.2    Prenatal modifiable factors and behaviors associated with overweight or obesity in children[a].

| Modifiable factor | Direction of association to overweight or obesity in children | Potential action for obesity prevention |
|---|---|---|
| Maternal preconception BMI | Higher maternal pre-pregnancy BMI[b] has been consistently and positively associated with overweight in infancy and childhood. | Educate and support parents on healthy parental weight and healthy lifestyle habits. |
| Paternal preconception BMI | Limited data suggest paternal BMI is positively associated with increased risk of overweight or obesity in infancy and childhood. | |
| Gestational weight gain | Excess gestational weight gain[c] has been consistently and positively associated with birth weight and risk for infant/child overweight. | Educate and support pregnant women on maintaining adequate gestational weight and glucose control during gestation. |
| Gestational glucose control | Gestational diabetes is consistently and positively associated with the likelihood of infants being LGA, and with subsequent development of overweight or obesity. | |
| Maternal (and paternal) prenatal smoking and alcohol exposure | Prenatal maternal tobacco smoking has been positively associated with increased risk of adiposity during childhood. Paternal smoking may also be associated with increased childhood weight and adiposity. | Educate and support parents on avoidance of smoking and maternal avoidance of alcohol during gestation. |
| Mode of birth | Birth by cesarean section has been associated with increased risk of child adiposity and BMI, although data have not been consistent. | Educate parents and health providers on consequences of birth by cesarean section, and use only when medically indicated. |
| Perinatal antibiotic exposure | Limited but consistent data suggest maternal exposure to antibiotics during pregnancy is associated with overweight or obesity in childhood. | Educate parents and health providers on consequences of antibiotic use and indicate them only when appropriate. |

[a] See text for supporting literature.
[b] BMI, body mass index.
[c] Weight Gain During Pregnancy Guidelines (IOM, 2009).

## 18.3.1 Maternal nutrition and gestational factors associated with obesity

### 18.3.1.1 Maternal nutrition and gestational weight gain

Systematic reviews and meta-analyses show a robust correlation between maternal pre-conception obesity and subsequent childhood obesity, with risk increases of 200%–400% (Heslehurst et al., 2019; Voerman et al., 2019). Prenatal exposure to maternal overnutrition, including maternal preconception overweight status and excess gestational weight gain (GWG) have been consistently and independently identified to associate with higher infant birth weight or childhood overweight (Woo Baidal et al., 2016; Larqué et al., 2019). In addition, women with excessive preconception weight (overweight or obese at the start of pregnancy) are also at increased risk of developing gestational diabetes mellitus (GDM) and of requiring higher rates of cesarean section delivery, each of which has been independently associated with later childhood risk for overweight.

Furthermore, women with overweight and GDM were 2.8 times as likely, and women with obesity and GDM were 5.5 times as likely to have an infant that was large for gestational age (LGA), compared to women within a healthy weight category without GDM (Black et al., 2013). A large meta-analysis reported significantly higher fat mass in infants of mothers with GDM, with the effect being higher in boys than in girls, even after controlling for maternal BMI (Logan et al., 2017). Infants born as LGA, in turn, have an independent risk factor for later childhood obesity. A large cohort study documented a relative risk (RR) of obesity of 1.55 among adolescents who had been large for gestational age at birth, compared to their peers born at an average birth weight category.

However, even in the absence of GDM, studies have consistently reported a positive association of maternal BMI with infant birth weight or future childhood obesity risk. Some of these effects may be mediated by excess GWG, which is associated with increased fat mass and percentage of neonatal body fat (Starling et al., 2014), as well as increase the risk of childhood obesity measured up to 5–18 years of age (Mamun et al., 2013). In a large Chinese study, the risk of overweight at 3–6 years was doubled in children whose mothers were overweight or obese before pregnancy and experienced excess GWG, compared to children of women with adequate preconception weight and recommended (Guo et al., 2015). In a large North American cohort, infants born vaginally to overweight or obese mothers were three times more likely to become overweight at age 1 year (Tun et al., 2018).

Excess GWG also has subsequent effects on the mother. GWG, above the recommended levels, was associated with a threefold higher risk of the mother becoming overweight after pregnancy, even among women who were under or average weight before pregnancy (Gunderson, 2009), perpetuating the likelihood of women entering a subsequent pregnancy at a higher than recommended weight. Timing of dietary influence may also be important. Higher maternal dietary glycemic index and total dietary glycemic load in early (11 weeks), but not in late pregnancy (34 weeks), has been associated with greater adiposity in offspring at 4 and 6 years of age (Okubo et al., 2014). Finally, emerging evidence suggests that independent of maternal pre-pregnancy BMI, and total energy intake, poor maternal diet quality, as assessed by 24h dietary recall and a healthy eating index score, can also increase neonatal adiposity (Shapiro et al., 2016). Further work is needed to identify specific macronutrient ranges associated with the most desirable in utero growth.

In addition, although the data are much more limited, several studies have found that increased paternal BMI is associated with increased childhood BMI (Campbell and McPherson, 2019). It has been postulated that metabolic changes due to parental overweight/obesity may affect epigenetic markers in oocytes and sperm and, in this way, influence epigenetic programming during embryogenesis. Further studies are needed to understand the relationship and mechanisms of paternal influence on child BMI and metabolic outcomes (Hieronimus and Ensenauer, 2021).

Lastly, maternal diet may influence childhood dietary patterns in other ways. Recent evidence shows that sensory experiences related to food can begin in utero and could play a role in establishing food preferences. A variety of flavors can be transmitted from the mother's diet to amniotic fluid, and this experience can modify their future acceptance of similarly flavored foods. In particular, garlic flavors transferred to amniotic fluid or breast milk lead to infant responses if their mothers ate garlic during the last month of pregnancy or ate garlic while breastfeeding. And experiences with garlic flavor during the last month of pregnancy resulted in greater acceptance of garlic-flavored foods by children at 8 to 9 years of age (Spahn et al., 2019). The consequences and potential interventions derived from these observations await further research.

### 18.3.1.2 Birth weight

Prematurity, low birth weight, and being small for gestational age have been associated with risk of increased adiposity and obesity in later life. Conversely, infants born large for gestational age also show increased risk. While the mechanisms are not clear, there is good evidence that there is an association between birth weight and subsequent BMI and overweight in young adults and children, which is linear and positive in some studies and J- or U-shaped in others (Rogers and EURO-BLCS Study Group, 2003). This association between birth weight and abdominal adiposity in later childhood and adolescence suggests that fetal nutrition, as reflected by birth weight, may have a programming effect on abdominal adiposity later in life, which leads to increased obesity and cardiometabolic risk in infants with low birth weight. Elevated weight, whether > 4 kg at birth or children born large for their gestational age, has consistently been shown to correlate with adolescent and subsequent obesity (Yu et al., 2011, (Geserick et al., 2018). While these associations appear clear, ultimately, birthweight is a consequence of the process of gestation and the factors influencing it, some of which can be modified. Thus, it can be considered more a marker than a causal factor for obesity development.

## 18.3.2 Non-nutritional maternal and perinatalfactors associated with obesity

### 18.3.2.1 Smoking and alcohol

The data on smoking and alcohol consumption during pregnancy are limited but appears consistent. In a European cross-sectional study, children whose mothers smoked during pregnancy had higher adiposity levels than children of non-smokers (Li et al., 2016). Several meta-analyses have reported an association between maternal smoking during pregnancy and obesity, with odds ratios of obesity ranging from 1.52 to 1.55 in the offspring (Ino, 2010; Rayfield and Plugge, 2017). Other meta-analyses have corroborated the associations between maternal smoking and paternal smoking, independently, with childhood overweight and/ or obesity (Riedel et al., 2014; Philips et al., 2020). A recent cohort study in the Netherlands documented an increased risk of overweight and adiposity in children exposed to maternal and paternal smoking, as well as to maternal and paternal cannabis use, also with a greater impact of maternal exposure (Cajachagua-Torres et al., 2022). In most of these studies, maternal influence is uniformly greater, suggesting a direct intrauterine effect. However, family social and environmental factors and confounders could partially explain these relationships.

The effect of alcohol consumption during pregnancy on short- and long-term developmental and neuropsychological outcomes has been well documented. However, we cannot identify adequate studies—observational or other—that document the association of alcohol consumption during pregnancy and childhood or later obesity. Obesity risk to the infant may be an additional potential complication of alcohol consumption during pregnancy. And although important in this regard, it only adds to other major associated complications (stillbirth, low birth weight, birth defects, sudden infant death syndrome, fetal alcohol syndrome, and neurocognitive delays).

While the literature on smoking and obesity risks appears consistent, even if still limited, and studies on alcohol consumption and similar risks are not available, the complications from smoking and alcohol exposure seem sufficient to avoid them during pregnancy.

### 18.3.2.2 *Microbiota-related factors: Antibiotic exposure, and mode of birth*

Over the last decade, increasing attention has been paid to the interaction between the host and its microbiota (the microbial ecosystems associated with the skin, respiratory tract, and the gut) and its microbiome (the collective genetic composition of the microbiota). The major roles that the microbiota plays regarding host health have been increasingly better described; and these include key influence over digestive, protective and immunologic, metabolic, and neurologic functions (Buccigrossi et al., 2013; Rinninella et al., 2019), the details of which are beyond the scope of this paper.

Evidence from animal models, clinical trials, and observational cohort studies supports the hypothesis that inadequate development of the microbiota (particularly, the gut microbiota) in early life can program the host and lead to the development of acute and chronic disease in the long term (Stinson, 2020). These microbial changes have been linked to an increased risk of obesity and other chronic NCDs (Calatayud et al., 2019; Kalliomäki et al., 2008). Therefore, environmental factors, including medical interventions such as cesarean section versus vaginal delivery, perinatal use of antibiotics, and use of alternatives to breastfeeding (discussed below), could potentially affect the maternal and infant microbiome, and in turn, increase the risk of overweight and obesity in later life (Mueller et al., 2015a). Critical factors in determining the development of an infant's "healthy" microbiota include vaginal birth and breastfeeding; and birth by cesarean section and use of infant formula, as well as maternal and perinatal use of antibiotics, have been identified as major disruptors of normal gut microbiota development in an infant (Mueller et al., 2015a; Yasmin et al., 2017).

#### Maternal antibiotic exposure

Antibiotics can disrupt maternal microbiota, which is a significant determinant of the normal development of the microbiota in the infant. Increasing evidence points to perinatal and maternal exposure to antibiotics as an independent risk for obesity in the offspring. Some studies suggest that maternal exposure to antibiotics during the second or third trimester has been associated with increased risk of overweight and obesity in school-aged children (Mor et al., 2015) and increased BMI, waist circumference, and body fat, as well as higher risk (up to 80% higher) of obesity in later childhood (Mueller et al., 2015b). The disruption of microbiota in infants, including that caused by the use of antibiotics in early life, as a risk factor for obesity, is discussed further below.

#### Cesarean section

Evidence from recent studies suggests an association between obesity risk and birth by cesarean section. A large cohort study revealed that children born by cesarean section had a higher average BMI and around 30% higher risk of overweight or obesity than children born vaginally. Within-family analysis showed that children born by cesarean section had a 2.7-fold higher risk of overweight/obesity than their peers born vaginally (Martín-Calvo et al., 2020). In a large international cohort study, the adjusted risk ratio for obesity among children delivered via cesarean section vs vaginally was 1.15. And it increased to 1.3 for cesarean delivery without known clinical indications. Furthermore, within-family analysis showed individuals born by cesarean section had 64% higher odds of obesity than did their siblings born via vaginal delivery (Yuan et al., 2016). And in yet another cohort, birth by cesarean section was associated with a 46% higher offspring risk of childhood obesity. Associations were similar for elective and non-elective CS (Mueller et al., 2015b). There also appears to be an interplay between maternal overweight and mode of birth, as exemplified by findings in a large ethnically diverse cohort in the United States. In this study, the odds of overweight or obesity were highest in children up to 5 years of age born by cesarean delivery to obese mothers (OR 2.8), followed by children born by cesarean delivery to overweight mothers (OR 2.2), then children born vaginally to obese mothers (OR 1.8) and finally children born vaginally to overweight mothers (OR 1.7) (Mueller et al., 2017).

At least three systematic meta-analyses appear to confirm the association between birth by cesarean section and the risk of obesity. In one, the overall pooled odds ratio of overweight/obesity for offspring delivered by cesarean section was 1.33 (1.32 for children, 1.24 for adolescents, and 1.50 for adults) (Li et al., 2013). Two other meta-analyses estimated a relative obesity risk of 1.34 (Kuhle et al., 2015) and 1.35 (Słabuszewska-Jóźwiak et al., 2020) in children born by cesarean section; and a third meta-analysis placed the risk of obesity with cesarean birth at an odds ratio of 1.59 in children below 5 years of age (Keag et al., 2018).

These findings suggest a possible mechanistic biological effect. Cesarean section and perinatal use of antibiotics clearly lead to alterations in the microbial ecosystem (dysbiosis). Furthermore, this aberrant microbiota, through various pathways, can affect energy intake and utilization. Several mechanisms have been advanced to explain these relationships, including increased microbial harvest of energy, microbial-related neurohormonal mediators of appetite and satiety, and inflammatory mediators affecting adipose tissue and insulin secretion (Mueller et al., 2015a; Davis et al., 2017). A large cohort study showed that intrapartum antibiotics in cesarean and vaginal delivery are associated with infant gut microbiota dysbiosis, and breastfeeding modifies some of these effects (Azad et al., 2016). In a large prospective cohort, children born to overweight or obese mothers were three times more likely to become overweight at 1 and 3 years. In this study, maternal and infant gut microbiota analysis showed that birth mode and infant gut microbiota sequentially mediated the association between maternal pre-pregnancy overweight and childhood overweight at ages 1 and 3 years (Tun et al., 2018). Similar microbiota-related mechanisms may operate for feeding of breast-milk alternatives versus breastfeeding and are discussed below.

However, a recent UK cohort study did not report a positive association of C section and adiposity in children (Ralphs et al., 2021), nor did one in the US extracting data from a large clinical database and assessing BMI at 5 years (Rifas-Shiman et al., 2018). A recent cohort study from Belarus (Rifas-Shiman et al., 2021) found cesarean delivery was associated with higher child BMI, and adiposity at 6.5 and 11.5 years of age, but not at 16 years; but further adjustment for maternal BMI substantially attenuated these associations.

In summary, while the association of birth by cesarean section and later BMI and obesity appears directionally consistent in many studies, significant confounding by interrelated factors, particularly maternal BMI, cannot be ignored, and limits the strength of the association.

## 18.4 Modifiable factors in early infancy associated with obesity

Following birth, diet, and behaviors related to feeding are under the immediate control of an infant's caregivers. The first 2 years provide a single and unique opportunity in life to take advantage of this control, since they are also characterized by infants' remarkable plasticity and learning ability, and thus the potential for programming and shaping an infant's eventual childhood and adult eating patterns. The process of parental, well-guided adoption of healthy eating choices, and behaviors by an infant has a much higher chance for effectiveness than attempts to change eating behaviors in later life. Lastly, women who just become mothers are motivated and eager to learn to do what is in the best interest of their newborns. Thus, based on what we have learned so far, addressing those postnatal "modifiable factors" associated with healthy growth through adoption of feeding practices, diet, and related behaviors in the first 2 years of life, is a unique opportunity to shape the future health of the individual.

This section addresses those approaches which can influence a child's healthy growth, with a focus on the prevention of an accelerated rate of weight gain during infancy, increased weight for length, BMI, or measures of adiposity during the first 24 months of life and through the toddler age, and the development of healthy eating behaviors. The potentially modifiable factors or exposures discussed below are consistent with those identified and reviewed by others (Dattilo et al., 2012; Dattilo, 2017); Woo Baidal et al., 2016; Larqué et al., 2019; Koletzko et al., 2020).

These factors are also fully consistent with the WHO Report of the Commission on Ending Childhood Obesity (WHO, 2016b), and specifically, the call to "Provide guidance on, and support for, healthy diet, sleep, and physical activity in early childhood to ensure children grow appropriately and develop healthy habits."

Table 18.3 summarizes the feeding and related behavioral modifiable factors in the first 2 years of life associated with overweight or obesity in later childhood; and potential actions for preventive interventions, as discussed below.

### 18.4.1 Diet-related childhood factors associated with obesity

Humans are the only mammals who feed their infants complementary foods before weaning from the breast, and the only primates that wean their offspring before they can forage independently. Thus, infants are most dependent on feeding by their parents and caregivers than any other mammalian species (Borowitz, 2021). Part of the effort in optimizing infant feeding and controlling obesity requires development and dissemination of science-based guidelines and guidance for parents and caregivers on diet, nutrition, and physical activity. It is remarkable, however, that historically, in most countries and geographies, comprehensive science-based dietary guidelines, which help drive nutrition and health strategies, have existed (in varying degrees) for adults and older children, but not for infants. Within the past few years, several high-income countries, including Australia, Canada, New Zealand, and

**TABLE 18.3** Feeding and related behavioral modifiable factors in the first 2 years of life associated with overweight or obesity in later childhood[a].

| Modifiable factor | Direction of association to overweight or obesity in children | Action |
|---|---|---|
| *Breastfeeding and formula feeding* | | |
| Breastfeeding or feeding infant formula | Breastfeeding, and breastfeeding duration and/or exclusivity has been inversely and consistently associated (infant formula feeding positively associated) with rate of weight gain, adiposity, and risk of overweight and obesity in children. | Promote and support exclusive breastfeeding from birth, and continued breastfeeding with complementary food introduction. |
| Bottle feeding | Limited but consistent evidence suggests that bottle feeding per se, whether infant formula or breastmilk may increase the risk of overweight or obesity in infancy or childhood (potentially mediated by frequency, response to hunger cues, schedule and related behaviors). | Use responsive feeding behaviors (see below) when bottle feeding. |
| *Foods and diet quality and quantity* | | |
| Time of introduction of complementary foods and beverages | Introduction to complementary foods < 4 months of age, particularly in formula fed infants, has been positively although inconsistently associated with rapid of weight gain, adiposity, and overweight or obesity in children. | Introduce developmentally appropriate solids after 4 months and not later than 6 months of age. |
| Energy and nutrient density; macronutrient intake | High total energy intake has been positively associated with higher risk or prevalence of overweight in children. | Introduce solids conforming to a nutrient dense diet, encouraging fruits, and vegetables which decreased energy density.[b] |
| Protein intake | High protein intake, from infant formulas as well as complementary foods has been positively associated with increased risk of higher weight gain, overweight, and obesity in childhood. | Encourage breastfeeding, use of lower protein formulas (below 2 g/dL). No consensus for specific total protein intake recommendations at this time. |
| Intake of sweetened beverages | Higher intakes of added sugars, sugar-sweetened beverages, and possibly juices have been positively but inconsistently associated with measures of adiposity, overweight, or obesity in children. | Limit intake of added sugars[c] and juice and avoid sugar-sweetened beverages under 2 years of age. |

**Feeding practices and other behaviors**

| Feeding practices and other behaviors | | |
|---|---|---|
| Attention to "hunger and satiety cues." | Parental inattention to a child's "hunger or satiety cues" has been positively associated with overfeeding or overweight in infants. | Use responsive feeding behaviors for bottle feeding and feeding of complementary foods. |
| Responsive feeding parenting behaviors | Parental use of "controlling," "rewarding," "indulgent," or "restrictive" feeding practices has been associated with the child's food intake, weight gain during infancy, and overweight or obesity in preschool age children. Depending on the parental feeding practice and child's age, the direction of the association has not been consistently reported. | |
| Sleep duration | Shorter sleep duration has been inversely and consistently associated with increased adiposity, overweight, and obesity in children. | Encourage adequate sleep duration[d] |
| Screen viewing time | Hours of TV or screen time viewing has been positively associated with overweight or obesity in toddler and preschool age children. | Limit screen viewing time[e] and discourage eating or snacking with screen time. |
| Physical activity. Active play/sedentary time | Time spent during physical activity or active play has been inversely associated with measures of adiposity or risk of overweight among infant, toddler, and preschool age children. | Discourage sedentary times, encourage active platy and tummy time. |
| Shared family meals/maternal diet/ eating out of home | Limited but consistent data support an inverse association between frequency of shared family meals and diet quality or BMI and overweight in children. However, data in infants are scarce. | Encourage shared family meal occasions. |
| Antibiotic exposure in early life | Limited but consistent data support a positive association between antibiotic exposure in infants and increased risk of subsequent overweight and obesity. | Utilize appropriate antibiotics only when medically indicated. |

[a] See text for supporting literature.
[b] USDA Dietary Guidelines for Infants (USDA, 2020).
[c] WHO recommends < 10% total energy intake from added sugars.
[d] The American Academy of Sleep Medicine recommends 12–16 h of daily sleep for infants 4–12 months old, 11–14 h for toddlers till 1–2 years, and 10–13 h for children 3–5 years of age (Paruthi et al., 2016).
[e] AAP Council on Communications & Media recommends: For children < 18 months discourage screen viewing other than video-chatting, for 18–24 months, limit to below an hour a day, for older than 2–6 years limit to 1 h or less/day, of high-quality programming (AAP, 2016).

the United Kingdom, began developing comprehensive guidance on infant and young child feeding. In the United States, the Dietary Guidelines for Americans (DGA) f.or the first time included guidelines for infants below 2 years in the year 2020.

It is also important to mention that historically most guidelines focused on "what to feed" (diet-related) and either ignored or minimized the importance of guidelines on "how to feed" infants and young children (feeding-related behaviors). Increasingly, these guidelines include components of parental and caregiver feeding and infant activity-related behaviors, and the DGA committee has recommended that "how to feed" be specifically addressed in the 2025 update to dietary guidelines for infants from birth-24 months of age within the United States (National Academies of Sciences, Engineering, and Medicine (NAS), 2020; Pérez-Escamilla et al., 2017).

### 18.4.1.1 Breastfeeding and formula feeding

Breastfeeding is the ideal sole source of nutrition for all human infants in their first few months of life. It is beyond the focus of this paper to outline the numerous benefits of breast-feeding in optimizing infant health. The impact of exclusive breastfeeding on child growth, development, and health is well documented. Moreover, exclusive breastfeeding is critical in decreasing early morbidity and mortality in low- and middle-income countries, particularly when inappropriate breastmilk substitutes are commonly used. That said, almost universally and exclusively, studies assessing the risk of obesity in infants who "breastfed or partially breastfed" have compared it to infants receiving some or all their feedings with infant formulas in the first months of life. We will discuss the "protective effects" of breastfeeding as typically addressed in the literature: versus infant formulas (sometimes concurrent with inappropriate feeding alternatives and practices). However, it must be noted that it is actually the *increase* in risk associated with formula feeding which is being addressed.Infant formulas have dramatically changed in the last 50 years, and continue changing. Thus, breastfeeding is the standard, and RR should be calculated for the alternatives, not the other way around. However, most research assessing risk-related benefits of breastfeeding estimate a RR starting with a RR of "1.0" for formula feeding and calculate a particular potential "risk reduction" with breastfeeding. E.g., a RR of 0.5 of a disease means a 50% risk reduction when breastfeeding (compared to formula feeding). However, if breastfeeding is considered as having a RR of 1.0 (the standard), in that same study, with the same data, a risk related to formula feeding would be 2.0 (double the risk). This contraposition goes beyond semantics since a level of relative risk of an intervention (e.g. formula feeding) is more clinically relevant when compared to the standard breastfeeding.

The global prevalence of exclusive breastfeeding increased from 36% in 2000 to 43% in 2015, and the prevalence of early initiation of breastfeeding was 45% (UNICEF, 2016). The latest FAO estimates, based on UNICEF data of exclusive breastfeeding until 6 months reveal 41.6% of infants under 6 months being exclusively breastfed in 2018. These rates are higher in the least developed countries, and higher also in rural areas than in urban babies. And these rates are uniformly lower in high income countries (FAO et al., 2019). Unfortunately, while initiation of breastfeeding has risen globally, with few exceptions, breastfeeding duration is still shorter than desirable, in both low and high-income countries. More importantly, only 37% of children younger than 6 months of age are exclusively breastfed in low- and middle-income countries (Victora et al., 2016). In these settings, the lack of exclusive breastfeeding, inappropriate breast milk substitutes, and early and inappropriate introduction of complementary feedings in unsanitary conditions all contribute to significant morbidity and mortality. Most of the burden and the related costs to society are born by low- and middle-income countries (Walters et al., 2019). The multiple nutritional and other clinical benefits of breastfeeding are discussed in various reviews (Victora et al., 2016; AAP, 2012). Here, we will discuss the relationship between breastfeeding and breastfeeding alternatives with overweight and obesity as it relates to otherwise healthy infants.

The growth trajectory in the first months of life in breastfed infants is different, with typically lower weight gain and less percent body fat, than their infant formula-fed counterparts (Dewey, 1998). Breastfed infants tend to be leaner and gain weight more slowly throughout infancy than formula-fed infants, particularly after 3 months of age. Since rapid and/or excessive weight gain during the first year of life is a major predictor of obesity risk (Ong and Loos, 2006), breastfeeding constitutes a first major postnatal modifiable factor in reducing obesity risk.

The great majority of studies on the topic show varying degrees of an inverse association between breastfeeding and obesity risk at various ages. Several meta-analyses show that breastfeeding is associated with a consistent decrease in risk reduction for later obesity, with rates of reduction estimated between 13% and 22% (Arenz et al., 2004; Weng et al., 2012; Horta et al., 2015). In addition, several other meta-analyses show that the duration of breastfeeding is inversely associated with the risk of overweight and obesity in later life, with a significant dose-response effect (Harder et al., 2005; Yan et al., 2014; Qiao et al., 2020). Each month of breastfeeding has been estimated to decrease obesity risk by approximately 4.0% (Harder et al., 2005; Qiao et al., 2020).

Recent studies reinforce earlier meta-analyses, showing a breastfeeding benefit. In a study in 11 high-income countries, breastfeeding for at least 3 months is associated with a significantly lower likelihood of rapid weight gain and an elevated BMI until school age, as well as of high BMI, skinfold thickness, and fat mass up to the age of 20 years (Rzehak et al., 2017). A 6-year follow-up study in the United States showed that infants who experienced rapid increases in bottle-feeding frequency (and decreased breastfeeding) during the first 6 months, versus low bottle-feeding frequency, had a significantly greater change in weight/age, and this predicted greater risk for obesity at age 6 years (Ventura et al., 2020). Several cohort studies confirm a risk reduction benefit, particularly with exclusive breastfeeding for 4 months, and a somewhat lesser effect with more prolonged breastfeeding (Pluymen et al., 2018; Kim et al., 2021; Aris et al., 2018; Pattison et al., 2019).

Other large studies also support a dose-related effect. In a lower-income US population, obesity risk at 4 years of age was lowest for infants exclusively breastfed for 7 months (27% reduction) and 13 months (37% reduction) (Anderson et al., 2020). Another cohort study in the United States found the occurrence of overweight or obesity was 38%, 27%, 20% for infants who were never breastfed, breastfed 0–6 months, and breastfed > 6 months, respectively (Pattison et al., 2019). In a large Danish cohort study, each additional month of breastfeeding was associated with less weight gain in the first year, a lower BMI score, and lower odds of being overweight by 1 year of age (Gubbels et al., 2011). In another large 12 country cross-sectional study, exclusive breastfeeding was associated with lower odds of obesity (24% reduction) and lower body fat (40% reduction) compared with exclusive formula feeding. The reduction in obesity risk was 26%, 30%, and 40% for children breastfed 1–6, 6–12, and > 12 months, respectively, with similar trends for body fat (Ma et al., 2020). And a study including populations from 22 participating countries, the WHO European COSI study, the odds of being obese were higher among children never breastfed (22% higher) or breastfed for a shorter period (12% higher) in 6- to 9-year-olds (Rito et al., 2019).

Prospective or randomized studies are not possible to assess the effect of breastfeeding, and because breastfeeding per se is significantly associated with other factors that can also affect growth, adiposity, and obesity. Therefore, care must be taken when assessing breastfeeding and breastfeeding duration as potential independent or causal factors, or relative contributors, to obesity. For example, complementary food introduction < 4 months seems to increase and/or mediate the risk of overweight and obesity seen with breastfeeding (Aris et al., 2018; Pluymen et al., 2018) and is often not controlled for. In a large cohort study in Canada that used multiple approaches to address confounding bias, breastfeeding was inversely associated with weight gain velocity, BMI, and overweight risk in the first year of life. These associations were dose-dependent (stronger with more prolonged and more exclusive breastfeeding) and independent of maternal BMI and socioeconomic status. After controlling for multiple confounders, breastfeeding cessation before 6 months was associated with a two-fold increased risk of rapid weight gain and a threefold increased risk of overweight, compared with exclusive breastfeeding past 6 months. The findings were also consistent with evidence that exclusively bottle-fed infants gained more weight than infants fed at the breast, regardless of the milk type (breast milk or formula) in the bottle. The authors conclude their findings suggest that shorter breastfeeding duration, feeding bottled breast milk, and formula supplementation all independently influence infant weight gain, BMI, and overweight risk (Azad et al., 2018). Not all findings show risk reduction of overweight or obesity with breastfeeding. In a large prospective cohort study with very high breastfeeding rates, breastfeeding was not found to be associated with a lower risk of later obesity, either at 6 or at 16 years of age (Martin et al., 2017).

Quite often, multiple confounders are not always taken into consideration in individual studies. Moreover, not all confounders are well known or easily measurable, and some are emerging, like birth by cesarean and gut microbiota, which are rarely addressed. Indeed, in many studies, adjustments to major confounding factors, including maternal obesity and smoking, and socioeconomic status, were shown to markedly reduce the inverse association between breastfeeding and lower BMI (Owen et al., 2005). And a recent systematic review and meta-analysis showed that consuming human milk is associated with a lower risk of overweight and obesity at ages 2 years and older, particularly if the duration of human milk consumption is > 6 months. However, the authors also concluded that residual confounding could not be ruled out, mainly because the great majority of included studies identified did not control for all of the key confounders. The authors noted that only a few studies account for complementary feeding practices and childhood diet, both of which are correlated with breastfeeding. Based on these limitations, the authors concluded that there was insufficient evidence to determine the relationship between the duration of any human milk consumption and overweight and/or obesity at age 2 years and older (Dewey et al., 2021). This is consistent with another recent systematic review of systematic reviews, which concluded there was a consistent association of breastfeeding with a reduction in the risk of later overweight and obesity in childhood and adulthood (the odds decreased by 13% based on high-quality studies), and suggested that although breastfeeding of very short duration may be less protective than breastfeeding of longer duration, confounding cannot be excluded (Patro-Gołąb et al., 2016).

In summary, the risk reduction benefit relative to overweight and obesity associated with breastfeeding (versus use of infant formula) is significant, and directionally very consistent. A "dose effect" relationship and quantification of the independent contribution to this risk reduction is still limited by multiple confounders. Additional work, for example, using sibling paired studies and triangulating evidence across study designs that do not share the same biases, may help unravel these relationships (Smithers et al., 2015). And further work on the mechanisms by which breastfeeding may reduce risk, discussed below, may shed light on future approaches in this line of research.

### Feeding with a bottle

Independent of breastfeeding vs feeding formula, bottle feeding per se and its related practices (e.g., "on-demand vs scheduled feeding," "bottle to bed," "bottle emptying," etc.), independent of what milk is used (breast vs formula), appears to contribute to differences between breastfed infants versus those that are not. Breastfeeding is a direct physiologic maternal-child interaction that goes beyond providing nutrition. Bottle feeding, whether human milk or infant formula, requires other conscious behaviors and actions that can influence the ultimate delivery of nutrients and has increasingly been identified as a potential independent risk factor for greater weight gain and adiposity (Appleton et al., 2018). Infant self-regulation of intake has been proposed as a plausible explanation for differences in energy intake between breastfed and formula-fed infants (Dewey and Lonnerdal, 1986). Compared with the natural maternal-child bidirectional feedback mechanisms of breastfeeding, bottle feeding by parents, and caregivers can easily override infants' satiety signals if they are not familiar with, educated in, or attentive to their infant's hunger and satiety cues. An infant's milk intake during feeding is strongly associated with the interaction between the infant and parent/caregiver and is likely to affect their ability to self-regulate milk intake (Kotowski et al., 2020).

Thus, increased intake and rapid weight gain in infants, which are risk factors for later overweight and obesity, can be influenced by the type of milk or formula provided and the mode of feeding and associated behaviors. Using a large bottle, for example, has been found to contribute to greater weight gain by 6 months of age. After adjusting for some confounders, infants fed with a 6 oz bottle had more weight gain between 2 and 6 months than infants fed with a smaller one (Wood et al., 2016). In mothers who breastfed, and also bottle-fed their own milk, a greater percent of bottle-feeding predicted greater intake during feeding with the bottle compared with breastfeeding (Ventura et al., 2021). Infants who feed only by bottle have been found to gain more weight per month when fed non-human milk only or human milk only, compared to infants fed at the breast. Weight gain has been negatively associated with the proportion of breast milk feedings, but positively associated with the proportion of bottle feedings among those who receive mostly breast milk in a bottle (Li et al., 2012). In one cross-sectional study, infants who often emptied bottles in early infancy seem more likely than those who rarely emptied bottles to have excess weight during late infancy, although maternal encouragement to empty the bottle did not seem to be a mediator (Li et al., 2008). Furthermore, in a cohort study, infants who received part of their breast milk in a bottle were found to have higher BMI and weight gain velocities than infants fed exclusively at the breast, but lower than infants receiving formula (Azad et al., 2018). In a cohort study in the United States, prolonged feeding with a bottle, up to 24 months, compared to shorter use, was found to also be significantly associated with increased risk of obesity at 5 years of age. And bedtime use of the bottle further increased the risk (Gooze et al., 2011).

Bottle feeding "on schedule" versus "on demand" has been assessed in terms of infant weight gain, with equivocal findings. Some identify a positive association with feeding on schedule and rapid weight gain in the first year of life (Mihrshahi et al., 2011) others not (Saxon et al., 2002; Gubbels et al., 2011). However, the different methodologies, schedules, and other confounders make it difficult to draw conclusions. In a review of the topic, the practice of putting an infant to bed with a bottle (which would be contraindicated for safety and other reasons) and its relationship to weight gain has been reviewed, showing equivocal findings (Appleton et al., 2018). Parents or caregivers may be motivated for their infant or young child to empty the bottle in the mistaken belief that rapid weight gain is desirable, to soothe or encourage the infant to sleep longer, or to avoid wasting formula (Kavanagh et al., 2008). Bottle emptying encouraged by mothers in early infancy increased the likelihood of mothers pressuring their 6-year-old child to eat and children's low satiety responsiveness (Li et al., 2014). Another study also identified a pressuring feeding style to be positively associated with increased infant intake (Ventura et al., 2021). The adequate reading on infant hunger and satiety cues appears critical in determining intake in bottle-fed babies; however, the extent to which mothers perceive and rely upon infant hunger and fullness cues to initiate and terminate feeding vary widely (Hodges et al., 2008). These responsive feeding behaviors as associated with infant growth are discussed below.

Thus, bottle-feeding per se and related practices appear to be an independent and modifiable risk factor for rapid infant weight gain and later obesity, and this may be independent of the milk in the bottle. It is important to note that causality or level of contribution is difficult to ascertain due to the multiple confounders associated with mode of feeding, like those discussed for exclusive breastfeeding and duration of breastfeeding. Surprisingly little research has been done in this area of feeding practices.

### 18.4.1.2 Potential mechanisms for the effect of breast vs formula feeding on obesity risk

Mechanisms that may mediate the association between formula feeding (vs breastfeeding) and risk of overweight and obesity include: The nutritional composition of the feeding (particularly protein content), bottle-feeding per se (discussed above), microbiota-related mechanisms (dysbiosis in formula-fed infants), hormonal effects of breastmilk (adipokines), breastmilk-related epigenetic programming, and potential effects of breastfeeding (vs formula) on later feeding or eating behaviors (flavor preference, "picky eating").

#### Energy and protein

Historically, infant formulas have been uniformly higher in energy density and protein content than human milk. In addition, the levels of energy and protein in breastmilk vary over time, not in infant formula. Protein levels of human milk gradually decrease over the first months of life, while exclusively infant formula-fed infants receive a consistently high level of protein throughout the first year. The relatively excessive levels of protein in infant formulas, compared to those present in breast milk, have been proposed as an obesogenic factor for a long time (Heinig et al., 1993; Koletzko et al., 2009a). The protein levels used in infant formulas have been high, in part, to compensate for the lower nutritional quality of bovine protein sources compared to human protein. As technology allows improving the nutritional quality of bovine proteins used in infant formulas, it is increasingly possible to lower the excess protein content of breast milk substitutes while ensuring adequate growth. For many decades, infant formulas have had more than 2 g protein/100 kcal, often close to 2.9 g/100 kcal. For "follow on" formulas intended for infants 6–12 months of age and older, protein levels have been as high as 4.4 g/100 kcal, while mature human milk has a protein content closer to 1.5 g/100 kcal, around 1 g/dL.

Several large prospective studies comparing infant formulas with lower protein content versus conventional formula point to a benefit in reducing adiposity and overweight and obesity. A randomized trial comparing infant formulas containing 1.77 vs 2.2 g protein/100 kcal for the first 6 months, and 2.9 and 4.4 g protein/100 kcal after 6 months of age showed a significantly higher weight gain in the first 2 years of life with higher protein levels, and no effect on length. In addition, higher protein content of infant formula has been associated in some studies with higher branched-chain amino acids, IGF-I, and urinary C-peptide: creatinine ratio after 6 months, all of which can contribute to insulinogenic effects and adiposity (Koletzko et al., 2009b; Socha et al., 2011). Another large study assessed infant formulas with cow milk protein of 2.05 compared with 1.25 g/dL in initiation formula and 3.2 compared with 1.6 g/dL in the follow-up formula. Consumption of higher protein formulas in the first year was found to be associated with fat mass deposition from 2 years onward and doubled the risk for excess body fat at 6 years, compared with lower protein formula (Weber et al., 2014; Totzauer et al., 2018).

Several smaller studies using infant formulas with 1.8 g of protein per 100 kcal, compared to 2.7 g protein per 100 kcal, have shown similar results and document adequate growth, comparable to the WHO growth standards and close to breastfed infants with the lower protein concentration (Putet et al., 2016; Alexander et al., 2016). Another small trial in older infants randomized healthy 1-year-old children to standard cows' milk or to a reduced protein milk formula (3.1 and 1.7 g/dL) until the second year of life, as part of their regular diet, and showed that a lower protein intake led to a small reduction (2%) of body fat at the age of 2 years (Wall et al., 2019).

In summary, convincing evidence has accumulated that excess protein intake in the first years of life is detrimental to body composition and increases the risk of adiposity and obesity. Maintaining protein in infant formula at levels lower than 2 g/dL, probably at around 1.25 g/dL or 1.8 g/100 kcal, appears to be protective, warranted that each product is shown to support adequate linear growth.

### Microbiota-associated effects of breastfeeding

Breastfeeding and breastmilk are key drivers and modulators of the development and the profile of the gut microbial ecosystem in the first months of life. This is, in turn, is a major programming determinant of health, including metabolic and immune functions, which, when disrupted, can lead to increased risk of inflammatory and metabolic disease, including allergic conditions, functional GI disorders, and overweight and obesity. Postnatally, formula feeding and infant antibiotic exposure are significant disruptors of gut microbiota development of dysbiosis. Moreover, dysbiosis has been associated with multiple health-related conditions, including pediatric allergy and asthma, functional GI disorders, as well as overweight and obesity (Davis et al., 2017; Stinson, 2020; Rinninella et al., 2019), the latter which we discuss below.

*Early feeding as determinant of the infant microbiota*    Breastmilk provides multiple factors that shape microbial colonization in infants. These include the breastmilk's own microbes (breast milk has a rich microbiota itself), as well as growth substrates for specific microbial species (Pannaraj et al., 2017; Davis et al., 2017). Gut microbiota develops quickly after birth and stabilizes in the first 2–3 months in breastfed infants, and changes again with the introduction of complementary food, stabilizing again at around 3 years of age (Laursen et al., 2017).

The fecal microbiota of breastfed infants is generally more stable over time, characterized by a lower diversity, and has a predominance of the genus *Bifidobacterium*, compared with that of formula-fed infants (Davis et al., 2017). And the effect of breastfeeding on microbial composition appears to follow a dose-dependent mode, even after the introduction of solid foods (Gomez-Gallego et al., 2016; Fehr et al., 2020). Low colonization with bifidobacteria is one of the most common markers of dysbiosis. Human milk contains growth factors that foster the growth of bifidobacteria; one of the most frequently studied is human milk oligo-saccharides (HMOs). HMOs are a family of structurally diverse carbohydrates synthesized in the mammary gland by sequential addition of monosaccharides to lactose, and various gly-cosidic linkages to *n*-acetyl glucosamine, fucose, and sialic acid. After lactose and fat, HMOs are the third largest component by weight in human milk. These sugars are not digested by human enzymes and have no nutritional value to the infant, but they are selectively used as substrate by bifidobacteria in the GI lumen of infants, i.e., they have a "prebiotic" effect. Until recently, infant formulas did not contain HMOs. The presence and quantity of several HMOs, through their effects on the infant microbiota as well as through some direct mucosal and systemic mechanisms, is responsible for several protective and immune-related benefits of human milk (Donovan and Comstock, 2016; Moossavi et al., 2018; Bode, 2020), and poten-tially for metabolic or obesity-related effect.

*Linking the microbiota to the risk of overweight and obesity*    Multiple mechanisms by which the microbiota can exert changes in the host that lead to metabolic disease, obesity, diabetes, and related inflammatory changes have been proposed. Animal studies, for example, indicate that the microbiome of obese animals has an increased capacity to harvest energy from the diet. Furthermore, this trait is transmissible; colonization of germ-free mice with an "obese microbiota" results in a significantly greater increase in total body fat than colonization with a "lean microbiota." Potential mechanisms to explain this effect include increased harvest of energy by the microbiota, neurohormonal mediators of appetite and satiety either from mi-crobial metabolites or modulating orexigenic (appetite-related) gut hormones, and inflamma-tory mediators affecting adipose tissue and insulin secretion (Davis, 2016; Fan and Pedersen, 2021; Mohammadkhah et al., 2018).

Many observational human studies have found associations between varying microbi-ota profiles in adolescents, children, and infants with overweight and obesity (Abenavoli et al., 2019; Kalliomäki et al., 2008; Balamurugan et al., 2010; Abdallah Ismail et al., 2011; Payne et al., 2011; Vael et al., 2011). The microbiome of the first-pass meconium, for exam-ple, predicted subsequent overweight at the age of 3 years (Korpela et al., 2020). Microbial composition and diversity in the first months of life have been associated with child-hood weight gain and BMI after 2 years of age (Scheepers et al., 2015; Stanislawski et al., 2018; Alderete et al., 2021), and early (vs later) introduction to solid foods, modified by breastfeeding duration, has been associated with altered gut microbiota composition and BMI in early childhood (Differding et al., 2020). A recent North American cohort study showed a significant interplay between breastfeeding, infant formula, and microbiota profiles, noting a stronger association with microbiota profiles at 3 months vs 12 months of age on later risk of overweight (Forbes et al., 2018). Additional evidence for the relationship between infant microbiota alterations and obesity comes from studies linking antibiotic use in infants, discussed below.

### Breast milk adipokines

A growing number of non-nutritive functional components with hormonal and metabolic functions are being described in human milk, which have the potential to influence orexigenic or anorexigenic-appetite-related-pathways, energy balance, and adiposity. These include leptin, adiponectin, ghrelin, resistin, obestatin, insulin-like growth factor-1, and nesfatin-1. Of these, the better studied so far are the adipokines or adipocytokines (cell signaling proteins) leptin and adiponectin, and the hormone ghrelin.

Leptin and adiponectin are primarily secreted by adipose tissue, but are also found in many other tissues and organs. The concentration of leptin in maternal serum and breastmilk is proportional to an individual's adiposity. Adiponectin concentration in serum, on the other hand, is inversely related to adiposity, but the amount of adiponectin in breastmilk is positively associated with maternal adiposity. Both leptin and adiponectin can be absorbed in the infant gut, and infant serum adiponectin has been found to correlate with concentrations in human milk. Leptin concentrations in breastmilk have been negatively correlated with infant BMI, overall weight gain, and risk of overweight over the first 2 years of life, suggesting that human milk leptin can contribute to the regulation of weight gain among breastfed infants. And breastmilk adiponectin concentrations have been negatively correlated with infant weight-for-age and weight-for-length, and risk of overweight in the first 2 years of life (Savino et al., 2009; Kratzsch et al., 2018; Young, 2017), although the effect in preschool-age or beyond may not be sustained (Meyer et al., 2017).

Ghrelin is an orexigenic appetite-regulating hormone secreted mainly in the GI tract, also found in breastmilk. Ghrelin receptors are present in the intestinal mucosa, and small initial studies have shown a negative association with weight gain only among breastfed infants, suggesting that ghrelin may contribute to infant appetite regulation and growth (Badillo-Suárez et al., 2017; Kratzsch et al., 2018). Finally, breastmilk could also influence the expression of infant genes associated with appetite by inducing epigenetic changes in infants. A recent study suggests that breastfeeding can influence infant DNA methylation levels of genes, such as those associated with lipid metabolism, including the Retinoid X Receptor Alpha (RXRA) and leptin genes (LEP). Thus, longer breastfeeding could influence childhood obesity development mediated by an upregulation of RXRA and a downregulation of LEP up to a year of age (Pauwels et al., 2019).

In summary, based on limited data so far, breastmilk adipokines and hormones appear to play a role in energy intake, weight gain, and adiposity, and via hormonal and/or epigenetic mechanisms, can directly or indirectly contribute to the development of overweight and obesity. The exact contribution of these factors still needs to be further elucidated (Badillo-Suárez et al., 2017; Kratzsch et al., 2018).

### Breastfeeding effects on later food-related behaviors

Some observational studies suggest that exclusive breastfeeding may influence food preferences in later childhood. Lower odds of picky eating behaviors, and higher daily intake of vegetables have been reported in exclusively breastfed infants until age 4–5 months compared to exclusively breastfed for 0–1 month (Specht et al., 2018). A recent meta-analysis found limited evidence suggesting that a longer duration of exclusive breastfeeding is associated with a lower risk of parent-reported feeding difficulties in children, although the differences were small (Bąbik et al., 2021). While a potential effect of breastfeeding on the risk of obesity via these food preference and behavior shaping or programming mechanisms is plausible, the number and complexity of confounders and the methodological challenges with these studies currently preclude firm conclusions.

### 18.4.1.3 Time of introduction of complementary foods

"Early" introduction of complementary feeding using a 4-month age cut-off has been a subject of debate as to its contribution to this risk. The timing of introduction to complementary foods and beverages in the first year of life has long been studied as a factor in determining growth, adiposity, and risk for overweight or obesity. Developmentally, to initiate solid foods safely, infants should have sufficient truncal strength and stability to allow sitting in an upright position with little or no support. This typically occurs between 4 and 7 months of age. By this time also, sucking, rooting, and oral motor and exclusion primitive reflexes will normally have diminished, and oral motor skills to handle non-liquid foods should emerge. Thus, developmentally, children under 4 months should be breastfed or bottle-fed only breastmilk or infant formula.

Several systematic reviews have found that introduction (at or before 4 months), rather than at 4–6 months or more than 6 months of age, may increase the risk of childhood overweight (Pearce et al., 2013; Wang et al., 2016; English et al., 2019a). While the evidence is limited and confounded by many other factors, there appears to be sufficient consistency among the observational studies reporting higher odds of overweight/obesity or weight when comparing feeding below 4 months to later introduction of complementary foods and beverages (English et al., 2019b). This increased risk is likely mediated by increased energy intake (Ong et al., 2006).

Some of the limitations in drawing conclusions relate to multiple confounders, some of which are addressed in studies and meta-analyses, many of which are not. Data from a large prospective survey in the United States showed the odds of obesity were higher among infants introduced to solid foods before 4 months compared to those introduced at 4–6 months (OR 1.66) in unadjusted analysis; however, this relationship was no longer significant after adjustment for covariates (Barrera et al., 2016). In particular, the interplay of solid food introduction and the duration of breastfeeding seem to be important in determining obesity risk. In another US cohort study, obesity at 2 years was highest among children introduced to solid foods before 4 months, compared with solid food introduction at 4–5 months or after 6 months, regardless of whether they were breastfed or not, and the obesity percentages were highest at 2 years for never-breastfed children than those who received formula (Moss and Yeaton, 2014). In an Australian cohort study, the odds of overweight or obesity were double among infants introduced to formula or solids at ≤ 4 months compared to those introduced at > 4 months. For those fed solid foods before 4 months, the risk doubled if they started formula around that age versus those who continued breastfeeding (Mannan, 2018). Similarly, in a large European cross-sectional study, early solid food introduction (< 4 months of age) was associated with a lower prevalence of overweight/obesity, but primarily among children that also ceased exclusive breastfeeding (and started infant formula) earlier than 4 months (Papoutsou et al., 2018). Formula feeding and the very early introduction of solids appear to be independent risk factors, which may also act synergistically. Of note, these differences in obesity risk are better documented in children 2–4 years of age but appear to become less significant for older children (Moss and Yeaton, 2014; Barrera et al., 2016).

Introduction of complementary foods between 4 and 6 months of age has not been consistently associated with increased risk of overweight or obesity in later infancy, or during early childhood, when compared to the introduction of infant feeding at 6 months of age (Grote et al., 2012; Pearce et al., 2013). A recent meta-analysis concluded that moderate evidence suggests that the introduction of complementary foods and beverages between 4 and 5 months compared with ~ 6 months is not associated with weight status, body composition, body circumferences, weight, or length (English et al., 2019a). The effect of delaying solid food introduction beyond 6 or 7 months and its influence on overweight or obesity risk has been less well studied. Interestingly, in a large European study, late solid food introduction (≥ 7 months of age) was also associated with an increased prevalence of later childhood overweight/obesity among exclusively breastfed children (Papoutsou et al., 2018). Overall, there appears to be too little evidence regarding the effects of solid food introduction after 7 months of age (English et al., 2019b). Additional studies are needed to adequately address the multiple confounders and manage a greater number of covariates, to assess better the relative contribution of each of the many factors contributing to growth and adiposity in early and later childhood.

Independent of these studies, solid food introduction is not recommended before 4 months of age, as infants have not yet developed the necessary gross motor skills (head, neck, and truncal control) to sit with or without support, nor the appropriate oral motor skills (tongue, mastication, and swallowing) to safely manage solid food introduction. What drives parents to the early introduction of complementary solid foods in infancy? In many countries, social and culturally established practices play a significant role. And varying social and economic realities can significantly impact the differences in feeding practices between high- and low-income populations.

In studies in the United States, the introduction of solid foods before age 4 months has been more often reported in infants who are not initially breastfed, those who are not breastfed until 6 months of age, and those born of less educated, single, young mothers (Clayton et al., 2013; Fein et al., 2008; Grummer-Strawn et al., 2008). In these studies, among the most common reasons cited by 70%–90% of mothers for early introduction of solid food are "my baby was old enough to begin to eat solid food." "My baby seemed hungry a lot of the time." "It would help my baby sleep longer at night." Regrettably, 55% of mothers reported that "a doctor or health care professional said my baby should begin eating solid food." Similar reasons ("the baby was hungry," "was *old enough*" or was "*ready for solids*") are given in other studies identifying predictors of solid food introduction (Scott et al., 2009).

Addressing these feeding barriers and misconceptions could have a meaningful impact on prolonging the duration of exclusive breastfeeding, and potential prevention of excess energy intake and rate of weight gain among young infants, given associated issues with diet quality discussed below. In low-income countries and populations, the challenges are different from those of higher income, or those of emerging economies that deal with the double burden of obesity and malnutrition. In these situations, the inappropriate introduction of solid foods and beverages in early infancy has contributed to undernutrition. The resulting inadequate diet, often of poor nutrient quality, is magnified by poor sanitation, which can perpetuate a cycle of poor growth, poor immunity, chronic inflammation, and ultimately chronic malnutrition and stunting. In these scenarios, nutrition education interventions are needed; and they should be combined with the provision of complementary foods that are affordable, particularly in food-insecure countries, coupled with initiatives that tackle the underlying conditions of poverty and poor sanitation that contribute to child malnutrition (Dewey and Adu-Afarwuah, 2008; Lassi et al., 2013).

In summary, the introduction of complementary solid foods below 4 months of age is not ideal from the developmental point of view. Notwithstanding the numerous confounders, there is consistent evidence indicating that such early introduction increases the risk of overweight and obesity in childhood. This effect is compounded in infants who do not breastfeed or are breastfed for shorter periods and fed with infant formulas. Solid food introduction between 4 and 6 months of age or after 6 months do not appear to be associated with increased obesity risk.

### 18.4.1.4 Energy and macronutrient composition of complementary foods

Obesity occurs when energy intake is in excess requirements. One goal of prevention is feeding of energy to an infant within the range of requirements and using a diet and feeding practices to develop adequate eating behaviors later. However, reliable data on the quantity and/or excess of energy intake (with or without adequacy of other macro- and micronutrients) in the first 2 years of life is exceedingly scarce. Furthermore, although excessive energy intake has been associated clinically with higher BMI during childhood, very limited data are available which specifically assess energy intake from complementary feeding on subsequent overweight status in children (Grote et al., 2012; Pearce et al., 2013). The great majority of observational studies, many of which find associations between obesity and breastfeeding, formula feeding, or timing of introduction of solids, neither quantify nor control for energy intake, which is in many cases, if not all, is likely the mediator of the effect.

#### Energy

Adequate global or regional dietary surveys estimating energy intake in infants and toddlers are extremely scarce, particularly for low- or middle-income countries. In high-income countries, elevated energy intakes are common, but not always well documented. The 2016 Feeding Infants and Toddlers Study (FITS) is the most comprehensive dietary survey done in the United States (Bailey et al., 2018). This nationally representative survey showed that infants from birth to 24 months had greater energy intakes than average estimated requirements. The mean reported intake of energy for infants 0–6 and 6–12 months of age, sexes combined, was about 25% higher than the estimated energy requirements for the children in the 50th percentile for these two age ranges (Stan et al., 2021) and about 30% higher than requirements for 12–24-month-olds.

Reliable data on energy intakes across populations remains sparce. As would be expected, there is great geographic and socioeconomically driven variation. A study in young children 1–3 years of age from 19 countries, showed energy intakes varied greatly between populations. In Bangladesh, China, India, and the Philippines, mean energy intake was below 800 kcal/day, which is lower than the FAO/WHO lowest energy intake recommendation of 950 for boys and 850 for girls aged 1–3 years (Suthutvoravut et al., 2015). Undoubtedly, within-country disparities account for the wide range of intakes and consequent occurrence of both undernutrition and obesity in many low- and middle-income countries.

## Protein

In the same global review of published energy and nutrient intakes of children aged 12–36 months, where energy intake fell short in many, protein intake exceeded WHO reference values in 16 of 17 studies analyzed (Suthutvoravut et al., 2015). Other studies confirm that excess protein intake by 1 year of age and after, when infants receive most of their energy from solid foods and other beverages (outside breast milk or infant formula), is associated with higher BMI and obesity. In fact, there is better data on the protein content of diets of infants and young children as related to growth and weight gain in the first 2 years of age than there is for energy intakes and ranges. As discussed above, the protein content of infant formulas vs breastmilk leads to excess protein intake in infants in the first year of life and has been consistently associated with increased weight gain and obesity in later childhood (Koletzko et al., 2009a; Socha et al., 2011; Weber et al., 2014; Totzauer et al., 2018).

In most developed populations, the macronutrient composition of solid foods becomes important after 4–6 months of age. A longitudinal European study showed that high-protein intake at 12 months (14.8% of energy) and between 18 and 24 months (13.8% of energy), but not at 6 months of age, was independently related to an increased mean BMI and body fat percentage at 7 years of age (Gunther et al., 2007). Data from a large Danish cohort showed that a 10 g higher intake of protein/day, especially animal protein at 1 year of age, was associated with a greater height, weight, BMI, and higher body fat mass, but not fat-free mass at age 6, and a small difference in BMI which persisted up to 9 years of age. The association with increased fat mass was stronger in girls than in boys, for animal than for vegetable protein intake, but did not differ between dairy and non-dairy animal protein (Voortman et al., 2016; Braun et al., 2016).

A large prospective twin cohort showed a higher protein intake (~ 16% of total energy) at 21 months was associated with higher weight gain and higher BMI (but not height) between 21 and 36 months, and 21 and 60 months, compared with lower intakes, with no evidence of diminution over time. The investigators estimated that 16% of energy from protein was equivalent to ~ 4-g/kg/day protein intake between 18 and 24 months, and that a 1% greater energy from protein at 21 months was associated with a greater BMI and a greater weight on average at any time point, all the way to 60 months. There was a trend toward an association of higher protein intake at 21 months and the odds of overweight or obesity at 36 months, but the difference was lost at 5 years of age (Pimpin et al., 2016). One systematic review found some association between high protein intakes at 2–12 months of age and higher body mass index (BMI) or body fatness in childhood, but noted results were not always consistent (Pearce et al., 2013). And two extensive and detailed reviews on the topic conclude that higher protein intake in infancy and early childhood, especially when it exceeds 15% of energy consumption, and particularly in the first 2 years of life, is associated with increased growth and higher BMI in childhood, but the exact level of protein intake above which there is an increased risk for being overweight later in life is yet to be established (Hornell et al., 2013; Rolland-Cachera et al., 2016).

Based on the above, high protein intakes are common globally and, in most populations. In high-income countries, they are several-fold higher than requirements for infants and young children. Higher protein intakes in the first 2 years of life consistently correlate with higher BMI in later childhood. While maintaining protein intake below 15% of energy seems reasonable at this time, further work needs to be done to establish protein amounts at which obesity risk may increase.

### Fat

Although data is scarce for infants, most studies have not identified fat intake during infancy or complementary feeding as an independent risk factor for overweight and obesity in later childhood. In fact, some studies have recognized that young children's diets in settings with significant rates of obesity, like the United States, contain less than dietary recommendations for total fat intake (Butte et al., 2010; Siega-Riz et al., 2010). A prospective French cohort study examined fat intake at 10 months of age and adiposity at 20 years. It found that a lower fat intake in early life was negatively associated with body fat (particularly at the trunk site) and serum leptin concentration at 20 years, suggesting that early low-fat intake could increase the susceptibility to develop overweight and leptin resistance at later ages (Rolland-Cachera et al., 2013).

However, a larger recently reported UK cohort study which assessed diet at 8 and 18 months and body composition at 9 and 17 years found a positive association between fat intake (% energy) at 18 months and fat mass at 9 years, primarily in boys, and not in girls (Jones et al., 2021). An Italian study examining diets at 1 year of age and anthropometry at 5 years found that children in the upper centiles of the 5-year BMI had a significantly higher protein intake at the 1 year of age. However, no associations were found with fat intakes at 1 year (Agostoni et al., 2000). Finally, a 2016 systematic review of systematic reviews reported finding no conclusive evidence of a relationship between fat intake up to 3 years of age and childhood overweight and obesity (Patro-Gołąb et al., 2016).

A recent meta-analysis concluded that moderate evidence suggests that consuming complementary foods with different fats and fatty acid compositions does not significantly affect growth or body composition (English et al., 2019a). There is still too little and equivocal evidence in infants regarding fat intakes and intakes of PUFA, MUFA, or saturated fat on long-term risk of overweight or obesity.

### Sugar

Over the last decades, much attention has been placed on sugar, particularly sugars added to infant diets as a risk factor for obesity. The term "free sugars" as defined by WHO includes all mono- and disaccharides added to foods and beverages in their processing and preparation, plus sugars naturally present in honey, syrups, fruit juice, and fruit juice concentrates, but not in fruit or milk (WHO, 2015). The European Food Safety Authority (EFSA) defines "sugars," and the US Department of Agriculture (USDA) defines "total sugars," as all sugars—including those added during processing and preparation plus those naturally present in foods (fruits, vegetables) and lactose in milk. And both EFSA and the USDA define "added sugars" as those added to foods during processing and preparation, excluding sugar naturally occurring in juices or milk (EFSA, 2010; USDA, 2019). The variable terminology used between agencies has resulted in difficulties for research (Newens and Walton, 2016), and has consequently complicated adequate and comparable estimates of consumption, research reporting, regulation, labeling, and communication to parents, consumers, and the public.

The literature has grown relative to sugar consumption and its effects in older children, adolescents, and adults. However, few studies to date have investigated the association between consumption of sugar or sugar-sweetened beverages (SSBs) in the first 2 years of life and overweight or obesity in later life. A US study found obesity prevalence at 6 years among children who consumed SSBs below a year of age to be 17% vs 8.6% in non-SSB consumers (Pan et al., 2014). In another study, high juice intake ($\geq$ 16 oz per day) at 1 year was associated with increased juice intake, SSB intake, and BMI in mid-childhood (Sonneville, 2015). Some studies in preschool children also suggest an association with later childhood weight gain and obesity (Dubois et al., 2007; Linardakis et al., 2008; Fiorito et al., 2009). And SSB consumption has also been found to correlate with other modifiable obesogenic factors: TV viewing/screen time and snack consumption, formula milk feeding, early introduction of solids, parental use of food as rewards (Mazarello Paes et al., 2015). A recent US cohort study found that higher fruit juice intake in infancy at 1 year was associated with greater abdominal adiposity in mid-childhood and early adolescence (Wu et al., 2021).

However, several other more recent studies have not replicated these findings in infants. A German cohort study showed that higher added sugar intake at 1 year was related to a lower BMI at age 7 years, and an increase in total added sugar during the second year of life tended to be associated with a higher BMI, although no associations were found with body fat percentage. In this study, higher intakes after a year of age had a greater negative effect (Herbst et al., 2011). In a study in which participants were introduced to SSBs before 24 months of age (the majority exposed before 12 months), SSB consumption before 12 months was not associated with increased odds of obesity, and there was no association between SSB introduction with risk of obesity at age 8–14 years. However, when considering only the highest tertile of cumulative consumption of SSB, there was a threefold increase in obesity by 8–14 years of age (Cantoral et al., 2016). In another small cohort study, the introduction of SSB under 18 months of age (excluding juice) was not associated with BMI at 8 years (Garden et al., 2011) or 11.5 years (Garden et al., 2012). Similarly, in a longitudinal ethnic cohort in the United Kingdom, researchers found no significant association between the introduction of SSBs, before 17 weeks and BMI at 3 years of age (Santorelli et al., 2014).

Two recent systematic reviews and meta-analyses have addressed the association between intake of SSB and overweight and obesity. A meta-analysis of meta-analyses concluded there was no consistent evidence of an association of the age of introducing complementary foods or SSB consumption with later overweight/obesity (Patro-Gołąb et al., 2016). A more recent systematic review concluded that there is "limited evidence" suggesting that SSB consumption during the complementary feeding period is associated with increased obesity risk in childhood, but is not associated with other measures of growth, size, or body composition. In addition, it noted limited evidence showing a positive association between juice intake and infant weight-for-length and child BMI (English et al., 2019a).

Independent of sugar and total energy consumption with SSB, the inclusion of added sugar, including juice very early, could theoretically play a role in shaping long-term food preferences, and in this way contribute to later sugar and energy intake excesses and obesity. Two key factors may play a role in the development of these unhealthy eating patterns. One is the innate (less modifiable) evolutionarily driven human taste preference for sweet and rejection for bitter tastes. Early environments likely drove this with limited nutrient availability and led to preference for energy and carbohydrate-rich and sodium-rich foods and rejection for bitter, potentially toxic plants and vegetables. The other factor, which can be modified, relates to lack of exposure (early feeding) of a variety of flavors and textures of safe, healthier, less energy-dense foods, including vegetables in early life (Mennella and Ventura, 2011; Trabulsi and Mennella, 2012; Forestell and Mennella, 2015; Mennella and Bobowski, 2015).

Overall, there appears to be evidence for a directionally negative effect of early introduction and higher amounts of SSB (including juice) in infancy and later risk of overweight or obesity. However, the evidence so far is limited and not strong nor consistent, especially regarding later risk of obesity. Eliminating confounders and longer follow up in future studies may help affirm a causal relationship. In summary, SSB, including juices, especially in large amounts, can provide significant amounts of energy, decrease nutrient density, and potentially promote preference for high sugar intake later; thus, limiting intake seems appropriate.

Currently, the WHO recommends, for children at any age, that the intake of free sugars should be < 10% of the total energy intake; however, these recommendations are based on the relationship of sugar with dental caries only and not related to growth or metabolism. The European Society for Pediatric Gastroenterology, Hepatology and Nutrition recommends that intake of free sugars be < 5% of total energy intake for children 2–18 years, and even lower for infants and toddlers (Fidler-Mis et al., 2017). The recently published US Dietary Guidelines recommend that added sugars be less than 10% of energy intake per day starting at age 2, and avoidance altogether of foods and beverages with added sugars for those younger than age 2 (USDA, 2020).

### Foods and food group introduction

For most infants, although with geographic and cultural variation, the period between 3 and 4 months and 6–7 months of age is exceptionally dynamic in both the amount and the variety of solid foods typically introduced to an infant in this brief period of the life cycle. In North America, at the beginning of this period, 20% of infants have already been exposed to complementary foods; within four additional weeks, this figure rises to 40%, and by 6 months, more than 90% of infants are receiving some solid food (Fein et al., 2008; Grummer-Strawn et al., 2008; Saavedra et al., 2013). In North America, grains tend to be the first food introduced, with the gradual addition of vegetables, fruits and juices, meats, dairy products, sweets, sweetened beverages, and desserts. Detailed nutritional surveys that are broadly representative are lacking, and there are likely wide geographic and cultural variations. However, poor patterns in terms of food group consumptions are becoming similar as urbanization and dietary "western patterns" take hold.

In the United States, 25%–30% of children aged 6 months and older do not eat a fruit serving on a given day (Roess et al., 2018). The same data show that on average, by 24 months and through 4 years, less than 10% of the energy comes from fruits and vegetables. A consequence of this low intake is that fiber intake remains very low in infants and toddlers, which directly correlates with an increased energy density (by volume) of the diets consumed during this age range. In general, the higher the fiber intake, particularly when fruits and vegetables are consumed as fresh, pureed, or whole produce, rather than extracts, juices, or beverages, the energy density of the diet significantly goes down, curtailing excess energy intake.

Following a period of rapid changes with the introduction of various food groups starting at 4–6 months, the relative energy contribution of each food group (grains, dairy, meats, fruits, vegetables, sweets) becomes constant by 20–24 months of age. It is this period of development of food acceptance, taste and texture preferences, and satiety patterns, where we may have the greatest opportunity to set the right course toward later patterns. Despite changes in absolute energy consumption and a growing variety and number of food group options with age, the relative energy contribution of each food group to total calories remains the same. For example, 10% energy from fruits and vegetables at 20 months remains constant till 4 years; and this, in turn, is similar to the adult average contribution to the adult diet in the United States. It appears that the ultimate eating patterns of adults, in fact, become established far earlier than commonly thought (Saavedra et al., 2013).

Coupled with the low intake of fruits and vegetables, which increases the energy density of the diet, by their first birthday, in many countries, children are fed some type of sweet or sweetened beverages regularly. In the United States, this is 70%–90% of infants, and on a given day, a toddler is more likely to be fed a sweet or sweetened beverage than a serving of fruit or vegetables. More than a third of the calorie increase from ages 6 months to 4 years is attributable to sweets and sweetened beverages, including candy, ice cream, sweet rolls, pie, cake, and cookies. And for children 1-4 years old age sugar intake is high, and more than one third of children do not reach a minimum acceptable amount of energy from fat (Fox et al., 2010; Bailey et al., 2018). Infrequent intake of fruits and vegetables during late infancy is associated with infrequent intake of these foods at 6 years of age. These findings highlight the importance of infant feeding guidance that encourages intake of fruits and vegetables and the need to examine barriers to fruit and vegetable intake during infancy (Grimm et al., 2014). Longer breastfeeding duration was consistently related to higher fruit and vegetable intake in young children, whereas the associations with age of introduction to fruit and vegetable intake were weaker and less consistent across the cohorts (de Lauzon-Guillain et al., 2013).

While the introduction of different food groups in the first 2 years, in part, determines ultimate energy and nutrient consumption, associations with these and the risk of overweight and obesity are difficult to find. Two systematic reviews have found inadequate evidence or no association between specific food group intakes and overweight or obesity (Pearce et al., 2013; Patro-Gołąb et al., 2016). A more recent systematic review stated that based on available data, no conclusions could be made about the relationship between specific complementary foods (vegetables, fruit, dairy products and/or cow milk, cereal-based products, milk-cereal drink, and/or categories such as "ready-made foods") and growth, size, body composition, and/or prevalence/incidence of overweight or obesity (English et al., 2019b). Ultimately, better data on frequency, amounts, and portion sizes, plus relative and total energy contribution, will be necessary to draw conclusions on food group specificity (if any) in terms of contribution to obesity or metabolic risk.

## 18.4.2 Infant and caregiver behaviors associated with obesity

As discussed previously, most work and effort has been so far in better defining and providing guidance to parents on "what to feed" their infant (diet-related guidance). It is clear "how to feed" infants and young children (feeding-related behaviors) are as important and critical to the development of healthy diet habits. This has been increasingly recognized, but such organized guidance or guidelines with any broad consensus are yet to be defined and developed. The Dietary Guidelines Advisory Committee of the Departments of Agriculture and Health and Human Services, which recently put forth the first ever set of dietary guidelines for infants from birth-24 months in the United States, recommended that "how to feed" the be addressed in 2025, in the next update to these guidelines (Perez Escamilla, 2017). The modifiable behaviors related to feeding which have been associated with overweight and obesity are summarized in Table 18.3 and discussed below.

### 18.4.2.1 Sleep

While causality has been hard to demonstrate, cross-sectional studies show a consistent increased risk of obesity among children and adults who sleep shorter times. Multiple observational studies have documented an inverse relationship between sleep duration and measures of adiposity, overweight, or obesity in infants, toddlers, and preschool-age children (Anderson and Whitaker, 2010; Monasta et al., 2011; Tian et al., 2010). In the last few years, several longitudinal and cohort studies have all found varying levels of inverse association between sleep time and BMI or adiposity for various pediatric ages (Collings et al., 2017; Baird et al., 2016; Diethelm et al., 2011; Reilly et al., 2005). In a US cohort, preschool-aged children with early weekday bedtimes were one-half as likely as children with late bedtimes to be obese as adolescents (Anderson et al., 2016).

In a large cohort of infants and toddlers in the United States, sleeping less than 12 h per day in infancy was related to a higher BMI and increased risk of obesity at 3–5 years of age (Taveras et al., 2008). And by 7–9 years, the highest prevalence of obesity was seen among those who had insufficient sleep across infancy and early childhood (Taveras et al., 2014). However, a large Danish study assessing sleep duration at 9, 18, and 36 months did not find a relationship to adiposity at 3 years of age (Klingenberg et al., 2012). A more recent study in another Danish cohort assessing sleep duration at ages 2, 6, 24, and 36 months, reported that shorter sleep duration at 2 months, but not at later ages, predicted higher BMI and fat mass at 6 years of age (Derks et al., 2017).

Several systematic reviews focused on children, some including infants, have been published in the last few years. A systematic review of 29 studies conducted in 16 countries suggests that short sleep is associated with an increased risk for being or becoming overweight or obese or having increased body fat. Late bedtimes were also found to be a risk factor for overweight/obesity in older children and adolescents (Hart et al., 2011). A systematic narrative review concluded that overall, shorter sleep duration was associated with higher adiposity and weight for length (in 20/31 studies) in children aged 0 to 4 years. And longer sleep duration was generally associated with better body composition (Chaput et al., 2017). Another systematic review and meta-analysis of longitudinal studies and incidence of obesity concluded that "short sleep duration" is a risk factor or marker of the development of obesity in infants, children, and adolescents. In this study, overall, short sleep increased the risk of overweight or obesity for all ages (RR: 1.58), and in pooled analysis, there was a change in BMI per hour of decrease in sleep (RR: − 0.03). For infants up to 3 years of age, with follow up times varying from 1 to 5 years, short sleep was associated with a RR 1.40; for overweight and obesity, with a high significance (Miller et al., 2018a). The same research group found similar results in a meta-analysis focusing only on preschool children (Miller et al., 2021). Finally, a meta-analysis of only prospective cohorts concluded that short sleep duration was associated with significant changes in BMI. Moreover, long sleep duration was identified as a protective factor for childhood obesity. In dose-response analyses, short sleep duration was significantly associated with obesity in toddlers (1–2 years) (RR = 1.20) and preschool children (3–5 years) (Deng et al., 2021). On the other hand, 1 systematic review, selecting 19 studies addressing sleep duration concluded that the evidence regarding sleep duration in the first 2 years of life and healthier body composition during childhood was inconsistent, primarily due to methodological quality and variability between studies (Harskamp-van Ginkel et al., 2020).

The mechanisms underlying the potential relationship between sleep and overweight are likely varied, multifactorial, and interrelated. Potential mediators include interaction with feeding practices and amounts, associations with screen time and sedentary activities, and hormonal changes affected by sleep. A recent systematic review addressed the evidence on the association of sleep duration and obesity and the underlying potential mediating mechanisms for all pediatric ages, including mostly school-age children and adolescents. It concluded there was stronger evidence so far for a link between short sleep duration and the development of insulin resistance, sedentarism, and unhealthy dietary patterns. But the role of other mediators like physical activity, screen time, and change in ghrelin and leptin levels remained unclear (Felso et al., 2017).

In adults, poor sleep has been associated with increases in ghrelin and insulin and a reduction in leptin (Al-Disi et al., 2010; Motivala et al., 2009; Lin et al., 2020); such relationships have yet to be studied in infants. In addition, in the first months of life, sleep patterns and feeding practices are closely intertwined. Feeding, especially bottle feeding and early introduction of complementary food (Wasser et al., 2011) is often be used as a "sleep aid" by parents seeking to soothe or calm a crying or fussy infant (Kavanagh et al., 2008; Scott et al., 2009), thus inadvertently leading to excess energy intake, and potentially programming a shift in satiety patterns. Sleep time could also interact with screen time, briefly discussed below. Data making these links in infants remains scarce. Recent interventions that promote alternative approaches to feeding for soothing a fussy infant or increasing nocturnal sleep duration have reported encouraging results (Taveras et al., 2010a; Paul et al., 2010) but need further corroboration.

The American Academy of Sleep Medicine recommends 12–16 h of daily sleep for infants 4–12 months old, 11–14 h for toddlers till 1–2 years, and 10–13 h for children 3–5 years of age, all including naps (Paruthi et al., 2016). Obviously, adequate sleep in infancy and childhood is important for developmental, psychosocial, and health reasons beyond growth and body composition. Based on the available data, these recommended sleep time ranges are consistent with sleep times that may decrease the risk of overweight or obesity in later childhood.

### 18.4.2.2 Screen time and activity

There is strong observational evidence that increased screen time has been associated with overweight, obesity, or adiposity, particularly in preschool children within multiple cohorts, various geographic and ethnic groups, mostly associated with "TV viewing" until a decade ago (Dennison et al., 2002; Janz et al., 2002; Jiang et al., 2006; LaRowe et al., 2010; Ariza, 2004; Mendoza et al., 2007; Anderson and Whitaker, 2010; Kimbro et al., 2011; Lumeng et al., 2006). The impact was particularly higher for 2–5-year-olds and underprivileged groups, and minorities. However, some studies did not show an association (Heppe et al., 2012), and very little data were available for infants under 2 years.

For older children, television viewing (or sedentary, passive screen time) may increase the risk of obesity-related not only to the sedentary aspect of the activity but also to the quality and quantity of foods consumed while watching television, which has been associated with higher intakes of calories, SSBs, fast food, and less fruit and vegetable consumption (Miller et al., 2008), especially when television watching happens during meals (Horodynski et al., 2010; Matheson et al., 2004; Feldman et al., 2007).

However, technology and the increased access to tablets and mobile devices can no longer be compared to older traditional TV viewing patterns of children. Until a decade ago, most "screen time" included or was defined as time and activity spent watching television or videotapes, video games, and home computer. Today, "screen time" is often defined as activities associated with watching television, videotapes, digital video discs, game devices, computers, cell phones, smartphones, tablets, electronic readers, and children's learning devices (Chen and Adler, 2019). In 1997, the average daily screen time in the United States was estimated at 1.32 h for children aged 0 to 2 years and 2.47 h/day for children aged 3 to 5 years. In 2014, screen time had doubled to 3.05 h/day for children 0 to 2 years and remained steady at 2.56 h/day for 3–5-year-olds. Television time still accounted for most of total screen time in children under 5 years of age (Chen et al., 2019). Screen time also correlates with poorer sleep outcomes and longer sedentary times, particularly in infants and toddlers (up to 2 years of age), but less significantly in preschoolers, as reported in a meta-analysis focusing on children under 5 years of age (Janssen et al., 2020).

A few reviews have been published on the subject of screen times and other sedentary behaviors in infants and toddlers. A systematic narrative review concluded that screen time use in children under 3-years-old was positively and consistently associated with BMI (Duch et al., 2013). A more recent systematic review and meta-analysis in children 1–7 years of age found screen time was associated with overweight and obesity and shorter sleep duration among toddlers. Overall, in 22 studies, excessive screen time was related to an increased risk of overweight/obesity and/or BMI or various measures of adiposity. Metanalysis of 9 showed that excessive screen time (> 1 h/day) was associated with twice the risk of obesity (effects size 1.99) and that screen time and sleep interacted significantly. Children with excessive screen time also had more than twice the risk of shorter sleep duration (effect size 2.2) (Li et al., 2020). A systematic narrative review focused on 0–4 years of age found a positive association between screen time and higher adiposity (20/31 studies) and an inverse association with longer screen times (5/5 studies) in 0–4 year olds (Chaput et al., 2017).

It is worth noting that not all sedentary times should be considered equal. A systematic review examining the relationships between sedentary behavior and health indicators in children 0–4 years of age concluded that associations between screen-based sedentary behaviors as well as time spent seated (e.g., in baby seats, car seats, highchairs, or strollers) or in the supine position and health indicators (adiposity, motor or cognitive development, and psychosocial health) were largely unfavorable or not significant. However, associations between reading or storytelling (also sedentary behaviors) and cognitive development were favorable or not significant. It also noted that when objectively measured total sedentary times were assessed (e.g., with the use of accelerometers worn by infants), the associations with health indicators (adiposity and motor development) were predominantly not significant (Poitras et al., 2017).

Data to support specific approaches to activity, play, "tummy time," or similar approaches in infants and their relation to risk of overweight are lacking. In addition, changing technologies will continue requiring further adaptation of our definitions for sedentary and non-sedentary screen time. Unraveling primary drivers and mutually confounding interactions between these factors will remain challenging. Nevertheless, overall, the literature supports the importance of minimizing screen and promoting healthy sleep time in infants for disease prevention and health promotion, including healthy growth in the early years. Decreasing sedentary non-interactive behaviors and fostering activity are also reasonable approaches to health beyond their effects on growth and obesity risk. In addition, not all sedentary time is the same. Interactive non-screen-based activities such as reading and storytelling have potential cognitive benefits.

The American Academy of Pediatrics Council on Communications and Media issued a Policy statement with screen time recommendations in 2016. For children younger than 18 months, it discouraged use of screen media other than video-chatting. For parents of children 18 to 24 months of age, the recommendations were to limit it to below an hour a day and to choose high-quality programming. And in children older than 2 years, to limit media to 1 h or less per day of high-quality programming. It recommended no screen viewing during meals and for 1 h before bedtime. No specific limit was included for children 6 and older, as long as screen time does not interfere with sleep, physical activity, and other healthy habits (AAP, 2016). WHO recently published guidelines on sedentary behaviors and screen time for children under 5 years of age (WHO, 2019). It recommended, for less than 1-year-olds, interactive floor-based play at least 30 min in prone position (tummy time), and not to be restrained more than 1 h at a time, and to get 14 to 17 h (0–3 months of age) or 12 to 16 h (4–11 months of age) of good quality sleep, including naps. For 1–2-year-olds, it recommended spending at least 180 min in various types of physical activities and having 11 to 14 h of good quality sleep, with no screen time recommended for 0–2 years.

### 18.4.2.3 Family meals/out of home meals

The potential link between family meals and family meal settings with infants and toddlers' participation in obesity has not been well studied so far. Some indicators are apparent. A large cross-sectional study of more than 8000 4-year-old children reported that those who engaged in family meals at five or more evenings per week were at a 16% decreased risk of obesity, compared to those consuming fewer family meals together (Anderson and Whitaker, 2010). But the data for these relationships in younger infants and toddlers are scant. The US FITS study from 2008 revealed that 33% of infants between 12 and 24 months, and 41% between 2 and 4 years ate at a fast-food restaurant 1–2 times per week. Family mealtime in the right setting may positively contribute to healthier choices and variety for preschool-age and older children. However, data and documentation on educational approaches are still lacking to improve diet quality and choices both in and outside the home. Data from school-age children and adolescents suggest that the frequency of family meals has an inverse association and snacking frequency and a positive association with childhood overweight or obesity (Lee et al., 2016; Murakami and Livingstone, 2016). A recent meta-analysis showed a positive association between family meal frequency and consumption of fruits, vegetables, lower SSBs, and better measures of diet quality in 2–18-year-olds. There was less clear evidence of this relation in snacks, fast food, and consumption of desserts (Robson et al., 2020). Another meta-analysis showed positive associations between family meal frequency, overall diet quality, and lower BMI. Child's age, country, number of family members present at meals, and meal type (i.e., breakfast, lunch, or dinner) did not change the relationship of meal frequency with healthy diet, unhealthy diet, or BMI (Dallacker et al., 2018). Data for infants and toddlers in this regard remain very scarce.

### 18.4.2.4 Responsive feeding

Infant self-regulation of feedings that aligns energy needs with energy intake is critical to minimize the risk for rapid weight gain and risk for overweight or obesity in childhood or later life. Human infants are entirely dependent on their mother and other caregivers with regard to what food and liquids they are offered. How they are fed, including the appropriate reading and response to their hunger and satiety cues has the potential to undermine their ability to self-regulate, if there is a mismatch between the infant's needs and the caregiver's feeding behaviors. The development of an adequate infant-caregiver feeding interaction is mediated by various factors, including the child's neuro-cognitive physiology and development (including vagal responses), environment, and social interactions, as well as the caregiver's behaviors related to feeding the infant. Therefore, the development of "discordant" feeding responsiveness by caregivers can lead to a mismatch between a caregiver's feeding behaviors and the infant's needs, such as overfeeding (Hodges et al., 2020; Wood et al., 2020). For example, lessened sensitivity to the infants' cues with a tendency to overfeed is predictive of weight gain at 6–12 months, particularly in bottle-fed infants, and parental inattention to an infant's hunger and satiety cues has been associated with weight gain at 4–5 months (Worobey et al., 2009; Kavanagh et al., 2008). However, moderate evidence supports that maternal education specific to hunger and satiety cue responsiveness may be protective of healthy weight gain or weight status among infants and young children (Spill et al., 2019).

The feeding choices, patterns, and routines set by the infants' immediate caregivers are an inextricable component of parenting. Responsive parenting entails prompt, appropriate responses to a child's behaviors, needs, and cues or signals, beyond the appropriate food choices (DiSantis et al., 2011; Black and Aboud, 2011; Sleddens et al., 2011; Grote and Theurich, 2014; Dattilo, 2017, 2022). Recent systematic reviews suggest that providing "responsive feeding guidance" to mothers and caregivers, particularly in the first 2 years, may support appropriate growth (Spill et al., 2019). The relevance, the importance, and the consequences of appropriate responsive feeding behaviors and how they fit within the overall context of parenting practices are major, and cannot be overstated. It is expected that future science-based guidance and guidelines for feeding in early life emphasize responsive feeding behaviors and other aspects of "how to feed" as much as "what to feed a child."

Appropriate responsive feeding behaviors, therefore, constitute a significant modifiable factor in approaches to the prevention of overweight and obesity in childhood and beyond.

### 18.4.2.5 Exposure to antibiotics in infancy

As discussed above, dysbiosis, or disruption of the development of a healthy microbiota in infants, has been associated with the risk of overweight or obesity in infants born by cesarean section or fed infant formulas. Similarly, early exposure to antibiotics can lead to dysbiosis and similar increases in risk. Two recent meta-analyses concluded that antibiotic exposure in infants aged < 24 months (Miller et al., 2018), and especially in the first 6 months of age

(Rasmussen et al., 2018), was associated with an increased risk of subsequent overweight and obesity. While increasing, the literature linking body weight and BMI outcomes of microbiota changes in early life is still limited. Specific species, varying profiles, and varying levels of microbial diversity are clearly different between obese and non-obese children, and some of these findings may precede obesity development (suggesting a causal connection). Effect sizes appear to vary significantly between studies and with age (Iozzo and Sanguinetti, 2018), and no single species or bacterial group or method to express bacterial profiles or diversity has consistently been well documented to date. Future work will be needed to demonstrate causality.

## 18.5 Summary: Modifiable factors for obesity prevention in early life

Tables 18.2 and 18.3 summarize the modifiable factors associated with obesity that have surfaced as relevant and potentially causally related to early weight gain and subsequent risk of overweight and obesity. These are consistent with other general and systematic reviews which identify them as potential targets for risk reduction of obesity in early life (Larqué et al., 2019; Dattilo, 2017; Woo Baidal et al., 2016; Koletzko et al., 2020). We note here that some researchers consider "early (infant) rapid weight gain" as a "risk factor" for later obesity. We consider this more of a "marker" of the trajectory toward obesity, resulting from the other potentially causal factors mentioned. Prevention and management of obesity in children beyond infancy requires addressing different modifiable factors which are not the focus of this discussion.

The relative strength of support and the relative contribution of each of these factors to obesity risk are very variable, and the relative contribution of each factor remains to be further well documented. No single factor has or would be expected to "cause" infant or childhood obesity. It is relevant and obvious that the interdependency and interaction of all these modifiable factors increase the difficulty in statistically demonstrating which factors have, and to which degree they have, a greater relative influence. As discussed above, for example, the timing of "complementary" food introduction is inextricably linked to what these foods are "complementing," whether exclusive breastfeeding, breast milk in a bottle, varying amounts of infant formula, and the many combinations thereof. Thus, the relative contribution of what and how much a child ingests, and the "how" they are fed, which is in turn influenced by which foods are provided, are interactions difficult to untangle. Lastly, these modifiable factors have a cumulative effect (Hu et al., 2020), which increases the complexity of identifying specific RR contributions. Sorting out each factor's relative and quantitative causal contributions will take longer, larger, and more detailed prospective work.

Interestingly, the subsequent influences that can mediate eating behaviors after infancy can modify the associations between early risks and subsequent outcomes found in observational cohort studies, thus explaining some inconsistencies in various studies. A recent cohort study examined whether cumulated risk factors in the first 1000 days (maternal pre-pregnancy and paternal overweight, excessive GWG, raised fasting plasma glucose during pregnancy, short breastfeeding duration, and early introduction of solid foods) were associated with adiposity at 6 years of age. A higher composite risk score was predictive of BMI and adiposity and was associated with larger self-served food portions, faster eating rates, and larger lunch intakes. However, the cumulative risk factors were not predictive of adiposity in those children who selected smaller food portions, ate slower, and consumed less energy (Fogel et al., 2020).

There are several reasons for which past as well as future research is hindered or may be limited. First, the contribution of one or other modifiable factors can be modified by genetic and epigenetic influences, which vary from individual to individual and possibly between populations. These are hard to account for. Second, some emerging risk factors are not accounted for in most studies so far, e.g., birth by cesarean section or prior use of antibiotics. Third, most of these factors are likely interdependent, as mentioned above. Hence, the number of confounders that need to be accounted for in any analysis is large and keeps growing, demanding even larger studies. Fourth, many of these factors are continuous variables. For example, breastfeeding and formula feeding and timing of solid food introduction are often characterized or considered as dichotomous variables, rather than a spectrum requiring segmentation for analysis. Fifth, some of these factors, cannot be studied in prospective intervention studies (e.g., breastfeeding and cesarean section) due to ethical and practical issues, requiring larger and longer cohort or observational studies to strengthen associations. Finally, non-immediately modifiable social and environmental factors can mitigate or exacerbate the relative contribution of one or another factor, which can limit generalization.

Nevertheless, despite the limitations, the factors summarized above still appear to "break through" the noise and help lay down a roadmap. Addressing these factors holistically appears to be the best approach for preventive action.

## 18.6 Intervention

### 18.6.1 Developing approaches for obesity prevention in early life

Tackling the global epidemic of obesity requires addressing the causal factors of the condition, and given prevention is always more desirable, addressing those related to early life is critical. In the narrative above, we have reviewed factors so far identified which appear to play such a role in the first 1000 days of life, and which are modifiable in an infant's immediate environment. These include factors modulating the in-utero circumstances (which are potentially modifiable by an infant's mother), and the food, diet, and nutrition factors determined by what and how an infant is fed by their parents and caregivers. Addressing these factors can be significantly affected by other broader environmental influences beyond the maternal, family, and home environment.

Beyond the immediate modifiable factors discussed, these environmental influences can contribute to an "obesogenic environment" that promotes high energy intake and sedentary behaviors (WHO, 2016b). These broader contributors remain critical to fighting the obesity epidemic but are not the topic of this paper. They include the larger community, society, and factors which challenge or facilitate addressing the epidemic, such as agriculture and food systems, health and education systems, and all the activity sectors which can play a role—communities, academia, the private sector, media, non-government organizations, and government actions and policies. Thus, addressing the epidemic will require multisectoral will and participation.

Nevertheless, from the nutritional point of view, it is the energy provided to the infant as part of a healthy diet that determines the risk for subsequent overweight and obesity. And this, in turn, is determined by a child's mother, family, and immediate home environment. Table 18.3 summarizes those modifiable factors (what and how an infant is fed) which have such potential causal relationships to the underlying energy mismatch. Given the highly dependent nature of human infants for their care and feeding, practically all factors are also highly dependent on parental and primarily maternal behaviors toward the infant. When addressing these modifiable and potentially causal factors (whether directly food and diet-related or feeding behavior-related), parental understanding and development of capabilities to feed the infant become critical. Thus, educational (not simply informational) strategies, directed to and executed by parents and caregivers, are necessary and fundamental to shape an infant's diet and related behaviors (Dattilo and Saavedra, 2020).

An overarching objective to help parents and families nourish their infants could be expressed as follows: *To develop science-based parental and caregiver recommendations, as well as nutrition education interventions, that help build parental capabilities towards a healthy infant diet accompanied with healthy related experiences, which leads to ultimate long-term adoption of food choices and related dietary behaviors and habits conducive to the long-term health and wellness of the individual.* This needs to be accompanied by the communal and societal support and systems that facilitate the execution and implementation of these parental and caregiver capabilities.

As mentioned above, these modifiable factors are interrelated and can be cumulative in terms of increasing obesity risk (Hu et al., 2020; Aris et al., 2018). Therefore, most or all factors need to be addressed concurrently. This has led to the critical concept of "multicomponent" approaches (Dattilo et al., 2012) to simultaneously address these multiple risk factors (Dattilo, 2017; Dattilo and Saavedra, 2020; Fornari et al., 2021). The development of strategies addressing those factors that can be modified entails identification of objectives (e.g., addressing multiple modifiable factors), educational efforts to build capabilities (e.g., multicomponent content and programs for nutrition education for behavior adoption), including the appropriate vehicles for implementation (e.g., in-person, digital, health and nutrition professionals, community approaches), and the right metrics and efficacy measures.

The educational approaches for this purpose should be designed based on applicable theory of health behavior and address various mediators (motivators and barriers) relevant to acting on these modifiable behaviors. This includes identifying the specific behavioral targets, addressing behavior mediating variables (underlying determinants that precede behavior adoption such as attitudes, beliefs, social norms which need to be addressed or overcome), and applying specific models for behavior adoption or change, such as the health belief model, theory of planned behavior, or the more often used social-cognitive theory. Incorporating these models allows for understanding individuals' actions and helps explain why some target behaviors are adopted, and others are not. A combination of health behavior models and theories for nutrition behavior change or adoption has been proposed to address the modifiable factors associated with healthy growth during the first 1000 days (Uesugi et al., 2016; Dattilo and Saavedra, 2020).

To be effective, the approaches above will require (a) addressing concurrently most of the modifiable potentially causative factors, (b) doing so in the first 1000 days, (c) through educational approaches broad enough to reach all segments of society, and (d) with the support of all sectors of society (including community, school, government, non-government organizations, the private sector, and academia).

## 18.6.2 Intervention studies

Over the last few years, there has been an increasing number of interventional studies toward obesity prevention and treatment. Some have addressed pre- and peri-natal factors, and the vast majority address postnatal ones. Even so, many addressed postnatal factors after the first 2 years of age, in preschool and school-age children, rather than the first 2 years of life. Furthermore, most studies have targeted a limited number of modifiable factors, often only one or two, mostly in older children, very few starting in pregnancy, the minority in infants, and mostly in high-income countries (Ash et al., 2017).

A few reviews address these studies. A 2016 systematic review assessed the effectiveness of interventions in the 0–2-year age group. Most interventions focused on individual and family level modifiable factors, providing guidance to parents on breastfeeding, complementary feeding, healthy diet, sleep, and physical activity. Most interventions addressed one or two modifiable factors, and the delivery of interventions varied widely, from home visits to individual counseling, group sessions in clinical settings, community settings, and a combination of these. The authors concluded that there are still very few effective interventions in the first 1000 days, and many target individual-level behaviors of parents and infants (Blake-Lamb et al., 2016). A recent systematic review of multicomponent randomized trials identified only six trials, whose interventions incorporated education to promote breastfeeding (four trials), responsive feeding (two trials), and healthy diet, increasing fruit and vegetables and limiting unhealthy snacks (five trials), delivered through home visits or at baby health clinics. Most reported relative reductions in BMI at the end of intervention, but two trials with follow-up to 1–3 years showed benefits were not maintained (Koplin et al., 2019).

Another review focused on physical activity as intervention, and identified only eight studies, all of which had multicomponent approaches and included adiposity, weight, or BMI as outcomes. They assessed study characteristics versus efficacy and concluded that effective interventions tended to target multiple levels of the socio-ecological model they used to assess studies (this model focuses on the interrelationships between individuals and the social, physical, and policy environment) (Reilly et al., 2019). Another narrative review analyzed interventions for childhood obesity prevention. It concluded that promoting breastfeeding, reducing protein content of formulated milks, and addressing the diet of the first 12–24 months are promising strategies or targets for reducing the risk of obesity. For older children, involving family and schools in interventions that promote physical activity and a healthy diet may be beneficial (Fornari et al., 2021).

In a recent review, we assessed intervention studies targeting growth, BMI, or adiposity in the first 2 years of postnatal life. Of 15 unique cohort studies and 5 follow-up studies, the great majority addressed several modifiable factors for obesity risk, and most included both dietary as well as behavioral aspects in the intervention. Most also use some type of behavioral change technique, and several interventions reported utilizing more than one nutrition education theory or theoretical construct. The majority of original cohort studies reported significant intervention effects on one or more modifiable dietary or feeding-related behavior outcomes, with half of the studies reporting significant differences related to growth and anthropometrics. Sustained effects on adiposity or overweight require to be better documented. Only one trial reported no significant outcomes for any of the multi-component intervention target behaviors or anthropometric changes (Dattilo and Saavedra, 2020). One additional major underlying weakness of the overall efforts to date is the fact that most have been done in high-income countries, and the literature regarding risk factors as well as potential interventions in low-income populations remains extremely scarce.

In summary, while still scarce, the number of intervention trials for obesity prevention is growing. Directionally, most work today suggests that targeting multiple modifiable risk factors described above, guided by a theory of health behavior, can significantly affect one or more dietary or feeding-related parental or caregiver behaviors associated with the healthy growth of infants. Multiple challenges remain to be addressed in future studies. These include better identification of target behaviors and the number of behaviors targeted, the means of delivery (healthcare personnel, community settings, digital approaches), defining the necessary "intensity" and duration of interventions, identifying ideal timing of initiation of intervention, standardization of minimal outcomes for specific behaviors as well as clinical outcomes (specific behaviors, weight gain, adiposity), scalability, and cost-effectiveness. In addition, given that effective prevention requires a broad reach to the general population, serious consideration should be given to the use of technology and digitally based programs, which can significantly improve reach, scalability (including lower-income segments), frequency (and potentially intensity), and cost-effectiveness. This is particularly relevant to the new generations of parents who are "digital natives."

## 18.7 Future directions

Much progress has been made in identifying the underlying potentially causal factors that lead to childhood and later obesity. However, unraveling the relative contribution of these remains challenging, due to their interdependence and mutual confounding. This is further complicated by the fact that some approaches to test interventions in infants are not possible for ethical or practical reasons. Observational efforts such as cohort studies need to continue, but they must be designed to address the increasingly growing variables and confounders identified, and the multiple interactions between them. Using within-family analyses, sibling paired studies, and triangulating studies with different gaps or biases may help.

Interventions need to focus on our best understanding of causes and mechanisms. Addressing most modifiable factors in early life (using a multicomponent approach) using behavioral theory based models in infancy appear to be critical. However, other less immediate environmental and socio-ecological factors cannot be overlooked, and these become increasingly important as children become older and more socially integrated. This includes family and environmental interventions that support food access, nutrition literacy, physical activity, and other factors (using multilevel strategies to intervene in the prevention of obesity). Resources need to be further prioritized to interventions that address multiple potentially causative factors as mentioned above and take advantage of technology to broaden reach and acceptance by future younger parents and families. Interventions, which need to be educational, must start early.

Given the transgenerational nature of obesity, this means starting prenatally, with parental education before conception and during pregnancy, as well as supporting adequate screening and prenatal care. Postnatally, the fact that most modifiable causative factors are under parent and caregiver control in the first 2 years of life, underscores the need to study the effect of holistic, multicomponent educational approaches that take advantage of this critical window of opportunity by holistically addressing these factors. *Developing and shaping behaviors* in infancy is likely to have a greater return on our efforts than attempting to *change behaviors* later in life.

## 18.8  Conclusion

Given the current epidemic, obesity prevention is critical and necessary for the well-being of individuals, families, and society. Early life events are a major determinant of future growth and health of the individual. Early life is also the most plastic time for shaping future behaviors (including food, and diet related). Moreover, because of an infant's complete dependency on their parents and immediate environment, the first 1000 days are a major opportunity to shape their future. Thus, early life preventive interventions have the greatest potential for efficacy and return on investment.

The potentially causative factors leading to obesity, which are modifiable in the immediate environment of the infant—can be addressed by the parents and caregivers if provided the education and support to empower them by building those capabilities for what and how to feed their infants. This education must be science-based, underpinned by effective educational theories, provided through accessible and cost-effective vehicles, supported by environmental systems and policies (including health and food systems), and reach all segments of society.

The challenge seems huge, but the opportunity for shaping healthier generations is more so.

## Sources of additional information

American Academy of Pediatrics (AAP), Clinical report: the role of the pediatrician in primary prevention of obesity. Daniels SR, Hassink SG; COMMITTEE ON NUTRITION. The Role of the Pediatrician in Primary Prevention of Obesity. Pediatrics. 2015 Jul;136(1):e275–92. doi: https://doi.org/10.1542/peds.2015-1558. Epub 2015 Jun 29. PMID: 26122812.

Dattilo AM 2022. Early Parent Feeding Behaviors to Promote Long-Term Health. In Saavedra, J.M. Dattilo, A. M., (Eds.), Early Nutrition and Long-term Health: Mechanisms, Consequences, and Opportunities, Second Edition. Elsevier, Oxford, (Chapter 20).

Federation of International Societies of Paediatric Gastroenterology, Hepatology and Nutrition (FISPGHAN) 2020. Koletzko B, Fishbein M, Lee WS, Moreno L, Mouane N, Mouzaki M, Verduci E. Prevention of Childhood Obesity: A Position Paper of FISPGHAN. J Pediatr Gastroenterol Nutr. 2020 May;70(5):702–710.

Gianni L. et al., 2022. Early Nutrition: Effects on Infants' Growth and Body Composition. In Saavedra, J.M. Dattilo, A. M., (Eds.), Early Nutrition and Long-term Health: Mechanisms, Consequences, and Opportunities, Second Edition. Elsevier, Oxford, (Chapter 4)

Institute of Medicine 2015. Examining a Developmental Approach to Childhood Obesity: The Fetal and Early Childhood Years: Workshop Summary. Washington, DC: The National Academies Press. https://doi.org/10.17226/21782.

Ludwig DS. Epidemic Childhood Obesity: Not Yet the End of the Beginning. Pediatrics. 2018 Mar;141(3):e20174078. doi: https://doi.org/10.1542/peds.2017-4078. PMID: 29483198; PMCID: PMC5847089.

Vickers M.H. 2022. Early Life Nutrition and its Effect on the Development of Obesity and Type-2 Diabetes. In Saavedra, J.M. Dattilo, A. M., (Eds.), Early Nutrition and Long-term Health: Mechanisms, Consequences, and Opportunities, Second Edition. Elsevier, Oxford, (Chapter 11).

World Health Organization, 2016. WHO Report of the commission on ending childhood obesity. Available from: http://apps.who.int/iris/bitstream/10665/204176/1/9789241510066_eng.pdf

WHO. Taking Action on Childhood Obesity. https://apps.who.int/iris/bitstream/handle/10665/274792/WHO-NMH-PND-ECHO-18.1-eng.pdf

# References

AAP Section on Breastfeeding, 2012. Breastfeeding and the use of human milk. Pediatrics 129 (3), e827–e841. https://doi.org/10.1542/peds.2011-3552. Epub 2012 Feb 27 22371471.

AAP Council on Communications and Media, 2016. Media and young minds. Pediatrics 138 (5), e20162591.

Abdallah Ismail, N., Ragab, S.H., Abd Elbaky, A., Shoeib, A.R., Alhosary, Y., Fekry, D., 2011. Frequency of Firmicutes and Bacteroidetes in gut microbiota in obese and normal weight Egyptian children and adults. Arch. Med. Sci. 7 (3), 501–507. https://doi.org/10.5114/aoms.2011.23418. Epub 2011 Jul 11 22295035. PMC3258740.

Abenavoli, L., Scarpellini, E., Colica, C., Boccuto, L., Salehi, B., Sharifi-Rad, J., Aiello, V., Romano, B., De Lorenzo, A., Izzo, A.A., Capasso, R., 2019. Gut microbiota and obesity: a role for probiotics. Nutrients 11 (11), 2690. https://doi.org/10.3390/nu11112690. PMID: 31703257; PMCID: PMC6893459.

Agostoni, C., Riva, E., Scaglioni, S., Marangoni, F., Radaelli, G., Giovannini, M., 2000. Dietary fats and cholesterol in italian infants and children. Am. J. Clin. Nutr. 72 (5 Suppl), 1384S–1391S. https://doi.org/10.1093/ajcn/72.5.1384s. 11063482.

Al-Disi, D., Al-Daghri, N., Khanam, L., Al-Othman, A., Al-Saif, M., Sabico, S., Chrousos, G., 2010. Subjective sleep duration and quality influence diet composition and circulating adipocytokines and ghrelin levels in teen-age girls. Endocr. J. 57 (10), 915–923.

Alderete, T.L., Jones, R.B., Shaffer, J.P., Holzhausen, E.A., Patterson, W.B., Kazemian, E., Chatzi, L., Knight, R., Plows, J.F., Berger, P.K., Goran, M.I., 2021. Early life gut microbiota is associated with rapid infant growth in Hispanics from Southern California. Gut Microbes 13 (1), 1961203. https://doi.org/10.1080/19490976.2021.1961203. 34424832. PMC8386720.

Alexander, D.D., Yan, J., Bylsma, L.C., Northington, R.S., Grathwohl, D., Steenhout, P., Erdmann, P., Spivey-Krobath, E., Haschke, F., 2016. Growth of infants consuming whey-predominant term infant formulas with a protein content of 1.8 g/100 kcal: a multicenter pooled analysis of individual participant data. Am. J. Clin. Nutr. 104 (4), 1083–1092. https://doi.org/10.3945/ajcn.116.130633. Epub 2016 Sep 7 27604774.

Anderson, S.E., Whitaker, R.C., 2010. Household routines and obesity in US preschool-aged children. Pediatrics 125 (3), 420–428. https://doi.org/10.1542/peds.2009-0417. Epub 2010 Feb 8 20142280.

Anderson, S.E., Andridge, R., Whitaker, R.C., 2016. Bedtime in preschool-aged children and risk for adolescent obesity. J. Pediatr. 176, 17–22. https://doi.org/10.1016/j.jpeds.2016.06.005. Epub 2016 Jul 14 27426836. PMC5003745.

Anderson, C.E., Whaley, S.E., Crespi, C.M., Wang, M.C., Chaparro, M.P., 2020. Every month matters: longitudinal associations between exclusive breastfeeding duration, child growth and obesity among WIC-participating children. J. Epidemiol. Community Health 74 (10), 785–791. https://doi.org/10.1136/jech-2019-213574.

Appleton, J., Russell, C.G., Laws, R., Fowler, C., Campbell, K., Denney-Wilson, E., 2018. Infant formula feeding practices associated with rapid weight gain: a systematic review. Matern. Child Nutr. 14 (3). https://doi.org/10.1111/mcn.12602, e12602.

Arenz, S., Rückerl, R., Koletzko, B., von Kries, R., 2004. Breast-feeding and childhood obesity—a systematic review. Int. J. Obes. Relat. Metab. Disord. 28 (10), 1247–1256. https://doi.org/10.1038/sj.ijo.0802758. 15314625.

Aris, I.M., Bernard, J.Y., Chen, L.W., Tint, M.T., Pang, W.W., Soh, S.E., Saw, S.M., Shek, L.P., Godfrey, K.M., Gluckman, P.D., Chong, Y.S., Yap, F., Kramer, M.S., Lee, Y.S., 2018. Modifiable risk factors in the first 1000 days for subsequent risk of childhood overweight in an Asian cohort: significance of parental overweight status. Int. J. Obes. (Lond) 42 (1), 44–51. https://doi.org/10.1038/ijo.2017.178. Epub 2017 Jul 28 28751763. PMC5671338.

Ariza, A., 2004. Risk factors for overweight in five- to six-year-old Hispanic-American children: a pilot study. J. Urban Health 81 (1), 150–161.

Ash, T., Agaronov, A., Young, T., Aftosmes-Tobio, A., Davison, K.K., 2017. Family-based childhood obesity prevention interventions: a systematic review and quantitative content analysis. Int. J. Behav. Nutr. Phys. Act. 14 (1), 113. https://doi.org/10.1186/s12966-017-0571-2. 28836983. PMC5571569.

Azad, M.B., Konya, T., Persaud, R.R., Guttman, D.S., Chari, R.S., Field, C.J., Sears, M.R., Mandhane, P.J., Turvey, S.E., Subbarao, P., Becker, A.B., Scott, J.A., Kozyrskyj, A.L., CHILD Study Investigators, 2016 May. Impact of maternal intrapartum antibiotics, method of birth and breastfeeding on gut microbiota during the first year of life: a prospective cohort study. BJOG 123 (6), 983–993. https://doi.org/10.1111/1471-0528.13601. Epub 2015 Sep 28. 26412384.

Azad, M.B., Vehling, L., Chan, D., Klopp, A., Nickel, N.C., JM, M.G., Becker, A.B., Mandhane, P.J., Turvey, S.E., Moraes, T.J., Taylor, M.S., Lefebvre, D.L., Sears, M.R., Subbarao, P., CHILD Study Investigators, 2018. Infant Feeding and Weight Gain: Separating Breast Milk From Breastfeeding and Formula From Food. Pediatrics 142 (4), e20181092. https://doi.org/10.1542/peds.2018-1092. 30249624.

Bąbik, K., Patro-Gołąb, B., Zalewski, B.M., Wojtyniak, K., Ostaszewski, P., Horvath, A., 2021. Infant feeding practices and later parent-reported feeding difficulties: a systematic review. Nutr. Rev. 79 (11), 1236–1258. https://doi.org/10.1093/nutrit/nuaa135. 33486523.

Badillo-Suárez, P.A., Rodríguez-Cruz, M., Nieves-Morales, X., 2017. Impact of metabolic hormones secreted in human breast milk on nutritional programming in childhood obesity. J. Mammary Gland Biol. Neoplasia 22 (3), 171–191. https://doi.org/10.1007/s10911-017-9382-y. Epub 2017 Jun 27 28653126.

Bailey, R.L., Catellier, D.J., Jun, S., Dwyer, J.T., Jacquier, E.F., Anater, A.S., Eldridge, A.L., 2018. Total usual nutrient intakes of US children (under 48 months): findings from the feeding infants and toddlers study (FITS) 2016. J. Nutr. 148 (9S), 1557S–1566S. https://doi.org/10.1093/jn/nxy042. 29878255. PMC6126633.

Baird, J., Hill, C.M., Harvey, N.C., Crozier, S., Robinson, S.M., Godfrey, K.M., Cooper, C., Inskip, H., SWS Study Group, 2016. Duration of sleep at 3 years of age is associated with fat and fat-free mass at 4 years of age: the Southampton Women's Survey. J. Sleep Res. 25 (4), 412–418. https://doi.org/10.1111/jsr.12389. Epub 2016 Feb 23 26909889. PMC4979987.

Balamurugan, R., George, G., Kabeerdoss, J., Hepsiba, J., Chandragunasekaran, A.M., Ramakrishna, B.S., 2010. Quantitative differences in intestinal Faecalibacterium prausnitzii in obese Indian children. Br. J. Nutr. 103 (3), 335–338. https://doi.org/10.1017/S0007114509992182. Epub 2009 Oct 23 19849869.

Barrera, C., Perrine, C., Li, R., Scanlon, K., 2016. Age at introduction to solid foods and child obesity at 6 years. Child. Obes. 12 (3), 188–192.

Black, M., Aboud, F., 2011. Responsive feeding is embedded in a theoretical framework of responsive parenting. J. Nutr. 141 (3), 490–494.

Black, M., Sacks, D., Xiang, A., Lawrence, J., et al., 2013. The relative contribution prepregnancy overweight and obesity, gestational weight gain, and IADPSG-defined gestational diabetes mellitus to fetal overgrowth. Diabetes Care 36, 56–62. Response to comment on: Black.

Blake-Lamb, T.L., Locks, L.M., Perkins, M.E., Woo Baidal, J.A., Cheng, E.R., Taveras, E.M., 2016. Interventions for childhood obesity in the first 1,000 days a systematic review. Am. J. Prev. Med. 50, 780–789.

Bode, L., 2020. Human milk oligosaccharides: structure and functions. Nestle Nutr. Inst. Workshop Ser. 94, 115–123. https://doi.org/10.1159/000505339. Epub 2020 Mar 11 32160614.

Borowitz, S.M., 2021. First bites-why, when, and what solid foods to feed infants. Front. Pediatr. 9, 654171. https://doi.org/10.3389/fped.2021.654171.

Braun, K.V., Erler, N.S., Kiefte-de Jong, J.C., Jaddoe, V.W., van den Hooven, E.H., Franco, O.H., Voortman, T., 2016. Dietary intake of protein in early childhood is associated with growth trajectories between 1 and 9 years of age. J. Nutr. 146 (11), 2361–2367. https://doi.org/10.3945/jn.116.237164. Epub 2016 Oct 12 27733529.

Buccigrossi, V., Nicastro, E., Guarino, A., 2013. Functions of intestinal microflora in children. Curr. Opin. Gastroenterol. 29 (1), 31–38. https://doi.org/10.1097/MOG.0b013e32835a3500. 23196853.

Buoncristiano, M., Spinelli, A., Williams, J., et al., 2021. Childhood overweight and obesity in Europe: changes from 2007 to 2017. Obes. Rev. 22 (Suppl. 6). https://doi.org/10.1111/obr.13226, e13226.

Butte, N., Fox, M., Briefel, R., Siega-Riz, A., Dwyer, J., Deming, D., Reidy, K., 2010. Nutrient intakes of US infants, toddlers, and preschoolers meet or exceed dietary reference intakes. J. Am. Diet. Assoc. 110 (12), S27–S37.

Cajachagua-Torres, K.N., El Marroun, H., Reiss, I.K.M., Santos, S., Jaddoe, V.W.V., 2022. Foetal tobacco and cannabis exposure, body fat and cardio-metabolic health in childhood. Pediatr. Obes. 17 (3). https://doi.org/10.1111/ijpo.12863, e12863.

Calatayud, M., Koren, O., Collado, M.C., 2019. Maternal microbiome and metabolic health program microbiome development and health of the offspring. Trends Endocrinol. Metab. 30 (10), 735–744. https://doi.org/10.1016/j.tem.2019.07.021. Epub 2019 Sep 5 31493988.

Campbell, J.M., McPherson, N.O., 2019. Influence of increased paternal BMI on pregnancy and child health outcomes independent of maternal effects: a systematic review and meta-analysis. Obes. Res. Clin. Pract. 13 (6), 511–521. https://doi.org/10.1016/j.orcp.2019.11.003.

Cantoral, A., Téllez-Rojo, M.M., Ettinger, A.S., Hu, H., Hernández-Ávila, M., Peterson, K., 2016. Early introduction and cumulative consumption of sugar-sweetened beverages during the pre-school period and risk of obesity at 8-14 years of age. Pediatr. Obes. 11 (1), 68–74. doi: 10.1111/ijpo.12023. Epub 2015 Apr 17. PMID: 25891908; PMCID: PMC5482497.Guideline: Sugars Intake for Adults and Children. Geneva: World Health Organization; 2015 25905159.

Chaput, J.P., Gray, C.E., Poitras, V.J., Carson, V., Gruber, R., Birken, C.S., MacLean, J.E., Aubert, S., Sampson, M., Tremblay, M.S., 2017. Systematic review of the relationships between sleep duration and health indicators in the early years (0-4years). BMC Public Health 17 (Suppl 5), 855. https://doi.org/10.1186/s12889-017-4850-2. 29219078. PMC5773910.

Chen, W., Adler, J.L., 2019. Assessment of screen exposure in young children, 1997 to 2014. JAMA Pediatr. 2019, 391–393.

Clayton, H., Li, R., Perrine, C., Scanlon, K., 2013. Prevalence and reasons for introducing infants early to solid foods: variations by milk feeding type. Pediatrics 131 (4), e1108–e1114.

Collings, P.J., Ball, H.L., Santorelli, G., West, J., Barber, S.E., McEachan, R.R., Wright, J., 2017. Sleep duration and adiposity in early childhood: evidence for bidirectional associations from the born in bradford study. Sleep 40 (2). https://doi.org/10.1093/sleep/zsw054, zsw054. 28364513. PMC5804981.

Crowder, S.L., Beckie, T., Stern, M., 2021. A review of food insecurity and chronic cardiovascular disease: implications during the COVID-19 pandemic. Ecol. Food Nutr. 60 (5), 596–611. https://doi.org/10.1080/03670244.2021.1956485.

Cunningham, S.A., Kramer, M.R., Narayan, K.M., 2014. Incidence of childhood obesity in the United States. N. Engl. J. Med. 370 (17), 1660–1661. https://doi.org/10.1056/NEJMc1402397.

Dallacker, M., Hertwig, R., Mata, J., 2018. The frequency of family meals and nutritional health in children: a meta-analysis. Obes. Rev. 19 (5), 638–653. https://doi.org/10.1111/obr.12659. Epub 2018 Jan 15 29334693.

Dattilo, A.M., 2017. Modifiable risk factors and interventions for childhood obesity prevention within the first 1,000 days. Nestle Nutr. Inst. Workshop Ser. 87, 183–196. https://doi.org/10.1159/000448966. Epub 2017 Mar 17 28315898.

Dattilo, A.M., 2022. Early parent feeding behaviors to promote long-term health. In: Saavedra, J.M., Dattilo, A.M. (Eds.), Early Nutrition and Long-term Health: Mechanisms, Consequences, and Opportunities, second ed. Elsevier, Oxford (Chapter 20).

Dattilo, A.M., Saavedra, J.M., 2020. Nutrition education: application of theory and strategies during the first 1,000 days for healthy growth. Nestle Nutr. Inst. Workshop Ser. 92, 1–18. https://doi.org/10.1159/000499544. Epub 2019 Nov 28 31779004.

Dattilo, A., Birch, L., Krebs, N., Lake, A., Taveras, E., Saavedra, J., 2012. Need for early interventions in the prevention of pediatric overweight: a review and upcoming directions. J. Obes. 2012, 1–18.

Davis, C.D., 2016. The gut microbiome and its role in obesity. Nutr. Today 51 (4), 167–174. https://doi.org/10.1097/NT.0000000000000167.

Davis, E.C., Wang, M., Donovan, S.M., 2017. The role of early life nutrition in the establishment of gastrointestinal microbial composition and function. Gut Microbes 8 (2), 143–171. https://doi.org/10.1080/19490976.2016.127810 4. Epub 2017 Jan 9 28068209. PMC5390825.

De Kroon, M., Renders, C., Van Wouwe, J., Van Buuren, S., Hirasing, R., 2010. The Terneuzen birth cohort: BMI changes between 2 and 6 years correlate strongest with adult overweight. PLoS One 5 (2), e9155.

de Lauzon-Guillain, B., Jones, L., Oliveira, A., Moschonis, G., Betoko, A., Lopes, C., Moreira, P., Manios, Y., Papadopoulos, N.G., Emmett, P., Charles, M.A., 2013. The influence of early feeding practices on fruit and vegetable intake among preschool children in 4 European birth cohorts. Am. J. Clin. Nutr. 98 (3), 804–812. https://doi.org/10.3945/ajcn.112.057026. Epub 2013 Jul 17. Erratum in: Am J Clin Nutr. 2014 Feb;99(2):423 23864537.

Deal, B.J., Huffman, M.D., Binns, H., Stone, N.J., 2020. Perspective: childhood obesity requires new strategies for prevention. Adv. Nutr. 11 (5), 1071–1078. https://doi.org/10.1093/advances/nmaa040. 32361757. PMC7490151.

Deng, X., He, M., He, D., Zhu, Y., Zhang, Z., Niu, W., 2021. Sleep duration and obesity in children and adolescents: evidence from an updated and dose-response meta-analysis. Sleep Med. 78, 169–181. https://doi.org/10.1016/j.sleep.2020.12.027. Epub 2020 Dec 29 33450724.

Dennison, B., Erb, T., Jenkins, P., 2002. Television viewing and television in bedroom associated with overweight risk among low-income preschool children. Pediatrics 109 (6), 1028–1035.

Derks, I.P.M., Kocevska, D., Jaddoe, V.W.V., Franco, O.H., Wake, M., Tiemeier, H., Jansen, P.W., 2017. Longitudinal associations of sleep duration in infancy and early childhood with body composition and cardiometabolic health at the age of 6 years: the generation R study. Child. Obes. 13 (5), 400–408. https://doi.org/10.1089/chi.2016.0341. Epub 2017 Jun 12 28604071.

III. Promoting long-term health: Taking action in the first 1000 days

Dewey, K., 1998. Growth characteristics of breast-fed compared to formula-fed infants. Neonatology 74 (2), 94–105.

Dewey, K.G., Adu-Afarwuah, S., 2008. Systematic review of the efficacy and effectiveness of complementary feeding interventions in developing countries. Matern. Child Nutr., 24–85.

Dewey, K., Lonnerdal, B., 1986. Infant self-regulation of breast milk intake. Acta Paediatr. Scand. 75 (6), 893–898.

Dewey, K.G., Güngör, D., Donovan, S.M., Madan, E.M., Venkatramanan, S., Davis, T.A., Kleinman, R.E., Taveras, E.M., Bailey, R.L., Novotny, R., Terry, N., Butera, G., Obbagy, J., de Jesus, J., Stoody, E., 2021. Breastfeeding and risk of overweight in childhood and beyond: a systematic review with emphasis on sibling-pair and intervention studies. Am. J. Clin. Nutr. 114 (5), 1774–1790. https://doi.org/10.1093/ajcn/nqab206. 34224561.

Di Cesare, M., Sorić, M., Bovet, P., Miranda, J.J., Bhutta, Z., Stevens, G.A., Laxmaiah, A., Kengne, A.P., Bentham, J., 2019. The epidemiological burden of obesity in childhood: a worldwide epidemic requiring urgent action. BMC Med. 17 (1), 212. https://doi.org/10.1186/s12916-019-1449-8. 31760948. PMC6876113.

Diethelm, K., Bolzenius, K., Cheng, G., Remer, T., Buyken, A.E., 2011. Longitudinal associations between reported sleep duration in early childhood and the development of body mass index, fat mass index and fat free mass index until age 7. Int. J. Pediatr. Obes. 6 (2-2), e114–e123. https://doi.org/10.3109/17477166.2011.566338. Epub 2011 May 23 21604964.

Differding, M.K., Doyon, M., Bouchard, L., Perron, P., Guérin, R., Asselin, C., Massé, E., Hivert, M.F., Mueller, N.T., 2020. Potential interaction between timing of infant complementary feeding and breastfeeding duration in determination of early childhood gut microbiota composition and BMI. Pediatr. Obes. 15 (8), e12642. https://doi.org/10.1111/ijpo.12642. Epub 2020 Apr 29 32351036. PMC7923600.

DiSantis, K., Hodges, E., Johnson, S., Fisher, J., 2011. The role of responsive feeding in overweight during infancy and toddlerhood: a systematic review. Int. J. Obes. Relat. Metab. Disord. 35 (4), 480–492.

Donovan, S.M., Comstock, S.S., 2016. Human milk oligosaccharides influence neonatal mucosal and systemic immunity. Ann. Nutr. Metab. 69 (Suppl 2), 42–51. https://doi.org/10.1159/000452818. Epub 2017 Jan 20 28103609. PMC6392703.

Dubois, L., Farmer, A., Girard, M., Peterson, K., 2007. Regular sugar-sweetened beverage consumption between meals increases risk of overweight among preschool-aged children. J. Am. Diet. Assoc. 107 (6), 924–934.

Duch, H., Fisher, E.M., Ensari, I., Harrington, A., 2013. Screen time use in children under 3 years old: a systematic review of correlates. Int. J. Behav. Nutr. Phys. Act. 23 (10), 102. https://doi.org/10.1186/1479-5868-10-102. 23967799. PMC3844496.

EFSA, 2010. Scientific opinion on dietary reference values for carbohydrates and dietary fibre. EFSA Panel on Dietetic Products, Nutrition, and Allergies (NDA)European Food Safety Authority (EFSA). EFSA J. 8 (3), 1462.

English, L.K., Obbagy, J.E., Wong, Y.P., Butte, N.F., Dewey, K.G., Fox, M.K., Greer, F.R., Krebs, N.F., Scanlon, K.S., Stoody, E.E., 2019a. Types and amounts of complementary foods and beverages consumed and growth, size, and body composition: a systematic review. Am. J. Clin. Nutr. 109 (Suppl_7), 956S–977S. https://doi.org/10.1093/ajcn/nqy281. Erratum in: Am J Clin Nutr. 2019 Oct 1;110(4):1041 30982866.

English, L.K., Obbagy, J.E., Wong, Y.P., Butte, N.F., Dewey, K.G., Fox, M.K., Greer, F.R., Krebs, N.F., Scanlon, K.S., Stoody, E.E., 2019b. Timing of introduction of complementary foods and beverages and growth, size, and body composition: a systematic review. Am. J. Clin. Nutr. 109 (Suppl_7), 935S–955S. https://doi.org/10.1093/ajcn/nqy267. 30982863.

Fan, Y., Pedersen, O., 2021. Gut microbiota in human metabolic health and disease. Nat. Rev. Microbiol. 19 (1), 55–71 Epub 2020 Sep 4 doi:10.1038/s41579-020-0433-9.

FAO, IFAD, UNICEF, WFP, WHO, 2019. The State of Food Security and Nutrition in the World 2019. Safeguarding Against Economic Slowdowns and Downturns. Rome, FAO. Licence: CC BY-NC-SA 3.0 IGO.

Fehr, K., Moossavi, S., Sbihi, H., Boutin, R.C.T., Bode, L., Robertson, B., Yonemitsu, C., Field, C.J., Becker, A.B., Mandhane, P.J., Sears, M.R., Khafipour, E., Moraes, T.J., Subbarao, P., Finlay, B.B., Turvey, S.E., Azad, M.B., 2020. Breastmilk feeding practices are associated with the co-occurrence of bacteria in mothers' milk and the infant gut: the CHILD Cohort study. Cell Host Microbe 28 (2), 285–297.e4. https://doi.org/10.1016/j.chom.2020.06.009. Epub 2020 Jul 10 32652062.

Fein, S., Labiner-Wolfe, J., Scanlon, K., Grummer-Strawn, L., 2008. Selected complementary feeding practices and their association with maternal education. Pediatrics 122 (Suppl), S91–S97.

Feldman, S., Eisenberg, M., Neumark-Sztainer, D., Story, M., 2007. Associations between watching TV during family meals and dietary intake among adolescents. J. Nutr. Educ. Behav. 39 (5), 257–263.

Felso, R., Lohner, S., Hollódy, K., Erhardt, É., Molnár, D., 2017. Relationship between sleep duration and childhood obesity: Systematic review including the potential underlying mechanisms. Nutr. Metab. Cardiovasc. Dis. 27 (9), 751–761. https://doi.org/10.1016/j.numecd.2017.07.008. Epub 2017 Jul 25 28818457.

Fidler-Mis, N., Braegger, C., Bronsky, J., Campoy, C., Domellöf, M., Embleton, N.D., Hojsak, I., Hulst, J., Indrio, F., Lapillonne, A., Mihatsch, W., Molgaard, C., Vora, R., Fewtrell, M., ESPGHAN Committee on Nutrition, 2017. Sugar in infants, children and adolescents: a position paper of the European Society for paediatric gastroenterology, hepatology and nutrition committee on nutrition. J. Pediatr. Gastroenterol. Nutr. 65 (6), 681–696. https://doi.org/10.1097/MPG.0000000000001733. 28922262.

Fiorito, L., Marini, M., Francis, L., Smiciklas-Wright, H., Birch, L., 2009. Beverage intake of girls at age 5 y predicts adiposity and weight status in childhood and adolescence. Am. J. Clin. Nutr. 90 (4), 935–942.

Fogel, A., McCrickerd, K., Aris, I.M., et al., 2020. Eating behaviors moderate the associations between risk factors in the first 1000 days and adiposity outcomes at 6 years of age. Am. J. Clin. Nutr. 111 (5), 997–1006. https://doi.org/10.1093/ajcn/nqaa052.

Forbes, J.D., Azad, M.B., Vehling, L., Tun, H.M., Konya, T.B., Guttman, D.S., Field, C.J., Lefebvre, D., Sears, M.R., Becker, A.B., Mandhane, P.J., Turvey, S.E., Moraes, T.J., Subbarao, P., Scott, J.A., Kozyrskyj, A.L., Canadian Healthy Infant Longitudinal Development (CHILD) Study Investigators, 2018. Association of exposure to formula in the hospital and subsequent infant feeding practices with gut microbiota and risk of overweight in the first year of life. JAMA Pediatr. 172 (7), e181161. https://doi.org/10.1001/jamapediatrics.2018.1161. Epub 2018 Jul 2. Erratum in: JAMA Pediatr. 2018 Jul 1;172(7):704 29868719. PMC6137517.

Forestell, C., Mennella, J., 2015. The ontogeny of taste perception and preference throughout childhood. In: Doty, R.L. (Ed.), Handbook of Olfaction and Gustation, third ed. Wiley-Liss, New York, pp. 795–827.

Fornari, E., Brusati, M., Maffeis, C., 2021. Nutritional strategies for childhood obesity prevention. Life (Basel) 11 (6), 532. https://doi.org/10.3390/life11060532. 34201017. PMC8227398.

Fox, M., Condon, E., Briefel, R., Reidy, K., Deming, D., 2010. Food consumption patterns of young preschoolers: are they starting off on the right path? J. Am. Diet. Assoc. 110 (12), S52–S59.

Garden, F.L., Marks, G.B., Almqvist, C., Simpson, J.M., Webb, K.L., 2011. Infant and early childhood dietary predictors of overweight at age 8 years in the CAPS population. Eur. J. Clin. Nutr. 65 (4), 454–462.

Garden, F.L., Marks, G.B., Simpson, J.M., WebbKL., 2012. Body mass index (BMI) trajectories from birth to 11.5 years: relation to early life food intake. Nutrients 4 (10), 1382–1398.

Geserick, M., Vogel, M., Gausche, R., et al., 2018. Acceleration of BMI in early childhood and risk of sustained obesity. N. Engl. J. Med. 379 (14), 1303–1312. https://doi.org/10.1056/NEJMoa1803527.

Gibbs, B.G., Forste, R., 2014. Socioeconomic status, infant feeding practices and early childhood obesity. Pediatr. Obes. 9 (2), 135–146. https://doi.org/10.1111/j.2047-6310.2013.00155.x.

Gomez-Gallego, C., Garcia-Mantrana, I., Salminen, S., Collado, M.C., 2016. The human milk microbiome and factors influencing its composition and activity. Semin. Fetal Neonatal Med. 21 (6), 400–405. https://doi.org/10.1016/j.siny.2016.05.003. Epub 2016 Jun 7 27286644.

Gooze, R.A., Anderson, S.E., Whitaker, R.C., 2011. Prolonged bottle use and obesity at 5.5 years of age in US children. J. Pediatr. 159 (3), 431–436. https://doi.org/10.1016/j.jpeds.2011.02.037. Epub 2011 May 4 21543085.

Grimm, K.A., Kim, S.A., Yaroch, A.L., Scanlon, K.S., 2014. Fruit and vegetable intake during infancy and early childhood. Pediatrics 134 (Suppl 1), S63–S69. https://doi.org/10.1542/peds.2014-0646K. 25183758. PMC4258845.

Grote, V., Theurich, M., 2014. Complementary feeding and obesity risk. Curr. Opin. Clin. Nutr. Metab. Care 17 (3), 273–277.

Grote, V., Theurich, M., Koletzko, B., 2012. Do complementary feeding practices predict the later risk of obesity? Curr. Opin. Clin. Nutr. Metab. Care 15 (3), 293–297.

Grummer-Strawn, L., Scanlon, K., Fein, S., 2008. Infant feeding and feeding transitions during the first year of life. Pediatrics 122 (Suppl. 2), S36–S42.

Gubbels, J.S., Thijs, C., Stafleu, A., van Buuren, S., Kremers, S.P., 2011. Association of breast-feeding and feeding on demand with child weight status up to 4 years. Int. J. Pediatr. Obes. 6 (2-2), e515–e522. https://doi.org/10.3109/17477166.2010.514343. Epub 2010 Sep 22 20858157.

Gunderson, E.P., 2009. Childbearing and obesity in women: weight before, during, and after pregnancy. Obstet. Gynecol. Clin. North Am. 36 (2), 317–332. https://doi.org/10.1016/j.ogc.2009.04.001.

Gunther, A.L., Buyken, A.E., Kroke, A., 2007. Protein intake during the period of complementary feeding and early childhood and the association with body mass index and percentage body fat at 7 y of age. Am. J. Clin. Nutr. 85 (6), 1626–1633. https://doi.org/10.1093/ajcn/85.6.1626. 17556702.

Guo, L., Liu, J., Ye, R., Liu, J., Zhuang, Z., Ren, A., 2015. Gestational weight gain and overweight in children aged 3–6 years. J. Epidemiol. 25 (8), 536–543.

Harder, T., Bergmann, R., Kallischnigg, G., Plagemann, A., 2005. Duration of breastfeeding and risk of overweight: a meta-analysis. Am. J. Epidemiol. 162 (5), 397–403. https://doi.org/10.1093/aje/kwi222. Epub 2005 Aug 2 16076830.

Harskamp-van Ginkel, M.W., Chinapaw, M.J.M., Harmsen, I.A., Anujuo, K.O., Daams, J.G., Vrijkotte, T.G.M., 2020. Sleep during infancy and associations with childhood body composition: a systematic review and narrative synthesis. Child. Obes. 16 (2), 94–116. https://doi.org/10.1089/chi.2019.0123. Epub 2019 Nov 20 31692365.

Hart, C., Cairns, A., Jelalian, E., 2011. Sleep and obesity in children and adolescents. Pediatr. Clin. North Am. 58 (3), 715–733.

Headey, D., Heidkamp, R., Osendarp, S., et al., 2020. Impacts of COVID-19 on childhood malnutrition and nutrition-related mortality. Lancet 396 (10250), 519–521. https://doi.org/10.1016/S0140-6736(20)31647-0.

Heinig, M.J., Nommsen, L.A., Peerson, J.M., Lonnerdal, B., Dewey, K.G., 1993. Energy and protein intakes of breast-fed and formula-fed infants during the first year of life and their association with growth velocity: the DARLING Study. Am. J. Clin. Nutr. 58 (2), 152–161.

Heppe, D., Kiefte-de Jong, J., Durmus, B., Moll, H., Raat, H., Hofman, A., Jaddoe, V., 2012. Parental, fetal, and infant risk factors for preschool overweight: the generation R study. Pediatr. Res. 73 (1), 120–127.

Herbst, A., Diethelm, K., Cheng, G., Alexy, U., Icks, A., Buyken, A.E., 2011. Direction of associations between added sugar intake in early childhood and body mass index at age 7 years may depend on intake levels. J. Nutr. 141 (7), 1348–1354. https://doi.org/10.3945/jn.110.137000. Epub 2011 May 11 21562234.

Heslehurst, N., Vieira, R., Akhter, Z., Bailey, H., Slack, E., Ngongalah, L., Pemu, A., Rankin, J., 2019. The association between maternal body mass index and child obesity: a systematic review and meta-analysis. PLoS Med 6. https://doi.org/10.1371/journal.pmed.1002817, e1002817.

Hieronimus, B., Ensenauer, R., 2021. Influence of maternal and paternal pre-conception overweight/obesity on offspring outcomes and strategies for prevention. Eur. J. Clin. Nutr. 75 (12), 1735–1744. https://doi.org/10.1038/s41430-021-00920-7.

Hodges, E., Hughes, S., Hopkinson, J., Fisher, J., 2008. Maternal decisions about the initiation and termination of infant feeding. Appetite 50 (2–3), 333–339.

Hodges, E.A., Propper, C.B., Estrem, H., Schultz, M.B., 2020. Feeding during infancy: interpersonal behavior, physiology, and obesity risk. Child Dev. Perspect. 14 (3), 185–191. https://doi.org/10.1111/cdep.12376. Epub 2020 Jul 14 34707686. PMC8547759.

Hornell, A., Lagström, H., Lande, B., Thorsdottir, I., 2013. Protein intake from 0 to 18 years of age and its relation to health: a systematic literature review for the 5th nordic nutrition recommendations. Food Nutr. Res. 23, 57. https://doi.org/10.3402/fnr.v57i0.21083. 23717219. PMC3664059.

Horodynski, M., Stommel, M., Brophy-Herb, H., Weatherspoon, L., 2010. Mealtime television viewing and dietary quality in low-income African American and Caucasian mother–toddler dyads. Matern. Child Health J. 14 (4), 548–556.

Horta, B.L., Loret de Mola, C., Victora, C.G., 2015. Long-term consequences of breastfeeding on cholesterol, obesity, systolic blood pressure and type 2 diabetes: a systematic review and meta-analysis. Acta Paediatr. 104 (467), 30–37. https://doi.org/10.1111/apa.13133. 26192560.

Hu, J., Aris, I.M., Lin, P.D., Rifas-Shiman, S.L., Perng, W., Woo Baidal, J.A., Wen, D., Oken, E., 2020. Longitudinal associations of modifiable risk factors in the first 1000 days with weight status and metabolic risk in early adolescence. Am. J. Clin. Nutr. 113 (1), 113–122. https://doi.org/10.1093/ajcn/nqaa297. Epub ahead of print 33184628. PMC7779210.

Iguacel, I., Gasch-Gallén, Á., Ayala-Marín, A.M., De Miguel-Etayo, P., Moreno, L.A., 2021. Social vulnerabilities as risk factor of childhood obesity development and their role in prevention programs. Int. J. Obes. (Lond) 45 (1), 1–11. https://doi.org/10.1038/s41366-020-00697-y. Epub 2020 Oct 8 33033393.

Ino, T., 2010. Maternal smoking during pregnancy and offspring obesity: meta-analysis. Pediatr. Int. 52 (1), 94–99. https://doi.org/10.1111/j.1442-200X.2009.02883.x. Epub 2009 Apr 27 19400912.

IOM National Research Council, 2009. Weight Gain During Pregnancy: Reexamining the Guidelines. The National Academies Press, Washington, DC, https://doi.org/10.17226/12584.

Iozzo, P., Sanguinetti, E., 2018. Early dietary patterns and microbiota development: still a way to go from descriptive interactions to health-relevant solutions. Front. Nutr. 2018, 5.

Janssen, X., Martin, A., Hughes, A.R., Hill, C.M., Kotronoulas, G., Hesketh, K.R., 2020. Associations of screen time, sedentary time and physical activity with sleep in under 5s: a systematic review and meta-analysis. Sleep Med. Rev. 49, 101226. https://doi.org/10.1016/j.smrv.2019.101226. Epub 2019 Nov 1 31778942. PMC7034412.

Janz, K., Levy, S.M., Burns, T.L., Torner, J.C., Willimg, M.C., Warren, J.J., 2002. Fatness, physical activity, and television viewing in children during the adiposity rebound period: the Iowa bone development study. Prev. Med. 35 (6), 563–571.

Jiang, J., Rosenqvist, U., Wang, H., Greiner, T., Ma, Y., Michael Toschke, A., 2006. Risk factors for overweight in 2- to 6-year-old children in Beijing, China. Int. J. Pediatr. Obes. 1 (2), 103–108.

Jones, L.R., Emmett, P.M., Hays, N.P., Shahkhalili, Y., Taylor, C.M., 2021. Association of nutrition in early childhood with body composition and leptin in later childhood and early adulthood. Nutrients 13 (9), 3264. https://doi.org/10.3390/nu13093264. 34579140. PMC8466313.

Kalliomäki, M., Collado, M.C., Salminen, S., Isolauri, E., 2008. Early differences in fecal microbiota composition in children may predict overweight. Am. J. Clin. Nutr. 87 (3), 534–538. https://doi.org/10.1093/ajcn/87.3.534. 18326589.

Kavanagh, K., Cohen, R., Heinig, M., Dewey, K., 2008. Educational intervention to modify bottlefeeding behaviors among formula-feeding mothers in the WIC Program: impact on infant formula intake and weight gain. J. Nutr. Educ. Behav. 40 (4), 244–250.

Keag, O.E., Norman, J.E., Stock, S.J., 2018. Long-term risks and benefits associated with cesarean delivery for mother, baby, and subsequent pregnancies: systematic review and meta-analysis. PLoS Med. 15 (1). https://doi.org/10.1371/journal.pmed.1002494, e1002494. 29360829. PMC5779640.

Kharas, H., et al., 2018. Assessing Current Trajectories on the Sustainable Development Goals. Brookings Global Economy and Development Working Paper No. 123.

Kim, J.H., Lee, S.W., Lee, J.E., Ha, E.K., Han, M.Y., Lee, E., 2021. Breastmilk feeding during the first 4 to 6 months of age and childhood disease burden until 10 years of age. Nutrients 13 (8), 2825. https://doi.org/10.3390/nu13082825. 34444985. PMC8400284.

Kimbro, R., Brooks-Gunn, J., McLanahan, S., 2011. Young children in urban areas: links among neighborhood characteristics, weight status, outdoor play, and television watching. Soc. Sci. Med. 72 (5), 668–676.

Klingenberg, L., Christensen, L., Hjorth, M., Zangenberg, S., Chaput, J., Sjödin, A., Mølgaard, C., Michaelsen, K., 2012. No relation between sleep duration and adiposity indicators in 9-36 months old children: the SKOT cohort. Pediatr. Obes. 8 (1), e14–e18.

Koletzko, B., von Kries, R., Closa, R., Escribano, J., Scaglioni, S., Giovannini, M., Beyer, J., Demmelmair, H., Gruszfeld, D., Dobrzanska, A., Sengier, A., Langhendries, J., Rolland Cachera, M., Grote, V., 2009a. Lower protein in infant formula is associated with lower weight up to age 2 y: a randomized clinical trial. Am. J. Clin. Nutr. 89 (6), 1836–1845.

Koletzko, B., von Kries, R., Monasterolo, R., Subias, J., Scaglioni, S., Giovannini, M., Beyer, J., Demmelmair, H., Anton, B., Gruszfeld, D., Dobrzanska, A., Sengier, A., Langhendries, J., Rolland Cachera, M., Grote, V., 2009b. Can infant feeding choices modulate later obesity risk? Am. J. Clin. Nutr. 89 (5), 1502S–1508S.

Koletzko, B., Fishbein, M., Lee, W.S., Moreno, L., Mouane, N., Mouzaki, M., Verduci, E., 2020. Prevention of childhood obesity: a position paper of the global federation of international societies of paediatric gastroenterology, hepatology and nutrition (FISPGHAN). J. Pediatr. Gastroenterol. Nutr. 70 (5), 702–710. https://doi.org/10.1097/MPG.0000000000002708. 32205768.

Koplin, J.J., Kerr, J.A., Lodge, C., Garner, C., Dharmage, S.C., Wake, M., Allen, K.J., 2019. Infant and young child feeding interventions targeting overweight and obesity: a narrative review. Obes. Rev. 20 (Suppl 1), 31–44. https://doi.org/10.1111/obr.12798. 31419047.

Korpela, K., Renko, M., Vänni, P., Paalanne, N., Salo, J., Tejesvi, M.V., Koivusaari, P., Ojaniemi, M., Pokka, T., Kaukola, T., Pirttilä, A.M., Tapiainen, T., 2020 Nov. Microbiome of the first stool and overweight at age 3years: a prospective cohort study. Pediatr. Obes. 15 (11). https://doi.org/10.1111/ijpo.12680, e12680. Epub 2020 Jul 7 32638554.

Kotowski, J., Fowler, C., Hourigan, C., Orr, F., 2020. Bottle-feeding an infant feeding modality: an integrative literature review. Matern. Child Nutr. 16 (2), e12939. https://doi.org/10.1111/mcn.12939. Epub 2020 Jan 6 31908144. PMC7083444.

Kratzsch, J., Bae, Y.J., Kiess, W., 2018. Adipokines in human breast milk. Best Pract. Res. Clin. Endocrinol. Metab. 32 (1), 27–38. https://doi.org/10.1016/j.beem.2018.02.001. Epub 2018 Feb 6. 29549957.

Kuhle, S., Tong, O.S., Woolcott, C.G., 2015. Association between caesarean section and childhood obesity: a systematic review and meta-analysis. Obes. Rev. 16 (4), 295–303. https://doi.org/10.1111/obr.12267. Epub 2015 Mar 5 25752886.

LaRowe, T., Adams, A., Jobe, J., Cronin, K., Vannatter, S., Prince, R., 2010. Dietary intakes and physical activity among preschool-aged children living in rural American Indian communities before a family-based healthy lifestyle intervention. J. Am. Diet. Assoc. 110 (7), 1049–1057.

Larqué, E., Labayen, I., Flodmark, C.E., Lissau, I., Czernin, S., Moreno, L.A., Pietrobelli, A., Widhalm, K., 2019. From conception to infancy—early risk factors for childhood obesity. Nat. Rev. Endocrinol. 15 (8), 456–478. https://doi.org/10.1038/s41574-019-0219-1. Epub 2019 Jul 3 31270440.

Lassi, Z.S., Das, J.K., Zahid, G., Imdad, A., Bhutta, Z.A., 2013. Impact of education and provision of complementary feeding on growth and morbidity in children less than 2 years of age in developing countries: a systematic review. BMC Public Health 13 (Suppl. 3), S13. https://doi.org/10.1186/1471-2458-13-S3-S13.

Laursen, M.F., Bahl, M.I., Michaelsen, K.F., Licht, T.R., 2017. First foods and gut microbes. Front. Microbiol. 6 (8), 356. https://doi.org/10.3389/fmicb.2017.00356. 28321211. PMC5337510.

Lee, H.J., Lee, S.Y., Park, E.C., 2016. Do family meals affect childhood overweight or obesity?: nationwide survey 2008-2012. Pediatr. Obes. 11 (3), 161–165. https://doi.org/10.1111/ijpo.12035. Epub 2015 Jun 10 26061428.

Li, R., Fein, S.B., Grummer-Strawn, L.M., 2008. Association of breastfeeding intensity and bottle-emptying behaviors at early infancy with infants' risk for excess weight at late infancy. Pediatrics 122 (Suppl 2), S77–S84. https://doi.org/10.1542/peds.2008-1315j. 18829835.

Li, R., Magadia, J., Fein, S., Grummer Strawn, L., 2012. Risk of bottle-feeding for rapid weight gain during the first year of life. Arch. Pediatr. Adolesc. Med. 166 (5), 431–436.

Li, H.T., Zhou, Y.B., Liu, J.M., 2013. The impact of cesarean section on offspring overweight and obesity: a systematic review and meta-analysis. Int. J. Obes. (Lond) 37 (7), 893–899. https://doi.org/10.1038/ijo.2012.195. Epub 2012 Dec 4 23207407.

Li, R., Scanlon, K., May, A., Rose, C., Birch, L., 2014. Bottle-feeding practices during early infancy and eating behaviors at 6 years of age. Pediatrics 134 (Suppl. 1), S70–S77.

Li, L., Peters, H., Gama, A., Carvalhal, M.I., Nogueira, H.G., Rosado-Marques, V., Padez, C., 2016. Maternal smoking in pregnancy association with childhood adiposity and blood pressure. Pediatr. Obes. 11 (3), 202–209. https://doi.org/10.1111/ijpo.12046. Epub 2015 Jul 14 26178147. PMC4949567.

Li, C., Cheng, G., Sha, T., Cheng, W., Yan, Y., 2020. The relationships between screen use and health indicators among infants, toddlers, and preschoolers: a meta-analysis and systematic review. Int. J. Environ. Res. Public Health 17 (19), 7324. https://doi.org/10.3390/ijerph17197324. 33036443. PMC7579161.

Lin, J., Jiang, Y., Wang, G., Meng, M., Zhu, Q., Mei, H., Liu, S., Jiang, F., 2020 Nov. Associations of short sleep duration with appetite-regulating hormones and adipokines: a systematic review and meta-analysis. Obes. Rev. 21 (11). https://doi.org/10.1111/obr.13051, e13051. Epub 2020 Jun 15 32537891.

Linardakis, M., Sarri, K., Pateraki, M., Sbokos, M., Kafatos, A., 2008. Sugar-added beverages consumption among kindergarten children of Crete: effects on nutritional status and risk of obesity. BMC Public Health 8 (1), 279.

Logan, K.M., Gale, C., Hyde, M.J., Santhakumaran, S., Modi, N., 2017. Diabetes in pregnancy and infant adiposity: systematic review and meta-analysis. Arch. Dis. Child. Fetal Neonatal Ed. 102 (1), F65–F72. https://doi.org/10.1136/archdischild-2015-309750. Epub 2016 May 26 27231266. PMC5256410.

Lumeng, J., Rahnama, S., Appugliese, D., Kaciroti, N., Bradley, R., 2006. Television exposure and overweight risk in preschoolers. Arch. Pediatr. Adolesc. Med. 160 (4), 417–422.

Mărginean, C.O., Mărginean, C., Meliţ, L.E., 2018. New insights regarding genetic aspects of childhood obesity: a minireview. Front. Pediatr. 6, 271. https://doi.org/10.3389/fped.2018.00271. 30338250. PMC6180186.

Ma, J., Qiao, Y., Zhao, P., Li, W., Katzmarzyk, P.T., Chaput, J.P., Fogelholm, M., Kuriyan, R., Lambert, E.V., Maher, C., Maia, J., Matsudo, V., Olds, T., Onywera, V., Sarmiento, O.L., Standage, M., Tremblay, M.S., Tudor-Locke, C., Hu, G., ISCOLE Research Group, 2020. Breastfeeding and childhood obesity: a 12-country study. Matern. Child Nutr. 16 (3). https://doi.org/10.1111/mcn.12984, e12984. Epub 2020 Mar 5 32141229. PMC7296809.

Mamun, A., Mannan, M., Doi, S., 2013. Gestational weight gain in relation to offspring obesity over the life course: a systematic review and bias-adjusted meta-analysis. Obes. Rev. 15 (4), 338–347.

Mannan, H., 2018. Early infant feeding of formula or solid foods and risk of childhood overweight or obesity in a socioeconomically disadvantaged region of australia: a longitudinal cohort analysis. Int. J. Environ. Res. Public Health 15 (8), 1685. https://doi.org/10.3390/ijerph15081685. 30087304. PMC6121544.

Martin, R.M., Kramer, M.S., Patel, R., Rifas-Shiman, S.L., Thompson, J., Yang, S., Vilchuck, K., Bogdanovich, N., Hameza, M., Tilling, K., Oken, E., 2017. Effects of promoting long-term, exclusive breastfeeding on adolescent adiposity, blood pressure, and growth trajectories: a secondary analysis of a randomized clinical trial. JAMA Pediatr. 171 (7). https://doi.org/10.1001/jamapediatrics.2017.0698, e170698. Epub 2017 Jul 3 28459932. PMC5576545.

Martín-Calvo, N., Martínez-González, M.Á., Segura, G., Chavarro, J.E., Carlos, S., Gea, A., 2020. Caesarean delivery is associated with higher risk of overweight in the offspring: within-family analysis in the SUN cohort. J. Epidemiol. Community Health 74 (7), 586–591. https://doi.org/10.1136/jech-2019-213724. Epub 2020 Apr 24 32332117. PMC7293569.

Matheson, D.M., Killen, J.D., Wang, Y., Varady, A., Robinson, T.N., 2004. Children's food consumption during television viewing. Am. J. Clin. Nutr. 79 (6), 1088–1094.

Mazarello Paes, V., Hesketh, K., O'Malley, C., Moore, H., Summerbell, C., Griffin, S., van Sluijs, E., Ong, K., Lakshman, R., 2015. Determinants of sugar-sweetened beverage consumption in young children: a systematic review. Obes. Rev. 16 (11), 903–913.

Mendoza, J., Zimmerman, F., Christakis, D., 2007. Television viewing, computer use, obesity, and adiposity in US preschool children. Int. J. Behav. Nutr. Phys. Act. 4 (1), 44.

Mennella, J., Bobowski, N., 2015. The sweetness and bitterness of childhood: insights from basic research on taste preferences. Physiol. Behav. 152, 502–507.

Mennella, J., Ventura, A., 2011. Early feeding: setting the stage for healthy eating habits. Nestle Nutr. Workshop Ser. Pediatr. Program. 68, 153–163.

Meyer, D.M., Brei, C., Stecher, L., Much, D., Brunner, S., Hauner, H., 2017. The relationship between breast milk leptin and adiponectin with child body composition from 3 to 5 years: a follow-up study Pediatr. Obes., 125–129.

Mihrshahi, S., Battistutta, D., Magarey, A., Daniels, L.A., 2011. Determinants of rapid weight gain during infancy: baseline results from the NOURISH randomised controlled trial. BMC Pediatr. 11, 99. https://doi.org/10.1186/1471-2431-11-99. 22054415. PMC3226648.

Miller, S., Taveras, E., Rifas-Shiman, S., Gillman, M., 2008. Association between television viewing and poor diet quality in young children. Int. J. Pediatr. Obes. 3 (3), 168–176.

Miller, S.A., Wu, R.K.S., Oremus, M., 2018. The association between antibiotic use in infancy and childhood overweight or obesity: a systematic review and meta-analysis. Obes. Rev. 19 (11), 1463–1475. https://doi.org/10.1111/obr.12717. Epub 2018 Jul 23 30035851.

Miller, M.A., Kruisbrink, M., Wallace, J., Ji, C., Cappuccio, F.P., 2018a. Sleep duration and incidence of obesity in infants, children, and adolescents: a systematic review and meta-analysis of prospective studies. Sleep 1, 41(4). https://doi.org/10.1093/sleep/zsy018. 29401314.

Miller, M.A., Bates, S., Ji, C., Cappuccio, F.P., 2021. Systematic review and meta-analyses of the relationship between short sleep and incidence of obesity and effectiveness of sleep interventions on weight gain in preschool children. Obes. Rev. 22 (2). https://doi.org/10.1111/obr.13113, e13113. Epub 2020 Aug 15 33237635.

Mohammadkhah, A.I., Simpson, E.B., Patterson, S.G., Ferguson, J.F., 2018. Development of the gut microbiome in children, and lifetime implications for obesity and cardiometabolic disease. Children (Basel) 5 (12), 160. https://doi.org/10.3390/children5120160. 30486462. PMC6306821.

Monasta, L., Batty, G., Cattaneo, A., Lutje, V., Ronfani, L., Van Lenthe, F., 2011. Early-life determinants of overweight and obesity: a review of systematic reviews. Obes. Metabol. 2, 76–77.

Moossavi, S., Miliku, K., Sepehri, S., Khafipour, E., Azad, M.B., 2018. The prebiotic and probiotic properties of human milk: implications for infant immune development and pediatric asthma. Front. Pediatr. 24 (6), 197. https://doi.org/10.3389/fped.2018.00197. 30140664. PMC6095009.

Mor, A., Antonsen, S., Kahlert, J., Holsteen, V., Jørgensen, S., Holm-Pedersen, J., Sørensen, H.T., Pedersen, O., Ehrenstein, V., 2015. Prenatal exposure to systemic antibacterials and overweight and obesity in Danish schoolchildren: a prevalence study. Int. J. Obes. (Lond.) 39 (10), 1450–1455. https://doi.org/10.1038/ijo.2015.129.

Moss, B., Yeaton, W., 2012. U. S. children's preschool weight status trajectories: patterns from 9-month, 2-year, and 4-year early childhood longitudinal study–birth cohort data. Am. J. Health Promot. 26 (3), 172–175.

Moss, B., Yeaton, W., 2014. Early childhood healthy and obese weight status: potentially protective benefits of breastfeeding and delaying solid foods. Matern. Child Health J. 18 (5), 1224–1232.

Motivala, S., Tomiyama, A., Ziegler, M., Khandrika, S., Irwin, M., 2009. Nocturnal levels of ghrelin and leptin and sleep in chronic insomnia. Psychoneuroendocrinology 34 (4), 540–545.

Mueller, N.T., Bakacs, E., Combellick, J., Grigoryan, Z., Dominguez-Bello, M.G., 2015a. The infant microbiome development: mom matters. Trends Mol. Med. 21 (2), 109–117. https://doi.org/10.1016/j.molmed.2014.12.002. Epub 2014 Dec 11 25578246. PMC4464665.

Mueller, N.T., Whyatt, R., Hoepner, L., Oberfield, S., Dominguez-Bello, M.G., Widen, E.M., Hassoun, A., Perera, F., Rundle, A., 2015b. Prenatal exposure to antibiotics, cesarean section and risk of childhood obesity. Int. J. Obes. (Lond) 39 (4), 665–670. https://doi.org/10.1038/ijo.2014.180. Epub 2014 Oct 9 25298276. PMC4390478.

Mueller, N.T., Mao, G., Bennet, W.L., Hourigan, S.K., Dominguez-Bello, M.G., Appel, L.J., Wang, X., 2017. Does vaginal delivery mitigate or strengthen the intergenerational association of overweight and obesity? Findings from the Boston Birth Cohort. Int. J. Obes. (Lond) 41 (4), 497–501. https://doi.org/10.1038/ijo.2016.219. Epub 2016 Nov 30 27899809. PMC5380521.

Murakami K., Livingstone M.B., 2016 Associations between meal and snack frequency and overweight and abdominal obesity in US children and adolescents from National Health and Nutrition Examination Survey (NHANES) 2003-2012 Br. J. Nutr. 2016 1819-1829.

National Academies of Sciences, Engineering, and Medicine (NAS), 2020. Feeding Infants and Children from Birth to 24 Months: Summarizing Existing Guidance. The National Academies Press, Washington, DC.

NCD Risk Factor Collaboration (NCD-RisC), 2017. Worldwide trends in body-mass index, underweight, overweight, and obesity from 1975 to 2016: a pooled analysis of 2416 population-based measurement studies in 128·9 million children, adolescents, and adults. Lancet 390 (10113), 2627–2642. https://doi.org/10.1016/S0140-6736(17)32129-3. Epub 2017 Oct 10 29029897. PMC5735219.

Newens, K.J., Walton, J., 2016. A review of sugar consumption from nationally representative dietary surveys across the world. J. Hum. Nutr. Diet. 29 (2), 225–240. https://doi.org/10.1111/jhn.12338. Epub 2015 Oct 10 26453428. PMC5057348.

Ogden, C., Carroll, M., Kit, B., Flegal, K., 2014. Prevalence of childhood and adult obesity in the United States, 2011-2012. JAMA 311 (8), 806.

Okubo, H., Crozier, S., Harvey, N., Godfrey, K., Inskip, H., Cooper, C., Robinson, S., 2014. Maternal dietary glycemic index and glycemic load in early pregnancy are associated with offspring adiposity in childhood: the Southampton Women's Survey. Am. J. Clin. Nutr. 100 (2), 676–683.

Ong, K., Loos, R., 2006. Rapid infancy weight gain and subsequent obesity: systematic reviews and hopeful suggestions. Acta Paediatr. 95 (8), 904–908.

Ong, K.K., Emmett, P.M., Noble, S., Ness, A., Dunger, D.B., ALSPAC Study Team, 2006. Dietary energy intake at the age of 4 months predicts postnatal weight gain and childhood body mass index. Pediatrics 117 (3), e503–e508. https://doi.org/10.1542/peds.2005-1668. 16510629.

Owen, C.G., Martin, R.M., Whincup, P.H., Davey-Smith, G., Gillman, M.W., Cook, D.G., 2005. The effect of breast-feeding on mean body mass index throughout life: a quantitative review of published and unpublished observational evidence. Am. J. Clin. Nutr. 82 (6), 1298–1307.

Pan, L., Li, R., Park, S., Galuska, D., Sherry, B., Freedman, D., 2014. A longitudinal analysis of sugar sweetened beverage intake in infancy and obesity at 6 years. Pediatrics, S29–S35.

Pannaraj, P.S., Li, F., Cerini, C., Bender, J.M., Yang, S., Rollie, A., Adisetiyo, H., Zabih, S., Lincez, P.J., Bittinger, K., Bailey, A., Bushman, F.D., Sleasman, J.W., Aldrovandi, G.M., 2017. Association between breast milk bacterial communities and establishment and development of the infant gut microbiome. JAMA Pediatr. 171 (7), 647–654. https://doi.org/10.1001/jamapediatrics.2017.0378. 28492938. PMC5710346.

Papoutsou, S., Savva, S.C., Hunsberger, M., et al., 2018. Timing of solid food introduction and association with later childhood overweight and obesity: The IDEFICS study. Matern. Child Nutr. 14 (1). https://doi.org/10.1111/mcn.12471, e12471.

Paruthi, S., Brooks, L.J., D'Ambrosio, C., Hall, W.A., Kotagal, S., Lloyd, R.M., Malow, B.A., Maski, K., Nichols, C., Quan, S.F., Rosen, C.L., Troester, M.M., Wise, M.S., 2016. Recommended amount of sleep for pediatric populations: a consensus statement of the american academy of sleep medicine. J. Clin. Sleep Med. 12 (6), 785–786. https://doi.org/10.5664/jcsm.5866. 27250809. PMC4877308.

Patro-Gołąb, B., Zalewski, B.M., Kołodziej, M., Kouwenhoven, S., Poston, L., Godfrey, K.M., Koletzko, B., van Goudoever, J.B., Szajewska, H., 2016. Nutritional interventions or exposures in infants and children aged up to 3 years and their effects on subsequent risk of overweight, obesity and body fat: a systematic review of systematic reviews. Obes. Rev. 17 (12), 1245–1257. https://doi.org/10.1111/obr.12476. Epub 2016 Oct 17. Erratum in: Obes Rev. 2018 Nov;19(11):1620 27749991. PMC5325317.

Pattison, K.L., Kraschnewski, J.L., Lehman, E., Savage, J.S., Downs, D.S., Leonard, K.S., Adams, E.L., Paul, I.M., Kjerulff, K.H., 2019. Breastfeeding initiation and duration and child health outcomes in the first baby study. Prev. Med. 118, 1–6. https://doi.org/10.1016/j.ypmed.2018.09.020. Epub 2018 Oct 1 30287329. PMC6322935.

Paul, I., Savage, J., Anzman, S., Beiler, J., Marini, M., Stokes, J., Birch, L., 2010. Preventing obesity during infancy: a pilot study. Obesity 19 (2), 353–361.

Pauwels, S., Symons, L., Vanautgaerden, E.-L., Ghosh, M., Duca, R.C., Bekaert, B., Freson, K., Huybrechts, I., Langie, S.A.S., Koppen, G., Devlieger, R., Godderis, L., 2019. The influence of the duration of breastfeeding on the infant's metabolic epigenome. Nutrients 11 (6), 1408. https://doi.org/10.3390/nu11061408.

Payne, A.N., Chassard, C., Zimmermann, M., Müller, P., Stinca, S., Lacroix, C., 2011. The metabolic activity of gut microbiota in obese children is increased compared with normal-weight children and exhibits more exhaustive substrate utilization. Nutr. Diabetes 1 (7). https://doi.org/10.1038/nutd.2011.8, e12. 23154580. PMC3302137.

Pearce, J., Taylor, M., Langley-Evans, S., 2013. Timing of the introduction of complementary feeding and risk of childhood obesity: a systematic review. Int. J. Obes. Relat. Metab. Disord. 37 (10), 1295–1306.

Pérez-Escamilla, R., Segura-Pérez, S., Lott, M., 2017. On behalf of the RWJF HER expert panel on best practices for promoting healthy nutrition, feeding patterns, and weight status for infants and toddlers from birth to 24 months. In: Feeding Guidelines for Infants and Young Toddlers: A Responsive Parenting Approach. Healthy Eating Research, Durham, NC.

Philips, E.M., Santos, S., Trasande, L., Aurrekoetxea, J.J., Barros, H., et al., 2020. Changes in parental smoking during pregnancy and risks of adverse birth outcomes and childhood overweight in Europe and North America: an individual participant data meta-analysis of 229,000 singleton births. PLoS Med. 17 (8). https://doi.org/10.1371/journal.pmed.1003182, e1003182.

Pimpin, L., Jebb, S., Johnson, L., Wardle, J., Ambrosini, G.L., 2016. Dietary protein intake is associated with body mass index and weight up to 5 y of age in a prospective cohort of twins. Am. J. Clin. Nutr. 103 (2), 389–397. https://doi.org/10.3945/ajcn.115.118612. Epub 2015 Dec 30 26718416. PMC4733258.

Pluymen, L.P.M., Wijga, A.H., Gehring, U., Koppelman, G.H., Smit, H.A., van Rossem, L., 2018. Early introduction of complementary foods and childhood overweight in breastfed and formula-fed infants in the Netherlands: the PIAMA birth cohort study. Eur. J. Nutr. 57 (5), 1985–1993. https://doi.org/10.1007/s00394-018-1639-8. Epub 2018 Feb 22 29470690. PMC6060808.

Poitras, V.J., Gray, C.E., Janssen, X., Aubert, S., Carson, V., Faulkner, G., Goldfield, G.S., Reilly, J.J., Sampson, M., Tremblay, M.S., 2017. Systematic review of the relationships between sedentary behaviour and health indicators in the early years (0-4years). BMC Public Health 17 (Suppl 5), 868. https://doi.org/10.1186/s12889-017-4849-8. 29219092. PMC5773886.

Putet, G., Labaune, J.M., Mace, K., Steenhout, P., Grathwohl, D., Raverot, V., Morel, Y., Picaud, J.C., 2016. Effect of dietary protein on plasma insulin-like growth factor-1, growth, and body composition in healthy term infants: a randomised, double-blind, controlled trial (Early Protein and Obesity in Childhood (EPOCH) study). Br. J. Nutr. 115 (2), 271–284. https://doi.org/10.1017/S0007114515004456. Epub 2015 Nov 20 26586096. PMC4697297.

Qiao, J., Dai, L.J., Zhang, Q., Ouyang, Y.Q., 2020. A meta-analysis of the association between breastfeeding and early childhood obesity. J. Pediatr. Nurs. 53, 57–66. https://doi.org/10.1016/j.pedn.2020.04.024. Epub 2020 May 25 32464422.

Ralphs, E., Pembrey, L., West, J., Santorelli, G., 2021. Association between mode of delivery and body mass index at 4-5 years in White British and Pakistani children: the Born in Bradford birth cohort. BMC Public Health 21 (1), 987. https://doi.org/10.1186/s12889-021-11009-y. 34039335. PMC8152119.

Rasmussen, S.H., Shrestha, S., Bjerregaard, L.G., Ängquist, L.H., Baker, J.L., Jess, T., Allin, K.H., 2018. Antibiotic exposure in early life and childhood overweight and obesity: a systematic review and meta-analysis. Diabetes Obes. Metab. 20 (6), 1508–1514. https://doi.org/10.1111/dom.13230. Epub 2018 Feb 25 29359849.

Rayfield, S., Plugge, E., 2017. Systematic review and meta-analysis of the association between maternal smoking in pregnancy and childhood overweight and obesity. J. Epidemiol. Community Health 71 (2), 162–173. https://doi.org/10.1136/jech-2016-207376. Epub 2016 Aug 1 27480843.

Reilly, J.J., Armstrong, J., Dorosty, A.R., Emmett, P.M., Ness, A., Rogers, I., Steer, C., Sherriff, A., Avon Longitudinal Study of Parents and Children Study Team, 2005. Early life risk factors for obesity in childhood: cohort study. BMJ 330 (7504), 1357. https://doi.org/10.1136/bmj.38470.670903.E0. Epub 2005 May 20 15908441. PMC558282.

Reilly, J.J., Hughes, A.R., Gillespie, J., Malden, S., Martin, A., 2019. Physical activity interventions in early life aimed at reducing later risk of obesity and related non-communicable diseases: a rapid review of systematic reviews. Obes. Rev. 20 (Suppl 1), 61–73. https://doi.org/10.1111/obr.12773. 31419046.

Riedel, C., Schönberger, K., Yang, S., Koshy, G., Chen, Y.C., Gopinath, B., Ziebarth, S., von Kries, R., 2014. Parental smoking and childhood obesity: higher effect estimates for maternal smoking in pregnancy compared with paternal smoking – a meta-analysis. Int. J. Epidemiol. 43 (5), 1593–1606. https://doi.org/10.1093/ije/dyu150.

Rifas-Shiman, S.L., Gillman, M.W., Hawkins, S.S., Oken, E., Taveras, E.M., Kleinman, K.P., 2018. Association of cesarean delivery with body mass index z score at age 5 years. JAMA Pediatr. 172 (8), 777–779. https://doi.org/10.1001/jamapediatrics.2018.0674.

Rifas-Shiman, S.L., Huh, S.Y., Martin, R.M., Kramer, M., Patel, R., Bogdanovich, N., Vilchuck, K., Thompson, J., Oken, E., 2021. Delivery by caesarean section and offspring adiposity and cardio-metabolic health at ages 6.5, 11.5 and 16 years: results from the PROBIT cohort in Belarus. Pediatr. Obes. 16 (9). https://doi.org/10.1111/ijpo.12783, e12783.

Rinninella, E., Raoul, P., Cintoni, M., Franceschi, F., Miggiano, G.A.D., Gasbarrini, A., Mele, M.C., 2019. What is the healthy gut microbiota composition? A changing ecosystem across age, environment, diet, and diseases. Microorganisms 7 (1), 14. https://doi.org/10.3390/microorganisms7010014. 30634578. PMC6351938.

Rito, A.I., Buoncristiano, M., Spinelli, A., Salanave, B., Kunešová, M., et al., 2019. Association between characteristics at birth, breastfeeding and obesity in 22 countries: the WHO European childhood obesity surveillance initiative—COSI 2015/2017. Obes. Facts 12 (2), 226–243. https://doi.org/10.1159/000500425. Epub 2019 Apr 26 31030194. PMC6547266.

Robson, S.M., McCullough, M.B., Rex, S., Munafò, M.R., Taylor, G., 2020. Family meal frequency, diet, and family functioning: a systematic review with meta-analyses. J. Nutr. Educ. Behav. 52 (5), 553–564. https://doi.org/10.1016/j.jneb.2019.12.012. Epub 2020 Jan 23 31982371.

Roess, A.A., Jacquier, E.F., Catellier, D.J., Carvalho, R., Lutes, A.C., Anater, A.S., Dietz, W.H., 2018. Food consumption patterns of infants and toddlers: findings from the feeding infants and toddlers study (FITS) 2016. J. Nutr. 148 (suppl_3), 1525S–1535S. https://doi.org/10.1093/jn/nxy171. 30247583. PMC6126630.

Rogers, I., EURO-BLCS Study Group, 2003. The influence of birthweight and intrauterine environment on adiposity and fat distribution in later life. Int. J. Obes. Relat. Metab. Disord. 27 (7), 755–777. https://doi.org/10.1038/sj.ijo.0802316. 12821960.

Rolland-Cachera, M.F., Maillot, M., Deheeger, M., Souberbielle, J.C., Péneau, S., Hercberg, S., 2013. Association of nutrition in early life with body fat and serum leptin at adult age. Int. J. Obes. (Lond) 37 (8), 1116–1122. https://doi.org/10.1038/ijo.2012.185. Epub 2012 Nov 13 23147117.

Rolland-Cachera, M.F., Akrout, M., Péneau, S., 2016. Nutrient intakes in early life and risk of obesity. Int. J. Environ. Res. Public Health 13 (6), 564. https://doi.org/10.3390/ijerph13060564. 27275827. PMC4924021.

Rzehak, P., Oddy, W.H., Mearin, M.L., Grote, V., Mori, T.A., Szajewska, H., Shamir, R., Koletzko, S., Weber, M., Beilin, L.J., Huang, R.C., Koletzko, B., 2017. WP10 working group of the Early Nutrition Project. Infant feeding and growth trajectory patterns in childhood and body composition in young adulthood. Am. J. Clin. Nutr. 106 (2), 568–580. https://doi.org/10.3945/ajcn.116.140962. Epub 2017 Jun 28 28659295.

Słabuszewska-Jóźwiak, A., Szymański, J.K., Ciebiera, M., Sarecka-Hujar, B., Jakiel, G., 2020. Pediatrics consequences of caesarean section—a systematic review and meta-analysis. Int. J. Environ. Res. Public Health 17 (21), 8031. https://doi.org/10.3390/ijerph17218031. 33142727. PMC7662709.

Saavedra, J., Deming, D., Dattilo, A., Reidy, K., 2013. Lessons from the feeding infants and toddlers study in North America: what children eat, and implications for obesity prevention. Ann. Nutr. Metab. 62 (s3), 27–36.

Santorelli, G., Fairley, L., Petherick, E.S., Cabieses, B., Sahota, P., 2014. Ethnic differences in infant feeding practices and their relationship with BMI at 3 years of age—results from the Born in Bradford birth cohort study. Br. J. Nutr. 111 (10), 1891–1897.

Savino, F., Fissore, M.F., Liguori, S.A., Oggero, R., 2009. Can hormones contained in mothers' milk account for the beneficial effect of breast-feeding on obesity in children? Clin. Endocrinol. (Oxf) 71 (6), 757–765. https://doi.org/10.1111/j.1365-2265.2009.03585.x. Epub 2009 Mar 19 19302580.

Saxon, T.F., Gollapalli, A., Mitchell, M.W., Stanko, S., 2002. Demand feeding or schedule feeding: Infant growth from birth to 6 months. J. Reprod. Infant Psychol. 20, 89–99. https://doi.org/10.1080/02646830220134586.

Scheepers, L.E., Penders, J., Mbakwa, C.A., Thijs, C., Mommers, M., Arts, I.C., 2015. The intestinal microbiota composition and weight development in children: the KOALA Birth Cohort Study. Int. J. Obes. (Lond) 39 (1), 16–25. https://doi.org/10.1038/ijo.2014.178. Epub 2014 Oct 9 25298274.

Scott, J., Binns, C., Graham, K., Oddy, W., 2009. Predictors of the early introduction of solid foods in infants: results of a cohort study. BMC Pediatr. 9 (1), 60.

Shapiro, A., Kaar, J., Crume, T., Starling, A., Siega-Riz, A., Ringham, B., Glueck, D., Norris, J., Barbour, L., Friedman, J., Dabelea, D., 2016. Maternal diet quality in pregnancy and neonatal adiposity: the healthy start study. Int. J. Obes. Relat. Metab. Disord. 40 (7), 1056–1062.

Siega-Riz, A., Deming, D., Reidy, K., Fox, M., Condon, E., Briefel, R., 2010. Food consumption patterns of infants and toddlers: where are we now? J. Am. Diet. Assoc. 110 (12), S38–S51.

Silventoinen, K., Jelenkovic, A., Sund, R., Hur, Y.M., Yokoyama, Y., Honda, C., et al., 2016. Genetic and environmental effects on body mass index from infancy to the onset of adulthood: an individual-based pooled analysis of 45 twin cohorts participating in the COllaborative project of Development of Anthropometrical measures in Twins (CODATwins) study. Am. J. Clin. Nutr. 104 (2), 371–379. https://doi.org/10.3945/ajcn.116.130252. Epub 2016 Jul 13 27413137. PMC4962159.

Sleddens, E., Gerards, S., Thijs, C., de Vries, N., Kremers, S., 2011. General parenting, childhood overweight and obesity-inducing behaviors: a review. Int. J. Pediatr. Obes. 6 (2–2), e12–e27.

Smithers, L.G., Kramer, M.S., Lynch, J.W., 2015. Effects of breastfeeding on obesity and intelligence: causal insights from different study designs. JAMA Pediatr. 169 (8), 707–708. https://doi.org/10.1001/jamapediatrics.2015.0175. 26053565.

Socha, P., Grote, V., Gruszfeld, D., Janas, R., Demmelmair, H., Closa-Monasterolo, R., Subías, J.E., Scaglioni, S., Verduci, E., Dain, E., Langhendries, J.P., Perrin, E., Koletzko, B., European Childhood Obesity Trial Study Group, 2011. Milk protein intake, the metabolic-endocrine response, and growth in infancy: data from a randomized clinical trial. Am. J. Clin. Nutr. 94 (6 Suppl), 1776S–1784S. https://doi.org/10.3945/ajcn.110.000596. Epub 2011 Aug 17 21849603.

Sonneville, K.R., 2015. Juice and water intake in infancy and later beverage intake and adiposity: could juice be a gateway drink? Obesity, 170–176.

Spahn, J.M., Callahan, E.H., Spill, M.K., Wong, Y.P., Benjamin-Neelon, S.E., Birch, L., Black, M.M., Cook, J.T., Faith, M.S., Mennella, J.A., Casavale, K.O., 2019. Influence of maternal diet on flavor transfer to amniotic fluid and breast milk and children's responses: a systematic review. Am. J. Clin. Nutr. 109 (Suppl_7), 1003S–1026S. https://doi.org/10.1093/ajcn/nqy240. 30982867.

Specht, I.O., Rohde, J.F., Olsen, N.J., Heitmann, B.L., 2018. Duration of exclusive breastfeeding may be related to eating behaviour and dietary intake in obesity prone normal weight young children. PLoS One 13 (7). https://doi.org/10.1371/journal.pone.0200388, e0200388. 29995949. PMC6040730.

Spill, M.K., Callahan, E.H., Shapiro, M.J., Spahn, J.M., Wong, Y.P., Benjamin-Neelon, S.E., Birch, L., Black, M.M., Cook, J.T., Faith, M.S., Mennella, J.A., Casavale, K.O., 2019. Caregiver feeding practices and child weight outcomes: a systematic review. Am. J. Clin. Nutr. 109 (Suppl_7), 990S–1002S. https://doi.org/10.1093/ajcn/nqy276. 30982865.

Stan, S.V., Grathwohl, D., O'Neill, L.M., Saavedra, J.M., Butte, N.F., Cohen, S.S., 2021. Estimated energy requirements of infants and young children up to 24 months of age. Curr. Dev. Nutr. 5 (11). https://doi.org/10.1093/cdn/nzab122, nzab122. 34761158. PMC8575726.

Stanislawski, M.A., Dabelea, D., Wagner, B.D., Iszatt, N., Dahl, C., Sontag, M.K., Knight, R., Lozupone, C.A., Eggesbø, M., 2018. Gut microbiota in the first 2 years of life and the association with body mass index at age 12 in a norwegian birth cohort. MBio 9 (5). https://doi.org/10.1128/mBio.01751-18, e01751-18. 30352933. PMC6199494.

Starling, A., Brinton, J., Glueck, D., Shapiro, A., Harrod, C., Lynch, A., Siega-Riz, A., Dabelea, D., 2014. Associations of maternal BMI and gestational weight gain with neonatal adiposity in the healthy start study. Am. J. Clin. Nutr. 101 (2), 302–309.

Stettler, N., Iotova, V., 2010. Early growth patterns and long-term obesity risk. Curr. Opin. Clin. Nutr. Metab. Care 13 (3), 294–299.

Stinson, L.F., 2020. Establishment of the early-life microbiome: a DOHaD perspective. J. Dev. Orig. Health Dis. 11 (3), 201–210. https://doi.org/10.1017/S2040174419000588. Epub 2019 Oct 11 31601287.

Suthutvoravut, U., Abiodun, P., Chomtho, S., Chongviriyaphan, N., Cruchet, S., Davies, P., Fuchs, G., Gopalan, S., van Goudoever, J., Nel, E., Scheimann, A., Spolidoro, J., Tontisirin, K., Wang, W., Winichagoon, P., Koletzko, B., 2015. Composition of follow-up formula for young children aged 12–36 months: recommendations of an international expert group coordinated by the nutrition association of Thailand and the early nutrition academy. Ann. Nutr. Metab. 67 (2), 119–132.

Taveras, E., Rifas-Shiman, S., Oken, E., Gunderson, E., Gillman, M., 2008. Short sleep duration in infancy and risk of childhood overweight. Arch. Pediatr. Adolesc. Med. 162 (4), 305.

Taveras, E., Blackburn, K., Gillman, M., Haines, J., McDonald, J., Price, S., Oken, E., 2010a. First steps for mommy and me: a pilot intervention to improve nutrition and physical activity behaviors of postpartum mothers and their infants. Matern. Child Health J. 15 (8), 1217–1227.

Taveras, E., Gillman, M., Kleinman, K., Rich-Edwards, J., Rifas-Shiman, S., 2010b. Racial/ethnic differences in early-life risk factors for childhood obesity. Pediatrics 125 (4), 686–695.

Taveras, E.M., Gillman, M.W., Peña, M.-M., Redline, S., Rifas-Shiman, S.L., 2014. Chronic sleep curtailment and adiposity. Pediatrics 133 (6), 1013–1022.

Tian, Z., Ye, T., Zhang, X., Liu, E., Wang, W., Wang, P., Liu, G., Yang, X., Hu, G., Yu, Z., 2010. Sleep duration and hyperglycemia among obese and nonobese children aged 3 to 6 years. Arch. Pediatr. Adolesc. Med. 164 (1), 46–52.

Totzauer, M., Luque, V., Escribano, J., Closa-Monasterolo, R., Verduci, E., ReDionigi, A., Hoyos, J., Langhendries, J.P., Gruszfeld, D., Socha, P., Koletzko, B., Grote, V., European Childhood Obesity Trial Study Group, 2018. Effect of lower versus higher protein content in infant formula through the first year on body composition from 1 to 6 years: follow-up of a randomized clinical trial. Obesity (Silver Spring) 26 (7), 1203–1210. https://doi.org/10.1002/oby.22203. 29932518.

Trabulsi, J., Mennella, J., 2012. Diet, sensitive periods in flavour learning, and growth. Int. Rev. Psychiatry 24 (3), 219–230.

Tun, H.M., Bridgman, S.L., Chari, R., Field, C.J., Guttman, D.S., Becker, A.B., Mandhane, P.J., Turvey, S.E., Subbarao, P., Sears, M.R., Scott, J.A., Kozyrskyj, A.L., Canadian Healthy Infant Longitudinal Development (CHILD) Study Investigators, 2018. Roles of birth mode and infant gut microbiota in intergenerational transmission of overweight and obesity from mother to offspring. JAMA Pediatr. 172 (4), 368–377. https://doi.org/10.1001/jamapediatrics.2017.5535. 29459942. PMC5875322.

Uesugi, K., Dattilo, A.M., Black, M., Saavedra, J.M., 2016. Design of a digital-based, multi-component nutrition guidance system for prevention of early childhood obesity. J. Obes. 2016, 12.

United Nations Children's Fund (UNICEF), 2016. From the First Hour of Life. A New Report on Infant and Young Child Feeding. October 2016: New York, NY https://data.unicef.org/resources/first-hour-life-new-report-breastfeeding-practices/.

United Nations Children's Fund (UNICEF), 2019. The State of the World's Children 2019. Children, Food and Nutrition: Growing well in a changing world. UNICEF, New York. ISBN:978-92-806-5003-7.

United Nations Children's Fund (UNICEF), World Health Organization, International Bank for Reconstruction and Development/The World Bank, 2021. Levels and Trends in Child Malnutrition: Key Findings of the 2021 Edition of the Joint Child Malnutrition Estimates. World Health Organization, Geneva. Licence: CC BY-NC-SA 3.0 IGO.

USDA, 2019. What are Added Sugars? https://ask.usda.gov/s/article/What-are-added-sugars.

USDA, 2020. U.S. Department of Agriculture and U.S. Department of Health and Human Services. Dietary Guidelines for Americans, 2020-2025, ninth ed. December 2020 DietaryGuidelines.gov.

Vael, C., Verhulst, S.L., Nelen, V., Goossens, H., Desager, K.N., 2011. Intestinal microflora and body mass index during the first three years of life: an observational study. Gut Pathog. 3 (1), 8. https://doi.org/10.1186/1757-4749-3-8. 21605455. PMC3118227.

Ventura, A.K., Li, R., Xu, X., 2020. Associations between bottle-feeding during infancy and obesity at age 6 years are mediated by greater infancy weight gain. Child. Obes. 16 (5), 316–326. https://doi.org/10.1089/chi.2019.0299. Epub 2020 Jun 4 32498550.

Ventura, A., Hupp, M., Lavond, J., 2021. Mother-infant interactions and infant intake during breastfeeding versus bottle-feeding expressed breast milk. Matern. Child Nutr. 17 (4), e13185. https://doi.org/10.1111/mcn.13185. Epub 2021 May 3 33939269. PMC8476436.

Victora, C., Bahl, R., Barros, A., França, G., Horton, S., Krasevec, J., Murch, S., Sankar, M., Walker, N., Rollins, N., 2016. Breastfeeding in the 21st century: epidemiology, mechanisms, and lifelong effect. Lancet 387 (10017), 475–490.

Voerman, E., Santos, S., Patro Golab, B., Amiano, P., Ballester, F., et al., 2019. Maternal body mass index, gestational weight gain, and the risk of overweight and obesity across childhood: an individual participant data meta-analysis. PLoS Med. 16 (2). https://doi.org/10.1371/journal.pmed.1002744, e1002744.

Voortman, T., Braun, K.V., Kiefte-de Jong, J.C., Jaddoe, V.W., Franco, O.H., van den Hooven, E.H., 2016. Protein intake in early childhood and body composition at the age of 6 years: the generation R study. Int. J. Obes. (Lond) 40 (6), 1018–1025. https://doi.org/10.1038/ijo.2016.29. Epub 2016 Feb 15 26975442.

Wall, C.R., Hill, R.J., Lovell, A.L., Matsuyama, M., Milne, T., Grant, C.C., Jiang, Y., Chen, R.X., Wouldes, T.A., Davies, P.S.W., 2019. A multicenter, double-blind, randomized, placebo-controlled trial to evaluate the effect of consuming Growing Up Milk "Lite" on body composition in children aged 12-23 mo. Am. J. Clin. Nutr. 109 (3), 576–585. https://doi.org/10.1093/ajcn/nqy302. 30831579.

Walters, D.D., Phan, L.T.H., Mathisen, R., 2019. The cost of not breastfeeding: global results from a new tool. Health Policy Plan. 34 (6), 407–417. https://doi.org/10.1093/heapol/czz050. 31236559. PMC6735804.

Wang, J., Wu, Y., Xiong, G., Chao, T., Jin, Q., Liu, R., Hao, L., Wei, S., Yang, N., Yang, X., 2016. Introduction of complementary feeding before 4months of age increases the risk of childhood overweight or obesity: a meta-analysis of prospective cohort studies. Nutr. Res. 36 (8), 759–770. https://doi.org/10.1016/j.nutres.2016.03.003. Epub 2016 Mar 3 27440530.

Wasser, H., Bentley, M., Borja, J., Davis Goldman, B., Thompson, A., Slining, M., Adair, L., 2011. Infants perceived as "fussy" are more likely to receive complementary foods before 4 months. Pediatrics 127 (2), 229–237.

Weber, M., Grote, V., Closa-Monasterolo, R., Escribano, J., Langhendries, J., Dain, E., Giovannini, M., Verduci, E., Gruszfeld, D., Socha, P., Koletzko, B., 2014. Lower protein content in infant formula reduces BMI and obesity risk at school age: follow-up of a randomized trial. Am. J. Clin. Nutr. 99 (5), 1041–1051.

Weng, S.F., Redsell, S.A., Swift, J.A., Yang, M., Glazebrook, C.P., 2012. Systematic review and meta-analyses of risk factors for childhood overweight identifiable during infancy. Arch. Dis. Child. 97 (12), 1019–1026. https://doi.org/10.1136/archdischild-2012-302263. Epub 2012 Oct 29 23109090. PMC3512440.

Winter, J., Langenberg, P., Krugman, S., 2010. Newborn adiposity by body mass index predicts childhood overweight. Clin. Pediatr. 49, 866–870.

Woo Baidal, J.A., Locks, L.M., Cheng, E.R., Blake-Lamb, T.L., Perkins, M.E., Taveras, E.M., 2016. Risk Factors for Childhood Obesity in the First 1,000 Days: A Systematic Review. Am. J. Prev. Med. 50 (6), 761–779. https://doi.org/10.1016/j.amepre.2015.11.012. Epub 2016 Feb 22 26916261.

Wood, C., Skinner, A., Yin, H., Rothman, R., Sanders, L., Delamater, A., Perrin, E., 2016. Bottle size and weight gain in formula-fed infants. Pediatrics 138 (1), e20154538.

Wood, A.C., Blissett, J.M., Brunstrom, J.M., Carnell, S., Faith, M.S., Fisher, J.O., Hayman, L.L., Khalsa, A.S., Hughes, S.O., Miller, A.L., Momin, S.R., Welsh, J.A., Woo, J.G., Haycraft, E., American Heart Association Council on Lifestyle and Cardiometabolic Health, Council on Epidemiology and Prevention, Council on Lifelong Congenital Heart Disease and Heart Health in the Young, Council on Cardiovascular and Stroke Nursing, Stroke Council, 2020. Caregiver influences on eating behaviors in young children: a scientific statement from the American Heart Association. J. Am. Heart Assoc. 9 (10). https://doi.org/10.1161/JAHA.119.014520, e014520.

World Food Program (WFP), 2020. COVID-19 will double number of people facing food crises unless swift action is taken Reference: WFP April 21, 2020, https://www.wfp.org/news/ (accessed November 2021).

World Health Organization (WHO), 2015. Guideline: Sugars Intake for Adults and Children. World Health Organization, Geneva, p. 2015. 25905159.

World Health Organization (WHO), 2016a. WHO Obesity and overweight Fact sheet. Available from: http://www.who.int/mediacentre/factsheets/fs311/en/.

World Health Organization (WHO), 2016b. WHO Report of the Commission on Ending Childhood Obesity. Available from: http://apps.who.int/iris/bitstream/10665/204176/1/9789241510066_eng.pdf.

World Health Organization (WHO), 2019. Guidelines on Physical Activity, Sedentary Behaviour and Sleep for Children Under 5 Years of Age. World Health Organization. https://apps.who.int/iris/handle/10665/311664.

World Health Organization (WHO), 2021. Obesity. In: WHO Health Topics. https://www.who.int/health-topics/obesity#tab=tab_1.

Worobey, J., Islas Lopez, M., Hoffman, D., 2009. Maternal behavior and infant weight gain in the first year. J. Nutr. Educ. Behav. 41 (3), 169–175.

Wu, A.J., Aris, I.M., Rifas-Shiman, S.L., Oken, E., Taveras, E.M., Hivert, M.F., 2021. Longitudinal associations of fruit juice intake in infancy with DXA-measured abdominal adiposity in mid-childhood and early adolescence. Am. J. Clin. Nutr. 114 (1), 117–123. https://doi.org/10.1093/ajcn/nqab043.

Yan, J., Liu, L., Zhu, Y., Huang, G., Wang, P.P., 2014. The association between breastfeeding and childhood obesity: a meta-analysis. BMC Public Health 14, 1267. https://doi.org/10.1186/1471-2458-14-1267. 25495402. PMC4301835.

Yasmin, F., Tun, H.M., Konya, T.B., Guttman, D.S., Chari, R.S., Field, C.J., Becker, A.B., Mandhane, P.J., Turvey, S.E., Subbarao, P., Sears, M.R., CHILD Study Investigators, Scott, J.A., Dinu, I., Kozyrskyj, A.L., 2017. Cesarean section, formula feeding, and infant antibiotic exposure: separate and combined impacts on gut microbial changes in later infancy. Front. Pediatr. 5, 200. https://doi.org/10.3389/fped.2017.00200. 29018787. PMC5622971.

Young, B.E., 2017. Breastfeeding and human milk: short and long-term health benefits to the recipient infant, chapter 2. In: Saavedra, J.M., Dattilo, A.M. (Eds.), Early Nutrition and Long-Term Health. Woodhead Publishing, ISBN: 9780081001684, pp. 25–53.

Yu, Z.B., Han, S.P., Zhu, G.Z., Zhu, C., Wang, X.J., Cao, X.G., Guo, X.R., 2011. Birth weight and subsequent risk of obesity: a systematic review and meta-analysis. Obes. Rev. 12 (7), 525–542. https://doi.org/10.1111/j.1467-789X.2011.00867.x. Epub 2011 Mar 28 21438992.

Yuan, C., Gaskins, A.J., Blaine, A.I., Zhang, C., Gillman, M.W., Missmer, S.A., Field, A.E., Chavarro, J.E., 2016. Association between cesarean birth and risk of obesity in offspring in childhood, adolescence, and early adulthood. JAMA Pediatr. 170 (11). https://doi.org/10.1001/jamapediatrics.2016.2385, e162385. Epub 2016 Nov 7 27599167. PMC5854473.

Zemrani, B., Gehri, M., Masserey, E., Knob, C., Pellaton, R., 2021. A hidden side of the COVID-19 pandemic in children: the double burden of undernutrition and overnutrition. Int. J. Equity Health 20 (1), 44. https://doi.org/10.1186/s12939-021-01390-w.

# 19

# Establishing healthy eating patterns in infancy

*Cristiana Berti and Carlo Agostoni*

Fondazione IRCCS Ca' Granda Ospedale Maggiore Policlinico, Pediatric Unit, Milano, Italy

## CHAPTER LEARNING OBJECTIVES

- To acquired update and consistent knowledge about healthy feeding in early infancy
- Early nutrition is part of a complex interrelationships between genetics, environment, acquisition of external relationships, and developmental milestones

possibly influencing health at medium- and long-term

- Pediatricians should collaborate with parents and caregivers to raise responsive behavior also in the context of nutrition as a part of a *holistic* individualized approach

## 19.1 Introduction

### 19.1.1 Importance of healthy feeding in early infancy

There is consensus that the first months of life represent the first opportunity to influence the offspring's health and potential (Young et al., 2012). Early nutritional insults likely have short- and long-term consequences on the individual's health and well-being until adulthood by modulating the differentiation of tissues and organs (Berti et al., 2017).

The World Health Organization (WHO) recommends that infants should be exclusively breastfed for the first 6 months to achieve optimal growth, development, and health, with the introduction of appropriate complementary foods thereafter and continued breastfeeding (BF) up to 2 years or beyond (WHO, 2003). BF is acknowledged to exhibit beneficial effects for infants given that human milk is a combination of a balanced supply of nutrients, bioactive proteins and indigestible oligosaccharides, and bifidogenic bacteria (Collado et al., 2012; Çatlı et al., 2014; Berti et al., 2017). Exclusive BF provides adequate nutrition up to 6 months of age for the majority of infants; however, some infants may need complementary foods in addition to BF before 6 months but not before 4 months (Fewtrell et al., 2017). According to the European Society for Pediatric Gastroenterology and Nutrition (ESPGHAN), "exclusive or full BF should be promoted for at least 4 months (17 weeks, beginning of the 5th month of life) and exclusive or predominant BF for approximately 6 months (26 weeks, beginning of the 7th month) is a desirable goal. Complementary foods (solids and liquids other than breast-milk or infant formula) should not be introduced before 4 months but should not be delayed beyond 6 months" (Fewtrell et al., 2017). During this period, basics for future eating patterns are also established as infants learn about what, when, and how much to eat through both the experience itself of eating and the observation of others' eating behaviors, that is the transmission of cultural and familial beliefs, attitudes, and practices around food and eating (Savage et al., 2007). Setting up healthy eating behaviors may be crucial in light of the dramatic increase in prevalence of pediatric overweigh and obesity, non-communicable diseases and micronutrient deficiencies occurring worldwide. Universally, the marked and rapid shifts of contemporary food patterns toward a diet dominated by higher intake of ultra-processed foods, have likely contributed for an obesogenic environment to be established (Popkin, 2006; Scaglioni et al., 2018). Consequently, understanding of factors that shape eating behaviors, i.e., food selection, food preferences, and regulation of food intake in this age group may help improve dietary patterns and health status.

### 19.1.1.1 Complementary feeding and implication for infant health

"Inappropriate feeding practices—sub-optimal or no BF and inadequate complementary feeding—remain the greatest threat to child health and survival globally" (*Innocenti Declaration on Infant and Young Child Feeding*, 2005). Despite recommendations of International Authorities, BF rates and duration remain suboptimal across countries, both low-income (LIC) and high-income countries (HIC) (Rollins et al., 2016), with complementary feeding (CF) introduced to infants aged 4 months or younger (Schiess et al., 2010; Arabi et al., 2012; Barrera et al., 2018). Complementary foods are often nutritionally inadequate (Dewey, 2013) with potential strikingly different implications on anthropometry that is stunting and over-weight in LIC and HIC, respectively (de Onis et al., 2010; Hardwick and Sidnell, 2014; Yang and Huffman, 2013; Young et al., 2012). In LIC and disadvantages populations, CF diets are usually typified by cereal-based porridges with low nutrient-density, poor dietary diversity, and mineral bioavailability (Dewey, 2013; Faber et al., 2016; Lessa et al., 2017). HIC diets exhibit a fall-off of nutrient-density and food variety, too, with high consumption in snacks, sweets, sweetened beverages while low in fruits and vegetables but their energy, protein, sodium, and saturated fat intakes are higher than recommended (Butte et al., 2010; Saavedra et al., 2013).

Mounting body of evidence suggests associations between variations in infant feeding, mainly depending on BF duration and dose (exclusive vs partial), and a range of health outcomes both in the short-medium and long-term ("Programming effects of infant feeding") (Przyrembel, 2012; Robinson and Fall, 2012; Hörnell et al., 2013; Pauwels et al., 2019). Briefly:

✓ BF is associated with lower rates of overall infections up to 1 year of age. BF exclusively at least by 4 months and partially thereafter seems protective for lower respiratory and gastrointestinal infections until the age of 6 months, and for respiratory tract infections between the ages of 7 and 12 months as well (Duijts et al., 2010). During the first half year of life, exclusive BF is more protective toward gastrointestinal infection than partial BF (Feachem and Koblinsky, 1984; Kramer et al., 2003), and partial BF is more protective compared to no BF (Feachem and Koblinsky, 1984). Recently, the EDEN mother–child prospective cohort study evidenced that BF was related to a lower risk of diarrhea events in early infancy and infrequent occurrence of bronchitis/bronchiolitis up to 2 years, and predominant BF duration negatively to the risk of diarrhea events in late infancy, infrequent otitis occurrence, and repeated bronchitis/bronchiolitis events throughout infancy (Davisse-Paturet et al., 2020). In particular, protection against diarrhea and ear infections seems to be afforded in a dose–response manner, that is, the more breast-milk infants receive in the first 6 months of life, the less likely they develop diarrhea or ear infection (Scariati et al., 1997)

✓ A positive association exists between BF and reduced risk of asthma/wheezing as evidenced by a meta-analysis of studies published between 1983 and 2012 (Dogaru et al., 2014) in children population from Europe, North America, South America, Australia, and New Zealand. In particular, children longer breastfed had a lower risk of developing asthma with the strongest association in children 0–2 years of age. The probability of respiratory illness occurring at any time during childhood is significantly reduced if the child is fed exclusively breast-milk for 15 weeks and no solid foods are introduced during this time. Interestingly, children fed a "Western" diet early in life are likely to suffer from wheeze and shortness of breath at 3–4 years of age (Tromp et al., 2012)

✓ BF imparts a protective effect against obesity relative to formula feeding, despite complex and confounded relationships between early life feeding practices and later child obesity risk (Dattilo et al., 2012; Farrow et al., 2013; Young et al., 2012; Dieterich et al., 2013). Overall, exclusive BF for longer than 4 months is associated with lower weight gain and body mass index (BMI) during the second half of the first year of age (Hörnell et al., 2013; Baird et al., 2008). Infants breast-fed from birth to 6 months gain weight, length and adiposity more slowly, and are of smaller size in infancy than the ones fed on formula-milks, independently of the timing of solids introduction (Baird et al., 2008; Moorcroft et al., 2011). Afterwards, this beneficial effect likely disappeared (Schack-Nielsen et al., 2010; DiSantis et al., 2011). Regarding the potential for BF to contribute to a reduction in later obesity, more detailed research is required (Agostoni et al., 2019). Interestingly, cow milk-formula (CMF) can accelerate weight-gain trajectories with respect to protein-hydrolyzed formula (PHF) (Table 19.1) maybe due to differences in their protein content or aminoacid profile (Mennella et al., 2011a, 2018). Indeed, free aminoacid and small peptides found in hydrolyzed formulas are acknowledged as satiation signalers and modulators of gastroduodenal motor functioning (Ventura et al., 2012). In particular free-glutamate likely accounted for the milk intake and satiation differences (Ventura et al., 2015), i.e., signals satiation sooner and satiate on lower volumes observed when infants fed PHF vs CMF, probably through its ability to trigger satiation when detected by glutamate-receptors in the gastrointestinal tract (Hartley et al., 2019)

✓ Direct BF during the first half-year of infancy is related to greater appetite regulation both in the second half-year (Li et al., 2010) and later in childhood (DiSantis et al., 2011) than bottle-feeding, regardless the type of milk in the bottle (either human milk or formula)

**TABLE 19.1** Effect of complementary feeding practices on appetite regulation.

| Study | Aim | Result | Reference |
|---|---|---|---|
| Infant Feeding Practices Study II (population-based longitudinal study conducted collaboratively by the Food and Drug Administration and the Centers for Disease Control and Prevention), USA: $n = 1250$ infants followed until 12 months. Bottle-emptying = indicator of self-regulation assessed from the seventh month | To explore whether infant's self-regulation of milk intake in the second half-year of infancy is affected by feeding mode (bottle vs breast) in the first half-year and the type of milk in the bottle (formula vs expressed BM) | – Emptied bottle/cup in the second half-year according to early: Exclusive BF: 27%; Exclusive BF + expressed BM: 47%; BF + formula: 55%; Exclusive BF + expressed BM + formula: 58%; Only expressed BM: 67%; Expressed BM + formula: 65%; Only formula: 68%<br>– Dose-response relationship between first half-year bottle-feeding and second half-year self-regulation: 10% increase of bottle-feeding intensity = 9% increased rate of infant-led emptying | Li et al. (2010) |
| Retrospective cohort design, USA: $n = 109$ children | To evaluate whether feeding BM from the breast (direct BF) in the first 3 months has a more optimal association with child appetite regulation behaviors and growth at age of 3–6 years, when compared to bottle-feeding (either BM or formula) | Children fed bottled BM 67% less likely to have high SR compared to directly breastfed children, after controlling for several variables; no association of bottle-feeding with young children's food responsiveness and enjoyment of food | DiSantis et al. (2011) |
| Within-subject experimental study, USA: $n (\leq 4\text{-month-old infants}) = 41$. CMF; CMF enriched with free amino-acid glutamate (CMF + Glu) | To determine whether timing, frequency and types of behaviors displayed differ when feeding isocaloric formulas different in satiation properties; infants are consistent in their display of these behaviors, regardless of amount consumed; the relationship between maternal feeding styles and infant self-regulation of intake and behavioral displays | Infants consumed less CMF + Glu and for shorter periods of time | Ventura et al. (2015) |
| Flavor-learning randomized study, USA: $n = 64$. Infants randomly assigned to be fed CMF ($n = 35$) or PHF ($n = 29$) between 0.5 and 7.5 months of age; monthly weighed and measured for 7 months | To examine whether healthy infants fed an extensively PHF would differ in feeding behavior and growth from those fed cow-milk formula | Infants fed PHF consumed less formula to satiation across the study period | Mennella et al. (2011a) |

| Sample and design | Objective | Key findings | Reference |
|---|---|---|---|
| RCT, USA: $n = 113$. Formula-fed infants randomly assigned to either CMF or PHF from 0.75 to 12.5 months of age. Monthly anthropometric measurements and diet records; energy balance assessments at 0.75, 3.5, and 12.5 months | To determine the direct impact of two types of infant isocaloric formula (PHF vs CMF) on growth and energy balance | Infants fed PHF consumed fewer calorie/day, fewer calories per kilogram of body weight/day, less formula per feed; at 12.5 months, more calories from other foods with similar calories from formula | Mennella et al. (2018) |
| Secondary analysis of cross-sectional data from an ethnically-diverse sample, USA: $n = 154$ mothers of infants (aged 7–11 months) and toddlers (aged 12–24 months) | To evaluate the association of BF duration with a wide range of maternal feeding approaches later in infancy and toddlerhood, including pressuring, restrictive, responsiveness, indulgence, and laissez-faire feeding styles | – Mothers of infants who breastfed for longer durations tended to report greater responsiveness to infant satiety cues and reduced pressuring in feeding complementary foods <br> – Mothers of toddlers who breastfed for longer durations tended to report reduced pressuring in feeding complementary foods | DiSantis et al. (2013) |
| Longitudinal cohort (Iron deficiency anemia preventive trial), Chile: $n = 576$ adolescents. Ad libitum breakfast followed after 20 min by SR assessment, and "Eating in the absence" (EAH) procedure (subjects invited to help themselves) | To assess whether sex, BMI, and duration of BF during infancy predicted SR and eating behavior at 16 years | Being breastfed for <6 months related to higher odds of both being in the 'not responsive' or 'still hungry' profile; 2.2 times more likely to eat during the EAH snack | Reyes et al. (2014) |
| BLISS RCT commencing in late pregnancy, consisting of a 12-month intervention phase with outcomes at 12 months of age and follow up at 2 years of age, New Zealand. BLISS group = 105 mother-infant dyads; Traditional Spoon-feeding group = 101 mother-infant dyads. All mothers received standard well-child care. BLISS mothers received lactation consultant support to 6 months, and educational sessions about BLISS (5.5, 7, and 9 months). Three-day weighed diet records collected at 7, 12, and 24 months | To determine whether allowing infants to control their own food intake by feeding themselves solid foods using a baby-led approach to complementary feeding (BLISS) results in differences in BMI-z-scores, energy self-regulation, eating behaviors, and energy intake at 12 and 24 months of age, compared with Traditional Spoon-feeding | BLISS infants vs Traditional Spoon-feeding infants: <br> – Exclusively breastfed for longer (21.7 weeks vs 17.3 weeks); introduced to solid foods later (24.6 weeks vs 22.6 weeks) with 64.6% (compared to 18.1%) meeting WHO guideline of delaying solids after 26 weeks of age <br> – At 12 months of age, greater food enjoyment; estimated energy intake difference = 55 kJ <br> – At 24 months, lower satiety responsiveness, and less food fussiness; estimated energy intake difference = 143 kJ <br> – No differences in BMI-z-scores | Taylor et al. (2017) |

BF, breastfeeding; BM, breast-milk; BMI, body mass index; CMF, cow-milk formula; PHF, protein hydrolysate-formula; RCT, randomized controlled trial; SR, satiety responsiveness.

(Table 19.1) to suggest the importance of maternal–infant interactions (see "Impacts of feeding practices and styles on child's skills for self-regulation of food") in infants' eating behavior, along with the milk composition (Karatas et al., 2011; Savino et al., 2011; Becerra-Bulla et al., 2015)

✓ Long-term BF likely plays a beneficial role on child neuropsychological development, including cognitive, intellectual, and behavioral outcomes. However, genetic variations in fatty acid metabolism and other factors may modulate the association between BF and brain development (Agostoni et al., 2017). Furthermore, increasing data show that gut microbiota and microbiome exert several functions which are able to influence neurodevelopment, body-weight regulation and immune function, through the "Microbiota-Gut-Brain Axis" (Agostoni et al., 2017; Cryan et al., 2019; Gupta et al., 2020). The neonatal period after birth is crucial for the establishment of the wider microbial community over time, with breast-milk modulating beneficially the infant gut microbiota composition (Berti et al., 2017; Dalby and Hall, 2020).

In spite of the plethora of findings, the real long-lasting influence of either qualitative or quantitative differences in early dietary intakes has not fully firmly established yet, as emerged by a recent review of meta-analyses and systematic reviews investigating the effects of different nutritional exposures during the first 2 years of age on health outcomes (Agostoni et al., 2019). Based on data, the authors concluded that only BF exerts a beneficial effect, which is nevertheless limited to few outcome measures, while effective type and duration are still unclear; as regards CF no strong effects of different dietary interventions are evident at follow up. Thereby, further research is needed to address some knowledge gaps.

There is also an urgent call for better understanding feeding requirements for formula-fed infants and revising recommendations accordingly (Bloomfield and Agostoni, 2020). A computational simulation model (i.e., the "Virtual Infant" agent-based model representing infant–caregiver pairs) aimed at testing whether several US established formula-feeding guidelines resulted in appropriate patterns of infant weight gain from birth to 6 months, identified that even for the minimum recommended amounts of daily formula infants moved into the overweight/obese weight category (Ferguson et al., 2020).

Alongside the nutritional aspects of BF and timely CF, other features assume a great importance in nutrition care, such as the caregiver-child interaction. Indeed, adequate feeding practices must also comprise optimal feeding's frequency and responsive styles (Engle et al., 1999) which should rely on: (1) adaptation of feeding methods to child's characteristics such as psycho-motor abilities (e.g., self-feeding or feeding by others; spoon holding, etc.) and appetite; (2) responsiveness to feeding situation by interacting positively with the child, that is, being sensitive to child's hunger and satiety cues (e.g., feeding when the child is hungry), encouraging a child to eat without forcing her/him, recognizing possible low appetite, balancing child vs caregiver control of eating, using an affectionate or warm style; (3) appropriateness of feeding, that is, creating a satisfactory feeding situation by reducing distractions, developing a consistent feeding schedule, and supervising and protecting children during eating.

## 19.2 Learning how to eat: Developmental stages and factors in infants' and toddlers' eating skill and behaviors

The development of eating behavior is a complex process which depends on interaction between biological systems (i.e., homeostatic mechanisms, neural reward systems, and child motor, sensory and socio-emotional capability) and environmental-behavioral factors (i.e., parenting, social influences, and food context) (Gahagan, 2012). Humans eat not only to satisfy their appetite but also for sensory hedonics and sensory stimulation, social pressure, etc. (Blundell, 1999).

Fig. 19.1 schematizes stages and factors involved in the development of infants' eating behavior from birth to toddlerhood and beyond. Even though being a long-life process, it evolves dramatically during the first 2 years of life as a consequence of both the child's neuromotor-cognitive development, and the transition from consuming an entirely milk-based diet to family foods. In this stage, children learn about food through "Familiarization", "Association", and "Observation" (Birch and Doub, 2014). The relationship the child establishes with food during the milk-feeding (*nursing period*), the introduction of CF (*transitional-feeding period*), and the transition to family-foods (*modified adult-feeding period*) is crucial for health and development, and has long-term consequences (Birch et al., 2007; Gahagan, 2012) with food preference and acceptance acquired in childhood tending to be long-lasting (Mennella and Trabulsi, 2012).

### 19.2.1 Nutritional and developmental appropriateness of introduction of foods

Morphological, physiological, and functional adaptations allow the child to cope with changes in the diet. Shortly after birth, milk is the only food an infant may consume with BF being the optimal form of nutrition for healthy infants. BF is a unique way of providing both immune protection and optimal nutrition for the healthy growth, functioning, and development of infants (Jeurink et al., 2013; Berti et al., 2017). Afterwards, breast-milk alone is no longer sufficient to meet energy and nutrition requirements (Agostoni and Przyrembel, 2013). Furthermore, infants start to show a very interest in foods other than milk based on their sensory perceptions thus becoming familiar with new foods in relation to their appearance, taste, and name as they are introduced to them (Aldridge et al., 2009; Mura Paroche et al., 2017). As a result, timely introduction of complementary foods becomes necessary both for nutritional and developmental reasons, and to enable the transition from milk-feeding to culturally appropriate family foods. Eating a variety of foods is essential to achieve adequate coverage of macro- and micronutrient needs. The time span during which transitional foods are introduced is a sensitive and dynamic period during which infants and toddlers undergo increasing and changing nutrient requirements, rapid growth, physiological maturation, and development. Generally, adequate growth, "defined by appropriate weight gain in early infancy and for the first few years of life" is a measure of successful feeding (Delaney and Arvedson, 2008). This process must be gradual and requires age-appropriate foods of the correct consistency from the form of purees through mashed foods to lumpy textured foods which need chewing, and then to family foods, depending on the child's maturation of the neuromuscular, digestive, renal, and defense systems (WHO, 2005; Lu and Ni, 2015; Fewtrell et al., 2017).

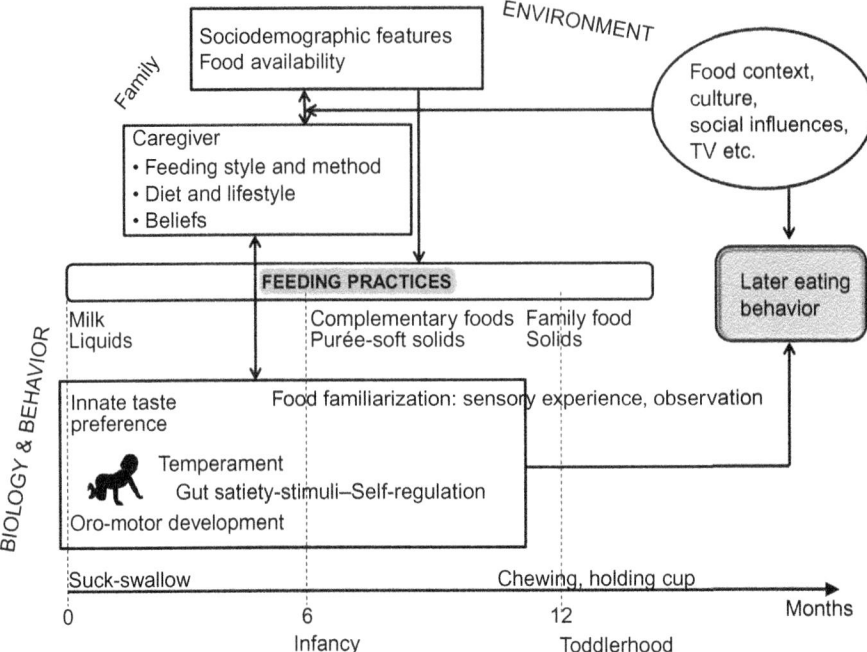

**FIG. 19.1** Factors influencing the early development of eating behavior as a long-life process as eating patterns established in infancy and toddlerhood continue into childhood and beyond. Eating habits, including food preferences, progress during the first 2 years of post-natal life as biological, cognitive (i.e., neurophysiology of eating regulation/homeostatic mechanisms, neural reward systems, and child motor, sensory and socio-emotional capability), and environmental (i.e., parenting, social influences and food context) processes are directed toward meeting requirements for health and growth. Diet undergoes radical changes moving from a single food (milk) to an increasing variety of foods which are required to meet nutritional needs. Morphological, physiological, and functional adaptations allow the child to cope with changes in the diet. Infants' ability to eat food and drink relies on achievement of general oro-motor skills by progressing from a basic suck-swallow mechanism to a chew-swallow mechanism. Infants and toddlers learn to trust and like food flavors and textures through sensory experiences guiding them from the innate preference for sweet and salt tastes to the acceptance of new foods as a consequence of early-life repeated exposure to variety. Infants also learn to eat through interactions with their caregiver(s). Child and caregiver(s) influence and react to one another's eating behavior. "What, when and how much" children eat, is fostered through the interaction between child's cues of hunger, emotional states, and temperament, caregiver's recognition of and responsiveness to these cues, and caregiver's beliefs and attitudes regarding nutrition and child-rearing. The relationship established with food by infants also reflects family features, social influences, cultural customs, and food context (i.e., food availability at home, parents' diet quality, sociodemographic factors, culture). (↔): reciprocal interaction.

### 19.2.1.1 Oral-motor development and (self-) feeding stages

"Self-regulation [...] ability to comply with a request, to initiate and cease activities according to situational demands, to modulate the intensity, frequency, and duration of verbal and motor acts in social and educational settings, to postpone acting upon a desired object or goal, and to generate socially approved behavior in the absence of external monitors" (Kopp, 1982). Children self-regulation evolves through: (1) neuro-physiological modulation (birth to 2–3 months), i.e., neuro-physiological and reflexive adaptations to the environment; (2) sensory-motor modulation (3 to 9+ months), i.e., sensory-motor adaptations in response to perceptual or motivational cues; (3) control (12 to 18+ months), self-control (24+ months), and self-regulation (36+ months), i.e., use of cognitive abilities to intentionally control their own behavior with an awareness of caregiver wishes and expectations.

Regarding infant ability to eat food and drink, it relies on the achievement of general oro-motor skills by progressing from a basic suck-swallow mechanism to a chew-swallow mechanism (Vereijken et al., 2011). The swallowing-mastication apparatus includes bones, muscles, tongue, pharynx, larynx, teeth, etc., and is not static over the course of a child's development (Le Révérend et al., 2014):

- Shortly after birth, neonates can only suck and swallow liquids as the anatomic configuration of oral and pharyngeal structures underlies and facilitates nipple feeding, thus supporting the act of suckling (Delaney and Arvedson, 2008). This apparently simple action represents a very active effort by infants as efficient eating requires coordinated sucking, swallowing, and breathing sequence via integration of multiple afferent and efferent systems within the central nervous system (Delaney and Arvedson, 2008). A strong bond exists between motor-skill achievement and child's responsive behavior (Gahagan, 2012). The small volume of colostrum decreases the chance of choking and regurgitation, and as coordinated sucking and swallowing rapidly improve, the volume of transitional milk gradually increases over the first 4–10 days (Gahagan, 2012).

Afterwards, anatomic changes occur in the oral-pharyngeal complex which allows the transition from the early pattern of suckling to sucking and the introduction of spoon feeding (Delaney and Arvedson, 2008):

✓ around 4–6 months of age, food is mashed by the tongue through an upward/downward motion (Le Révérend et al., 2014)
✓ by around 6 months, most infants can "sweep a spoon" with their upper lip (Agostoni et al., 2008). However, before introducing solid foods it is important to monitor the ability of the infant to accept non-liquid food without choking, gagging, or tongue thrusting (Gahagan, 2012)
✓ by around 8 months they have sufficient tongue flexibility to chew and swallow more solid lumpier foods in larger portions
✓ from 9 to 12 months, most infants have acquired manual skills to feed themselves and drink from a cup using both hands, so that usually, by 1 year of age, children are physically capable of eating family foods cut into bite-sized portions and eaten from a spoon, or as finger foods (Agostoni et al., 2008).

Eating maturity for purée and soft solids is likely accomplished at 6 and 8 months of age, respectively, whereas for more solid textures, an increase in efficiency continued after 24 months of age, suggesting that for example cereal-like textures may still challenge the mastication abilities of children (Le Révérend et al., 2014). Recently, a prospective study demonstrated that children likely accepted most textures earlier than expected, despite their feeding behaviors depends on age, with food texture and acceptance of hard textures being related to the development of chewing (Demonteil et al., 2019). The study was designed to investigate the evolution of food texture acceptance and feeding behaviors from 6 to 18 months in a challenging situation for a child, namely, by offering a large variety of food textures (i.e., smooth and rough purees; soft cooked pieces such as baby food pasta and shredded chicken; hard foods such as baby biscuit; double textures such as baby food muesli; sticky foods such as banana and cheese) at an earlier age than the common feeding practices. Results showed that pureed and double textures were highly accepted at 6 months, and cooked pieces at 8; up to 10 months, the acceptance of more complex textures increased strongly with age as did chewing behavior; and at 12 months, most food textures were accepted, with chewing behavior predominant over sucking.

A sort of reciprocal relationship seems to exist between children mastication efficiency and food consistency. On one side, the development of the mastication apparatus influences the oral food processing determining the gradual introduction of foods based on the correct consistency. On the other side, diet consistency can likely influence the oro-facial growth, that is to say, a diet with harder textures may enhance bone- and muscle-growth, which could indirectly lead to better mastication efficiency (Simione et al., 2018).

Indeed, newborns show a very strong compensation-ability to self-modulate their energy intake. Infants may in fact consume more or less of milk (from both breast and bottle) depending on the total energy intake and previous preloads (Olsen et al., 2013). They are very sensitive to unlearned internal hunger and satiety cues. Complex neurophysiologic pathways are involved in eating regulation and energy homeostasis. Hypothalamus and brain stem, gastrointestinal tract, pancreas, and adipose tissue interact and integrate their signals through neuro-endocrine feedback loops. Peripheral signals arising from selection, ingestion, digestion, and absorption of food, are anatomically localized to oro-gastrointestinal signals (including mechanical stimuli), circulating factors, metabolic signals, nutrient stores, and sensory capabilities of the nervous system (Stubbs, 1999; de Graaf et al., 2004). Energy status, sensation of gastric (un)filling, desire to suckle, food-neurophysiology interactions are likely involved in self-modulating the intake. However, this innate ability diminishes with age (Olsen et al., 2013).

## 19.2.2 Familiarity at the origin of food preferences

Infants learn to prefer foods available in their family context through sensory experiences (Aldridge et al., 2009). Taste is a strong determinant of food choice, because human beings derive pleasure and reward from eating (Gahagan, 2012; Møller, 2015), and children appear to be guided by their taste sensitivity to a greater extent than adults (Olsen et al., 2013). Table 19.2 shows the influence of feeding practices and strategies on the development of taste and food acceptance. On the whole, available literature about the development of flavor/food preference in infants and toddler is limited as most of the existing studies regard children aged ≥ 2 years.

Flavor and food preferences depend on a combination of genetic, familiar, and environmental factors (Wardle and Cooke, 2008). Infants learn about flavors before any taste of foods by the means of a "flavor bridge" (Mennella and Trabulsi, 2012). The recognition of tastes and odors develops in utero via swallowing the amniotic fluid flavored by the mother's diet (Mennella, 2014). Capacities for perceiving flavor sensations apparently begin as a consequence of the morphological development and early functioning of fetal gustatory and olfactory systems that are functionally mature by the end of gestation (Ventura and Worobey, 2013). It continues after birth with infants still exposed to flavors from milk (Beauchamp and Mennella, 2009).

Taste (sweet, sour, salty, bitter, umami, or savory) preferences (i.e., the predispositions to form flavor preference) have a strong inborn component with sweet, umami, and salty substances innately preferred, whereas bitter and sour substances innately disliked (Birch, 1999). Broadly, sweet taste is preferred from birth to 4–6 months with a marginal decrease by the

**TABLE 19.2** Effect of feeding practices and strategies on taste and food acceptance.

| Study | Aim | Result | Reference |
|---|---|---|---|
| OPALINE Programme, France: $n = 122$ | To examine impact of exclusive BF duration (DEB) on taste acceptance at 6 and 12 months of age | – 6 months: infants preferred sweet, salty and umami solutions over water; indifferent to sour and bitter solutions. Association between DEB and umami taste acceptance<br>– 12 months: infants preferred sweet and salty solutions over water; indifferent to sour, bitter, and umami solutions | Schwartz et al. (2013) |
| Western Australian Pregnancy Cohort (Raine) Study, Australia: $n = 1905$ children 2-year-old.<br>Core food variety score (CFVS); Fruit and vegetable variety score (FVVS) | To investigate association of BF duration and food variety at 2 years | BF duration directly associated with CFVS and FVVS, independently of maternal demographic characteristics known to predict food variety in toddlers | Scott et al. (2012) |
| Hertfordshire Cohort Study, United Kingdom: $n = 3217$ adults aged between 59 and 73 years.<br>Early life type of milk-feeding: 'Breast-Fed only', 'Breast & Bottle-Fed', or 'Bottle-fed only' | To investigate association between BF and a beneficial profile of health behaviors in later life | Key dietary pattern = 'prudent' pattern, describing compliance with 'healthy' eating recommendations. Independent associations between feeding type and prudent diet score in adults, with higher scores associated with being breast fed | Robinson et al. (2013) |
| Intervention trial, USA.<br>Infants aged 0.5 months randomly allocated to six groups starting at different months:<br>- from the age of 0.5 months and fed for 7 months = 2 CGs: CMF ($n = 12$) and PHF ($n = 12$)<br>- from the age of 1.5 months = 2 groups ($n = 11$, each) fed PHF for either 1 or 3 months and CMF otherwise<br>- from the age of either 2.5 or 3.5 months = 2 groups ($n = 11$, each) fed PHF for 1 month and CMF otherwise | To determine effects of timing and duration of early-life exposure on acceptance of PHF compared to CMF | – PHF acceptance in 1-month exposure infants based on timing of PHF-exposure: on first day, less PHF than CMF intake in all age-groups (favoring their familiar CMF), and less PHF intake in the 3.5 months-group (greater rejection)<br>– PHF acceptance at 7.5 months based on duration of PHF-exposure (started at 1.5 months): greater in infants fed for 1 and 3 months vs no-exposure (CMF-CG), lower vs 7 months-exposure (PHF-CG)<br>– PHF acceptance at 7.5 months based on timing of 1-month exposure to PHF: higher relative PHF than CMF intake within infants PHF-fed before 3.5 months. Patterns of maternal perceptions and frequency of distaste/rejection behaviors consistent with timing-related difference in intake | Mennella et al. (2011b) |

*Continued*

TABLE 19.2 Effect of feeding practices and strategies on taste and food acceptance—cont'd

| Study | Aim | Result | Reference |
|---|---|---|---|
| Within- and between-subjects design study, USA: MF-fed infants (n =50); protein PHF-fed infants (n =24). Infants ranged from 6 to 11 months of age | To test hypothesis that the flavor of formula fed to infants modifies their acceptance of some foods | PHF-fed infants more likely to be feeding meats; consuming less broccoli/cauliflower in terms of both grams and calories relative to carrots (evident also when expressed as intake (g)/infants' BMI); reported not to enjoy feeding the broccoli/cauliflower | Mennella et al. (2006) |
| Intervention trial, USA. Age: 4–9 months. Infants fed BM: n =37; Infants fed MFs: n =16; Infants fed hydrolyzed casein formulas (HCFs) fed group: n =13. Infant food = cereal mixed with: water = plain cereal; D-lactose solution = sweet cereal; sodium chloride solution = salty cereal; urea solution = bitter cereal; citric acid solution = sour cereal; Monosodium Glutamate Solution = savory cereal | To compare effects of HCFs (pronounced bitter, sour, and savory tastes), BM and MFs on responses to basic taste compounds in a familiar infant food (rice, oatmeal, or barley) | — Intake: HCF infants ate significantly more savory, bitter, and sour and plain cereals than did BM or MF<br>— Liking: HCF infants displayed fewer facial expressions of distaste with bitter and savory cereals; HCF and BM infants were more likely to smile while eating savory | Mennella et al. (2009) |
| OPALINE Programme, France: n =203 | To study whether maternal feeding practices in the first year (exclusive BF duration, age of initiation of weaning, *variety* of new foods) impacted infants' later acceptance of new foods from beginning of weaning to age of 15 months | — Exclusive BF duration: no impact<br>— Age of weaning: impact on vegetable acceptance as the earlier vegetables were introduced, the higher the acceptance of new ones was<br>— Variety: new food acceptance correlated with number of different foods in the first 2 months of weaning | Lange et al. (2013) |
| ALSPAC, United Kingdom: n (age 2 years) =7269; EDEN, France: n (age 2 years) =1302; Generation XXI, Portugal: n (age 2 years) =800; EuroPrevall, Greece: n (age 4 years) =556 | To examine whether early feeding practices (e.g., BF duration and timing of CF) influence later fruit and vegetable (FV) intake in 2–4 years old children | — Longer BF duration consistently related to higher fruit and mainly vegetable intake with maternal fruit-vegetable intake not substantially attenuating the relation<br>— Weaker and less consistent associations with age of introduction to FV<br>— Large differences in early feeding practices across cohorts | de Lauzon-Guillain et al. (2013) |
| Cohort study (data from Healthy Start primary intervention study, Danish Medical Birth registry and Danish Health Visitor's Child Health Database), Denmark: n =236 children aged 2–6 years. Infant feeding registered up to 4 times: from few days-old to 10-months-old | To investigate if exclusive BF duration was associated with pickiness or dietary intake of vegetables, fruit, starchy foods or sugar sweetened beverages in later childhood among obesity prone normal weight children | — Lower odds of picky eating behavior when exclusively breastfed until age 4-5months compared to exclusively breastfed for 0–1month.<br>— Exclusively breastfed until age 6–10months associated with higher daily intake of vegetables | Specht et al. (2018) |

| Design/Sample | Objective | Findings | Reference |
|---|---|---|---|
| Intervention trial, France: n = 95. Pre-exposure cross-over test (basic artichoke purée and control carrot purée) + random Exposure Period (three groups, each exposed 10 times to a differently flavored artichoke purée) + Post-exposure cross-over test (basic artichoke purée and control carrot purée) + tests at 2-week (basic artichoke purée, cross-over 3-months, and cross-over 6-months follow-ups) | To compare learning mechanisms, i.e., repeated exposure (RE), flavor-flavor learning (FFL), flavor-nutrient learning (FNL) at increasing artichoke acceptance in infants at CF; to measure the stability of learning effect in short- and middle-term; to examine impact of infants feeding history on artichoke acceptance | – Between pre- and post-exposure: intake of the basic artichoke increased in RE and FFL groups; liking increased in the RE group. After exposure: artichoke as much consumed and liked as carrot in RE group<br>– Learning of artichoke acceptance stable up to 3 months post-exposure<br>– Initial artichoke intake significantly related to number of vegetables offered before the study | Remy et al. (2013) |
| Intervention trial, United Kingdom. IG: n = 18; CG: n = 18. IG: 12 daily exposures to vegetable puree added to milk, then 12 × 2 daily exposures to vegetable puree added to rice at home, 11 daily exposures to vegetable puree; CG: Plain milk and rice, then 11 daily exposures to vegetable puree | To test step-by-step exposure to vegetables in milk then rice during CF, on intake and liking of vegetables (carrots, green beans, spinach, broccoli, parsnip) | IG infants ate more of target vegetables (carrots and green beans) and more rapidly than the CG infants. Intake, liking and pace of eating greater for IG than CG infants. Intake and liking of carrots were greater than green beans. However, at 6 months then 18 months follow-up, vegetable (carrot > green beans) but not group differences were observed | Hetherington et al. (2015) |
| 8-day home exposure period, USA. Age: 6–9 months.<br>Study A. Green Bean Group (GBG): n = 11; Between-Meal Vegetable Variety Group (BMVG): n = 12; Between-Meal and Within-Meal Vegetable Variety Group (BM-WM): n = 12. GBG fed only green beans; BMVG fed one vegetable (green beans, peas, spinach, squash, carrots) each day, with green and orange vegetables alternated daily; BM-WM fed two vegetables each day (one green, one orange).<br>Study B. Pear Group (PG): n = 20; Between-Meal Fruit Variety Group (BFMG): n = 19. PG fed only pears; BM fed a fruit (peach, prune, apple) different than the one experienced during the previous 2 days | Study A: To determine whether experience with a variety of pureed vegetables both within a meal and between meals leads to greater acceptance of vegetables. Study B: To examine the effects of repeated experience with either one pureed fruit or a variety of pureed fruits on infants' acceptance of pureed pears and green beans | *Study A*<br>– Exposure to vegetable variety both between and within meals: increased acceptance of green beans, carrots and spinach<br>– Exposure to green beans alone and variety of vegetables between meals: increased green beans' intake of after the exposure<br>*Study B*<br>Exposure to pears or a variety of fruits between meals resulted in greater consumption of pears | Mennella et al. (2008) |
| Prospective cohort study Project Viva, USA: n = 1162 children | To identify patterns of CF behaviors around 1 year and examine associations with diet quality in early childhood (median age 3.1 year). | – "Breast milk and delayed sweets and fruit juice" class: the highest later Youth Healthy Eating Index (YHEI) scores<br>– "Picky eaters" class: the lowest later YHEI scores<br>– "Late flavor introduction and delayed sweets" and "Early flavor introduction and more fruit juice" classes: moderate scores. | Switkowski et al. (2020) |

Continued

TABLE 19.2 Effect of feeding practices and strategies on taste and food acceptance—cont'd

| Study | Aim | Result | Reference |
|---|---|---|---|
| OTIS portfolio RCT, Sweden: $n=250$ (aged 4–6 months). Infants, breast- or formula-fed at study start, randomly allocated to either a Nordic-diet group (IG) or a Conventional-diet group (CG). IG following a systematic taste portions schedule of home-made purées of Nordic foods for 24 days; then supplied with baby food products and homemade baby food recipes based on Nordic ingredients with reduced protein content. CG advised to follow current Swedish CF recommendation. Five-day food records collected at 6 and 9 months of age; anthropometric data and blood samples collected at baseline and 9 months | To compare a protein-reduced complementary diet based on Nordic foods (i.e., systematic introduction of taste portions with repeated exposures of a variety of fruits/berries and vegetables) to regular Swedish complementary diet on growth, measures of iron status and intake of fruits and vegetables up to 9 months of age | IG infants had higher intake of fruits and vegetables: $225 \pm 109\,g/day$ vs $156 \pm 77\,g/day$; similar energy intake, but lower protein intake (compensated for by higher intake of carbohydrate from fruits and vegetables); no differences in growth or iron status | Johansson et al. (2019) |
| ALSPAC, United Kingdom: $n=9360$ Infants introduced to lumps before 6 months of age; Infants introduced between 6 and 9 months; Infants introduced at or after 10 months | To document infants' dietary patterns and development of perceived feeding difficulties at 15 months according to age of lumpy solids' introduction | Infants introduced at 10 months or later: more difficult to feed and with more definite likes and dislikes at 15 months; less likely to be having family foods at 15 months compared to those introduced between 6 and 9 months | Northstone et al. (2001) |
| ALSPAC, United Kingdom: $n=7821$ | To investigate long-term impact of timing of introduction of lumpy foods on children's eating behavior and food intake at 7 years of age | Children introduced to lumpy solids after 9 months of age: more feeding problems at 7 years by eating less of many of the food groups, fewer types, and portions of fruit and vegetables than the rest of the sample | Coulthard et al. (2009) |
| ALSPAC, United Kingdom: $n=821$ | To examine whether fruit and vegetable feeding practices at 6 months predict children's intake at 7 years | – Raw fruit, home-cooked fruit and vegetable: higher frequency at 6 months strongly associated with a higher frequency of consumption at 7 years of age<br>– Older age of introduction and low frequency of home-cooked vegetables: infants more likely to eat fewer vegetables at 7 years | Coulthard et al. (2010) |

| Sample/design | Aim | Findings | Reference |
|---|---|---|---|
| Survey, United Kingdom: $n = 155$ children (aged 20–78 months) | To examine if the weaning method "Baby-led weaning" vs the traditional "Spoon feeding" influences food preferences, BMI, and picky eating in early childhood | – "Baby-led" infants: increased liking for carbohydrates "Spoon feeding" infants: increased liking for sweet foods <br> – No difference in picky eating between the groups | Townsend and Pitchford (2012) |
| BLISS RCT commencing in late pregnancy (a modified version of "Baby-led weaning" to prevent iron deficiency), New Zealand. BLISS Group (IG) = 105 mother-infant dyads; Traditional Spoon-feeding Group (CG) = 101 mother-infant dyads. For details, see Table 19.1 | To determine the impact of BLISS method on iron status of infants from 7 to 12 months of age, and on food and nutrient intake from 7 to 24 months of age as well | IG vs CG: <br> – More sodium and fat at 7 months, less saturated fat at 12 months; no difference at 24 months <br> – Higher intake of "grains and cereals", "meat and meat alternatives", "milk and milk products", and "miscellaneous foods" at 7 months; no differences by 12 months <br> – At 7 months, feeding themselves of their food on average 40% (25th, 75th percentile: 27%, 51%) vs 9% (0%, 31%); at 12 months, less likely to be fed by an adult (0 vs 7%) <br> – at 7 months, 2–4 times as likely to eat meals with family and to consume the same foods; at 12 months still twice as likely to be eating the same foods as the family at lunch and evening meals <br> – No differences on iron status | Williams Erickson et al. (2018); Daniels et al. (2018) |
| Longitudinal cohort (the Infant Feeding Practices Study II and the Follow-Up Study), USA: $n = 1333$ | To examine whether sugar-sweetened beverage (SSB) intake during infancy predicts SSB intake at 6 years of age | Adjusted odds of consuming SSBs at age 6 years $\geq 1$ time/day associated with any SSB intake during infancy, age at SSB introduction (aOR = 2.33 for age $\geq 6$ months, 2.01 for age < 6 months vs never), mean SSB intake during age 10 to 12 months (aOR = 2.72 for 1 to < 2 times/week, 2.57 for $\geq 3$ times/week vs none) | Park et al. (2014) |
| Multicenter intervention trial: United Kingdom, $n = 108$, aged 6–36 months; France, $n = 123$, aged 4–8 months; Denmark, $n = 172$, aged 6–36 months. Between 5 and 10 exposures to a novel vegetable (artichoke puree) in one of three versions (basic, sweet or added-energy): intake of basic artichoke puree measured before and after the exposure period | To understand individual characteristics predicting different responses (i.e., initial acceptance, patterns of acceptance-intake over time; effectiveness) to repeated exposure of a novel vegetable | – Patterns of eating behavior during exposure: "Learners" (40%) increasing intake over time; "Plate-clearers" (21%) consuming >75% offered; "Non-eaters" (16%) <10 g by the 5th exposure; "Others" (23%) with highly variable pattern. <br> – Age: positively correlated with satiety responsiveness and food enjoyment. Youngers consumed more artichoke, enjoyed food more, had lower satiety responsiveness, were less fussy and more likely to be "Learners" and "Plate clearers"; older children were more likely to be "Non-eaters" <br> – Intake over time: the smallest change in added-energy condition | Caton et al. (2014) |

12th month; preference for high levels of salty taste develops undoubtedly after 4 months of age maybe as a consequence of the progressive replacement of milk with CF; acceptance for umami emerges at 6 months (Ventura and Worobey, 2013; Schwartz et al., 2017). Regardless of "dislike" or "distaste" facial expressions in response to bitter and sour tastes, infants do not systematically reject their ingestion (Birch, 1999). The OPALINE Programme aimed at understanding the formation of food preferences from birth until the age of 2 years, highlighted that between 5 and 7 months of age, the most bitter- or sour-tasting foods were not rejected; the specific taste profile of a food influenced its acceptance (for example, vegetables added with salt or a salty ingredient more accepted than plain vegetables); the taste acceptance played a critical role in new food acceptance with a higher acceptance for a taste associated to an enhanced acceptance of foods bearing this taste (for example, sweet taste acceptance with Cereal&Dessert and SweetFruit acceptance; sour taste acceptance with SourFruit acceptance; umami taste acceptance with SaltyUmamiVeg and MildSweet&BitterVeg acceptance) (Schwartz et al., 2011). Similarly, a study investigating infants' acceptance for extreme sour tastes and its relation to fruit intake found that at ages of 15–20 months some infants could accept high concentrations of sourness; infants who accepted the most sour solutions had a higher fruit intake at 6 months, a significantly higher increase in fruit intake from 12 to 18 months, as well as a significantly higher fruit intake, variety, and frequency of consumption at 18 months than those who rejected the highly sour taste (Blossfeld et al., 2007).

The innate taste preferences predispose children to favor acceptance of sweet- and salty-tasting foods and beverages possibly as an evolutionary adaptive response to uncertain substances which is the basic need to correctly discriminate energy-dense and nutrient-rich foods from toxic or poisonous ones (Ventura and Worobey, 2013). For example, a longitudinal cohort analysis of 1333 children revealed that sugar-sweetened beverage intake during infancy significantly increased the likelihood of consuming these types of drink $\geq$ time/day at 6 years of age (Park et al., 2014). Alarmingly, the current food context (i.e., Western Diet), characterized by availability of too much inexpensive, palatable, high-calorie foods, fits perfectly in these predispositions (Birch and Anzman, 2010). Discouraging innate preference for sweetness early in life may have a persistent influence on diet quality as observed in the Project Viva prospective study finding that a delayed introduction of sweets and fruit juice at 1 year predicted a less frequent consumption of these foods and a higher diet quality approximately 2 years later (Switkowski et al., 2020).

### 19.2.2.1 The importance of nursing period, transitional-feeding period, and modified adult-feeding period

Children are not genetically restricted to a narrow range of foodstuff as the innate tendencies can be modified by pre- and post-natal experiences based upon the process of learning (Mennella, 2014; Mura Paroche et al., 2017). Infants and toddlers gain trust and liking of food flavor and texture by repeated exposure to nutritious foods and flavor variety due to an inherent plasticity in the development of the chemical senses, which interact with early-life experiences (Mennella, 2014). During the post-natal period the developing human brain is characterized by a very functional flexibility that makes it strongly sensitive to environmental influences (i.e., external cues). The early environment is likely able to shape neural circuits, determining structural and functional aspects of the brain, and hence behaviors. This suggests the ability for children and adolescents to memorize and modify food likes and dislikes based on experience, i.e., familiarization (Aldridge et al., 2009; Mennella and Trabulsi, 2012).

Across life there is, in fact, a shift from primarily hedonic-based preferences early in life to learned preferences that involve consideration of health, social, and economic impacts of foods later in life (Savage et al., 2007; Ventura and Worobey, 2013).

Type, timing and duration of milk-feeding regimen (breast vs formula) in early post-natal life likely exerts different effects on flavor learning and establishment of food preference which appear to be long-lived (Beauchamp and Mennella, 2009; Mennella et al., 2011b; Schwartz et al., 2013). Existing data suggest that prolonged BF may affect the initial acquisition of acceptance/preference of tastes such as umami (probably relate to the higher free-glutamate content of human milk compared with formula-milk) and foods, facilitating the transition to modified-adult foods (Mennella et al., 2009; Schwartz et al., 2013). Breastfed children likely, in fact, more willing to try novel foods than formula-feds (Mennella, 2014). It may be postulated that unlike milk-formulas characterized by a constant and plain flavor which makes milk-feeding a monotonous experience, human milk carrying a unique and transient variety of flavors (depending on maternal diet) exposes breast-fed infants to a wide range of sensory experiences, providing them with opportunities to learn to like new flavors (Nicklaus, 2017). Consistent with this, greater exposure to breast-milk is linked to healthier dietary patterns both in 2- to 6-year-old children in different cultural contexts (Scott et al., 2012; de Lauzon-Guillain et al., 2013; Specht et al., 2018) and in adult life (Robinson et al., 2013).

The type (milk formula vs hydrolysate formulas) and composition of formula appear to be involved in shaping flavor's preferences, too, plausibly because of remarkable differences in the flavor profile exists among the different formulas. In general, formula-fed infants tend to prefer foods containing the distinctive flavors of the formula they are provided with (Mennella and Beauchamp, 2005). Compared with milk formula-fed infants, hydrolysate formula-feds displayed more positive responses to savory, bitter, and sour food matrices (Liem and Mennella, 2002; Mennella et al., 2006, 2009) probably because of their more pronounced savory, bitter, and sour tastes and stronger odors due to the high content of free-glutamate and sulfur volatiles (Mennella, 2014; Ventura et al., 2015).

Given that acceptance of new tastes emerges between 4 and 6 months of age, and that of solid textures from 6 to 12 months, types, variety and frequency of foods offered have a crucial impact in acquisition of food preferences (Vereijken et al., 2011). Clearly, CF represents a favorable time-frame for caregivers to promote familiarity toward untasted or disliked foods such as vegetables (Aldridge et al., 2009; Nicklaus, 2016). Infants and young children are generally readily more accepting of novel foods (for example, they are less fussy, enjoy food more, have low satiety responsiveness) until the age of 18 months (Olsen et al., 2013; Caton et al., 2014). Afterwards, they begin to indicate avoidance/fear, an overall reluctance to try new foods (neophobia) (Brown and Harris, 2012). Neophobia is minimal at infancy and sometimes peaks between 2 and 6 years but it is not a permanent condition (Brown and Harris, 2012). Available data demonstrate that both repeatedly exposing (around 10 times) infants to a particular fruit/vegetable, and applying daily variety in rotation schemes of fruits/vegetables are effective strategies to enhance fruit/vegetable liking and consumption in the short-term and later at 2–7 years of age (Mennella et al., 2008; Remy et al., 2013; Coulthard et al., 2010; Johansson et al., 2019). In particular, feeding systematically and gradually less appealing foods along with familiar ones, such as milk or baby-cereals, may be adopted as an approach to progressively accustom infants to novel foods (Hetherington et al., 2015). Moreover, encouraging acceptance of unfamiliar or rejected foods through gradually exposure or modeling may help counteract neophobia (Aldridge et al., 2009; Brown and Harris, 2012). Data from

Australian studies indicated that neophobia was associated with a lower variety of fruits and vegetables and higher energy intake from discretionary foods at 24 months (Perry et al., 2015).

Food texture also plays a large role in how foods are perceived (Szczesniak, 2002; Werthmann et al., 2015) with food textural properties being the most influential in eliciting disgust (Brown and Harris, 2012). Offering appropriate textures at the recommended ages is important, as children are more likely to accept textures that they are able to process, and early exposure to a range of textures facilitates the acceptance of foods of various textures in middle childhood (Le Révérend et al., 2014). It was observed that differences in food acceptance and problematic eating occurred and persisted according to the age at which they began to have lumps in their food. Children exposed from 10 months of age, were reported to be more difficult to feed (i.e., not eating sufficient amounts, being choosy with food, refusing to eat foods) when they were both 15 months (Northstone et al., 2001) and 7 years old (Coulthard et al., 2009) than those introduced to lumps between 6 and 9 months. Furthermore, they consumed less fruits and vegetables. In contrast, infants fed lumpy solids before 6 months, were more likely to eat certain categories of fruit and vegetables including green leafy vegetables and citrus fruits, suggesting that they accept more readily bitter or sour tastes (Coulthard et al., 2009). An effect of age seems to exist on vegetable acceptance, too, with the earlier vegetables are introduced, the higher the acceptance of new vegetables is (Lange et al., 2013). Moreover, infants consumed a greater variety of family foods (i.e., bread, biscuits, meat, fish, potatoes, raw fruit, and vegetables) at the age of 6 months (Northstone et al., 2001).

## 19.3 Child-caring in child eating behavior formation, nutrition, and growth: The role of food parenting practices and styles

"Care refers to the behaviours and practices of caregivers (mothers, siblings, fathers and childcare providers) that provide the food, health care, stimulation and emotional support necessary for children's healthy growth and development" (Engle et al., 2000). Parenting refers to the general approaches dealing with the task of care and feeding one's children (Savage et al., 2007). Caregivers and their child reciprocally learn to recognize and interpret both verbal and non-verbal communication signals from one another (Larsen et al., 2015). This process is pivotal to the child's healthy social–emotional functioning (Black and Aboud, 2011). "Parenting styles" refer to the emotional climate within which parenting practices are applied, and are defined by how demanding and responsive parents are in relationship to child behaviors (Blissett, 2011; Gahagan, 2012). They are recognized as important environmental determinants of child emotional maturity, self-regulation, and behavioral inhibition. Responsive parenting reflects reciprocity between child and caregiver, and is typified by prompt, emotionally supportive, contingent, and developmentally appropriate behaviors (Black and Aboud, 2011). According to the dimensions of warmth or responsiveness, and behavioral-control or demandingness exhibited by parents/caregivers, they are classified as (Blissett, 2011; Gahagan, 2012) "Authoritative" (demanding and responsive, high levels of control and warmth); "Authoritarian" (low warmth and responsiveness, highly demanding expectations and control of the child); "Permissive-Indulgent" (high levels of warmth and responsiveness, low demands); "Uninvolved/Neglectful Permissive" (neither demanding nor responsive, low levels of warmth).

## 19.3.1 Caregiver's feeding practices and styles

Caregivers play a critical role in shaping the children eating environment, as infants and toddlers are fully dependent on them for nutrition and feeding practices (Birch and Doub, 2014; Daniels, 2019). As well-explained by Engle et al. (2000) "feeding requires much more from the caregiver than food selection and preparation". Caregivers have the responsibility to decide when and under what circumstances to feed child, how to deal with children who are not interested in food or refuse it, that is, to encourage intake with praise or use demands or threats, etc. They also serve as models for dietary choices and patterns that children learn to emulate (i.e., modeling) (Birch et al., 2007). Hence, the first 2 years of life represent a critical time period where parents should intervene to encourage and launch healthy patterns that may last a lifetime and could help curb the obesity trend (Saavedra et al., 2013; Daniels, 2019). Fig. 19.2 illustrates *Food parenting practices* and *Feeding styles*.

### 19.3.1.1 *The caregiver-child feeding context: Responsive and non-responsive feeding*

Family-care the child received together with food availability and access to healthcare services affects children's nutritional status (Engle and Pelto, 2011). Responsive Feeding (RF) is listed among the family-care behaviors necessary for child survival, and incorporated into International infant feeding guidelines and recommendations by UNICEF, PAHO, and WHO (WHO, 2005; Hromi-Fiedler et al., 2020).

– **RF** consists of a mutual relationship between an infant or child and his/her caregiver: the caregiver creates routine, structure and emotional context that promote interaction; the child communicates feelings of hunger and satiety through motor actions, facial expressions, or vocalization; the caregiver immediately responds by providing appropriate and nutritious food in an emotionally and developmentally supportive manner, while maintaining an appropriate feeding environment; the child experiences predictable responses (Harbron et al., 2013; Black and Aboud, 2011). Scientific evidence indicates that RF is associated with ideal growth standards, optimal nutrient intake, and long-term regulation of weight, suggesting that RF may help the development of healthy eating behavior and optimal skills for self-regulation and self-control of food intake (Birch et al., 2007; Dattilo et al., 2012; Harbron et al., 2013; Balantekin et al., 2020).
– **Non-Responsive Feeding (NRF)** is typified by a lack of reciprocity between the caregiver and child: Indulgence Feeding (the child controls the feeding situation), Pressuring-Controlling-Restricting Feeding (the caregiver takes excessive control and dominates the feeding situation), and Uninvolved Feeding (the caregiver ignores the child during meals).

## 19.3.2 Impacts of feeding practices and styles on child's skills for self-regulation of food

Many child-feeding practices evolved across human history to protect children by food scarcity. For this reason "traditional feeding practices" include feeing frequently and quickly in response to crying and distress (*feeding to soothe*), offering possibly preferred foods, encouraging children to eat as much as possible by pressure and force feeding (Birch and Doub, 2014; Savage et al., 2007). Despite awareness that the contemporary food environment poses the opposite threat, that is, food surfeit, traditional feeding practices and beliefs that "a chubby baby is a

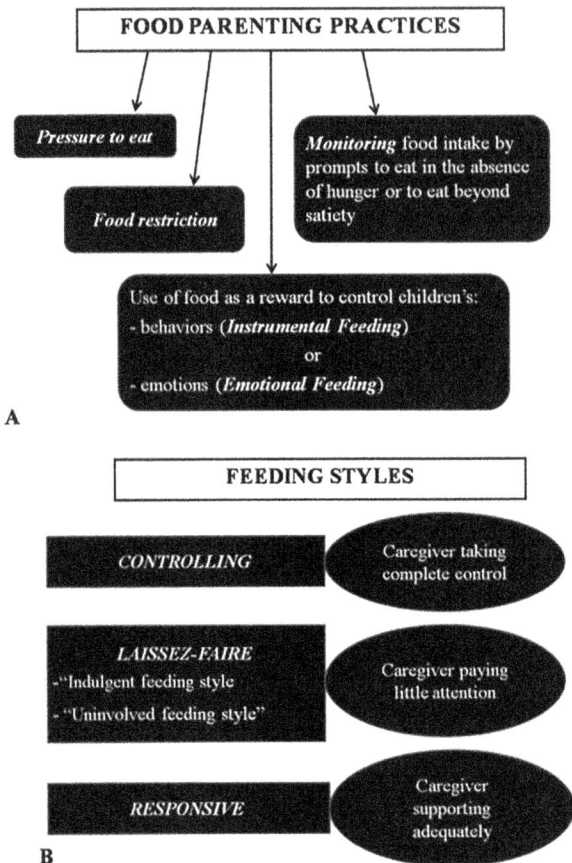

**FIG. 19.2** Parenting and feeding: linkage between approaches chosen to feed and emotional environments established by the caregiver(s), and the child's food preferences and appetite regulation. (A) Food parenting practices regarded as active processes, are specific strategies or behaviors usually used to manage *how much, when, and what* children eat (Blissett, 2011; Jansen et al., 2012; Larsen et al., 2015). (B) Feeding styles refer to how the parent/caregiver interacts with the child when it comes to feeding, i.e., the type of feeding interactions which takes place (Jansen et al., 2012; Engle et al., 2000; Thompson et al., 2009): *Controlling.* The caregiver takes the complete control of when and how much the child eats (i.e., forcing/pressuring or restricting). The child may be unable to develop mechanisms for learning to regulate their intake. *Laissez-faire.* The caregiver makes little effort to encourage eating or limit infant diet quality or quantity by expecting the child to make decisions around meals on his/her own at an early age, and shows little interaction with the infant during feeding. The *indulgent attitude* may be detrimental with low-appetite children, and at the same time problematic because of the infants' genetic predispositions to prefer sweet and salty tastes. *Uninvolved feeders* have limited knowledge on child feeding recommendations, and may be unaware of what or when their toddler is eating. *Responsive.* The caregiver responds to the child's hunger cues in reasonable time, feeding by encouragement and praise. This attitude may help the child develop a mechanisms for food-intake regulation.

healthy baby" still persist, particularly among low-income and ethnic groups (Anzman et al., 2010). Their persistence may be problematic as promoting excessive energy intake, overeating, and overweight in low-income groups, considering the lower costs of junk foods.

A systematic review in HIC evidenced that the majority of existing studies were cross-sectional, and explored the relationship between NRF and weight outcomes rather than the efficacy of RF interventions (Hurley et al., 2011). Similar remarks were drawn from studies carried out in low- and middle-income countries (LAMI) (Bentley et al., 2011) to indicate a general call for either longitudinal or repeated-measure designs to both understand causality and test the efficacy of RF interventions. Moreover, while a number of research studies have been conducted in pre-school and older children, studies among infants and toddlers are still very limited (Hurley et al., 2011; Birch and Doub, 2014). Some examples are reported in Table 19.3. To date, there are few obesity prevention studies which focus on maternal feeding practices and commence very early in child's life, namely, the Australian primary prevention program for childhood obesity (NOURISH) randomized control trial (Daniels et al., 2012, 2013, 2020), and the American Intervention Nurses Start Infants Growing on Health Trajectories (INSIGHT) randomized control trial (Savage et al., 2016, 2018; Paul et al., 2018; Ruggiero et al., 2020). Both show significantly evident guidance-to-RF effects on maternal feeding practices (Table 19.4).

Findings suggest that NRF, especially *controlling feeding practices* including food *restriction and pressure-to-eat*, is the aspect of food parenting most consistently associated with less healthy weight gain trajectories during early life, food preferences and dietary habits (Clark et al., 2007; Savage et al., 2007; Daniels et al., 2013). The most frequent relation found in HIC was between restriction and higher BMI and/or overweight/obesity, and between pressure and lower BMI/weight gain (Hurley et al., 2011). Typically, caregivers limit children's access to palatable foods that are high in sugar, salt, and fat, whereas they insist on consumption of healthy foods such as fruit and vegetable (Anzman et al., 2010). They tend to pressure infants who are lighter and have a smaller appetite, and restrict infants with larger appetites or perceive to be at risk for overweight (Fildes et al., 2015; Black and Aboud, 2011; Harbron et al., 2013).

In contrast, **RF** likely promotes children's interest in eating, attention to internal cues of hunger, and satiety (satiety responsiveness), ability to communicate needs to their caregiver with meaningful signals leading children to progress to independent feeding (see Engle and Zeitlin, 1996; Aboud et al., 2008; Dearden et al., 2009; Daniels et al., 2013, 2014 in Table 19.3). *Parent responsivity* has a central role in BF (see studies in Table 19.1), as mothers learn to recognize their infants' signals of hunger and satiety, and to feed or stop accordingly, with long-lasting effects on CF, too, as demonstrated by a secondary analysis of cross-sectional data from an ethnically diverse sample (DiSantis et al., 2013). Moreover, when infants were fed human milk in a bottle, they exhibited a higher consumption of milk (Li et al., 2010) and a lower satiety responsiveness (DiSantis et al., 2011) than those directly breastfed, to suggest that BF itself rather than breast-milk is related to greater appetite regulation both in the short- and medium-term. Bottle-feeding likely provides visual cues which might lead to mothers/caregivers to feed in response to the amount in the bottle rather than feeding responsively to their infants' cues.

Studies in Table 19.3 also demonstrated that providing social interaction through voice, touch, facial expression, and looking at the infant's face and eyes exerts strong immediate impacts on suckling in terms of both volume-intake of milk and total sucks (Lumeng et al., 2007). Again, positive verbalization including encouragement by caregivers was seen to be associated with higher rates of acceptance of food in older children, while threatening verbalization was associated with higher rates of rejection (Ha et al., 2002; Dearden et al., 2009). Mothers which were not worried too much and kept calm when confronted with toddlers' food refusal at mealtime, hence creating a positive atmosphere at mealtime, were found negatively associated with toddlers' food neophobia (An et al., 2020). These findings are consistent with data collected from LAMI countries (Bentley et al., 2011). *Responsive/authoritative feeding style* is associated with better nutritional status and weight-related outcomes (Nti and Lartey, 2008; Larsen et al., 2015),

**TABLE 19.3**  Effect of parental feeding practices and styles on infants' eating behavior and health.

| Study | Aim | Result | Reference |
|---|---|---|---|
| Gemini twin cohort, United Kingdom: $n = 1920$ mothers | To investigate association between differences in maternal use of restriction and pressure at early stage and infant appetite and weight; to test whether mothers respond differently according to feeding method (breast- and bottle-feeding); to test the hypothesis that pressure and restriction would be higher, and less child-responsive, for bottle-fed infants | – Pressure: associated with lower birth weight, greater concern about underweight, lower infant appetite <br> – Restriction associated with higher appetite and bottle feeding <br> – Interaction with feeding method: mothers who bottle-fed their infants restricted more in response to a heartier infant appetite | Fildes et al. (2015) |
| Observational study part of a prospective, randomized community intervention trial, Vietnam: $n = 91$ mother/child pairs, children aged 12 and 17 months | To test whether caregiver encouragement, caregiver's and child's behaviors, and other feeding characteristics were associated with acceptance of food | – Caregiver's positive and mechanical/direct verbalization associated with odds of a child accepting the offered bite (children 2.4 times as likely to accept bites) <br> – Force feeding positively associated with acceptance <br> – Children feeding themselves more likely to accept bites <br> – 12-months-olds: in the caregiver's arms or lap less likely to accept bites; crawling during feeding 2.8 times as likely to accept bites <br> – 17-months-olds playing less likely to accept bites <br> – Comparison between ages: 17-months-olds sitting on a lap, on the floor, on a chair, stool or bed, or being in the caregiver's arms more likely to accept bites | Dearden et al. (2009) |
| Follow-up to the Technological University Dublin (DIT)-Coombe Hospital birth cohort study, Ireland: $n = 205$ mother/child pairs, toddler aged 1.5 to 3.4 years | To explore the associations between maternal feeding practices, mealtime emotions, and toddlers' food neophobia | – Maternal practice of coaxing the children to eat at refusal positively associated with higher degree of child food neophobia <br> – Unpleasant emotions at mealtime (e.g., stressful or hectic for mothers, or tearful for children) associated with higher degree of child food neophobia <br> – Mothers not worrying about child's food refusal negatively associated with toddlers' food neophobia | An et al. (2020) |

| Sample/Design | Aim | Results | Reference |
|---|---|---|---|
| Randomized trial, USA: $n = 25$ healthy, full term, 7- to 14-week-old infants. Bottle-fed their own formula twice by their mothers plus four experimental conditions with a $2 \times 2$ design: (a) held, provided social interaction (through voice, touch, facial expression, looking at infant's face and eyes); (b) held, without interaction; (c) not held (infant seated in an infant seat), provided social interaction; (d) not held, denied social interaction. Volume-intake from a bottle (VI), total sucks, infant gaze direction, and time elapsed since the last feeding assessed | To investigate social influences on human suckling behavior | Social interaction increased VI by 43% independently of holding; VI was linearly related to the time since the last feeding in held infants; total sucks and VI highly correlated with privation length when infants did not look at the feeder and when fed by the mother | Lumeng et al. (2007) |
| Within-subject experimental study, USA: $n$ ($\leq$ 4-months-old infants) $= 41$. CMF; CMF enriched with free amino-acid glutamate (CMF + Glu) | To determine whether timing, frequency and types of behaviors displayed differ when feeding isocaloric formulas; infants are consistent in their display of these behaviors, regardless of amount consumed; the relationship between maternal feeding styles and infant self-regulation of intake and behavioral displays | – Maternal feeding styles: the less responsive the mother's feeding style, the less consistent the infant displayed behaviors across the formula meals<br>– Infant behavior: Infants who spat up consumed more formula and had mothers who scored lower in food responsiveness | Ventura et al. (2015) |
| Survey as part of a larger study of positive deviance, Nicaragua: $n = 80$ children aged 12–19 months. | To examine association of caregivers' feeding behavior with young children's anthropometric status | – Meal type: more active feeding at the midday meal (more encouragement, threats to finish, orders to eat, offers of additional food, talks)<br>– Mothers: more likely to offer encouragement for eating, to serve the midday meal vs snacks<br>– Active feeding negatively associated with child's demand and interest for bottle feeds<br>– Height-for-age and weight-for-age positively associated with Child Demand Scale for bottle feeds | Engle and Zeitlin (1996) |
| Community-based longitudinal, Ghana: $n = 100$ mothers with infants aged 6–12 months | To assess how parental practices influence nutritional status of young children | Caregivers with positive deviant children provided good quality diets from highly diversified sources, and exhibited high responsiveness during feeding | Nti and Lartey (2008) |

*Continued*

**TABLE 19.3** Effect of parental feeding practices and styles on infants' eating behavior and health—cont'd

| Study | Aim | Result | Reference |
|---|---|---|---|
| Cluster randomized field trial, Bangladesh. Mothers with 12- to 24-months-olds. IG: $n = 102$ attending 6-sessions within an educational programme emphasizing practice of child self-feeding and maternal responsiveness; CG: 100 receiving sessions on foods to feed. Outcomes assessed at pre-test, 2-week post-intervention and at 5-month postintervention | To test the hypotheses that IG children would show more self-feeding, more mouthfuls of food taken, and greater weight gain than the CG ones; to test the hypothesis that IG mothers would show more responsive behaviors | – IG child weight, weight gain and self-feeding higher<br>– IG mothers gave their children more vegetables, and spontaneously recalled more feeding messages at the 5-month follow-up | Aboud et al. (2008) |
| Observational study within a large randomized intervention trial, the ViSION project, Vietnam: $n = 40$ child/mother pairs; children aged 12 or 18 months | To investigate feeding styles of rural caregivers for their young children | – Children 12 months: more likely to be fed semi-solid puddings, porridges, or noodles<br>– Caregivers: providing physical help to eat nearly all of the time in the younger children, and about 70% of the time among 18 months olds; verbalizing during only 30% of intended bites with only half of these verbalizations being responsive in tone or words; positive behaviors associated with higher child's food acceptance, non-RF behaviors associated with food rejection | Ha et al. (2002) |

*BMI, body mass index; CG, control group; CMF, cow-milk formula; IG, Intervention group; RF, responsive feeding.*

**TABLE 19.4** Effects of obesity prevention intervention studies focusing on maternal feeding practice and commencing in the child's first weeks of life.

| Study | Aim | Result | Reference |
|---|---|---|---|
| Community-based early feeding intervention, (NOURISH) RCT, Australia: $n = 698$ mothers with healthy term infants aged ($4.3 \pm 1.0$ months) months at baseline. CG: self-directed access to usual care; IG: attendance to two 6-session interactive group education modules providing guidance on early feeding practices. Outcomes assessed at infant age $13.7 \pm 1.3$ months | To evaluate a universal obesity prevention intervention, which commenced at infant age 4–6 months, using outcome data assessed 6 months after completion of the first of two intervention modules and 9 months from baseline | – CG infants: at follow-up, higher BMI-for-age z-score, more likely to show rapid weight gain from baseline<br>– CG mothers: more likely to report using non-RF practices such as encouraging eating by using food as a reward or using games | Daniels et al. (2012) |
| NOURISH RCT, Australia. Outcomes assessed at 2 years of age | To report impact evaluation of the NOURISH intervention on child eating behavior, food preferences, dietary intake, and parenting practices | – IG mothers: using RF more and overall less controlling feeding practices (i.e., lower levels of instrumental, emotional feeding, and greater use of "autonomy encouragement"; more likely to interpret food refusal as a signal of satiety, less to use non-responsive/coercive practices such as insisting or offering rewards)<br>– IG Children: rated higher on satiety responsiveness, and lower on emotional overeating, fussiness, and food responsiveness; "liked" more fruits, and fewer non-core foods and beverages<br>– No differences in health outcomes | Daniels et al. (2013); Daniels et al. (2014) |
| Secondary analysis of data from a NOURISH RCT subsample of mother–father dyads, Australia: $n = 70$ | To compare feeding practices within parent dyads and explore whether the positive intervention impact on maternal feeding practices generalized to any indirect effect on fathers' feeding practices | Fathers whose partners were allocated to the IG group used less pressure and were more willing to let the child decide how much to eat | Daniels et al. (2020) |

*Continued*

**TABLE 19.4** Effects of obesity prevention intervention studies focusing on maternal feeding practice and commencing in the child's first weeks of life—cont'd

| Study | Aim | Result | Reference |
|---|---|---|---|
| INSIGHT RCT, USA: $n = 291$ primiparous mother-newborn dyads. Home visits by research nurses at 3 weeks, 16 weeks, 28 weeks, and 40 weeks; a research center visit at 1 year. IG = received messages about infant feeding, sleep hygiene, active social play, emotion regulation, and growth record education CG = received a developmentally appropriate home safety intervention | To explore the effect of the responsive parenting intervention on infant weight gain between birth and 28 weeks and overweight status at age 1 year, and on parents' infant feeding practices in the first year after birth as well. | – IG infant: mean conditional weight gain score lower, reflecting a slower weight gain, independently of feeding mode (predominantly fed breast-milk or not); lower mean weight-for-length percentiles at 1 year, and less likely to be overweight at age 1 year (5.5% vs 12.7%). <br> – IG mothers: more likely to use of structure-based feeding practices; less likely to use non-RF practices such as pressuring their infant to finish the bottle/food, and using food to soothe propping the bottle (between 4 and 8 months), and putting baby to bed with a bottle at age 1 year <br> – Few differences in what specific foods infants were fed | Savage et al. (2016); Savage et al. (2018) |
| INSIGHT RCT, USA: $n = 232$ mother–child dyads | To examine the effect of INSIGHT intervention on children's weight outcomes at 3 years | IG children had a lower mean BMI-z-scores; no significant difference in mean BMI percentiles; odds ratios for overweight or obesity 0.51 (95% CI = 0.25 to 1.06, $P = 0.07$) and 0.32 (95% CI = 0.08 to 1.20, $P = 0.09$), respectively, compared with CG children | Paul et al. (2018) |
| Observation-only ancillary study of INSIGHT, USA: $n = 117$ mother-secondborn dyads ($n$ from IG = 57; $n$ from CG = 60) | To assess the spillover effect of INSIGHT intervention on maternal feeding practices with their secondborn infants, and to test the moderating effect of spacing of births risk of obesity and other co-morbidities throughout life course | IG mothers used more consistent feeding routines; less non-responsive, controlling feeding practices; no difference in bottle-feeding practices such as putting to bed with a bottle/sippy cup or adding cereal to the bottle | Ruggiero et al. (2020) |

BMI, body mass index; CG, control group; IG, intervention group; RCT, randomized controlled trial; RF, responsive feeding.

as well as with better fruit and vegetable consumption in the childhood years accompanied by practices such as modeling consumption, increasing availability at home, encouraging children to try them and so on (Blissett, 2011).

In *controlling styles of feeding*, caregiver potentially override the child's internal hunger/fullness regulatory cues interfering with his/her ability to self-regulate their energy and food intake, thus increasing responsiveness to external, contextual cues (Engle et al., 2000; Black and Aboud, 2011). By misinterpreting child's refusal to accept food as a sign of poor appetite, rather than a signal for autonomy, the mealtime may lead child to frustration, inattention to internal cues, lack of interest in communicating to the caregiver, and food refusal (Engle and Zeitlin, 1996; Ha et al., 2002; Black and Aboud, 2011; Ventura et al., 2015; An et al., 2020). Several findings demonstrated that children *pressured or offered with rewards* to eat a certain food may exhibit a decreased preference for the target food later on, even though an immediate increase of the target-food intake is observed during the eating occasion where the practice is used (Ventura and Worobey, 2013; Larsen et al., 2015). According to Ventura and Worobey (2013), such practices devalue the target food conveying the child the unintentional message that a target food is not preferable in itself. Moreover, *instrumental and/or emotional feeding* was found positively correlated with intake of palatable high-energy-density foods, and associated with overeating (Lo et al., 2015; Larsen et al., 2015). Attempts at *restricting* access to forbidden foods also seems to be counterproductive, as findings evidenced that children exhibited a clear interest/preference for and a high consumption of restricted foods when subsequently available (Savage et al., 2007; Ventura and Worobey, 2013). To summarize, high levels of both parental control and pressure to eat are associated with low fruit and vegetable intakes, and high intakes of fats (Savage et al., 2007; Blissett, 2011; Birch and Doub, 2014).

Similarly, *indulgent feeding styles* and high levels of *inattention* to a child's "hunger or satiety cues" may result in overfeeding (Dattilo et al., 2012; Bentley et al., 2011), or high risk of childhood overweight (Dattilo et al., 2012; Mitchell et al., 2013; Larsen et al., 2015).

### 19.3.3 Other determinants in the progression of children's eating behaviors and dietary patterns

Beyond genetic factors, a number of factors, including child's appetite and temperament (Russell and Russell, 2018), caregiver's behavioral eating traits and ecology may promote overeating and obesity in children (Larsen et al., 2015; Costa et al., 2018; Monteiro et al., 2018; Scaglioni et al., 2018).

- *Family context.* As the early experiences of eating occur in the home food environment, it is reasonable that family features shape the context in which eating occurs (Mura Paroche et al., 2017; Dattilo et al., 2020), as also shown in findings displayed in Table 19.5. In this context, it may be interesting to cite the "Gemini cohort" study involving 1216 twins aged 21 months aimed at testing the hypothesis that diet in early childhood was primarily determined by the environment rather than by genes (Pimpin et al., 2013). The authors found that shared environmental influences were the predominant drivers of dietary intake contributing between 66% (milk-based desserts) and 97% (juice) of the variation vs genetic factors which accounted for between 4% (savory snacks) and 18% (bread) of dietary intake variation, suggesting the importance of factors such as home food environment and parental behaviors. Parents are responsible for both availability and easy accessibility of specific foods (e.g., healthy foods) at

**TABLE 19.5** Impact of several family variables, including parents' dietary patterns, sociodemographic factors, culture on infants' feeding patterns.

| Study | Aim | Result | Reference |
|---|---|---|---|
| Cross-sectional survey. Children design between 6 and 36 months: United Kingdom, $n=71$; Denmark, $n=70$. Mothers received questionnaires including vegetables available in national supermarkets and main grocery stores (United Kingdom, $n=54$, Denmark, $n=41$; France, $n=52$) | To examine pre-school children's experience with vegetables across three European countries in order to assess cultural differences, effects of age, and culinary practices | – Children: effect of nationality and age on both number of vegetables introduced and frequency those were offered; mothers: effect of nationality on familiarity with vegetables and preparation techniques <br> – Age (significant effect on liking and preparation techniques, too) <br> – Children aged 6–12 months: offered vegetables more frequently; higher reported liking for these vegetables; more likely to receive pureed or mashed vegetables. Children aged 25–36 months: introduced to the greatest number of vegetables <br> – Nationality <br> – UK: children = introduced higher number and offered more frequently than French, liking related to frequency of maternal intake and frequency of offering; mothers = recognized more vegetables; steaming more vegetables than Danish. France: preparing more vegetables by steaming, stewing, pureeing or mashing. Denmark: children = introduced the greatest number and offered vegetables more frequently; mothers = familiar with lower of "common" vegetables than French; offering more vegetables raw and boiled | Ahern et al. (2013) |
| Two observational cohorts, SKOT I (non-obese mothers) and SKOT II (obese mothers), Denmark: $n=374$ infants of 9 months of age | To investigate association between family and child indicators and adherence to dietary patterns for infants aged 9 months | Two patterns: "Family Food" (transition) = *BreastMilk* and *Formula* the lowest loadings while *Meat*, *FatsAnimal*, *RyeBread* and *Milk* the highest; "Health-Conscious Food" = *SweetsCake* and *SugaryDrink* the lowest loadings while *Potato*, *FatsVegetable*, *Fruit* and *Vegetable* the highest. <br> – Lower "Family Food" score: higher BMI-z-scores at 9 months; infants with immigrant/descendant parents, parents sharing cooking responsibilities <br> – Lower "Health-Conscious Food" score: higher maternal BMI, greater numbers of children in the household, higher BMI-z-scores at 9 months | Andersen et al. (2015) |

| Study | Aim | Findings | Reference |
|---|---|---|---|
| EDEN mother–child cohort, France: $n = 1004$. Feeding practices assessed at birth, 4, 8 and 12 months | To identify patterns of feeding in the first year of life and examine associations with family features | – "Late CF introduction and use of ready-prepared baby foods": related to high family income, maternal age and education, and low parity; mothers more often recruited in urban centers<br>– "Longer BF, late CF introduction and use of home-made foods" (the closest to infant feeding guidelines): mothers likely to be older, to have high education level and less likely to be obese, more often recruited in rural centers<br>– "Use of adults' foods" (a less age-specific diet for the infants): associated with low maternal age, being multiparous, mothers more often recruited in urban centers | Betoko et al. (2013) |
| Prospective, observational study, Ireland: $n = 401$ pregnant women followed up at 6 weeks and 6 months postpartum | To assess compliance with WHO recommendation and examine weaning practices, including the timing of weaning of infants; to investigate factors predicting weaning at ≤12 weeks and 6 months post-partum | – Weaning at ≤12 weeks: mothers' age ≤24 years, low education (primary and secondary level), smoking in pregnancy; mothers more likely to engage in other sub-optimal weaning practices such as adding non-recommended condiments (ordinary gravy, butter, sauces, vegetable stock, salt and sugar/honey), solids to infants' bottled feeds, offering non-recommended snacks (chocolates, biscuits, crisps, and ice cream)<br>– Predictive factors of weaning at ≤12 weeks: antenatal reporting on infants to be weaned onto solids at ≤12 weeks, and to be formula fed at 12 weeks; reporting of maternal grandmother as principal source of feeding advice<br>– Predictive factors of weaning at >12 weeks: mothers' reporting of public health nurse as principal source of feeding advice; positive correlation between mothers' antenatal reporting on weaning time and actual weaning time<br>– Mothers' reasons weaning at ≤12 weeks: perception of infant hunger and sleep promotion | Tarrant et al. (2010) |

Continued

**TABLE 19.5** Impact of several family variables, including parents' dietary patterns, sociodemographic factors, culture on infants' feeding patterns—cont'd

| Study | Aim | Result | Reference |
|---|---|---|---|
| Population-based, prospective birth-cohort study, the Netherlands: n = 2420 children aged 14 months | To identify common dietary patterns in toddlers and explore parental and child indicators | – "Health conscious" (pasta, fruits, vegetables, oils, legumes, fish): inversely associated with maternal co-morbidity, alcohol consumption in pregnancy, and female sex of child; positively associated with single parenthood, folic-acid use and dietary fiber intake in pregnancy<br>– "Western" (savory snacks, confectionery, animal fats, sugar-based beverages): positively associated with low paternal education, low income, parental smoking, multiparity, maternal BMI, maternal carbohydrate intake and television-watching of child; inversely associated with parental age, dietary fiber intake in pregnancy, introduction of solids after 6 months and female sex of child | Kiefte-de Jong et al. (2013) |
| Type 1 Diabetes Prediction and Prevention Nutrition Study, Finland: mothers = 4862; 1-year-olds = 719, in 3-years-olds = 708, in 6-years-olds = 841 | To describe dietary clusters of pre-school children and their mothers, and analyze similarity of dietary clusters within child–mother pairs | – Patterns based on age: "Healthy" (skimmed milk, whole-grain bread, vegetables) and "Traditional" (dairy spread, high-fat milk) in all three age groups; "Ready-to-eat baby foods" (infant formulas, manufactured baby foods) in 1-year-olds; "Fast foods, sweet" (sugars-sweetened beverages, fried potatoes, chips, nuts, dried fruit) in >1-year-olds<br>– Some familial dependence between dietary clusters of mother–child pairs observed in 6-years-olds<br>– Mother younger age and lower educational level associated with "Fast foods, sweet" in 3-years-olds | Ovaskainen et al. (2009) |
| Southampton Women's Survey, United Kingdom: n = 1434 | To describe dietary patterns of a general population sample of infants aged 6 and 12 months, and consider maternal and family factors associated | Infants' patterns identified: "Infant guidelines" (fruit, vegetables, home-prepared foods); "Adult foods" (bread, savory snacks, biscuits, chips).<br>Dietary pattern scores<br>– Correlated with infant age ("Infant guidelines" at 6 months; "Adult foods" at 12 months)<br>– Associated with maternal level of education and diet quality: Women complying with dietary recommendations, high intakes of fruit, vegetables, wholemeal bread, rice and pasta, more likely to have high 'infant guidelines' scores' infants; women with low "Prudent diet" scores and high intake of chips, white bread, crisps and sweets, more likely to have high "Adult foods" scores' infants | Robinson et al. (2007) |

| Study details | Aim | Findings | Reference |
|---|---|---|---|
| Gemini cohort, England and Wales: families with twins = 2402; dietary diaries available = 1216. Twins aged 21 months | To test the hypothesis that diet in early childhood is primarily determined by the environment rather than by genes; to characterize the early childhood diet | Diet of the children at 21 months of age consisted predominantly of small portions of common family foods.<br>– Shared environment: the predominant determinant of dietary intake, contributing between 66% (milk-based desserts) and 97% (juice) of the variation<br>– Genetic factors: account for between 4% (savory snacks) and 18% (bread) of dietary intake variation | Pimpin et al. (2013) |
| A cross-sectional study design, USA: n = 80 African American first-time mother with 12–18 months-olds | To assess association between objective measures of fruits and vegetables at home with reported infant and maternal diet in low income African Americans | Homes in the highest tertile of availability of fruits and vegetables: associations with infant diet; strongest for infant consumption of fruit (103.3 vs 42.5g) | Bryant et al. (2011) |
| Infant Care, Feeding and Risk of Obesity Study = Observational cohort, USA: n = 217 low-income, African-American mother–infant dyads, followed from 3 to 18 months postpartum | To examine non-maternal involvement (NMC) in feeding during the first 2 years of life and association with BF duration, early introduction of CF, and dietary intakes of selected foods and beverages | Longitudinal models adjusted for confounding variables.<br>– NMC associated with a 95% decrease in BF; increased odds of infant or toddler consuming any whole fruit as well as any juice (twice the recommended level)<br>– Mother's characteristics: a one-unit increase in age associated with 0.05 more servings of whole fruit; any maternal college with fewer servings of fried potatoes, sweetened beverages, salty snacks; maternal depression with more servings of salty snacks | Wasser et al. (2013) |
| Cross-sectional study (data from the Early Food for Future Health randomized controlled trial), Norway: n = 715 mother–infant dyads.<br>Web questionnaire to assess daily food consumption, BF duration, and timing of introduction to solid food completed at child age 5.5 months | To explore potential associations between timing of solid foods' introduction and a wide range of maternal and infant characteristics | Solid food introduction before 4 months of age associated with infant less often exclusive breastfed the first month and more often receiving only formula milk at 3 months; mother being younger, not married/cohabitant, smoking, less educated and having more economic difficulties<br>– Not being introduced to solid food at 5.5 months associated with infant being a girl, being exclusive breastfed the first month, receiving only breast-milk at 3 months; mother being older, married, and having 3 or more children | Helle et al. (2018) |
| Cross-sectional data from the BeeBOFT study, The Netherlands: n = 2157.<br>Data on CF practices and potential determinants obtained by questionnaire at infant's age of 6 months | To investigate factors associated with introduction of CF before age 4 months, and factors associated with infants consumption of non-recommended foods, including sweet beverages and snack foods | 21.4% of infants had received CF before 4 months of age; at 6 months, 20.2% of all infants were consuming sweet beverages daily and 16.5% snack foods daily<br>– Younger maternal age, lower maternal educational level, absence or shorter duration of BF, parental conviction that "my child always wants to eat when he/she sees someone eating", not attending day-care independently associated with both early introduction of CF and consumption of non-recommended foods | Wang et al. (2019) |

*BF*, Breastfeeding; *CF*, complementary feeding; *BMI*, body mass index.

home (Bryant et al., 2011), and infants' feeding practices as well. In addition, they influence their children's eating behavior by modeling their own behavior, taste preferences, and food choices (Kral and Rauh, 2010). Lifestyle, dietary habits, education and financial background of the caregivers, especially mothers, have been shown to play a significant role in the development of dietary patterns with adherence to unhealthy dietary patterns and feeding practices in infants being linked to caregivers' unfavorable lifestyles (i.e., smoking, longer television watching, and so on) and low sociodemographic background (i.e., low educational level, low income, and so on) (Robinson et al., 2007; Ovaskainen et al., 2009; Betoko et al., 2013; Kiefte-de Jong et al., 2013; Wasser et al., 2013; Helle et al., 2018). Also the maternal age has been observed as a predictive factor of the compliance with WHOs recommendation for CF with younger mothers more likely to deviate from recommendations, for example, by weaning their infants at $\leq 12$ weeks of age (Helle et al., 2018; Tarrant et al., 2010; Wang et al., 2019).

- *Ecological context*. Child feeding practices are influenced by additional macro-environmental features, such as the cost and availability of food. Moreover, their nutritional appropriateness and styles, in terms of food type and preparation, age of introduction, feeding style, frequency and schedules, and feeding environment reflect differences in ethnic and cultural patterns (Engle et al., 2000; Van Esterik, 2002; Pelto et al., 2003; Black and Aboud, 2011; Grote et al., 2011; Ahern et al., 2013). It is acknowledged that food choices or child feeding practices are responsive to the ecological contexts in which they are practiced (Kumanyika, 2008). Thus, despite healthy infant feeding practices are promoted by health clinicians as well as by numerous national and international organizations, in fact, mothers and caregivers base their infant feeding decisions on their experiences, family demands, socioeconomic circumstances, cultural taboos, and religious beliefs (Marquis et al., 1998; Pelto et al., 2003; Steinman et al., 2010; Bentley et al., 2011; Harrison et al., 2017; Agho et al., 2019; Tully et al., 2019). Grandmothers likely play a central role as both advisers to younger women and caregivers of children on nutrition and health issues (Aubel, 2012; Tarrant et al., 2010). Tradition and culture, i.e., social norms within the caregiver's environment seem mostly to shape parental infant feeding beliefs and perceptions about when to begin CF, and what first foods to be offered (Dattilo et al., 2020). For example, among several ethnic groups and traditional communities, in the first few days after birth infants are fed with liquids other than breast-milk because colostrum is considered "evil", while sugared water, tea, oils, etc. are considered newborn's gut cleaners (Pak-Gorstein et al., 2009); in the Middle East and some African countries, mixed milk feeding is a common practice (Monge-Montero et al., 2020); the feeding laissez-faire *style* is the most adopted, as feeding children from 6 to 24 months is considered time-consuming, while interactive feeding does not seem culturally normative (Pelto et al., 2003).

## 19.4 Future trends and research

Feeding guidelines need to be implemented and reappraised based on current evidence and best practice (Vereijken et al., 2011; Bloomfield and Agostoni, 2020; Matvienko-Sikar et al., 2019). The new models reflecting infants' and young children's neurobehavioral responses to prolonged BF even while introducing solids may have a higher impact in establishing dietary habits, personal taste, and choices than believed before.

"Addressing nutrition through the life-course also requires a more holistic view and integrated provision of health and nutrition services by health-care systems in all settings" (WHO, 2019). Fig. 19.3 shows that through-the-life-course education and translational research to enable people to establish healthy dietary practices, if integrated into multisector programs and starting from early age as an entry point, may have important implications for the prevention of long-term health (Berti et al., 2017; Black et al., 2017). In particular, interventions promoting responsive parenting behaviors should be implemented right at the start of a new life in order to prevent not only the use of some NRF practices but also the risk of child's obesity (see Table 19.4).

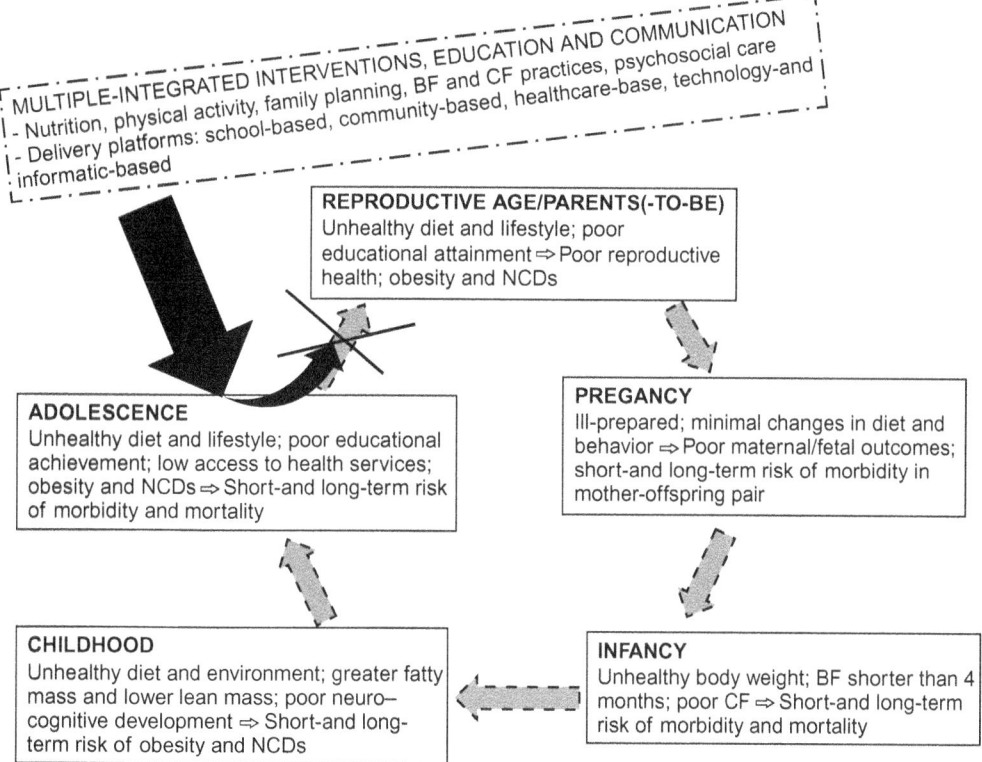

FIG. 19.3 Early age as the "entry-point" to break the intergenerational cycle of malnutrition and noncommunicable diseases. Malnourished and poor educated parents are at higher risk of poor nutritional status, reproductive health, and adverse fetal growth, with long-lasting negative consequences on the overall health and social development of the parent-infant pair. By breaking this vicious cycle, multiple-integrated nutrition and lifestyle programs, including health literacy, aimed at today pediatric groups may have transformative impact on nutritional status, health and well-being of the current and succeeding generations. Better nourished and educated youth may be more healthier and attentive upcoming parents and have healthier children. School, community, communication, and information technology, specialized health-services are the most effective platforms to deliver interventions on nutrition, physical activity, reproductive health-education, and lifestyle. *BF:* breastfeeding; *CF:* complementary feeding; *NCDs:* non-communicable diseases.

In the meantime, some practical points on CF may be recalled (Alvisi et al., 2015; Fewtrell et al., 2017):

- The start of CF should be defined on an individual basis, accommodating to infant competences. The limit of 6 months of age (WHO, 2001) still remains a desirable goal also in Western societies. Nevertheless, the "not before 4 completed month neither beyond 6 completed months" paradigm may be useful for the few breastfed subjects possibly requiring some more energy in 4–6 month period
- Continued BF is recommended along with the introduction of CF
- It is not advisable to delay the introduction of potentially allergenic foods nor of gluten with the purpose of preventing the development of allergic diseases; at the same time, there is no ideal timing for gluten introduction in relation with the onset of celiac disease, despite consumption of large quantities should be avoided during the first weeks after gluten introduction and later during infancy
- Parents should be encouraged to respond to their infant's hunger and satiety cues, and avoid feeding as a relief or a reward.

## 19.5 Conclusion

The satisfaction of the infant's curiosity and requests with repeatedly small tastings of food should be promoted, starting to offer ground, chopped, or finger food only once the child has developed the necessary postural and oral-motor skills. At the same time, parents and caregivers should be encouraged to respect every child's self-regulatory capacity, that is, to respond to infants' cues of appetite or satiety. However, for parents and caregivers to best feed infants and toddler appropriately and adequately, they must be guided, motivated, and educated. Pediatricians have the responsibility to provide clear and consistent knowledge or advice about nutrition and practices (i.e., alternating new food with a highly liked food or presenting it together with familiar tastes to increase acceptance) in a step-by-step way that can be easily translated into practice (Vereijken et al., 2011; Larsen et al., 2015; Brambilla et al., 2020). But probably the most important, not quantifiable, rule is that solid introduction should privilege family, traditional, and ethnic habits (Alvisi et al., 2015).

## Sources of further information

https://www.unicef.org/media/60806/file/SOWC-2019.pdf

https://healthyeatingresearch.org/research/feeding-guidelines-for-infants-and-young-toddlers-a-responsive-parenting-approach/

https://cesni-biblioteca.org/archivos/UNICEF_Programming_Guidance_Complementary_Feeding.pdf

http://www.unicef.org/nutrition/index_breastfeeding.html

https://www.who.int/news-room/fact-sheets/detail/infant-and-young-child-feedinghttp://www.espghan.org/guidelines/nutrition/

https://efsa.onlinelibrary.wiley.com/doi/10.2903/j.efsa.2019.5780https://www.nal.usda.gov/fnic/complementary-feeding-and-baby-foods

# References

Aboud, F.E., Moore, A.C., Akhter, S., 2008. Effectiveness of a community-based responsive feeding programme in rural Bangladesh: a cluster randomized field trial. Matern. Child Nutr. 4 (4), 275–286.

Agho, K.E., Ezeh, O.K., Ghimire, P.R., Uchechukwu, O.L., Stevens, G.J., Tannous, W.K., Fleming, C., Ogbo, F.A., Global Maternal And Child Health Research Collaboration GloMACH, 2019. Exclusive breastfeeding rates and associated factors in 13 "Economic Community of West African States" (ECOWAS) countries. Nutrients 11 (12), 3007. https://doi.org/10.3390/nu11123007.

Agostoni, C., Przyrembel, H., 2013. The timing of introduction of complementary foods and later health. World Rev. Nutr. Diet. 108, 63–70.

Agostoni, C., Decsi, T., Fewtrell, M., Goulet, O., Kolacek, S., Koletzko, B., Michaelsen, K.F., Moreno, L., Puntis, J., Rigo, J., Shamir, R., Szajewska, H., Turck, D., van Goudoever, J., ESPGHAN Committee on Nutrition, 2008. Complementary feeding: a commentary by the ESPGHAN committee on nutrition. J. Pediatr. Gastroenterol. Nutr. 46 (1), 99–110.

Agostoni, C., Mazzocchi, A., Leone, L., Ciappolino, V., Delvecchio, G., Altamura, C.A., Brambilla, P., 2017. The first model of keeping energy balance and optimal psycho affective development: breastfed infants. J. Affect. Disord. 224, 10–15.

Agostoni, C., Guz-Mark, A., Marderfeld, L., Milani, G.P., Silano, M., Shamir, R., 2019. The long-term effects of dietary nutrient intakes during the first 2 years of life in healthy infants from developed countries: an umbrella review. Adv. Nutr. 10 (3), 489–501.

Ahern, S.M., Caton, S.J., Bouhlal, S., Hausner, H., Olsen, A., Nicklaus, S., Møller, P., Hetherington, M.M., 2013. Eating a rainbow. Introducing vegetables in the first years of life in 3 European countries. Appetite 71, 48–56.

Aldridge, V., Dovey, T.M., Halford, J.C.G., 2009. The role of familiarity in dietary development. Dev. Rev. 29, 32–44.

Alvisi, P., Brusa, S., Alboresi, S., Amarri, S., Bottau, P., Cavagni, G., Corradini, B., Landi, L., Loroni, L., Marani, M., Osti, I.M., Povesi-Dascola, C., Caffarelli, C., Valeriani, L., Agostoni, C., 2015. Recommendations on complementary feeding for healthy, full-term infants. Ital. J. Pediatr. 41, 36. https://doi.org/10.1186/s13052-015-0143-5.

An, M., Zhou, Q., Younger, K.M., Liu, X., Kearney, J.M., 2020. Are maternal feeding practices and mealtime emotions associated with toddlers' food neophobia? A follow-up to the DIT-Coombe Hospital birth cohort in Ireland. Int. J. Environ. Res. Public Health 17 (22), E8401.

Andersen, L.B., Mølgaard, C., Michaelsen, K.F., Carlsen, E.M., Bro, R., Pipper, C.B., 2015. Indicators of dietary patterns in Danish infants at 9 months of age. Food Nutr. Res. 59, 27665.

Anzman, S.L., Rollins, B.Y., Birch, L.L., 2010. Parental influence on children's early eating environments and obesity risk: implications for prevention. Int. J. Obes. 34 (7), 1116–1124.

Arabi, M., Frongillo, E.A., Avula, R., Mangasaryan, N., 2012. Infant and young child feeding in developing countries. Child Dev. 83 (1), 32–45.

Aubel, J., 2012. The role and influence of grandmothers on child nutrition: culturally designated advisors and caregivers. Matern. Child Nutr. 8 (1), 19–35.

Baird, J., Poole, J., Robinson, S., Marriott, L., Godfrey, K., Cooper, C., Inskip, H., Law, C., the Southampton Women's Survey Study Group, 2008. Milk feeding and dietary patterns predict weight and fat gains in infancy. Paediatr. Perinat. Epidemiol. 22 (6), 575–586.

Balantekin, K.N., Anzman-Frasca, S., Francis, L.A., Ventura, A.K., Fisher, J.O., Johnson, S.L., 2020. Positive parenting approaches and their association with child eating and weight: a narrative review from infancy to adolescence. Pediatr. Obes. 15 (10), e12722.

Barrera, C.M., Hamner, H.C., Perrine, C.G., Scanlon, K.S., 2018. Timing of introduction of complementary foods to US infants, National Health and Nutrition Examination Survey 2009–2014. J. Acad. Nutr. Diet. 118 (3), 464–470.

Beauchamp, G.K., Mennella, J.A., 2009. Early flavor learning and its impact on later feeding behavior. J. Pediatr. Gastroenterol. Nutr. 48 (suppl 1), S25–S30.

Becerra-Bulla, F., Bonilla-Bohorquez, L., Rodriguez-Bonilla, J., 2015. Leptina y lactancia materna: beneficios fisiológicos. Rev. Fac. Med. 63 (1), 119–126.

Bentley, M.E., Wasser, H.M., Creed-Kanashiro, H.M., 2011. Responsive feeding and child undernutrition in low- and middle-income countries. J. Nutr. 141 (3), 502–507.

Berti, C., Agostoni, C., Davanzo, R., Hyppönen, E., Isolauri, E., Meltzer, H.M., Steegers-Theunissen, R.P., Cetin, I., 2017. Early-life nutritional exposures and lifelong health: immediate and long-lasting impacts of probiotics, vitamin D, and breastfeeding. Nutr. Rev. 75 (2), 83–97.

Betoko, A., Charle, M.A., Hankard, R., Forhan, A., Bonet, M., Saurel-Cubizolles, M.J., Heude, B., de Lauzon-Guillain, B., EDEN mother-child cohort study group, 2013. Infant feeding patterns over the first year of life: influence of family characteristics. Eur. J. Clin. Nutr. 67 (6), 631–637.

Birch, L.L., 1999. Development of food preferences. Annu. Rev. Nutr. 19, 41–62.

Birch, L.L., Anzman, S.L., 2010. Learning to eat in an obesogenic environment: a developmental systems perspective on childhood obesity. Child Dev. Perspect. 4 (2), 138–143.

Birch, L.L., Doub, A.E., 2014. Learning to eat: birth to age 2 y. Am. J. Clin. Nutr. 99 (suppl), 723S–728S.

Birch, L., Savage, J.S., Ventura, A., 2007. Influences on the development of children's eating behaviours: from infancy to adolescence. Can. J. Diet. Pract. Res. 68 (1), s1–s56.

Black, M.M., Aboud, F.E., 2011. Responsive feeding is embedded in a theoretical framework of responsive parenting. J. Nutr. 141 (3), 490–494.

Black, M.M., Walker, S.P., Fernald, L.C.H., Andersen, C.T., DiGirolamo, A.M., Lu, C., McCoy, D.C., Fink, G., Shawar, Y.R., Shiffman, J., Devercelli, A.E., Wodon, Q.T., Vargas-Barón, E., Grantham-McGregor, S., 2017. Early childhood development coming of age: science through the life course. Lancet 389 (10064), 77–90.

Blissett, J., 2011. Relationships between parenting style, feeding style and feeding practices and fruit and vegetable consumption in early childhood. Appetite 57, 826–831.

Bloomfield, F.H., Agostoni, C., 2020. The potential impact of feeding formula-fed infants according to published recommendations. Pediatr. Res. 88 (4), 526–528.

Blossfeld, I., Collins, A., Boland, S., Baixauli, R., Kiely, M., Delahunty, C., 2007. Relationships between acceptance of sour taste and fruit intakes in 18-month-old infants. Br. J. Nutr. 98, 1084–1091.

Blundell, J.E., 1999. The control of appetite: basic concepts and practical implications. Schweiz. Med. Wochenschr. 129, 182–188.

Brambilla, P., Giussani, M., Picca, M., Bottaro, G., Buzzetti, R., Milani, G.P., Agostoni, C., Becherucci, P., 2020. Do the opinions of pediatricians influence their recommendations on complementary feeding? Preliminary results. Eur. J. Pediatr. 179 (4), 627–634.

Brown, S.D., Harris, G., 2012. A theoretical proposal for a perceptually driven, food-based disgust that can influence food acceptance during early childhood. Int. J. Child Health Nutr. 1, 1–10.

Bryant, M., Stevens, J., Wang, L., Tabak, R., Borja, J., Bentley, M.E., 2011. Relationship between home fruit and vegetable availability and infant and maternal dietary intake in African American families: evidence from the exhaustive home food inventory. J. Am. Diet. Assoc. 111 (10), 1491–1497.

Butte, N.F., Fox, M.K., Briefel, R.R., Siega-Riz, A.M., Dwyer, J.T., Deming, D.M., Reidy, K.C., 2010. Nutrient intakes of US infants, toddlers, and preschoolers meet or exceed dietary reference intakes. J. Am. Diet. Assoc. 110 (12 suppl), S27–S37.

Çatlı, G., Dündar, N.O., Dündar, B.N., 2014. Adipokines in breast milk: an update. J. Clin. Res. Pediatr. Endocrinol. 6 (4), 192–201.

Caton, S.J., Blundell, P., Ahern, S.M., Nekitsing, C., Olsen, A., Møller, P., Hausner, H., Remy, E., Nicklaus, S., Chabanet, C., Issanchou, S., Hetherington, M.M., 2014. Learning to eat vegetables in early life: the role of timing, age and individual eating traits. PLoS One 9 (5), e97609.

Clark, H.R., Goyder, E., Bissell, P., Blank, L., Peters, J., 2007. How do parents' child-feeding behaviours influence child weight? Implications for childhood obesity policy. J. Public Health 29 (2), 132–141.

Collado, M.C., Cernada, M., Baüerl, C., Vento, M., Pérez-Martínez, G., 2012. Microbial ecology and host-microbiota interactions during early life stages. Gut Microbes 3 (4), 352–365.

Costa, C.S., Del-Ponte, B., Assunção, M.C.F., Santos, I.S., 2018. Consumption of ultra-processed foods and body fat during childhood and adolescence: a systematic review. Public Health Nutr. 21 (1), 148–159.

Coulthard, H., Harris, G., Emmett, P., 2009. Delayed introduction of lumpy foods to children during the complementary feeding period affects child's food acceptance and feeding at 7 years of age. Matern. Child Nutr. 5 (1), 75–85.

Coulthard, H., Harris, G., Emmett, P., 2010. Long-term consequences of early fruit and vegetable feeding practices in the United Kingdom. Public Health Nutr. 13 (12), 2044–2051.

Cryan, J.F., O'Riordan, K.J., Cowan, C.S.M., Sandhu, K.V., Bastiaanssen, T.F.S., Boehme, M., Codagnone, M.G., Cussotto, S., Fulling, C., Golubeva, A.V., Guzzetta, K.E., Jaggar, M., Long-Smith, C.M., Lyte, J.M., Martin, J.A., Molinero-Perez, A., Moloney, G., Morelli, E., Morillas, E., O'Connor, R., Cruz-Pereira, J.S., Peterson, V.L., Rea, K., Ritz, N.L., Sherwin, E., Spichak, S., Teichman, E.M., van de Wouw, M., Ventura-Silva, A.P., Wallace-Fitzsimons, S.E., Hyland, N., Clarke, G., Dinan, T.G., 2019. The microbiota-gut-brain axis. Physiol. Rev. 99 (4), 1877–2013.

Dalby, M.J., Hall, L.J., 2020. Recent advances in understanding the neonatal microbiome. F1000Res 9. https://doi.org/10.12688/f1000research.22355.1. F1000 Faculty Rev.-422.

Daniels, L.A., 2019. Feeding practices and parenting: a pathway to child health and family happiness. Ann. Nutr. Metab. 74 (suppl 2), 29–42.

Daniels, L.A., Mallan, K.M., Battistutta, D., Nicholson, J.M., Perry, R., Magarey, A., 2012. Evaluation of an intervention to promote protective infant feeding practices to prevent childhood obesity: outcomes of the NOURISH RCT at 14 months of age and 6 months post the first of two intervention modules. Int. J. Obes. 36 (10), 1292–1298.

Daniels, L.A., Mallan, K.M., Nicholson, J.M., Battistutta, D., Magarey, A., 2013. Outcomes of a nearly feeding practices intervention to prevent childhood obesity. Pediatrics 132 (1), e109–e118.

Daniels, L.A., Mallan, K.M., Battistutta, D., Nicholson, J.M., Meedeniya, J.E., Bayer, J.K., Magarey, A., 2014. Child eating behavior outcomes of an early feeding intervention to reduce risk indicators for child obesity: the NOURISH RCT. Obesity (Silver Spring) 22 (5), E104–E111.

Daniels, L., Taylor, R.W., Williams, S.M., Gibson, R.S., Fleming, E.A., Wheeler, B.J., Taylor, B.J., Haszard, J.J., Heath, A.M., 2018. Impact of a modified version of babyled weaning on iron intake and status: a randomised controlled trial. BMJ Open 8 (6), e019036.

Daniels, L.A., Mallan, K.M., Jansen, E., Nicholson, J.M., Magarey, A.M., Thorpe, K., 2020. Comparison of early feeding practices in mother–father dyads and possible generalization of an efficacious maternal intervention to fathers' feeding practices: a secondary analysis. Int. J. Environ. Res. Public Health 17 (17), 6075.

Dattilo, A.M., Birch, L., Krebs, N.F., Lake, A., Taveras, E.M., Saavedra, J.M., 2012. Need for early interventions in the prevention of pediatric overweight: a review and upcoming directions. J. Obes. 2012, 123023.

Dattilo, A.M., Carvalho, R.S., Feferbaum, R., Forsyth, S., Zhao, A., 2020. Hidden realities of infant feeding: systematic review of qualitative findings from parents. Behav. Sci. 10 (5), 83.

Davisse-Paturet, C., Adel-Patient, K., Forhan, A., Lioret, S., Annesi-Maesano, I., Heude, B., Charles, M.A., de Lauzon-Guillain, B., 2020. Breastfeeding initiation or duration and longitudinal patterns of infections up to 2 years and skin rash and respiratory symptoms up to 8 years in the EDEN mother-child cohort. Matern. Child Nutr. 16 (3), e12935.

de Graaf, C., Blom, W.A., Smeets, P.A., Stafleu, A., Hendriks, H.F., 2004. Biomarkers of satiation and satiety. Am. J. Clin. Nutr. 79 (6), 946–961.

de Lauzon-Guillain, B., Jones, L., Oliveira, A., Moschonis, G., Betoko, A., Lopes, C., Moreira, P., Manios, Y., Papadopoulos, N.G., Emmett, P., Charles, M.A., 2013. The influence of early feeding practices on fruit and vegetable intake among preschool children in 4 European birth cohorts. Am. J. Clin. Nutr. 98 (3), 804–812.

de Onis, M., Blössner, M., Borghi, E., 2010. Global prevalence and trends of overweight and obesity among preschool children. Am. J. Clin. Nutr. 92 (5), 1257–1264.

Dearden, K.A., Hilton, S., Bentley, M.E., Caulfield, L.E., Wilde, C., Bich Ha, P., Marsh, D., 2009. Caregiver verbal encouragement increases food acceptance among Vietnamese toddlers. J. Nutr. 139, 1387–1392.

Delaney, A.L., Arvedson, J.C., 2008. Development of swallowing and feeding: prenatal through first year of life. Dev. Disabil. Res. Rev. 14, 105–117.

Demonteil, L., Tournier, C., Marduel, A., Dusoulier, M., Weenen, H., Nicklaus, S., 2019. Longitudinal study on acceptance of food textures between 6 and 18 months. Food Qual. Prefer. 71, 54–65.

Dewey, K.G., 2013. The challenge of meeting nutrient needs of infants and young children during the period of complementary feeding: an evolutionary perspective. J. Nutr. 143 (12), 2050–2054.

Dieterich, C.M., Felice, J.P., O'Sullivan, E., Rasmussen, K.M., 2013. Breastfeeding and health outcomes for the mother-infant dyad. Pediatr. Clin. N. Am. 60 (1), 31–48.

DiSantis, K.I., Collins, B.N., Fisher, J.O., Davey, A., 2011. Do infants fed directly from the breast have improved appetite regulation and slower growth during early childhood compared with infants fed from a bottle? Int. J. Behav. Nutr. Phys. Act. 8, 89.

DiSantis, K.I., Hodges, E.A., Fisher, J.O., 2013. The association of breastfeeding duration with later maternal feeding styles in infancy and toddlerhood: a cross-sectional analysis. Int. J. Behav. Nutr. Phys. Act. 10, 53.

Dogaru, C.M., Nyffenegger, D., Pescatore, A.M., Spycher, B.D., Kuehni, C.E., 2014. Breastfeeding and childhood asthma: systematic review and meta-analysis. Am. J. Epidemiol. 179 (10), 1153–1167.

Duijts, L., Jaddoe, V.W., Hofman, A., Moll, H.A., 2010. Prolonged and exclusive breastfeeding reduces the risk of infectious diseases in infancy. Pediatrics 126 (1), e18–e25.

Engle, P.L., Pelto, G., 2011. Responsive feeding: implications for policy and program implementation. J. Nutr. 141 (3), 508–511.

Engle, P.L., Zeitlin, M., 1996. Active feeding behavior compensates for low interest in food among young Nicaraguan children. J. Nutr. 126, 1808–1816.

Engle, P.L., Menon, P., Haddad, L., 1999. Care and nutrition: concepts and measurement. World Dev. 27 (8), 1309–1337.

Engle, P.L., Bentley, M., Pelto, G., 2000. The role of care in nutrition programmes: current research and a research agenda. Proc. Nutr. Soc. 59 (1), 25–35.

Faber, M., Laubscher, R., Berti, C., 2016. Poor dietary diversity and low nutrient density of the complementary diet for 6 to 24 month old children in urban and rural KwaZulu-Natal, South Africa. Matern. Child Nutr. 12 (3), 528–545.

Farrow, C., Haycraft, E., Mitchell, G., 2013. Milk feeding, solid feeding, and obesity risk: a review of the relationships between early life feeding practices and later adiposity. Curr. Obes. Rep. 2, 58–64.

Feachem, R.G., Koblinsky, M.A., 1984. Interventions for the control of diarrhoeal diseases among young children: promotion of breast-feeding. Bull. World Health Organ. 62 (2), 271–291.

Ferguson, M.C., O'Shea, K.J., Hammer, L.D., Hertenstein, D.L., Syed, R.M., Nyathi, S., Gonzales, M.S., Domino, M.S., Siegmund, S., Randall, S., Wedlock, P., Adam, A., Lee, B.Y., 2020. Can following formula-feeding recommendations still result in infants who are overweight or have obesity? Pediatr. Res. 88 (4), 661–667.

Fewtrell, M., Bronsky, J., Campoy, C., Domellöf, M., Embleton, N., Fidler Mis, N., Hojsak, I., Hulst, J.M., Indrio, F., Lapillonne, A., Molgaard, C., 2017. Complementary feeding: a position paper by the European Society for Paediatric Gastroenterology, hepatology, and nutrition (ESPGHAN) committee on nutrition. J. Pediatr. Gastroenterol. Nutr. 64 (1), 119–132.

Fildes, A., van Jaarsveld, C.H., Llewellyn, C., Wardle, J., Fisher, A., 2015. Parental control over feeding in infancy. Influence of infant weight, appetite and feeding method. Appetite 91, 101–106.

Gahagan, S., 2012. The development of eating behavior - biology and context. J. Dev. Behav. Pediatr. 33 (3), 261–271.

Grote, V., Schiess, S.A., Closa-Monasterolo, R., Escribano, J., Giovannini, M., Scaglioni, S., Stolarczyk, A., Gruszfeld, D., Hoyos, J., Poncelet, P., Xhonneux, A., Langhendries, J.P., Koletzko, B., European Childhood Obesity Trial Study Group, 2011. The introduction of solid food and growth in the first 2 y of life in formula-fed children: analysis of data from a European cohort study. Am. J. Clin. Nutr. 94 (6 suppl), 1785S–1793S.

Gupta, A., Osadchiy, V., Mayer, E.A., 2020. Brain-gut-microbiome interactions in obesity and food addiction. Nat. Rev. Gastroenterol. Hepatol. 17 (11), 655–672.

Ha, P.B., Bentley, M.E., Pachón, H., Sripaipan, T., Caulfield, L.E., Marsh, D.R., Schroeder, D.G., 2002. Caregiver styles of feeding and child acceptance of food in rural Viet Nam. Food Nutr. Bull. 23 (4 suppl), 95–100.

Harbron, J., Booley, S., Najaar, B., Day, C.E., 2013. Responsive feeding: establishing healthy eating behaviour early on in life. S. Afr. J. Clin. Nutr. 26 (3 suppl), S141–S149.

Hardwick, J., Sidnell, A., 2014. Infant nutrition—diet between 6 and 24 months, implications for paediatric growth, overweight and obesity. Nutr. Bull. 39, 354–363.

Harrison, M., Brodribb, W., Hepworth, J., 2017. A qualitative systematic review of maternal infant feeding practices in transitioning from milk feeds to family foods. Matern. Child Nutr. 13 (2), e12360.

Hartley, I.E., Liem, D.G., Keast, R., 2019. Umami as an 'Alimentary' taste. A new perspective on taste classification. Nutrients 11 (1), 182.

Helle, C., Hillesund, E.R., Øverby, N.C., 2018. Timing of complementary feeding and associations with maternal and infant characteristics: a Norwegian cross-sectional study. PLoS One 13 (6), e0199455.

Hetherington, M.M., Schwartz, C., Madrelle, J., Croden, F., Nekitsing, C., Vereijken, C.M., Weenen, H., 2015. A step-by-step introduction to vegetables at the beginning of complementary feeding. The effects of early and repeated exposure. Appetite 84, 280–290.

Hörnell, A., Lagström, H., Lande, B., Thorsdottir, I., 2013. Breastfeeding, introduction of other foods and effects on health: a systematic literature review for the 5th nordic nutrition recommendations. Food Nutr. Res. 57. https://doi.org/10.3402/fnr.v57i0.20823.

Hromi-Fiedler, A.J., Carroll, G.J., Tice, M.R., Sandow, A., Aryeetey, R., Pérez-Escamilla, R., 2020. Development and testing of responsive feeding counseling cards to strengthen the UNICEF infant and young child feeding counseling package. Curr. Dev. Nutr. 4 (9), nzaa117.

Hurley, K.M., Cross, M.B., Hughes, S.O., 2011. A systematic review of responsive feeding and child obesity in high-income countries. J. Nutr. 141 (3), 495–501.

Anon., 2005. Innocenti Declaration on Infant and Young Child Feeding. http://www.unicef.org/nutrition/files/innocenti2005m_FINAL_ARTWORK_3_MAR.pdf.

Jansen, E., Daniels, L., Nicholson, J., 2012. The dynamics of parenting and early feeding—constructs and controversies: a viewpoint. Early Child Dev. Care 182 (8), 967–981.

Jeurink, P.V., van Bergenhenegouwen, J., Jiménez, E., Knippels, L.M., Fernández, L., Garssen, J., Knol, J., Rodríguez, J.M., Martín, R., 2013. Human milk: a source of more life than we imagine. Benefic. Microbes 4 (1), 17–30.

Johansson, U., Öhlund, I., Hernell, O., Lönnerdal, B., Lindberg, L., Lind, T., 2019. Protein-reduced complementary foods based on Nordic ingredients combined with systematic introduction of taste portions increase intake of fruits and vegetables in 9 month old infants: a randomised controlled trial. Nutrients 11 (6), 1255.

Karatas, Z., Durmus Aydogdu, S., Dinleyici, E.C., Colak, O., Dogruel, N., 2011. Breastmilk ghrelin, leptin, and fat levels changing foremilk to hindmilk: is that important for self-control of feeding? Eur. J. Pediatr. 170 (10), 1273–1280.

Kiefte-de Jong, J.C., de Vries, J.H., Bleeker, S.E., Jaddoe, V.W., Hofman, A., Raat, H., Moll, H.A., 2013. Socio-demographic and lifestyle determinants of 'Western-like' and 'health conscious' dietary patterns in toddlers. Br. J. Nutr. 109 (1), 137–147.

Kopp, C.B., 1982. Antecedents of self-regulation: a developmental perspective. Dev. Psychol. 18 (2), 199–214.

Kral, T.V.E., Rauh, E.M., 2010. Eating behaviors of children in the context of their family environment. Physiol. Behav. 100 (5), 567–573.

Kramer, M.S., Guo, T., Platt, R.W., Sevkovskaya, Z., Dzikovich, I., Collet, J.P., Shapiro, S., Chalmers, B., Hodnett, E., Vanilovich, I., Mezen, I., Ducruet, T., Shishko, G., Bogdanovich, N., 2003. Infant growth and health outcomes associated with 3 compared with 6 mo of exclusive breastfeeding. Am. J. Clin. Nutr. 78 (2), 291–295.

Kumanyika, S.K., 2008. Environmental influences on childhood obesity: ethnic and cultural influences in context. Physiol. Behav. 94, 61–70.

Lange, C., Visalli, M., Jacob, S., Chabanet, C., Schlich, P., Nicklaus, S., 2013. Maternal feeding practices during the first year and their impact on infants' acceptance of complementary food. Food Qual. Prefer. 29, 89–98.

Larsen, J.K., Hermans, R.C., Sleddens, E.F., Engels, R.C., Fisher, J.O., Kremers, S.P., 2015. How parental dietary behavior and food parenting practices affect children's dietary behavior. Interacting sources of influence? Appetite 89, 246–257.

Le Révérend, B.J., Edelson, L.R., Loret, C., 2014. Anatomical, functional, physiological and behavioural aspects of the development of mastication in early childhood. Br. J. Nutr. 111 (3), 403–414.

Lessa, A.C., Fonseca, L.B., Nobre, L.N., Assis, A.M.O., 2017. Dietary patterns of children during the first year of life: a cohort study. Food Nutr. Sci. 8, 1001–1011.

Li, R., Fein, S.B., Grummer-Strawn, L.M., 2010. Do infants fed from bottles lack self-regulation of milk intake compared with directly breastfed infants? Pediatrics 125 (6), e1386–e1393.

Liem, J.A., Mennella, D.G., 2002. Sweet and sour preferences during childhood: role of early experiences. Dev. Psychobiol. 41 (4), 388–395.

Lo, K., Cheung, C., Lee, A., Tam, W.W., Keung, V., 2015. Associations between parental feeding styles and childhood eating habits: a survey of Hong Kong pre-school children. PLoS One 10 (4), e0124753.

Lu, C.-Y., Ni, Y.-H., 2015. Gut microbiota and the development of pediatric diseases. J. Gastroenterol. 50 (7), 720–726.

Lumeng, J.C., Patil, N., Blass, E.M., 2007. Social influences on formula intake via suckling in 7 to 14-week-old-infants. Dev. Psychobiol. 49 (4), 351–361.

Marquis, G.S., Díaz, J., Bartolini, R., Creed de Kanashiro, H., Rasmussen, K.M., 1998. Recognizing the reversible nature of child-feeding decisions: breastfeeding, weaning, and relactation patterns in a shanty town community of Lima, Peru. Soc. Sci. Med. 47 (5), 645–656.

Matvienko-Sikar, K., Griffin, C., McGrath, N., Toomey, E., Byrne, M., Kelly, C., Heary, C., Devane, D., Kearney, P.M., 2019. Developing a core outcome set for childhood obesity prevention: a systematic review. Matern. Child Nutr. 15 (1), e12680.

Mennella, J.A., 2014. Ontogeny of taste preferences: basic biology and implications for health. Am. J. Clin. Nutr. 99 (suppl), 704S–711S.

Mennella, J.A., Beauchamp, G.K., 2005. Understanding the origin of flavor preferences. Chem. Senses 30 (suppl 1), i242–i243.

Mennella, J.A., Trabulsi, J.C., 2012. Complementary foods and flavor experiences: setting the foundation. Ann. Nutr. Metab. 60 (suppl 2), 40–50.

Mennella, J.A., Kennedy, J.M., Beauchamp, G.K., 2006. Vegetable acceptance by infants: effects of formula flavours. Early Hum. Dev. 82 (7), 463–468.

Mennella, J.A., Nicklaus, S., Jagolino, A.L., Yourshaw, L.M., 2008. Variety is the spice of life: strategies for promoting fruit and vegetable acceptance during infancy. Physiol. Behav. 94 (1), 29–38.

Mennella, J.A., Forestell, C.A., Morgan, L.K., Beauchamp, G.K., 2009. Early milk feeding influences taste acceptance and liking during infancy. Am. J. Clin. Nutr. 90 (3), 780S–788S.

Mennella, J.D., Ventura, A.K., Beauchamp, G.K., 2011a. Differential growth patterns among healthy infants fed protein hydrolysate or cow-milk formulas. Pediatrics 127, 110–118.

Mennella, J.A., Lukasewycz, L.D., Castor, S.M., Beauchamp, G.K., 2011b. The timing and duration of a sensitive period in human flavor learning: a randomized trial. Am. J. Clin. Nutr. 93, 1019–1024.

Mennella, J.A., Inamdar, L., Pressman, N., Schall, J.I., Papas, M.A., Schoeller, D., Stallings, V.A., Trabulsi, J.C., 2018. Type of infant formula increases early weight gain and impacts energy balance: a randomized controlled trial. Am. J. Clin. Nutr. 108 (5), 1015–1025.

Mitchell, G.L., Farrow, C., Haycraft, E., Meyer, C., 2013. Parental influences on children's eating behaviour and characteristics of successful parent-focussed interventions. Appetite 60 (1), 85–94.

Møller, P., 2015. Satisfaction, satiation and food behaviour. Curr. Opin. Food Sci. 3, 59–64.

Monge-Montero, C., van der Merwe, L.F., Papadimitropoulou, K., Agostoni, C., Vitaglione, P., 2020. Mixed milk feeding: a systematic review and meta-analysis of its prevalence and drivers. Nutr. Rev. 78 (11), 914–927.

Monteiro, C.A., Moubarac, J.C., Levy, R.B., Canella, D.S., Louzada, M.L.D.C., Cannon, G., 2018. Household availability of ultra-processed foods and obesity in nineteen European countries. Public Health Nutr. 21 (1), 18–26.

Moorcroft, K.E., Marshall, J.L., McCormick, F.M., 2011. Association between timing of introducing solid foods and obesity in infancy and childhood: a systematic review. Matern. Child Nutr. 7 (1), 3–26.

Mura Paroche, M., Caton, S.J., Vereijken, C.M.J.L., Weenen, H., Houston-Price, C., 2017. How infants and young children learn about food: a systematic review. Front. Psychol. 8, 1046.

Nicklaus, S., 2016. Complementary feeding strategies to facilitate acceptance of fruits and vegetables: a narrative review of the literature. Int. J. Environ. Res. Public Health 13 (11), 1160.

Nicklaus, S., 2017. The role of dietary experience in the development of eating behavior during the first years of life. Ann. Nutr. Metab. 70 (3), 241–245.

Northstone, K., Emmett, P., Nethersole, F., ALSPAC Study Team. Avon Longitudinal Study of Pregnancy and Childhood, 2001. The effect of age of introduction to lumpy solids on foods eaten and reported feeding difficulties at 6 and 15 months. J. Hum. Nutr. Diet. 14 (1), 43–54.

Nti, C.A., Lartey, A., 2008. Influence of care practices on nutritional status of Ghanaian children. Nutr. Res. Pract. 2 (2), 93–99.

Olsen, A., Møller, P., Hausner, H., 2013. Early origins of overeating: early habit formation and implications for obesity in later life. Curr. Obes. Rep. 2, 157–164.

Ovaskainen, M.L., Nevalainen, J., Uusitalo, L., Tuokkola, J.J., Arkkola, T., Kronberg-Kippilä, C., Veijola, R., Knip, M., Virtanen, S.M., 2009. Some similarities in dietary clusters of pre-school children and their mothers. Br. J. Nutr. 102 (3), 443–452.

Pak-Gorstein, S., Haq, A., Graham, E.A., 2009. Cultural influences on infant feeding practices. Pediatr. Rev. 30 (3), e11–e21.

Park, S., Pan, L., Sherry, B., Li, R., 2014. The association of sugar-sweetened beverage intake during infancy with sugar-sweetened beverage intake at 6 years of age. Pediatrics 134 (suppl 1), S56–S62.

Paul, I.M., Savage, J.S., Anzman-Frasca, S., Marini, M.E., Beiler, J.S., Hess, L.B., Loken, E., Birch, L.L., 2018. Effect of a responsive parenting educational intervention on childhood weight outcomes at 3 years of age: the INSIGHT randomized clinical trial. JAMA 320 (5), 461–468.

Pauwels, S., Symons, L., Vanautgaerden, E.L., Ghosh, M., Duca, R.C., Bekaert, B., Freson, K., Huybrechts, I., Langie, S.A.S., Koppen, G., Devlieger, R., Godderis, L., 2019. The influence of the duration of breastfeeding on the infant's metabolic epigenome. Nutrients 11 (6), 1408.

Pelto, G.H., Levitt, E., Thairu, L., 2003. Improving feeding practices: current patterns, common constraints, and the design of interventions. Food Nutr. Bull. 24 (1), 45–82.

Perry, R.A., Mallan, K.M., Koo, J., Mauch, C.E., Daniels, L.A., Magarey, A.M., 2015. Food neophobia and its association with diet quality and weight in children aged 24 months: a cross sectional study. Int. J. Behav. Nutr. Phys. Act. 12, 13.

Pimpin, L., Ambrosini, G.L., Llewellyn, C.H., Johnson, L., van Jaarsveld, C.H., Jebb, S.A., Wardle, J., 2013. Dietary intake of young twins: nature or nurture? Am. J. Clin. Nutr. 98 (5), 1326–1334.

Popkin, B.M., 2006. Global nutrition dynamics: the world is shifting rapidly toward a diet linked with noncommunicable diseases. Am. J. Clin. Nutr. 84, 289–298.

Przyrembel, H., 2012. Timing of introduction of complementary food: short- and long-term health consequences. Ann. Nutr. Metab. 60 (suppl 2), 8–20.

Remy, E., Issanchou, S., Chabanet, C., Nicklaus, S., 2013. Repeated exposure of infants at complementary feeding to a vegetable purée increases acceptance as effectively as flavor-flavor learning and more effectively than flavor-nutrient learning. J. Nutr. 143, 1194–1200.

Reyes, M., Hoyos, V., Martinez, S.M., Lozoff, B., Castillo, M., Burrows, R., Blanco, E., Gahagan, S., 2014. Satiety responsiveness and eating behavior among Chilean adolescents and the role of breastfeeding. Int. J. Obes. 38 (4), 552–557.

Robinson, S., Fall, C., 2012. Infant nutrition and later health: a review of current evidence. Nutrients 4 (8), 859–874.

Robinson, S., Marriott, L., Poole, J., Crozier, S., Borland, S., Lawrence, W., Law, C., Godfrey, K., Cooper, C., Inskip, H., Southampton Women's Survey Study Group, 2007. Dietary patterns in infancy: the importance of maternal and family influences on feeding practice. Br. J. Nutr. 98 (5), 1029–1037.

Robinson, S., Ntani, G., Simmonds, S., Syddall, H., Dennison, E., Sayer, A.A., Barker, D., Cooper, C., Hertfordshire Cohort Study Group, 2013. Type of milk feeding in infancy and health behaviours in adult life: findings from the Hertfordshire cohort study. Br. J. Nutr. 109 (6), 1114–1122.

Rollins, N.C., Bhandari, N., Hajeebhoy, N., Horton, S., Lutter, C.K., Martines, J.C., Piwoz, E.G., Richter, L.M., Victora, C.G., Lancet Breastfeeding Series Group, 2016. Why invest, and what it will take to improve breastfeeding practices? Lancet 387 (10017), 491–504.

Ruggiero, C.F., Hohman, E.E., Birch, L.L., Paul, I.M., Savage, J.S., 2020. The intervention nurses start infants growing on healthy trajectories (INSIGHT) responsive parenting intervention for firstborns impacts feeding of second-borns. Am. J. Clin. Nutr. 111 (1), 21–27.

Russell, C.G., Russell, A., 2018. Biological and psychosocial processes in the development of children's appetitive traits: insights from developmental theory and research. Nutrients 10 (6), 692.

Saavedra, J.M., Deming, D., Dattilo, A., Reidy, K., 2013. Lessons from the feeding infants and toddlers study in North America: what children eat, and implications for obesity prevention. Ann. Nutr. Metab. 62 (suppl 3), 27–36.

Savage, J.S., Orlet Fisher, J., Birch, L.L., 2007. Parental influence on eating behavior: conception to adolescence. J. Law Med. Ethics 35 (1), 22–34.

Savage, J.S., Birch, L.L., Marini, M., Anzman-Frasca, S., Paul, I.M., 2016. Effect of the INSIGHT responsive parenting intervention on rapid infant weight gain and overweight status at age 1 year: a randomized clinical trial. JAMA Pediatr. 170 (8), 742–749.

Savage, J.S., Hohman, E.E., Marini, M.E., Shelly, A., Paul, I.M., Birch, L.L., 2018. INSIGHT responsive parenting intervention and infant feeding practices: randomized clinical trial. Int. J. Behav. Nutr. Phys. Act. 15 (1), 64.

Savino, F., Petrucci, E., Lupica, M.M., Nanni, G.E., Oggero, R., 2011. Assay of ghrelin concentration in infant formulas and breast milk. World J. Gastroenterol. 17 (15), 1971–1975.

Scaglioni, S., De Cosmi, V., Ciappolino, V., Parazzini, F., Brambilla, P., Agostoni, C., 2018. Factors influencing Children's eating behaviours. Nutrients 10 (6), 706.

Scariati, P.D., Grummer-Strawn, L.M., Fein, S.B., 1997. A longitudinal analysis of infant morbidity and the extent of breastfeeding in the United States. Pediatrics 99, e5.

Schack-Nielsen, L., Sørensen, T.I., Mortensen, E.L., Michaelsen, K.F., 2010. Late introduction of complementary feeding, rather than duration of breastfeeding, may protect against adult overweight. Am. J. Clin. Nutr. 91 (3), 619–627.

Schiess, S., Grote, V., Scaglioni, S., Luque, V., Martin, F., Stolarczyk, A., Vecchi, F., Koletzko, B., European Childhood Obesity Project, 2010. Introduction of complementary feeding in 5 European countries. J. Pediatr. Gastroenterol. Nutr. 50 (1), 92–98.

Schwartz, C., Chabanet, C., Lange, C., Issanchou, S., Nicklaus, S., 2011. The role of taste in food acceptance at the beginning of complementary feeding. Physiol. Behav. 104 (4), 646–652.

Schwartz, C., Chabanet, C., Laval, C., Issanchou, S., Nicklaus, S., 2013. Breast-feeding duration: influence on taste acceptance over the first year of life. Br. J. Nutr. 109 (6), 1154–1161.

Schwartz, C., Chabanet, C., Szleper, E., Feyen, V., Issanchou, S., Nicklaus, S., 2017. Infant acceptance of primary tastes and fat emulsion: developmental changes and links with maternal and infant characteristics. Chem. Senses 42 (7), 593–603.

Scott, J.A., Chih, T.Y., Oddy, W.H., 2012. Food variety at 2 years of age is related to duration of breastfeeding. Nutrients 4 (10), 1464–1474.

Simione, M., Loret, C., Le Révérend, B., Richburg, B., Del Valle, M., Adler, M., Moser, M., Green, J.R., 2018. Differing structural properties of foods affect the development of mandibular control and muscle coordination in infants and young children. Physiol. Behav. 186, 62–72.

Specht, I.O., Rohde, J.F., Olsen, N.J., Heitmann, B.L., 2018. Duration of exclusive breastfeeding may be related to eating behaviour and dietary intake in obesity prone normal weight young children. PLoS One 13 (7), e0200388.

Steinman, L., Doescher, M., Keppel, G.A., Pak-Gorstein, S., Graham, E., Haq, A., Johnson, D.B., Spicer, P., 2010. Understanding infant feeding beliefs, practices and preferred nutrition education and health provider approaches: an exploratory study with Somali mothers in the USA. Matern. Child Nutr. 6 (1), 67–88.

Stubbs, R.J., 1999. Peripheral signals affecting food intake. Nutrition 15, 614–625.

Switkowski, K.M., Gingras, V., Rifas-Shiman, S.L., Oken, E., 2020. Patterns of complementary feeding behaviors predict diet quality in early childhood. Nutrients 12 (3), 810.

Szczesniak, A.S., 2002. Texture is a sensory property. Food Qual. Prefer. 13, 215–225.

Tarrant, R.C., Younger, K.M., Sheridan-Pereira, M., White, M.J., Kearney, J.M., 2010. Factors associated with weaning practices in term infants: a prospective observational study in Ireland. Br. J. Nutr. 104 (10), 1544–1554.

Taylor, R.W., Williams, S.M., Fangupo, L.J., Wheeler, B.J., Taylor, B.J., Daniels, L., Fleming, E.A., McArthur, J., Morison, B., Erickson, L.W., Davies, R.S., Bacchus, S., Cameron, S.L., Heath, A.M., 2017. Effect of a baby-led approach to complementary feeding on infant growth and overweight: a randomized clinical trial. JAMA Pediatr. 171 (9), 838–846.

Thompson, A.L., Mendez, M.A., Borja, J.B., Adair, L.S., Zimmer, C.R., Bentley, M.E., 2009. Development and validation of the infant feeding style questionnaire. Appetite 53 (2), 210–221.

Townsend, E., Pitchford, N.J., 2012. Baby knows best? The impact of weaning style on food preferences and body mass index in early childhood in a case-controlled sample. BMJ Open 2 (1), e000298.

Tromp, I.I., Kiefte-de Jong, J.C., de Vries, J.H., Jaddoe, V.W., Raat, H., Hofman, A., de Jongste, J.C., Moll, H.A., 2012. Dietary patterns and respiratory symptoms in pre-school children: the generation R study. Eur. Respir. J. 40 (3), 681–689.

Tully, L., Allen-Walker, V., Spyreli, E., McHugh, S., Woodside, J.V., Kearney, P.M., McKinley, M.C., Dean, M., Kelly, C., 2019. Solid advice: complementary feeding experiences among disadvantaged parents in two countries. Matern. Child Nutr. 15 (3), e12801.

Van Esterik, P., 2002. Contemporary trends in infant feeding research. Annu. Rev. Anthropol. 31, 257–278.

Ventura, A.K., Worobey, J., 2013. Early influences on the development of food review preferences. Curr. Biol. 23, R401–R408.

Ventura, A.K., San Gabriel, A., Hirota, M., Mennella, J.A., 2012. Free amino acid content in infant formulas. Nutr. Food Sci. 42 (4), 271–278.

Ventura, A.K., Inamdar, L.B., Mennella, J.A., 2015. Consistency in infants' behavioural signalling of satiation during bottle-feeding. Pediatr. Obes. 10 (3), 180–187.

Vereijken, C.M., Weenen, H., Hetherington, M.M., 2011. Feeding infants and young children. From guidelines to practice-conclusions and future directions. Appetite 57 (3), 839–843.

Wang, L., van Grieken, A., van der Velde, L.A., Vlasblom, E., Beltman, M., L'Hoir, M.P., Boere-Boonekamp, M.M., Raat, H., 2019. Factors associated with early introduction of complementary feeding and consumption of non-recommended foods among Dutch infants: the BeeBOFT study. BMC Public Health 19 (1), 388. https://doi.org/10.1186/s12889-019-6722-4.

Wardle, J., Cooke, L., 2008. Genetic and environmental determinants of children's food preferences. Br. J. Nutr. 99 (suppl 1), S15–S21.

Wasser, H.M., Thompson, A.L., Siega-Riz, A.M., Adair, L.S., Hodges, E.A., Bentley, M.E., 2013. Who's feeding baby? Non-maternal involvement in feeding and its association with dietary intakes among infants and toddlers. Appetite 71, 7–15.

Werthmann, J., Jansen, A., Havermans, R., Nederkoorn, C., Kremers, S., Roefs, A., 2015. Bits and pieces. Food texture influences food acceptance in young children. Appetite 84, 181–187.

WHO, 2001. The Optimal Duration of Exclusive Breastfeeding: Report of an Expert Consultation. World Health Organization, Geneva. Available from: http://www.who.int/nutrition/publications/optimal_duration_of_exc_bfeeding_report_eng.pdf.

WHO, 2003. Global Strategy for Infant and Young Child Feeding. Available from http://www.who.int/nutrition/publications/gs_infant_feeding_text_eng.pdf.

WHO, 2005. Guiding Principles for Feeding Non-breastfed Children 6–24 Months of Age. WHO Library Cataloguin-in-Publication Data. WHO Press, Geneva, Switzerland.

WHO, 2019. Essential Nutrition Actions: Mainstreaming Nutrition through the Life-Course. World Health Organization, Geneva. Licence: CC BY-NC-SA 3.0 IGO. Available from: https://apps.who.int/iris/handle/10665/326261.

Williams Erickson, L., Taylor, R.W., Haszard, J.J., Fleming, E.A., Daniels, L., Morison, B.J., Leong, C., Fangupo, L.J., Wheeler, B.J., Taylor, B.J., Te Morenga, L., McLean, R.M., Heath, A.M., 2018. Impact of a modified version of baby-led weaning on infant food and nutrient intakes: the BLISS randomized controlled trial. Nutrients 10 (6), 740.

Yang, Z., Huffman, S.L., 2013. Nutrition in pregnancy and early childhood and associations with obesity in developing countries. Matern. Child Nutr. (suppl. 1), 105–119.

Young, B.E., Johnson, S.L., Krebs, N.F., 2012. Biological determinants linking infant weight gain and child obesity: current knowledge and future directions. Adv. Nutr. 3 (5), 675–686.

# Early parent feeding behaviors to promote long-term health

*Anne M. Dattilo*

Nutrition Research and Practice Service, Hollywood, FL, United States

## CHAPTER LEARNING OBJECTIVES

1. To describe links among responsive feeding practices and parental feeding styles as they relate to the promotion of infant self-regulation of energy intake for healthy growth and development.

2. To discuss the influence of parent responsiveness to hunger and satiety cues, and infant clarity of displaying these cues, within the reciprocal feeding relationship among the mother-infant dyad with breastfeeding and bottle use.

3. To identify parent feeding practices associated with the introduction of novel complementary foods, and the influence of parent feeding behaviors on the immediate, and potential long-term dietary intake of infants and young children.

4. To recognize gaps/challenges within current parent feeding behavior literature and advantages of future evidence-based guidance and recommendation development and dissemination.

## 20.1 Introduction

The period from birth, through the first several months of life, characterizes a unique time when caregivers or parents (hereafter referred to as parents), make essentially all decisions about their healthy infant or young child's diet regarding what, when, where, and how the child will be offered foods and beverages. Ideally, the parent supports the child's autonomy by allowing the child to decide whether, or not, they will eat what the parent has offered, and the quantity they will consume. This division of responsibility between the parent and child (Lohse and Satter, 2021) promotes young children's innate self-regulatory capacity for energy intake, based on their hunger, satiety, and interoceptive signals (Boswell, 2021). Although inherent individual differences in appetite and self-regulation of energy intake are known, the expression of children's eating tendencies may also be moderated by *how* children are offered foods and beverages (Wood et al., 2020). Questions of "how to feed" are of critical importance with regard to establishing healthy eating habits, beginning at birth, that can be maintained throughout life (DGAC, 2020; NASEM, 2020; Perez-Escamilla et al., 2017; Wood et al., 2020).

Responsive feeding is one component of "how to feed" infants and young children ≤ 2 years of age, as compared to a second important, category of "what to feed" (NASEM, 2020). Recently, the construct of responsive feeding has been defined from an interdisciplinary perspective as "feeding practices that encourage the child to eat autonomously and in response to physiological and developmental needs, which may encourage self-regulation in eating and support cognitive, emotional and social development" (Pérez-Escamilla et al., 2021). Parent feeding behaviors while offering food and liquid, also referred to as feeding practices, and ways in which they engage with children at eating occasions, shape how children develop their own feeding behaviors and are inclusive within a responsive feeding construct. Responsive feeding, opposed to non-responsive feeding, reflects parenting behaviors that promptly respond to a child's signals/communications of hunger and satiety, or the parent's best interpretation of the child's cues, in an emotionally supportive, and developmentally appropriate fashion.

Parent application of responsive feeding behaviors has been positively associated with immediate and long-term benefits related to infant and young child's dietary intake, healthy growth, and child development (Black and Aboud, 2011; Dattilo, 2017a,b; Disantis et al., 2011a; Hurley et al., 2011; Redsell et al., 2021; Spill et al., 2019b; Wood et al., 2020). Parent feeding behaviors have also been implicated to infant and young child appetitive traits and food-related behaviors such as satiety responsiveness, food responsiveness, food fussiness, and eating in the absence of hunger (Llewellyn et al., 2011; Mallan et al., 2014; Sleddens et al., 2011) that can have lifelong influences on eating behaviors.

The aims of this chapter are to describe early parent feeding behaviors, with infants and young children ≤ 2 years of age, specific to outcomes of dietary intakes or healthy growth. A historical overview of parenting and feeding behaviors, related to responsive feeding, is provided. Tools and questionnaires utilized to assess parent feeding behaviors, parent responsiveness to infant hunger and satiety cues, the use of food to soothe a crying infant, and pressuring/restrictive practices at the start of complementary feeding are included. Existing guidance and recommendations available for implementation about "how to feed" infants and young children are provided.

It is recognized that the majority of published studies that assess parent attitudes, beliefs, and behaviors associated with infant and young child feeding are conducted in high-income countries, and enroll only mother and child dyads. One qualitative systematic review of 73 global studies concluded that how infants and young children ≤ 2 years of age are offered food is primarily a maternal decision (Dattilo et al., 2020). As such, within this chapter, the term parent is nearly always the mother as the primary caretaker of infants regarding the care of the child with food. It is acknowledged that results may be different among studies that include fathers, grandparents, and other caretakers in the home or within early education facilities.

In addition, parent feeding behaviors that meet descriptions and criteria for responsive feeding practices describe *how* infants and young children are *offered* food and beverages. Throughout this text, terminology consistent with responsive feeding principles is used. Terms such as "bottle fed infants," or "spoon-fed children" implies that the parent, rather than the child or a reciprocal relationship between the parent and child, controls the feeding interaction. Such statements have been amended to "infants who are offered bottles," or "children who were offered complementary foods by spoon." It is hopeful that adoption of such language may have practical implications in the pediatric clinic or public health setting. Teaching parents that "the baby is showing signs of hunger; time to offer him a feeding," rather than "time for you to feed your baby," may serve an unmet nutrition education opportunity related to attitudes, beliefs, and parent feeding behaviors.

## 20.2 Responsive parenting and feeding behaviors

The act of "parenting" refers to parenting *behaviors*, ways of engaging, or approaches to child-rearing that shape how a child develops (IOM, 2016). Responsive parenting, opposed to non-responsive parenting, reflects parenting behaviors in which prompt, emotionally supportive, and developmentally appropriate responses are provided by the parent, contingent upon the child's signals or communications (Black and Aboud, 2011). Secure emotional attachment during infancy, setting the stage for subsequent emotional development, is strongly associated with responsive parenting, and clear benefits for the child such as better health outcomes and enhanced cognitive, language, and psychosocial development have consistently been identified (IOM, 2016).

From a historical developmental psychology perspective (Baumrind, 1971; Darling and Steinberg, 1993; Maccoby and Martin, 1983), parent feeding behaviors have roots within attitudes, beliefs, and behaviors that describe how a parent will interact with a child across domains of parenting. Parenting styles, thought to develop within the first years of the parenting journey, and which remain stable over time, are identified by the relative extent to which parents are responsive to their child's needs (responsiveness), and controlling of their child's behaviors (demandingness). Responsiveness is a parenting style that fosters the development of infant and young children's self-regulation of dietary intake (Spill et al., 2019b).

Within the spectrum of demandingness and responsiveness, four traditional parenting styles have been described as authoritative, authoritarian, indulgent, and neglectful (Maccoby and Martin, 1983). Baumrind (Baumrind, 1971) developed one of the first validated measures for parenting style assessment, and since that time, an authoritative parenting style has been so consistently linked across a number of healthy childhood outcomes that it is often considered as the reference style in which other parenting styles are compared (Shloim et al., 2015). Based on the aforementioned general categorical dimensions of parenting styles, parental feeding styles have been identified as following a similar spectrum of demandingness and responsiveness within a feeding context (Hughes et al., 2005). As such, parental feeding styles are a component of responsive feeding in which a balance of responsiveness and demandingness, related to feeding, is realized.

Authoritative parents are characterized by having high demands for maturity and self-control from their children, yet also show high responsiveness, such as child-centeredness, acceptance, care, empathy, and nurturance. Parents with a dominant authoritative feeding style, utilize responsive feeding practices in which they offer foods or beverages when their child shows signs of hunger, or at predictable times when they anticipate their child will be hungry. Mealtime rules and routines are established, yet in a positive feeding environment based on nurture and support. A consistent meal schedule is established, yet parents offer meals and snacks, frequently throughout the day (NASEM, 2020). Parents encourage a child to try a taste of novel foods with a limited number of prompts within an authoritative parental feeding environment whereas parents use more frequent, and more pressure type of prompts to get their children to eat within an authoritarian parenting domain (Edelson et al., 2016). The authoritarian parental phenotype is also described as having high demands for rules and expectations, but with less responsiveness or sensitivity to the child's needs. Authoritarian parents use more "intrusive" behaviors at mealtimes (Hughes et al., 2011), such as insisting that the child eat a predetermined quantity of a food, or percentage of the plate of food offered, or stay at a mealtime for an extended time period until these parent goals are met.

Indulgent (or permissive) parenting is described by less emphasis on demands and rules, but high responsiveness. Parents rated as strong within an indulgent feeding style spectrum are categorized as using permissive behaviors, with little guidance for regular mealtime routines, and parents typically offer foods they think their young children will prefer. One study (Chaidez and Kaiser, 2011) with 94 mothers of infants aged 12–24 months identified that diets of children from parents scoring high within the indulgent feeding styles were greater in energy intakes, as well as higher in total fat, saturated fat, and sweetened beverages, compared to diets of children with more authoritative feeding style mothers. In an additional study by this group (Chaidez et al., 2014) of 67 similarly aged infants and their mothers, baseline data on feeding styles, dietary intake, and anthropometry were compared to a 6-month follow-up. Parent indulgent feeding scores were positively associated with child weight change z scores and contributed to a greater change in weight-for-height ($P = .03$), body mass index (BMI) ($P = .05$), and weight-for-age ($P = .04$), relative to authoritative feeding style scores. Higher indulgent scores were positively related, and authoritative scores negatively associated with dietary fat and sweetened beverage intake.

These results, similar to findings with older children from multiple countries, indicated that a parent indulgent feeding style was associated with a child's higher weight or BMI z-scores and lower diet quality (Hurley et al., 2011; Shloim et al., 2015; Vollmer and Mobley, 2013;), compared to authoritative feeding styles. One study noted the longitudinal nature of the association of indulgent feeding styles, compared to authoritative feeding styles, with childhood overweight 3 years later, even after controlling for the child's weight at baseline (Olvera and Power, 2010). A dominant indulging parenting style may be established as early as 1 year after a child's birth, and from limited data, at least this feeding style may persist during the toddler ages.

Parents with high scores on the neglectful (uninvolved) feeding style scale are neither demanding nor responsive. They may engage in bottle propping, not be present or engage with their child at mealtime or supervise their young child's eating. Few mealtime routines are held. A widely used tool to assess parent feeding styles was developed by Hughes and colleagues (Hughes et al., 2005), originally validated in 3–5-year-old children. Tools have since been developed for parents of infants and children ≤ 2 years that assess similar constructs (Chaidez and Kaiser, 2011; Hodges et al., 2013; Hurley et al., 2013; Thompson et al.,

2009; Wood et al., 2016). Application of these questionnaires within intervention studies, and nutrition education efforts, can enhance parents' awareness of their existing feeding styles. Behavior adoption of characteristics within an authoritative feeding style, via an anticipatory guidance framework, may be useful to guide parents of very young infants toward responsive feeding behaviors (Uesugi et al., 2016). Additional longitudinal studies addressing parent feeding styles as part of a responsive feeding approach, particularly with infants and toddler age populations, are needed.

## 20.3 Parenting feeding practices and behaviors

Within the concept of responsive feeding, parent feeding practices refer to specific *behaviors* used by parents to support or influence their child's dietary intake. Responsive behaviors are those in which parents strive for their child to eat in response to physiological and developmental needs, with a goal of regulatory capacity and feeding autonomy (Pérez-Escamilla et al., 2021). As such, parents accept that the children have capabilities to eat, or to stop eating, based on their internal satiation signals. Responsive feeding behaviors require that parents are present at mealtimes, both physically and emotionally, and design the feeding occasion to have few distractions.

Attention to a child's signals or cues of hunger and satiety, and appropriate parental response to these signals, is one parent behavior consistently promoted within responsive feeding interventions (Daniels et al., 2012; Paul et al., 2011; Savage et al., 2016) and within nutrition education programs for early childhood education professionals (Savage et al., 2019). As responsive feeding is a reciprocal relationship in which children need to communicate their needs in order for parents to respond, more recently, attention to the child's clarity of expressing hunger and satiety cues has been explored (Ventura, 2017; Ventura et al., 2019; Ventura and Hernandez, 2019). Non-responsive feeding practices of using food to soothe a distressed or unhappy child in the absence of hunger (Ma et al., 2015; Jansen et al., 2019; Stifter et al., 2011; Stifter and Moding, 2015; Temmen et al., 2021), or rewarding children with food (or rewarding children for consuming foods) can lead to children's diminished ability to regulate intake, which may then lead to increased emotional overeating (Powell et al., 2017). Parent feeding behaviors are often described as overly encouraging a child to eat more (pressuring practices) or influencing a child to eat less (restrictive practices), both of which are inconsistent with responsive feeding principles.

Parent feeding behaviors may differ across children within the same family, depending on the child age, gender, eating behavior, skill development for eating, child's appetite, temperament, or birth order compared to siblings (Black and Aboud, 2011; Ruggiero et al., 2021; Thompson et al., 2013). Behaviors are also influenced by parental factors such as attitudes, beliefs, norms within their culture, and access to affordable and healthy food (Dattilo et al., 2020). Parenting feeding style (described above as authoritarian, authoritative, indulgent, or uninvolved) is associated with specific feeding behaviors, and how the parent interprets the child's actual or perceived weight is predictive of excess use of pressuring or restrictive feeding behaviors. Given the interactions between the child's and parent's characteristics and behaviors, the relationship between parent feeding practices and child dietary intake is bidirectional in nature (Ventura and Birch, 2008).

## 20.4 Existing guidance for how to feed

The underlying concepts of responsive feeding transcend across feeding interactions of parents with their infants and children in all global regions, despite economic status. Parental responsive feeding behaviors have been incorporated into global policy statements and/or promoted by multiple international agencies and pediatric-related organizations (DGAC, 2020; NASEM, 2020; UNICEF, 2016; WHO, 2003, 2009) for at least the past 20 years. More recently, a resurgence of literature has begun to identify associations with parent feeding behaviors and children's diet and healthy growth, with emphasis on prevention of overnutrition, rather than undernutrition (Perez-Escamilla et al., 2017; Redsell et al., 2021; Spill et al., 2019b; Wood et al., 2020).

Surprisingly, within the recently released Scientific Report of the 2020 Dietary Guidelines Advisory Committee (DGAC, 2020) the concept of responsive feeding was not selected as a topic for inclusion within dietary guidelines for infants and young children from birth through 2 years of age. However, a recent consensus study report from the United States, National Academies of Sciences, Engineering, and Medicine (NASEM, 2020) reviewed existing global feeding recommendations from government agencies and authoritative international organization documents for infants and children from birth to 24 months. The aim of this report was to compare existing guidance and recommendations for consistency across sources, not to systematically review the literature to identify evidence-based recommendations to update current guidance, or for the establishment of new recommendations.

Results were categorized by the committee (NASEM, 2020) as recommendations related to "what to feed" and "how to feed." A summary of the findings has been recently published within journals designed for dietitian nutritionists (Jimenez et al., 2021), and other pediatric healthcare professionals (Atkinson et al., 2021; Pérez-Escamilla et al., 2021). Based on 23 of 43 guideline documents reviewed, 8 topic areas emerged as existing guidance and recommendations on how to feed infants and young children (Table 20.1).

Responsive feeding recommendations were based on nine source documents, primarily narrative reviews, from high-income countries, although documents from the World Health Organization were also included. After synthesis of findings, recommendations were rated as consistent (alignment across guidance) or generally consistent (the recommendation tended to provide similar guidance, yet there were some differences in wording or details across recommendations.) The three recommendations within the topic area of responsive feeding included encouragement of self-feeding and self-regulation, a pleasant and nurturing feeding environment, and repeated exposure to novel foods.

The one hunger and satiety cue recommendation of "…emphasizing the importance of using hunger and satiety cues to guide infant and child feeding" was rated as generally consistent among documents reviewed, suggesting that at least one of the source documents reviewed did not include, or reliably agree, with this statement. The remaining topic areas within the category of "how to feed" addressed food safety, bottle/cup recommendations, timing of introduction to complementary foods, food texture, and meal frequency. Although these recommendations are highly relevant, there is need to identify evidence-based responsive feeding recommendations (Atkinson et al., 2021; Jimenez et al., 2021), especially for low-and-middle income countries (Pérez-Escamilla et al., 2021), and incorporate responsive feeding guidance into infant and young child feeding recommendations. More specific

**TABLE 20.1**  Existing guidance and recommendations on how to feed infants and young children.

1. Responsive feeding: Consistent findings (CF) identified that repeated exposure is needed for acceptance of new foods. Recommendations were generally consistent (GC) that self-feeding and self-regulation be encouraged and that the feeding environment be pleasant and include nurturing behaviors by caregivers.

2. Hunger and satiety cues: GC findings emphasized the importance of using hunger and satiety cues to guide feeding.

3. Meal frequency: GC findings recommended that several eating occasions, for both meals and snacks, are needed each day and a consistent meal schedule be established.

4. Introduction of complementary foods: CF identified that new foods be gradually introduced and that first foods offered be iron rich or iron fortified. GC findings recommended that foods not be introduced < 4 months of age, nor > 6 months of age. However, guidance was not consistent (NCF) if age of introduction be a range of 4–6 months, or at approximately 6 months.

5. Food consistency and texture: CF among recommendations identified that consistency and texture advance as the child gets older, and be tailored to the child's developmental needs.

6. Bottle use: GC findings identified that bottle use be discontinued at about 12 months of age, certain foods and fluids not be added to bottles, and that infants not go to bed or sleep with a bottle. CF recommended that bottle propping not be used.

7. Cup use: GC findings identified that infants 6–12 months of age transition to cup use, and that milk be offered to toddler age children in a cup.

8. Food safety: CF identified that infants and young children be supervised while eating and advice about risk of choking be provided to caregivers. CF recommendations identified that milk, milk products, and juice offered to children be pasteurized, and honey not be ingested by children < 1 year of age. GC findings identified that raw or undercooked eggs not be consumed.

Consistent findings (CF) are those with alignment across the source documents reviewed; generally consistent findings (GC) tended to provide similar guidance, although some differences in wording or details were identified among recommendations reviewed; not consistent findings (NCF) indicated that recommendations within documents reviewed provided different guidance.
*Adapted from NASEM. National Academies of Science, Engineering and Medicine, 2020. Feeding Infants and Children from Birth to 24 Months: Summarizing Existing Guidance. The National Academies Press, Washington, DC.*

guidance is likely to enhance adoption by the professional pediatric community, and support communication and dissemination of the guidance for parents. Systematic literature reviews (Appleton et al., 2018; Dattilo et al., 2020; Hurley et al., 2011; McNally et al., 2016; Matvienko-Sikar et al., 2019; Redsell et al., 2021; Spill et al., 2019a,b; Ventura, 2017) and detailed narrative reviews (Perez-Escamilla et al., 2017; Wood et al., 2020) provide, in part, a literature base to help draw future meaningful recommendations about responsive feeding behaviors for parents with infants and young children ≤ 2 years of age.

## 20.5  Measures of parent feeding behaviors

Parent feeding practices or behaviors, in conjunction with parent attitudes and beliefs surrounding these practices, are ways in which responsive feeding variables are operationalized for assessment (Dattilo and Saavedra, 2020). Within clinical and research settings, both parent and child feeding behaviors are observed and/or video-recorded, and subsequently coded and assessed by trained investigators. This approach, with the aid of reliable and valid tools such as the Nursing Child Assessment Satellite Training (NCAST), Parent Child Interaction Feeding and Teaching Scales, and various sub-scales (Sumner and Spieta, 1994), have become more frequently applied to assess parent-child feeding interactions. The clarity of infant hunger/satiety cues and mother's sensitivity to these cues, as well as maternal engagement during feeding (Golen and Ventura, 2015; Shloim et al., 2017; Ventura and Golen, 2015; Ventura and Hernandez, 2019; Whitfield and Ventura, 2019) have been assessed by NCAST tools.

Several questionnaires, validated for use within infants and children through 24 months of age that aim to assess parent feeding and infant and young child eating behaviors related to growth have been previously described (Dattilo, 2017b). Questionnaire items are often developed after identification of mediating variables, defined as underlying determinants associated with a specific parent feeding behavior (e.g., attitude, belief, perception, self-efficacy, skills, etc. (Uesugi et al., 2016). Although it can be argued that consensus on how parent feeding constructs are defined or operationalized is still evolving (O'Connor et al., 2016), and that questionnaires do not comprehensively measure parent or child feeding behaviors, per se (Lohse and Satter, 2021), questionnaires can serve as surrogates to some aspects of direct observation for assessment of food-related behaviors of children and parents. However, it is important to acknowledge that results of self-reported questionnaire items and conclusions from direct observations have reported various levels of congruence (Bergmeier et al., 2015).

Two of the more widely used parent-report scales include the Infant Feeding Styles Questionnaire (IFSQ), validated in children age 3–18 months (Thompson et al., 2009) and the Infant Feeding Questionnaire (IFQ) (Baughcum et al., 2001), validated for children age 11–23 months. Of questionnaires with satisfactory internal consistency (Cronbach's alpha within the 0.70 to 0.90 limit), designed for parents of infants and young children from birth to < 24 months of age, several sub-scales measure parent feeding practices such as pressuring or restriction (Chaidez and Kaiser, 2011; Thompson et al., 2009; Wood et al., 2016;), and others delineate between parental behaviors related to feeding, or beliefs and attitudes about feeding (Thompson et al., 2009; Wood et al., 2016). In addition, measures of responsive feeding constructs applicable to this age group, such as feeding to soothe (Stifter et al., 2011), feeding to a routine (Brown and Lee, 2013; Lakshman et al., 2011), acceptance of foods and mealtime behaviors (Horodynski and Stommel, 2005), provision of rewards for behavior or eating (Jansen et al., 2014), assessment of food and satiety responsiveness (Llewellyn et al., 2011; Mallan et al., 2014), and maternal perceptions of hunger and satiety (Baughcum et al., 2001; Gross et al., 2010; Ma et al., 2015; Thompson et al., 2009) have been utilized. For longitudinal assessment of feeding practices across childhood, one questionnaire has been developed to measure authoritative parent feeding practices related to responsiveness for children ≤ 2 years (Jansen et al., 2016) which can be used in conjunction with an original version designed for parents of children > 2 years (Jansen et al., 2014).

Within some of the scales, intercorrelations between distinct feeding constructs have been reported, suggesting that feeding practices may not be parental categorical traits, but rather, parents simultaneously reported using different feeding practices. For example, if mothers were concerned about their child's intake at a particular meal, or appetite on a given day, they may vacillate between increasing their control (pressuring or restrictive) or relaxing the control (indulgence, food reward) to try to influence their child's intake (Hurley et al., 2013). Despite limitations, based on studies with parents and their children ≤ 2 years of age, parental feeding practice associations with child weight or diet provide learnings that may be unique to this age group and can be incorporated within scale-up responsive feeding interventions or nutrition education programs.

## 20.6 Hunger and satiety cues

Parenting behaviors of responding to infant and young child hunger and satiety cues throughout an infant feeding interaction is a primary component, if not a hallmark, of responsive feeding behaviors. Within a comprehensive literature review of the barriers and enablers to caregiver responsive feeding (Redsell et al., 2021), parents' ability to recognize their child's feeding cues and signals was identified as an overarching skill of responsive feeding. Parent feeding practices that are unresponsive to infant hunger or fullness cues have been suggested to influence an infant's ability to self-regulate energy intake and thought to contribute to overnutrition by promoting eating in the absence of hunger or eating beyond fullness (Disantis et al., 2011a; Hodges et al., 2013; Hurley et al., 2011).

Observational studies of healthy infant and young children's behaviors demonstrating hunger and fullness signals, cues, or ways of communicating are limited. Results from a systematic review of 27 publications that aimed to identity how these cues are expressed within infants and toddlers concluded that feeding cues are diverse, variable across and within the children, and caregiver perception of such is influenced by the child's age, gender, temperament, and feeding method (McNally et al., 2016). From the limited number of observational reports of infants under controlled conditions before, during, and after a feeding within the review ($n = 3$), hand-mouth movements as well as infant sucking and motor activity reportedly varied with hunger and satiation, yet the precise pattern was inconsistent and differed within ranges of infant age.

Hodges and colleagues (Hodges et al., 2013) identified 20 hunger cues and 28 fullness cues while developing an observational scoring tool to assess parental responsiveness to child feeding cues. Infant feeding cue behaviors were categorized into early (mouthing, increased alertness, sucking on hands), active (excitatory limb movements, leaning toward foods), and late (fussing/crying) cue categories. Parent responsiveness was defined by the latency of response to the infant's cue across the course of a feeding, with those responding earlier and to more subtle cues being rated as having higher attentiveness to feeding cues than those who responded to later or more overt cues.

## 20.7 Parent assessment of hunger and satiety cues

To assess maternal perceptions of infant hunger and satiety, 4 statements were proposed to 368 mothers of 4–5-month-old infants (Gross et al., 2010). When asked about perception of infant feeding cues, most of the mothers believed that infant sucking on hands indicated hunger (66%) and that head turning indicated satiety (91%). Although the vast majority (93%) believed that infants could sense their own satiety, over half the mothers rated high on a pressuring feeding scale, as assessed by response to "If you give a baby a bottle, you should always make sure he finishes it." In addition, 72% believed that if their infant was crying, he must be hungry, a statement significantly associated with pressuring feeding style in multivariate analysis (OR = 2.59). Thus, it appeared there was some disconnect to what mothers reportedly believed about infants being able to sense satiation, and the actual behaviors they used.

In another study by the same group (Gross et al., 2014), the authors assessed beliefs of 412 mothers ($n = 204$ low income, primarily Hispanic [high-risk group], and $n = 208$ high income, primarily Caucasian [low-risk group]) about their 2 week to 6-month-old infant's hunger and satiety by using four statements from the Infant Feeding Questionnaire (Baughcum et al., 2001), a scale validated for children within the age range of 11–24-month-olds. Specifically, mothers replied on a 4-point scale to statements such as "you know when the baby is hungry," "you know when the baby is full," "the baby knows when he or she is hungry," and "the baby knows when he or she is full." After adjusting for infant age, gender, birth order, and maternal age, results indicated that the sample of mothers within the high-risk group was more likely to believe in their ability to know when the infant was hungry and full, and less likely to believe that the infant knew their own hunger and satiety. Consistent with these findings, the high-risk group was significantly more likely to engage in both pressuring and restrictive feeding practices, as well as the early introduction of juice and the practice of adding cereal to the infant bottle. The potential influence of lack of availability of healthy and affordable food for infants was not specifically addressed, yet the high-risk group infants were enrolled in the Supplemental Program for Women, Infants, and Children (WIC).

In addition, within an ethnically diverse sample of 7–24-month-old children and their mothers ($n = 144$) (Hodges et al., 2013), 75% of mothers were responsive or highly responsive to child hunger cues, yet only 45% were observed to be similarly responsive to fullness cues ($P < .001$). The general responsiveness of the mother and child during feeding appeared reciprocal. Overall, more responsive mothers had more responsive children, as assessed by the child's visual attentiveness and expressiveness during the feeding. Responsiveness was not associated with child weight-for-length in this sample. However, the study may not have been adequately powered to determine such, as less than 5% of the infants or toddlers were obese.

To assess maternal sensitivity to infant cues at multiple time points, within a natural setting, 96 mother-infant dyads were observed during home visits when the infants were 3 and 6 months of age; weight was measured at both these times, and at 12 months (Worobey et al., 2009). The feeding subscale of the Nursing Child Assessment Satellite Training Feeding Scale was used to rank the caregiver during a feeding interaction on 16 behaviors, such as slowing, pausing, or terminating the feeding when the infant disengaged or showed satiety cues. All infants were offered infant formula, by bottle. After controlling on birth weight, maternal BMI, and infant weight gain from 3 to 6 months, mothers who were less sensitive to satiety cues had infants who gained more weight between 6 and 12 months ($P = .002$). Within this study, a high prevalence of obesity (40% at 12 months) was noted.

Parents have often reported their desire to learn how to recognize and respond to the child's hunger and fullness cues (Redsell et al., 2021); however, not all infants are effective communicators during infant feeding interactions, particularly in the number and types of cues to signal satiation (Shloim et al., 2017) which highlights the possibility that responsive feeding may be more difficult for some parents than others. Infant clarity of communicating hunger and satiation cues, and parental sensitivity and responsiveness, was explored among 86 mother-infant dyads at 4 months of age (Ventura et al., 2019). After video-recording of a feeding session, trained raters coded findings using the Nursing Child Assessment Parent-Child Interaction Feeding Scale's Infant Clarity of Cues and Maternal Sensitivity to Cues subscales. Consistent with previous findings (Hodges et al., 2013), greater clarity of cues by infants was strongly associated with the observed maternal sensitivity to these cues ($P = .001$), suggesting a positive maternal-infant reciprocal and bidirectional nature of communication. Infants consuming breast milk or infant formula exhibited similar clarity of cues ($P = .06$) and clue clarity was not associated with infant sex, age, or temperament. However, lower clarity of infant cues was associated with greater weight-for-age $z$ score change among infants that consumed formula, compared to breastfeeding infants.

Taken together, these results indicate that parental interpretation of infant cues, and responding appropriately, can be difficult for some parents. Mothers appear better skilled at recognizing hunger cues, and less so at identifying cues of satiety. Infants with greater clarity of their hunger and satiety cues tend to have mothers with higher sensitivity and responsiveness to these cues. Limited research suggests that misinterpretation of satiety cues is related to rate of weight gain among infants, although findings are confounded by limited sample size and lack of long-term follow-up. Identification of underlying beliefs that mothers are better at knowing an infant's hunger and satiety than the infant himself, as well as guidance on early and late external appetite cues across infancy (Hodges et al., 2016) provide opportunities for nutrition education. In fact, one recent systematic literature review (Spill et al., 2019b) concluded that there is moderate evidence from randomized controlled intervention trials to suggest that teaching mothers to recognize and respond appropriately to a child's hunger and satiety cues can lead to normal weight gain and weight status in children $\leq 2$ years, compared with children whose mothers did not receive this guidance.

## 20.8 Using food to soothe during infancy

Parenting use of food, and more often the offering of milk during early infancy, for non-nutritive purposes such as to soothe an infant that is upset, crying, distressed, anxious, or angry is described by the construct of using food to soothe (Stifter et al., 2011). One distinction with offering food to soothe (FTS), rather than the broader construct of attention to hunger and satiety cues, is highlighted by the parent's desire to calm a crying/fussing child with food, regardless if they recognize that their infant or child is not hungry, or unlikely to be hungry. Also referred to as "emotional feeding," this non-responsive approach of offering food or beverages to an infant when he/she is upset for reasons other than hunger is often successful in immediately calming an infant's negative affect (Hamburg et al., 2014), which may explain, in part, its frequent use as a feeding strategy by parents (Jansen et al., 2019).

Without having other soothing strategies readily available to calm a distressed infant, parents may offer breastfeeding, infant formula, or food, finding relief that their infant is quickly calmed. Through the repeated practice of using FTS, it is postulated that children may learn that eating in the absence of hunger will soothe their distress (Farrow et al., 2015), and this type of emotional eating may override innate hunger and satiety responses. As infants acclimate to eating in response to non-hunger cues, they may develop obesogenic eating behaviors, such as high responsiveness to food, lower satiety responsiveness, greater enjoyment and faster eating speed, all of which have been implicated to infant weight (Mallan et al., 2014).

However, one recent intervention to decrease the use of FTS (Savage et al., 2018) has shown promising results as evident by a randomized controlled trial with 279 mother-infant dyads. As part of a responsive parenting education program delivered when infants were 8, 16, 32, and 44 weeks of age, mothers within the education group used FTS significantly fewer times ($P < .01$) than those in the control group.

The Basic Baby Needs Questionnaire (BBNQ) (Stifter et al., 2011) has been utilized to assess FTS within a 13-question scale that includes parental report of the frequency of offering food or liquid to soothe their child in a given time frame (e.g., per week) and how likely a parent was to use FTS infant distress in various locations (e.g., grocery store, doctor's waiting room, religious service) and when the parent was stressed, tired, or found nothing else to work to soothe their infant. Rated on a 5-point scale, these items provide a unique way to operationalize the FTS construct. Previous studies have demonstrated that greater use of FTS during infancy has been associated with higher infant weight status (Morris et al., 1982; Saxon et al., 2002) and greater increase in infant weight from 6 to 18 months (Stifter and Moding, 2015). Within one recent study that addressed the use of FTS during infancy (Temmen et al., 2021), the use of more frequent maternal FTS infants at 2 months of age was related to their infant's greater responsiveness to food at 6 months, which was then related to more frequent maternal FTS at 6 months. In addition, greater satiety responsiveness, faster eating speed, and greater responsiveness to food in infants at 6 months were related to more maternal use of FTS at 12 months. These results suggest that FTS and infant appetite behaviors may be bidirectionally linked and underscore that maternal feeding practices may influence the development of obesogenic eating as early as the first year of life.

In addition, within a study with 3960 children from the Generation R, population-based birth cohort (Jansen et al., 2019), the more frequent use of FTS at 6 months of age (assessed by a single-item question) was significantly associated with higher levels of children's emotional overeating at ages 4 and 10 years, compared with children whose parents reported never using FTS during infancy. The more frequent use of FTS at 6 months predicted a higher BMI at age 6 years, and a BMI z score 0.13 units higher at age 10 years (95% CI, 0.03, 0.22). Although the observational nature of this study design cannot infer causality, this study was the first to report, via a longitudinal population-based study, that FTS during infancy was associated with unhealthy weight development during childhood (Jansen et al., 2019).

## 20.9 Breastfeeding, expressed human milk, and responsive feeding

Through breastfeeding, the infant first communicates hunger cues, and with appropriately interpreted and prompt maternal responses, the infant latches and a positive responsive feeding relationship begins. It has long been suggested that the infant-centered nature of breastfeeding supports healthy self-regulation of energy intake during infancy (Li et al., 2010; Wright et al., 1980). Direct breastfeeding (rather than offering expressed breast milk in a bottle) relies on the infant's satiety response to end a feeding, with little influence from the mother to recognize common satiety signals with milk intake (e.g., reduced sucking, infant relaxed state, change in infant posture or drowsiness) (Hodges et al., 2016). As such, the inherent nature of breastfeeding is consistent with responsive feeding practices that encourage the child to eat in response to physiological and developmental needs, which encourages self-regulation.

The practice of expressing breast milk has increased in recent years among women with healthy term infants, yet limited data are available with this subset of women (Johns et al., 2013). Previous research indicated that when infants consumed expressed human milk, they gained significantly more weight (88.8 g/month) compared to a sub-set of infants that fed directly from the breast (Li et al., 2010). Moreover, after controlling for known covariates, children who consumed expressed human milk during the first 3 months of life were 67% less likely to have high satiety responsiveness at the age of 3–6 years when compared to children who directly breastfed (Disantis et al., 2011b), suggesting that early maternal feeding behaviors with milk may influence appetite regulation in latter childhood. More recently, within a small study (Whitfield and Ventura, 2019) of mother-infant dyads, mothers were rated as more responsive to infant cues when directly breastfeeding their 6-month-old infants than when infants consumed their expressed breast milk. Offering an infant expressed human milk, provides a precise visual confirmation to the parent about the amount of milk remaining in the bottle, which may lead to pressuring feeding practices (e.g., encouraging bottle emptying), resulting in interference with infants' continuing developing abilities to self-regulate intake, poor satiety responsiveness, risk for overfeeding, and rapid weight gain during infancy (Ventura and Hernandez, 2019).

To assess feeding practices of mothers that breastfeed, Brown and Lee (Brown and Lee, 2013) developed and validated one of the first Infant Milk Feeding Questionnaires for application with mothers of infants from birth to 6 months of age. Within their study of 384 mother-infant dyads, mothers who exclusively breastfed at birth ($n = 140$) reported more responsive feeding practices compared to those that offered milk in a bottle (primarily infant formula) ($n = 185$). Specifically, mothers that breastfed scored significantly lower on scales that measured excess encouraging of feeding, limiting feeding, weight concerns of their infants, feeding to a routine, and monitoring feeding, compared to mothers who used bottles. Mothers who used a combination of feeding approaches (e.g., both breastfeeding and offering infant formula in a bottle, $n = 63$), were more likely to feed to a routine and monitor feeding compared to those that exclusively breastfed. Moreover, these feeding practices of mothers during infancy may have long-term effects on child eating behaviors. For example, within a 6 year follow-up study of 1117 mother-infant pairs (Li et al., 2014), infant bottle drinking patterns, and caregiver reported encouragement of their infant to finish a bottle was initially recorded during infancy, and subsequent maternal feeding styles 6 years later were assessed. Frequent bottle emptying encouragement by mothers during infancy doubled the odds that mothers would encourage their child to eat all the food on their plate (OR: 2.37; 95% CI: 1.65–3.41), make sure their child ate enough (OR: 1.62; 95% CI: 1.14–2.31) and increased the odds that the child actually ate all the food on their plate at 6 years of age (OR: 2.01; 95% CI: 1.05–3.83). These findings suggest that parental feeding practices with bottle use displayed during infancy continue through at least early childhood.

Additional responsive feeding associations between breastfeeding and maternal responsiveness to infant cues have been evaluated by a systematic review (Ventura, 2017) that included 43 cross-sectional observational studies. Greater responsiveness with feeding among mothers that reported breastfeeding, compared to mothers using infant formula/bottle feeding was apparent, although the mechanisms underlying this association were not clear. Some, but not all, studies identified that mothers who reported longer breastfeeding durations showed greater responsiveness to infant and child satiety cues at 7–24 months and reported using more authoritative feeding styles and responsive feeding practices with offering complementary foods through 24 months (DiSantis et al., 2013; Hodges et al., 2013; Jansen et al., 2016). Although distinct attitudes, beliefs, and perceptions of infant feeding from mothers that breastfeed, and those that could not or chose not to breastfeed have been identified via systematic review (Dattilo et al., 2020), offering milk within a bottle does not unequivocally promote overfeeding (Ventura and Mennella, 2017). Providing responsive feeding education to mothers has been shown to promote healthy weight status within their children, at least through the first 2 years of life (Spill et al., 2019b).

## 20.10 Consideration when offering milk in a bottle

Via a systematic review of 18 studies (Appleton et al., 2018) that examined associations between infant formula intake and rapid weight gain during infancy, several potential recommendations for best practices with bottle use emerged. The authors concluded that offering formula with a lower protein concentration, not adding cereals to bottles, not putting a baby to bed with a bottle, and not overfeeding (e.g., using responsive feeding behaviors), may be protective of rapid or excess weight gain associated with bottle use and formula. As a mother that is breastfeeding does not know how much milk her infant has consumed, or little about the rate with which the infant is drinking, it has been postulated that these factors could help explain why direct breastfeeding may be associated with less maternal control during infant feeding and more responsiveness to infant feeding cues than with bottle use. Moreover, within healthy term infants, the anatomical actions used during either breastfeeding or bottle feeding are similar (Kotowski et al., 2020). However, bottle and teat characteristics (bottle size, bottle weight, use of opaque bottles, flow rate, teat material, shape, hole size) may be implicated to milk intake and subsequent rate of weight gain and growth (Kotowski et al., 2020).

The hypothesis that bottle characteristics may influence infant milk intake, and parent responsive feeding behaviors, was tested among studies that compared bottle size, color, and weight. Based on 298 infants offered exclusively formula, infants whose parents used large bottles ($\geq$ 180 mL size) at 2 months of age realized a 0.21 kg (95% CI: 0.05 to 0.37) greater weight change, 0.24 U (95% CI: 0.07 to 0.41) higher change in WAZ, and 0.31 U (95% CI: 0.08 to 0.54) larger change in WLZ at 6 months, compared to infants consuming milk from bottles holding less than 180 mL (Wood et al., 2016). Although no volume of milk intake or parental feeding behaviors were recorded, this association is noteworthy in that it suggests that bottle size alone may be associated with parent feeding practices.

To examine mothers' feeding practices, infant intake of milk, and a potential effect of an opaque weighted bottle, compared to a conventional clear bottle type on an infant feeding experience, a pilot study (Ventura and Golen, 2015) enrolled 25 mother-infant dyads of whom used exclusively ($n = 22$) or predominantly (> 80% of feeds; $n = 3$) infant formula. No infants had been introduced to solid foods. Maternal sensitivity and responsiveness to infant cues were observed using the Nursing Child Assessment Feeding Scale (NCAFS), and pressuring feeding practice was recorded. Overall, mothers were significantly more responsive to infant cues when they used opaque, compared to clear, bottles ($P = .04$), yet mothers' pressuring feeding practice mediated the effects. Mothers with higher levels of pressuring feeding were significantly more responsive to their infants' cues ($P = .02$) and their infants consumed significantly less formula when using opaque versus clear bottles ($P = .01$). In contrast, mothers with lower levels of pressuring feeding behaviors showed no differences in responsiveness or infant intake when using opaque versus clear bottles.

To expand testing of the hypothesis that opaque, weighted bottles may have an effect on mothers' feeding practices and infant milk intake, a similar study (Ventura and Hernandez, 2019), with 76 mother-infant dyads, examined maternal responsive feeding practices and infant milk consumption outcomes. When using opaque, compared with clear bottles, mothers exhibited significantly greater sensitivity to infant hunger and satiety cues ($P = .04$), and their infants consumed less milk ($P = .049$), at a significantly slower rate ($P = .009$). Although these results were not mediated by bottle contents (expressed breast milk or infant formula), infant clarity of cues was a significant moderator of effects of bottle type on milk intake ($P = .028$). Infants who exhibited greater clarity of hunger and satiety cues consumed less during the opaque bottle testing, compared to clear bottles, whereas infants who exhibited poorer clarity of cues consumed similar amounts during both conditions. Collectively, these studies suggest that when a mother does not readily see or feel the amount of milk her infant has consumed throughout a feeding, her feeding behaviors increase in responsiveness. Although additional studies are needed for confirmation, these findings may offer a practical approach to improving bottle use by parents of young infants, particularly within infants of whom are less clear in communicating their hunger and satiety cues.

Many healthy infants have the developmental motor skills needed to drink from a cup at about 8–10 months (Ross, 2017) and some have mastered this skill beginning at 6 months of age. After 12 months of age, bottle use is discouraged (NASEM, 2020). Prolonged bottle use is a documented risk for childhood obesity (Bonuck et al., 2014), and each additional month of bottle use beyond a 12–15 age range has been associated with increased odds of moving to a higher weight category (e.g., < 85th percentile, to > 85th, to > 95th percentile of BMI). In a study of approximately 7000 children, 24-month-old children using bottles realized a 33% risk of obesity at 5.5 years (Gooze et al., 2011). Bedtime bottle use was associated with a near twofold increased risk of obesity among 3-year-old children (Kimbro et al., 2007). Recommendations stress that infants or toddler age children should not be put to sleep or go to bed with a bottle (Perez-Escamilla et al., 2017; NASEM, 2020), not only for safety and oral hygiene reasons, but for the potential of fostering infant self-soothing habits with oral intake, and excess energy intake. Potential mechanisms with prolonged bottle use and rate of weight gain, or excess weight gain include high protein intake from infant formula (Koletzko et al., 2009), and/or excessive total energy intake, as identified in one study of 12–13 month aged children of whom had a median energy intake of nearly 1100 kcal/day with consumption of complementary foods and 4 bottles/day of primarily infant formula and whole milk (Bonuck et al., 2014). The authors reported no difference in bottle use among overweight and healthy weight children in this study, yet 35% of the children were > 85th percentile of weight-for-length.

## 20.11 Parent feeding practices and introduction of complementary foods

The maternal diet provides an opportunity for first teachings with flavor familiarity in utero, and during lactation (Mennella et al., 2017). One recent systematic literature review reconfirmed that limited, yet consistent, evidence supports the fact that specific flavors from the maternal diet during pregnancy or lactation can transfer to amniotic fluid or breast milk (Spahn et al., 2019). Infant acceptance of similarly flavored foods during complementary feeding, and potentially throughout childhood, may result. However, much of the early learnings about flavors in foods occurs within the family setting, after birth, and repeated exposure to novel foods is recommended as one responsive feeding behavior to promote acceptance of new foods (NASEM, 2020). One systematic literature review of 21 studies (Spill et al., 2019a) identified moderate evidence to support the conclusion that 8–10 daily tastes of a novel fruit or vegetable are likely to increase acceptability of that food among 4–24-month-old children, and the effect of repeated exposure on acceptability is likely to generalize to other foods within the same food category. In addition, another study showed that children who had tried more fruits and vegetables at 14 months of age, enjoyed a wider range of fruits and vegetables at 3–4 years of age (Mallan et al., 2016), suggesting that the effect of early repeated exposure and tasting may last during early childhood.

It is well recognized that a child needs to actually taste a food multiple times before acceptance is expected, and that simply offering or presenting a novel food to a child, particularly a strongly flavored vegetable, is unlikely to be successful in a child tasting it. Unfortunately, foods are most often offered to infants and young children for a limited number of times (typically less than five times) before the parent decides that the infant dislikes this food (Nicklaus, 2016). Parents may resort to non-responsive behaviors of overtly pressuring or reward-based approaches to reach the goal of having their child taste and accept new foods.

Unlike pressuring a young child to eat, moderate encouragement for children to taste a novel food can be beneficial. Among a small study ($n = 60$, 1–3-year-old children) (Edelson et al., 2016), the way parents urged, or encouraged, their toddlers to try a new food was assessed. Results suggested that words of encouragement, when used in moderation, may help when introducing new foods. On average, it required about 2.5 encouragements before a child would try a new food. Children who ate the most vegetables had parents who used words of reasoning (e.g., try the carrots because they are good for you) as encouragement rather than rewards or undue pressure. These results with toddler age children are inspiring in that infants 6–12 months of age typically accepted more tastes and were rated by caregivers as liking a strongly flavored vegetable more than older toddlers ($\geq$ 18 months of age) (Johnson et al., 2021). Repeated exposure is more likely to be effective during the first year, when new tastes are more easily accepted.

Although it has not been adequately studied, infants and young children are likely to respond to multiple tastes with foods (e.g., acceptance and liking) from other food categories, particularly palatable energy-dense, high sugar, snack, or dessert foods. From a purely nutritional perspective, there is a strong rationale for limiting, or omitting such foods from infant and young children's diets. On the other hand, it is well established that restricting specific foods from pre-school age children results in increased desire for restricted foods (Shloim et al., 2015). Moreover, restrictive feeding practices by parents of pre-school age and older children have been associated with children eating in the absence of hunger, eating in response to negative emotions, as well as increased body weight or measures of adiposity (Faith et al., 2004; Farrow et al., 2015; Rollins et al., 2014; Ventura and Birch, 2008).

Little is known about the use of restrictive feeding practices regarding the quality of an infant or young toddler's diet and long-term outcomes with these parental practices. Restricting a child's diet, with regard to foods that parents perceive as poor quality, was assessed in a sample ($n = 2578$) of mothers (Gubbels et al., 2009) by asking "Are there specific foods that you do not allow your child to eat or drink?" When children were 2 years of age, 42.9% of the mothers disallowed soft drink intake, and fewer reported restricting other types of sweets, cookies, cakes, sugar, or crisps. Overall, reported maternal restriction of the energy-dense, poorer quality foods was related to less consumption of the items, and a higher consumption of items considered to be healthy. Similarly, within a study of 217 mother-infant pairs (Thompson et al., 2013), infant dietary intake and maternal response to sub-scale questions within the Infant Feeding Style Questionnaire (Thompson et al., 2009) related to diet quality were assessed. Results indicated that higher restrictive diet scores were associated with better quality infant diets. In addition, a poor diet in 2-year-old children was highly associated with their mothers reporting of being unlikely to restrict sweets (OR=21.63, 95% CI 2.70, 173.30) (Crombie et al., 2009). Taken together, restricting the intake of some foods within a young age group (3–24 months) appears to improve diet quality, without increased weight-for-length or other measures of anthropometry that have been previously associated with "restriction feeding practices" among older children. Restriction for younger children may be more comparable to "covert" control that is not apparent to the child. As children become older, parental imposed diet restrictions may be more recognizable, resulting in increased desire for the restricted food(s).

In addition to the commonly assessed parent behavior of restricting foods from children's diets, a greater pressuring to eat score has been reported by mothers of smaller infants (Brown and Lee, 2013; Thompson et al., 2013), compared to infants of healthy or higher weights. Parental ranking as high about concerns that their child did not eat enough (indicative of pressuring) also increased the odds of a poor diet among 2-year-old children (OR=2.37, 95% CI 1.09–5.16) (Crombie et al., 2009). Previous research with older children has rather consistently shown that pressuring a child to eat was associated with fussier eating and lower child consumption of pressured foods (which are often healthy foods such as fruit and vegetables) (Galloway et al., 2006).

Finally, within a small dietary and feeding practice survey ($n = 60$) (Gregory et al., 2011), pressuring feeding practices by mothers of 1-year-old children, as assessed by the Child Feeding Questionnaire (Birch et al., 2001) was inversely related to fruit consumption at 2 years of age. Child frequency of vegetable consumption approached significance for less frequent use of pressure to eat, yet was significantly predicted by more frequent maternal use of healthy dietary modeling. As dietary patterns of infants and young children become established prior to 2 years of age (Deming et al., 2014; Reidy and Squatrito, 2017; Saavedra et al., 2013), a balance of responsive feeding practices by parents with setting limits, yet not overly pressuring young children to eat could have a long-lasting influence on a child's diet quality.

## 20.12 Parent feeding practices and child weight outcomes

One systematic review (Matvienko-Sikar et al., 2019) that aimed to identify a set of core outcomes for developing a future childhood intervention addressing healthy growth searched relevant published infant feeding literature for outcomes in infants through age 12 months.

Studies meeting inclusion criteria were not limited to those with outcomes addressing anthropometrics. Studies of infant feeding interventions within observational, quasi-experimental, and randomized control designs were included in the 126 publications meeting final inclusion criteria. The majority addressed breastfeeding and infant feeding ($n = 104$), followed by introduction of solids ($n = 81$), dietary intake ($n = 66$), and child weight-related outcomes ($n = 64$). Caregiver feeding practices were addressed in 28 studies, indicating that there are a number of studies including this modifiable parental feeding behavior within infant age populations that could be useful when designing future interventions that promote healthy growth during infancy. Responsive feeding education has been included in several clinical trials with encouraging results. For example, one recent systematic literature review (Spill et al., 2019b) of 8 controlled trials and 19 longitudinal cohort studies examined the relationship between maternal feeding practices in children from birth to 24 months of age and child weight gain, size, or body composition in both infancy and childhood. The authors concluded there is moderate evidence from randomized controlled trials to suggest that providing responsive feeding guidance, to teach mothers to recognize and respond appropriately to a child's hunger and satiety cues, can lead to normal weight gain and weight status in children $\leq 2$ years, compared with children whose mothers did not receive responsive feeding guidance.

Further systematic review questions (Spill et al., 2019b) assessed if feeding behaviors of parents influenced infant and young child weight status. The authors concluded that moderate evidence indicated an association between maternal feeding practices and a child's weight status and/or weight gain, but the direction of the effect was not adequately identified. Four RCT's (Daniels et al., 2012; Kavanagh et al., 2008; Paul et al., 2011; Savage et al., 2016) were included in the review, and several of these original trials had multiple follow-up publications. All had interventions focusing on responsive feeding practices within their multicomponent interventions, and three (e.g., Daniels et al., 2012; Paul et al., 2011; Savage et al., 2016) were effective in influencing at least one weight-related outcome of rapid weight gain, overweight status, weight-for-age, or BMI through 24 months of age. One trial (Kavanagh et al., 2008) had participants in the intervention group gain more weight than the control, yet this study had > 60% attrition rate, and was likely not adequately powered from enrollment. Another trial (Daniels et al., 2012) did not find sustained differences on weight gain indicators at 20 months, or at 4.5 year follow-up. Longitudinal results are awaited for the other studies.

Evidence suggests that parent's feeding behaviors with infants and young children are strongly influenced by the actual or perceived assessment of the child's size, weight status, or concern about the child's body weight. Mothers of smaller infants tend to use more pressuring feeding practices, and those with larger infants use more restrictive practices. For example, within one longitudinal study design (Dinkevich et al., 2015) with 169 mother-infant dyads, the Infant Feeding Questionnaire (Baughcum et al., 2001) with minor modifications (Dinkevich et al., 2015) was provided to mothers of 6–12-month-old infants. Anthropometrics were assessed at baseline and recorded for up to 30 months. Results indicated that pressuring to eat was associated with lower overall weight, and restrictive feeding with higher weight, in the first year of life, and that the relationship with restriction was partly explainable by maternal concerns about child eating and weight. Restrictive feeding scores and concern about child overeating/weight were significantly correlated ($r = 0.22$, $P < .01$). Similarly, pressuring to eat and concern about undereating/weight ($r = 0.25$, $P < .01$) were related. A higher pressuring score at enrollment was associated with lower overall weight-for-length z (WLZ) assessed at multiple time points through to toddlerhood. However, there was no association between pressuring to eat and infant weight trajectories throughout the course of the study. For restrictive feeding, higher scores were associated with higher WLZ at enrollment as well as through toddlerhood, but as with pressuring to eat, there were no discernible effects on infant weight trajectory.

These results are consistent with another study (Rifas-Shiman et al., 2011) of 837 mother infant pairs that investigated the relationship of reported maternal restriction on multiple measures of growth and adiposity. Maternal restriction was measured at 1 year using only one item from the Child Feeding Questionnaire (CFQ) (Birch et al., 2001) that was modified to read: "I have to be careful not to feed my child too much." Feeding restriction score at the age of 1 year was associated with higher BMI and greater sum of skinfolds at age 3 years, but the relationship was no longer significant after adjusting for weight-for-length at the age of 1 year. In another study, assessment of maternal feeding practices and behaviors, by use of the Toddler Feeding Behavior Questionnaire (Hurley et al., 2013), identified that higher restrictive feeding scores of mothers of infants with an average age of 20 months ($n = 297$) were positively associated with toddler overweight (OR = 1.58). The study design did not allow for longitudinal assessment. It is possible that mothers of larger and heavier infants utilized more restrictive practices due to concern of their child's current weight.

In contrast, results from a smaller study ($n = 62$ mother-infant pairs) (Farrow and Blissett, 2008) that assessed maternal feeding practices with the pressuring, restricting, and monitoring subscales of the Child Feeding Questionnaire (Birch et al., 2001) reported that after controlling for infant weight at 1 year, greater restriction at 1 year of age was associated with lower child weight at the age of 2 years. And, within a study of 217 mother-infant pairs (Thompson et al., 2013), dietary intake and maternal feeding practice scores, as assessed by the Infant Feeding Style Questionnaire (Thompson et al., 2009) showed that higher restriction scores measured at multiple times throughout the 3–18-month-old infants were positively associated with weight-for-age and larger sum of skinfolds within the longitudinal study.

One important distinction within the above studies is the difference in assessment of restrictive feeding, for each of the studies used a different tool. Restricting total amount of food or volume of milk offered to an infant or young child is a relatively different practice than restricting energy-dense, typically high sugar, snack, or dessert foods. Given that both dietary patterns and growth trajectories are established early, there is need for increased attention to responsive feeding approaches as a means for obesity prevention (IOM, 2011) beginning at birth. The bidirectional relationship, supported by findings that mothers of smaller infants apply more pressuring feeding practices, whereas parents of larger infant size tend to utilize more restrictive practices, may be present within the first year of parenting. As parenting feeding practices do not have a direct effect on a child's weight, per se, but instead, the effect of parenting behaviors on a child's weight is mediated by effects of parenting practices on a child's eating (Ventura and Birch, 2008), additional investigation into the effect of responsive feeding practices on dietary intake are needed.

## 20.13 Conclusions

Parent feeding behaviors are ways in which parents engage with their infant or young child at eating occasions. These behaviors tend to ladder-up to general parenting styles that parents utilize for child-rearing. Among studies with infants and toddlers, limited evidence suggests that an indulgent feeding style, compared to an authoritative style, is associated with a lower diet quality, and greater rate of weight gain during the toddler years. One major goal of responsive feeding behaviors is to promote energy-regulatory capacity of the child, and ultimately, feeding autonomy. Responsive feeding includes behaviors by parents that are attentive to an infant or child's hunger or satiety cues, by accurately interpreting the cue, and providing a prompt and ultimately predictable response. Like responsive feeding behaviors, unresponsive feeding practices (e.g., controlling, pressuring, restrictive) may be established within the first year of life and be stable throughout toddlerhood.

To date, few studies have empirically assessed child feeding cues within the first 2 years of life. Data to assess parent responsiveness, and immediate or long-term outcomes for the child regarding diet quality, healthy growth, or development are incomplete. The majority of data are based on a few studies from high-income countries that assess or describe only maternal child feeding interactions, without addressing other caretakers. Recently, more attention to the bidirectional relationship of the feeding interaction has brought light to the fact that some infants and young children are less clear within exhibiting hunger and satiety cues. Mothers often resort to using feeding to soothe young infants, as well as pressuring or restrictive feeding practices based on their interpretation of their child's current weight. These finding can further enhance education programs by teaching parents about the subtlety within early infant cues, encourage parents to accept that their healthy infant has the self-regulatory skills needed to eat in response to physiological and developmental needs, and potentially set the stage for a more responsive feeding relationship.

There is need from the professional pediatric and nutrition community to expand research with the birth-24-month age population related to "how to feed" concepts. As evidence-based guidance and recommendations emerge, these can enhance both future interventions, as well as infant and young child nutrition education and recommendations within global populations.

## 20.14 Future research needs

Additional research is needed to understand the relationships between parent responsive feeding behaviors, children's dietary intake, and weight status. In particular, longitudinal designs, beginning at birth and extending into middle childhood and beyond, would provide knowledge about the developmental trajectories and processes that are causally linked. Studies designed to identify the direction of associations and investigate if feeding styles and practices, and their effects, are stable throughout early childhood are warranted. Continued and extended validation of feeding practice questionnaires, and assessment of their concordance with observational data will help strengthen the confidence of results.

Identification of factors associated with parents that utilize specific feeding practices (mother compared to father, first time parent, maternal BMI, post-partum depression, breastfeeding exclusivity and duration), as well as characteristics of their children (infant BMI, temperament, satiety responsiveness, enjoyment of food, slowness in eating) are needed. Multivariate analyses to identify the degree of difference in dietary intake or growth associated with or explainable by specific responsive feeding behaviors would enhance understandings. Finally, randomized control testing of the efficacy of responsive feeding interventions, and the application, to scale, of specific successful intervention components are needed to provide education about how parents can optimally engage with infants and young children as they offer nutrient dense, safe, and developmentally appropriate food and liquids.

## Sources of additional information

1. American Academy of Pediatrics (AAP), the AAP Parenting Website. Available at: http://healthychildren.org.
2. Perez-Escamilla, R., Segura-Perez, S., Lott M, on behalf of the RWJF HER Expert Panel on Best Practices for Promoting Healthy Nutrition, Feeding Patterns, and Weight Status for Infants and Toddlers from Birth to 24 Months. Feeding Guidelines for Infants and Young Toddlers: A Responsive Parenting Approach. Durham, NC: Healthy Eating Research, 2017. Available at: http://healthyeatingresearch.org.
3. United Nations Children's Fund (UNICEF) UK. (2016). Responsive feeding: Supporting close and loving relationships. Available at: https://www.unicef.org.uk/babyfriendly/wpcontent/uploads/sites/2/2017/12/Responsive-Feeding-Infosheet-Unicef-UK-Baby-Friendly-Initiative.pdf.

# References

Appleton, J., Russell, C.G., Laws, R., Fowler, C., Campbell, K., Denney-Wilson, E., 2018. Infant formula feeding practices associated with rapid weight gain: a systematic review. Matern. Child Nutr. 14 (3), 12602.

Atkinson, S.A., Jimenez, E.Y., Pérez-Escamilla, R., 2021. Evidence gaps and research needs in current guidance on feeding children from birth to 24 months. Appl. Physiol. Nutr. Metab. 46 (3), 294–297.

Baughcum, A., Powers, S., Johnson, S., et al., 2001. Maternal feeding practices and beliefs and their relationships to overweight in early childhood. J. Dev. Behav. Pediatr. 22, 391–408.

Baumrind, D., 1971. Current patterns of parental authority. Dev. Psychol. Monogr. 4, 101–103.

Bergmeier, H., Skouteris, H., Haycraft, E., et al., 2015. Reported and observed controlling feeding practices predict child eating behavior after 12 months. J. Nutr. 145, 1311–1316.

Birch, L.L., Fisher, J.O., Grimm-Thomas, K., Markey, C.N., Sawyer, R., Johnson, S.L., 2001. Confirmatory factor analysis of the child feeding questionnaire: a measure of parental attitudes, beliefs and practices about child feeding and obesity proneness. Appetite 36, 201–210.

Black, M.M., Aboud, F.E., 2011. Responsive feeding is embedded in a theoretical framework of responsive parenting. J. Nutr. 141 (3), 490–494.

Bonuck, K., Avraham, S.B., Hearst, M., Kahn, R., Hyden, C., 2014. Is overweight at 12 months associated with differences in eating behaviour or dietary intake among children selected for inappropriate bottle use? Matern. Child Nutr. 10 (2), 234–244.

Boswell, N., 2021. Complementary feeding methods-a review of the benefits and risks. Int. J. Environ. Res. Public Health 4 (13), 7165.

Brown, A., Lee, M., 2013. Breastfeeding is associated with a maternal feeding style low in control from birth. PLoS One 8 (1), e54229.

Chaidez, V., Kaiser, L.L., 2011. Validation of an instrument to assess toddler feeding practices of Latino mothers. Appetite 57, 229–236.

Chaidez, V., McNiven, S., Vosti, S., Kaiser, L., 2014. Sweetened food purchases and indulgent feeding are associated with increased toddler anthropometry. J. Nutr. Educ. Behav. 46 (4), 293–298.

Crombie, I., Kiezebrink, K., Irvine, L., et al., 2009. What maternal factors influence the diet of 2-year-old children living in deprived areas? A cross-sectional survey. Public Health Nutr. 12 (8), 1254–1260.

Daniels, L.A., Mallan, K.M., Battistutta, D., Nicholson, J.M., Perry, R., Magarey, A., 2012. Evaluation of an intervention to promote protective infant feeding practices to prevent childhood obesity: outcomes of the NOURISH RCT at 14 months of age and 6 months post the first of two intervention modules. Int. J. Obes. 36 (10), 1292–1298.

Darling, N., Steinberg, L., 1993. Parenting style as context: an integrative model. Psychol. Bull. 113, 487–496.

Dattilo, A.M., 2017a. Modifiable risk factors and interventions for childhood obesity prevention within the first 1,000 days. Nestle Nutr. Inst. Workshop Ser. 87, 183–196.

Dattilo, A.M., 2017b. Programming long-term health: Effect of parent feeding approaches on long-term diet and eating patterns. In: Saavedra, J.M., Dattilo, A.M. (Eds.), Early Nutrition and Long-Term Health, Mechanisms, Consequences and Opportunities. Elsevier Ltd., United Kingdom, pp. 471–495.

Dattilo, A.M., Saavedra, J.M., 2020. Nutrition education: application of theory and strategies during the first 1000 days for healthy growth. Nestle Nutr. Inst. Workshop Ser. 92, 1–18.

Dattilo, A.M., Carvalho, R.S., Feferbaum, R., Forsyth, S., Zhao, A., 2020. Hidden realities of infant feeding: systematic review of qualitative findings from parents. Behav. Sci. 10 (5), 83.

Deming, D.M., Briefel, R.R., Reidy, K.C., 2014. Infant feeding practices and food consumption patterns of children participating in WIC. J. Nutr. Educ. Behav. 46, S29–S37.

DGAC. Dietary Guidelines Advisory Committee, 2020. Scientific Report of the 2020 Dietary Guidelines Advisory Committee: Advisory Report to the Secretary of Agriculture and the Secretary of Health and Human Services. U.S. Department of Agriculture, Agricultural Research Service, Washington, DC.

Dinkevich, E., Leid, L., Pryor, K., et al., 2015. Mothers' feeding behaviors in infancy: do they predict child weight trajectories? Obesity 23, 2470–2476.

DiSantis, K.I., Hodges, E.A., Johnson, S.L., Fisher, J.O., 2011a. The role of responsive feeding in overweight during infancy and toddlerhood: a systematic review. Int. J. Obes. 35 (4), 480–492.

DiSantis, K.I., Collins, B.N., Fisher, J.O., Davey, A., 2011b. Do infants fed directly from the breast have improved appetite regulation and slower growth during early childhood compared with infants fed from a bottle? Int. J. Behav. Nutr. Phys. Act. 17 (8), 89.

DiSantis, K.I., Hodges, E.A., Fisher, J.O., 2013. The association of breastfeeding duration with later maternal feeding styles in infancy and toddlerhood: a cross-sectional analysis. Int. J. Behav. Nutr. Phys. Act. 10, 53–65.

Edelson, L., Mokdad, C., Martin, N., 2016. Prompts to eat novel and familiar fruits and vegetables in families with 1-3 year-old children: relationships with food acceptance and intake. Appetite 99, 138–148.

Faith, M.S., Scanlon, K.S., Birch, L.L., Francis, L.A., Sherry, B., 2004. Parent-child strategies and their relationships to child eating and weight status. Obes. Res. 12, 1711–1722.

Farrow, C., Blissett, J., 2008. Controlling feeding practices: cause or consequence of early child weight? Pediatrics 121 (1), e164–e169.

Farrow, C.V., Haycraft, E., Blissett, J.M., 2015. Teaching our children when to eat: how parental feeding practices inform the development of emotional eating—a longitudinal experimental design. Am. J. Clin. Nutr. 101 (5), 908–913.

Galloway, A.T., Fiorito, L.M., Francis, L.A., Birch, L.L., 2006. 'Finish your soup': counterproductive effect of pressuring children to eat on intake and affect. Appetite 46, 318–323.

Golen, R.B., Ventura, A.K., 2015. Mindless feeding: is maternal distraction during bottle-feeding associated with overfeeding? Appetite 91, 385–392.

Gooze, R.A., Anderson, S.E., Whitaker, R.C., 2011. Prolonged bottle use and obesity at 5.5 years of age in US children. J. Pediatr. 159 (3), 431–436.

Gregory, J., Paxton, S., Brozovic, A., 2011. Maternal feeding practices predict fruit and vegetable consumption in young children. Results of a 12-month longitudinal study. Appetite 57 (1), 167–172.

Gross, R., Fierman, A., Mendelsohn, A., et al., 2010. Maternal perceptions of infant hunger, satiety, and pressuring feeding styles in an urban Latina WIC population. Acad. Pediatr. 10, 29–35.

Gross, R., Mendelsohn, A., Fierman, A., et al., 2014. Maternal infant feeding behaviors and disparities in early child obesity. Child. Obes. 10 (2), 145–152.

Gubbels, J., Kremers, S., Stafleu, A., et al., 2009. Diet-related restrictive parenting practices. Impact on dietary intake of 2-year-old children and interactions with child characteristics. Appetite 52, 423–429.

Hamburg, M.E., Finkenauer, C., Schuengel, C., 2014. Food for love: the role of food offering in empathic emotion regulation. Front. Psychol. 5, 1–9.

Hodges, E.A., Johnson, S.L., Hughes, S.O., et al., 2013. Development of the responsiveness to child feeding cues scale. Appetite 65, 210–219.

Hodges, E.A., Wasser, H.M., Colgan, B.K., Bentley, M.E., 2016. Development of feeding cues during infancy and toddlerhood. a2 41, 244–251.

Horodynski, M.A., Stommel, M., 2005. Nutrition education aimed at toddlers: an intervention study. Pediatr. Nurs. 31, 364–372.

Hughes, S.O., Power, T.G., Orlet Fisher, J., Mueller, S., Nicklas, T.A., 2005. Revisiting a neglected construct: parenting styles in a child-feeding context. Appetite 44, 83–92.

Hughes, S.O., Power, T.G., Papaioannou, M.A., Cross, M.B., Nicklas, T.A., Hall, S.K., et al., 2011. Emotional climate, feeding practices, and feeding styles: an observational analysis of the dinner meal in head start families. Int. J. Behav. Nutr. Phys. Act. 10 (8), 60.

Hurley, K.M., Cross, M.B., Hughes, S.O., 2011. A systematic review of responsive feeding and child obesity in high-income countries. J. Nutr. 141, 495–501.

Hurley, K.M., Pepper, M.R., Candelaria, M., et al., 2013. Systematic development and validation of a theory-based questionnaire to assess toddler feeding. J. Nutr. 143, 2044–2049.

IOM, Institutes of Medicine, 2011. Committee on obesity prevention policies for young children. In: Institute of Medicine (Ed.), Early Childhood Obesity Prevention Policies. The National Academies Press, Washington, DC.

IOM, Institutes of Medicine, 2016. National Academies of Sciences, Engineering, and Medicine. Parenting Matters: Supporting Parents of Children Age 0–8. The National Academies Press, Washington, DC.

Jansen, E., Mallan, K.M., Nicholson, J.M., et al., 2014. The feeding practices and structure questionnaire: construction and initial validation in a sample of Australian first-time mothers and their 2-year olds. Int. J. Behav. Nutr. Phys. Act. 11, 72.

Jansen, E., Mallan, K.M., Byrne, R., et al., 2016. Breastfeeding duration and authoritative feeding practices in first-time mothers. J. Hum. Lact. 32 (3), 498–506.

Jansen, P.W., Derks, I.P.M., Batenburg, A., Jaddoe, V.W.V., Franco, O.H., Verhulst, F.C., et al., 2019. Using food to soothe in infancy is prospectively associated with childhood BMI in a population-based cohort. J Nutr. 149 (5), 788–794.

Jimenez, E.Y., Perez-Escamilla, R., Atkinson, S.A., 2021. Existing guidance on feeding infants and children from birth to 25months: implications and next steps for registered dietitian nutritionists. J. Am. Diet. Assoc. 121 (4), 647–654.

Johns, H.M., Forster, D.A., Amir, L.H., et al., 2013. Prevalence and outcomes of breast milk expressing in women with healthy term infants: a systematic review. Pregnancy Childbirth 13, 212.

Johnson, S.L., Moding, K.J., Grimm, K.J., Flesher, A.E., Bakke, A.J., Hayes, J.E., 2021. Infant and toddler responses to bitter-tasting novel vegetables: findings from the good tastes study. J. Nutr. 151 (10), 3240–3252.

Kavanagh, K.F., Cohen, R.J., Heinig, M.J., Dewey, K.G., 2008. Educational intervention to modify bottle-feeding behaviors among formula-feeding mothers in the WIC program: impact on infant formula intake and weight gain. J. Nutr. Educ. Behav. 40 (4), 244–250.

Kimbro, R.T., Brooks-Gunn, J., McLanahan, S., 2007. Racial and ethnic differentials in overweight and obesity among 3-year-old children. Am. J. Public Health 97, 298–305.

Koletzko, B., von Kries, R., Monasterolo, R.C., Subias, J.E., Scaglioni, S., Giovannini, M., et al., 2009. Infant feeding and later obesity risk. Adv. Exp. Med. Biol. 646, 15–29.

Kotowski, J., Fowler, C., Hourigan, C., Orr, F., 2020. Bottle-feeding an infant feeding modality: an integrative literature review. Matern. Child Nutr. 16 (2), e12939.

Lakshman, R.R., Landsbaugh, J.R., Schill, A., et al., 2011. Development of a questionnaire to assess maternal attitudes toward infant growth and milk feeding practices. Int. J. Behav. Nutr. Phys. Act. 8, 35.

Li, R., Fein, S.B., Grummer-Strawn, L.M., 2010. Do infants fed from bottles lack self-regulation of milk intake compared with directly breastfed infants? Pediatrics 125 (6), e1386–e1393.

Li, R., Scanlon, K., May, A., et al., 2014. Bottle-feeding practices during infancy and eating behaviors at 6years of age. Pediatrics 134, S70–S77.

Llewellyn, C.H., van Jaarsveld, C.H., Johnson, L., et al., 2011. Development and factor structure of the baby eating behavior questionnaire in the german birth cohort. Appetite 57, 388–396.

Lohse, B., Satter, E., 2021. Use of an observational comparative strategy demonstrated construct validity of a measure to assess adherence to the Satter division of responsibility in feeding. J. Acad. Nutr. Diet. 121 (6), 1143–1156.

Ma, J.Q., Zhou, L.L., Hu, Y.Q., Liu, S.S., Sheng, X.Y., 2015. Association between feeding practices and weight status in young children. BMC Pediatr. 15, 97.

Maccoby, E.E., Martin, J.A., 1983. Socialization in the context of the family: parent–child interaction. In: Hetherington, E. (Ed.), Handbook of Child Psychology: Socialization, Personality and Social Development. Wiley, New York, NY, pp. 1–101.

Mallan, K.M., Daniels, L.A., de Jersey, S.J., 2014. Confirmatory factor analysis of the baby eating behavior questionnaire and associations with infant weight gain, gender and feeding mode in an Australian sample. Appetite 82, 43–49.

Mallan, K.M., Fildes, A., Magarey, A.M., et al., 2016. The relationship between number of fruits, vegetables, and noncore foods tried at age 14months and food preferences, dietary intake patterns, fussy eating behavior, and weight status at age 3.7years. J. Acad. Nutr. Diet. 116 (4), 630–637.

Matvienko-Sikar, K., Griffin, C., McGrath, N., Toomey, E., Byrne, M., Kelly, C., et al., 2019. Developing a core outcome set for childhood obesity prevention: a systematic review. Matern. Child Nutr. 15 (1), e12680.

McNally, J., Hugh-Jones, S., Caton, S., et al., 2016. Communicating hunger and satiation in the first 2years of life: a systematic review. Matern. Child Nutr. 12 (2), 205–228.

Mennella, J.A., Daniels, L.M., Reiter, A., R., 2017. Learning to like vegetables during breastfeeding: a randomized clinical trial of lactating mothers and infants. Am. J. Clin. Nutr. 106 (1), 67–76.

Morris, S.S., Farrier, S.C., Rogers, C.S., Taper, L.J., 1982. Feeding behaviors, food attitudes, and body fatness in infants. J. Am. Diet. Assoc. 80 (4), 330.

NASEM. National Academies of Science, Engineering and Medicine, 2020. Feeding Infants and Children from Birth to 24Months: Summarizing Existing Guidance. The National Academies Press, Washington, DC.

Nicklaus, S., 2016. Complementary feeding strategies to facilitate acceptance of fruits and vegetables: a narrative review of the literature. Int. J. Environ. Res. Public Health 13 (11), 1160.

O'Connor, T.M., Pham, T., Watts, A.W., Tu, A.W., Hughes, S.O., Beauchamp, M.R., et al., 2016. Development of an item bank for food parenting practices based on published instruments and reports from Canadian and US parents. Appetite 1 (103), 386–395.

Olvera, N., Power, T.G., 2010. Brief report: parenting styles and obesity in Mexican American children: a longitudinal study. J. Pediatr. Psychol. 35, 243–249.

Paul, I.M., Savage, J.S., Anzman, S.L., Beiler, J.S., Marini, M.E., Stokes, J.L., et al., 2011. Preventing obesity during infancy: a pilot study. Obesity 19 (2), 353–361.

Perez-Escamilla, R., Segura-Perez, S., Lott, M., 2017. Feeding Guidelines for Infants and Young Toddlers: A Responsive Parenting Approach. Healthy Eating Research, Durham, NC.

Pérez-Escamilla, R., Jimenez, E.Y., Dewey, K.G., 2021. Responsive feeding recommendations: Harmonizing integration into dietary guidelines for infants and young children. Curr. Dev. Nutr. 5 (6).

Powell, E.M., Frankel, L.A., Hernandez, D.C., 2017. The mediating role of child self-regulation of eating in the relationship between parental use of food as a reward and child emotional overeating. Appetite 113, 78–83.

Redsell, S.A., Slater, V., Rose, J., Olander, E.K., Matvienko-Sikar, K., 2021. Barriers and enablers to caregivers' responsive feeding behavior: a systematic review to inform childhood obesity prevention. Obes. Rev. 22 (7), e13228.

Reidy, K.C., Squatrito, C., 2017. Programming long-term health: nutrition and diet in toddlers. In: Saavedra, J.M., Dattilo, A.M. (Eds.), Early Nutrition and Long-Term Health, Mechanisms, Consequences and Opportunities. Elsevier Ltd, United Kingdom, pp. 537–560.

Rifas-Shiman, S., Sherry, B., Scanlon, K., et al., 2011. Does maternal feeding restriction lead to childhood obesity in a prospective cohort study? Arch. Dis. Child. 96, 265–269.

Rollins, B.Y., Loken, E., Savage, J.S., et al., 2014. Maternal controlling feeding practices and girls' inhibitory control interact to predict changes in BMI and eating in the absence of hunger from 5 to 7years. Am. J. Clin. Nutr. 99, 249–257.

Ross, E., 2017. Eating development in young children: understanding the complex interplay of developmental domains. In: Saavedra, J.M., Dattilo, A.M. (Eds.), Early Nutrition and Long-Term Health, Mechanisms, Consequences and Opportunities. Elsevier Ltd, United Kingdom, pp. 229–262.

Ruggiero, C.F., McHale, S.M., Paul, I.M., Savage, J.S., 2021. Learned experience and resource dilution: conceptualizing sibling influences on parents' feeding practices. Int. J. Environ. Res. Public Health 18 (11), 5739.

Saavedra, J., Deming, D., Dattilo, A., Reidy, K., 2013. Lessons from the feeding infants and toddlers study in North America: what children eat, and implications for obesity prevention. Ann. Nutr. Metab. 62 (s3), 27–36.

Savage, J.S., Birch, L.L., Marini, M., Anzman-Frasca, S., Paul, I.M., 2016. Effect of the INSIGHT responsive parenting intervention on rapid infant weight gain and overweight status at age 1year: a randomized clinical trial. JAMA Pediatr. 170 (8), 742–749.

Savage, J.S., Hohman, E.E., Marini, M.E., Shelly, A., Paul, I.M., Birch, L.L., 2018. INSIGHT responsive parenting intervention and infant feeding practices: Randomized clinical trial. Int. J. Behav. Nutr. Phys. Act. 15 (1), 64.

Savage, J., Hess, L., Dattilo, A., Sigman-Grant, M., Ward, D.S., Shuell, J., 2019. Formative evaluation of an online responsive feeding training program for early childhood education professionals. Curr. Dev. Nutr. 3 (Suppl 1), P11-068-19.

Saxon, T.F., Gollapalli, A., Mitchell, M.W., Stanko, S., 2002. Demand feeding or schedule feeding: infant growth from birth to 6months. J. Reprod. Infant Psychol. 20 (2), 89–99.

Shloim, N., Edelson, L., Martin, N., et al., 2015. Parenting styles, feeding styles, feeding practices and weight status in 4–12year-old children: a systematic review of the literature. Front. Psychol. 6, 1849.

Shloim, N., Vereijken, C., Blundell, P., Hetherington, M.M., 2017. Looking for cues—Infant communication of hunger and satiation during milk feeding. Appetite 108, 74–82.

Sleddens, E.F., Gerards, S.M., Thijs, C., de Vries, N.K., KRemers, S.P., 2011. General parenting, childhood overweight and obesity-inducing behaviors: a review. Int. J. Pediatr. Obes. 6 (2–2), e12–e27.

Spahn, J.M., Callahan, E.H., Spill, M.K., Wong, Y.P., Benjamin-Neelon, S.E., Birch, L., et al., 2019. Influence of maternal diet on flavor transfer to amniotic fluid and breast milk and children's responses: a systematic review. Am. J. Clin. Nutr. 109 (Suppl 7), 1003S–1026S.

Spill, M.K., Johns, K., Callahan, E.H., Shapiro, M.J., Wong, Y.P., Benjamin-Neelon, S.E., et al., 2019a. Repeated exposure to food and food acceptability in infants and toddlers: a systematic review. Am. J. Clin. Nutr. 1109 (Suppl 7), 978S–989S.

Spill, M.K., Callahan, E.H., Shapiro, M.J., Spahn, J.M., Wong, Y.P., Benjamin-Neelon, S.E., et al., 2019b. Caregiver feeding practices and child weight outcomes: a systematic review. Am. J. Clin. Nutr. 109 (Suppl 7), 990S–1002S.

Stifter, C.A., Moding, K.J., 2015. Understanding and measuring parent use of food to soothe infant and toddler distress: a longitudinal study from 6 to 18months of age. Appetite 95, 188–196.

Stifter, C.A., Anzman-Frasca, S., Birch, L.L., Voegtline, K., 2011. Parent use of food to soothe infant/toddler distress and child weight status. An exploratory study. Appetite 57 (3), 693–699.

Sumner, G., Spieta, A., 1994. NCAST Caregiver/Parent–Child Interaction Teaching Manual. NCAST Publications, University of Washington, School of Nursing, Seattle, pp. 1–168.

Temmen, C.D., Lipsky, L.M., Faith, M.S., Nansel, T.R., 2021. Prospective relations between maternal emotional eating, feeding to soothe, and infant appetitive behaviors. Int. J. Behav. Nutr. Phys. Act. 18 (1), 105.

Thompson, A., Mendez, M., Borja, J., et al., 2009. Development and validation of the infant feeding style questionnaire. Appetite 53, 210–221.

Thompson, A., Adair, L., Bentley, M., 2013. Pressuring and restrictive parenting styles influence infant feeding and size among a low-income African-American sample. Obesity 21 (3), 562–571.

Uesugi, K., Dattilo, A.M., Black, M., Saavedra, J.M., 2016. Design of a digital-based, multi-component nutrition guidance system for prevention of early childhood obesity. J. Obes. 2016, 5,067,421.

UNICEF. United Nations Children's Fund, 2016. Responsive Feeding: Supporting Close and Loving Relationships.

Ventura, A.K., 2017. Associations between breastfeeding and maternal responsiveness: a systematic review of the literature. Adv. Nutr. 8 (3), 495–510.

Ventura, A.K., Birch, L.L., 2008. Does parenting affect children's eating and weight status? Int. J. Behav. Nutr. Phys. Act. 5, 15.

Ventura, A.K., Golen, R.P., 2015. A pilot study comparing opaque, weighted bottles with conventional, clear bottles for infant feeding. Appetite 85, 178–184.

Ventura, A.K., Hernandez, A., 2019. Effects of opaque, weighted bottles on maternal sensitivity and infant intake. Matern. Child Nutr. 15 (2), 1–9.

Ventura, A.K., Mennella, J.A., 2017. An experimental approach to study individual differences in infants' intake and satiation behaviors during bottle-feeding. Child. Obes. 13 (1), 44–52.

Ventura, A.K., Sheeper, S., Levy, J., 2019. Exploring correlates of infant clarity of cues during early feeding interactions. J. Acad. Nutr. Diet. 119 (9), 1452–1461.

Vollmer, R.L., Mobley, A.R., 2013. Parenting styles, feeding styles, and their influence on child obesogenic behaviors and body weight: a review. Appetite 71, 232–241.

Whitfield, K.C., Ventura, A.K., 2019. Exploration of responsive feeding during breastfeeding versus bottle feeding of human milk: a within-subject pilot study. Breastfeed. Med. 14 (7), 482–486.

Wood, C.T., Perreira, K.M., Perrin, E.M., et al., 2016. Confirmatory factor analysis of the Infant feeding styles questionnaire in latino families. Appetite 100, 118–125.

Wood, A.C., Blissett, J.M., Brunstrom, J.M., Carnell, S., Faith, M.S., Fisher, J.O., et al., 2020. Caregiver influences on eating behaviors in young children: a scientific statement from the American Heart Association. J. Am. Heart Assoc. 9 (10), e014520.

World Health Organization, 2003. Guiding Principles on Complementary Feeding of the Breastfed Child. World Health Organization, Geneva.

World Health Organization, 2009. Infant and Young Child Feeding: Model Chapter for Textbooks for Medical Students and Allied Health Professionals. World Health Organization, Geneva.

Worobey, J., Lopez, M., Hoffman, D., 2009. Maternal behavior and infant weight gain in the first year. J. Nutr. Educ. Behav. 41, 169–175.

Wright, P., Fawcett, J., Crow, R., 1980. The development of differences in the feeding behavior of bottle and breast-fed human infants from birth to two months. Behav. Process. 5, 1–20.

# Programming long-term health: Nutrition and diet in infants aged 6 months to 1 year

*Hermann Kalhoff*[a,b] *and Mathilde Kersting*[b]

[a]Pediatric Clinic, Dortmund, Germany [b]Research Institute of Child Nutrition, University Clinic Bochum, Bochum, Germany

## LEARNING OBJECTIVES

1. To understand that nutrition changes fundamentally and more dramatically in the first year of life than in any other later period due to nutritional needs and neuromotor development.

2. To understand the complexities involved in the transition from exclusive milk feeding to complementary feeding.

3. To understand that in many affluent countries, it is recommended that complementary feeding be introduced within an age window.

4. To understand that the total daily diet in the second half of infancy should be conceived as a modular system of complementary meals and residual breastfeeding, taking into account national habits.

## 21.1 Introduction

Transition from milk feeding to complementary feeding and family diet

The World Health Organization (WHO) recommends exclusive breastfeeding for the first 6 months of life. Complementary foods are defined by the WHO as any food or liquid other than breast milk. However, as many infants receive human milk substitutes from the first weeks of life, other authorities have suggested that the term complementary foods should be applied to foods other than breast milk or infant formula introduced to an infant to provide nutrients, thus complementing milk feeding.

After 6 months of age, it becomes increasingly difficult for breastfed infants to meet their nutritional needs (energy, iron, zinc, protein, and some fat-soluble vitamins) from human milk alone (Fewtrell et al., 2017). Therefore, complementary foods should provide adequate energy density, and the diet should include good sources of iron, zinc, and protein. The introduction of complementary feeding (CF) is an important process during infancy, most likely playing a major role for the child's future development and health. Introduction of complementary food helps infants finally and gradually to acquire their family's diet model (EFSA et al., 2019; Fewtrell et al., 2017).

What is the optimal age for introduction of complementary foods? There is agreement that exclusive breastfeeding is desirable in situations where there is lack of clean drinking water or of safe complementary foods, but there is less consensus regarding infants in developed countries or in higher income settings, respectively. Overall, there is evidence to support the WHO recommendation to introduce complementary foods at 6 months, but depending on the infant's readiness for solid food introduction could be started around 4 months already (EFSA et al., 2019). One of the main concerns is that the rate of iron deficiency anemia (IDA) in breastfed infants might be positively altered by earlier introduction of solids (Qasem et al., 2015).

Thus, in many affluent countries, it is recommended to introduce complementary foods in an age window. The European Society for Pediatric Gastroenterology, Hepatology, and Nutrition (ESPGHAN) recommends introducing complementary foods between 17 and 26 weeks of age. The European Food Safety Authority concluded that for healthy full-term infants in the European Union complementary foods may be safely introduced between 4 and 6 months of age (WHO, 2002; Fewtrell et al., 2017; EFSA et al., 2019).

During sensitive periods of infancy, nutritional, and metabolic factors may have a long-term programming effect on health and well-being in later age. This has been intensively studied during the prenatal and postnatal periods, where programming effects may be assumed most effective. In affluent countries, infants are unlikely to experience deficiencies of macronutrients during the CF period. However, there is still some discussion, if nutrition at variance from the recommendations exceeding upper limits, for example, for protein and/or energy in the early months might have long-term consequences on later health outcome, for example, related to adiposity during childhood (Koletzko et al., 2016).

Usually around the end of the first year of life, infants are ready to participate more and more in the family diet, where the food choice and meal composition often depend to a great extent on sociocultural traditions. As risks of an inadequate nutrition decrease as the child gets older, optimal diet and specific recommendations for this age are less often in the scientific focus.

This chapter starts with addressing nutritional needs (nutrient based) in a physiological context. Second, we address nutritional needs, first qualitatively, and then, quantitatively (food, meal based), additionally considering a sociocultural context. Furthermore, we comment on the evidence base for recommendations, on knowledge gaps and need for future research. Finally, we attempt a holistic summary and conclusions for feeding the infant from 6 to 12 months of age.

## 21.2 Basic nutritional needs

### 21.2.1 Nutrient requirements

The dietary requirement of a nutrient is the amount, which must be consumed on a regular basis to maintain health in an otherwise healthy individual, on the assumption that the requirements for energy and all other nutrients have already been satisfied, taking into account extra needs related to intensive growth during infancy.

Several concepts are in use to describe nutritional requirements of a population group. Dietary reference intakes (DRIs), introduced by the Food and Nutrition Board of the Institute of Medicine, guide nutrient intake in a variety of settings. The DRIs are actually a set of several reference values that include values related to both adequate intakes and upper levels of intakes. The (estimated) *average requirement (E) AR* is defined as the nutrient intake value that is estimated to meet the requirement of half the healthy individuals in a group. In order to estimate a recommended intake that will safely meet the nutritional requirements of almost all healthy individuals in the group, the EAR is increased by two standard deviations to obtain the RDA for this nutrient. When a population reference intake cannot be firmly established (because an AR cannot be determined), the *adequate intake (AI)* is estimated, based on experimentally determined approximations or estimates of nutrient intakes by a group of apparently healthy individuals. For energy and macronutrients, the *reference intake range (RI)* describes intakes that are adequate for maintaining health and associated with a low risk of selected chronic diseases (IOM, 2005a,b; Yates, 2006; EFSA, 2010, 2013a; American Academy of Pediatrics, Committee on Nutrition., 2019a).

Most of the references for nutrient intake covering the first 4–6 months are based on exclusive breastfeeding and average composition of breast milk of well-nourished mothers. Afterward, recommendations for infants and children are based on assumptions, sometimes in analogy to data from adults (e.g., per kilogram bodyweight, per energy intake). Here, energy and nutrient needs in the second half of infancy are presented according to the conceptual basis of relevant DRIs, depending on the scientific evidence of the existing data necessary to maintain a healthy state.

*Energy*: Energy requirement is the amount of food energy to balance energy expenditure needed to maintain body mass, body composition, and a level of physical activity consistent with long-term good health. In children, this includes the energy for optimal growth and development of children (IOM, 2005a,b; EFSA, 2013a). The energy requirements in infants are based on total energy expenditure (TEE) established by Butte and adding energy requirements for growth (for methods, see EFSA, 2010, 2013b; Deutsche Gesellschaft für Ernährung, 2015) (Tables 21.1–21.3).

*Protein*: Dietary protein supplies the body with nitrogen and amino acids as well as other nonprotein metabolically active nitrogenous substances. The requirement of dietary protein is composed of two components: maintenance and growth. It may be defined as the (minimum) intake of high-quality protein (i.e., containing all essential amino acids) that provides the means for maintaining an appropriate body composition and permitting growth at a normal rate for age (assuming normal physical activity).

Estimation of protein intakes from breast milk is difficult in the first 6 months because of the nonprotein nitrogen fraction and changing composition of the protein fraction of breast

**TABLE 21.1** Energy—European Union: intakes of energy considered adequate for infants from 7 to 12 months of age (EFSA, 2013b).

| Age (months) | AR (kcal/day) | | AR (kcal/kg body weight per day) | |
|---|---|---|---|---|
| | Boys | Girls | Boys | Girls |
| 6 to <7 | 599 | 546 | 76 | 75 |
| 7 to <8 | 634 | 572 | 76 | 76 |
| 8 to <9 | 661 | 597 | 77 | 76 |
| 9 to <10 | 698 | 628 | 77 | 76 |
| 10 to <11 | 724 | 655 | 79 | 77 |
| 11 to <12 | 742 | 674 | 79 | 77 |

**TABLE 21.2** Energy—German, Austrian, and Swiss reference values (DACH, 2018).

| Age (months) | RI (kcal/day) |
|---|---|
| 4 to <12 months | Boys: 700 Girls: 600 |

**TABLE 21.3** Energy—United States and Canada dietary reference intakes (IOM, 2005a,b).

| Age (months) | RI (kcal/day) | |
|---|---|---|
| | Boys | Girls |
| 6 to <7 | 645 | 593 |
| 7 to <8 | 668 | 608 |
| 8 to <9 | 710 | 643 |
| 9 to <10 | 746 | 678 |
| 10 to <11 | 793 | 717 |
| 11 to <12 | 817 | 742 |

milk with time. For older infants, the EAR is calculated by a factorial method including data form nitrogen balance studies (requirement for maintenance) and estimation for protein deposition derived from body composition analysis and the efficiency of protein utilization for each age group (requirement for growth) (Tables 21.4–21.6).

**TABLE 21.4** Water—European Union: intake of water considered adequate for infants from 7 to 12 months of age (EFSA, 2017).

| Age (months) | AI (mL/day) |
|---|---|
| 7–11 | 800–1000 |

TABLE 21.5 Water—German, Austrian, and Swiss reference values (DACH, 2018).

| | RI water intake via | | | |
| | Fluids | Solids | Metabolism | Total water intake |
| Age (months) | (mL/day) | (mL/day) | (mL/day) | (mL/day) |
|---|---|---|---|---|
| 4 to <12 months | 400 | 500 | 100 | 1000 |

TABLE 21.6 Water—United States and Canada dietary reference intakes (IOM, 2005a,b).

| Age (months) | AI (L/day) |
|---|---|
| 6<12 | 0.8 |

*Fat*: Fat is an important energy source. Moreover, it supplies essential fatty acids and facilitates the absorption of fat-soluble dietary components (e.g., vitamins).

Energy requirements remain high during the second half of infancy. The recommendations for fat intake are based on the assumption to enable the transition from high fat intake with breast milk (up to 50% of energy intake) to the moderate fat intake in children (about 30%–35%), considered as primary prevention for later development of adiposity. However, the range of optimal fat intake during infancy is still under discussion and the recommendations of different bodies vary considerably. Qualitatively, the consumption of saturated fats (mainly found in foods of animal origin) should be limited, while unsaturated fats (found mainly in foods of vegetable and fish origin) should be preferred.

Based on practical considerations (as current levels of intake and achievable dietary patterns) the EFSA panel decided to define only an RI value for intake of total fat (40%, EFSA, 2013a).

*Fatty acids* (n-3/n-6 fatty acids): In human nutrition, two polyunsaturated fatty acids (PUFA), linoleic acid (LA, C18:2 n-6) and alpha-linoleic acid (ALA, C18:3 n-3) are essential. They regulate membrane fluidity and act as precursors for the long-chain n-3 polyunsaturated fatty acids (LC-PUFA) arachidonic acid, eicosapentaenoic acid, and docosahexaenoic acid. The AIs for LA and ALA were based on the lowest estimated mean intakes of various population groups from a number of European countries where there is no overt deficiency of these fatty acids (EFSA, 2010, 2013a, 2017) (Tables 21.4–21.6).

*Carbohydrates*: The main glycemic carbohydrates are the monosaccharides glucose and fructose, the disaccharides sucrose and lactose, maltooligosaccharides, and the polysaccharide starch. They mainly provide carbohydrate (glucose) to the body cells. Dietary references for the intake of glycemic carbohydrates are based on the recommended intake values of the two other macronutrients, fat and protein, respectively (Tables 21.7–21.10).

*Critical nutrients*: We focus on iron, and iodine, as data from studies show that intake is below recommendations in a considerable portion of infants in underdeveloped countries and in developed countries as well. Furthermore, some biomarkers are indicative to describe the adequacy of the nutritional status (EFSA, 2013a).

*Iron*: Iron has important metabolic functions in oxygen-transfer and in oxygen-mediated redox reactions. Insufficient intake results in anemia; moreover, iron deficiency is suggested to impair psychomotor development, cognitive performance, and immune function. Infants in the second 6 months of life are at a high risk of ID and IDA because of extraordinary requirements

**TABLE 21.7** Protein—European Union: intakes of protein considered adequate for infants from 7 to 12 months of age (EFSA, 2013a).

| Age (months) | AR (g/day) | |
|---|---|---|
| | Boys | Girls |
| 6 to <7 | 9 | 8 |
| 7 to <8 | 11 | 10 |
| 8 to <9 | 11 | 10 |
| 9 to <10 | 11 | 10 |
| 10 to <11 | 11 | 10 |
| 11 to <12 | 11 | 10 |

**TABLE 21.8** Fat (essential fatty acids, PUFA)—European Union: intakes of fat, essential fatty acids, and LC-PUFAs considered adequate for infants from 7 to 12 months of age (EFSA, 2017).

| Age (months) | Total fat (E%) | LA (E%) | ALA (E%) | DHA (mg/day) | DHA+EPA (mg/day) | ARA (mg/day) |
|---|---|---|---|---|---|---|
| 7–11 | 40 | 4 | 0.5 | 100 | – | – |

**TABLE 21.9** Protein and fat (essential fatty acids, PUFA)—German, Austrian, and Swiss reference values (DACH, 2018).

| Age (months) | Protein (g/kg birth weight per day) | Total fat (E%) | Ess FA (E%) |
|---|---|---|---|
| 4 to <12 | 1.3 | | |
| 4 to <12 | | 35–45 | n-6: 3.5 n-3: 0.5 |

**TABLE 21.10** Protein and fat (essential fatty acids, PUFA)—United States and Canada dietary reference intakes (IOM, 2005a,b).

| Age (months) | Protein (g/day) | Total Fat (E%) | n-6 PUFA (g/day) | n-3 PUFA (g/day) |
|---|---|---|---|---|
| 7 to <12 | 11.0 | 30 | 4.6 | 0.5 |

for growth (Domeloff, 2007; Kalhoff et al., 2010). In 2014, the ESPGHAN Committee on Nutrition stated, that from the age of 6 months, all infants and toddlers should receive iron-rich (complementary) foods, including meat products and/or iron-fortified foods (Domellöf et al., 2014).

One way to estimate required alimentary iron intake is to combine the amount of iron needed in the body with iron content of foods and estimations of iron absorption. In 2013, the EFSA panel decided to take the reference values of the DACH as a basis, which were based on observed intakes of infants at the end of the first year of life who did not develop ID (EFSA, 2013a; DACH, 2018).

In 2015, the EFSA Panel concluded that in infants aged 7–11 months, the requirement for absorbed iron is 0.79 mg/day to replace obligatory losses (0.19 mg/day) and increase hemoglobin mass, tissue iron, and storage iron (0.6 mg/day). Assuming 10% absorption, this gives an AR of 8 mg/day and, based on a coefficient of variation (CV) of 20%, which allows for high individual variation relating to growth rate, iron losses, absorption, and dietary pattern, the population reference intake (PRI) was set as 11 mg/day (EFSA, 2015). *Iodine*: The most important physiological function of iodine seems to be the normal metabolism of thyroid hormones (thyroid gland). Iodine deficiency is associated with goiter, hypothyroidism, mental retardation, and increased neonatal and infant mortality. On insufficient iodine intake, levels of T4 and T3 are low and thyroid-stimulating hormone (TSH) is high, due to loss of feedback inhibition on TSH synthesis. The increased TSH levels lead to hyperplasia and hypertrophy of the thyroid gland, with visible and palpable thyroid gland enlargement, known as goiter (Zimmermann et al., 2008). More recently, studies demonstrated that even a mild iodine deficiency during the first years of life adversely affects brain development (Remer et al., 2010).

As AI for infants in the second half of the first year of life, the EFSA panel decided to take the midpoint of recent reference values for iodine of other scientific or authoritative bodies (range of 50–130 µg/day) (EFSA, 2013a).

## 21.3 Major foods in the CF period

*Eating skills:* Bodies like ESPGHAN and the Nutrition Committee of the German Pediatric Society recommend exclusive breastfeeding during the first 4–6 months, followed by partial breastfeeding along with CF. Thus, CF should be introduced between the beginning of the 5th and 7th month (Fewtrell et al., 2017; Ernährungskommission der Deutschen Gesellschaft für Kinder- und Jugendmedizin, 2014; EFSA et al., 2019).

There are milestones of development an infant reach, when it is ready to consume complementary foods. When an infant is able to sit with support and has good head and neck control, it usually has achieved other skills like adequate truncal control and the ability to propel pureed foods to the posterior pharynx for swallowing (American Academy of Pediatrics, 2019b).

Once thin purees are tolerated and the infant can sit independently and tries to grasp food, thicker foods can be introduced. By around 8 months of age, infants have developed sufficient tongue flexibility to chew and swallow food with more texture. By 8–10 months of age, infants develop skills like sitting independently, eye-hand coordination needed to grasp and manipulate food, and the ability to chew and swallow. By the time the infant is around 12 months of age, the hand grasp further matures to a fine pincer grasp. At this developmental stage, finely chopped soft foods and foods that dissolve easily can be offered as finger foods. In parallel, many infants learn to drink from a standard cup using their two hands and eat family food with minor adaptations (e.g., cut into bite-sized portions) (American Academy of Pediatrics, 2019b; Fewtrell et al., 2017; EFSA et al., 2019).

Generally, there is variation in the ages at which an infant will achieve new developmental stages, determined, for example, by his or her innate abilities and interaction with the environment. That is a major reason why a time span is recommended in population based guidance for the introduction of CF as well as for transition to family food instead of a fixed age.

*Milk*: Continued breastfeeding is recommended along with the introduction of CF in the second 6 months of life. Breastfeeding may continue beyond the first year as long as mutually desired by mother and infant (EK-DGKJ). In addition to or instead of breast milk, infant or follow-up formula may be used, composed according to scientific recommendations on the essential composition (e.g., EFSA, 2014; EU (European Union), 2016). As infant formula is adequate as milk, as part of the diet along with CF, and there is no fundamental nutritional need to switch to follow-on formula for healthy young infants in the CF period.

Regarding cow's milk, the AAP Committee on Nutrition recommends to avoid the consumption of whole, unmodified cow's milk during the first year of life because of the high renal solute load and the increased risk of iron deficiency due to low iron content (American Academy of Pediatrics, 2019).

The ESPGHAN Committee on Nutrition suggests not using cow's milk as the main drink before 12 months of age; small volumes of cow's milk may be added to complementary foods (Fewtrell et al., 2017). Generally, plant-based milks (like soy, rice, almond, or coconut) should be avoided due to insufficient caloric and nutrient content.

For any choices of milk substitutes, the major differences between the composition of human breast milk and milk from different animal species have to be considered (Fig. 21.1).

*Cereals*: Single-grain infant cereals are good choices for the first supplemental food as they supply additional energy, may be enriched with microminerals, for example, iron or combined with vitamin C. In many countries, rice is offered first because it is easily accessible (some concerns have been raised however regarding the potential contamination of rice cereals with arsenic which might be harmful, if given high amounts of consumption (American Academy of Pediatrics, 2014)). Another option is to start with wheat cereals (Ziegler et al., 2006) or oat flakes, which are rich in iron and easily available. Whole grain cereals (often available as instant products) are preferable as they are higher in nutrient and fiber content than refined products. To enhance oral motor function and to prevent overnutrition, some guidelines recommend that cereals should not be added to the bottles, but preferably fed with a spoon.

*Vegetables and fruits*: Vegetables and fruits provide infants and children with vitamins (especially provitamin A, C, folate), minerals, and fiber. Fruits in addition provide carbohydrates, for example, fructose or saccharose. Due to low glycemic load and energy density and

| Per 100 mL | Sheep | Horse | Goat | Cow | Human |
|---|---|---|---|---|---|
| Energy (kcal) | 96 | 47 | 67 | 64 | 69 |
| Protein (g) | 5.3 | 2.2 | 3.7 | 3.3 | 1.1 |
| Carbohydrates | 6.3 | 1.5 | 3.9 | 3.6 | 4.0 |
| Minerals, total | 4.6 | 6.2 | 4.2 | 4.6 | 7.0 |
| Calcium | 0.86 | 0.36 | 0.79 | 0.74 | 0.21 |
| Vit. A (Retinol) | 183 | 110 | 127 | 120 | 32 |
| Folat | 50 | 12 | 68 | 28 | 69 |
| Vit. C | * | * | 0.8 | 6.4 | 8.5 |
| | 4 | 15 | 2 | 2 | 4 |

FIG. 21.1    Features of the composition of milk of different species in comparison to human milk. *, not applicable.

high fiber content, in particular vegetables are generally regarded as healthy food. However, to children, vegetables are less appealing as they often taste bitter. As the acceptance of vegetables may be increased by an early exposure, some groups promote the idea of an early introduction of various vegetables and fruit (either in commercial or in homemade meals) during CF (Hetherington et al., 2015; Kalhoff et al., 2021).

*Vegetable oils*: Introduction of complementary food usually leads to decreasing intakes of LC-PUFA compared to full breastfeeding. However, during later infancy the n-3 LC-PUFA requirements for brain growth are still high. In the randomized controlled Dortmund intervention trial for optimization of infant nutrition, DINO, we observed, that usage of rapeseed oil (high in n-3 alpha linolenic acid, ALA) in complementary meals (concordant to EU legislation for commercial meals) instead of corn oil (high in n-6 linoleic acid, LA) enhanced endogenic synthesis and DHA-status (Schwartz et al., 2009). In the follow-up study, PINGU rapeseed oil addition resulted in an increased EPA status but not in DHA status (Libuda et al., 2016). Thus, improving the ratio of linoleic acid to alpha-linoleic acid in CF may be considered as one dietary strategy to support n-3 LC-PUFA metabolism in infants (Schwartz et al., 2010).

*Fish*: Modern societies have adapted to a diet, rich in n-6 FA acids and poor in n-3 FA. There are just a few food sources with relevant amounts of preformed n-3 LC-PUFA, such as oily fish. Our PINGU trial, showed that regular fish (salmon) consumption during CF improved the infants EPA and DHA status at 10 months of age (Libuda et al., 2016), but did not affect visual or cognitive development of these term infants (Kalhoff et al., 2020). However, although fish consumption with complementary meals could be a major source of omega-3 polyunsaturated fatty acid in infants from 6 to 12 months of age, a recent nationwide consumer survey in Germany revealed still low consumption in infants and their mothers (Stimming et al., 2014).

*Eggs*: Eggs can be introduced safely to infants as former assumptions about an increased risk to develop hypersensitivity after early introduction were not substantiated. Recent findings suggest that an early exposure to dietary antigens may be more protective toward allergy than a later introduction (Agostoni and Lacuini, 2014). Moreover, in a randomized controlled trial, early regular oral egg exposure in infants with eczema (starting from 4 to 8 months of age) could be shown to induce immune tolerance pathways and a reduction in egg allergy incidence with 12 months of age (Palmer et al., 2013; EFSA et al., 2019).

Eggs, in particular egg yolk, is rich in nutrients such as vitamin A, D, E, B12, folate, zinc, and iron but bioavailability of iron is low. All eggs and egg-rich foods must be carefully handled and properly prepared to reduce the possibility of bacterial contamination (e.g., salmonella or other bacteria).

*Salt, sugar*: At birth, human infants are either insensitive or indifferent to salty taste, with the development of the ability to detect and respond to salty tastes thought to occur over the first 6 months of life (Beauchamp et al., 1986). As early dietary experience during infancy and early childhood are suggested to shape the salty taste responses later in life, early salt intake may be a predictor of future sodium intake, blood pressure, or other health-related outcomes (Stein et al., 2012; Strazzullo et al., 2012).

With the introduction of solid foods, all types of carbohydrates may be introduced into the diet, for example, through cereals, potatoes, fruits, and vegetables. An observational study evaluating associations between added sugar intake during early childhood (1 year of age) and body fat at age of 7 years Dortmund Nutritional and Anthropometic Longitudinally

Designed (DONALD) study reported, that added sugar at low intake levels during early childhood did not appear to be critical for BMI and body fat age 7 years (Herbst et al., 2011). Another study found an association between the consumption of sugar-sweetened beverages during infancy and increased risk of obesity at the age of 6 years (Pan et al., 2014).

Hence, the addition of sugar and salt to complementary food is discouraged. Low sugar and salt intake during infancy may help to set a lower threshold for sweet and salty tastes later in life (Beauchamp and Mennella, 2009).

*Beverages*: Water is the most essential nutrient (Manz et al., 2002). Only few dietary reference systems comprise water up to now. Water is the main constituent of the human body, around 60% in infants between 6 and 12 months of age. It is involved in practically all body functions. Water homeostasis is controlled by mechanisms modifying excretion and, to some lesser extent, water intake. Total water intake with the diet comprises water content of food and beverages, including drinking water.

Maintenance of body water is a regulated balance of intakes and outputs mediated by physiologic mechanisms coupled to regulation of electrolytes. The needs for water are influenced by thermoregulation (especially in hot environments) and physical activity. The high water content of the newborn (about 70%–80% of body weight) decreases throughout infancy, but is still quite high with 1 year of age (about 65% of BW) (Kalhoff et al., 2015).

For the second half of infancy, the AI for water was based on estimates of total dietary water intake from human milk (or formula), complementary food, and beverages. Following German recommendations based on calculations considering alimentary water intake, renal solute load, water losses with urine and stools, and the concept of positive free urine volume as a marker of euhydration (Manz et al., 2002), additional water intake during the second half of infancy is not needed in the German food-based dietary guidelines, until all three recommended daily complementary meals are introduced (Ernährungskommission der Deutschen Gesellschaft für Kinderund Jugendmedizin, 2014) (Tables 21.4–21.6).

Tap water is often culturally assumed to be drinking water, especially in developed countries. Usually it is potable, although water quality problems are not rare. One concern raised in developed countries is the possible intake of lead with drinking water. Lead can enter drinking water when service pipes that contain lead corrode, especially where the water has high acidity or low mineral content that corrodes pipes and fixtures (Brown and Margolis, 2012).

In Germany, drinking water quality is governed by a law known as the "Trinkwasserverordnung," as well as by other regulations—plus various guidelines, recommendations, and directives (e.g., EU directive, 2020).

### 21.3.1 Meals in complementary feeding

#### 21.3.1.1 *Principles of food and meal-based dietary guidelines*

Food selection and even more the combination of foods in meals reflect socioculturally determined dietary habits within a population, starting already with CF. In contrast, the fundamental nutrient requirements and consequently nutrient reference values are physiologically determined and can therefore be the same, for example, across European countries.

To make nutrient based recommendations applicable in dietary practice and dietary advice, for example, by pediatric counseling, they need to be translated into Food Based Dietary

Guidelines (FBDG) (EFSA). We suggest that also country specific meal-based dietary guidelines should be available starting from the CF period to ease translation of nutrients into practice.

Hence, CF recommendations and practices are generally not evidence based and vary between countries as most current guidelines are based upon cultural factors and food availability (Grammatikaki et al., 2019; Kersting et al., 2020). In developing countries, the focus is still on providing adequate nutrients to support growth and development, whereas in affluent countries it may be more important to achieve a balanced (optimized) intake of nutrients, avoiding deficiencies as well as excess. However, in spite of easy access to macronutrients with foods, sufficient intake of some micronutrients during the second half of infancy may still remain critical in affluent countries as well.

The AAP Committee on Nutrition suggests that infant cereals and pureed meats may be offered as first complementary foods, because they provide iron and zinc, which are the nutrients most likely deficient in the diets of infants in the Unites States (Briefel et al., 2006; Krebs et al., 2006, 2012). Pureed meats in addition increase the absorption of nonheme iron (Engelmann et al., 1998). Once, the infants accept these foods, strained or pureed fruits and vegetables may be added, at least once per day in late infancy (Jones et al., 2010; American Academy of Pediatrics, 2019b).

### 21.3.1.2 Exemplary modular system

In line with scientific recommendations, we propose two modular systems of meals starting with a "dietary schedule for the first year of life" and smoothly perpetuating into an "optimized mixed-diet" (OMD) for children that is easy to adopt in the family setting (Kersting et al., 2017, 2020). This concept translates the nutrient-related recommendations into food- and meal-based dietary guidelines, considering national or traditional dietary habits in Germany. Using this approach, it is possible to evaluate the potential of common (unfortified) foods to achieve an adequate nutrient intake and to disclose "critical" nutrients for which modes of an additional supply by fortification or supplementation are needed. The EFSA Panel on Dietetic Products, Nutrition, and Allergies has recommended this total-diet concept and modular system as an example for the establishment of food-based dietary guidelines for infants, children, and adolescents (EFSA, 2013a).

Food-based dietary guidelines for the first year of life in Germany consider ESPGHAN food-based recommendations for CF and translate them into the German feeding tradition. As recommend, CF is introduced between the beginning of the fifth and the seventh month and should be accompanied by breastfeeding or formula. Variation of food (esp. vegetables) in complementary meals is recommended; both home preparation and commercial complementary food is possible, including deep-frozen menus if available (Fig. 21.2; Maier-Nöth et al., 2016; Kalhoff et al., 2021).

In Germany, the first complementary meal which is commonly introduced is a vegetable-potato-meal (Fig. 21.3), including meat with highly bioavailable iron and zinc (5–6 times per week) or fish with omega-3 LC-PUFA, iron and iodine (once per week). Potatoes may be alternated with noodles, rice, preferably as whole grain, in variation.

In about monthly intervals, additional meals [a cereal-milk meal with some fruit (juice) and a fruit-cereal meal] follow. From the age of about 10 months, (soft) bread may be offered, along with drinking milk from a cup, thus beginning the transition to family diet. There is no

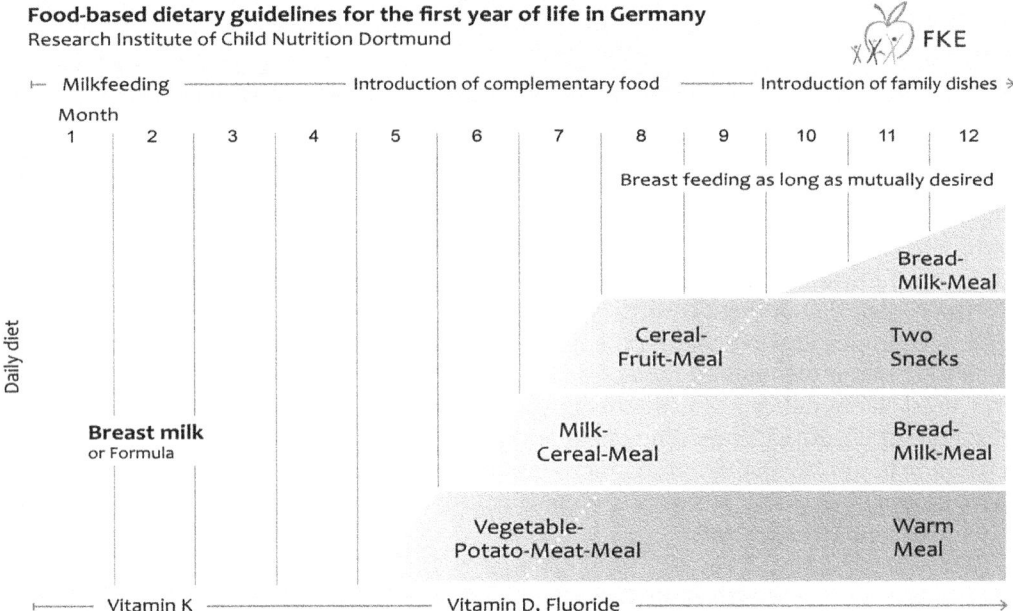

**FIG. 21.2**    Dietary Scheme for the 1st year of life with transition from milk to complementary feeding and the family diet. *Kersting, M., Kalhoff, H., Voss, S., Jansen, K., Lücke, T., 2020. Translating European child nutrition guidelines into practice—the German Dietary Scheme for the first year of life. J. Pediatr. Gastroenterol. Nutr. 71(4), 550–556.*

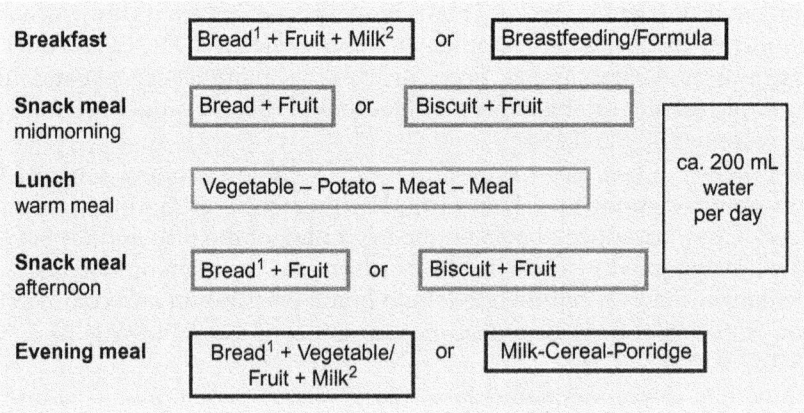

**FIG. 21.3**    Types of meals in the transition period from complementary feeding to the family diet, as recommended in Germany. *1*, about 50% as wholegrain products; *2*, whole cow's milk (cup).

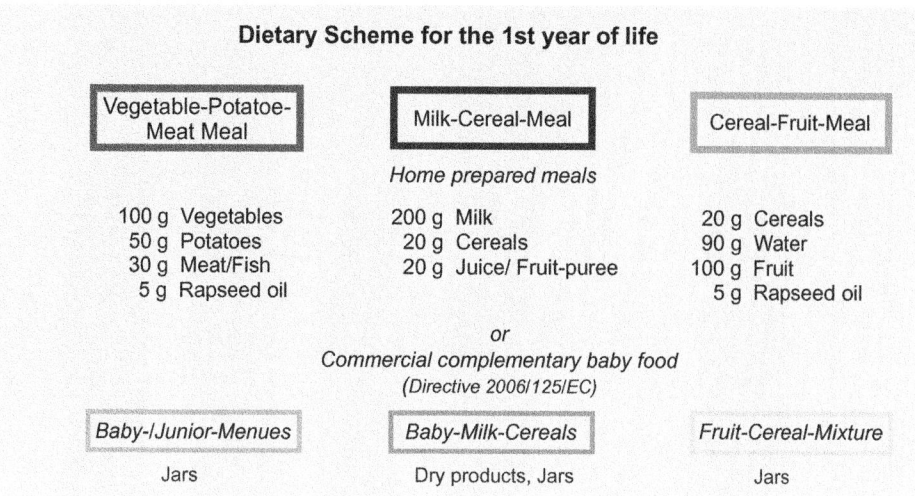

**Dietary Scheme for the 1st year of life**

| Vegetable-Potatoe-Meat Meal | Milk-Cereal-Meal | Cereal-Fruit-Meal |

*Home prepared meals*

| 100 g Vegetables | 200 g Milk | 20 g Cereals |
| 50 g Potatoes | 20 g Cereals | 90 g Water |
| 30 g Meat/Fish | 20 g Juice/ Fruit-puree | 100 g Fruit |
| 5 g Rapseed oil | | 5 g Rapseed oil |

*or*
*Commercial complementary baby food*
*(Directive 2006/125/EC)*

| Baby-/Junior-Menues | Baby-Milk-Cereals | Fruit-Cereal-Mixture |
| Jars | Dry products, Jars | Jars |

**FIG. 21.4**  Recipes for complementary meals as home prepared and alternative commercial complementary baby food, as recommended in Germany.

need to offer liquid (water) in addition to breast milk or formula prior to reaching the three solid food meals per day, except in cases of fever, vomiting, or diarrhea.

The modular system during CF proposes recipes for the three meals to be home prepared and suggests suitable commercial product types (Fig. 21.4).

The following figure shows the distribution of macronutrients (Fig. 21.5) between the meals following the "Dietary Scheme for the 1st Year of Life." Together with the intake of breast milk/formula, the recipes for complementary meals ensure a sufficient intake of energy and nutrients according to guidelines, only with the exception of iron and iodine (see Section 21.4.2.2).

Infants have an innate ability to self-regulate energy intake to a certain extent. However, this self-regulation may be influenced by factors, such as restriction of intake, coercive feeding, or other environmental cues (Fox et al., 2006). Offering finger foods among the first complementary foods was proposed to encourage self-feeding, thus taking advantage of the critical period for oral and motor development and transferring the principle of feeding-on-demand from breastfeeding to CF (Rapley, 2011). Common concerns about self-feeding include the mess created and food waste (e.g., Brown and Lee, 2011). Moreover, up to now a reliable calculation of the nutrient intake is missing, so that intake of important nutrient rich food might be low following this concept, thus endangering sufficient intake of energy and nutrients.

### 21.3.1.3 Homemade or commercial meals

Complementary food can be homemade or bought as ready-to-eat or ready-to-mix commercial products. Parents may choose to prepare complementary food at home for a variety of reasons (e.g., freshness, cost, increased variety and texture, avoidance of preservatives) (Mesch et al., 2014). In contrast to the tight nutrient-related regulation by law of infant and follow-on formula, only a few specifications are set for CF, for example, in the EC Directive (COMMISSION DIRECTIVE 2006/125/EC of December 5, 2006 on processed cereal-based

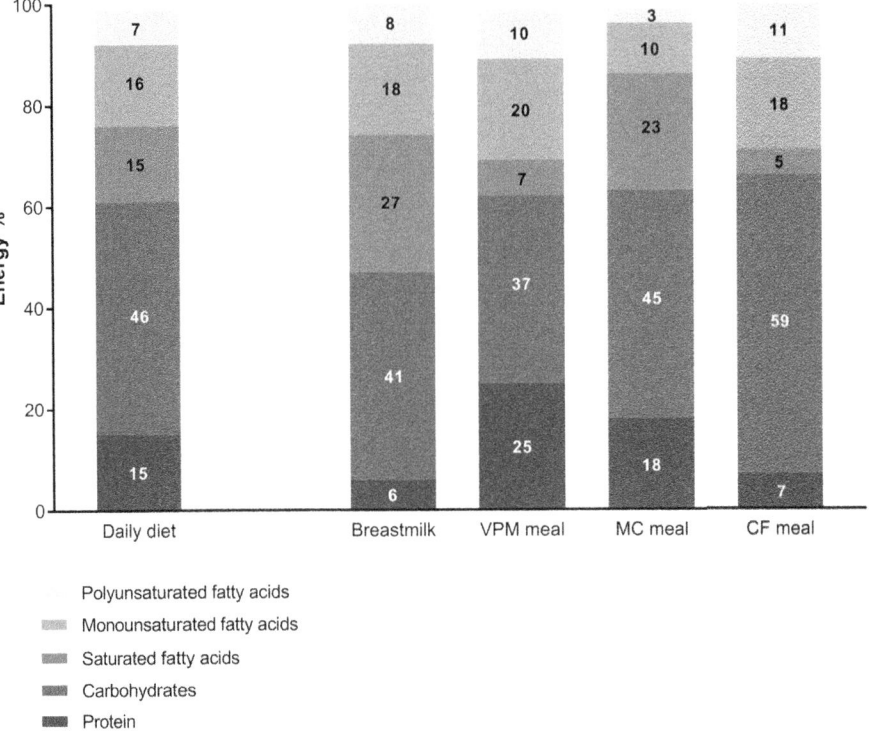

**FIG. 21.5** Distribution of protein, fat, and carbohydrates (as percentage of energy content) in the daily meals and in the total diet of the German Dietary Scheme for the 1st year of life. *Kersting, M., Kalhoff, H., Voss, S., Jansen, K., Lücke, T., 2020. Translating European child nutrition guidelines into practice—the German Dietary Scheme for the first year of life. J. Pediatr. Gastroenterol. Nutr. 71(4), 550–556.*

foods and baby foods for infants and young children). Specification exists, for example, for protein and fat content in meals or sugar content in foods containing fruit. Regarding safety aspects, such as minimizing pesticide residues, the strict EC regulations are almost the same for formula and commercial food. Nevertheless, common food is regarded to be suitable in homemade CF. Overarching international food standards are harmonized by the Codex Alimentarius or "Food Code," established by FAO and the World Health Organization in 1963, thus protecting consumer health and promoting fair practices in food trade worldwide.

The preparation of homemade complementary meals is the responsibility of caregivers in some observational studies home-prepared foods were found low in some nutrients (Melø et al., 2008). A study comparing the composition of commercial and homemade complementary meals as eaten by healthy German infants recently did not find any serious nutrient inadequacies in homemade complementary food (Hilbig et al., 2015).

### 21.3.1.4 Food selection—Vegetarian diets

Vegetarian type diets during the second half of infancy are typically found in poor countries, where meat (and fish) is scare and not (regularly) available for many families. If infants receive a vegetarian diet, it is important that diets include a sufficient amount of milk and dairy products (lacto-vegetarian diet). A variety of nutrient-dense foods should be introduced during CF.

In affluent countries, vegetarian diets are often linked with a life style assumed to decrease risk for common diseases of adulthood, like adiposity, cardiovascular problems, or cancer. Thus, it is difficult to disentangle the potential favorable health effects of the vegetarian diet from other life style influences. Parents on a vegetarian diet often decide to raise their infants on a vegetarian diet as well.

In vegetarian diets for infants, critical nutrients whose adequacy should be monitored include vitamin B12, calcium, vitamin D, iron, iodine, omega-3 fatty acids, and zinc. Combination of iron-rich plant-based food (e.g., cereals) and vitamin C-rich food increases iron bioavailability. Fig. 21.6 shows iron content of foods that might be used in CF. Carefully planned mixed (ovo-)lacto-vegetarian diets (with milk and eggs) are thought to be providing sufficient energy, protein, and most nutrients. However, restrictive or unbalanced vegetarian diets (vegan diets) can result in growth failure and in serious nutrient deficiencies (Van Winckel et al., 2011; Kersting et al., 2017; Kalhoff et al., 2019).

For the first 4–6 months, infants on vegetarian diets should solely receive breast milk or a commercial infant formula (just like all infants) and continued along with adequate complementary food. Iron is the first nutrient to get critical after exclusive breastfeeding or formula feeding in the first 4–6 months. Meat or fortified infant cereal is an appropriate first complementary food. Instead of meat, a complementary meal can be made of wholegrain iron-rich cereals combined with vitamin C-rich vegetables or fruit to improve the low iron bio-availability. An example is the meat exchange by cereals in the German vegetable-potato-meat meal (Fig. 21.7). Additional foods are introduced with timing similar to that for nonvegetarians. Growth should be monitored cautiously (Mangels and Driggers, 2012).

| Food | Iron (mg/100g) |
|---|---|
| Bioavailability high | |
| Pork | 1.0 |
| Poultry | 1.3 |
| Beef | 3.0 |
| Fish | 0.7 |
| Bioavailability low | |
| Cow's milk | <0.1 |
| Egg yolk | 7.2 |
| Rice | 0.8 |
| Wheat, whole grain | 3.2 |
| Oat flakes | 5.8 |
| Carrot, cauliflower | 0.5 |
| Zucchini | 1.0 |
| Apple | 0.3 |

FIG. 21.6  Iron content of potential foods for complementary feeding.

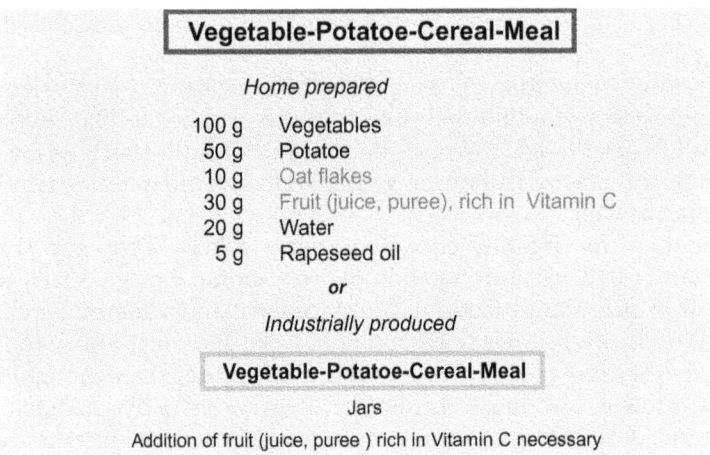

**FIG. 21.7** Recipe for a vegetarian complementary meal and alternative industrially produced products in the German dietary Scheme for the 1st year of life.

Vegan diets without micronutrient supplementation should be discouraged in infancy, especially because of the risk of vitamin B12 deficiency, which can affect neurodevelopment. Fortified soy-based infant formula or follow-on formula can provide substantial parts of nutrient supply. As manifestations of vegetarian diets are often blurred in dietary practice, individual dietary advice after a detailed dietary history and monitoring in pediatric care of vegan infants is advisable.

### 21.3.1.5 Eating habits

Health clinicians and numerous national and international organizations promote healthy infant feeding practices, including breastfeeding and timely introduction of complementary foods. However, mothers decision on feeding their infant is based on a number of factors, including own experiences, family demands, socioeconomic circumstances, and cultural beliefs (Pak-Gorstein et al., 2009). Thus, the types of food presented to infants are influenced by culture, tradition, and individual preference (Agostoni et al., 2008; Menella, 2014). While country-specific cultural barriers to appropriate infant feeding may vary, there are key decision points along the child's growth development and nutrient requirements that can be focused on and effectively addressed (USAID'S infant and young child nutrition project, 2011).

Sensory experiences during infancy may contribute to the development of food preferences in children and thus may have a role in increasing the probability of later development of obesity (Benton, 2004; Hendricks et al., 2006). Some authors suggest that early learning may influence eating behavior and food preferences (e.g., Birch and Doub, 2014), and that feeding practices and preferences established during infancy appear to persist in early childhood (Park et al., 2014; Grimm et al., 2014; Kersting et al., 2015).

The CF period offers the possibility to expose the infant to a variety of flavors. During the second half of infancy, food textures are broadened from fluids to pureed and lumpy food until solid common food of the family table are eaten.

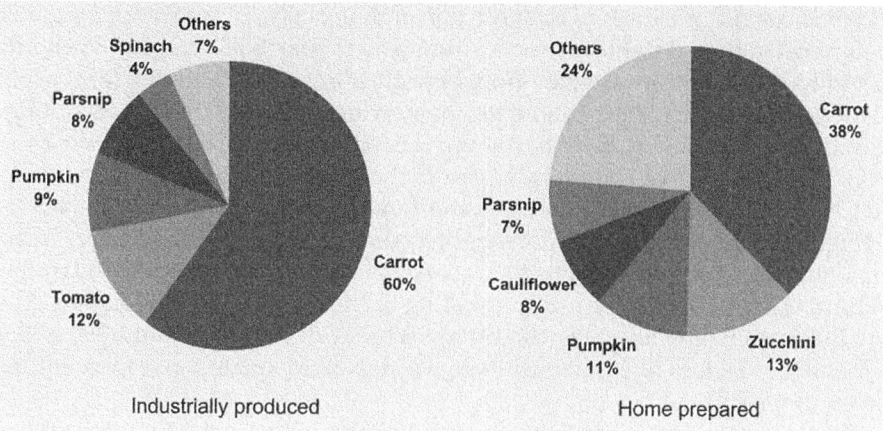

**FIG. 21.8** Proportion of different types of vegetables in complementary vegetable-potato-meat-meals as industrially produced or home prepared in Germany. *Mesch, C.M., Stimming, M., Foterek, K., Hilbig, A., Alexy, U., Kersting, M., Libuda, L., 2014. Food variety in commercial and homemade complementary meals for infants in Germany. Market survey and dietary practice. Appetite 76, 113–119.*

Infants have a particular preference for sweet taste and developing around the introduction of CF also for salty and umami tastes, while rejecting bitter and sour, according to the universal pattern of the human species (Menella, 2014). However, these preferences are hardly compatible with the recommendations for infant nutrition. In the period of the introduction of complementary food, variation in food offered may increase acceptance of new food even several months later (Kalhoff et al., 2021). On the other hand, initial rejection of previously unknown food can be overridden by repeated, unforced presentation (Forestell and Mennella, 2007).

German data from dietary practice shows that it is necessary to promote these advantages of a food variety in early infancy as vegetable choices in both home preparation and industrial production of complementary meals obviously is still dominated by the classical vegetables, while others make up a small proportion only in homemade meals (Mesch et al., 2014) (Fig. 21.8). Nevertheless, up to now, evidence from long-term follow-up studies confirming an imprinting of food preferences by early sensory experiences is still missing (Kersting et al., 2015).

## 21.4 Poor nutrition

### 21.4.1 Energy, macronutrients

#### 21.4.1.1 *Undernutrition*

The second half of infancy is a critical period of growth during which nutrient deficiencies and illnesses particularly contribute to higher rates of undernutrition among children under 5 years of age worldwide (WHO, 2002; Black et al., 2008; Victora et al., 2021). Contaminated water and food are major causes of malnutrition and mortality in the developing world, particularly among children. Infants are most vulnerable to diarrheal illnesses when introduced to fluids and foods as they are weaned from breastfeeding to a mixed diet (Marino, 2007).

Based on anthropometric measurements, malnutrition can be classified as stunting, wasting, and underweight. Height (length) for age is used to assess stunting (Z score $< -2$ based on the WHO child growth charts); it is the result of chronic malnutrition (Black et al., 2013b). Weight for height (length) is used for assessing wasting, which is the result of acute malnutrition. Weight for age measures underweight, indicating the combined effect of acute and chronic malnutrition. Undernutrition, that is, low weight for age, can be caused by low height for age (stunting), low weight for height (wasting or thinness), or a combination.

*Energy:* Primary malnutrition, as commonly seen in developing countries, is due to the combined effect of factors like low birth weight, lack of adequate food, frequent infections, and often enteropathy.

Severe protein-energy malnutrition is associated with either marasmus (characterized by wasting of muscle mass and depletion of body fat stores, but without edema) or kwashiorkor (characterized by marked muscle atrophy with normal or increased body fat and peripheral edema) (Balint, 1998; Jahoor et al., 2008).

*Protein:* Normal growth parameters at birth with subsequent deceleration in weight, followed by deceleration in stature (stunting) and finally deceleration in head circumference is characteristic of inadequate alimentary protein intake. As stunting develops, the weight-for-length may return toward normal (Black et al., 2008; Frank, 2011).

*Fat:* Dietary lipids are important for infants not only to meet their high energy needs, but also to fulfill numerous metabolic and physiological functions critical to their growth, development, and health.

*Water:* In developing countries, the access to safe (clean) water may be limited, resulting in an increased risk for morbidity and mortality from diarrhea associated with water intake. Undernutrition is an underlying cause of much of the diarrhea related mortality in these infants.

### 21.4.1.2 Overnutrition—Overweight/adiposity

Different cut-off points for prediction of risk of overweight and adiposity in adolescents and young adults have been proposed (Kartiosuo et al., 2019). Rapid weight gain during the first 2 years of life may promote the risk of developing overweight and associated metabolic disorders in childhood; and during adolescence and adulthood as well (Monteiro and Victora, 2005; Black et al., 2013b).

However, analyses on participants of the DONALD study showed, that in early life (0–2 years), faster weight gain was associated with an only moderately higher fat mass index and fat free mass index in young adulthood in women. Faster weight gain during other life periods, for example, mid-childhood and puberty may be more relevant for adult fat mass (Cheng et al., 2015).

*Protein:* High protein intake during the transition to the family diet at 12 months of age was shown to be associated with an unfavorable body composition at the age of 7 years (Günther et al., 2007). In total, the role of protein intake as a whole or protein intake from specific foods such as cow's milk in complementary and toddler feeding on obesity development is still unknown (EFSA, 2013a).

*Fat:* An EFSA panel recommended that fat should constitute 40% of energy intake from 6 to 12 months, including 4% of energy from linoleic acid, 0.5% from alpha-linolenic acid, and 100 mg/day from docosahexaenoic acid (DHA) (EFSA, 2013a, 2017; Fewtrell et al., 2017). Reference nutrient intakes suggest a range of 30%–40% of energy from fat in the second half of the first year of life (Tables 21.8–21.10) and a moderate decrease from the high fat breast milk diet to a lower fat intake in complementary and toddler feeding.

In countries with high rates of childhood obesity, it may be advisable to accustom children to low-fat products with an optimized fatty acid composition from an early age. In the Special Turku Coronary Risk Factor Intervention Project (STRIP) study, saturated fat was replaced by unsaturated fat in the child's diet starting in infancy (moreover favoring use of vegetables, fruits, and wholegrain products while reducing intake of salt) and cardiovascular health data was collected until 20 years of age. This intervention, which was embedded in close meshed dietary advice and supervision has led to outcomes like lower LDL cholesterol and blood pressure, improved insulin sensitivity, and diminished clustering of other risk factors for atherosclerosis (e.g., Qi et al., 2015) without showing negative consequences for health and development.

## 21.4.2 Critical micronutrients

### 21.4.2.1 Poor countries

Micronutrient deficiencies are common in infants and children with undernutrition (Ahmed et al., 2012). In addition to insufficient intake from the diet, factors like impaired intestinal uptake or nutrient utilization, and enhanced wastage of nutrients and destruction of vitamins may all confer to micronutrient deficiency states. The resulting (multiple) micronutrient deficiencies account for a substantial number of child deaths, child undernutrition, wasting, and stunting as well as delayed child development (Bhutta et al., 2009). There is evidence, that about 12% of the global deaths of children <5 years of age can be attributed to the deficiencies in five common micronutrients (vitamins A and D, iron, zinc, and iodine) singly or in combination (Bhutta et al., 2008).

In populations with widespread micronutrient deficiencies, food fortification or micronutrient supplementation interventions could be shown to be effective measures (Bhutta et al., 2013). CF interventions are usually targeted at the age range of 6–24 months, which is the time of peak incidence of growth faltering, micronutrient deficiencies, and infectious illnesses in developing countries (Dewey and Adu-Afarwuah, 2008).

*Iron:* IDA is the most prevalent form of nutritional anemia. It accounts for approximately half of the global anemia cases and increases the risk of child mortality (Ahmed et al., 2012). The most familiar feature of ID is a microcytic, hypochromic anemia. However, this is the extreme end of a spectrum of deficiency. Other features include weakness and even lethargy (Lozoff et al., 1998, 2000; Black, 2003; Larson et al., 2017).

In developing countries, heme iron intake is very low and most dietary iron intake is from nonheme food sources with low bioavailability. More than 90% of the iron requirements during the CF period of a breastfed infant have to be provided by complementary foods. These foods, however, often have poor bio-availability of the nonheme iron because of the presence of phytate, which chelates iron and decreases its absorption (Fig. 21.6). Strategies to achieve that intake include complementary food rich in bioavailable iron, such as meat, iron-fortified complementary foods or formula, combination of iron-rich cereals with vitamin C-rich food (Fig. 21.7) or supplements.

In order to promote iron absorption, at least one feeding per day should contain foods rich in vitamin C (Shah et al., 2003). When starting during the second half of infancy, home fortification of foods with multiple micronutrient powders was shown to be an effective intervention to reduce anemia and ID in children (De-Regil et al., 2013). Cow's milk is a poor iron source, not recommended as the main drink during infancy (see Section 21.3.1.4).

*Iodine*: Iodine deficiency still remains a major public health issue in parts of the world where its incorporation into diet has been unsuccessful. Globally, iodine deficiency remains among the most common micronutrient deficiencies (Zimmermann et al., 2008). It is suggested that approximately 1.9 billion individuals suffer from iodine deficiency (Black et al., 2013a,b), which is supposed to impair infant growth and brain development, and increase infant mortality.

In regions where <90% of households use iodized salt and the median urinary iodine concentration in children is <100 μg/L, WHO recommends iodine supplementation in pregnancy and lactation (250 μg daily) (WHO Secretariat et al., 2007).

*Zinc*: Along with iron, iodine, and vitamin A, zinc deficiency is one of the most important micronutrient deficiencies globally, probably with even increased prevalence in infants and small children (Wessels and Brown, 2012). However, zinc nutrition is essential for adequate growth, immunocompetence, and neurobehavioral development. As zinc is a critical nutrient when exclusive breastfeeding is prolonged, lasting longer than 6 months, infants in the second 6 months of life need age appropriate zinc rich food such as meat in addition to breastfeeding to meet the requirements (Krebs et al., 2012). An alternate mode could be adding a micronutrient powder to local complementary foods, starting in infants with 6 months of age (Ariff et al., 2014).

Preventive zinc supplementation was shown to be associated with a reduction in morbidity from childhood diarrhea and decreased the severity of lower respiratory infections; it may also contribute to improved growth in populations where diarrhea is high (Brown et al., 2009). Recently, a Cochrane review concluded, that in children starting at the age of 6 months, the benefits of preventive zinc supplementation outweigh possible risks in areas with high risk of zinc deficiency (Mayo-Wilsin et al., 2014).

*Vitamin D*: Vitamin D is important for regulating calcium and phosphorus metabolism; in infancy vitamin D deficiency leads to rickets. Vitamin D (cholecalciferol) is synthetized in skin cells upon exposure to sunlight. It can also be obtained through the diet from natural sources, such as fish, egg yolk, or milk, which are, however, mostly not sufficient. In some countries, fortified foods are available. Supplementation during infancy is recommended, either by fortification or by supplements both in poor and rich countries.

### 21.4.2.2 Developed countries

Recently, the European Food Safety Authority concluded that dietary intakes of some unsaturated fatty acids, iron, vitamin D, and iodine (in some European countries) are low in infants and young children living in Europe, when compared to reference intake data (EFSA, 2013a,b). Nutrient intake of infants fed according to the German pediatric Food-Based Dietary Guidelines (Dietary Scheme for the 1st Year of Life) (Fig. 21.4) was evaluated by the Research Department of Child Nutrition. Together with the remaining intake of breast milk/formula, the recipes for complementary meals ensure a sufficient intake of energy and nutrients, only with the exception of iron and iodine (Fig. 21.9).

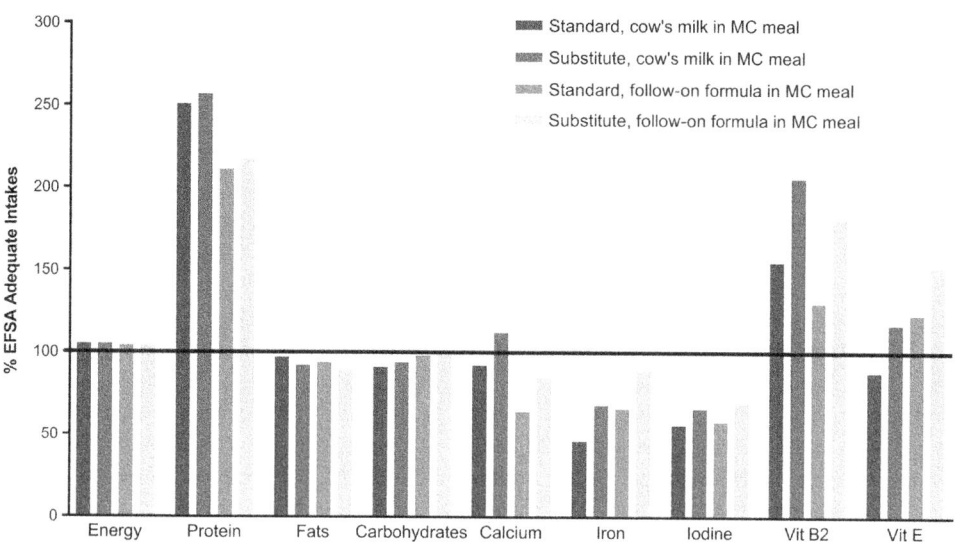

**FIG. 21.9** Daily intake of selected nutrients in different assumptions of the milk part in the dietary scheme as percentage of actual EFSA reference values. MC = milk cereal meal (Kersting et al., 2020).

Vitamin D supplementation is well-established in Germany throughout the first year of life and in the winter months after the first birthday. This leads to a sufficient Vitamin D status [serum 25-Hydroxy-Vitamin-D (25-OHD)] in infants, and decreasing values and insufficiency in large proportions of toddlers and older children (Thierfelder et al., 2007).

*Iron:* The prevalence of ID reported in European studies was described to be 1.4%–20% in infancy, the prevalence of IDA to be <2% during the first half of infancy, 2%–3% between 6 and 9 months, and 3%–9% between 1 and 3 years of age (EFSA, 2013a,b; Domellöf et al., 2014). Similarly, rates of low iron intake and of ID were reported to vary between 2% and 25% in infants of 6–12 months of age in Europe (Eussen et al., 2015). However, different definitions of ID according to the relevant blood parameters as well as their cut-off values make a comparison of study results difficult (EFSA, 2013a).

Several other studies suggest that the time of introduction of complementary foods influences the rate of IDA in breastfed infants (Chantry et al., 2007; Jonsdottir et al., 2012). Recently, rice-based complementary food products were shown to be effective to improve iron status during the second half of infancy (Skau et al., 2015).

Results of the Dortmund Intervention Trial for Optimization of Infant Nutrition (DINO) suggested that the risk of ID and IDA in the second half of infancy while fed in accordance with German pediatric Food-Based Dietary Guidelines (and low iron intake) might be higher in infants fully breastfed for 4–6 months compared to formula fed infants (Dube et al., 2010a,b). A second analysis of dietary intake and markers of iron status in the dietary intervention study, PINGU 5 years later than DINO confirmed that iron intake was considerably below German (8 mg/day) and even more below the latest EFSA iron intake reference value as well as the IOM value (11 mg/day). Up to 30% of infants presented with ID at the age of 10 months. No general effects of the mode of milk feeding in the first 4 months (breast milk, formula) or the time of CF introduction (within the age window 4–6 months) on most markers of iron status could be discerned. However, in infants with mainly breastfeeding, new functional markers (Schoorl et al., 2015) like the range of variation of erythrocyte volume (RDW-CV) possibly indicated incipient iron depletion (Kalhoff and Kersting, 2017). Recently, EFSA confirmed the recommendation of timely introduction of iron-rich complementary foods for the healthy development of children (EFSA et al., 2019).

Several strategies, for example, optimized dietary choices, fortification of milk or complementary foods, or supplements could be discussed as options to enhance iron intake during infancy.

*Iodine:* To assure a sufficient intake of iodine, fortification of complementary food is recommended and practiced in Germany and other European countries. Among scenarios of iodine intake of an infant in the second half of the first year of life, receiving breast milk or formula and three complementary meals per day according to the German "Dietary Scheme for the 1st year of life," it turned out that a partially breast-fed infant getting homemade complementary meals reached less than 50% of the recommended iodine intake (Fig. 21.10). As infants should not yet receive salt (see Section 21.3) population based strategies of iodized salt to overcome iodine deficiency do not cover the infant diet yet. As sufficient iodine intake is essential for optimal brain development, iodine fortification of complementary food

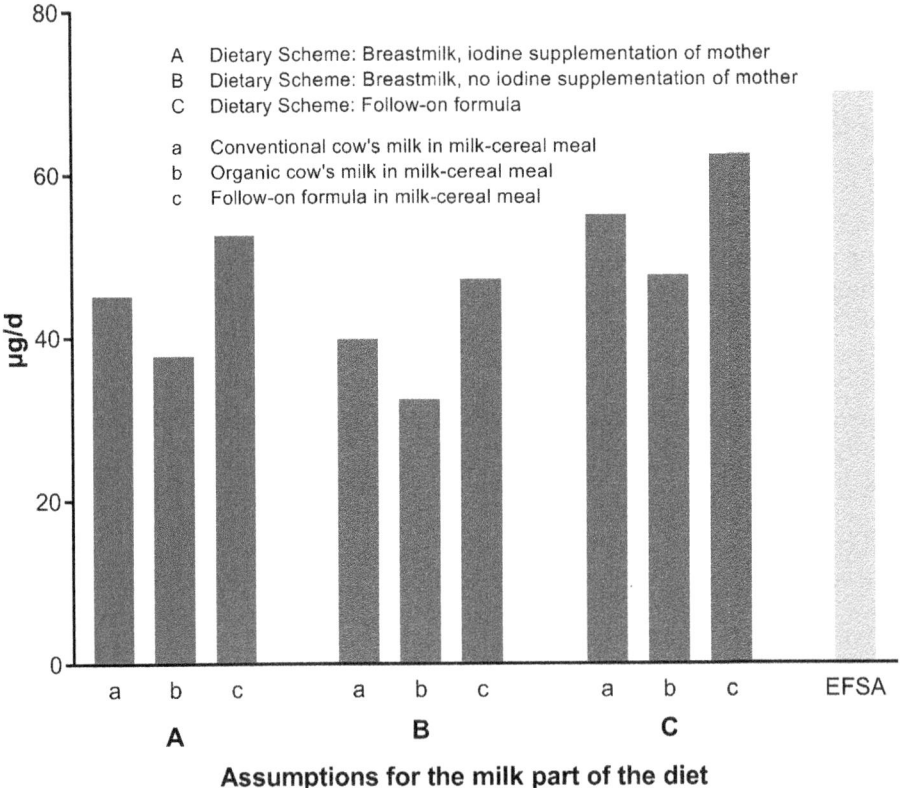

**FIG. 21.10** Potential daily iodine intakes with different assumptions for the milk part in the Dietary Scheme for the 1st year of life in Germany. *Kersting, M., Kalhoff, H., Voss, S., Jansen, K., Lücke, T. 2020. Translating European child nutrition guidelines into practice—the German Dietary Scheme for the first year of life. J. Pediatr. Gastroenterol. Nutr. 71(4), 550–556.*

(e.g., one iodine-fortified cereal-milk complementary meal), the use of iodine fortified formula, or iodine supplements seem to be practicable options to achieve an adequate iodine supply in the second 6 months of life (Remer and Johner, 2014).

## 21.5 Selected food-related health outcomes

Early-life development factors play a central role in determining an individual's later susceptibility to noncommunicable diseases, such as type 2 diabetes and cardiovascular disease. This new understanding of health-programming during early child development may offer the hope of developing novel intervention strategies to reduce the risk for later morbidity (e.g., Hanson et al., 2011).

Generally, evidence for effects of nutrition in early life on later health outcomes seems to be best when considering the prenatal and early postnatal period (Koletzko et al., 2016). Moreover, studies testing the effect of interventions during the CF period are rare. In conclusion, the possible health effects of nutrition during the second half of infancy may often only be derived from analyses of observational cohort studies.

### 21.5.1 Overweight—Adiposity

Early childhood feeding seems to be a major contributor to childhood obesity. The rate of weight gain during infancy may be linked to weight status in later childhood and to cardiovascular risk factors as well (Stettler et al., 2002).

During infancy, dietary intake may have a greater impact on nutrient balance and hormone responses than energy expenditure. In a large prospective cohort study, dietary energy intake during infancy determined infant weight gain and seemed to influence obesity risk during childhood. This could be shown at least among formula- and mixed-fed infants (Ong et al., 2006; Ong and Loos, 2006). Recently, weight-gain from birth to the age of 1 year among children was observed to be associated with greater adiposity in early adulthood, pointing to modifiable determinants of later weight gain during infancy (Salgin et al., 2015). Overall, high consumption of complementary foods with high energy density may promote high weight gain in infancy, with the long-term implications for future obesity risk still under discussion (Monteiro and Victora, 2005; Ong and Loos, 2006; EFSA et al., 2019; Usheva et al., 2021).

Delayed introduction of solid food was discussed to reduce the odds of overweight in children (Yew et al., 2009); however, a literature review could not find this association (Karaolis-Danckert et al., 2007). When considering these issues in 2009, the EFSA Panel stated, that the age of introduction of CF did not seem to have a strong impact on growth and other health outcomes. Thus, the available evidence so far has not answered this issue sufficiently (Barrera et al., 2016; EFSA et al., 2019).

There is some evidence suggesting, that high protein intake during the first years of life, starting just postnatally, is associated with an increased risk of developing overweight and adiposity later in life (Michaelsen and Greer, 2014; Koletzko et al., 2016; see Section 21.4.1.2). A lower prevalence of obesity at 6 years of age was reported in a cohort that had received formula with lower protein content than in a cohort fed formula with higher protein content (Thorisdottir et al., 2013).

## 21.5.2 Neurodevelopment—Cognition

Worldwide, severe malnutrition is a leading cause of death among children younger than 5 years of age. Among those who survive, impaired intellectual or cognitive and motor development is common. There is evidence that impaired growth during infancy is associated with impaired mental development and that insufficient intake of specific nutrients during the vulnerable periods of most rapid development may have a persistent effect on the nervous system (Perrin et al., 2003; Corbett and Drewett, 2004; Bergen, 2008). A higher score of length for age at 2 years is associated with better cognitive scores in later childhood (Fisher Walker et al., 2012), and early head-growth is associated with later intelligence as well (Gale et al., 2006).

*LC-PUFA*: The supply with LC-PUFA during infancy is considered to play an important role in visual and cognitive development in infancy (Agostoni et al., 2008). However, meta-analyses on studies testing effects of postnatal LC-PUFA supply on infant's visual and cognitive development are still inconsistent (Simmer et al., 2011; Qawasmi et al., 2012). Studies on LC-PUFA and cognition in the CF period are rare. In the recent randomized controlled intervention trial PINGU, examining the effects of adding n-3 ALA-rich rapeseed oil or DHA-rich salmon to commercial complementary food on endogenous fatty acid status and developmental status (Libuda et al., 2016; Kalhoff et al., 2020), we could not observe discernible effects in cognitive or visual development, when tested in infants at 10 months age.

*Iron*: IDA is the most prevalent form of nutritional anemia (see Section 21.2.1). In the second year of life, IDA can produce development delays until at least 10 years of age (Lozoff et al., 2000; Larson et al., 2017). The cognition of children aged >5 years with IDA benefited from iron supplementation, but studies of children <3 years were not that convincing (Black et al., 2013a,b; Bhutta et al., 2013).

*Zinc* is another critical micronutrient considering neurodevelopment; zinc deficiency is associated with delayed motor- and cognitive development during childhood (Black, 1998).

## 21.5.3 Sensitization—Allergy—Celiac disease

Timing of exposure to potential allergens seems to modulate the induction of tolerance and the risk for sensitization. For decades, allergy prevention guidelines emphasized late exposure to food to prevent allergy. However, an increasing body of evidence now seems to suggest that oral tolerance is probably best achieved by introducing several possible antigens early in life. Thus, highly allergenic complementary foods may be introduced between 4 and 6 months of age, once a few typical complementary foods have been fed and tolerated (Fleischer et al., 2013).

Delaying the introduction of solid foods beyond the 6th month of life or even beyond the age of 4 months does not seem to have a protective effect. It may even increase the risk of subsequent allergic diseases (Zutavern et al., 2008; Heine, 2014; Nwaru et al., 2013; EFSA et al., 2019).

In contrast to data from earlier observational studies, the findings from several recent randomized trials have shown that the age at introduction of gluten does not seem to influence the risk of developing celiac disease (Vriezinga et al., 2014; Lionetti et al., 2014; Aronsson et al., 2016). Just recently, the ESPGHAN provided an updated recommendation stating that gluten may be introduced into the infant's diet anytime between 4 and 12 completed months of age and proposed that consumption of large quantities of gluten should be avoided during the first weeks after gluten introduction (Szajewska et al., 2016).

## 21.5.4 Cardiovascular health—Metabolic syndrome

Infant feeding practices are suggested to influence later cholesterol levels (Owen et al., 2002). Some studies favor a protective effect of early dietetic intervention in infants on markers of cardiovascular health in later life (Guardamagna et al., 2012; Kaikkonen et al., 2014). As an example, counseling parents on saturated versus unsaturated fat in diet during infancy in the STRIP project, proved to result in lower rate of markers for metabolic syndrome in adolescence (Nupponen et al., 2015).

## 21.5.5 Immune function

In marasmus, a variety of immune functions are diminished (Sauerwein et al., 1997). Thus, the severely malnourished child is at high risk for infection because of diminished immune defenses, and is typically exposed to infection because of inadequate sanitation and impaired access to clean water and safe food.

In children with severe malnutrition, diarrhea is common and often is a serious, sometimes fatal event. Management of these children must also focus on their malnutrition and treatment of other infections (WHO, 2013) (Tables 21.11–21.13).

TABLE 21.11 Iron, iodine, zinc, vitamin D—European Union: reference intakes of iron, iodine, zinc, vitamin D for infants from 7 to 12 months of age (EFSA, 2017).

| Age (months) | Iron (mg/day) | Iodine (µg/day) | Zinc (mg/day) | Vitamin D (µg/day) |
| --- | --- | --- | --- | --- |
| 7 to 11 | 11 | 70 | 2.9 | 10 |

TABLE 21.12 Iron, iodine, zinc, vitamin D—German, Austrian, and Swiss reference values (DACH, 2018) (Iodine: Germany, Austria).

| Age (months) | Iron (mg/day) | Iodine (µg/day) | Zinc (mg/day) | Vitamin D (µg/day) |
| --- | --- | --- | --- | --- |
| 6 to <12 | 8 | 80 | 2.5 | 10 |

TABLE 21.13 Iron, iodine, zinc, vitamin D—United States and Canada dietary reference intakes (IOM, 2005a,b).

| Age (months) | Iron (mg/day) | Iodine (µg/day) | Zinc (mg/day) | Vitamin D (µg/day) |
| --- | --- | --- | --- | --- |
| 6 to <12 | 11 | 130 | 3 | 10 |

## 21.6 Future trends and research

The etiology of many diseases is multifactorial and is influenced by both environmental and genetic factors. One of the most important environmental factors is the food our infants consume. Evidence is accumulating that proper infant nutrition is not only a prerequisite for adequate growth, but is a significant part of environmental factors affecting the incidence of various diseases (Elenberg and Shoul, 2014).

Important goals in infant nutrition in underdeveloped countries are to eradicate hunger and insufficient nutrient intake and to ensure access to safe water. In affluent countries, perspectives on CF may imply not only sufficient intake of (some still critical) micronutrients, but the compositional quality of macronutrients like carbohydrates (e.g., Augustin et al., 2015), lipids (Delplanque et al., 2015), and proteins (Lönnerdal, 2014) as well. As early diet and lifestyle are increasingly recognized to modulate the composition and the metabolic activity of the human gut microbiota, the impact of diet during the second half of infancy on microbial gut profiles could be a further promising research trend (Conlon and Bird, 2015). Moreover, the risks and benefits of prebiotics and probiotics in infant nutrition will probably be deeper addressed in future research (Stiemsma and Michels, 2018; Ryan et al., 2019).

Development of modern technologies for metabolic assessment may help better to characterize the individual's nutritional and health status (Dessi et al., 2014) and may thus address the composition of new (functional) food for infants. However, as the industry for infant food is increasingly globalized, there is growing need not only for cooperation and guidance, but for monitoring and regulation as well (Kent, 2015).

An important new aspect is the sustainability of nutritional habits for the protection of our environment, especially in the light of the climate crisis and the protection of the next generation. Global warming, which is now recognized as a crisis, places particularly high demands on fluid balance and thus on the special challenges of nutrition in early childhood (Smith, 2019; Helldén et al., 2021).

Finally, it is a special task for nutritionists and pediatricians as well to deliver important new findings and recommendations for healthy infant feeding to the families. Only with repeated information and supported by an increased use of several information technologies, parents will get enough support to choose a healthy diet for their infants. In this context, digital media applications are increasingly being used worldwide and show promise in combination with traditional guidance and counseling options.

## 21.7 Summary and conclusions

Since the CF period is characterized by rapid growth and infants are susceptible to nutrient deficiencies and excesses, it is plausible that timing, content or method of CF might improve later health and development. However, there are complexities associated with study design, nutritional variants, feeding, behavioral, social, and psychological factors associated with CF. In conclusion, available evidence relating timing and content of CF to later health and development is limited.

Experts agree in recommending easy to adopt dietary strategies to help families feeding their infants according to nutrient based guidelines. The Research department for child nutrition developed a food-guided modular system translating scientific recommendations into an dietary scheme for the first year of life (Kersting et al., 2020), followed by food-based dietary guidelines, named Optimized Mixed Diet, for children and adolescents, applicable also for the transition period from infancy to family diet (Kersting et al., 2017). As these two concepts fully and comprehensively meet the requirements for sustainable nutrition, they are also guiding principles for the promotion of future healthy and environmentally friendly child nutrition.

## Sources of additional information

**(1)** European Commission—foods for infants and young children. http://ec.europa.eu/ food/safety/labelling_nutrition/special_groups_food/children/index_en.htm.
**(2)** European Food Safety Authority. http://www.efsa.europa.eu/.
**(3)** European Journal of Nutrition. http://www.springer.com/food+science/journal/394.
**(4)** European Society for Paediatric Gastroenterology, Hepatology and Nutrition. http:// www.espghan.org/.
**(5)** Research Department of Child Nutrition, Ruhr-University Bochum, Germany. www. fke-bo.de.
**(6)** Healthy start-young family network. Infant nutrition and nutrition for breastfeeding mothers. https://www.gesund-ins-leben.de/fileadmin/SITE_MASTER/content/ Dokumente/Downloads/Medien/3291_2013_he_saeug-linge_englisch.pdf.

# References

Agostoni, C., Decsi, T., Fewtrell, M., et al., 2008. Complementary feeding: a commentary by the ESPGHAN Committee on Nutrition. J. Pediatr. Gastroenterol. Nutr. 46, 99.

Agostoni, C., Lacuini, E., 2014. Early exposure to allergens: a new window of opportunity for non-communicable disease prevention in complementary feeding. Int. J. Food Sci. Nutr. 61 (1), 1–2.

Ahmed, T., Hossain, M., Sanin, K.I., 2012. Global burden of maternal and child undernutrition and micronutrient deficiencies. Ann. Nutr. Metab. 61 (Suppl. 1), 8–17.

American Academy of Pediatrics, 2014. Arsenic in Food Products. Available from: http://www.aap.org/en-us/ about-the-aap/aap-press-room/Pages/Arsenic-in-Food-Products.aspx.

American Academy of Pediatrics, 2019b. Feeding the infant. In: Kleinman, R.E., Greer, F.R. (Eds.), Pediatric Nutrition, eighth ed. American Academy of Pediatrics, Itasca, IL, p. 189.

American Academy of Pediatrics, Committee on Nutrition, 2019a. Appendix E1. Dietary reference intakes. In: Kleinman, R.E., Greer, F.R. (Eds.), Pediatric Nutrition, eighth ed. American Academy of Pediatrics, Itasca, IL, p. 1531.

Ariff, S., Krebs, N.F., Soofi, S., Westcott, J., Bhatti, Z., Tabassum, F., Bhutta, Z.A., 2014. Absorbed zinc and exchangeable zinc pool size are greater in Pakistani infants receiving traditional complementary food with zinc-fortified micronutrient powder. J. Nutr. 144 (1), 20–26.

Aronsson, C.A., Lee, H.S., Koletzko, S., Uusitalo, U., Yang, J., Virtanen, S.M., Liu, E., Lernmark, Å., Norris, J.M., Agardh, D., TEDDY Study Group, 2016. Effects of gluten intake on risk of celiac disease: a case-control study on a Swedish Birth Cohort. Clin. Gastroenterol. Hepatol. 14, 403–409.

Augustin, L.S.A., Kendall, C.W.C., Jenkinds, D.J.A., et al., 2015. Glycemic index, glycemic load and glycemic response: an international scientific consensus summit from the international carbohydrate quality consortium (ICQC). Nutr. Metab. Cardiovasc. Dis. 25 (9), 795–815.

Balint, J.P., 1998. Physical findings in nutritional deficiencies. Pediatr. Clin. North Am. 45, 245.

Barrera, C.M., Perrine, C.G., Li, R., Scanlon, K.S., 2016. Age at introduction to solid foods and child obesity at 6 years. Child. Obes. 12 (3), 188–192. https://doi.org/10.1089/chi.2016.0021.

Beauchamp, G.K., Mennella, J.A., 2009. Early flavor learning and its impact on later feeding behaviour. J. Pediatr. Gastroenterol. Nutr. 48, S25–S30.

Beauchamp, G.K., Cowart, B.J., Moran, M., 1986. Developmental changes in slat acceptability in human infants. Dev. Psychobiol. 19, 17–25.

Benton, D., 2004. Role of parents in the determination of the food preferences of children and the development of obesity. Int. J. Obes. Relat. Metab. Disord. 28, 858.

Bergen, D.C., 2008. Effects of poverty on cognitive function: a hidden neurologic epidemic. Neurology 71, 447.

Bhutta, Z., Ahmed, T., Black, R.E., et al., 2008. What works? Interventions for maternal and child undernutrition and survival. Lancet 371, 417–440.

Bhutta, Z.A., Rizvi, A., Razza, F., et al., 2009. A comparative evaluation of multiple micronutrient and deficiencies and iron-folic acid supplementation during pregnancy in Pakistan: impact on pregnancy outcomes. Food Nutr. Bull. 30 (suppl. 4), S496–S505.

Bhutta, Z.A., Das, J.K., Rizvi, A., et al., 2013. Evidence-based interventions for improvement of maternal and child nutrition: what can be done and at what cost? Lancet 382, 452–477.

Birch, L.L., Doub, A.E., 2014. Learning to eat: birth to age 2y. Am. J. Clin. Nutr. 99 (3), 723S–728S.

Black, M.M., 1998. Zinc deficiency and child development. Am. J. Clin. Nutr. 68 (2 Suppl), 464S–469S.

Black, M., 2003. Micronutrient deficiencies and cognitive functioning. J. Nutr. 133 (11 Suppl. 2), 3927S–3931S.

Black, R.E., Allen, L.H., Bhutta, Z.A., Caulfield, L.E., de Onis, M., Ezzati, M., Mathers, C., Rivera, J., Maternal and Child Undernutrition Study Group, 2008. Maternal and child undernutrition: global and regional exposures and health consequences. Lancet 371, 243–260.

Black, R.E., Aldeman, H., Bhutta, Z.A., Maternal and Child Nutrition Study Group, et al., 2013a. Maternal and child nutrition: building momentum for impact. Lancet 382, 372–375.

Black, R.E., Victora, C.G., Walker, S.P., et al., 2013b. Maternal and child undernutrition and overweight in low income and middle-income countries. Lancet 382, 427–451.

Briefel, R., Ziegler, P., Novak, T., Ponza, M., 2006. Feeding infants and toddlers study: characteristics and usual nutrient intake of Hispanic and non-Hispanic infants and toddlers. J. Am. Diet. Assoc. 106, S84.

Brown, A., Lee, M., 2011. A descriptive study investigating the use and nature of baby led weaning in a UK sample of mothers. Matern. Child Nutr. 7 (1), 34–47.

Brown, M.J., Margolis, S., 2012. Lead in drinking water and human blood lead levels in the United States. MMWR Suppl. 61, 1–9.

Brown, K.H., Peerson, J.M., Baker, S.K., et al., 2009. Preventive zinc supplementation among infants, preschoolers, and older children. Food Nutr. Bull. 30 (1 Suppl), S12–S40.

Chantry, C.J., Howard, C.R., Auinger, P., 2007. Full breastfeeding duration and risk for iron deficiency in U.S. infants. Breastfeed. Med. 2 (2), 63–73.

Cheng, G., Bolzenius, K., Joslowski, G., Güntzzher, A.L., Kroke, A., Heinrich, J., Buyken, A.E., 2015. Velocities of weight, height and fat mass gain during potentially critical periods of growth are decisive for adult body composition. Eur. J. Clin. Nutr. 69 (2), 262–268.

Conlon, M.A., Bird, R.B., 2015. The impact of diet and lifestyle on gut microbiota and human health. Nutrition 7, 17–44.

Corbett, S.S., Drewett, R.F., 2004. To what extent is failure to thrive in infancy associated with poorer cognitive development? A review and meta-analysis. J. Child Psychol. Psychiatry 45, 641.

DACH. Deutsche Gesellschaft für Ernährung. Österreichische Gesellschaft für Ernährung. Schweizerische Gesellschaft für Ernährung, 2018. D-A-CH Referenzwerte für die Nährstoffzufuhr. Umschau/Braus Verlag Franfurt a.M. (2. Auflage 2015) 4. aktualisierte Auflage.

Delplanque, B., Gibson, R., Koletzko, B., et al., 2015. Lipid quality in infant nutrition: current knowledge and future opportunities. J. Pediatr. Gastroenterol. Nutr. 61 (1), 8–17.

De-Regil, L.M., Suchdev, P.S., Vist, G.E., Walleser, S., Pena-Rosas, J.P., 2013. Home fortification of foods with multiple micronutrient powders for health and nutrition in children under two years of age (review). Evid. Based Child Health 8 (1), 112–201.

Dessi, A., Marincola, F.C., Masili, A., et al., 2014. Clinical metabolomics and nutrition: the new frontier in neonatology and pediatrics. Biomed. Res. Int. https://doi.org/10.1155/2014/981219.

Deutsche Gesellschaft für Ernährung, 2015. Ausgewählte Fragen und Antworten zur Energiezufuhr.

Dewey, K.G., Adu-Afarwuah, S., 2008. Systematic review of the efficacy and effectiveness of complementary feeding interventions in developing countries. Matern. Child Nutr. 4, 24–85.

Domellöf, M., Braegger, C., Campoy, C., et al., 2014. (ESPGHAN Committee on Nutrition). Iron requirements of infants and toddlers. J. Pediatr. Gastroenterol. Nutr. 58 (1), 119–129.

Domeloff, M., 2007. Iron requirements, absorption and metabolism in infancy and childhood. Curr. Opin. Clin. Nutr. Metab. Care 10, 329–335.

Dube, K., Schwartz, J., Mueller, M.J., Kalhoff, H., Kersting, M., 2010a. Iron intake and iron status status in breast-fed infants during the first year of life. Clin. Nutr. 29 (6), 773–776.

Dube, K., Schwartz, J., Mueller, M.J., Kalhoff, H., Kersting, M., 2010b. Complementary food with low (8%) or high (12%) meat content as source of dietary iron: a double-blinded randomized controlled trial. Eur. J. Nutr. 49, 11–18.

EFSA (European Food Safety Authority), 2017. Dietary Reference Values for nutrients. Summary Report. EFSA Supporting Publication, p. e15121. 98 pp.

EFSA NDA Panel (EFSA Panel on Dietetic Products, Nutrition and Allergies), 2013a. Scientific opinion on nutrient requirements and dietary intakes of infants and young children in the European Union. EFSA J. 11 (10), 3408. 103.

EFSA NDA Panel (EFSA Panel on Dietetic Products, Nutrition and Allergies), 2013b. Scientific opinion on dietary reference values for energy. EFSA J. 11 (1), 3005. 81.

EFSA NDA Panel (EFSA Panel on Dietetic Products, Nutrition and Allergies), 2014. Scientific opinion on the essential composition of infant and follow-on formulae. EFSA J. 12 (7), 3760. 106.

EFSA NDA Panel (EFSA Panel on Dietetic Products, Nutrition and Allergies), 2015. Scientific opinion on dietary reference values for iron. EFSA J. 13 (10), 4254. 115.

EFSA Panel on Dietetic Products, Nutrition, and Allergies (NDA), 2010. Scientific opinion on principles for deriving and applying dietary reference values. EFSA J. 8 (3), 1458.

EFSA Panel on Nutrition, Novel Foods and Food Allergens (NDA), Castenmiller, J., de Henauw, S., Hirsch-Ernst, K.I., et al., 2019. Appropriate age range for introduction of complementary feeding into an infant's diet. EFSA J. 17 (9), e05780.

Elenberg, Y., Shoul, R., 2014. The role of infant nutrition in the prevention of future disease. Front. Pediatr. 21 (2), 7.

Engelmann, M.D., Davidsson, L., Sandström, B., et al., 1998. The influence of meat on nonheme iron absorption in infants. Pediatr. Res. 43, 768.

Ernährungskommission der Deutschen Gesellschaft für Kinder- und Jugendmedizin (DGKJ), Bührer, C., Genzel-Boroviczeny, O., Jochum, F., Kauth, T., Kersting, M., Koletzko, B., Mihatsch, W., Przyrembel, H., Reinehr, T., Zimmer, P., 2014. Nutrition of healthy infants. Recommendations of the nutrition committee oft the German Pediatric Society. Monatsschr. Kinderheilkd., 527–538.

EU (European Union), 2016. Commission Delegated Regulation 2016/127 of 25 September 2015 supplementing Regulation (EU) No 609/2013 of the European Parliament and of the Council as Regards the Specific Compositional and Information Requirements for Infant Formula and Follow-on Formula and as Regards Requirements on Information Relating to Infant and Young Child Feeding. Available at: https://eur-lex.europa.eu/legal-content/EN/TXT/?uri=uriserv%3AOJ.L_.2016.025.01.0001.01.ENG.

EU (European Union), 2020. Directive 2020/2184 of the European Parliament and of the Council of 16 December 2020 on the Quality of Water Intended for Human Consumption. https://eur-lex.europa.eu/eli/dir/2020/2184/oj.

Eussen, S., Alles, M., Uijterschout, L., Brus, F., van der Horst-Graat, J., 2015. Iron intake and status of children aged 6-36 months in Europe: a systematic review. Ann. Nutr. Metab. 66, 80–92.

Fewtrell, M., Bronsky, J., Campoy, C., et al., 2017. Complementary feeding: a position paper by the ESPGHAN Committee on Nutrition. J. Pediatr. Gastroenterol. Nutr. 64 (1), 119–132.

Fisher Walker, C.L., Lamberti, L., Adair, L., et al., 2012. Does childhood diarrhea influence cognition beyond the diarrhoea-stunting pathway? PLoS One 7, e47908.

Fleischer, D.M., Spergel, J.M., Assa'ad, A.H., Pongracic, J.A., 2013. Primary prevention of allergic disease through nutritional interventions: guidelines for healthcare professionals. J. Allergy Clin. Immunol. Pract. 1, 29–36.

Forestell, C.A., Mennella, J.A., 2007. Early determinants of fruit and vegetable acceptance. Pediatrics 120, 1247.

Fox, M.K., Devaney, B., Reidy, K., et al., 2006. Relationship between portion size and energy intake among infants and toddlers: evidence of self-regulation. J. Am. Diet. Assoc. 106, S77.

Frank, D., 2011. Failure to thrive. In: Augustyn, M., Zuckerman, B., Caronna, E.B. (Eds.), The Zuckerman Parker Handbook of Developmental, Behavioral Pediatrics for Primary Care, third ed. Lippincott Williams & Wilkins, Philadelphia, p. 204.

Gale, C.R., O'Callaghan, F.J., Bredow, M., Martyn, C.N., 2006. The influence of head growth in fetal life, infancy and childhood on intelligence at the ages of 4 and 8 years. Pediatrics 118, 1486–1492.

Grammatikaki, E., Wollgast, J., Caldeira, S., 2019. Feeding infants and young children. In: A Compilation of National Food-Based Dietary Guidelines and Specific Products Available in the EU Market; PUBSY No. 115583.

Grimm, K.A., Kim, S.A., Yaroch, A.L., Scanlon, K.S., 2014. Fruit and vegetable intake during infancy and early childhood. Pediatrics 134 (Suppl. 1), S63.

Guardamagna, O., Abello, F., Cagliero, P., et al., 2012. Impact of nutrition since early life on cardiovascular prevention. Ital. J. Pediatr. 38, 73.

Günther, A.L., Remer, T., Kroke, A., Buyken, A.E., 2007. Early protein intake and later obesity risk: which protein sources at which time points throughout infancy and childhood are important for body mass index and body fat percentage at 7 y of age? Am. J. Clin. Nutr. 86 (6), 1765–1772.

Hanson, M.A., Low, F.M., Gluckman, P.D., 2011. Epigenetic epidemiology: the rebirth of soft inheritance. Ann. Nutr. Metab. 58 (suppl. 2), 8–15.

Heine, R.G., 2014. Preventing atopy and allergic disease. Nestle Nutr. Inst. Workshop Ser. 78, 141–153.

Helldén, D., Andersson, C., Nilsson, M., Ebi, K.L., Friberg, P., Alfvén, T., 2021. Climate change and child health: a scoping review and an expanded conceptual framework. Lancet Planet. Health, e164–e175.

Hendricks, K., Briefel, R., Novak, T., Ziegler, P., 2006. Maternal and child characteristics associated with infant and toddler feeding practices. J. Am. Diet. Assoc. 106, S135.

Herbst, A., Diethelm, K., Cheng, G., Alexy, U., Icks, A., Buyken, A.E., 2011. Direction of associations between added sugar intake in early childhood and body mass index atr age 7 years may depend on intake levels. J. Nutr. 141 (7), 1348–1354.

Hetherington, M.M., Schwartz, C., Madrelle, J., Croden, F., Nekitsing, C., Vereijken, C.M.J.L., Weenen, H., 2015. A step-by-step introduction to vegetables at the beginning of complementary feeding. The effects of early and repeated exposure. Appetite 84, 280–290.

Hilbig, A., Foterek, K., Kersting, M., Alexy, U., 2015. Home-made and commercial complementary meals in German infants: results of the DONALD study. J. Hum. Nutr. Diet. 28, 613–622.

IOM (Institute of Medicine), 2005a. Dietary Reference Intakes for Energy, Carbohydrate, Fiber, Fat, Fatty Acids, Cholesterol, Protein and Amino Acids. The National Academies Press.

IOM (Institute of Medicine), 2005b. Dietary Reference Intakes for Water, Potassium, Sodium, Chloride, and Sulfate. The National Academies Press.

Jahoor, F., Badaloo, A., Reid, M., Forrester, T., 2008. Protein metabolism in severe childhood malnutrition. Ann. Trop. Paediatr. 28, 87.

Jones, L.R., Steer, C.D., Rogers, I.S., Emmett, P.M., 2010. Influences on child fruit and vegetable intake: sociodemographic, parental and child factors in a longitudinal cohort study. Public Health Nutr. 13, 1122.

Jonsdottir, O.H., Thorsdottir, I., Hibberd, P.L., et al., 2012. Timing of the introduction of complementary foods in infancy: a randomized controlled trial. Pediatrics 130, 1038.

Kaikkonen, J.E., Mikkilä, V., Raitakari, O.T., 2014. Role of childhood food patterns on adult cardiovascular disease risk. Curr. Atheroscler. Rep. 16 (19), 443.

Kalhoff, H., Dube, K., Kersting, M., 2010. Iron deficiency in infants fully breastfed for 6 months may not be transitory: first observations during the second half of infancy. (Letter to the editor). Public Health Nutr. 13 (12), 2130–2131.

Kalhoff, H., Hilbig, A., Libuda, L., 2015. Fluid intake- what to drink and how much? Physiology and practice from infancy to adolescence. Kinder- Jugendmed. 15, 7–12.

Kalhoff, H., Kersting, M., 2017. Breastfeeding and formula feeding and iron status in the second 6 months of life. A critical role for complementary feeding. J. Pediatr. 187, 333.

Kalhoff, H., Lücke, T., Kersting, M., 2019. Practical counseling and care for vegetarian child nutrition. Recommendations from the Research Department for Child (Article in German). Monatsschr. Kinderheilkd. 167, 803–812.

Kalhoff, H., Mesch, C.M., Stimming, M., Israel, A., Spitzer, C., Beganovi, C.L., Perez, R.E., Koletzko, B., Warschburger, P., Kersting, M., Libuda, L., 2020. Effects of LC-PUFA supply via complementary food on infant development—a food based intervention (RCT) embedded in a total diet concept. Eur. J. Clin. Nutr. 74, 682–690.

Kalhoff, H., Schmidt, I.V., Heindl, I., Kunert, J., Kersting, M., 2021. Influence of feeding frozen complementary foods on food acceptance in infants: the randomized intervention trial Baby Gourmet. Nutr. Res. 87, 49–56.

Karaolis-Danckert, N., Günther, A.L., Kroke, A., Hornberg, C., Buyken, A.E., 2007. How early dietary factors modify the effect of rapid weight gain in infancy on subsequent body-composition development in term children whose birth weight was appropriate for gestational age. Am. J. Clin. Nutr. 86 (6), 1700–1708.

Kartiosuo, N., Ramakrishnan, R., Lemeshow, S., et al., 2019. Predicting overweight and obesity in young adulthood from childhood body-mass index: comparison of cutoffs derived from longitudinal and cross-sectional data. Lancet Child Adolesc. Health 3 (11), 795–802.

Kent, G., 2015. Global infant formula: monitoring and regulating the impacts to protect human health. Int. Breastfeed. J. 23, 10.

Kersting, M., Disse, S., Hilbig, A., 2015. Infant nutrition and taste imprinting. Impact of early sensory experiences on childhood nutrition. Monatsschr. Kinderheilkd. 163, 783–789.

Kersting, M., Hilbig, A., Hohoff, E., Alexy, U., Kalhoff, H., Lücke, T., 2017. Von Nährstoffen zu Lebensmitteln und Mahlzeiten: das Konzept der Optimierten Mischkost für Kinder und Jugendliche in Deutschland. Aktuel. Ernährungsmed. 42, 304–315.

Kersting, M., Kalhoff, H., Voss, S., Jansen, K., Lücke, T., 2020. Translating European child nutrition guidelines into practice—the German Dietary Scheme for the first year of life. J. Pediatr. Gastroenterol. Nutr. 71 (4), 550–556.

Koletzko, B., Demmelmair, H., Grote, V., Hellmuth, C., Kirchberg, F., Uhl, O., Weber, M., Prell, C., 2016. Long-term impact on health by infant nutrition. Monatsschr. Kinderheilkd. 164, 114–121.

Krebs, N.F., Westcott, J.E., Butler, N., et al., 2006. Meat as a first complementary food for breastfed infants: feasibility and impact on zinc intake and status. J. Pediatr. Gastroenterol. Nutr. 42, 207.

Krebs, N.F., Westcott, J.E., Culbertson, D.L., et al., 2012. Comparison of complementary feeding strategies to meet zinc requirements of older breastfed infants. Am. J. Clin. Nutr. 96, 30–35.

Larson, L.M., Phiri, K.S., Pasricha, S.R., 2017. Iron and cognitive development: what is the evidence? Ann. Nutr. Metab. 71 (suppl 3), 25–38.

Libuda, L., Mesch, C.M., Stimming, M., Demmelmair, H., Koletzko, B., Warschburger, P., Blanke, K., Reischl, E., Kalhoff, H., Kersting, M., 2016. Fatty acid supply with complementary foods and LC-PUFA status in healthy infants: results of a randomised controlled trial. Eur. J. Nutr. 55, 1633–1644.

Lionetti, E., Castellanetta, S., Francavilla, R., et al., 2014. Introduction of gluten, HLA status, and the risk of celiac disease in children. N. Engl. J. Med. 371, 1295–1303.

Lönnerdal, B., 2014. Infant formula and infant nutrition: bioactive proteins of human milk and implications for the composition of infant formulas. Am. J. Clin. Nutr. 99 (suppl), 712S–717S.

Lozoff, B., Klein, N.K., Nelson, E.C., et al., 1998. Behavior of infants with iron-deficiency anemia. Child Dev. 69, 24.

Lozoff, B., Jimenez, E., Hagen, J., et al., 2000. Poorer behavioral and developmental outcome more than 10 years after treatment for iron deficiency in infancy. Pediatrics 105, E51.

Maier-Nöth, A., Schaal, B., Leathwood, P., Issanchou, S., 2016. The lasting influences of early food-related variety experience: a longitudinal study of vegetable acceptance from 5 months to 6 years in two populations. PLoS One 11 (3). https://doi.org/10.1371/journal.pone.0151356, e0151356.

Mangels, R., Driggers, J., 2012. The youngest vegetarians. Vegetarian infants and toddlers. Infant Child Adolesc. Nutr. 4, 8–20.

Manz, F., Wentz, A., Sichert-Hellert, W., 2002. The most essential nutrient: defining the adequate intake of water. J. Pediatr. 141, 587–592.

Marino, D.D., 2007. Water and food safety in the developing world: global implications for health and nutrition of infants and young children. J. Am. Diet. Assoc. 107 (11), 1930–1934.

Mayo-Wilsin, E., Imdad, A., Junior, J., Dean, S., Bhutta, Z.A., 2014. Preventive zinc supplementation for children and the effect of additional iron: a systematic review and meta-Analysis. BMJ Open 4 (6), e004647.

Melø, R., Gellein, K., Evje, L., Syversen, T., 2008. Minerals and trace elements in commercial infant food. Food Chem. Toxicol. 46, 3339.

Menella, J.A., 2014. Ontogeny of taste preferences: basic biology and implications for health. Am. J. Clin. Nutr. 99 (Suppl), 704S–711S.

Mesch, C.M., Stimming, M., Foterek, K., Hilbig, A., Alexy, U., Kersting, M., Libuda, L., 2014. Food variety in commercial and homemade complementary meals for infants in Germany. Market survey and dietary practice. Appetite 76, 113–119.

Michaelsen, K.F., Greer, F.R., 2014. Protein needs early in life and long-term health. Am. J. Clin. Nutr. 99 (3), 718S–722S.

Monteiro, P.O., Victora, C.G., 2005. Rapid growth in infancy and childhood and obesity in later life—a systematic review. Obes. Rev. 6, 143.

Nupponen, M., Pahkala, K., Juonala, M., et al., 2015. Metabolic syndrome from adolescence to early adulthood: effect of infancy-onset dietary counseling of low saturated fat: the Special Turku Coronary Risk Factor Intervention Project (STRIP). Circulation 131, 605–613.

Nwaru, B.I., Takkinen, H.M., Niemelä, O., et al., 2013. Timing of infant feeding in relation to childhood asthma and allergic diseases. J. Allergy Clin. Immunol. 131, 78.

Ong, K.K., Loos, R.J., 2006. Rapid infancy weight gain and subsequent obesity: systematic reviews and hopeful suggestions. Acta Paediatr. 95, 904.

Ong, K.K., Emmett, P.M., Noble, S., et al., 2006. Dietary energy intake at the age of 4 months predicts postnatal weight gain and childhood body mass index. Pediatrics 117, e503.

Owen, C.G., Whincup, P.H., Odoki, K., Gilg, J.A., Cook, D.G., 2002. Infant feeding and blood cholesterol: a study in adolescents and a systematic review. Pediatrics 110, 597–608.

Pak-Gorstein, S., Haq, A., Graham, E.A., 2009. Cultural influences on infant feeding practices. Pediatr. Rev. 30, e11–e21.

Palmer, D.J., Metcalfe, J., Makrides, M., Gold, M.S., Quinn, P., West, C.E., Loh, R., Prescott, S.L., 2013. Early regular egg exposure in infants with eczema: a randomized controlled trial. J. Allergy Clin. Immunol. 132 (2), 387–392.

Pan, L., Li, R., Park, S., et al., 2014. A longitudinal analysis of sugar-sweetened beverage intake in infancy and obesity at 6 years. Pediatrics 134 (Suppl. 1), S29.

Park, S., Pan, L., Sherry, B., Li, R., 2014. The association of sugar-sweetened beverage intake during infancy with sugar-sweetened beverage intake at 6 years of age. Pediatrics 134 (Suppl. 1), S56.

Perrin, E., Frank, D., Cole, C., et al., 2003. Criteria for Determining Disability in Infants and Children: Failure to Thrive. Evidence Report/Technology Assessment No. 72. AHRQ Publication NO. 03-E026. Agency for Healthcare Research and Quality, Rockville, MD.

Qasem, W., Fenton, T., Friel, J., 2015. Age of introduction of first complementary feeding for infants: a systematic review. BMC Pediatr. 15, 107.

Qawasmi, A., Landeros-Weisenberger, A., Leckmann, J.F., Bloch, M.H., 2012. Meta-analysis of long-chain polyunsaturated fatty acid supplementation of formula and infant cognition. Pediatrics 129 (6), 1141–1149.

Qi, Q., Downer, M.K., Kilpeläinen, T.O., et al., 2015. Dietary intake, FTO genetic variants, and adiposity: a combined analysis of over 16,000 children and adolescents. Diabetes 64 (7), 2467–2476.

Rapley, G., 2011. Baby-led weaning: transitioning to solid foods at the baby's own pace. Community Pract. 84 (6), 20–23.

Remer, T., Johner, S., 2014. Critical nutrient iodine. Monatsschr. Kinderheilkd. 162, 5607–5615.

Remer, T., Johner, S.A., Gärtner, R., Thamm, M., Kriener, E., 2010. Iodine deficiency in infancy—a risk for cognitive development. Dtsch. Med. Wochenschr. 135 (31–32), 1551–1556.

Ryan, P.M., Stanton, C., Ross, R.P., et al., 2019. Paediatrician's perspective of infant gut microbiome research: current status and challenges. Arch. Dis. Child. 104, 701–705.

Salgin, B., Norris, S.A., Prentice, P., Pettifor, J.M., Richter, L.M., Ong, K.K., Dunger, D.B., 2015. Even transient rapid infancy weight gain is associated with higher BMI in young adults and earlier menarche. Int. J. Obes. (Lond) 39 (6), 939–944.

Sauerwein, R.W., Mulder, J.A., Mulder, L., et al., 1997. Inflammatory mediators in children with protein-energy malnutrition. Am. J. Clin. Nutr. 65, 1534.

Schoorl, M., Schoorl, M., van Pelt, J., Bartels, P.C.M., 2015. Application of innovative hemocytometric parameters and algorithms for improvement of microcytic anemia discrimination. Hematol. Rep. 7, 5843.

Schwartz, J., Dube, K., Sichert-Hellert, W., Kannenberg, F., Kunz, C., Kalhoff, H., Kersting, M., 2009. Modification of dietary PUFA via complementary food enhances n-3 LC-PUFA synthesis in healthy infants—a double blinded randomized controlled trial. Arch. Dis. Child. 94, 876–882.

Schwartz, J., Dube, K., Alexy, U., Kalhoff, H., Kersting, M., 2010. PUFA and LC-PUFA intake during the first year of life: can dietary practice achieve a guideline diet? Eur. J. Clin. Nutr. 64, 124–130.

Shah, M., Griffin, I.J., Lifschitz, C.H., Abrams, S.A., 2003. Effect of orange and apple juices on iron absorption in children. Arch. Pediatr. Adolesc. Med. 157, 1232.

Simmer, K., Patole, S.K., Rao, S.C., 2011. Long-chain polyunsaturated fatty acid supplementation in infants born at term. Cochrane Database Syst. Rev. 12, CD000376.

Skau, J.K., Touch, B., Chhoun, C., et al., 2015. Effects of animal source food and micronutrient fortification in complementary food products on body composition, iron status, and linear growth: a randomized trial in Cambodia. Am. J. Clin. Nutr. 101 (4), 742–751.

Smith, C.J., 2019. Pediatric thermoregulation: considerations in the face of global climate change. Nutrients 11 (9), 2010. 26.

Stein, L.J., Cowart, B.J., Beauchamp, G.K., 2012. The development of salty taste acceptance is related to dietary experience in human infants: a prospective study. Am. J. Clin. Nutr. 94, 123–129.

Stettler, N., Zemel, B.S., Kumanyika, S., Stallings, V.A., 2002. Infant weight gain and childhood overweight status in a multicenter, cohort study. Pediatrics 109, 194–199.

Stiemsma, L., Michels, K., 2018. The role of the microbiome in the developmental origins of health and disease. Pediatrics 141, e20172437.

Stimming, M., Mesch, C.M., Kersting, M., Kalhoff, H., Demmelmair, H., Koletzko, B., Schmidt, A., Boehm, V., Libuda, L., 2014. Vitamin E content and estimated need in German infant and follow-on formulae with and without long-chain polyunsaturated fatty acids (LC-PUFA) enrichment. J. Agric. Food Chem. 62 (41), 10153–10161.

Strazzullo, P., Campanozzi, A., Avallone, S., 2012. Does salt intake in the first two years of life affect the development of cardiovascular disorders in adulthood? Nutr. Metab. Cardiovasc. Dis. 22 (10), 787–792.

Szajewska, H., Shamir, R., Mearin, L., et al., 2016. Gluten introduction and the risk of coeliac disease: a position paper by the European Society for pediatric gastroenterology, hepatology, and nutrition. J. Pediatr. Gastroenterol. Nutr. 62 (3), 507–513.

Thierfelder, W., Dortschy, R., Hintzpeter, B., Kahl, H., Scheidt-Nave, C., 2007. Biochemical measures in the German Health Interview and Examination Survey for Children and Adolescents (KIGGS). Bundesgesundheitsblatt Gesundheitsforschung Gesundheitsschutz 50, 757–770.

Thorisdottir, B., Gunnarsdottir, I., Thorisdottir, A.V., et al., 2013. Nutrient intake in infancy and body mass index at six years in two population-based cohorts recruited before and after revision of infant dietary recommendations. Ann. Nutr. Metab., 145–151.

USAID'S infant & young child nutrition project, 2011. Summary of Sociocultural and Epidemiological Findings on Infant and Young Child Feeding in 11 Countries. JYCN, Washington DC.

Usheva, N., Galcheva, S., Cardon, G., et al., On behalf of The ToyBox-Study Group, 2021. Complementary feeding and overweight in european preschoolers: the toybox-study. Nutrients 13 (4), 1199.

Van Winckel, M., Vande Velde, S., De Bruyne, R., Van Biervliet, S., 2011. Vegetarian infant and child nutrition. Eur. J. Pediatr. 170, 1489–1494.

Victora, C.G., Christian, P., Vidaletti, L.P., et al., 2021. Revisiting maternal and child undernutrition in low-income and middle-income countries: variable progress towards an unfinished agenda. Lancet 397 (10282), 1388–1399.

Vriezinga, S.L., Aurichio, R., Bravi, E., et al., 2014. Randomizede feeding intervention in infants at high risk for celiac disease. N. Engl. J. Med. 371, 1304–1315.

Wessels, K.R., Brown, K.H., 2012. Estimating the global prevalence of zinc deficiency: results based on zinc availability in national food supplies and the prevalence of stunting. PLoS One 7 (11), e50568.

WHO, 2002. Complementary Feeding: Report of the Global Consultation, and Summary of Guiding Principles for Complementary Feeding of the Breastfed Child. Geneva. vol. 2002.

WHO, 2013. Guideline: Updates on the Management of Severe Acute Malnutrition in Infants and Children. Available from: http://apps.who.int/iris/bitstream/10665/95584/1/9789241506328_eng.pdf.

WHO Secretariat, Andersson, M., de Benoist, B., et al., 2007. Prevention and control of iodine deficiency in pregnant and lactating women and in children less than 2-years-old: conclusions and recommendations of the Technical Consultation. Public Health Nutr. 10, 1606.

Yates, A.A., 2006. Dietary reference intakes: concepts and approaches underlying protein and energy requirements. In: Rigo, J., Ziegler, E.E. (Eds.), Protein and Energy Requirements in Infancy and Childhood. Nestlé Nutrition Institute Workshop Series: Pediatric Program. vol. 58. Nestlé Ltd., Vevey/S. Karger AG, Basel, pp. 74–94.

Yew, K.S., Webber, B., Hodges, J., Carter, N.J., 2009. Clinical inquiries: are there any known health risks to early introduction of solids to an infant's diet? J. Fam. Pract. 58, 219–220.

Ziegler, P., Hanson, C., Ponza, M., et al., 2006. Feeding infants and toddlers study: meal and snack intakes of Hispanic and non-Hispanic infants and toddlers. J. Am. Diet. Assoc. 106, S107.

Zimmermann, M.B., Jooste, P.L., Pandav, C.S., 2008. Iodine-deficiency disorders. Lancet 372, 1251.

Zutavern, A., Brockow, I., Schaaf, B., et al., 2008. Timing of solid food introduction in relation to eczema, asthma, allergic rhinits, and food and inhalant sensitisation at the age of 6 years: results from a prospective birth cohort study. Pediatrics 121, e44–e52.

# Developing science-based dietary guidelines for infants and toddlers

*Lynda M. O'Neill[a] and Jennifer Orlet Fisher[b]*

[a]Nestlé Research Center, Lausanne, Switzerland [b]Temple University, Center for Obesity Research and Education, Philadelphia, PA, United States

## CHAPTER LEARNING OBJECTIVES

(1) Describe the role of milk feeding, nutrient requirements, and dietary patterns for the development of quantitative food-based dietary guidelines (FBDG) during complementary feeding

(2) Evaluate existing quantitative FBDG for infants and toddlers relative to energy and nutrient requirements, including overconsumed nutrients (i.e., saturated fats, free sugars and sodium)

(3) Identify challenges to and strategies for achieving adequate intakes of iron, calcium, and zinc among infants of 6–12 months and vitamin D among all children, including dietary supplements and fortified foods, which provide nutrients without additional energy

## Abbreviations

| | |
|---|---|
| **AAP** | American Academy of Pediatrics |
| **AI** | adequate intake |
| **DGAC** | Dietary Guideline Advisory Committee |
| **DHA** | docosahexaenoic acid |
| **EAR** | estimated average requirement |
| **EER** | estimated energy requirement |
| **EFSA** | European Food Standards Authority |
| **ESPGHAN** | European Society for Pediatric Gastroenterology Hepatology and Nutrition |
| **FAO** | Food and Agriculture Organization |

| FBDG | food-based dietary guideline |
| FITS | Feeding Infants and Toddlers Study |
| IOM | Institute of Medicine |
| LCPUFA | long chain polyunsaturated fatty acid |
| NASEM | National Academies of Sciences, Engineering and Medicine |
| NRV | nutrient reference value |
| OECD | Organization for Economic Co-operation and Development |
| RDA | recommended daily allowance |
| SSB | sugar sweetened beverage |
| WHO | World Health Organization |

## 22.1 Introduction

Optimal nutrition is essential to support growth and development during infancy and early childhood. Complementary feeding is a critical period for nutrient adequacy as children transition from an exclusively milk based diet to one in which nutrient requirements are met from all food groups. According to the World Health Organization (WHO), complementary feeding begins around 6 months of age and extends until 24 months of age (WHO, 2009). The types of foods that are introduced during complementary feeding should not only be aligned to meet nutrient requirements but should also be developmentally appropriate (Demonteil et al., 2019) and help to establish lifelong healthy eating habits (Forestell, 2017). Therefore, evidence-based guidance on complementary feeding is critical to population-based efforts to promote optimal nutrition and health in early development and beyond.

Food-based dietary guidelines (FBDG) are recommendations emphasizing the foods, food groups, and dietary patterns that provide required nutrients (FAO, 2020). FBDG are intended to advise the general public about consuming nutritious foods and living a healthier life (FAO, 2020). These guidelines translate nutrient targets and dietary goals, along with cultural and socio-economic considerations to specific actionable food-based recommendations, which should meet the nutrient needs of a given population (Andrade and Andrade, 2016). Another purpose of FBDG is to reduce lifetime risk of diet-related chronic diseases, such as obesity and cardiovascular disease. Indeed, poor dietary patterns that begin during complementary feeding show links to chronic disease in later life (Hu et al., 2020; Lanigan and Singhal, 2009).

FBDG can be qualitative or quantitative in nature. Qualitative guidelines on complementary feeding often include recommendations regarding the introduction of solid foods, the types of foods to offer at various ages, the introduction of increasingly complex textures with age, the avoidance of specific foods (e.g., cow's milk before 1 year of age), and responsive feeding practices (Critch et al., 2014). While such guidelines are essential, they lack critical information on portion sizes. Quantitative guidelines, in contrast, provide recommendations regarding specific amounts, or ranges, of each food group to be consumed daily. This degree of specificity is needed to ensure that the complementary diet is compatible with nutrient requirements, which is one of the main goals of FBDG. Many countries have some type of dietary guidance targeting infants and young children. A recent analysis of infant feeding guidelines in the WHO European region, revealed that 94% of 48 countries assessed had specific recommendations for the complementary feeding period (Koletzko et al., 2020). Currently however, there is no universal consensus on the optimal approach to developing recommendations around quantitative FBDG for complementary feeding. Furthermore, methodologies used to develop FBDG vary widely from expert opinion and consensus (Alvisi et al., 2015) to more rigorous quantitative approaches (Santika et al., 2009; Tharrey et al., 2017).

As such, the alignment of current quantitative FBDG for complementary feeding with nutrient requirements for growth and development is not well characterized. Therefore, in this chapter we discuss key considerations in developing quantitative FBDG for the complementary feeding period and evaluate the extent to which existing global quantitative FBDG can be translated to achieve nutrient adequacy during this life stage. Such FBDG can provide the basis for interventions, educational programs and health messages targeted to parents and caregivers of very young children.

## 22.2 Considerations for developing quantitative food based dietary guidelines for infants and toddlers

Throughout complementary feeding, energy, and nutrient needs are continuously evolving as the child grows and in parallel becomes less reliant on milk as the key source of nutrition. The shift from a solely milk-based to a more varied diet necessitates careful consideration of the types and amounts of various food groups that meet nutrient requirements, aligned with developmental readiness and are culturally acceptable. Simultaneously, this period is a critical window of opportunity to foster long-term healthy eating habits (Reidy et al., 2017). Below we review considerations of milk feeding, energy and nutrient requirements, and dietary patterns in the development of quantitative FBDG.

## 22.3 Milk feeding and energy requirements

The quantity of complementary foods required by children at different ages is largely driven by the energy gap between estimated energy requirements (EER) and energy consumed from milk, whether breast milk, a breast milk substitute, or cow's milk, in the case of toddlers. At 6 months, as complementary foods are introduced, milk provides the majority of the volume, energy, and nutrients consumed (WHO, 2009). From 6 months onward, however, the quantity of milk in the diet gradually declines, while the quantity of complementary foods progressively increases (Dewey, 2001). Usual intakes of human milk by age have been quantified in developing and industrialized countries (PAHO/WHO, 2003). Based on these assumptions and considering the energy contribution of human milk, the energy needs from complementary foods to provide the EER have been estimated at 163 kcal and 372 kcal, for infants 6 to 8 months and 9 to 11 months, respectively. Based on further observations studies, the WHO advised that the energy needed above and beyond human milk is approximately 200 kcal per day in infants 6 to 8 months, 300 kcal per day in infants 9 to 11 months, and 550 kcal per day in toddlers 12 to 23 months of age (WHO, 2009). In industrialized countries, where breast feeding beyond 12 months is less common, authoritative organizations recommend cow's milk at quantities of 480 ml (Gidding et al., 2006). Recommendations regarding cow's milk vary, with most organizations recommending whole cow's milk beginning at 12 months of age (Agostoni et al., 2008; Koletzko et al., 2008). Considering the significant quantity of milk consumed by children 6 to 24 months, quantitative guidelines on complementary feeding need to consider the energy and nutrient contribution of the relevant milk in the diet. As with energy, nutrients needed from complementary foods reflects the difference between the daily nutrient reference values (NRVs) and nutrients consumed from human milk for infants and cow's milk for toddlers (Butte et al., 2004).

## 22.4 Nutrient requirements during complementary feeding

In addition to consideration of energy requirements, quantitative FBDG must take in consideration the NRV of the target population (EFSA, 2010). Nutrient requirements of infants (6–12 months) and toddlers (12–24 months) have been established by various national and international authoritative organizations (e.g., WHO, Institute of Medicine (IOM) and European Food Standards Authority (EFSA)) and should form the basis of sound quantitative complementary feeding guidelines. The daily intake of calories should be correctly distributed among the various macronutrients (Alvisi et al., 2015). WHO recommendations on protein intake during complementary feeding amount to 5% to 6% of daily energy intake (WHO/FAO/UNU, 2002) when taking into account the recommended quantity per day based on median body weight. Guidance from the European Society of Pediatric, Gastroenterology, Hepatology and Nutrition (ESPGHAN), indicates that total protein should not exceed 15% of daily energy intake due to emerging evidence that elevated protein intakes at 12 months are associated with increased body mass index (BMI) later in childhood (Pimpin et al., 2016; Weber et al., 2014). Recommendations for total fat intakes are 40% to 60% of daily energy intake at the beginning of complementary feeding, with a gradual decline to 35% by the end of the second year of life (FAO, 2008). The type of fat is also important, with unsaturated fats being preferable and long-chain polyunsaturated fatty acids (LCPUFA), found in vegetable oils, some oily fish, and fish oils, being vital. LCPUFA include the omega-3 fatty acids, alpha-linolenic acid (ALA), and docosahexaenoic acid (DHA), which are considered essential and can only be obtained through the diet. Once protein and total fat requirements are fulfilled, the residual calories, by default, are contributed by carbohydrates, which amount to around 45% to 65% of daily energy. Complementary feeding recommendations advise that the consumption of rapidly absorbed carbohydrates should be limited, in favor of slowly absorbed, or low glycemic, carbohydrates (Zalewski et al., 2017). Free sugars should be restricted during complementary feeding given evidence of links with overweight/obesity, dental caries, and cardiometabolic disease as well as the more immediate impact of diluting the nutrient density of the diet and reducing dietary diversity (Fidler Mis et al., 2017). Sugar-sweetened beverages (SSBs) and fruit juices are particularly rich in free sugars. Dietary fiber, occurring in plant-based foods such as vegetables, fruits, legumes, and wholegrains, is important for its role in supporting digestive health and minimizing the risk of several chronic diseases in later life (Dahl and Stewart, 2015). However, there is a paucity of recommendations on the fiber requirements of infants and toddlers owing to the limited evidence available to derive such requirements for children (EFSA, 2010a).

NRV are a prerequisite to the development of FBDG (NASEM, 2018). However, given the uncertainty associated with the micronutrient requirements of infants, only, iron, and zinc have an estimated average requirements (EAR) and thus, a recommended daily allowance (RDA), according to the US dietary reference intakes (DRI). The remaining nutrients only have an adequate intake (AI) for infants. The WHO and EFSA have established requirements for some additional nutrients for infants, i.e., calcium and additionally vitamin A in the case of EFSA (O'Neill et al., 2020). The situation is only slightly better for toddlers, with EAR for a few more nutrients, but not as many as for the population over the age of 2 years. Given that the AI is based on estimations of usual intake from healthy Western populations, most of whom consume fortified foods, or on experimental data, the extent to which the AI overestimates true physiological requirements has been questioned (Young, 2003). Thus, the lack of well substantiated nutrient requirements for infants and toddlers is an intrinsic limitation of any exercise designed to establish quantitative FBDG for the complementary feeding period. Nevertheless, in the absence of more complete and proven data, the AI is considered an acceptable substitute for the RDA (Atkinson, 2011).

The consumption of nutrient dense foods is particularly critical during complementary feeding given the high nutrient requirements of infants and toddlers relative to their energy needs (Solomons and Vossenaar, 2013). Iron and zinc requirements are particularly challenging to achieve as their target nutrient density (the amount of the nutrient per kcal of food) is the highest when comparing the requirements for these nutrients relative to the expected energy from complementary foods (Dewey and Vitta, 2013). For this reason, it is highly advised that complementary feeding includes foods with high nutrient densities of these trace minerals, such as animal foods and fortified foods as well as mineral supplements, or some combination of these approaches to ensure the AI is satisfied (Dewey and Vitta, 2013; Krebs et al., 2014). Bioavailability is another important consideration around iron and zinc nutrition, as both minerals are susceptible to binding with phytates, which are intrinsic to plant-based foods, particularly cereals and legumes, and limit intestinal absorption (Gibson et al., 2010). The phytate content of the total diet, i.e., the quantity of plant-based foods in the diet is particularly important for zinc, as its ratio to phytates is thought to be a significant determinant of zinc requirements (Gibson et al., 2018) and a crude proxy for bioavailability (Ma et al., 2007). Alternatively, for iron, heme sources found in meats are absorbed more efficiently than non-heme iron sources. Iron absorption from plant-based and fortified non-heme sources can be improved by consuming those foods with vitamin C or heme iron (Theuer, 2008). Concerns around bioavailability of iron, however, are somewhat offset by evidence that the iron deficient infants show up-regulation of iron absorption from the diet (Krebs, 2014). Nevertheless, accounting for the bioavailability of both iron and zinc when planning FBDG during the complementary feeding period is important (Dewey et al., 2004; Santika et al., 2009).

## 22.5 Dietary patterns

The FAO/WHO strongly recommend that FBDG consider the typical dietary patterns of the target population (FAO, 2020). The USDA defines dietary patterns as the amounts, proportions, variety or combination of different foods and nutrients in diets, and the frequency with which they are habitually consumed (Essery Stoody et al., 2014). It is well established that dietary patterns, rather than individual nutrients, have a greater influence on health outcomes, therefore dietary recommendations or FBDG are often expressed as dietary patterns (Green, 2015). A critical window for the development of dietary patterns is the complementary feeding period, when the infant gradually transitions from an exclusively milk-based diet to one consisting of family foods. The Feeding Infants and Toddlers Study (FITS) from 2008 identified that the first 2 years of life are the most dynamic period in the exposure and introduction of foods to children's diets, and dietary patterns that emerge by 2 years of age are still evident at 4 years of age (Reidy et al., 2017). Although health benefits of fruits and vegetables are well-documented, most children fall short of the recommendations starting in early childhood. It has been identified that infrequent consumption of fruits and vegetables during infancy is associated with infrequent consumption of the same at 6 years of age (Grimm et al., 2014). A similar finding was identified with respect to SSBs, whereby intakes of these beverages during infancy increased the likelihood of consuming SSB at least once a day at 6 years of age (Park et al., 2014). Thus, the foods to which children are exposed during infancy have an influential role on the development of food acceptance and dietary intake patterns (Lange et al., 2013; Nicklaus, 2016). Therefore, it is critical to ensure the dietary patterns of infants and toddlers are appropriate, not only for short-term health, but also to shape long-term preferences and habits that persist into later life.

Even though dietary patterns in early life are critical for long-term diet and health, studies show that those observed during complementary feeding are suboptimal, even in affluent countries. For example, FITS 2016 found inadequate consumption of iron rich foods among infants, inadequate fruit and vegetables consumption among infants and toddlers, and a low variety within the vegetable group, in the United States. The study also found a high intake of SSB and 100% juice (Roess et al., 2018). A study aimed at characterizing the dietary patterns of Australian toddlers identified that two distinct patterns were evident at the ages of 14 and 24 months (Bell et al., 2013). One pattern consisted of "core foods" including fruits and vegetables, whereas the other pattern was characterized by "non-core" foods, such as white bread, ice cream, sweets, and SSB. The EU childhood obesity project (CHOP) investigated the major dietary patterns prospectively in young children at 1, 2, 3, 4, 5, and 8 years of age in five EU countries (Belgium, Germany, Italy, Poland, and Spain) and found that dietary patterns were established between the ages of 1 and 2 years and persisted to 8 years of age (Luque et al., 2018). The study also identified that unhealthy dietary patterns during early childhood, characterized by added sugars, unhealthy fats, and low intakes of vegetables, fruits, fish, and olive oil, were more likely to persist into mid-childhood. Therefore, early experience is critical in shaping eating behaviors and provides opportunities to promote the acceptance of healthful foods (Mennella and Ventura, 2011; Mennella and Trabulsi, 2012; Spill et al., 2019). These findings underscore of the role of FBDG in establishing healthy dietary patterns that can persist far beyond the complementary feeding period.

## 22.6 Methodologies for developing dietary guidelines

FBDG are largely derived by governmental or large authoritative organizations (FAO, 2020). Smitasiri and Uauy proposed that the development of FBDG should not only reflect nutrient recommendations but also take into consideration food composition, nutrient bioavailability, relevant nutritional problems, upper intake levels, current food intake, and food supply (Smitasiri and Uauy, 2007). Further, it is important that FBDG are culturally appropriate and, in the case of very young children, reflect local complementary feeding practices (Tuck, 2013). Nationally representative dietary intake data are key for characterizing local complementary feeding practices and identifying nutritional problems among infants and toddlers. A number of methods of varying rigor have been used to develop FBDG for infants and toddlers, including the use of expert opinion, menu planning, and mathematical modeling. Expert opinion, while providing consensus around existing evidence and prevailing views, generally does not provide rigorous formulation of quantitative guidance. Menu planning is an approach whereby different food combinations in different amounts are repeatedly tested in a menu plan with the aim of reaching an optimal complementary diet that meets energy and nutrient requirements based on the local food supply (Kersting et al., 2005). This empirical "trial and error" approach does not require modeling software nor biostatistics knowledge nor does it involve a nationally representative dietary intake dataset, but it does necessitate knowledge of local feeding practices and nutrient inadequacies. Moreover, the menu planning approach is time consuming, error prone and is generally not an efficient approach to understanding how to optimize the supply of nutrients from available complementary foods when energy requirements are limited relative to that from milk (Briend et al., 2003). Linear programming is a newer and more rigorous approach that uses mathematical models to optimize diets based on habitual dietary patterns while minimizing or maximizing multiple constraints (Briend et al., 2003). Nutritional constraints ensure the nutrient adequacy of the diet at the appropriate energy level, whereas food consumption constraints ensure that the diet consists of foods that are regularly consumed and included in quantities that are typical (Darmon et al., 2002). Food constraints are particularly important for ensuring that optimized diets are palatable and socially acceptable; for these reasons local dietary intake data are essential. When linear programming is applied to diet optimization in developing countries, a cost constraint is also introduced to avoid that the optimized diet is cost-prohibitive (Santika et al., 2009). Thus, the identification of appropriate constraints is critical to the development of robust linear models that ensure diverse, adequate, and culturally acceptable diets. Usually several iterations of the program are run, with new adjustments to the restrictions being introduced each time, so that acceptable diets are produced (Dewey et al., 2004).

## 22.7 A review of current quantitative food-based dietary guidelines from developed countries

Ensuring nutrient adequacy and exposure to a variety of healthy foods during complementary feeding is critical during the rapid growth and development that occur during this period. A few approaches have been applied to develop quantitative FBDG for this period, but there is little consensus as to which approach is optimal. Importantly, little is known about the extent to which existing quantitative FBDG achieve the goals of a nutritionally adequate and diverse diet. To address this gap, we evaluated the extent to which existing quantitative FBDG for infants (6–12 months old) and toddlers (12–24 months old) from developed populous countries address NRVs during complementary feeding. Quantitative FBDG that met pre-defined eligibility criteria were translated into 7-day menus and compared to country-specific and global reference values for energy, macronutrients, and selected micronutrients that have been previously identified as nutrients of concern for this life stage (O'Neill et al., 2020).

## 22.7.1 Review methods

### 22.7.1.1 FBDG selection

#### 22.7.1.1.1 Inclusion/exclusion criteria

For the purposes of assessing nutrient adequacy the review focused on FBDG from developed countries. For infants, guidelines were included if the age range was given as 6 to 12 months or 7 to 12 months. For toddlers, a broader definition was utilized because while complementary feeding extends from the age of 12 to 24 months (WHO, 2009), some guidelines were developed for 1 to 3 year or even 1 to 4-year-old children. Given the interest in evaluating nutrient adequacy of the total diet, qualitative guidelines were excluded (e.g., broad statements such as "Give your baby dark-green leafy vegetables and orange colored vegetables and fruit every day" without specifying an amount), guidelines that omitted one or more major food groups, or guidelines that combined multiple food groups of varying nutrient composition (e.g., combined recommendations for vegetables, legumes, and grains). However, guidelines that combined fruit and vegetables into a single food group were included considering the nutritional similarities between said food groups.

#### 22.7.1.1.2 Search strategy

Two approaches were taken to identify country specific quantitative FBDG for complementary feeding (Fig. 22.1). First, literature searches were performed using PubMed and Ovid Medline to identify relevant publications from June 2008 through June 2018 using the following search terms: "complementary feeding" OR "dietary guideline" AND "infant" OR "child" OR "young child feeding." Fifteen developed countries (Australia, Canada, Chile, Colombia, Germany, Great Britain, France, Italy, Korea, Mexico, Poland,

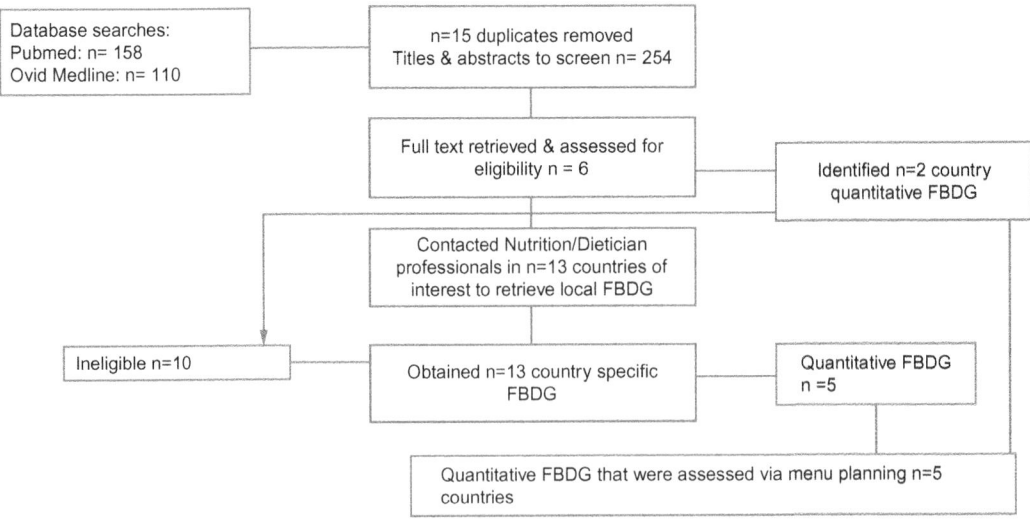

**FIG. 22.1**   Search strategy to identify country specific quantitative FBDG for complementary feeding.

South Africa, Spain, Turkey, and the United States) were identified based on Organization for Economic Cooperation and Development (OECD) membership (OECD, 2019) and population size ($n > 15$ million); these criteria were applied to identify large countries with medium to high levels of economic development, under assumptions that these countries would likely have the infrastructure and economic resources to formulate and implement dietary recommendations. Second, pediatric experts in the countries of interest were consulted to provide and translate their national government or nutrition society complementary feeding guidelines.

### 22.7.1.2 Translation of FBDG into 7-day menus

Registered Dietitians translated each FBDG into 7-day menus using Nutritionist-Pro (AXXYA Systems LLC., Stafford, TX, USA Systems, 2016). Seven days were chosen to allow for dietary intake variation over time (Lanigan et al., 2004). The country specific quantitative guidelines were followed verbatim to create the menus. For example, if 65 g of vegetables were recommended per day, then 65 g of a range of vegetables was included daily across the 7 days. The midpoint of the range was used when food quantity was recommended as a range. Menus were developed to emphasize whole foods, except in the case of grains and dairy products. For example, infant cereals were included as a source of grains, when specified by a recommendation, and yogurt and cheese were included as sources of dairy if such foods were proposed. Except for bananas, the nutrient compositions of fruits and vegetables were included as cooked, without added seasonings such as sugar or salt. In order to maximize comparisons, similar types of foods in each group were used across countries. Food diversity across the week within each food group was ensured, but foods not specified in the guidelines were not included and no extra foods were added. In general, leaner cuts of meat and poultry were chosen. If country specific FBDG included provisions for 100% fruit juice and/or an allowance for occasional foods, these were included in the corresponding menus.

### 22.7.1.3 Milk intake and composition

For infant menus, analyses were performed under assumptions of exclusive human milk feeding given that it is the biologic norm and the optimal milk source during the first year of life (Victora et al., 2016). Because formula is fortified with many nutrients (Dipasquale et al., 2020), in accordance with regulations, the evaluation of FBDG under assumptions of exclusive formula feeding would likely provide an upper limit of the nutritional adequacy of the complementary diet specified by the FBDG. In guidelines where no recommendations on milk intake were given for infants, WHO observational data (Dewey, 2001; Dewey et al., 2004) on human milk for infants 9 to 11 months old, were used and expressed as a percentage of energy that translated to 50% of daily energy from milk. Estimates were based on intakes of infants 9 to 11 months old, because the milk consumption of infants 6 to 8 months does not require appreciable energy from complementary foods to meaningfully carry out the analysis.

A global composition of mature human milk was derived by averaging data from food composition databases (Souci et al., 2015; USDA, 2016) as well as other published data on human milk composition (AAP, 2006; Giuffrida et al., 2016; Yang et al., 2014). The calculated average composition was comparable to published data from two systematic reviews on the energy and macronutrient content of human milk (Gidrewicz and Fenton, 2014; Hester et al., 2012). One of the reviews also contained data on the calcium content of the same (Hester et al., 2012) with which our data were consistent.

Cow's milk was the milk source included for toddler menus. The type (i.e., full fat or reduced fat) and amount was taken directly from the specific FBDG being assessed. The composition of the cow's milk applied in each weekly menu was from the specific food composition database of the country being evaluated.

### 22.7.1.4 Food composition databases

Country-specific food composition databases were used, or if unavailable, country-specific fortified foods were manually entered into Nutritionist Pro. This is important since wheat and other grains are fortified in many countries (Food Fortification Initiative, 2018), and cow's milk is fortified in some developed countries (Dror and Allen, 2014). If fortified grains were mentioned in a country specific guideline (e.g., iron-fortified infant cereal), fortified versions were included in that country's menu.

While some FBDG recommended the provision of specific supplements, the menus did not include dietary supplements since the intent was to see if existing FBDG could meet the nutrient needs of the population they were destined for solely through consumption of foods, including milk.

### 22.7.1.5 Country-specific and global nutrient reference values

The energy and nutrients provided by menus generated from each FBDG were compared to country and global NRV as well as WHO reference values for energy (FAO/WHO/UNU, 2001), protein (WHO/FAO/UNU, 2002), and fat and fatty acids (FAO, 2008). Given that WHO has not recommended a maximal limit for protein intake among infants and young children, we considered the limit suggested by the European Society for Pediatric Gastroenterology, Hepatology and Nutrition (ESPGHAN), which is 15% of total energy intake (Fewtrell et al., 2017). For sugars, the definition and limit proposed by the WHO (WHO, 2015) was applied. As free sugars cannot be assessed by Nutritionist Pro, the content of free sugars in the country-specific menus was manually calculated. Other overconsumed nutrients, namely saturated fatty acids (SFA) and sodium, were also evaluated. Given that there are no WHO standards for SFA, we applied the European Food Standards Authority (EFSA) recommendations in toddler diets (EFSA, 2010b). Harmonized global NRV for micronutrients of major concern to infants and young children, such as: potassium, calcium, iron, zinc, and vitamin D, were identified using previous reviews (NASEM, 2017; O'Neill et al., 2020). Vitamin A was also included as it has frequently been reported as a short-fall nutrient in early life (Hilger et al., 2015).

## 22.7.2 Review results

Fourteen FBDG from 15 OECD-member (OECD, 2019) countries (the United States, Mexico, Germany, Turkey, France, United Kingdom, Italy, South Africa, Korea, Colombia, Spain, Poland, Canada, Australia, and Chile) were identified. All addressed topics of responsive feeding, developmental appropriateness, age of introduction of allergens, and other pertinent topics. Table 22.1 presents the quantitative complementary feeding FBDG

**TABLE 22.1**  Eligible country-specific quantitative FBDG for infants and young children, nutrient databases, and country-specific NRV.

| Country | FBDG for infants and young children | Reference for NRVs | Nutrient database applied |
|---|---|---|---|
| Australia | National Health and Medical Research Council (NHMRC), Eat for Health; Educator guide (2013)(NHMRC, 2013) | National Health and Medical Research Council. Educator Guide. Canberra: National Health and Medical Research Council. (2013) | Imported data from AUSNUT 2011–2013, Food Standards Australia & New Zealand |
| Chile | Ministerio de Salud Chile (2015) Guideline of nutrition of children less than 2 years | Ministry of Health: Government of Chile. Guideline of nutrition before adolescence. 5th Edition. (2016) | As there is no national nutrient database for Chile, the USDA nutrient composition database was utilized and compositions for grain and dairy products from Chilean manufacturers were utilized |
| Germany | Hilbig et al. (2012) Einführung und Zusammensetzung der Beikost. Wissenschaftliche Evidenz und praktische Empfehlungen in Deutschland And | German Nutrition Society. New references values for energy intake. Ann Nutr Metab. (2015) DACH Reference Values for Nutritional Intakes, 2nd Edition, (2015) | Imported data from Souci et al. (2015) |
| Great Britain | British Dietetic Association: Clinical Pediatric Dietetics. 4th ed. (Shaw, 2014) | British Nutrition Foundation. Nutrition Requirements. (2016) | Composition of Foods Integrated Dataset (CoFID), (2015) |
| US Child and Adult Care Food Program (CACFP) | Murphy et al. (2011) Child and Adult Care Food Program: Aligning Dietary Guidance for all. National Academy of Sciences | DRIs: Otten JJ, Hellwig JP, Meyers LD. Institute of Medicine. The National Academies Press. (2006). Updated values for calcium and vitamin D: IOM (Institute of Medicine) (2011) updated values for sodium and potassium: NASEM (National Academies of Science Engineering and Medicine) (2019) | USDA Nutrient Database for Standard Reference 28, (2016) |

from five countries that met inclusion criteria. Quantitative FBDG from Australia, Chile, Germany, and Great Britain were targeted to health care providers and available on government websites and/or publications. In the absence of US federal dietary guidelines for children 0 to 24 months of age, prior to December 2020, quantitative guidelines from the federal Child and Adult Care Food Program (CACFP) were included. CACFP is a nutrition assistance program targeting low-income populations that provides reimbursements for nutritious meals and snacks for infants and young children in child-care (Institute of Medicine,

2011). The CACFP guidelines were developed by the Institute of Medicine (IOM) to be used for specific meals as well as across a whole day to align CACFP with current dietary recommendations from the American Academy of Pediatrics (AAP), encourage breast-feeding, and promote health by enabling children to meet nutrient requirements. Table 22.1 also indicates the food composition database applied for each country-specific menu analysis, and the corresponding country-specific NRV applied for evaluating the nutrient adequacy of the menus. The Australian guidelineswere developed using linear programming (NHMRC, 2011). The CACFP guidelines were established by assessing dietary intake, setting nutrient targets, developing meal patterns and food specifications, and using the criteria to iteratively evaluate and finalize the meal and snack requirements (Institute of Medicine, 2011). The Chilean (Castillo-Durán et al., 2013) and British guidelines (Shaw, 2014) appear to be based on expert opinion. While the German guidelines were developed based on a menu planning approach (Hilbig et al., 2012).

Table 22.2 shows the food groups and corresponding daily quantities recommended by the guidelines for infants. The quantity of fruit varies the most with 10 g being recommended in Australia and 100 g in both Chile and Germany. In Great Britain and the United States, the fruit and vegetable groups are combined into one group, with 60 to 80 g recommended by the former and 0 to 2 tbsp per feeding occasion, which could be up to 150 g per day for the latter. The quantities of vegetables being recommended by the other countries varies from 30 to 40 g of vegetables, including legumes, in Australia, and up to 100 g in Germany. Comparing the non-dairy protein recommendations, both Australia and Chile recommend 30 g of meat/fish/egg/day, while Germany recommends 20 to 30 g of meat/fish, and the British recommendation is for 20 to 40 g of meat/fish/eggs/pulses/nuts/seeds. All guidelines recommend around 60 to 80 g of grains and starches, like white potato, a day. The legume group differs to the greatest extent with some recommendations not mentioning them, others combining them with either the vegetable group or the non-dairy protein group, while the guideline from Chile considers them as an independent food group to be consumed twice a week at 70 to 80 g. There is no recommendation for fats and oils in Great Britain and the United States, whereas the guidelines from both Australia and Germany recommend up to 15 g. The Chilean and German guidelines don't mention dairy products, stating that breast milk or a substitute are sufficient, whereas small amounts of dairy products are recommended in Australia and Great Britain, but the guidelines from the United States mention that up to 56 g of cheese or 112 g of cottage cheese or yogurt could be offered once a day.

### 22.7.2.1 Nutrient content analysis of 7-day menus

#### 22.7.2.1.1 Infants

Table 22.3 shows an example of a 7-day menu based on the translation of the FBDG for breast-fed infants. The average daily energy and nutrient compositions of the menus created under assumptions of exclusive human milk-feeding are shown relative to local and global NRVs. The average daily energy contents of menus were relatively close to their respective energy targets, ranging from 90% of the target for the Chilean menus up to 120% of the target for the German menus. The protein contents of the menus tended to be higher than the targets and this was evident across all countries (Table 22.4). The fat contents were adequate, ranging from 92% of the global target in Chile, up to 115% of the global target in Australia. Similarly, deviations from the local fat targets were minor. Both iron and vitamin D daily contributions were below the global NRVs. Compared with the global NRVs, iron in all menus

TABLE 22.2  Daily quantitative FBDG for infants, which met the eligibility criteria.

| Country | Fruit | Vegetables | Grains/starches | Meat/fish/egg | Legumes | Breast milk (BM) or substitutes (BMS) and dairy products | Oil |
|---|---|---|---|---|---|---|---|
| Australia | 10g of fruit | 30–40g (veg and legumes/beans) | 20g infant cereal (un-reconstituted) and 60g of bread equivalents | 30g (lean meat/fish/tofu/eggs) | See vegetables | 600mL BM or BMS and 10mL of yogurt or 5g of cheese (3–4 × a week) | 4–15g oils or seed/nut paste |
| Chile | 100g fruit | 75g from 60g of colored veg & 15g of green veg | 10g cereal raw (maize rice, quinoa), 50g potato | 30g meat or fish or egg (meat 3 × a week, fish 2 × a week, egg 1–2 × a week) | 70–80g legumes (beans, chickpeas, lentils) 2 × a week | BM or BMS | 5g |
| Germany | 100–120g fruit | 90–100g of veg | 20g infant cereal 2 × a day and 40–60g of potato/rice/noodles. Toward the end of the first year, bread, preferably wholegrain, may replace cereal | 20–30g meat, 5–7 × a week (fish should be consumed 1–2 × a week) | No advice given | BM or BMS | 13–15g |
| Great Britain[a] | 3–4 (60–80g) servings of fruit and veg | | 3–4 servings a day (60–80g/day), i.e., bread, cereal, pasta (anything made with flour) | 1–2 servings (20–40g); 2–3 servings (40–60g) for vegetarians | 2–3 servings | About 500 to 600mL of BM or BMS and some yogurt and cheese | No advice given |
| United States[b] | Up to 10 tbsp (150g) of vegetables or fruit per day (or 0–2 tbsp per feeding occasion) including white potato but not juice | | Up to 4 tbsp (60g) of iron-fortified infant cereal per meal if no other protein or iron sources. 1/2 a slice of wholegrain bread or 2 wholegrain crackers may be served as snacks | 0–4 tbsp (60g)/main meal of meat/fish/egg/infant cereal | 0–4 tbsp (60g) | About 650 to 950mL. Up to 56g of cheese or 112g of cottage cheese or same amount of yogurt or a combination of the 2 at 1 of the 3 main meals per day | No advice given |

[a] Based on guidance from the Pediatric Group of the British Dietetic Association.
[b] US CACFP guidance is given per feeding occasion, based on 3 meals and 2 snacks and summing to get the daily recommendation. Guidance given in tablespoons and ounces was converted to grams based on the assumption that 1 tablespoon = 15g.

TABLE 22.3 Sample menu based on translation of the Australian[a] FBDG for infants.

| Feeding occasion | Sunday | Monday | Tuesday | Wednesday | Thursday | Friday | Saturday |
|---|---|---|---|---|---|---|---|
| Breakfast | Breast milk: 124 g<br>Infant cereal: 20 g<br>Sweet potato: 20 g | Breast milk: 124 g<br>Infant cereal: 20 g<br>Yogurt: 10 g<br>Mango: 10 g | Breast milk: 124 g<br>Infant cereal: 20 g<br>Apple: 10 g<br>Peanut butter: 10 g | Breast milk: 124 g<br>Infant cereal: 20 g<br>Yogurt: 10 g<br>Apricot: 10 g | Breast milk: 124 g<br>Infant cereal: 20 g<br>Banana: 10 g<br>Peanut butter: 10 g | Breast milk: 124 g<br>Infant cereal: 20 g<br>Yogurt: 10 g<br>Orange: 10 g | Breast milk: 124 g<br>Infant cereal: 20 g<br>Sweet potato: 20 g<br>Peanut butter: 10 g |
| Mid-morning | Breast milk: 124 g | Breast milk: 124 g | Breast milk: 124 g | Breast milk: 124 g | Breast milk: 124 g | Breast milk: 124 g | Breast milk: 124 g |
| Lunch | Breast milk: 124 g<br>Beef: 30 g<br>Asparagus: 15 g<br>Rice: 40 g<br>Canola oil: 10 g | Breast milk: 124 g<br>Chicken: 30 g<br>Zucchini: 15 g<br>Rice: 40 g<br>Canola oil: 10 g | Breast milk: 124 g<br>Salmon: 30 g<br>Rice: 80 g | Breast milk: 124 g<br>Turkey: 30 g<br>Pasta: 60 g<br>Canola oil: 10 g | Breast milk: 124 g<br>Egg: 30 g<br>Cheese: 5 g<br>Pasta: 40 g | Breast milk: 124 g<br>Salmon: 30 g<br>Quinoa: 45 g<br>Canola oil: 10 g | Breast milk: 124 g<br>Lamb: 30 g<br>Cauliflower: 15 g<br>Rice: 40 g |
| Mid-afternoon | Breast milk: 124 g | Breast milk: 124 g | Breast milk: 124 g | Breast milk: 124 g | Breast milk: 124 g | Breast milk: 124 g | Breast milk: 124 g |
| Dinner | Breast milk: 124 g<br>Yogurt: 10 g<br>Blueberries: 10 g<br>Muesli: 30 g | Breast milk: 124 g<br>Cheese: 5 g<br>Tomato: 20 g<br>Pasta: 60 g<br>Canola oil: 10 g | Breast milk: 124 g<br>Black beans: 20 g<br>Sweet corn: 15 g<br>Quinoa: 45 g | Breast milk: 124 g<br>Split peas: 20 g<br>Carrots: 15 g<br>Rice: 40 g | Breast milk: 124 g<br>Carrots: 20 g<br>Broccoli: 15 g<br>Rice: 40 g | Breast milk: 124 g<br>Chickpeas: 20 g<br>Avocado: 15 g<br>Bread: 40 g | Breast milk: 124 g<br>Yogurt: 10 g<br>Strawberries: 10 g<br>Muesli: 30 g |

[a] NHMRC (2013).

**TABLE 22.4** Energy and nutrient composition of an average day, based on a weekly menu plan, developed by translating FBDG for infants from five countries: compliance with global and country-specific NRVs.

| Nutrient | Australia | Chile | Germany | Great Britain | United States (CACFP) |
|---|---|---|---|---|---|
| Energy, kcal/day | 808 | 625 | 778 | 679 | 676 |
| % global RV[a] | 119% | 92% | 115% | 100% | 100% |
| % local RV | 113% | 90% | 120% | 100% | 98% |
| Protein, g/day | 24 | 18 | 24 | 23 | 25 |
| % global NRV[b] | 239% | 176% | 240% | 27% | 246% |
| % local NRV | 171% | 153% | 221% | 154% | 227% |
| Lipids, g/day | 37 | 28 | 28 | 29 | 33 |
| % global NRV[c,d] | 115% | 92% | 93% | 95% | 110% |
| % local NRV | 123% | – | 97% | – | 107% |
| ALA, g/day | 0.8 | 0.9 | 0.8 | 0.3 | 0.4 |
| % global NRV[c] | 203% | 349% | 213% | 75% | 107% |
| % local NRV | 163% | – | 220% | – | 80% |
| DHA, mg/day | 172 | 150 | 133 | 164 | 238 |
| % global NRV[c] | 179% | 163% | 145% | 178% | 259% |
| % local NRV | – | – | – | – | – |
| Sodium, mg/day | 193 | 131 | 184 | 190 | 292 |
| % global NRV[e] | 52% | 35% | 50% | 51% | 79% |
| % local NRV | 114% | 35% | 92% | 54% | 79% |
| Potassium, mg/day | 692 | 1035 | 1262 | 855 | 767 |
| % global NRV[e,f] | 99%[f] | 148% | 180% | 122% | 110% |
| % local NRV | – | 148% | 210% | 122% | 110% |
| Calcium, mg/day | 241 | 237 | 498 | 345 | 373 |
| % global NRV[e,g] | 60%[g] | 59%[g] | 125% | 86% | 93% |
| % local NRV | 88% | 91% | 151% | 66% | 143% |
| Iron, mg/day | 6.3 | 3.2 | 5.5 | 2.9 | 5.5 |
| % global NRV[e,h] | 64%[h] | 35%[h] | 59%[h] | 31%[h] | 59%[h] |
| % local NRV | 75% | 29% | 69% | 37% | 50% |
| Zinc, mg/day | 2.9 | 2.5 | 3.5 | 3.5 | 3.6 |
| % global NRV[e,i] | 71% | 62% | 85% | 85% | 88% |
| % local NRV | 97% | 84% | 175% | 70% | 120% |
| Vitamin A (RE), µg/day | 570 | 907 | 937 | 445 | 704 |
| % global NRV[e] | 143% | 227% | 234% | 111% | 176% |
| % local NRV | 133% | 181% | 156% | 127% | 141% |
| Vitamin D, µg/day | 0.8 | 1.6 | 4.3 | 0.6 | 1.0 |
| % global NRV[e] | 8%[j] | 16%[j] | 43%[j] | 6%[j] | 10%[j] |
| % local NRV | 16% | 16% | 43% | 7% | 10% |

[a] FAO reference value for energy (FAO/WHO/UNU, 2001).

[b] WHO reference value for protein (WHO/FAO/UNU, 2002).

[c] FAO reference value for fat and fatty acids (FAO, 2008).

[d] There are no published SFA limits for infants and free sugars were negligible in all infant diets.

[e] Harmonized nutrient reference values for micronutrients, based predominantly on WHO and NASEM recommendations (O'Neill et al., 2020).

[f] The minimum for potassium is 750 mg/day and is based on the adequate intake (AI) cited in (O'Neill et al., 2020) and based on EFSA (EFSA, 2016).

[g] The minimum for calcium is 260 mg/day and is based on the adequate intake (AI) cited in (O'Neill et al., 2020) and based on NASEM (NASEM, 2011).

[h] The minimum for iron is 6.9 mg/day and is based on the estimated average intake (EAR) cited in (O'Neill et al., 2020) and based on NASEM (formerly known as Institute of Medicine) recommendations (IOM, 2011).

[i] The minimum for zinc is 2.5 mg/day and is based on the estimated average intake (EAR) and the maximum is based on the tolerable upper intake level of zinc of 5.8 mg/day as cited in (O'Neill et al., 2020) and based on NASEM recommendations (IOM, 2001).

[j] The minimum for vitamin D is 10 µg/day and is cited in (O'Neill et al., 2020) and based on NASEM (formerly known as Institute of Medicine) recommendations (IOM, 2011).

was lower than the minimum, which was based on the EAR from the United States. On the other hand, vitamin A contents were generally close to or higher than global NRVs. Relative to the global NRVs, the same results indicated that calcium intakes, based on the Australian and the Chilean menus, were below the minimum. Additionally, potassium was below the minimum according to both the Australian and the US menus. The British menu contained only 66% of the local calcium NRV, but the other country-specific menus were very close to or higher than their country-specific and global NRVs, apart from the Australian menu, which yielded a sodium contribution close to the local NRV. In summary, all infant FBDG reached the local energy and lipid requirements they were designed to achieve, but far exceeded their local protein recommendations. In terms of the critical micronutrients, the Australian menu satisfied four of the six requirements considered (was no more than 20% short of the local NRV) and falls short only in terms of iron and vitamin D. On the other hand, the German and Great British menus fulfilled their local vitamin A requirements but failed to achieve the other five critical micronutrient recommendations (potassium, calcium, iron, zinc, and vitamin D).

#### 22.7.2.1.2 Toddlers

Table 22.5 provides the mean daily nutrients provided by each 7-day menu based on the translation of the FBDG for toddlers, relative to global and local requirements. Among these menus, the daily energy contributions came close to requirements in most countries, apart from the menu based on the British FBDG, which achieved 70% of the local energy target. The daily protein contributions were high ranging from 177% of the local NRV achieved in the British menu to 337% of the NRV in the US menu. In terms of lipids, the menus were relatively low in total lipids, especially compared with the local NRVs, particularly the German menu providing only 68% of the local NRV. Whereas the DHA levels were low in the Chilean, German, and US menus, but high in the Australian menu. Regarding local micronutrient NRV, the German menu met five of the six critical micronutrient requirements, under achieving only in terms of the vitamin D requirement. The Australian, United States, and Chilean menus for toddlers failed to meet local requirements for two micronutrients each, including vitamin D. While the British toddler menu was low in iron, zinc and vitamin D. With respect to the overconsumed nutrients, free sugars, saturated fats and sodium, the average daily contributions were well below the recommendations in all menus.

### 22.7.3 Discussion of review

The alignment of FBDG with nutrient needs is critical during complementary feeding to support growth and development. Yet, only 5 of 15 OECD-member countries had quantitative FBDG for complementary feeding with enough specificity to be translated into daily food plans/menus. Although these FBDG were developed in diverse cultures and using different methods, the results indicated that many similarities exist between them. For example, the quantity of non-dairy protein sources as well as grains and starches was the same across countries. The menu analysis indicated that most of the FBDG were adequate in energy and macronutrients. Protein, however, tended to be above the recommended 15% of total energy intake across all menus, but was lower than the upper end of the US Institute of Medicine's acceptable macronutrient distribution ratio (AMDR), which is 22% of energy for the general population (Meyers et al., 2006). A mean intake of 15% of energy from protein was suggested

**TABLE 22.5**  Energy and nutrient composition of an average day for 12 to 24-month old's, based on a weekly menu plan, developed by translating FBDG from five countries: compliance with global Nutrient Reference Values (NRVs) and country-specific NRV.

| Nutrient | Australia menu | Chile menu | German menu | Great Britain menu | United States (CACFP) menu |
|---|---|---|---|---|---|
| Energy, kcal/day | 911 | 1051 | 938 | 664 | 761 |
| % global RV[a] | 106% | 122% | 109% | 77% | 88% |
| % local RV | 100% | 99% | 78% | 70% | 88% |
| | | | | | |
| Protein, g/day | 46 | 43 | 32 | 26 | 37 |
| % global NRV[b] | 418% | 389% | 286% | 234% | 285% |
| % local NRV | 328% | 305% | 225% | 177% | 337% |
| | | | | | |
| Lipids, g/day | 30 | 33 | 31.7 | 30 | 25 |
| % global NRV[c] | 90% | 98% | 95% | 90% | 74% |
| % local NRV | – | – | 68% | – | 69% |
| | | | | | |
| ALA, g/day | 0.8 | 1.7 | 1.5 | 0.8 | 0.5 |
| % global NRV[c] | 152% | 358% | 314% | 16% | 103% |
| % local NRV | 159% | – | 226% | – | 79% |
| | | | | | |
| DHA, mg/day | 283 | 68 | 54 | 94 | 89 |
| % global NRV[c] | 244% | 59% | 47% | 81% | 77% |
| % local NRV | 708% | – | – | – | – |
| | | | | | |
| SFA, g/day | 9.1 | 11.2 | 10 | 12 | 10.6 |
| % global NRV[d] | 61% | 75% | 65% | 80% | 71% |
| % local NRV | – | – | – | – | – |
| | | | | | |
| Free sugars, g/day | 0 | 0.2 | 10 | 3.3 | 5.8 |
| % global NRV[e] | 0% | 1% | 47% | 15% | 26% |
| % local NRV | – | – | – | – | – |
| | | | | | |
| Sodium, mg/day | 377 | 466 | 314 | 352 | 685 |
| % global NRV[f] | 38% | 47% | 31% | 35% | 69% |
| % local NRV | 189% | 47% | 79% | 70% | 69% |
| | | | | | |
| Potassium, mg/ day | 1619 | 2251 | 1373 | 1175 | 1572 |
| % global NRV[f] | 81% | 75% | 46% | 39% | 52% |
| % local NRV | 81% | 75% | 125% | 147% | 52% |
| | | | | | |
| Calcium, mg/day | 452 | 883 | 488 | 543 | 856 |
| % global NRV[f] | 90% | 177% | 81% | 109% | 171% |
| % local NRV | 90% | 126% | 98% | 217% | 122% |
| | | | | | |
| Iron, mg/day | 6.9 | 9.1 | 7.1 | 2.9 | 7.8 |
| % global NRV[f,g] | 119% | 157% | 122% | 49%[g] | 136% |
| % local NRV | 77% | 130% | 89% | 41% | 113% |
| | | | | | |
| Zinc, mg/day | 5.6 | 7.8 | 4.8% | 3.2 | 6.7 |
| % global NRV[f] | 136% | 190% | 117% | 77% | 164% |
| % local NRV | 186% | 260% | 160% | 63% | 220% |

*Continued*

**TABLE 22.5**   Energy and nutrient composition of an average day for 12 to 24-month old's, based on a weekly menu plan, developed by translating FBDG from five countries: compliance with global Nutrient Reference Values (NRVs) and country-specific NRV—cont'd

| Nutrient | Australia menu | Chile menu | German menu | Great Britain menu | United States (CACFP) menu |
|---|---|---|---|---|---|
| Vitamin A (RE), µg/day | 773 | 1170 | 598 | 321 | 656 |
| % global NRV[f,h] | 193% | 293% | 150% | 80%[h] | 164% |
| % local NRV | 258% | 390% | 100% | 80% | 219% |
| Vitamin D, µg/day | 0.5 | 2.8 | 0.3 | 0.4 | 5.6 |
| % global NRV[f,i] | 3%[i] | 19%[i] | 2%[i] | 3%[i] | 37%[i] |
| % local NRV | 10% | 19% | 2% | 4% | 37% |

[a] FAO reference value for energy (FAO/WHO/UNU, 2001).
[b] WHO reference value for protein (WHO/FAO/UNU, 2002).
[c] FAO reference value for fat and fatty acids (FAO, 2008).
[d] EFSA recommendation on SFA (EFSA, 2010).
[e] WHO recommendation for free sugars (WHO, 2015).
[f] Harmonized nutrient reference values for micronutrients, based predominantly on WHO and NASEM recommendations (O'Neill et al., 2020).
[g] the minimum for iron is 3 mg/day for toddlers and is based on the estimated average intake (EAR) cited in (O'Neill et al., 2020) and based on NASEM (formerly known as Institute of Medicine) recommendations (IOM, 2011).
[h] the minimum for vitamin A is 400 mg/day and is based on the RNI from WHO cited in (O'Neill et al., 2020) and based on the WHO (2004).
[i] the minimum for vitamin D is 15 µg/day and is cited in (O'Neill et al., 2020) and based on NASEM (formerly known as Institute of Medicine) recommendations (IOM, 2011).

as a safe upper level during complementary feeding, as there is no risk of protein inadequacy at this level of intake (Fewtrell et al., 2017). However, this safety threshold has not been adopted by other authoritative groups such as the WHO or the AAP.

The global DHA requirement was met in infant menus as human milk contains this fatty acid. However, DHA was not achieved in toddler menus. This was because a limited number of FBDG for young children recommend oily fish, which is necessary to meet DHA requirements. In fact, all five FBDG mentioned fish in general, but only two of them (Germany and Great Britain) stressed that oily fish should constitute one feeding occasions due to its' provision of LC-PUFA. The lack of specific recommendations to consume oily fish in complementary feeding FBDG may be due to cultural, availability, or affordability reasons, or related to the risk of exposure to environmental contaminants, such as methylmercury. Among young children, oily fish consumption has been associated with increased levels of blood mercury (Avella-Garcia and Julvez, 2014). The addition of DHA to foods as a fortificant or the use of a dietary supplement may provide alternative ways to ensure that sufficient amounts are consumed.

None of the FBDG approached the maxima for the overconsumed nutrients (i.e., free sugars, sodium and saturated fats) based on the global NRVs. A free sugar content of 10% of energy was considered as an upper limit in this analysis, even though recent guidelines from the WHO specifically targeted to commercial complementary foods state that the addition of sugars to such foods should be completely avoided (WHO, 2019). Since the definition of free sugars includes those coming from 100% juice, the WHO guidelines imply that juice should be avoided during complementary feeding. The AAP has previously issued guidance to avoid juice during infancy and to limit consumption beyond the age of 12 months (Daniels and Hassink, 2015). Alternatively, the German FBDG state that juice can be offered to promote iron absorption, but it should be first diluted with water. A recent review of FBDG for complementary feeding from the European region identified that 7 out of 21 countries recommend juice consumption, whereas 10 countries advise that fruit juice should be limited (Grammatikaki et al., 2019). Sweet foods such as cakes, desserts, candy, and ice cream are another contributor to free sugars and all the FBDG assessed in the current study recommended that such foods be avoided during infancy. However, "tolerated foods" were permitted in FBDG for toddlers from Germany and Great Britain. The German guidelines allowed 10% of energy from low nutrient dense or non-core food such as confectionery, SSBs, and snacks. Alternatively, the British FBDG state that foods high in fat and sugar may be consumed in addition to, but not instead of, the other food groups, with specific portion sizes limits on such foods. Even with the inclusion of tolerated foods in the menus from these countries, the average daily free sugars compositions of both the German and British menus were below the limit. The US 2020 Dietary Guideline Advisory Committee (DGAC) recently adapted the food pattern modeling approach, to determine if dietary patterns could be established for infants and toddlers. The adapted food modeling failed to identify food patterns that meet the unique nutritional needs of some infants during CF, particularly for those who are breast-fed (DGAC, 2020). Nevertheless, the food pattern modeling exercise indicated that targeting nutrient adequacy for ages 6 to 24 months, leaves practically no residual energy for added sugars and little energy for solid fats, i.e., saturated and trans fatty acids (DGAC, 2020).

The Vitamin D composition of all menus, regardless of age, were low. Apart from Australia, FBDG recommend Vitamin D supplements for infants. Australian FBDG stated that "Casual sunlight exposure is believed to be adequate beyond 6 months to achieve the vitamin D requirement," given cutaneous synthesis of the vitamin upon sunlight exposure, which accounts for around 90% of vitamin D supplies (Munns et al., 2016; Wagner and Greer, 2008). Apart from Great Britain, however, none of the FBDG recommend vitamin D supplements for toddlers. This warrants further consideration given concerns about vitamin D status worldwide (Holick, 2012; Roth et al., 2018).

Many of the menus for infants provided inadequate amounts of other key micronutrients. For instance, iron was not achieved in any of the menus, when the results were compared with the country specific NRVs. Based on the comparison with the global NRVs, the Australian menu for breast-fed infants just fell short of the minimum iron requirement of 6.9 mg/day. Further, of the five FBDG assessed, only those from Chile and the United States recommended iron supplements for breast-fed infants. The German guidance indicated that iron supplements were not essential, citing evidence that the iron status of human milk-fed infants who obtained their iron from foods was not impaired though intake was below requirements (Kersting et al., 2016). Calcium was low in infant diets according to the Australian and Chilean menus. While zinc was low in the infant menu based on the British recommendations. Potassium was not achieved in either the Australian or in the US menus for infants. In the recent report from the US DGAC, nutritionally adequate food patterns for breast-fed infants could not be modeled; the most challenging nutrients to achieve were, iron, zinc, choline, LC-PUFA, and potassium. One of the main conclusions drawn from that work was the need to prioritize iron fortified infant cereal and animal source foods, as well as potassium-rich fruits and vegetables during infancy. However, modeling of adequate food patterns for toddlers fed whole cow's milk was successful, where key foods to reach adequacy included potassium-rich fruits and vegetables, seafood, predominantly wholegrains, and oils over solid fats (DGAC, 2020).

Several limitations of this analysis merit consideration, particularly those related to the translation of the FBDG into 7-day menus. First, some FBDG recommended wide ranges for a food or food groups per day; in these cases, we applied the mid-point. The widest ranges were given in the US CACFP guidelines. For instance, they suggested 0–2 tablespoons of fruit or vegetables per feeding occasion, with 5 feeding occasions per day. Given that 1 tablespoon is the equivalent of 15 g, this translates into 0 to 150 g of fruit or vegetables per day. Thus, we selected 75 g of these foods per day, but if we had selected a quantity closer to the minimum or the maximum of the range, different results would likely have been obtained. The second limitation is that results may be dependent on the specific foods selected within each food group. In order to maximize the potential of each FBDG to reach NRVs, the guidance on foods to be offered was followed precisely and most guidelines mentioned specific foods within each food group. The fact that the menus resulted in daily energy and macronutrients that were close to country-specific targets supports the assumptions and specifications that we used to translate FBDG to 7-day menus. Another limitation was that infant menus were constructed under assumptions of exclusive breast-feeding. As such, results are not directly applicable to formula-feeding or mixed milk-feeding. Considering that just 35% of infants are breast fed by the age of 12 months (CDC, 2020), would suggest that rates of formula-feeding are relatively high, at least in the United States. Nevertheless, our intent was to compare FBDG under similar conditions to provide an indication of the extent to which such guidelines align with nutrient requirements.

Despite the above limitations, we believe that this review has merit given that previous reviews of FBDG for complementary feeding in developed countries have focused on qualitative rather than quantitative guidelines. A previous study (Ferguson et al., 2019) compared four US-based guidelines (from the private sector) on complementary feeding based on a computational infant-simulation model. The study revealed that because these guidelines did not provide portion size recommendations, over-feeding may result, and infants would likely experience unhealthy weight gain by the age of 9 months. This finding underscores the importance of quantitative recommendations that provide guidance on the amounts of food from each food group to offer. To our knowledge the present analysis is the first to evaluate the nutritional adequacy by translating current quantitative FBDG to menu plans and evaluating the nutrient compositions of such plans against country specific as well as global NRV.

## 22.8 Conclusions and public health implications

In conclusion, there are multiple considerations associated with the establishment of quantitative FBDG for any population, and extra considerations are warranted in the case of infants and toddlers. Key among them are the residual energy and nutrients for complementary foods after the type and quantity of milk consumed are taken into account. Given the low energy and high nutrient needs from complementary food, the provision of nutrient dense foods during complementary feeding is critical, particularly for the breast-fed infant.

Across the 5 FBDG and age-groups considered, the main nutrients that fell short of the NRVs were iron, zinc, potassium, vitamin D, and DHA. The recent scientific report from the US DGAC, highlights the challenges of deriving dietary guidelines for children aged 6 to 24 months. They applied a food pattern modeling approach and concluded that the limiting nutrients were, iron, zinc, potassium, vitamin D, DHA, choline, and vitamin E (DGAC, 2020). This would suggest that iron, zinc, potassium, vitamin D, and DHA are indeed difficult to achieve nutrients, with vitamin E and choline being additional key nutrients to consider, which were out of scope for our analyses. Iron and zinc adequacy are particularly challenging to attain in the complementary diet due to the required density of these micronutrients per 100 kcal of food and due to their limited absorption from a diet rich in phytate, found in plant-based foods. The bioavailability of iron is hindered by the dietary source, with heme iron being more readily absorbed than non-heme. Inadequacies in any of these nutrients may lead to adverse health effects due to their critical roles in healthy growth and development.

While FBDG for the complementary feeding period have been widely adopted globally, our review indicates that few provide highly specific recommendations that can be translated to meet key nutrient requirements for growth and development. A relevant consideration when developing FBDG is the methodology applied. The Australian authorities applied a linear programming approach, which would explain why the infant menu based on their FBDG is reasonably close to the Australian NRVs. However, the FBDG from Chile and Great Britain appeared to be based on expert opinion, while those from Germany and the United States were established based on an iterative menu planning process, guided by experts. Overall, it appears that FBDG employing systematic methods, such as linear programming, may have better translation for achieving nutrient targets, particularly during infancy, since micronutrients can be difficult to achieve during this time given the energy limitation. Indeed, linear programming, has been recommended as the gold standard for developing nutritionally adequate FBDG with complex restrictions, such as the many restrictions associated with the complementary feeding period. The empirical menu planning approach applied in Germany worked particularly well in the second year of life.

The complementary feeding period is a critical window for achieving optimal nutrition and fostering healthy dietary patterns for short- and long-term health benefits. Thus, establishing nutritionally adequate FBDG for this life stage is key. Such guidelines can ultimately be translated into health messages and interventions for parents and caregivers to improve complementary feeding practices. Although nutritional adequacy is paramount, so is achieving a healthy dietary pattern for shaping children's long-term eating habits and preferences. Healthy eating practices learned during this life stage are sustained far beyond, where they may eventually lead to better health outcomes.

## 22.9 Future trends

Future development of FBDG should include consideration of alternative dietary patterns and special diets. The vegan diet, for instance, is not recommended for infants and toddlers by ESPGHAN (Fewtrell et al., 2017), as unless very carefully managed it will lead to micronutrient and LC-PUFA inadequacies. However, the lacto-ovo-vegetarian diet, which eliminates meat, fish, and poultry, but permits dairy products and eggs, is feasible, particularly from the second year of life. The recent scientific report of the US DGAC demonstrated the modeling of lacto-ovo-vegetarian diets for toddlers and found that most nutrient requirements could be achieved but that potassium, vitamin E, vitamin D, choline, and calcium required special attention and the selection of specific nutrient-rich foods was needed to avoid dietary gaps

(DGAC, 2020). Quantitative FBDG for the caregivers of lacto-ovo-vegetarian toddlers would be beneficial, as would such guidelines for any elimination diet, especially food allergies (e.g., peanut, eggs) and intolerances (e.g., gluten, lactose…), which are rising in prevalence (Acker et al., 2017; Tang and Mullins, 2017). Achieving a dietary pattern compatible with nutrient adequacy even when all food groups are permitted, is challenging during the complementary feeding period. Therefore, specific FBDG to address the needs of infants and toddlers with a significant dietary restriction, would be a valuable development.

## Sources of additional information

**(1)** American Academy of Pediatrics https://www.aap.org/Infant-Food-and-Feeding.aspx
**(2)** European Society for Pediatric Gastroenterology, Hepatology and Nutrition https://www.espghan.org
**(3)** USDA infant nutrition https://www.nal.usda.gov/fnic
**(4)** World Health Organization: complementary feeding https://www.who.int and Preparation and use of food based dietary guidelines

## Acknowledgments

We thank Lyndsey Huss, Nestlé Infant Nutrition R&D, and Carielle Nikkel for their support in translating the country-specific FBDG into 7-day menus.

## References

AAP, 2006. Breastfeeding Handbook for Physicians. AAP, Elk Grove Village, Il, USA.

Acker, W.W., Plasek, J.M., Blumenthal, K.G., Lai, K.H., Topaz, M., Seger, D.L., Goss, F.R., Slight, S.P., Bates, D.W., Zhou, L., 2017. Prevalence of food allergies and intolerances documented in electronic health records. J. Allergy Clin. Immunol. 140, 1587–1591.e1.

Agostoni, C., Decsi, T., Fewtrell, M., Goulet, O., Kolacek, S., Koletzko, B., Michaelsen, K.F., Moreno, L., Puntis, J., Rigo, J., 2008. Complementary feeding: a commentary by the ESPGHAN committee on nutrition. J. Pediatr. Gastroenterol. Nutr. 46, 99–110.

Alvisi, P., Brusa, S., Alboresi, S., Amarri, S., Bottau, P., Cavagni, G., Corradini, B., Landi, L., Loroni, L., Marani, M., 2015. Recommendations on complementary feeding for healthy, full-term infants. Ital. J. Pediatr. 41, 36.

Andrade, J., Andrade, J., 2016. Food-Based Dietary Guidelines: An Overview. Integrating Gender and Nutrition within Agricultural Extension Services and USAID, Washington.

Atkinson, S.A., 2011. Defining the process of dietary reference intakes: framework for the United States and Canada. Am. J. Clin. Nutr. 94, 655S–657S.

Avella-Garcia, C.B., Julvez, J., 2014. Seafood intake and neurodevelopment: a systematic review. Curr. Environ. Health Rep. 1, 46–77.

Bell, L., Golley, R., Daniels, L., Magarey, A., 2013. Dietary patterns of Australian children aged 14 and 24 months, and associations with socio-demographic factors and adiposity. Eur. J. Clin. Nutr. 67, 638–645.

Briend, A., Darmon, N., Ferguson, E., Erhardt, J.G., 2003. Linear programming: a mathematical tool for analyzing and optimizing children's diets during the complementary feeding period. J. Pediatr. Gastroenterol. Nutr. 36, 12–22.

Butte, N., Cobb, K., Dwyer, J., Graney, L., Heird, W., Rickard, K., 2004. The start healthy feeding guidelines for infants and toddlers. J. Am. Diet. Assoc. 104, 442–454.

Castillo-Durán, C., Balboa, P., Torrejón, C., Bascuñán, K., Uauy, R., 2013. Alimentación normal del niño menor de 2 años: Recomendaciones de la Rama de Nutrición de la Sociedad Chilena de Pediatría 2013. Rev. Chil. Pediatr. 84, 565–572.

CDC, 2020. Breastfeeding Report Card United States. CDC.

Critch, J.N., Society, C.P., Nutrition & Committee, G, 2014. Nutrition for healthy term infants, six to 24 months: an overview. Paediatr. Child Health 19, 547.

Dahl, W.J., Stewart, M.L., 2015. Position of the academy of nutrition and dietetics: health implications of dietary fiber. J. Acad. Nutr. Diet. 115, 1861–1870.

Daniels, S., Hassink, S., 2015. AAP Committee on nutrition. The role of the pediatrician in primary prevention of obesity. Pediatrics 136, e275–e292.

Darmon, N., Ferguson, E., Briend, A., 2002. Linear and nonlinear programming to optimize the nutrient density of a population's diet: an example based on diets of preschool children in rural Malawi. Am. J. Clin. Nutr. 75, 245–253.

Demonteil, L., Tournier, C., Marduel, A., Dusoulier, M., Weenen, H., Nicklaus, S., 2019. Longitudinal study on acceptance of food textures between 6 and 18 months. Food Qual. Prefer. 71, 54–65.

Dewey, K.G., 2001. Nutrition, growth, and complementary feeding of the breastfed infant. Pediatr. Clin. N. Am. 48, 87–104.

Dewey, K.G., Vitta, B.S., 2013. Strategies for Ensuring Adequate Nutrient Intake for Infants and Young Children during the Period of Complementary Feeding. Alive & Thrive, Washington, p. 7.

Dewey, K.G., Cohen, R.J., Rollins, N.C., 2004. Feeding of nonbreastfed children from 6 to 24 months of age in developing countries. Food Nutr. Bull. 25, 377–402.

DGAC, 2020. Scientific Report of the 2020 Dietary Guidelines Advisory Committee: Advisory Report to the Secretary of Agriculture and the Secretary of Health and Human Services. U.S. Department of Agriculture, Washington, DC.

Dipasquale, V., Serra, G., Corsello, G., Romano, C., 2020. Standard and specialized infant formulas in Europe: making, marketing, and health outcomes. Nutr. Clin. Pract. 35, 273–281.

Dror, D.K., Allen, L.H., 2014. Dairy product intake in children and adolescents in developed countries: trends, nutritional contribution, and a review of association with health outcomes. Nutr. Rev. 72, 68–81.

EFSA, 2010a. Scientific opinion on dietary reference values for carbohydrates and dietary fibre. EFSA J. 8, 1462.

EFSA, 2010b. Scientific opinion on dietary reference values for fats, including saturated fatty acids, polyunsaturated fatty acids, monounsaturated fatty acids, trans fatty acids, and cholesterol. EFSA J. 8, 1461.

EFSA, 2010. Scientific opinion on establishing fod based dietary guidelines. EFSA J. 8 (3), 1460.

EFSA, 2016. Dietary reference values for potassium. EFSA J. 14 (10), 4592.

Essery Stoody, E., Spahn, J., McGrane, M., MacNeil, P., Fungwe, T., Altman, J., Lyon, J., Obbagy, J., Wong, Y., 2014. A Series of Systematic Reviews on the Relationship Between Dietary Patterns and Health Outcomes. Evidence Analysis Library Division, Center for Nutrition, Alexandria, VA.

FAO, 2008. Fats and Fatty Acids in Human Nutrition: Report of an Expert Consultation. FAO, Rome.

FAO, 2020. Food-Based Dietary Guidelines. Food and Agriculture Organization of the United Nations, Rome. (Online). Available from: http://www.fao.org/nutrition/education/food-dietary-guidelines/background/en/. (Accessed 28 January 2020).

FAO/WHO/UNU, 2001. Human Energy Requirements: Report of a Joint Expert FAO/WHO/UNU Consultation. FAO, Rome.

Ferguson, M.C., O'shea, K.J., Hammer, L.D., Hertenstein, D.L., Schwartz, N.J., Winch, L.E., Siegmund, S.S., Lee, B.Y., 2019. The impact of following solid food feeding guides on BMI among infants: a simulation study. Am. J. Prev. Med. 57, 355–364.

Fewtrell, M., Bronsky, J., Campoy, C., Domellöf, M., Embleton, N., Mis, N.F., Hojsak, I., Hulst, J.M., Indrio, F., Lapillonne, A., 2017. Complementary feeding: a position paper by the European Society for paediatric gastroenterology, hepatology, and nutrition (ESPGHAN) committee on nutrition. J. Pediatr. Gastroenterol. Nutr. 64, 119–132.

Fidler Mis, N., Braegger, C., Bronsky, J., Campoy, C., Domellöf, M., Embleton, N.D., Hojsak, I., Hulst, J., Indrio, F., Lapillonne, A., 2017. Sugar in infants, children and adolescents: a position paper of the European Society for Paediatric Gastroenterology, hepatology and nutrition committee on nutrition. J. Pediatr. Gastroenterol. Nutr. 65, 681–696.

Food Fortification Initiative (2018) http://www.ffinetwork.org/global_progress/index.php. (Online). Available from: http://www.ffinetwork.org/global_progress/index.php. (Accessed).

Forestell, C.A., 2017. Flavor perception and preference development in human infants. Ann. Nutr. Metab. 70, 17–25.

Gibson, R.S., Bailey, K.B., Gibbs, M., Ferguson, E.L., 2010. A review of phytate, iron, zinc, and calcium concentrations in plant-based complementary foods used in low-income countries and implications for bioavailability. Food Nutr. Bull. 31, S134–S146.

Gibson, R.S., Raboy, V., King, J.C., 2018. Implications of phytate in plant-based foods for iron and zinc bioavailability, setting dietary requirements, and formulating programs and policies. Nutr. Rev. 76, 793–804.

Gidding, S.S., Dennison, B.A., Birch, L.L., Daniels, S.R., Gilman, M.W., Lichtenstein, A.H., Rattay, K.T., Steinberger, J., Stettler, N., Van Horn, L., 2006. Dietary recommendations for children and adolescents: a guide for practitioners. Pediatrics 117, 544–559.

Gidrewicz, D.A., Fenton, T.R., 2014. A systematic review and meta-analysis of the nutrient content of preterm and term breast milk. BMC Pediatr. 14, 216.

Giuffrida, F., Cruz-Hernandez, C., Bertschy, E., Fontannaz, P., Masserey Elmelegy, I., Tavazzi, I., Marmet, C., Sanchez-Bridge, B., Thakkar, S.K., De Castro, C.A., 2016. Temporal changes of human breast milk lipids of Chinese mothers. Nutrients 8, 715.

Grammatikaki, E., Wollgast, J., Caldeira, S., 2019. Feeding Infants and Young Children. A Compilation of National Food-Based Dietary Guidelines and Specific Products Available in the EU Market.

Green, H., 2015. Should foods or nutrients be the focus of guidelines to promote healthful eating? Nutr. Bull. 40, 296–302.

Grimm, K.A., Kim, S.A., Yaroch, A.L., Scanlon, K.S., 2014. Fruit and vegetable intake during infancy and early childhood. Pediatrics 134, S63–S69.

Hester, S.N., Hustead, D.S., Mackey, A.D., Singhal, A., Marriage, B.J., 2012. Is the macronutrient intake of formula-fed infants greater than breast-fed infants in early infancy? J. Nutr. Metab. 2012, 891201.

Hilbig, A., Lentze, M., Kersting, M., 2012. Einführung und Zusammensetzung der Beikost. Monatsschr. Kinderheilkd. 160, 1089–1095.

Hilger, J., Goerig, T., Weber, P., Hoeft, B., Eggersdorfer, M., Carvalho, N.C., Goldberger, U., Hoffmann, K., 2015. Micronutrient intake in healthy toddlers: a multinational perspective. Nutrients 7, 6938–6955.

Holick, M.F., 2012. The D-lightful vitamin D for child health. J. Parenter. Enter. Nutr. 36, 9S–19S.

Hu, J., Aris, I.M., Lin, P.-I.D., Rifas-Shiman, S.L., Perng, W., Woo Baidal, J.A., Wen, D., Oken, E., 2020. Longitudinal associations of modifiable risk factors in the first 1000 days with weight status and metabolic risk in early adolescence. Am. J. Clin. Nutr. 113, 113–122.

Institute of Medicine, 2001. Dietary Reference Intakes for Vitamin A, Vitamin K, Arsenic, Boron, Chromium, Copper, Iodine, Iron, Manganese, Molybdenum, Nickel, Silicon, Vanadium, and Zinc. National Academies Press, Washington DC.

Institute of Medicine, 2011. Child and Adult Care Food Program: Aligning Dietary Guidance for all. The National Academies Press, Washington DC.

Kersting, M., Alexy, U., Clausen, K., 2005. Using the concept of food based dietary guidelines to develop an optimized mixed diet (OMD) for German children and adolescents. J. Pediatr. Gastroenterol. Nutr. 40, 301–308.

Kersting, M., Alexy, U., Schürmann, S., 2016. Critical Dietary Habits in Early Childhood: Principles and Practice. Karger Publishers, Hidden Hunger.

Koletzko, B., Cooper, P., Makrides, M., Garza, C., Uauy, R., Wang, W., 2008. Pediatric Nutrition in Practice. Reinhardt Druck, Basel, Karger, pp. 285–291.

Koletzko, B., Hirsch, N.L., Jewell, J.M., Dos Santos, Q., Breda, J., Fewtrell, M., Weber, M.W., 2020. National recommendations for infant and Young child feeding in the World Health Organization European region. J. Pediatr. Gastroenterol. Nutr. 71, 672.

Krebs, N.F., 2014. Food based complementary feeding strategies for breastfed infants: what's the evidence that it matters? Nutr. Today 49, 271.

Krebs, N.F., Miller, L.V., Michael Hambidge, K., 2014. Zinc deficiency in infants and children: a review of its complex and synergistic interactions. Paediatr. Int. Child Health 34, 279–288.

Lange, C., Visalli, M., Jacob, S., Chabanet, C., Schlich, P., Nicklaus, S., 2013. Maternal feeding practices during the first year and their impact on infants' acceptance of complementary food. Food Qual. Prefer. 29, 89–98.

Lanigan, J., Singhal, A., 2009. Early nutrition and long-term health: a practical approach: symposium on 'early nutrition and later disease: current concepts, research and implications'. Proc. Nutr. Soc. 68, 422–429.

Lanigan, J., Wells, J., Lawson, M., Cole, T., Lucas, A., 2004. Number of days needed to assess energy and nutrient intake in infants and young children between 6 months and 2 years of age. Eur. J. Clin. Nutr. 58, 745–750.

Luque, V., Escribano, J., Closa-Monasterolo, R., Zaragoza-Jordana, M., Ferré, N., Grote, V., Koletzko, B., Totzauer, M., Verduci, E., Redionigi, A., 2018. Unhealthy dietary patterns established in infancy track to mid-childhood: the EU childhood obesity project. J. Nutr. 148, 752–759.

Ma, G., Li, Y., Jin, Y., Zhai, F., Kok, F., Yang, X., 2007. Phytate intake and molar ratios of phytate to zinc, iron and calcium in the diets of people in China. Eur. J. Clin. Nutr. 61, 368–374.

Mennella, J.A., Trabulsi, J.C., 2012. Complementary foods and flavor experiences: setting the foundation. Ann. Nutr. Metab. 60, 40–50.

Mennella, J.A., Ventura, A.K., 2011. Early feeding: setting the stage for healthy eating habits. In: Early Nutrition: Impact on Short-and Long-Term Health. 68, pp. 153–168.

Meyers, L.D., Hellwig, J.P., Otten, J.J., 2006. Dietary Reference Intakes: The Essential Guide to Nutrient Requirements. National Academies Press.

Munns, C.F., Shaw, N., Kiely, M., Specker, B.L., Thacher, T.D., Ozono, K., Michigami, T., Tiosano, D., Mughal, M.Z., Mäkitie, O., 2016. Global consensus recommendations on prevention and management of nutritional rickets. Horm. Res. Paediatr. 85, 83–106.

NASEM, 2017. Review of WIC Food Packages: Improving Balance and Choice. National Academies Press.

NASEM, 2018. Global Harmonization of Methodological Approaches to Nutrient Intake Recommendations: Proceedings of a Workshop. National Academies Press.

NHMRC, 2011. A Modelling System to Inform the Revision of the Australian Guide to Healthy Eating. National Health and Medical Research Council, Canberra.

NHMRC, 2013. Eat for Health: Educator Guide. National Health and Medical Research Council, Canberra.

Nicklaus, S., 2016. The role of food experiences during early childhood in food pleasure learning. Appetite 104, 3–9.

OECD, 2019. Organization for Economic co-operation and Development. OECD. (Online). Available from: https://www.oecd.org/about/members-and-partners/. (Accessed 6 January 2017).

O'Neill, L.M., Dwyer, J.T., Bailey, R.L., Reidy, K.C., Saavedra, J.M., 2020. Harmonizing micronutrient intake reference ranges for dietary guidance and menu planning in complementary feeding. Curr. Dev. Nutr. 4, nzaa017.

PAHO/WHO, 2003. Guiding Principles for Complementary Feeding of the Breastfed Child.

Park, S., Pan, L., Sherry, B., Li, R., 2014. The association of sugar-sweetened beverage intake during infancy with sugar-sweetened beverage intake at 6 years of age. Pediatrics 134, S56–S62.

Pimpin, L., Jebb, S., Johnson, L., Wardle, J., Ambrosini, G.L., 2016. Dietary protein intake is associated with body mass index and weight up to 5 y of age in a prospective cohort of twins, 2. Am. J. Clin. Nutr. 103, 389–397.

Reidy, K.C., Deming, D.M., Briefel, R.R., Fox, M.K., Saavedra, J.M., Eldridge, A.L., 2017. Early development of dietary patterns: transitions in the contribution of food groups to total energy—feeding infants and toddlers study, 2008. BMC Nutr. 3, 5.

Roess, A.A., Jacquier, E.F., Catellier, D.J., Carvalho, R., Lutes, A.C., Anater, A.S., Dietz, W.H., 2018. Food consumption patterns of infants and toddlers: findings from the feeding infants and toddlers study (FITS) 2016. J. Nutr. 148, 1525S–1535S.

Roth, D.E., Abrams, S.A., Aloia, J., Bergeron, G., Bourassa, M.W., Brown, K.H., Calvo, M.S., Cashman, K.D., Combs, G., De-Regil, L.M., 2018. Global prevalence and disease burden of vitamin D deficiency: a roadmap for action in low-and middle-income countries. Ann. N. Y. Acad. Sci. 1430, 44–79.

Santika, O., Fahmida, U., Ferguson, E.L., 2009. Development of food-based complementary feeding recommendations for 9-to 11-month-old peri-urban Indonesian infants using linear programming. J. Nutr. 139, 135–141.

Shaw, V.L., 2014. Clinical Paediatric Dietetics. Wiley Online Library.

Smitasiri, S., Uauy, R., 2007. Beyond recommendations: implementing food-based dietary guidelines for healthier populations. Food Nutr. Bull. 28, S141–S151.

Solomons, N., Vossenaar, M., 2013. Nutrient density in complementary feeding of infants and toddlers. Eur. J. Clin. Nutr. 67, 501–506.

Souci, W, Fachmann, H, Kraut, I, 2015. Food Composition and Nutrition Tables. Medpharm Scientific Publishers, Germany. (Online). Available from: https://www.sfk.online/#/home. (Accessed 29 November 2016).

Spill, M.K., Johns, K., Callahan, E.H., Shapiro, M.J., Wong, Y.P., Benjamin-Neelon, S.E., Birch, L., Black, M.M., Cook, J.T., Faith, M.S., 2019. Repeated exposure to food and food acceptability in infants and toddlers: a systematic review. Am. J. Clin. Nutr. 109, 978S–989S.

Tang, M.L., Mullins, R.J., 2017. Food allergy: is prevalence increasing? Intern. Med. J. 47, 256–261.

Tharrey, M., Olaya, G.A., Fewtrell, M., Ferguson, E., 2017. Adaptation of new Colombian food-based complementary feeding recommendations using linear programming. J. Pediatr. Gastroenterol. Nutr. 65, 667–672.

Theuer, R.C., 2008. Iron-fortified infant cereals. Food Rev. Int. 24, 277–310.

Tuck, C., 2013. Providing advice and guidance on complementary feeding. J. Health Visit. 1, 266–270.

USDA, 2016. National Nutrient Database for Standard Reference 28. (Online). Available from: https://ndb.nal.usda.gov/. (Accessed 29 November 2016).

Victora, C.G., Bahl, R., Barros, A.J., França, G.V., Horton, S., Krasevec, J., Murch, S., Sankar, M.J., Walker, N., Rollins, N.C., 2016. Breastfeeding in the 21st century: epidemiology, mechanisms, and lifelong effect. Lancet 387, 475–490.

Wagner, C.L., Greer, F.R., 2008. Prevention of rickets and vitamin D deficiency in infants, children, and adolescents. Pediatrics 122, 1142–1152.

Weber, M., Grote, V., Closa-Monasterolo, R., Escribano, J., Langhendries, J.-P., Dain, E., Giovannini, M., Verduci, E., Gruszfeld, D., Socha, P., 2014. Lower protein content in infant formula reduces BMI and obesity risk at school age: follow-up of a randomized trial. Am. J. Clin. Nutr. 99, 1041–1051.

WHO, 2009. Infant and Young Child Feeding: Model Chapter for Textbooks for Medical Students and Allied Health Professionals. WHO, Geneva.

WHO, 2015. Guideline: Sugars Intake for Adults and Children. World Health Organization.

WHO, 2019. Commercial foods for infants and Young children in the WHO European region. In: A Study of the Availability, Composition and Marketing of Baby Foods in Four European Countries. Author, Geneva, Switzerland.

WHO/FAO/UNU, 2002. Protein and Amino Acid Requirements in Human Nutrition: Report of a Joint WHO/FAO/UNU Expert Consultatiom. WHO Technical Report Series.

Yang, T., Zhang, Y., Ning, Y., You, L., Ma, D., Zheng, Y., Yang, X., Li, W., Wang, J., Wang, P., 2014. Breast milk macronutrient composition and the associated factors in urban Chinese mothers. Chin. Med. J. 127, 1721–1725.

Young, V.R., 2003. Setting Dietary Reference Intakes for micronutrients for healthy North American infants: a process of trials and errors. In: Nestle Nutrition Workshop Series. Karger, pp. 35–53.

Zalewski, B.M., Patro, B., Veldhorst, M., Kouwenhoven, S., Crespo Escobar, P., Calvo Lerma, J., Koletzko, B., Van Goudoever, J.B., Szajewska, H., 2017. Nutrition of infants and young children (one to three years) and its effect on later health: a systematic review of current recommendations (EarlyNutrition project). Crit. Rev. Food Sci. Nutr. 57, 489–500.

# Index

Note: Page numbers followed by *f* indicate figures and *t* indicate tables.

CPI Antony Rowe
Eastbourne, UK
April 22, 2024